Differential Diagnoses in Surgical Pathology Tumors and their Mimickers

A Volume in the Series Foundations in Diagnostic Pathology

Other books in this series

Busam: *Dermatopathology,* 2e
978-0-323-26191-3

Nucci and Parra-Herran: *Gynecologic Pathology*, 2e
978-0-323-35909-2

Folpe and Nielsen: *Bone and Soft Tissue Pathology*, 2e
978-0-323-75871-0

Hsi: *Hematopathology,* 3e
978-0-323-47913-4

Srivastava and Allende: *Gastrointestinal and Liver Pathology,* 3e
978-0-323-52794-1

Marchesvsky, Abdul-Karim, and Balzer: *Intraoperative Consultation*
978-1-455-74823-5

O' Malley, Pinder, and Mulligan: *Breast Pathology*, 2e
978-1-437-71757-0

Prayson: *Neuropathology*, 3e
978-0-3237-1344-3

Procop and Pritt: *Pathology of Infectious Diseases*
978-1-437-70762-5

Thompson: *Head and Neck*, 3e
978-0-323-47916-5

Zhou and Magi-Galluzzi: *Genitourinary Pathology*, 2e
978-0-323-18827-2

Zander: *Pulmonary Pathology,* 2e
978-0-323-39308-9

Differential Diagnoses in Surgical Pathology Tumors and their Mimickers

A Volume in the Series Foundations in Diagnostic Pathology

Fadi W. Abdul-Karim, MD, MEd
Professor Emeritus
Pathology
Case Western Reserve Univ/ Cleveland Clinic Lerner College of Medicine
Cleveland, Ohio
United States

Charles D. Sturgis, MD
Professor of Pathology & Pathology Residency Program Director
Laboratory Medicine & Pathology
Mayo Clinic
Rochester, Minnesota
United States

Series Editor
John R. Goldblum, MD, FCAP, FASCP, FACG
Chairman, Department of Anatomic Pathology
The Cleveland Clinic Foundation
Cleveland Clinic Lerner College of Medicine
Case Western Reserve University
Cleveland, Ohio
United States

ELSEVIER

Elsevier
1600 John F. Kennedy Blvd.
Ste 1800
Philadelphia, PA 19103-2899

DIFFERENTIAL DIAGNOSES IN SURGICAL PATHOLOGY TUMORS
AND THEIR MIMICKERS: A VOLUME IN THE SERIES FOUNDATIONS
IN DIAGNOSTIC PATHOLOGY

ISBN: 978-0-323-75611-2

Executive Content Strategist: Michael Houston
Content Development Manager: Ranjana Sharma
Publishing Services Manager: Shereen Jameel
Project Manager: Gayathri S
Design Direction: Margaret M. Reid

Printed in India

Last digit is the print number: 9 8 7 6 5 4 3 2 1

Working together
to grow libraries in
developing countries

www.elsevier.com • www.bookaid.org

List of Contributors

Fadi W. Abdul-Karim, MD, MEd
Professor Emeritus
Pathology
Case Western Reserve University/Cleveland Clinic
    Lerner College of Medicine
Cleveland, Ohio
United States

Scott W. Aesif, MD, PhD
Senior Associate Consultant
Department of Laboratory Medicine and Pathology
Mayo Clinic Florida
Jacksonville, Florida
United States

Omonigho Aisagbonhi, MD, PhD
Assistant Professor
Pathology
University of California San Diego
La Jolla, California
United States

Scott C. Bresler, MD, PhD
Assistant Professor
Departments of Pathology and Dermatology
Michigan Medicine, University of Michigan
Ann Arbor, Michigan
United States

May P. Chan, MD
Professor
Departments of Pathology and Dermatology
University of Michigan
Ann Arbor, Michigan
United States

Oluwole Fadare, MD
**Professor of Pathology and Chief of Anatomic
    Pathology**
Pathology
University of California San Diego
La Jolla, California
United States

Clifton G. Fulmer, MD, PhD
Staff
Robert J. Tomsich Pathology and Laboratory Medicine
    Institute
Cleveland Clinic
Cleveland, Ohio
United States

Toshi Ghosh, MD
Fellow Physician
Anatomic Pathology
Mayo Clinic
Rochester, Minnesota
United States

Sandra G. Gjeorgjievski, MD
Assistant Professor
Department of Pathology and Laboratory Medicine
Emory University
Atlanta, Georgia
United States

Christopher Griffith, MD, PhD
Staff
Anatomic Pathology
Cleveland Clinic Foundation
Cleveland, Ohio
United States

Paul W. Harms, MD, PhD
Associate Professor
Departments of Pathology and Dermatology
University of Michigan
Ann Arbor, Michigan
United States

Scott E. Kilpatrick, MD
**Director of Orthopedic Pathology & Co-Director
    of ePathology**
Anatomic Pathology
Cleveland Clinic
Cleveland, Ohio
United States

Keith K. Lai, MD
Staff Pathologist
Anatomic Pathology
Cleveland Clinic
Cleveland, Ohio
United States

Grace Lin, MD, PhD
Clinical Professor
Pathology
University of California San Diego Health
La Jolla, California
United States

Kelsey E. McHugh, MD
Staff Pathologist
Pathology and Laboratory Medicine Institute
Cleveland Clinic
Cleveland, Ohio
United States

Mohamed Amin Mustafa, MBBS
Assistant Professor
Department of Pathology and Laboratory Medicine
Indiana University School of Medicine
Indianapolis, Indiana
United States

Jane K. Nguyen, MD, PhD
Associate Staff
Robert J. Tomsich Pathology and Laboratory Medicine
    Institute
Cleveland Clinic
Cleveland, Ohio
United States

Raghavendra Pillappa, MBBS, MD
Assistant Professor
Department of Pathology
Virginia Commonwealth University Health
Richmond, Virginia
United States

Richard A. Prayson, MD, MEd
Head, Section of Neuropathology
Department of Anatomic Pathology
Cleveland Clinic;
Professor of Pathology
Cleveland Clinic Lerner College of Medicine
Cleveland, Ohio
United States

Mobeen Rahman, MD
Staff Pathologist
Robert J. Tomsich Pathology and Laboratory Medicine
    Institute
Cleveland Clinic
Cleveland, Ohio
United States

John D. Reith, MD
Staff Pathologist, Orthopedic Pathology
Pathology
Cleveland Clinic
Cleveland, Ohio
United States

Michael Rivera, MD
Assistant Professor
Pathology
Mayo Clinic
Rochester, Minnesota
United States

Daniel E. Roberts, MD
Assistant Professor
Department of Pathology
Cleveland Clinic Lerner College of Medicine
Cleveland, Ohio
United States

Michael Roh, MD, PhD
Consultant
Laboratory Medicine and Pathology
Mayo Clinic
Rochester, Minnesota
United States

Rajal B. Shah, MD
Dr. Charles T. Ashworth Professor of Pathology
Pathology
University of Texas Southwestern Medical Center
Dallas, Texas
United States

Malvika Solanki, MBBS, MPH, PhD
Senior Associate Consultant
Department of Laboratory Medicine and Pathology
Mayo Clinic
Rochester, Minnesota
United States

Charles D. Sturgis, MD
Professor of Pathology & Pathology Residency
    Program Director
Laboratory Medicine & Pathology
Mayo Clinic
Rochester, Minnesota
United States

Vera Vavinskaya, MD
Associate Clinical Professor
Pathology
University of California San Diego Health
La Jolla, California
United States

Preface

Historically, the Elsevier *Foundations in Diagnostic Pathology* series of textbooks has been organized in an organ system–based fashion, with each separate book covering the spectrum of disease states seen in an organ system. Our textbook is unique in this series in that the focus is on differential diagnoses, and this single text encompasses diseases encountered in routine surgical pathology practice from many organ systems. Leaders from numerous disciplines in anatomic pathology have authored excellent chapters for this book on the most important and commonly encountered differential diagnostic struggles and pitfalls in their multiple respective realms of expertise. Chapter authors were advised to consider their consultative practices, questions from residents and fellows, and inquiries from colleagues in selecting the topics to be covered in each organ system chapter. This text is meant to be practical, up to date, and user friendly. The chapters include concise summaries of clinical and pathologic findings for many of the most important differential diagnostics concepts encountered in routine practice. Side-by-side microphotographic illustrations of the highest quality accompany each entity and its differential diagnoses. Significance of and recommendations for ancillary testing are incorporated throughout, making this book a valuable adjunct in distinguishing specific entities from their histomorphologic and clinical mimics. Knowledge of differential diagnoses is essential to issuing accurate and nuanced anatomic pathology reports. It is our hope that this text will serve as a roadmap for residents, fellows, and practicing pathologists, as they both create and refine differential diagnoses, working through various considerations to arrive at single best unique interpretations.

Fadi W. Abdul-Karim, MD, MEd
Charles D. Sturgis, MD

Foreword

Surgical pathology continues to become increasingly complex and even more sophisticated, particularly over the past 10 years. It is simply not possible for any individual to master all of the skills and knowledge required to perform these tasks at the highest level. With virtually every case encountered, the pathologist is faced with a differential diagnosis, sometimes requiring the use of immunohistochemistry or molecular diagnostic techniques to arrive at a definitive diagnosis. Every other volume of the *Foundations in Diagnostic Pathology* series has focused on a particular organ or system. The current edition is unique in this entire series and is completely focused on the approach to differential diagnoses in surgical pathology. Drs. Fadi Abdul-Karim and Charles Sturgis, both colleagues of mine at some point in their career at the Cleveland Clinic, have edited an outstanding edition for this series on the topic of the approach to differential diagnoses in surgical pathology. This first edition is up-to-date with regard to our current understanding of the essentials of both non-neoplastic and neoplastic conditions in some of the most common areas of surgical pathology. Both Drs. Abdul-Karim and Sturgis are highly accomplished and experienced surgical pathologists who have provided an excellent framework for dealing with such a broad topic. The book is organized into 13 chapters which cover all of the major differential diagnoses in the most common specimens seen by practicing surgical pathologists, including the gastrointestinal tract, gynecologic tract, and genitourinary tract, among many others. There is uniformity in the organization of these chapters, each of which provides very practical information and numerous photomicrographs that emphasize the essential differential diagnostic points.

I extend my most sincere appreciation to Drs. Abdul-Karim and Sturgis, as well as all of the authors who have contributed to this outstanding first-of-its-kind edition in the Foundations in Diagnostic Pathology series. I am confident you will thoroughly enjoy this volume and find it useful in your everyday practice.

John R. Goldblum, MD, FCAP, FASCP, FACG

Dedications

To my husband, James E. Porter, Jr., without whom, essentially nothing would be possible.

-Charles D. Sturgis, MD

To my colleagues at the Pathology and Laboratory Medicine Institute at the Cleveland Clinic, Ohio, USA, with gratitude.

-Fadi W. Abdul-Karim, MD, MEd

Contents

1 Gastrointestinal Tract

Kelsey E. McHugh • Keith K. Lai

ESOPHAGUS

GASTROESOPHAGEAL REFLUX ESOPHAGITIS

DDX: eosinophilic esophagitis, lymphocytic esophagitis, lichen planus, squamous dysplasia

Clinical Features

Gastroesophageal reflux disease (GERD) is very common in Western countries, with a prevalence rate among adults in the United States estimated to be 20% to 40% based on symptomatology surveys. The etiology of GERD is reflux of gastric and/or duodenal contents (e.g., gastric acid, pepsin, bile, duodenal contents including pancreatic secretions) into the esophagus. Predisposing factors for GERD include anything that decreases the tone of the lower esophageal sphincter (e.g., alcohol, smoking, medications, hypothyroidism, pregnancy, scleroderma), interferes with the normal functionality of the lower esophageal sphincter (e.g., hiatal hernia, achalasia, nasogastric tube, obesity), or alters the emptying of gastric contents (e.g., obesity, diabetes mellitus, Roux-en-Y surgical procedure). Esophagitis secondary to GERD is diagnosed and graded via upper endoscopy, using the Los Angeles Classification comprised of four grades of severity (Grade A through D) based on the extent of erosions in the distal esophagus. Identification of reflux esophagitis is clinically relevant because of its associated morbidities, including increased risk of esophageal adenocarcinoma (by way of intestinal metaplasia) and esophageal rupture, amongst others.

Pathologic Features

GROSS FINDINGS

At upper endoscopy, the gross endoscopic findings are typically that of erythematous esophageal mucosa with varying degrees of associated erosion (mucosal breaks), depending on the severity of disease. These findings are generally restricted to the distal 8 to 10 cm of the esophagus, without proximal esophageal involvement.

MICROSCOPIC FINDINGS

Gastroesophageal reflux esophagitis is characterized by nonspecific reactive epithelial changes with or without associated intraepithelial inflammation. Reactive epithelial changes, including a thickened basal layer, increased length of rete pegs, and elongation of vascular papillae, represent squamous hyperplasia in response to repeated bouts of mucosal injury (Fig. 1.1). At initial description, a thickened basal layer was defined as basal cell and suprabasal cell hyperplasia resulting in expansion of the basal compartment to more than 15% of the epithelium's thickness. Accompanying lengthening of the rete pegs, elongation of lamina propria vascular papillae was defined as their extension into the upper one third of the squamous mucosa. Generally, in gastroesophageal reflux esophagitis, squamous hyperplasia is accompanied by intraepithelial inflammation which may include neutrophils, eosinophils, and/or lymphocytes. In association with intraepithelial inflammation, there may be spongiosis. This intercellular edema is characterized by exaggerated white spaces between keratinocytes, accentuating their spanning intercellular bridges. Depending on the phase of disease and the patient's treatment status, the constituents of intraepithelial inflammation may vary considerably, or intraepithelial inflammation may be completely absent. In rare instances, complications such as stricture formation may occur. Microscopically, strictures are composed of dense submucosal fibrosis with varying amounts of associated inflammation. Barrett's esophagus, the preneoplastic condition defined as the presence of biopsy-proven intestinal metaplasia accompanying endoscopic identification of abnormal mucosa extending at least 1 cm proximal to the gastroesophageal junction, is significantly associated with reflux symptoms and endoscopic evidence of esophagitis. The prevalence of Barrett's esophagus in patients with GERD is estimated to be 1% to 13%.

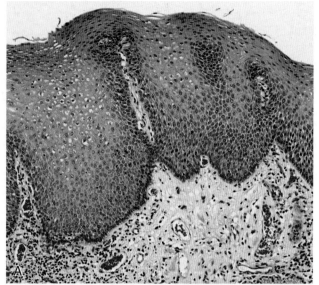

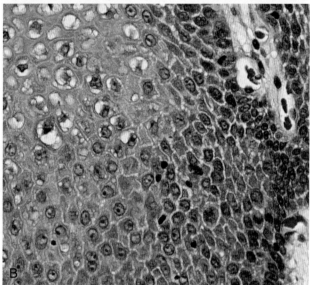

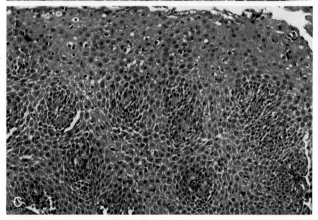

FIG. 1.1

Gastroesophageal reflux esophagitis. Low-power image of hyperplastic squamous mucosa with increased intraepithelial inflammation **(A)**. High-power review reveals mixed intraepithelial inflammation, including neutrophils, eosinophils, and lymphocytes **(B)**. In some instances, inflammation secondary to gastroesophageal reflux disease may be eosinophil-rich **(C)**.

Ancillary Studies

Immunohistochemistry (IHC) and histochemical stains are unnecessary in rendering a diagnosis of reflux esophagitis. Given the possibility of intraepithelial neutrophilic, eosinophilic, and/or mixed inflammation, the use of special stains and/or immunohistochemical stains to exclude the possibility of infectious etiologies may be warranted. Grocott's methenamine silver (GMS) or periodic acid–Schiff (PAS) special stain can be used to exclude the possibility of fungal organisms. In the esophagus, the most common etiology of fungal esophagitis is *Candida* sp., in which special stains highlight yeast and pseudohyphae. In the setting of erosion and/or ulceration, cytomegalovirus (CMV) and herpes simplex virus (HSV) immunohistochemical stains may be employed to exclude a viral-induced esophagitis. In addition to identification of viral cytopathic effect on routine H&E-stained slides, CMV and HSV immunohistochemical stains highlight intranuclear (HSV, CMV) and intracytoplasmic (CMV) viral inclusions composed of viral antigens.

Differential Diagnosis

GASTROESOPHAGEAL REFLUX ESOPHAGITIS VERSUS EOSINOPHILIC ESOPHAGITIS

Eosinophilic esophagitis (EOE) is a relatively uncommon allergic/immune-mediated disorder, with an estimated prevalence of approximately 26 to 57 cases per 100,000 persons per year among the US population. Patients with EOE typically present with symptoms of esophageal dysfunction including dysphagia, food impaction, heartburn, regurgitation, vomiting, and chest pain. While the pathogenesis of EOE is poorly understood, it is generally identified in patients with a history of atopy: allergy, asthma, drug sensitivity, peripheral eosinophilia, and elevated serum IgE levels, amongst other conditions. T-helper cell (Th2)–mediated immune response to food and/or aeroallergens exposure may play a role in the development of EOE. Prototypical endoscopic findings include esophageal rings ("trachealization" when fixed; "felinization" when transient), longitudinal furrows, white mucosal plaques or exudates, and a narrowing caliber of the esophagus. Histologic findings in EOE are that of esophageal eosinophilia. Diagnostic criteria set forth by the AGREE conference (2017) require that, in addition to a clinical presentation suggestive of EOE, biopsy material must demonstrate ≥15 intraepithelial eosinophils in a single high-power field (Fig. 1.2A). In all, EOE is a clinicopathologic diagnosis that requires clinical exclusion of non-EOE disorders that may cause or contribute to esophageal eosinophilia. In addition to the threshold

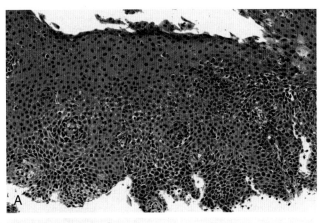

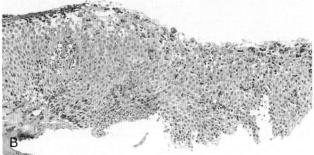

FIG. 1.2

Eosinophilic esophagitis. Squamous mucosa shows increased intraepithelial eosinophils **(A)**. Eosinophilic microabscess formation with superficial layering of eosinophils within squamous mucosa is common **(B)**.

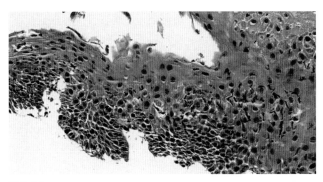

FIG. 1.3

Lymphocytic esophagitis. Esophageal squamous mucosa with increased intraepithelial inflammation comprised nearly exclusively of lymphocytes. These lymphocytes often appear "squiggly" as they infiltrate the mucosa. Associated spongiosis, seen as white spaces between keratinocyte junctions, is also appreciated.

⩾15 eosinophils in a single high-power field, other histologic findings suggestive of EOE include eosinophilic microabscesses (collection of four or more eosinophils), layering of eosinophils in the superficial squamous mucosa, eosinophil degranulation within squamous epithelium, and surface epithelial sloughing with admixed eosinophils (Fig. 1.2B). In addition to intraepithelial eosinophilia, accompanying hyperplastic squamous epithelial changes similar to those seen in GERD may be identified. As increased intraepithelial eosinophils can be seen in a variety of disease entities (e.g., GERD, drug hypersensitivity, infection, gluten-sensitive enteropathy, Crohn's disease [CD], vasculitis), these aforementioned histologic findings in concert with clinical presentation, endoscopic impression, and clinical exclusion of other etiologies of increased intraepithelial eosinophils are necessary to render a definitive diagnosis. Distribution of disease at endoscopy certainly plays an important role, as EOE generally most heavily involves the proximal and mid esophagus, whereas gastroesophageal reflux esophagitis is distal-predominant disease process. Patients with EOE generally respond well to steroid treatment. While it is now understood that a subset of EOE patients respond to proton pump inhibitor (PPI) therapy, those refractory generally respond to topical corticosteroids or budesonide and/or systemic corticosteroids. Younger patients may respond to dietary elimination, but this approach is generally

not well tolerated in adults. Of note, patients with EOE are at increased risk for complications secondary to endoscopic procedures, including esophageal tears and ruptures. This is due to the increased fragility of the esophageal wall secondary to full-thickness involvement by dense eosinophilic inflammation. There is no increased risk of preneoplasia or malignancy.

GASTROESOPHAGEAL REFLUX ESOPHAGITIS VERSUS LYMPHOCYTIC ESOPHAGITIS

Lymphocytic esophagitis is a pattern of injury rather than a specific disease entity. In various retrospective reviews, authors have found lymphocytic esophagitis to be associated with a variety of medical conditions, including reflux esophagitis, *Helicobacter pylori* gastritis, duodenal lymphocytosis, drug/medication-induced mucosal injury, hiatal hernia, celiac disease, CD, and lichen planus, amongst others. The histologic findings in lymphocytic esophagitis are a subjective increase in intraepithelial lymphocytes, generally in peripapillary epithelium and with associated spongiosis (Fig. 1.3). The exact number of "necessary" intraepithelial lymphocytes is not defined and pathologists generally rely on an overall gestalt. Authors who have attempted to quantify "too many" intraepithelial lymphocytes have suggested cutoffs of ⩾20 intraepithelial lymphocytes in a single high-power field within interpapillary epithelium or >50 to 55 intraepithelial lymphocytes per high-power field within peripapillary epithelium. It is important to remember that a "few" intraepithelial lymphocytes are considered normal in the esophagus. Dissimilar from gastroesophageal reflux esophagitis, the intraepithelial inflammation in lymphocytic esophagitis is nearly exclusively composed of lymphocytes, whereas in prototypical reflux esophagitis, the intraepithelial inflammation is mixed. The medical management of lymphocytic esophagitis depends upon the underlying etiology or association.

GASTROESOPHAGEAL REFLUX ESOPHAGITIS VERSUS LICHEN PLANUS

Lichen planus is a subacute to chronic inflammatory mucocutaneous condition that generally involves the skin, oral mucosa, genital mucosa, scalp, and/or nails. While esophageal lichen planus is reportedly rare, recent prospective studies suggest that 26% to 50% of patients with known lichen planus experience esophageal involvement, though it is often asymptomatic. Similar to EOE, patients with esophageal lichen planus typically present with persistent dysphagia. The endoscopic manifestations of lichen planus include mucosal denudation/sloughing, hyperemia, and submucosal plaques. Chronic complications include stricture. While the histology of cutaneous lichen planus includes acanthosis, hypergranulosis, hyperorthokeratosis, "saw-tooth" rete pegs, and a band-like lymphocytic infiltrate undermining squamous epithelium, esophageal lichen planus often lacks these well-developed features. Unlike gastroesophageal reflux esophagitis, the lymphocytic inflammation associated with lichen planus typically presents as it does cutaneously: as a band-like lymphocytic infiltrate undermining esophageal squamous mucosa with associated spilling of lymphocytes into the lower layers of squamous mucosa (Fig. 1.4). Similar to skin, occasional Civatte bodies (apoptotic keratinocytes) may be seen in the basal and suprabasal cell layers. The squamous mucosa of the esophagus may be variably acanthotic or atrophic. Given the lack of a granular cell layer in its "normal" physiologic state, esophageal mucosa involved by lichen planus typically has parakeratosis rather than hypergranulosis and hyperorthokeratosis. If material is collected in Michel's medium, biopsy material can be sent for direct immunofluorescence (DIF), which reveals fibrinogen deposition along the basement membrane. Unlike cutaneous and oral lichen planus, the risk of subsequent malignancy is not well established for esophageal lichen planus. Rare cases of subsequent well-differentiated squamous cell carcinoma and verrucous carcinoma have been reported. Given the relatively rare reports of esophageal lichen planus, there is no standardized therapeutic approach. Therapeutic options include intralesional steroid injection, systemic corticosteroids, cyclosporine, azathioprine, and systemic retinoids. Esophageal stricture, secondary to either repeated bouts of mucosal injury or repeated traumatic injury during esophageal dilatation, may be a chronic complication of untreated esophageal lichen planus.

GASTROESOPHAGEAL REFLUX ESOPHAGITIS VERSUS SQUAMOUS DYSPLASIA

Squamous dysplasia is a neoplastic alteration of the esophageal squamous mucosa that can occur anywhere within the esophagus, from proximal to distal. The prevalence of esophageal squamous dysplasia varies widely over different

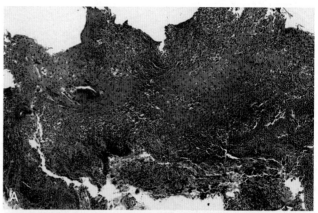
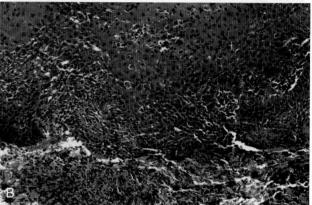

FIG. 1.4

Esophageal lichen planus. Low-power image shows a band of lymphocyte-rich inflammation undermining acanthotic squamous mucosa with increased intraepithelial lymphocytes **(A)**. High-power image of the squamous-stroma interface shows spillover of lymphocytes into squamous mucosa with scattered Civatte bodies (apoptotic keratinocytes) in the suprabasilar mucosa **(B)**.

geographic regions, ranging from approximately 3% to 38%. Risk factors for the development of esophageal squamous dysplasia include low socioeconomic status, tobacco use, alcohol consumption, hot beverage consumption, increased body mass index, genetic factors, and multiple associated medical conditions (e.g., achalasia, Plummer-Vinson syndrome) among other etiologies. In the United States, there is a significant male predominance, with an almost fourfold increased risk in comparison with female counterparts. Esophageal squamous dysplasia is most commonly diagnosed in patients in the fifth and sixth decades of life. Histologically, squamous dysplasia presents as combined cytologic and architectural atypia. It is graded as either low- or high-grade dysplasia. Cytologic atypia encompasses nuclear atypia such as nuclear enlargement, pleomorphism, hyperchromasia, membrane irregularity, loss of polarity, and overlapping. Architectural atypia is defined as atypical or disrupted epithelial maturation. In multiple settings, including pseudoepitheliomatous hyperplasia and ulceration, reactive epithelial changes accompanying reflux esophagitis may mimic squamous dysplasia. In the case of pseudoepitheliomatous hyperplasia, the homogeneity of the cytologic and architectural changes is a reassuring

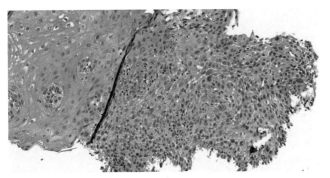

FIG. 1.5

Inflamed squamous dysplasia. While squamous dysplasia may be accompanied by intraepithelial inflammation, the hallmark of recognizing this neoplastic process is identifying the combination of cytologic atypia with accompanying full-thickness architectural disarray. In the right side of this photomicrograph, cytologic atypia characterized by nuclear enlargement, pleomorphism, variable hyperchromasia, nuclear membrane irregularities, and increased nuclear-to-cytoplasmic ratios is accompanied by epithelial disarray characterized by a jumbled appearance of the squamous mucosa without appreciable maturation. This is nicely contrasted with the adjacent nondysplastic squamous mucosa in the left half of the photomicrograph.

feature. In comparison, true squamous dysplasia is usually relatively heterogeneous, both in its identifiable cytologic atypia (e.g., variable nuclear membrane irregularity, hyperchromasia, enlargement) and in its patterns of architectural distortion (e.g., irregular rete peg length) (Fig. 1.5). In the setting of ulceration with associated neutrophilic inflammation, ulcer bed granulation tissue often contains scattered markedly abnormal fibroblasts and endothelial cells. Typically, these cells are markedly enlarged and show dramatic nuclear pleomorphism with increased nuclear-to-cytoplasmic ratios. The singly dispersed pattern of these atypical cells is characteristic of their reactive, rather than neoplastic, nature. Performance of a broad-spectrum cytokeratin immunohistochemical stain is reassuring, as it will be negative in these wildly atypical "ulcerocytes."

Prognosis and Therapy

The clinical management of gastroesophageal reflux esophagitis is typically minimization of the amount of refluxing gastric acid, generally through use of PPIs.

GASTROESOPHAGEAL REFLUX ESOPHAGITIS – DISEASE FACT SHEET

Definition
- ▶▶ Reflux of gastric and/or duodenal (including pancreatic) contents into the esophagus

Incidence and Location
- ▶▶ High prevalence in Western countries
- ▶ In the United States, there is a similar prevalence of GERD symptoms amongst the races
- ▶▶ Distal esophagus more severely affected than mid or proximal

Sex and Age Distribution
- ▶▶ Estimated to occur among 20% to 40% of US adults
- ▶▶ Can affect any age and any sex; no sex predilection in US populations
- ▶▶ Incidence generally thought to increase with age

Clinical Features
- ▶▶ Typical presentation is that of heartburn and effortless regurgitation
- ▶▶ Risk factors include anything that affects tone or integrity of the lower esophageal sphincter

Endoscopic Features
- ▶▶ Mucosal hyperemia with or without mucosal erosion
- ▶▶ Disease severity diminishes from distal to proximal esophagus

Prognosis and Therapy
- ▶▶ Most patients have recurrent but nonprogressive disease
- ▶▶ A subset of patients will go on to develop Barrett's esophagus (estimated 1%–13%)
- ▶▶ Therapeutic options to alleviate symptomatology include proton pump inhibitors and other acid inhibitors

---

GASTROESOPHAGEAL REFLUX DISEASE – PATHOLOGIC FEATURES

Gross Findings
- ▶▶ Mucosal hyperemia
- ▶▶ Mucosa erosions or ulcerations

Microscopic Findings
- ▶▶ Thickened basal layer
- ▶▶ Increased rete peg length
- ▶▶ Elongation of vascular papillae
- ▶▶ Intraepithelial inflammation: neutrophils, eosinophils, and/or lymphocytes
- ▶▶ Intercellular edema (spongiosis)

Pathologic Differential Diagnoses
- ▶▶ Eosinophilic esophagitis
- ▶▶ Lymphocytic esophagitis
- ▶▶ Lichen planus
- ▶▶ Squamous dysplasia

STOMACH

GASTRIC HYPERPLASTIC POLYP

DDX: fundic gland polyp, pyloric adenoma, gastric adenoma, hamartomatous/syndromic polyp

Clinical Features

Hyperplastic polyps are among the most common types of gastric polyps, occurring in about 2% of US patients who undergo upper endoscopy and accounting for approximately 17% of gastric polyps. There is no sex predilection and these polyps are typically identified in the sixth to seventh decade of life. They are thought to arise as a reactive/regenerative phenomenon secondary to ongoing background mucosal injury. Gastric hyperplastic polyps have only a slight predilection for the gastric antrum in comparison with the corpus and the fundus. Approximately 20% of the times, these polyps occur in multiples within the stomach.

Pathologic Features

GROSS FINDINGS

Endoscopically, all gastric polyps including gastric hyperplastic polyps present as projections protruding above the adjacent mucosal surface. The size of gastric polyps can vary significantly, ranging from < 1 mm to multiple centimeters in greatest diameter.

MICROSCOPIC FINDINGS

Gastric hyperplastic polyps are characterized by elongated, tortuous, branching, and dilated hyperplastic gastric foveolae (Fig. 1.6A). The foveolar-type epithelium lining these structures maintains their apical mucin cap. The associated stroma is typically edematous, congested, and inflamed. Often, a granulation tissue-type appearance to the stroma can be appreciated, particularly within the superficial compartment of the lamina propria or near sites of surface epithelial erosion/ulceration (Fig. 1.6B). Commensurate with the degree of inflammation/erosion, the surface gastric epithelium may demonstrate a spectrum of reactive cytologic changes including reduced cytoplasmic volume, increased nuclear size, and one to multiple conspicuous nucleoli. These reactive epithelial changes are often most striking in the "neck" of these dilated foveolae, as this is where the gastric epithelial "stem cells" responsible for reacting to mucosal injury are housed. Additionally, the gastric foveolar-type epithelium may also acquire a pronounced distended appearance to their apical mucin caps, mildly reminiscent of goblet cells. PAS/Alcian blue stain can be used to distinguish these "dystrophic" foveolar cells from true intestinal metaplasia, as the distended apical mucin caps are still composed of neutral mucin and thus will be positive for PAS and negative for Alcian blue (whereas the acid mucin in goblet cells will be stained by Alcian blue). A minority of gastric hyperplastic polyps are associated with true intestinal metaplasia (approximately 15%), epithelial dysplasia (2%–20%, with most studies citing an incidence between 4% and 10%), or carcinoma (2%) (Fig. 1.6C). Most typically, neoplasia or malignancy occurs in gastric hyperplastic polyps that exceed 1 cm in greatest dimension. Overall, while gastric hyperplastic polyps themselves are believed to be

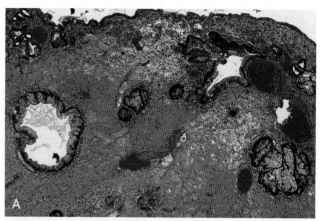

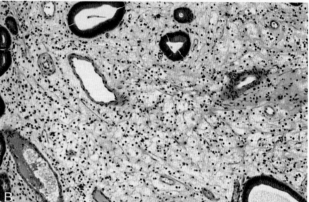

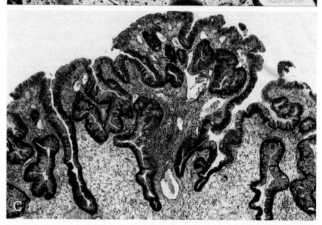

FIG. 1.6

Gastric hyperplastic polyp. Characteristic features include elongated, tortuous, branched, and dilated hyperplastic gastric foveolae in a background of expanded, edematous stroma **(A)**. The stroma shows mixed inflammation and abundant vascularity. If erosion is present, inflammation may be concentrated superficially, with associated granulation tissue-type stroma **(B)**. A minority of hyperplastic polyps may harbor dysplasia or carcinoma. In this example, foveolar-type low-grade dysplasia is characterized by nuclear elongation and pseudostratification **(C)**.

non-neoplastic based on molecular studies, these patients do have increased risk of synchronous or metachronous adenocarcinoma arising anywhere within their stomach. This is because of the association between gastric hyperplastic polyps and background ongoing mucosal injury, particularly atrophic gastritides, including autoimmune metaplastic atrophic gastritis (AMAG) and environmental etiologies (e.g., *H. pylori* infections).

Often, mutations in TP53, resulting in aberrant immunohistochemical p53 profiles (i.e. diffuse positivity or null pattern), are identified in sites of malignant transformation.

Ancillary Studies

Ancillary studies are not necessary in order to render a diagnosis of gastric hyperplastic polyp. Given the association of gastric hyperplastic polyps with background acute and chronic etiologies of gastritis, performing the *H. pylori* immunostain on a representative section of actively inflamed gastric mucosa may be of utility in investigating for the presence of *H. pylori* infection. Additionally, recommending biopsies of background non-polypoid gastric mucosa may be useful in encouraging clinical investigation as to the etiology of the gastric hyperplastic polyp(s).

Differential Diagnosis

GASTRIC HYPERPLASTIC POLYP VERSUS FUNDIC GLAND POLYP

Fundic gland polyps (FGPs) are the most common type of polyp of the stomach, accounting for 70% to 90% of gastric polyps submitted to pathology and occurring in approximately 7% of US patients who undergo upper endoscopy. Unlike gastric hyperplastic polyps, which can arise anywhere in the stomach though there is a slight predilection for the antrum, FGPs are restricted to the gastric body/corpus and fundus. Similar to gastric hyperplastic polyps, FGPs also arise secondary to glandular hyperplasia and dilatation (Fig. 1.7A). However, the dilated glands in FGPs are oxyntic glands, lined by parietal cells, chief cells, and variable numbers of mucus neck cells (Fig. 1.7B). These dilated glands arise in a background of oxyntic mucosa with a relatively preserved glandular architecture and are generally not associated with background gastritides. In fact, there is an inverse correlation between *H. pylori* infection and the presence of FGPs. FGPs are generally small (a few millimeters in size; rarely exceeding 1 cm) and may occur singly or in multiples. When ≥20 FGPs are identified at the time of upper endoscopy or when FGPs are identified with concurrent duodenal adenomas, a syndromic etiology must be considered. FGPs arise in two clinical scenarios: sporadically and in association with polyposis syndromes, most commonly familial adenomatous polyposis (FAP). FGPs have been reported to occur in the syndrome gastric adenocarcinoma and proximal polyposis of the stomach (GAPPS) as well. Sporadic FGPs are common, may occur at any age, have a female predominance in US populations, and are associated

with PPI use. These polyps are very rarely associated with epithelial dysplasia and there are no reported cases of progression to adenocarcinoma within the English language literature in the United States. Sporadic FGPs are associated with mutations in the *CTNNB1* gene (encoding beta-catenin; chromosome 3p22.1) rather than *APC* gene mutations (chromosome 5q21) as in FAP. In FAP or FAP variant (e.g., attenuated FAP, GAPPS) patients, FGPs are extremely common, reportedly identified in 13% to 84% of patients. The prevalence of FGPs in these patient cohorts increases with age. Unique presentations of FGPs in FAP patients include "carpeting" of the gastric fundus and body by polyposis (extremely rare in non-FAP patients) as well as FGPs arising in pediatric patients (again, extremely rare in non-FAP patients). FAP-associated FGPs demonstrate epithelial dysplasia in up to a quarter of cases and progression to adenocarcinoma is reported in the literature, though still markedly rare in the United States–based English language literature (Fig. 1.7C and D).

GASTRIC HYPERPLASTIC POLYP VERSUS PYLORIC GLAND ADENOMA

Unlike gastric hyperplastic polyps, which are non-neoplastic polyps with a predilection for the gastric antrum, pyloric gland adenomas (PGAs) are neoplastic proliferations that preferentially occur in the gastric corpus. They are less common than gastric hyperplastic polyps, accounting for approximately 3% of all gastric polyps. Gastric PGAs generally occur in older patients (median age in eighth decade) and have a female predominance. Similar to gastric hyperplastic polyps, gastric PGAs are frequently associated with background gastritides, most notably AMAG. Approximately one third of gastric PGAs occur in the clinical setting of AMAG and, in AMAG patients, gastric PGAs account for approximately 10% of identified polyps. Histologically, PGAs are characterized by closely packed pyloric-type glands lined by low cuboidal epithelial cells with pale to eosinophilic apical "ground glass"-type cytoplasm and small, round basally located nuclei without conspicuous nucleoli (Fig. 1.8A). Similar to hyperplastic polyps, these pyloric-type glands may be variably cystically dilated. Low-grade dysplasia, high-grade dysplasia, and carcinoma are reportedly estimated to occur in approximately 12%, 39%, and 10% to 15% of cases, respectively (Fig. 1.8B). Though not a common practice at our institution, one can use MUC special stains to aid in distinguishing PGA from gastric hyperplastic polyps and gastric adenomas. PGAs classically show coexpression of MUC5AC (foveolar mucin marker) and MUC6 (pyloric gland mucin marker), while lacking expression of MUC2 (intestinal mucin marker). Generally, as with adenomas identified at other gastrointestinal (GI) sites, PGAs should be completely excised and background non-polypoid gastric mucosa should be biopsied to evaluate etiologic entities that may be afflicting non-polypoid mucosa.

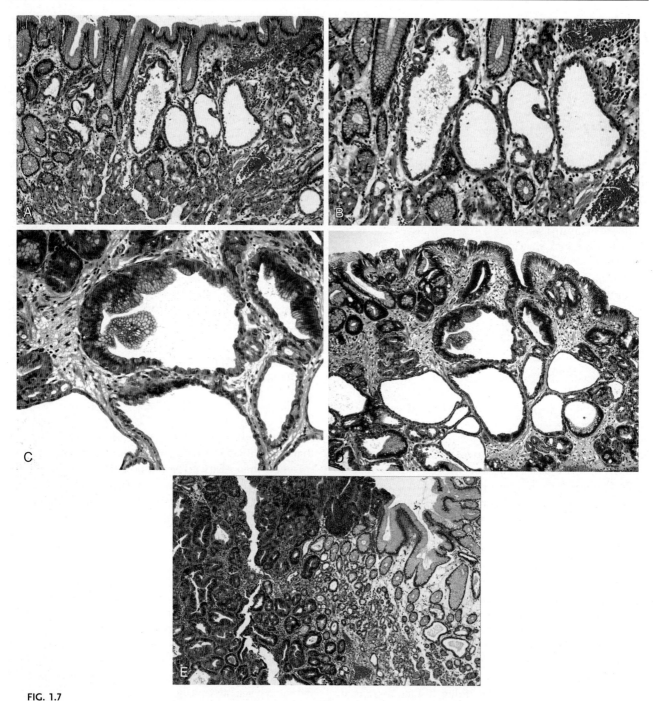

FIG. 1.7
Fundic gland polyp (FGP). The most common gastric polyp, they are composed of variably dilated oxyntic glands lined by parietal cells, chief cells, and mucus cells as seen in this low-power image **(A)**. The three distinct cell types, all of which have small round basally oriented nuclei, are better appreciated at high-power magnification **(B)**. More common in syndromic-related FGP than in sporadic, low-grade dysplasia characterized by nuclear elongation, hyperchromasia, and pseudostratification may develop. Pictured here deep within the glands **(C)**, dysplasia will extend to involve surface epithelium as well **(D)**. The characteristics of high-grade dysplasia include severe cytologic atypia (e.g., nuclear rounding, enlargement, loss of nuclear polarity) coupled with architectural complexity, including cribriforming as in this example **(E)**.

GASTRIC HYPERPLASTIC POLYP VERSUS GASTRIC ADENOMA

Gastric adenomas are the third most common polyp in the stomach, following FGPs and gastric hyperplastic polyps. Similar to gastric hyperplastic polyps, gastric adenomas are polypoid lesions that typically arise in a background inflammatory milieu with or without associated intestinal metaplasia. They are most typically solitary and can arise anywhere within the stomach, though they have a predilection for the most common sites of intestinal metaplasia in the stomach which includes the distal stomach and angularis incisura. Gastric adenomas are composed of crowded dysplastic tubules that form polyps. The two main histologic morphologies of gastric

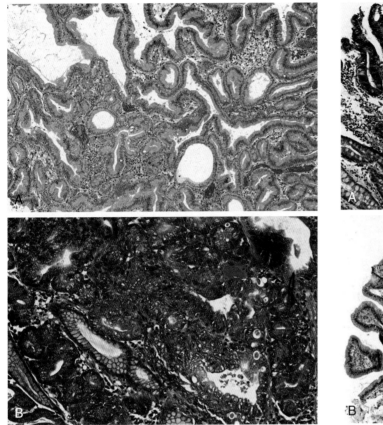

FIG. 1.8

Pyloric gland adenoma. Closely packed pyloric-type glands with variable degrees of glandular dilatation comprise these lesions. These glands are lined by low columnar to cuboidal epithelium with basally oriented round to ovoid nuclei. These cells have moderate amounts of lightly eosinophilic epithelium that lack developed apical mucin caps **(A)**. Up to half of cases show high-grade dysplasia characterized by severe cytologic atypia with accompanying architectural distortion **(B)**.

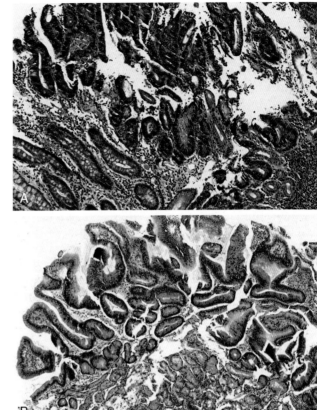

FIG. 1.9

Gastric adenoma. In gastric adenomas with intestinal-type dysplasia, the cytologic features recapitulate those seen in adenomas of the lower gastrointestinal tract, including columnar epithelium with hyperchromatic and pseudostratified nuclei as well as scattered goblet cells and Paneth cells **(A)**. In gastric adenomas with foveolar-type, similar nuclear changes are seen in gastric foveolar-type epithelium that maintains its apical mucin cap **(B)**.

adenomas are intestinal-type gastric adenomas and gastric foveolar-type adenomas. Intestinal-type gastric adenomas exceed foveolar-type gastric adenomas in frequency, >4:1. In intestinal-type adenomas, the tubules are lined by columnar epithelium with nuclear elongation and pseudostratification, akin to the cytomorphologic changes seen in colorectal tubular adenomas (Fig. 1.9A). Admixed goblet cells and Paneth cells are often seen. In foveolar-type gastric adenomas, the tubules are similarly lined by columnar epithelium with nuclear elongation and pseudostratification; however, a distinctive apical mucin cap can be appreciated, as can the paucity of intestinal metaplasia or Paneth cells (Fig. 1.9B). When a gastric adenoma is identified, care is taken to categorize the dysplasia as either low grade or high grade. A diagnosis of high-grade dysplasia requires severe cytologic atypia, characterized by enlarged, rounded, hyperchromatic nuclei with irregular nuclear contours, increased nuclear-to-cytoplasmic ratios, and loss of nuclear polarity. This cytologic atypia is generally accompanied by architectural complexity including dilated and cribriforming glandular structures. Careful

examination of the polypoid lesion as well as representative sections of background gastric mucosa is undertaken to exclude the presence of invasive adenocarcinoma, which has been reported in up to 15% of gastric adenomas. In US populations, intestinal-type gastric adenomas are significantly more likely to harbor high-grade dysplasia, and adenocarcinomas are frequently associated with intestinal metaplasia in background non-polypoid gastric mucosa, as well as background gastritis of some ilk. As with PGAs and adenomas at other anatomic sites within the GI tract, complete endoscopic removal of the polyp should be performed, as there is risk of neoplastic progression.

GASTRIC HYPERPLASTIC POLYP VERSUS HAMARTOMATOUS/SYNDROMIC POLYP

It can be impossible to distinguish gastric hyperplastic polyps from hamartomatous/syndromic polyps based on histology alone. Generally, correlation with clinical data is paramount in rendering an accurate interpretation. Additionally helpful in many scenarios is biopsy of background non-polypoid gastric mucosa, as we know gastric hyperplastic polyps are associated with myriad background gastritides, whereas most hamartomatous/syndromic polyps have unremarkable background gastric mucosa. Examples of syndromes that present with hamartomatous-type polyps in the stomach include Peutz-Jeghers syndrome, juvenile polyposis, Cowden disease, and Cronkhite-Canada syndrome. Peutz-Jeghers syndrome is caused by an autosomal dominant germline mutation in the *LBK1/STK11* gene on chromosome 19p13.3. Peutz-Jeghers polyps classically demonstrate an arborizing pattern on low-power microscopy due to prominent branching of the muscularis mucosae. This feature is less well-developed in Peutz-Jeghers polyps of the stomach compared with the more commonly identified small bowel polyps. The histology of gastric Peutz-Jeghers polyps includes dilated and branched mucus-filled pits generally associated with a more inconspicuous proliferation of smooth muscle (Fig. 1.10). Similar to gastric

hyperplastic polyps, patients with Peutz-Jeghers syndrome are at increased risk of adenocarcinoma arising anywhere within their stomach, though the hamartomatous polyps themselves are not generally secondary to increased risk of neoplasia/malignancy. Juvenile polyposis is a genetically heterogeneous condition in which a subset of affected patients have autosomal dominant germline mutations in the *DPC4* gene on chromosome 18q21. Histologically, juvenile polyps can essentially exactly recapitulate gastric hyperplastic polyps, composed of hyperplastic and dilated gastric foveolae set within abundantly edematous and inflamed lamina propria. The silhouette of juvenile polyps is often described as being rounded in contour on low-power microscopy compared with the more villiform to lobulated appearance of gastric hyperplastic polyps, though this is certainly a "soft" histologic feature. Unlike gastric hyperplastic polyps, a relatively high percentage (approximately 33%) of gastric juvenile polyps is associated with epithelial dysplasia or malignancy. Cowden disease is caused by an autosomal dominant germline mutation in the *PTEN* gene on chromosome 10q22-23. Similar to juvenile polyps, gastric polyps in Cowden disease are described as being histologically indistinguishable from gastric hyperplastic polyps. Similar to gastric hyperplastic polyps and unlike juvenile polyps, gastric polyps secondary to Cowden disease generally do not house associated epithelial dysplasia or malignancy. The molecular underpinning of Cronkhite-Canada syndrome, if any, has not yet been discerned. The typical clinical presentation is that of diffuse polyposis throughout the GI tract, with sparing of the esophagus, coupled with innumerable "ectodermal" abnormalities such as alopecia and onychodystrophy. Similar to juvenile polyps, Cowden disease polyps, and gastric hyperplastic polyps, the polyps of Cronkhite-Canada syndrome are characterized by cystic gastric glands and edematous lamina propria. Unlike the aforementioned polyps, Cronkhite-Canada polyps are typically sessile with a broad base, rather than pedunculated. Association of Cronkhite-Canada polyps with neoplasia/malignancy remains controversial.

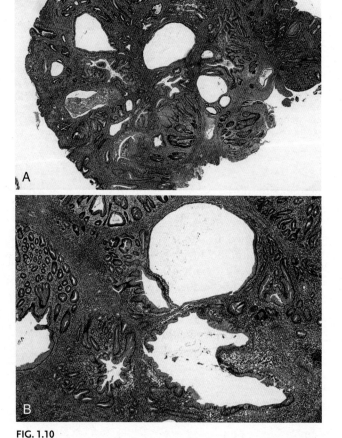

FIG. 1.10

Hamartomatous/syndromic polyp. Hamartomatous/syndromic polyps of the stomach encompass a spectrum of lesions, many of which have features similar to those pictured here, including cystically dilated gastric glands containing mucinous secretions set within a variably inflamed lamina propria **(A)**. In many of these polyps, bland bundles of smooth muscles can be seen traversing the lesion **(B)**.

Prognosis and Therapy

Due to the increased risk of associated neoplasia, complete endoscopic resection of gastric hyperplastic polyps with subsequent pathologic examination is recommended. As mentioned above, one of the most important clinical associations for gastric hyperplastic polyps is their high potential for associated background gastritides. Thus, if background flat mucosa is not sampled at the time of endoscopic biopsy/resection of gastric hyperplastic polyps, it is most prudent to include a recommendation for biopsy of flat fundic and antral mucosa in order to exclude atrophic, acute, chronic, and "chemical" forms of gastritis.

GASTRIC HYPERPLASTIC POLYP – DISEASE FACT SHEET

Definition
- ▸▸ Benign epithelial proliferation comprises elongated, tortuous, and dilated gastric foveolae
- ▸▸ Accounts for nearly 20% of gastric polyps

Incidence and Location
- ▸▸ Found in approximately 2% of those undergoing upper endoscopy
- ▸▸ Most commonly found in the gastric antrum
- ▸▸ Usually solitary, though can be multiple

Sex and Age Distribution
- ▸▸ Typically occur in the sixth or seventh decade of life
- ▸▸ No sex predilection

Clinical Features
- ▸▸ Typically asymptomatic
- ▸▸ If eroded, iron deficiency anemia may result
- ▸▸ If large and in the pyloric region, obstruction may occur

Endoscopic Features
- ▸▸ Small dome-shaped polyp, typically < 1 cm
- ▸▸ Can be large, lobulated, pedunculated, and/or eroded

Prognosis and Therapy
- ▸▸ Generally, extremely good prognosis as these polyps are not neoplastic
- ▸▸ Prevalence of associated dysplasia (1%–20%) or carcinoma (<2%) is low

---

GASTRIC HYPERPLASTIC POLYP – PATHOLOGIC FEATURES

Gross Findings
- ▸▸ Ovoid polypoid lesions
- ▸▸ Can be large, lobulated, pedunculated
- ▸▸ May show mucosal erosion

Microscopic Findings
- ▸▸ Elongated, tortuous, branched, cystically dilated hyperplastic foveolae
- ▸▸ Expanded edematous stroma with mixed inflammation and prominent vasculature
- ▸▸ Haphazard bundles of smooth muscle throughout lamina propria
- ▸▸ May harbor dysplasia or carcinoma in minority of cases

Pathologic Differential Diagnoses
- ▸▸ Fundic gland polyp
- ▸▸ Pyloric gland adenoma
- ▸▸ Gastric adenoma
- ▸▸ Hamartomatous/syndromic polyp

AMPULLA

INTRA-AMPULLARY PAPILLARY-TUBULAR NEOPLASM

DDX: invasive ampullary adenocarcinoma, adenoma of ampullary duodenum, poorly differentiated neuroendocrine carcinoma

Clinical Features

Intra-ampullary papillary-tubular neoplasms (IAPNs) are preneoplastic lesions that are localized to within the ampullary channel, with minimal to no involvement of the duodenal papilla, distal common bile duct, or pancreatic duct. These tumors are often asymptomatic lesions incidentally identified at the time of upper endoscopy. Alternatively, given their intra-ampullary location, patients may present with obstructive jaundice or, more rarely, cholangitis or pancreatitis. In general, these tumors are exceedingly rare in comparison with their colorectal counterparts, with an estimated prevalence of ampullary adenomas in autopsy series of 0.04% to 0.12%. It is important to note that the ampullary location is by far the most frequently involved small bowel region in regard to precursor and invasive adenocarcinoma. It is posited that the predilection for small bowel adenomas to arise within an intra-ampullary location is secondary to the effluence of bile acids through these channels, serving as a carcinogenic insult.

Pathologic Features

GROSS FINDINGS

IAPN presents as a compact, exophytic lesion localized to within the ampullary channel. These tumors often have a polypoid, nodular, or granular appearance grossly. Given their intra-ampullary location, prior to dissection they often present mucosa-covered elevations or subtle ulcers within the region of the ampulla. Polypoid, granular material may be seen protruding from within the ampulla itself.

MICROSCOPIC FINDINGS

IAPN has a microscopic appearance not dissimilar to intraductal papillary mucinous neoplasms (IPMNs) of the pancreas. Similar to IAPNs, IPMNs may be lined by epithelium with intestinal-, pancreatobiliary-, and/or gastric-type epithelium. They generally have a papillary, villous, or tubulovillous architecture, and the cells lining these structures are dysplastic, with greater than

80% of cases harboring a mixture of low- and high-grade dysplasia (Fig. 1.11A). The most typical of form of observed low-grade dysplasia is intestinal-type dysplasia in which the cells have elongated nuclei with inconspicuous nuclei that are pseudostratified within the cytoplasm of tall, columnar cells (Fig. 1.11B). Admixed Paneth cells, goblet cells, or endocrine cells may be seen. High-grade dysplasia is characterized by a combination of severe cytologic atypia coupled with architectural complexity. Cytology atypia includes a rounding and enlargement of the nuclei with coarse nuclear chromatin, variably conspicuous nucleoli, and nuclear stratification with loss of basal-oriented nuclear polarity. Architectural complexity encompasses back-to-back glandular, cribriforming, and sheeting configurations (Fig. 1.11). While the epithelium lining IAPNs may purely recapitulate any of the above-listed epithelial types, in more than half of cases, multiple types of epithelial differentiations coexist. The most common combination is that of intestinal-type and pancreatobiliary-type differentiation.

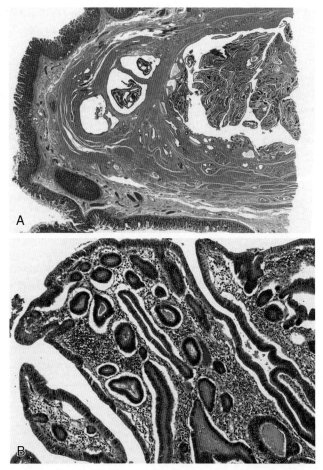

FIG. 1.11

Intra-ampullary papillary-tubular neoplasm. This lesion demonstrates an exophytic growth pattern composed of variably tubular, villous, and papillary growth patterns **(A)**. The majority of these lesions have an intestinal-type morphology, in which the neoplastic epithelium is composed of tall columnar with elongated, pseudostratified nuclei **(B)**.

Ancillary Studies

No ancillary studies are necessary to render a diagnosis of IAPN. Rather, careful gross evaluation is necessary to ensure the lesion's epicenter lies within the ampullary channel. Of course, similar to other sites within the digestive tract, the immunohistochemical profile of IAPN varies based on the type of epithelium comprising the lesion. Tumors with an intestinal phenotype express MUC2 and CDX2. Tumors with a pancreatobiliary phenotype express MUC1, MUC5AC, and MUC6. Discerning one phenotype from another is entirely unnecessary in regard to rendering an accurate diagnosis or prognosticating for the patient.

Differential Diagnosis

IAPN VERSUS INVASIVE AMPULLARY ADENOCARCINOMA

Invasive adenocarcinomas of the ampulla may arise out of IAPNs, and thus have a very similar clinical presentation, or may arise from flat dysplasia lining the ampullary duct. In either scenario, patients may present with biliary obstruction, jaundice, and weight loss. Grossly, tumors arising from IAPN show an infiltrative lesion underlying a nodular, polypoid excrescence projecting into the ampullary channel (Fig. 1.12A). In contrast, tumors arising from *in situ* dysplasia/neoplasia or the ampullary duct lining typically show a concentrically thickened duct with an ill-defined infiltrative lesion extending from it walls. Microscopically, the vast majority of invasive adenocarcinomas are tubule (gland) forming. The defining feature of invasive adenocarcinoma is the presence of at least submucosal invasion with its elicited desmoplastic stromal response microscopically (Fig. 1.12B). This is in contrast to IAPNs, in which the neoplasia is entirely restricted to the mucosal compartment, without disruption of the muscularis mucosae. The epithelium comprising these tumors is a hybrid of differentiations in up to 40% of the cases, which is logical given that the ampulla is a transitional zone between intestinal-type and pancreatobiliary-type epitheliums.

IAPN VERSUS ADENOMA OF AMPULLARY DUODENUM

In contrast to IAPN, adenomas of the ampullary duodenum present as exophytic, possibly ulcerated lesions arising from the surface mucosa surrounding the duodenal ampulla. Often, visualization of the ampulla is obscured secondary to these polypoid lesions. These adenomas typically have tubular or tubulovillous architecture and are lined by epithelial cells with intestinal-type low-grade dysplasia characterized by tall, columnar cells with elongated nuclei, inconspicuous nucleoli, and nuclear pseudostratification (Fig. 1.13). Identical to IAPN, tumors

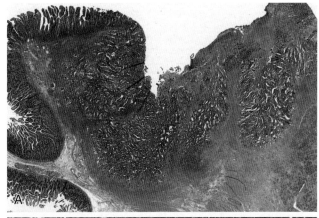

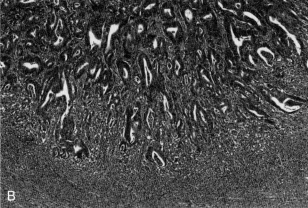

FIG. 1.12
Invasive ampullary adenocarcinoma. Low-power histologic view shows infiltrative adenocarcinoma with an associated desmoplastic stromal response, circumferentially surrounding one half of the ampullary duct **(A)**. On higher-power magnification, the infiltrative front of the tumor with its associated desmoplastic stromal response can be appreciated **(B)**.

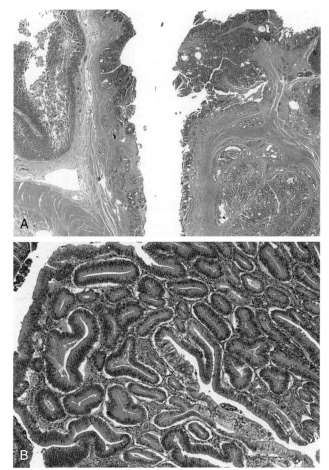

FIG. 1.13
Adenoma of ampullary duodenum. Location is often the only feature that distinguished adenoma of the ampullary duodenum from intra-ampullary papillary-tubular neoplasm. This low-power image highlights the localization of this exophytic lesion to the surface of the duodenal ampulla **(A)**. As adenomas of other sites within the lower gastrointestinal tract, the tumor has a tubular and villous architecture, with structures lined by columnar epithelial cells with elongated, hyperchromatic, and pseudostratified nuclei **(B)**.

with high-grade dysplasia show foci of marked cytologic atypia coupled with architectural complexity. Given that adenomas of the ampullary duodenal arise from the small intestinal mucosa surrounding the ampulla, they typically do not harbor pancreatobiliary- or gastric-type differentiation, which is dissimilar to IAPNs.

IAPN VERSUS POORLY DIFFERENTIATED NEUROENDOCRINE CARCINOMA

While neuroendocrine tumors occur throughout the entire small bowel, poorly differentiated neuroendocrine carcinomas are nearly exclusive to the ampulla. Similar to IAPNs and invasive adenocarcinomas, these tumors have their epicenter within the ampullary channel and patients may present with obstructive jaundice, cholangitis, or pancreatitis. Similar to invasive adenocarcinomas arising within ampulla, poorly differentiated neuroendocrine carcinomas are invasive tumors with an associated desmoplastic stromal response. They are high-grade carcinomas with tumor cells arranged in poorly formed nests, trabeculae, and sheets. These malignant cells may demonstrate small cell or large cell features. Small cell carcinomas have

increased nuclear-to-cytoplasmic ratios with nearly no visible cytoplasm. The tumor nuclei are enlarged and hyperchromatic with nuclear molding, extensive apoptosis, and frequent mitoses. Large cell carcinoma is characterized by enlarged cells that maintain a moderate amount of cytoplasm and have enlarged nuclei with coarse nuclear chromatin and prominent nucleoli (Fig. 1.14).

Prognosis and Therapy

The prognosis for pure IAPNs, without an associated invasive carcinoma component, is excellent with 100% 3-year and 5-year survival following complete excision. Importantly, up to 75% of IAPNs are associated with an invasive carcinoma and the prognosis in this setting is significantly diminished. Resected ampullary carcinomas have a 5-year survival rate of approximately 45%.

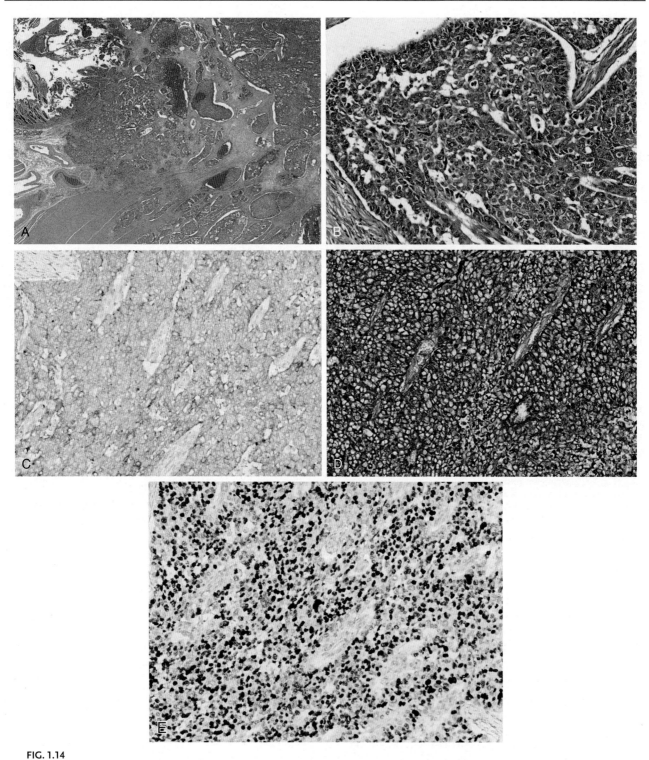

FIG. 1.14

Poorly differentiated neuroendocrine carcinoma of ampulla. This high-grade carcinoma of the ampulla is composed of sheets, trabeculae, and nests of tumor cells invading the ampullary wall **(A)**. This neuroendocrine carcinoma is the large cell type, with tumor cells that maintain a moderate amount of cytoplasm and have enlarged nuclei with coarse nuclear chromatin and prominent nucleoli **(B)**. Consistent with their neuro-endocrine line of differentiation, these tumors demonstrate positivity for neuroendocrine markers including synaptophysin **(C)**, chromogranin **(D)**, and INSM1 **(E)**.

**INTRA-AMPULLARY PAPILLARY-TUBULAR NEOPLASM –
DISEASE FACT SHEET**

Definition
▸▸ A polyp composed of dysplastic glandular epithelium occurring within the ampullary lumen, representing the confluence of the distal common bile duct and main pancreatic duct

Incidence and Location
▸▸ Relatively rare, with estimated prevalence of ampullary adenomas ⩽0.12% in autopsy series
▸▸ Over half of small bowel neoplasms occur in the duodenum, the majority around the ampulla
▸▸ It is posited that bile acids serve as a locoregional carcinogen

Sex and Age Distribution
▸▸ No well-defined sex predilection to date
▸▸ Typically diagnosed in adults, with mean age at diagnosis in the seventh decade of life

Clinical Features
▸▸ Often asymptomatic
▸▸ May present with symptoms related to biliary obstruction

Endoscopic Features
▸▸ Exophytic polypoid lesion with its epicenter within the ampullary channel
▸▸ Minimal involvement of the common bile duct, main pancreatic duct, or duodenal papilla

Prognosis and Therapy
▸▸ IAPNs lacking associated carcinoma are benign neoplasms with excellent prognosis
▸▸ Complete resection of IAPNs is recommended, as they have a higher rate of malignant transformation than adenomas of nonampullary small bowel sites
▸▸ In some series, invasive carcinomas are identified in up to 75% of resected IAPNs
▸▸ Invasive carcinoma arising from IAPN has a better prognosis than those from flat dysplasia

---

**INTRA-AMPULLARY PAPILLARY-TUBULAR NEOPLASM –
PATHOLOGIC FEATURES**

Gross Findings
▸▸ Compact, exophytic polypoid lesion centered within the ampulla

Microscopic Findings
▸▸ Variably tubular, tubulovillous, or papillary growth patterns
▸▸ Typically intestinal-type with tall columnar cells with elongated and pseudostratified nuclei
▸▸ Rarely pancreatobiliary-type with features of intraductal papillary mucinous neoplasm
▸▸ The majority of cases (>80%) show a mixture of low-grade and high-grade dysplasia
▸▸ High-grade dysplasia characterized by architectural complexity coupled with nuclear stratification and severe cytologic atypia

Pathologic Differential Diagnoses
▸▸ Adenoma of ampullary duodenum
▸▸ Invasive ampullary adenocarcinoma
▸▸ Poorly differentiated neuroendocrine carcinoma

APPENDIX

APPENDICEAL MUCINOUS NEOPLASM

DDX: mucinous adenocarcinoma, retention cyst, appendiceal diverticulum (ruptured), serrated epithelial lesions, mullerianosis

Clinical Features

Appendiceal mucinous neoplasms are rare tumors, but accurate diagnosis is essential as patients may require long-term follow-up or procedures such cryoreductive surgery with heated intraperitoneal chemotherapy in the setting of pseudomyxoma peritonei (PMP). Epidemiologic data has been difficult to assess due to inconsistencies in reporting and evolving definitions of the entity, but these lesions have been reported in adults of all ages with a peak incidence in the sixth decade, with a possible, slight female predominance. Clinically, patients often present with appendicitis, or may have nonspecific symptoms with lesions incidentally discovered on radiologic studies. Less commonly, patients may present with palpable abdominal masses, tumor-associated intestinal obstruction or intussusception, acute abdomen secondary to rupture, and in the setting of established PMP, malignant ascites.

Pathologic Features

GROSS FINDINGS

Appendiceal mucinous neoplasms are often associated with abundant luminal mucin and cystic dilation of the appendiceal wall. Calcifications may be felt. The serosal surface should be carefully inspected for mucin deposition in nonruptured specimens. In general, mucinous lesions of the appendix should be thoroughly sampled or entirely submitted for histologic examination when practicable.

MICROSCOPIC FINDINGS

A consensus paper from the Peritoneal Surface Oncology Group International (PSOGI) has sought to unify classification and reporting of mucinous appendiceal lesions. In this paper, appendiceal mucinous neoplasms are defined by cytologic atypia and any of the following features: (1) loss of muscularis mucosae, (2) submucosal fibrosis, (3) "pushing invasion (expansile or diverticular-type growth), (4) dissection of acellular mucin in wall, (5) undulating or flattened epithelial growth, (6) rupture of appendix, and (7) mucin and/or cells outside appendix. Importantly, an infiltrative pattern of invasion precludes mucinous neoplasm terminology, and is considered a diagnostic feature for classification as a mucinous adenocarcinoma. The degree of cytologic atypia differentiates between low-grade appendiceal mucinous neoplasms (LAMNs) and high-grade appendiceal mucinous neoplasms (HAMNs) (Fig. 1.15A–D). Classically, at low magnification, appendiceal mucinous neoplasms are most often recognized by a hypermucinous or attenuated surface layer that is associated with effacement of the lamina propria, the absence of normal crypt architecture, and submucosal fibrosis.

The cytologic atypia in LAMNs may be minimal, but is typically characterized by uniform, small, dark, basally oriented nuclei with moderate to abundant apical mucin. As such, the nuclear-to-cytoplasmic ratios are low. In contrast, the cytologic atypia in HAMNs is more pronounced with enlarged, hyperchromatic nuclei and high nuclear-to-cytoplasmic ratios, which may be associated with atypical mitotic figures, vesicular nuclei with prominent nucleoli, and increased architectural complexity, such as cribriform gland formation and loss of nuclear polarity. HAMNs, however, are rare, and HAMN itself is a new diagnostic category, recommended by the PSOGI consensus group and added to the 2019 WHO Blue Books on Digestive System Tumors, but there is little published data available. Molecular studies have shown that both LAMNs and HAMNs share a mutational profile, with both typically demonstrating *KRAS* mutations, as well as an increased rate of GNAS mutations, suggesting a common histogenesis. In a study by Liao et al., the majority of HAMNs also showed either mutations in TP53 and/or ATM, which may account for disease progression.

In the absence of clinically established disseminated disease, histopathologic features that have been associated with a risk of recurrent disease/PMP in LAMNs are extra-appendiceal mucin and extra-appendiceal neoplastic epithelium. LAMNs entirely confined within the muscularis propria of the appendix are thought to have no risk of recurrent disease, and simple appendectomy is considered curative. In this respect, the PSOGI recommendation to eliminate "(mucinous) adenoma" terminology in this setting of a benign lesion is controversial. In a study by Pai et al., LAMNs with extra-appendiceal acellular mucin had a relatively low risk of disease recurrence (~7%), whereas LAMNs with extra-appendiceal mucin with neoplastic epithelium had a high risk of recurrence (~78%). However, in regard to pathologic tumor staging, the eighth edition of the American Joint Committee on Cancer (AJCC) Cancer Staging Manual, does not intrinsically distinguish between LAMNs with extra-appendiceal acellular mucin and LAMNs with extra-appendiceal

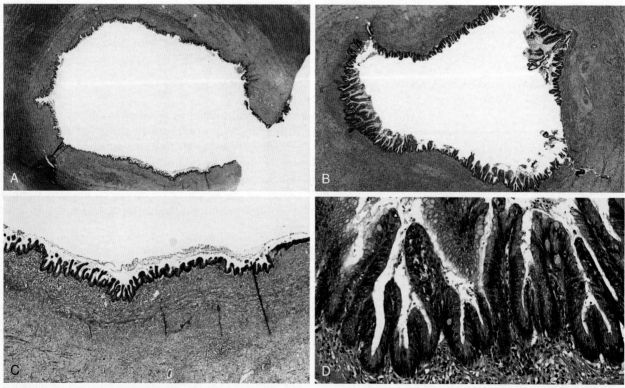

FIG. 1.15

At low magnification, low-grade appendiceal mucinous neoplasms (LAMNs) may show an attenuated, undulating, or hyperplastic-appearing surface epithelium **(A, B)**. Key to the diagnosis of LAMN is the destruction/replacement of the lamina propria and muscularis mucosae **(C)**. LAMNs also must show cytologic atypia, typically with hyperchromatic nuclei and a hypermucinous appearance **(D)**.

mucin and neoplastic epithelium. Instead, LAMNs entirely confined within the muscularis propria are considered pTis, and LAMNs with extracellular mucin with or without neoplastic epithelium are considered pT3 or pT4, depending on serosal involvement. Having said this, the AJCC recommends clearly stating the presence or absence of mucinous epithelial cells in extra-appendiceal mucin in surgical pathology reports. Also, in part due to their novelty as a distinct entity, HAMNs are not formally incorporated within the AJCC staging criteria. However, the WHO recommends staging HAMNs similarly to invasive adenocarcinomas.

Ancillary Studies

Ancillary immunohistochemical and molecular diagnostic studies have limited utility in the diagnosis of appendiceal mucinous neoplasms with classic histologic features.

Differential Diagnosis

APPENDICEAL MUCINOUS NEOPLASM VERSUS RETENTION CYST

Retention cysts are caused by obstructive dilation of the appendix and may occur as a result of a fecalith or following an inflammatory process, such as appendicitis. Grossly, retention cysts exhibit cystic dilation of the lumen and may be mucin-filled, mimicking an appendiceal mucinous neoplasm radiologically and grossly. Histologically, retention cysts are typically lined by an intact, colonic-type mucosa. While retention cysts may show areas with an attenuated epithelial lining and crypt dropout, particularly in the setting of inflammation, there are typically retained mucosal elements, including lamina propria and muscularis mucosae. Importantly, while reactive atypia is allowed commensurate to the degree of inflammation, the cytologic atypia characteristic of appendiceal mucinous neoplasms cannot be present (Fig. 1.16).

APPENDICEAL MUCINOUS NEOPLASM VERSUS RUPTURED APPENDICEAL DIVERTICULUM

Like retention cysts, ruptured appendiceal diverticula are a non-neoplastic mimic of appendiceal mucinous neoplasms. In cases of ruptured diverticula, mucin may be seen on the serosal surface of the appendix as well as on adjacent structures, raising concern for localized PMP intraoperatively. Grossly, diverticula may sometimes be appreciated by a careful prosector that identifies multiple luminal profiles, and, in contrast to appendiceal mucinous neoplasms or retention cysts, cases of

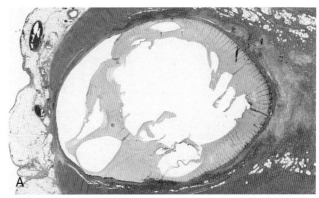
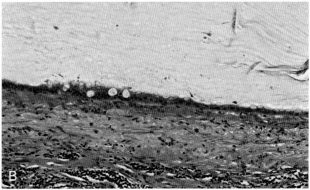

FIG. 1.16
While retention cysts may show an attenuated surface layer and a dilated, mucin-filled lumen mimicking a low-grade appendiceal mucinous neoplasm, cytologic atypia is not appreciated **(A, B)**.

ruptured diverticula are not typically associated with appendiceal dilation.

Histologically, the classical feature of a diverticulum is the herniation of mucosa through the muscularis propria. While there is often marked, suppurative inflammation associated with the rupture, there is retained mucosal architecture, including crypt formation and lamina propria. While the epithelium may exhibit hyperplastic-type and reactive changes, an undulating, villiform contour of the epithelium or neoplastic cytologic changes are not seen (Fig. 1.17).

APPENDICEAL MUCINOUS NEOPLASM VERSUS SERRATED POLYP

Serrated neoplasms of the appendix are common. While they may have an overlapping morphology with sessile serrated lesions in the colorectum, serrated lesions in the appendix appear to harbor different molecular alterations. Serrated lesions of the appendix are more likely to demonstrate KRAS mutations and less likely to exhibit BRAF mutations, raising the possibility that these serrated neoplasms may be precursor lesions for appendiceal mucinous neoplasms. Because of these molecular differences, the PSOGI consensus was to refer to tumors with serrated features confined to the mucosa as a "serrated polyp," with or without dysplasia.

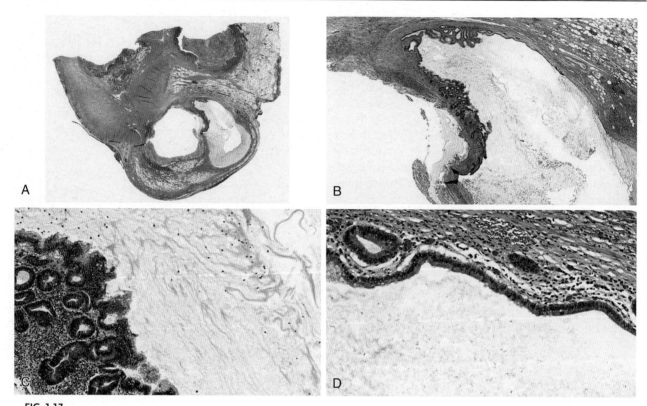

FIG. 1.17

Ruptured appendiceal diverticuli also mimic low-grade appendiceal mucinous neoplasms with the appearance of extra-appendiceal mucin **(A)**. However, the epithelium lining the mucin typically shows preservation of the lamina propria **(B, C)**, and the surface epithelium will not demonstrate significant atypia **(D)**.

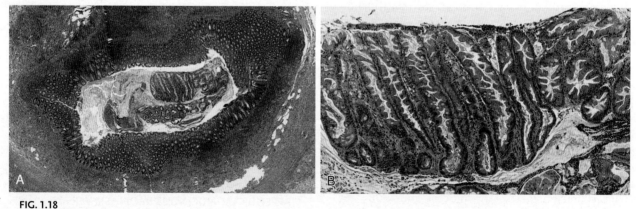

FIG. 1.18

Serrated polyps of the appendix will typically exhibit cytoarchitectural features resembling a sessile serrated polyp/adenoma. However, in contrast to counterparts in the colon, appendiceal serrated polyps do not typically harbor BRAF mutations, and their malignant potential is not well understood **(A, B)**.

LAMNs may histologically evoke serrated lesions in cases without conventional-type cytological dysplasia and where a villiform architecture mimics a serrated appearance. Serrated polyps of the appendix may also exhibit a hypermucinous appearance on low magnification. However, serrated polyps still demonstrate retained mucosal architecture with a lamina propria and well-defined submucosal layer (Fig. 1.18).

APPENDICEAL MUCINOUS NEOPLASM VERSUS ENDOMETRIOSIS WITH INTESTINAL METAPLASIA

Endometriosis of the appendix is readily distinguishable from appendiceal mucinous neoplasms histologically. However, when intestinal metaplasia is present as a component of the endometriosis, these cases may grossly and histologically resemble appendiceal mucinous neoplasms.

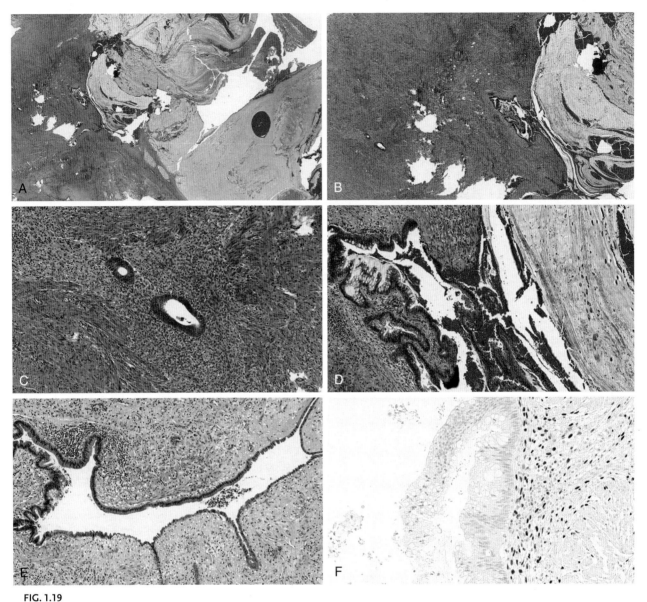

FIG. 1.19

Endometriosis may mimic low-grade appendiceal mucinous neoplasms when endometrial glands are rare/focal, particularly in cases where endometrial glands exhibit intestinal metaplasia. In this case, endometriosis can be readily appreciated **(A–C)**. The glands associated with luminal mucin appear intestinal and, importantly, maintain lamina propria **(D)**. In areas, some glands appear lined by both endometrial and intestinal-type epithelium **(E)**. Estrogen receptor stain highlights the stroma surrounding the intestinal-type epithelium, suggestive of intestinal metaplasia within an endometriosis **(F)**.

Clinically, in a case series presented by Misdraji et al., the patients most commonly presented with symptoms of acute appendicitis or for evaluation of an appendiceal or cecal mass, and a minority had a known history of endometriosis. Grossly, these lesions were associated with complex, cystic masses with mucin. Histologically, there was a variable amount of endometrial stroma present, and some cases displayed epithelial dysplasia in association with the intestinal metaplasia. Importantly, however, cases of appendiceal endometriosis with intestinal metaplasia appear to always have at least focal areas with classical endometrial-type glands. Immunohistochemical stains, such as Pax-8, may be helpful in establishing this diagnosis (Fig. 1.19).

APPENDICEAL MUCINOUS NEOPLASM – DISEASE FACT SHEET

Definition

▶▶ Neoplastic proliferation of mucinous epithelium, which may be filiform, villous, or attenuated, with associated extracellular mucin and a pushing front of invasion

Incidence and Location

▶▶ Always occur in the appendix, with variable involvement of the surrounding peritoneal cavity
▶▶ Relatively rare tumors, identified in approximately 0.3% of appendectomy specimens

(Continued)

APPENDICEAL MUCINOUS NEOPLASM – DISEASE FACT SHEET—cont'd

Sex and Age Distribution

▸▸ Tend to occur in adults, with peak incidence in the sixth decade of life
▸▸ Suggestion of a slight female predominance

Clinical Features

▸▸ Often an incidental finding with an asymptomatic presentation
▸▸ Can present with right lower quadrant pain/appendicitis or palpable abdominal mass
▸▸ If ruptured, may present with abdominal distension and/or features of acute abdomen
▸▸ Less commonly, can present with colicky abdominal pain or GI bleeding due to associated intussusception of the bowel

Endoscopic Features

▸▸ Dilated appendix
▸▸ Appendiceal orifice extruding extracellular mucin

Prognosis and Therapy

▸▸ Prognosis largely dependent on pathologic stage
▸▸ If tumor confined to appendix, prognosis is excellent
▸▸ If tumor associated with peritoneal dissemination, prognosis is worse and largely associated with the ability or lack thereof to successfully remove all macroscopically identifiable tumor in the abdomen

---

ANAL GLAND ADENOCARCINOMA – PATHOLOGIC FEATURES

Gross Findings

▸▸ Variable, though appendix often dilated by extracellular mucin
▸▸ Perforation with extrusion of mucin may be seen
▸▸ Appendiceal wall can be thinned due to dilatation or thickened with dystrophic calcifications, as part of the reactive milieu
▸▸ Appendix may also be grossly unremarkable

Microscopic Findings

▸▸ Replacement of normal appendiceal mucosa by a monolayered proliferation of mucinous epithelium
▸▸ Neoplastic epithelium typically demonstrates low-grade dysplasia with tall, columnar cells with bland basally located nuclei and abundant apical cytoplasmic mucin
▸▸ High-grade dysplasia characterized by combined severe cytologic atypia and architectural complexity
▸▸ If an infiltrative epithelial process, with an associated desmoplastic stromal response is identified, should be characterized as an invasive adenocarcinoma
▸▸ Neoplastic epithelium may be arranged in any of the following patterns: filiform, villous, undulating/scalloped, flattened/attenuated
▸▸ The tumor generally lacks an associated lamina propria, as it has been obliterated by its pushing front
▸▸ Appendiceal wall often fibrosed, hyalinized, and/or calcified
▸▸ Mucin may dissect through appendiceal wall, including to peritoneal surface

Pathologic Differential Diagnoses

▸▸ Mucinous adenocarcinoma
▸▸ Retention cyst
▸▸ Appendiceal diverticulum (ruptured)
▸▸ Serrated epithelial lesions
▸▸ Mullerianosis

COLON

CROHN'S COLITIS

DDX: ulcerative colitis, infectious colitis, ischemic colitis, medication-induced colitis, diverticular disease–associated colitis

Clinical Features

Crohn's disease (CD) is a chronic inflammatory condition of the GI tract that is episodic in nature, with bouts of chronic and/or active inflammation followed by periods of respite. Women are slightly more frequently affected than men (female-to-male ratio 1.3:1) and, geographically, CD is comparatively more common in Northern latitudes. The majority of patients with CD are diagnosed within the second to fourth decades of life, with a smaller peak of onset in the fifth through seventh decades. In the United States, the prevalence of CD in adults is estimated to be approximately 200 cases per 100,000 individuals. The prevalence is lower amongst pediatric cohorts, estimated to be approximately 40 cases per 100,000 adolescents. CD is categorized according to the Montreal classification, which takes into account the age at diagnosis, anatomic distribution of disease, and the clinical behavior. In distribution of disease, approximately 30% to 40% of patients have disease restricted to the small bowel, another 30% to 40% have ileocolonic involvement, and a final 10% to 20% have disease restricted to the colon. In patients with disease initially isolated to either the small bowel or the colon, approximately 20% of each cohort will go on to develop disease that affects both anatomic sites. In those patients with Crohn's colitis, right-sided colitis (approximately 50%) is more common than left-sided colitis (approximately 40%), with pancolitis (approximately 10%) being the least common scenario. The clinical presentation of CD is extremely variable, given the breadth of possibly involved anatomic sites within the GI tract and the myriad clinical behaviors of disease. A common clinical presentation of CD is that of diarrhea with or without blood. In pediatric patients, CD often presents with fever and weight loss. A relatively substantial subset of patients (up to 25%) present with perianal disease (e.g., skin tags, anal fissures, ulcers) prior to onset of GI symptoms. It is important to note that up to a quarter of patients with CD may present with extraintestinal manifestations of disease and that those patients with colonic involvement are at increased risk. Examples of extraintestinal disease manifestations include pauciarticular arthropathy, polyarticular arthropathy, peripheral arthralgias, granulomatous vasculitis, mucocutaneous lesions, episcleritis, uveitis, and primary sclerosing cholangitis (though this is more common amongst ulcerative colitis [UC] patients).

Pathologic Features

GROSS FINDINGS

When involving the colon, and also in its distribution throughout the entire GI tract, CD is characterized by a patchy or segmental distribution of disease. Characteristically, the inflammation and fibrosis in CD involves the bowel wall in a transmural manner, resulting in segmental thickening of the involved colon. Thus, at gross evaluation of a resection specimen, the bowel does not lie flat. Accompanying this thickening, other features of CD appreciable at the serosa include congestion, fibrinous exudate, and fat wrapping ("creeping fat") involving anti-mesenteric portions of the bowel surface. Upon opening the bowel, the mucosa is often described as "cobblestoning" secondary to discontinuous regions of ulceration adjacent to intact edematous mucosa. Ulcers often begin as relatively small, well-circumscribed aphthous ulcers which may have a hyperemic border. With disease progression, these ulcers elongate and connect to form longitudinal, serpiginous ulcers described as "bearclaw-type" furrows.

MICROSCOPIC FINDINGS

Both grossly and microscopically, CD is characterized by "skip lesions" in which affected bowel alternates with areas of bowel wall sparing. As discussed previously within the gross pathologic findings, CD generally elicits a varied combination of mucosal and mural changes in the bowel wall. As for all idiopathic inflammatory bowel disease (IBD), including UC, mucosal injury is generally characterized by the presence of chronic and/or active mucosal injury. Features of chronic mucosal injury include crypt architectural distortion (e.g., irregular crypt spacing, crypt branching, crypt foreshortening, crypt atrophy/dropout, villiform surface epithelium), basal lymphoplasmacytosis, diffused mixed lymphoplasmacytic inflammation throughout the lamina propria, metaplasia (e.g., Paneth cell metaplasia in the left colon, pyloric gland metaplasia), and basal lymphoid aggregates. Features of active mucosal injury include neutrophilic cryptitis, crypt abscess, erosion, ulceration, regenerative or degenerative epithelial changes, and necrosis. The combination of chronic and/or active mucosal injury gets descriptively bucketed into the following categories at the time of microscopic review: chronic inactive colitis, chronic active colitis, and active colitis. Additional mucosa-based findings characteristic of CD, though neither sensitive nor specific for the diagnosis, include well-formed non-necrotizing epithelioid granulomas and pyloric gland metaplasia (Fig. 1.20A). Non-necrotizing

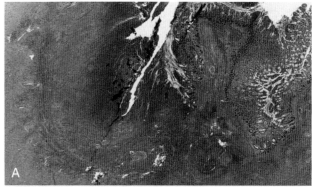
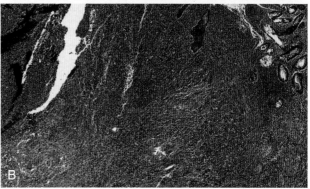

FIG. 1.20
Crohn's colitis. Low-power histologic image shows patchy chronic active colitis with associated transmural inflammation, including lymphoid aggregates within the submucosa, as well as noncaseating granulomas involving the mucosa and submucosa **(A)**. High-power histologic image highlights chronic active colitis with deep ulceration and associated granuloma **(B)**.

granulomas in CD are identified in up to 50% of biopsy specimens and up to 60% of resection specimens. Care must be taken to ensure these granulomas are not crypt rupture (mucin)–related granulomas commonly seen in UC. While pyloric gland metaplasia can be seen secondary to any form of chronic mucosal injury in the colon, it is more common in CD than in UC and, when seen, is most typically identified in the ileocecum or right colon. Regarding erosion and ulceration, as mentioned previously in discussion of the gross pathologic findings in CD, the most common type of mucosal ulceration associated with active CD are small, relatively superficial aphthous ulceration which, with time and persistence of activity, may coalesce to form the long, serpiginous "bearclaw-type" ulcers classic of CD. Microscopically, aphthous ulcers generally are superficial mucosal ulceration that overlie reactive lymphoid aggregates with or without admixed neutrophilic inflammation (Fig. 1.20B). Irregularly shaped crypts and low-cuboidal brightly eosinophilic regenerative-type epithelium with relatively increased nuclear-to-cytoplasmic ratios may be found at the periphery of these ulcers as they heal.

In resection specimens, mural-based changes of CD can be appreciated. Classic of CD are well-formed lymphoid aggregates with or without germinal centers, including away from sites of active mucosal ulceration. These lymphoid aggregates are commonly seen at the junction of the mucosa and the submucosa as well as transmural, beyond muscular propria in the subserosal adipose tissue (Fig. 1.20A). Lymphoid aggregates may or may not be accompanied by granulomatous inflammation. Additional typical mural findings include fissuring ulcers, which are knife-like ulcerations oriented perpendicular to the longitudinal axis of the bowel wall. These ulcers may extend through submucosa and muscularis propria and may be associated with sinus tract formation, fistulization, and pericolonic abscess formation. Accompanying these aforementioned mural insults are myriad of injury-response phenomena, including submucosal fibrosis, neural hypertrophy, hypertrophy of muscularis mucosae and propria, neural plexitis, perivascular lymphoid aggregates, and serositis.

Ancillary Studies

Ancillary studies specific to the pathology laboratory are not required to render a diagnosis of CD. Of course, careful clinical, serologic, and endoscopic correlation is generally required prior to a definitive diagnosis. In cases with florid granulomas or in which the granulomas are necrotizing, GMS and AFB stains should be performed to exclude the possibility of infection. Of greater sensitivity in this endeavor is also the option of polymerase chain reaction performed on the formalin-fixed paraffin-embedded tissue for bacterial and fungal elements. Of note, in areas of ulceration, especially if the patient is being managed on immunomodulating biologic agents, careful review for viral cytopathic effect is important. Immunostains to aid in identification of CMV infection or adenovirus infection can be used. Furthermore, in ulcerations rich in lymphocytes and plasma cells, Epstein-Barr virus chromogenic *in situ* hybridization (CISH) can be used to identify viral RNA.

Differential Diagnosis

CROHN'S DISEASE VERSUS ULCERATIVE COLITIS

Similar to CD, UC is also an idiopathic IBD with a relapsing and remitting clinical course. Similar to CD, UC has a predilection for clinical presentation in the second to third decades of life, with a secondary peak occurring in the seventh decade. In UC, the female-to-male ratio is essentially equal, with the incidence of UC greatest in Caucasians compared with other ethnic groups. Similar to CD, the prevalence of UC is geographically variable, with increased rates of occurrence in industrialized countries and urban settings. In the United States, the annual incidence of UC is estimated

to range from 5 to 20 cases per 100,000 individuals, with approximately 1% of the US population afflicted with UC in their lifetime. Clinical symptomatology in patients with UC is variable, depending on the severity of disease. Typical clinical symptoms include urgency, passing mucus, tenesmus, rectal bleeding, diarrhea (often bloody), abdominal pain, fever, and weight loss. While CD can involve any part of the GI tract, typically with a patchy or segmental distribution, untreated UC prototypically involves the rectum with variable continuous proximal extension depending on disease severity. The Montreal classification subdivides the extent of UC into the following categories: ulcerative proctitis (involves rectum only), left-sided or distal UC (involvement limited to colorectum distal to splenic flexure), and extensive UC or pancolitis (involvement of colon proximal to splenic flexure). At presentation, approximately 45% of patients present with ulcerative proctitis, 10% to 15% with distal UC, and 20% with pancolitis. Approximately 50% to 70% of patients who initially present with proctitis or distal UC ultimately develop pancolitis. In contrast, recall that only approximately one third of CD patients will have disease limited to the colon. Similar to CD, "skip lesions" are identified in up to 80% of untreated UC patients. These patients have appendiceal, periappendiceal, and/or cecal/ascending colon involvement despite lacking pancolitis. Of course, patchy disease distribution is also seen in the setting of treated UC. At gross pathologic examination, colon segments from UC patients generally lie flat, without evidence of wall thickening or fat wrapping. This is contrast to CD patients in which the bowel wall is thickened and stiff secondary to mural changes. In longstanding UC, strictures may form, which may or may not be associated with malignancy. Gross pathologic features typical of malignant strictures include location proximal to the splenic flexure; clinical findings are usually that of the stricture being symptomatic and the stricture arising in the setting of longstanding disease (e.g., >20 years). Microscopically, UC presents very similar to CD in that the prototypical histologic pattern in that of chronic active colitis (Fig. 1.21A and B). Depending on the extent of disease and the patient's treatment history, other histomorphologic patterns common to UC include chronic inactive (quiescent) colitis or active colitis without evidence of chronicity. When looking at biopsy specimens in untreated patients from areas of involvement, typically all tissue fragments demonstrate a similarly homogenous or diffuse pattern of injury. A more patchy disease distribution becomes apparent in the setting of treatment. When reviewing resection specimens, the distribution of disease in UC is typically restricted to the mucosa and superficial submucosa, with occasional extension into deep submucosa in areas of extensive ulceration. Generally, transmural inflammatory and fibrotic activity typical of CD is not present in UC. Similar to CD,

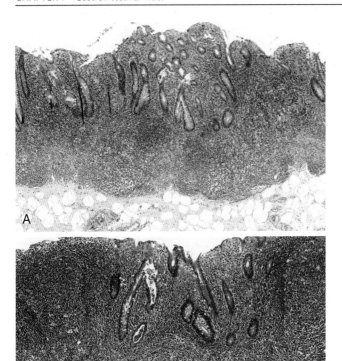

FIG. 1.21

Ulcerative colitis. Low-power histologic image shows a diffuse pattern of chronic active colitis, including crypt foreshortening, crypt branching, and scattered crypt microabscesses. The increased inflammation within the lamina propria shows a dense basal lymphoplasmacytosis and associated dense chronic inflammation in the superficial submucosa **(A)**. High-power histologic image highlights cryptitis with crypt microabscess formation, crypt architectural distortion, and superficial surface epithelial erosion **(B)**.

there is no curative treatment for UC and the focus of immunomodulating medical therapies is to quell active disease and prevent recurrence of disease in remission. Approximately 50% of patients respond to medical therapy alone. A small subset of patients, approximately 5% of patients in each cohort, are plagued by complications including toxic megacolon or colonic strictures. As up to a quarter of strictures are associated with malignancy, there should be a high index of suspicion for carcinoma in this clinical setting. In patients who are medically refractory, develop complications, or develop dysplasia or carcinoma, surgical intervention is indicated. Surgical options include subtotal colectomy with ileostomy, colectomy with ileorectal anastomosis, and proctocolectomy with ileal pouch-anal anastomosis.

CROHN'S DISEASE VERSUS INFECTIOUS COLITIS

Infectious colitis, also termed acute self-limited colitis, typically has a relatively abrupt clinical onset, with patients experiencing fever, abdominal tenderness, and bloody diarrhea. Common infectious etiologies include bacteria such as *Campylobacter jejuni*, *Salmonella* species,

Shigella species, *Escherichia coli*, and *Yersinia enterocolitica*. In the immunocompromised or immunosuppressed, viral colitides such as CMV colitis may be seen. In the hospital setting or in the context of recent antibiotic administration, a patient may present with *Clostridium difficile*–related colitis. Finally, less commonly, amoebiasis-related colitis, such as colitis secondary to *Entamoeba histolytica*, is also possible (Fig. 1.22A–E). Symptomatology is generally related to organisms invading the mucosa or to their generation of enterotoxins and, most typically, symptoms resolve within 2 to 4 weeks. While most patients with infectious colitis do not undergo routine endoscopy with biopsy early in their disease course, typical microscopic findings in early infectious colitides include prominent neutrophilic inflammation within the lamina propria, neutrophils infiltrating crypt and surface epithelium, crypt microabscesses, and lamina propria edema. Similar to idiopathic IBDs, erosions, ulcerations, and granulomas may be seen. In infectious colitis, granulomas are most typically of the crypt rupture–type within the basal half of the lamina propria. In contrast to CD (or idiopathic IBD in general), the acute and self-limited nature of infectious colitis precludes findings of chronic mucosal injury except in extremely rare instances. Thus, pertinent negatives include a lack of architectural distortion such as basal lymphoplasmacytosis, crypt foreshortening, crypt branching, and crypt dropout. In rare case reports in which longstanding infectious colitis results in crypt architectural distortion, distorted crypts are set within a relatively paucicellular lamina propria, in contrast to the increased cellularity of lamina propria typical of CD and UC. As endoscopy with biopsy is often not delayed until a few weeks of persistent symptoms, the resolving phase of infectious colitis may endoscopically mimic CD due to a patchy distribution of inflammation. Microscopically, findings are often whelming, most frequently characterized as "focal" or "patchy" active colitis with or without mucosal edema and regenerative epithelial changes. As implied with the moniker "self-limited," most infectious colitides, especially those bacterial in origin, can be managed conservatively without the use of antibiotics. Antibiotics are generally reserved for those cases with complication, such as sepsis.

CROHN'S DISEASE VERSUS DRUG/ MEDICATION-INDUCED COLITIS

Drug/medication-induced colitis can present with myriad patterns of injury, including acute and chronic patterns of mucosal injury that overlap with idiopathic IBD. General features of drug/medication-induced colitis that are similar to those of CD include the presence of focal activity (cryptitis), mild crypt architectural distortion, erosions or ulcers, and strictures. Increased epithelial apoptosis, pseudomembrane formation, and ischemic-type changes are additional patterns of injury more so suggestive of a drug/medication-induced etiology and also raising the

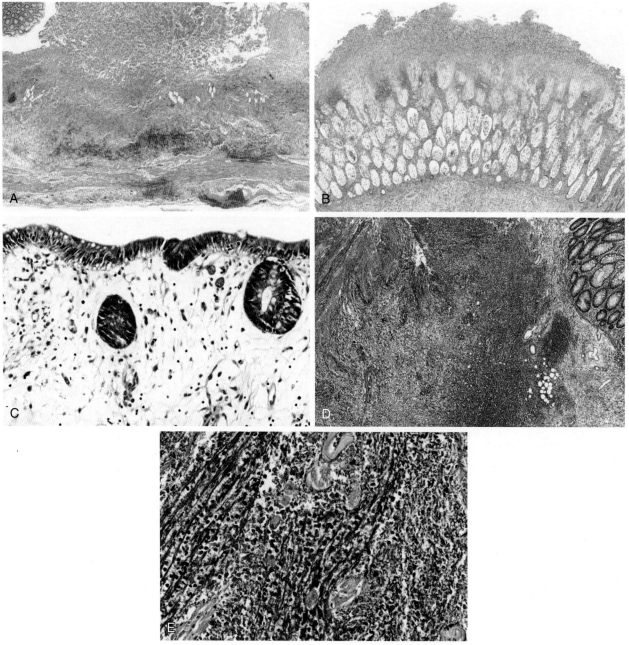

FIG. 1.22

Infectious colitis. Infectious colitides may occur secondary to myriad pathogens (e.g., bacteria, viral, parasitic) in a variety of clinicopathologic settings, including within the immunocompromised. Toxigenic *Clostridium* species bacteria classically cause eruptive-appearing "volcano-" or "mushroom-" type lesions with extensive mucosal necrosis **(A)**. Pseudomembranes composed of fibrin, mucin, and neutrophils line the mucosal surface and underlying degenerating glands show changes including ballooning, sloughed epithelium, neutrophils, and mucin **(B)**. Cytomegalovirus (CMV) infection in an immunocompromised host shows scattered CMV-infected mesenchymal cells in the superficial lamina propria. These infected cells are characterized by nuclear and cytoplasmic enlargement, with typical "owl's eye" intranuclear inclusions **(C)**. In advanced cases, protozoal infection by *Entamoeba histolytica* shows deep, extensive ulceration **(D)**. On high-power histologic image, scattered organisms have lightly eosinophilic foamy cytoplasm with round, eccentrically located nuclei that have peripherally marginated nuclear chromatin. In this advanced lesion, these organisms are embedded deep within the ulcer bed amongst abundant necrotic debris **(E)**.

possibility of infectious and primary ischemic origins. Relatively common etiologies of drug/medication-induced colitis include nonsteroidal anti-inflammatory drugs (NSAIDs), mycophenolate mofetil (MMF), and chemotherapy-associated colitis (e.g., 5-flurouracil, mitomycin, cisplatin, methotrexate, anti-PDL1 drugs). NSAID-related colitis typically involves the right colon more than the left and shows a patchy distribution of disease, with variably present erythema, friability, erosions, or ulceration. In acute NSAID-induced colitis, mild architectural distortion, neutrophilic cryptitis, focal erosions, and increased crypt apoptosis are common findings. In the setting of chronic NSAID-related mucosal injury, the crypt architectural distortion may be well-developed, with accompanying mild basal plasmacytosis, Paneth cell metaplasia, neutrophilic cryptitis, and crypt abscess formation. Generally, unlike CD, drug/medication-induced colitis lacks epithelioid granulomas and transmural lymphoid aggregates. Resolution of symptoms and mucosal changes after cessation of NSAIDs is the only way to confirm the diagnosis. Patients suffering from MMF toxicity with associated colitis frequently lack identifiable endoscopic or mucosal abnormalities. While the mucosal manifestations of MMF-associated colitis are vast, the most common histologic presentation is that of mild crypt architectural distortion, lamina propria edema, increased crypt epithelial apoptosis, and degenerative crypts with microcystic- and hypereosinophilic-type changes. Occasional cases of MMF-associated colitis mimic CD in that there is crypt architectural distortion, crypt dropout, Paneth cell metaplasia, and a lamina propria mildly expanded by a chronic lymphoplasmacytic inflammatory infiltrate. Lastly, chemotherapeutic drug–related injury is common for many of the aforementioned anti-metabolite drugs and, more recently, has been described as a consequence of immune checkpoint inhibitors in the setting of PDL1 blockade. Endoscopic evaluation in these patients reveals ulcerations in approximately one third of cases and nonulcerative inflammation, including erythema, edema, erosion, and altered vasculature, in approximately 40%. Microscopically, checkpoint inhibitor–induced colitis can present with acute, chronic, chronic active, or microscopic patterns of mucosal injury. The most common histologic finding is marked expansion of the lamina propria by mixed inflammation including neutrophils, lymphocytes, plasma cells, and eosinophils, with accompanying neutrophilic cryptitis, crypt abscess, crypt epithelial apoptosis, glandular destruction with crypt dropout, and erosion. Approximately half of patients have established evidence of chronic mucosal injury (e.g., basal lymphoplasmacytosis, crypt architectural

distortion) at the time of initial presentation, certainly mimicking idiopathic IBD. Interestingly, a diffuse pattern of inflammation is actually more common than patchy at initial onset. Also of note, crypt rupture–related granulomas have been reported in checkpoint inhibitor–induced colitis, certainly mimicking the findings in CD and even UC.

CROHN'S DISEASE VERSUS ISCHEMIC COLITIS

Similar to CD, ischemic colitis can present as an acute, active phenomenon or with features of chronicity. Colitis secondary to ischemic injury more commonly develops in women than in men, though men have a younger onset of disease than their female counterparts. Chronic ischemic colitis develops in approximately 25% of cases and most typically occurs in patients greater than 60 years of age. Chronic ischemic injury may mimic idiopathic IBD endoscopically and microscopically. Endoscopically, chronic ischemic injury often presents with mucosal granularity, pseudopolyp formation, congestion, edema, and ulceration. Disease distribution in ischemic colitis is left side predominant (75% of cases), with a subset of cases involving the splenic flexure (25%) or right colon (10%). Histologic features of chronic ischemic injury that share significant overlap with chronic active colitis in the setting of idiopathic IBD include crypt architectural distortion, Paneth cell metaplasia, a cellular lamina propria expanded by chronic lymphoplasmacytic inflammation with a basal predominance, neutrophilic cryptitis, and erosions or ulceration. Features more suggestive of an ischemic etiology to the chronic mucosal injury include withering crypts, lamina propria hyalinization, mucosal hemorrhage, hemosiderin-laden macrophages, and capillary microthrombi (Fig. 1.23A and B).

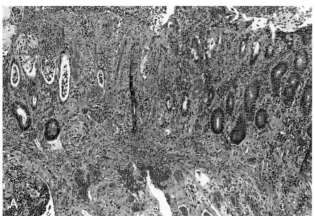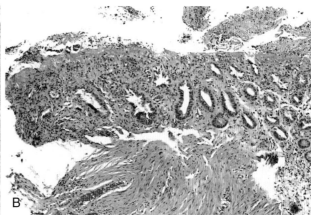

FIG. 1.23

Ischemic colitis. While histologic findings vary depending on the duration of disease, typical microscopic features include superficial mucosal necrosis, withering crypts, mucosal hemorrhage, and crypt microabscesses **(A)**. More long-standing cases show hyalinized lamina propria surrounding withered crypts with overlying superficial mucosal necrosis **(B)**.

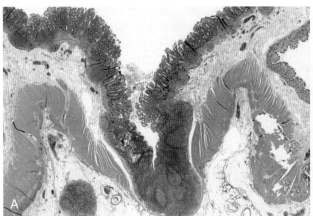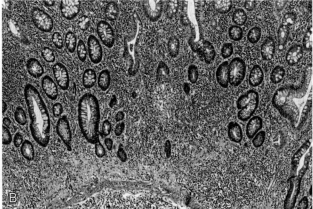

FIG. 1.24

Diverticular disease-associated colitis. Diverticular disease characterized by a blind protrusion of mucosa through muscularis propria **(A)**. As pictured, mucosal changes that can be seen in the setting of diverticular disease include increased lymphoid infiltrate within the lamina propria, mild cryptitis with crypt microabscess, and crypt architectural distortion which may mimic idiopathic IBD **(B)**.

CROHN'S DISEASE VERSUS DIVERTICULAR DISEASE–ASSOCIATED COLITIS

Similar to CD, diverticular disease–associated colitis can present with histologic changes of active or chronic mucosal injury, including cryptitis, crypt abscess, mild crypt architectural distortion, Paneth cell metaplasia, and expansion of the lamina propria by lymphocytes and plasma cells. Unique to diverticular disease–associated colitis, these findings are usually most pronounced deep within diverticula rather than at the mucosal surface (Fig. 1.24A and B). Often, there may be accompanying erosion or ulceration. The clinical context of mucosal involvement restricted to diverticula is paramount in rendering an accurate diagnosis. Generally, interdiverticular mucosa is spared in diverticular disease–associated colitis, unless there is extensive ulceration with abscess formation involving the colonic wall secondary to diverticular rupture. It is important to recall that greater than 90% of cases of diverticulosis involve the sigmoid colon, with cecum and ascending colon involvement uncommon (5% of cases), as is pancolonic involvement (15%). Gross pathologic features of diverticular disease–associated colitis include bowel wall thickening and shortening in the segmental region of disease distribution.

Prognosis and Therapy

The clinical course of CD is extremely variable. The goal of therapy in CD is to induce and maintain clinical remission. Medications used in this endeavor include aminosalicylates, antibiotics, prednisone, thiopurine analogs (e.g., azathioprine, 6-mercaptopurine), methotrexate, monoclonal anti-TNF antibodies (e.g., infliximab, adalimumab), and monoclonal anti-α_4-integrin (e.g., natalizumab). In long-term

follow-up studies conducted in the United States and Denmark, approximately 10% of patients remained in remission, 70% had a chronic intermittent disease course, and 20% experienced continuous chronicity and activity. Surgery is generally reserved for patients who are medically refractory or develop intra-abdominal abscess, intestinal obstruction, toxic megacolon, dysplasia, or malignancy. Features that increase a patient's risk for disease recurrence postsurgery include penetrating/fistulizing disease, young age at diagnosis, short duration of disease prior to surgical intervention, perianal disease, and ileocolonic disease. Importantly, CD patients are at increased risk for small bowel and colorectal adenocarcinoma, given the episodic chronic and active mucosal injury. Recent estimates of the 25-year risk of developing dysplasia in the setting of colonic CD range from 12% to 25%.

CROHN'S COLITIS – DISEASE FACT SHEET

Definition

▶▶ Episodic chronic inflammatory condition of the GI tract

Incidence and Location

▶▶ Incidence in adults roughly 0.2% (approximately 1 case per 500 individuals)
▶▶ Incidence in pediatric cohorts is lower, estimated at 0.04%
▶▶ More common in Northern latitudes

Sex and Age Distribution

▶▶ Slight female predominance (1.3:1)
▶▶ Majority of diagnoses occur in the second to fourth decades of life
▶▶ Smaller diagnostic peak in the fifth through seventh decades of life

Clinical Features

▶▶ Extremely variable clinical presentation
▶▶ Often diarrhea with or without blood in the stool

▸▸ Approximately one quarter of patients present with perianal disease prior to GI symptoms

▸▸ Pediatric presentation often with fever and weight loss

Endoscopic Features

▸▸ Patchy or segmental distribution of disease

▸▸ May involve any organ of the GI tract, from esophagus to anus

Prognosis and Therapy

▸▸ Extremely variable clinical course

▸▸ Goal of therapy, via medication, is to induce and maintain remission

▸▸ Some long-term follow-up studies show that only 10% of patients remain in remission, with the majority (approximately 70%) experiencing chronic intermittent disease flares

▸▸ Medically refractory patients are generally surgically managed

---

CROHN'S COLITIS – PATHOLOGIC FEATURES

Gross Findings

▸▸ "Cobblestoning" in which ulcered bowel mucosa sits adjacent to intact edematous mucosa

▸▸ Segmental thickening of the colon wall

▸▸ Bowel wall does not lie flat on the grossing bench

▸▸ Serosal fat wrapping ("creeping" fat) around anti-mesenteric side of bowel wall

▸▸ Small, well-circumscribed aphthous ulcers that progress to connected, longitudinal, serpiginous "bearclaw-type" furrows

Microscopic Findings

▸▸ "Skip lesions" in which unremarkable mucosa is interspersed amongst mucosa afflicted with chronic and/or active injury

▸▸ Chronic mucosal injury: crypt architectural distortion, basal lymphoplasmacytosis, diffuse lamina propria expansion by chronic lymphoplasmacytic inflammation, metaplasias, basal lymphoid aggregates

▸▸ Active mucosal injury: neutrophilic cryptitis, crypt abscess, erosions, ulcerations, necrosis

▸▸ Well-formed, non-necrotizing epithelioid granulomas

Pathologic Differential Diagnoses

▸▸ Ulcerative colitis

▸▸ Infectious colitis

▸▸ Ischemic colitis

▸▸ Diverticular disease–associated colitis

COLON

SESSILE SERRATED LESION

DDX: hyperplastic polyp, traditional serrated adenoma, unclassified serrated adenoma

Clinical Features

Sessile serrated lesions (SSLs), previously called sessile serrated adenomas (SSA) or sessile serrated polyps (SSPs), are typically asymptomatic polyps of the colon and rectum that are identified incidentally at the time of endoscopy. The majority of SSLs lack associated bleeding, so fecal occult blood–based screening methodologies are ineffective. While the incidence of SSLs varies greatly from study to study and has certainly expanded with its evolving definition, it is estimated that SSLs constitute approximately 10% of all colon polyps. Clinically, the majority (70%–80%) of SSLs present as sessile polyps with a predilection for the proximal colon. The identification of SSLs at the time of colonoscopy does alter the recommended colonoscopic screening interval, depending on the number of polyps identified and their respective sizes. Per the 2020 update to polypectomy surveillance recommendations sponsored by the US Multi-Society Task Force (US-MSTF) on Colorectal Cancer, individuals with SSLs <10 mm in size should undergo colonoscopy within 5 to 10 years if one to two polyps are identified and within 3 to 5 years if three or four polyps are found. The recommended screening interval is reduced to 3 years for patients with 5 to 10 SSLs, an SSL ≥10 mm in size or SSL with dysplasia.

Pathologic Features

GROSS FINDINGS

The classic endoscopic appearance of SSL is that of a pale, sessile polyp with a relatively smooth surface contour, surface mucus, and a surrounding rim of debris or bubbles imparting a "cloud-like" appearance. SSLs may have peripheral boundaries that are relatively ill-defined or indistinct from surrounding nonserrated mucosa. Commonly, these polyps easily flatten during bowel insufflation, making their endoscopic identification more challenging.

MICROSCOPIC FINDINGS

SSLs are characterized by cytologically bland epithelial cells forming prominent serrations that appear to involve the entire colonic crypt, from surface to base (Fig. 1.25A). The defining feature of SSLs is their architectural distortion, particularly distortions involving the basal portion (bottom one third) of the colonic crypts. These distortions result from the migration of the proliferative zone from the base of the crypts to a more lateral location along the crypt wall. Subsequent proliferation results in the base of the crypt growing or extending horizontally along the muscularis mucosae. People often liken these crypt bases to the shapes of an "inverted T," "L," or "boot" (Fig. 1.25B). Other forms of crypt architectural distortion common to SSLs include crypt base dilation and crypt branching. Per the 2019 WHO Classification of Digestive System Tumors, a diagnosis of SSL hinges on identification of at least one unequivocal architecturally distorted serrated crypt. It is important to note that one of the features of SSLs is maturation of epithelium from the basal aspect of the crypts through their surface. The cells on the surface of SSLs may on occasion appear crowded, but they are generally cytologically bland with small, round, basally oriented nuclei. Occasionally, one may observe a proliferation of bland, elongated spindle cells in the stroma surrounding SSLs. These cells resemble a perineurioma ("perineurioma-like stroma") and are believed to represent a reactive phenomenon with no clinical significance (Fig. 1.25C).

The development of epithelial dysplasia is SSLs occurs as part of the polyp's progression along the dysplasia-carcinoma pathway. Generally, the epithelial dysplasia is distinctly demarcated from the surrounding nondysplastic SSL. There are two main types of dysplasia that arise in SSLs: conventional adenomatous dysplasia and serrated dysplasia. Conventional adenomatous dysplasia resembles that observed in tubular adenomas: nuclear elongation, pseudostratification, and coarse nuclear chromatin (Fig. 1.25D). Serrated dysplasia is characterized by round atypical nuclei, prominent nucleoli, numerous mitoses, and eosinophilic cytoplasm (Fig. 1.25E). In areas of dysplasia within SSLs, there is often accompanying architectural distortion including diminishment or enhancement of the degree of epithelial serration, crypt elongation, crypt branching, crowding, and cribriforming. Due to relatively poor interobserver reproducibility, delineation of dysplasia into low-grade and high-grade categories is not recommended. Rather, a statement on the presence or absence of dysplasia is all that is necessary to dictate appropriate clinical management.

Ancillary Studies

Ancillary studies are generally unnecessary when rendering a diagnosis of SSL. Of note, Liu et al. have described a variant of SSLs that harbor MLH1 promoter hypermethylation, yet lack obvious cytologic dysplasia based on H&E findings. They have termed these lesions SSLs with minimal deviation dysplasia (Fig. 1.25F and G). Some groups advocate for performing MLH1 IHC on all SSLs in order to identify those which harbor mismatch repair (MMR) protein deficiency.

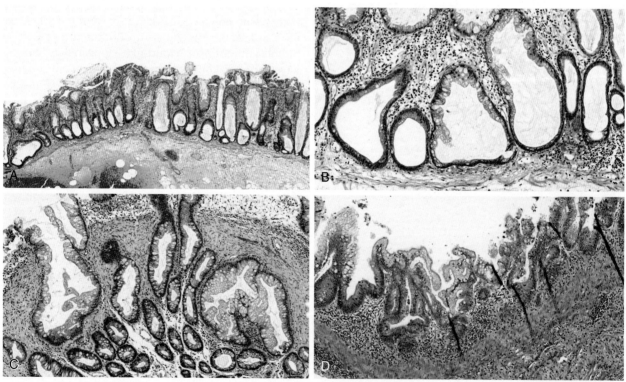

FIG. 1.25

Sessile serrated lesion. Low-power image of sessile serrated lesion with prominent serrations that appear to involve the entire colonic crypt, from surface to base **(A)**. High-power image highlights the distortion of the crypt bases, with obvious "inverted T" and "L" shaped forms **(B)**. An incidental finding in some sessile serrated lesions is the presence of a proliferation of bland, elongated spindle cells in the stroma, termed "perineurioma-like stroma" **(C)**. Sessile serrated lesions may go on to develop dysplasia, including conventional adenomatous-type dysplasia identical to that seen in tubular adenomas **(D)**.

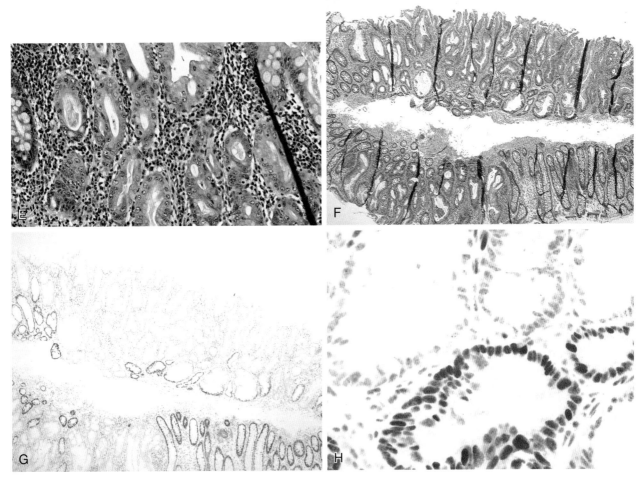

FIG. 1.25, cont'd
A more challenging form of dysplasia that may arise in sessile serrated lesions is serrated dysplasia, characterized by round atypical nuclei, prominent nucleoli, numerous mitoses, and eosinophilic cytoplasm **(E)**. An extremely cytologically subtle form epithelial dysplasia in a minority of sessile serrated lesions is termed minimal deviation dysplasia **(F)**. Minimal deviation dysplasia is best detected/confirmed by the presence of nuclear loss of MLH1 by immunohistochemistry within the dysplastic nuclei **(G)**. The loss of MLH1 in this case is the "dot-like" staining pattern that is a diagnostic pitfall, as it may errantly be interpreted as retained nuclear expression **(H)**.

Differential Diagnosis

SESSILE SERRATED LESION VERSUS HYPERPLASTIC POLYP

Hyperplastic polyps are typically small (<5 mm). In contrast to SSLs, the serrated epithelium in hyperplastic polyps is restricted to the superficial two thirds of the glands, without extension into crypt bases (Fig. 1.26A). The proliferative center is preserved in the central crypt base, preventing distorted crypt shapes. In contrast to the horizontal extension of crypts in SSLs, hyperplastic polyps have funnel-shaped crypts that lack dilatation or distortion (Fig. 1.26B). Rarely, crypt branching may be seen. In many ways, hyperplastic polyps are a diagnosis of exclusion, rendered after excluding crypt architectural distortion significant enough to warrant a diagnosis of SSL. Similar to SSLs, the epithelium in hyperplastic polyps is bland with complete surface maturation. The

cells have round, basally oriented nuclei. On cross section, crypts in hyperplastic polyps often have a stellate or star-like appearance. There are two main "subtypes" of hyperplastic polyps to be familiar with: microvesicular and goblet cell–rich. Microvesicular hyperplastic polyps lack substantial numbers of goblet cells, generally have well-developed epithelial serrations, and harbor *BRAF* mutations (70%–80%) as their predominant molecular signature. In contrast, goblet cell–rich hyperplastic polyps are typically more subtle, with elongated crypts, less pronounced epithelial serrations, and *KRAS* mutations (50%).

SESSILE SERRATED LESION VERSUS TRADITIONAL SERRATED ADENOMA

In contrast to SSLs, traditional serrated adenomas (TSAs) are more commonly large protuberant to pedunculated polyps that have a predilection for the

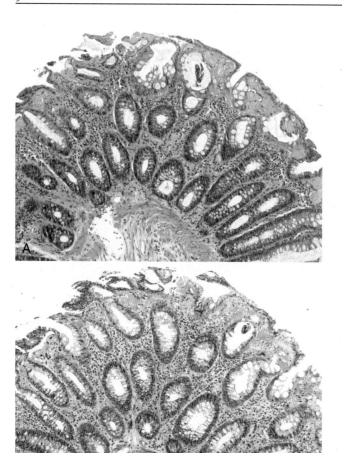

FIG. 1.26

Hyperplastic polyp. In contrast to sessile serrated lesions, hyperplastic polyps are generally smaller in size and have serrated epithelium restricted to the superficial two thirds of the glands. Given the lack of involvement of crypt bases, hyperplastic polyps have funnel-shaped crypts that lack distortion **(A)**. In some instances, hyperplastic polyps may be associated with an expanded subepithelial collagen table, appreciable on H&E and highlighted on trichrome stain **(B)**.

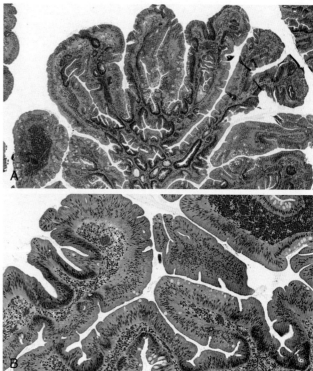

FIG. 1.27

Traditional serrated adenoma. At low power, traditional serrated adenomas typically have a papillary or villiform architecture with prominent "slit-like" serrations **(A)**. The epithelial cells lining traditional serrated adenoma are columnar, hypereosinophilic, and goblet cell depleted with basally oriented pencillate-type nuclei and arrangements within "ectopic crypt" type structures **(B)**.

left colon, particularly the sigmoid colon and rectum. Microscopically, they typically have a papillary or villiform architecture. The serrations in TSA are typically prominent and "slit-like," closely resembling the normal serration observed in unremarkable small bowel mucosa (Fig. 1.27A). The cells lining TSA villi and crypts are generally tall columnar cells with hypereosinophilic eosinophilic cytoplasm and basally oriented pencillate-type nuclei that have relatively open chromatin and low nuclear-to-cytoplasmic ratios (Fig. 1.27B). A characteristic feature of TSAs is the presence of "ectopic crypts," which are crypt-like structures that arise along the vertical axis of TSA villi, without anchorage to muscularis mucosae. Goblet cells are typically relatively depleted within TSAs, though rare "goblet cell–rich" forms have been described. One can observe conventional adenomatous or serrated-type dysplasia superimposed on the cytologic changes

classic of TSA. Generally, these additional forms of dysplasia should be documented, particularly if high-grade dysplasia is present, as these may represent more "advanced" lesions in regard to progression along the dysplasia-carcinoma pathway. Also of note, some authors report "precursor" hyperplastic polyps or SSLs are observed at the periphery of TSAs in up to half of cases. In contrast to the predominance of *BRAF* mutations and epigenetic hypermethylation in SSLs, TSAs have similar frequencies of *BRAF* mutations (20%–40%) and *KRAS* mutations (50%–70%). Approximately 10% of TSAs lack either of the two aforementioned mutations. The clinical management of TSAs is similar to that of SSLs, as they require complete endoscopic removal and a diminished screening interval. Similar to patients with five or more SSLs, an SSL ≥10 mm, or an SSL with dysplasia, the colonoscopy screening interval is reduced to 3 years when a TSA is identified.

SESSILE SERRATED LESION VERSUS CONVENTIONAL ADENOMA WITH SERRATED ARCHITECTURE

It is posited that conventional tubular, tubulovillous, or villous adenomas may demonstrate a superimposed serrated architecture through acquisition of *KRAS*

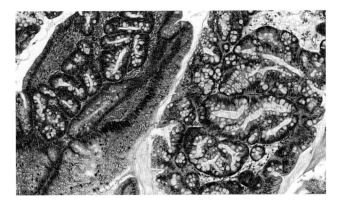

FIG. 1.28

Conventional adenoma with serrated architecture. In a conventional adenoma with serrated architecture, the dysplasia is a typical adenomatous-type dysplasia. The lack of a nondysplastic serrated component precludes characterization as a sessile serrated lesion that has acquired dysplasia.

given that their peripheral borders are often endoscopically ill-defined and that these lesions frequently flatten at the time of bowel insufflation. Given the increased risk of metachronous preneoplastic serrated polyps and of colorectal carcinoma in patients with identified SSLs, reduced screening intervals are recommended for patients with SSLs. In the United States, the US-MSTF recommends screening intervals are based on a multitude of factors including subtype of serrated polyp, number of polyps, polyp size, and the presence or absence of dysplasia. For SSLs, a 5-year screening interval is recommended if one or more SSLs <10 mm in greatest diameter are identified at colonoscopy. If any SSL is ≥10 mm in diameter or has epithelial dysplasia, the recommended screening interval is reduced to 3 years. Notably, screening recommendations for SSL vary by country.

mutations in addition to the already present chromosomal instability pathway alterations (e.g., *APC* gene mutations). The dysplastic features of conventional adenoma, including elongated "cigar"-shaped nuclei with coarse nuclear chromatin and nuclear stratification, should be relatively easily discerned from the cytologic alterations typical of SSLs or TSAs. Without the presence of a microscopically identified nondysplastic component of a serrated lesion, one must consider the possibility of a conventional adenoma with superimposed serrated features (Fig. 1.28). Often, it is challenging to definitively categorize these lesions. In the scenario where one does not feel confident in "bucketing" the polyp into a specific diagnostic category, the most important job of the pathologist is recognizing and communicating the presence or absence of dysplasia. Rendering a diagnosis of "unclassifiable serrated lesion" either with or without cytologic dysplasia is certainly a reasonable interpretation in these challenging cases.

Prognosis and Therapy

Approximately 30% of colorectal neoplasia is known to arise via the "serrated dysplasia" pathway, with SSLs and TSAs being the known precursor lesions. In SSLs, the epithelial dysplasia-carcinoma pathway begins with *BRAF* mutation and progresses through CpG island methylator phenotype (CIMP) resulting in accumulation of epigenetic hypermethylation. Critical in the progression to epithelial dysplasia and subsequent carcinoma is MLH1 promoter hypermethylation resulting in MMR protein deficiency, which occurs in approximately 75% of SSLs with epithelial dysplasia. The majority of the remaining 25% of dysplastic SSLs progress through the dysplasia-carcinoma sequence via *TP53* mutations. Given the preneoplastic nature of these polyps, SSLs certainly warrant complete endoscopic removal, which can be challenging

---

SESSILE SERRATED LESION – DISEASE FACT SHEET

Definition
▸▸ Sessile polyps characterized by epithelial proliferation arranged in a serrated (sawtooth or stellate) architecture

Incidence and Location
▸▸ Estimated to constitute approximately 10% of colon polyps
▸▸ Predilection for the proximal colon

Sex and Age Distribution
▸▸ May occur at any age
▸▸ There is no known sex predilection

Clinical Features
▸▸ Typically asymptomatic incidental findings at the time of colonoscopy

Endoscopic Features
▸▸ Small, pale, sessile polyp with a relatively smooth surface contour
▸▸ Often have a surrounding rim of debris or bubbles imparting a "cloud-like" appearance
▸▸ Can be easily flattened at the time of bowel insufflation, making identification challenging

Prognosis and Therapy
▸▸ Generally an excellent prognosis, particularly if the polyp is small (<10 mm)
▸▸ Large serrated polyps increase the risk of colorectal carcinoma and thus are associated with a decreased screening interval (to 3 years) if they are identified

---

SESSILE SERRATED LESION – PATHOLOGIC FEATURES

Gross Findings
▸▸ Small, pale, sessile polyp
▸▸ Relatively smooth surface contours, sometimes appear "cloud-like"
▸▸ May have ill-defined borders from surrounding nonpolypoid mucosa

(Continued)

SESSILE SERRATED LESION – PATHOLOGIC FEATURES—cont'd

Microscopic Findings

▸▸ Proliferation of cytologically bland epithelial cells with prominent serrations that appear to involve the entire colonic crypt

▸▸ Architectural distortion of crypt base resulting in "inverted T," "L," or "boot" configurations

▸▸ Need to identify at least one architecturally distorted crypt to render the interpretation of SSL

▸▸ Crypt dilatation and crypt branching also common

Pathologic Differential Diagnoses

▸▸ Hyperplastic polyp

▸▸ Traditional serrated adenoma

▸▸ Conventional adenoma with serrated architecture

ANUS

ANAL GLAND ADENOCARCINOMA

DDX: fistula-associated anal adenocarcinoma, HPV-related adenocarcinoma of the lower anogenital tract, mucosal-type anal adenocarcinoma, metastatic adenocarcinoma

Clinical Features

Anal cancers are relatively rare tumors, with <10,000 cases diagnosed per year in the United States. Squamous cell carcinomas constitute the vast majority of these tumors, with anal adenocarcinoma accounting for approximately 10% of these cancers. Risk factors for all anal adenocarcinomas include smoking, HIV infection, anoreceptive intercourse, anal CD, chronic anal fistula, and anal human papillomavirus (HPV) infection. Adenocarcinomas of the anus are divided into two major subtypes: mucosal and extramucosal. Mucosal-type adenocarcinomas are essentially indistinguishable from colorectal adenocarcinoma. Extramucosal anal adenocarcinomas are further subcategorized into anal gland adenocarcinoma, fistula-associated adenocarcinoma, and extramucosal anal canal adenocarcinoma non-anal gland and non-fistula–associated type. It is thought that mucosal, intestinal-type adenocarcinomas share carcinogenesis pathways with their morphologically identical colorectal adenocarcinoma counterparts. The pathogenesis of fistula-associated extramucosal adenocarcinoma, most commonly seen in the clinical setting of CD, is thought to be related to cytokines and transcriptional factors upregulated in this inflammatory microenvironment. As primary extramucosal anal gland adenocarcinoma is extremely rare, epidemiologic data is largely derived from case reports. Considering this caveat, there does appear to be a slight male predilection (1.7:1) for primary extramucosal anal gland adenocarcinoma.

Pathologic Features

GROSS FINDINGS

Anal gland adenocarcinomas arise within the anal glands or ducts. Thus, they often present clinically as firm infiltrative submucosal or mural-based mass in the anorectal region. In case series, the average tumor size is 2 to 5 cm. Associated reactive-type mucosal changes overlying the submucosal mass may be seen, including erosion or ulceration.

MICROSCOPIC FINDINGS

Though the histologic spectrum of anal gland adenocarcinomas is not sharply defined, the typical microscopic appearance of anal gland adenocarcinoma is that of haphazardly dispersed glands involving the wall of the anus (Fig. 1.29A). Confluent and anastomosing glands are often seen extending to involve the overlying squamous epithelium. These glands are generally lined by low-cuboidal epithelial cells with relatively depleted amounts of cytoplasmic mucin (Fig. 1.29B). Generally, these adenocarcinomas are nonmucinous in nature, though rare cases of mucin production–prominent tumors have been reported.

Ancillary Studies

Anal gland adenocarcinomas characteristically express CK7 and are negative for markers of intestinal-type differentiation, including CK20 and CDX2 (Fig. 1.29C). Markers typically expressed in non-neoplastic anal glands, including CK5/6 and p63, are conspicuously absent in anal gland adenocarcinoma.

Differential Diagnosis

ANAL GLAND ADENOCARCINOMA VERSUS FISTULA-ASSOCIATED ANAL ADENOCARCINOMA

Fistula-associated anal adenocarcinoma typically arises in the clinical setting of CD (in which there is a slight female predominance) or a chronic anal fistula (in which there is an overwhelming male predominance). Histologically, these tumors may be composed of anal gland-type epithelium similar to anal gland adenocarcinomas. Alternatively, the cells comprising these tumors may be transitional-type or intestinal-type epithelium (Fig. 1.30A). Generally, these tumors

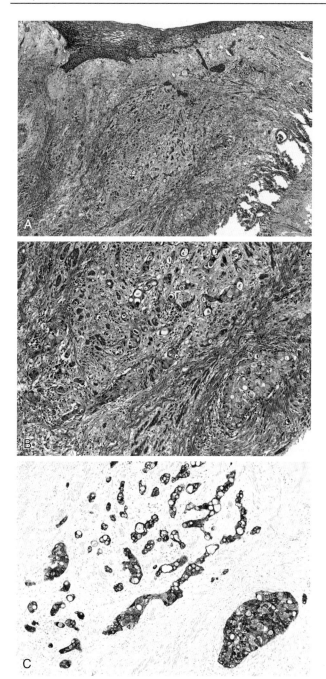

FIG. 1.29

Anal gland adenocarcinoma. At low power, these tumors are composed of haphazardly dispersed glands involving the wall of the anus and lacking an overlying precursor/*in situ* glandular component **(A)**. The glandular structures that comprise these tumors are typically lined by low-cuboidal epithelial cells with relatively depleted amounts of cytoplasmic mucin **(B)**. When immunohistochemistry is performed, these tumors are typically positive for CK7 **(C)**. They are negative for CK20 and CDX2.

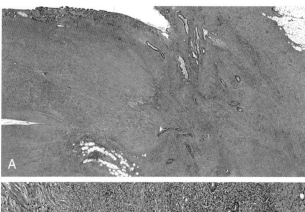

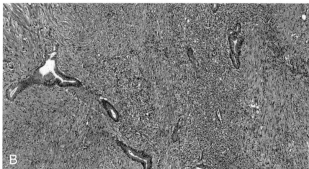

FIG. 1.30

Fistula-associated anal adenocarcinoma. These tumors are typically mucinous neoplasms with an intestinal-type morphology. On rare occasions, the tumor may have an anal adenocarcinoma morphology, making it extremely challenging to discern a fistula-associated anal adenocarcinoma from anal gland adenocarcinoma that has fistulized **(A)**. Clinical history of a long-standing fistula tract is paramount in helping discern between the two **(B)**.

are mucinous in nature and morphologically resemble mucinous colorectal adenocarcinoma. When of anal gland morphology, it can be extremely challenging to discern fistula-associated anal adenocarcinoma from mucin-producing anal gland adenocarcinoma (Fig. 1.30B). The presence of an *in situ* component favors a fistula-associated anal adenocarcinoma,

though surface colonization by anal gland adenocarcinoma can certainly mimic *in situ* neoplasia. The defining distinguishing feature is the presence of a pre-existing typically longstanding fistula tract. Of course, exclusion of colonization or involvement by an adenocarcinoma arising elsewhere, particularly the rectum or the colon, is certainly necessary.

ANAL GLAND ADENOCARCINOMA VERSUS HPV-RELATED ADENOCARCINOMA OF THE LOWER ANOGENITAL TRACT

In 2020, Voltaggio et al. described a rare series of adenocarcinomas of the lower anogenital tract that are associated with HPV infection in both men and women. Similar to mucosal-type anal adenocarcinomas, these tumors usually present as an exophytic mass lesion involving the anal mucosa. Histologically, the lesions have a papillary or villoglandular architecture. The glands are lined by cells that are described as resembling usual-type HPV-associated adenocarcinoma of the endocervix, in that the cells are tall columnar epithelial cells with crowded "cigar"-shaped to ovoid irregular nuclei and either mucinous or nonmucinous apical cytoplasm. Similar to anal gland adenocarcinoma, these tumors are strongly and diffusely positive for CK7.

CDX2 is reported to demonstrate patchy nuclear staining in some cases. In the few reported anal lesions, CK20 was negative. Differentiating itself from anal gland adenocarcinoma, these tumors are strongly and diffusely positive for p16, which correlates with the identification of high-risk HPV infection by *in situ* hybridization in 100% of cases.

ANAL GLAND ADENOCARCINOMA VERSUS MUCOSAL-TYPE ANAL ADENOCARCINOMA

Mucosal-type anal adenocarcinoma is the most common form of anal adenocarcinoma. Unlike anal gland adenocarcinomas, mucosal-type adenocarcinoma arises within luminal mucosa of the anus and thus typically presents as a mucosal-based mass lesion rather than within the submucosa. The histopathology of mucosal-type anal adenocarcinoma is essentially indistinguishable from colorectal adenocarcinoma in that the tumor has an intestinal-type morphology (Fig. 1.31A). In keeping with intestinal-type adenocarcinomas, these tumors can be mucinous (Fig. 1.31B) or nonmucinous. In fitting with the morphology, these tumors have a demonstrable intestinal-type immunophenotype, with tumor cells that are negative for CK7 and positive for CK20 and CDX2 (Fig. 1.31C and D).

ANAL GLAND ADENOCARCINOMA VERSUS METASTATIC ADENOCARCINOMA

Given the mural-based nature of the anal gland adenocarcinomas and the lack of an easily defined associated "*in situ*" neoplasia, one must always consider the possibility of metastatic adenocarcinoma to the anal canal within the differential diagnosis. Based on the classic histomorphologic appearance of anal gland adenocarcinomas, with low-cuboidal–type epithelium lining haphazardly distributed glands, main diagnostic considerations include metastatic adenocarcinoma of gynecologic, breast (Fig. 1.32A–F), or pancreatobiliary origin. Similar to anal gland adenocarcinomas, metastatic adenocarcinoma of gynecologic, breast, and pancreatobiliary origin will also express CK7. Adenocarcinomas of gynecologic and breast origin will also lack expression of CK20 and CDX2, whereas pancreatobiliary adenocarcinomas may demonstrate patchy cytoplasmic and nuclear positivity, respectively. When excluding metastases from extra-anal sites of origin, including correlation with the patient's known medical history and imaging studies, IHC for nuclear transcription factors specific to extra-anal sites of origin are of utility including GATA3 for breast and PAX8 for gynecologic tumors.

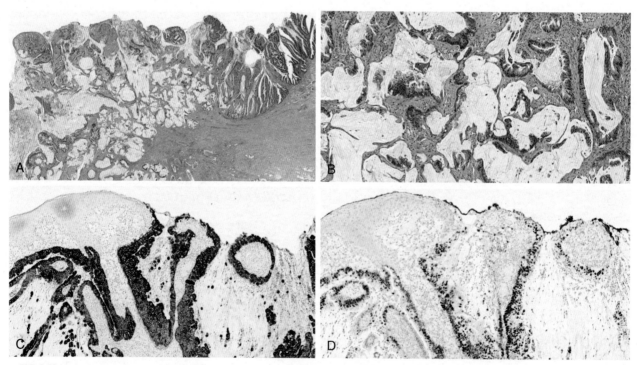

FIG. 1.31

Mucosal type anal adenocarcinoma. Mucosal-type adenocarcinoma arises from the intestinal-type epithelium that lines a portion of the anal canal, seen here adjacent to anal squamous mucosa on low power **(A)**. These tumors have a morphologic appearance indistinguishable from typical colorectal-type adenocarcinoma and can be mucinous, as in this example, or nonmucinous **(B)**. When immunohistochemistry is performed, these tumors are positive for CK20 **(C)** and CDX2 **(D)** in keeping with their colorectal-type morphology. They are typically negative for CK7.

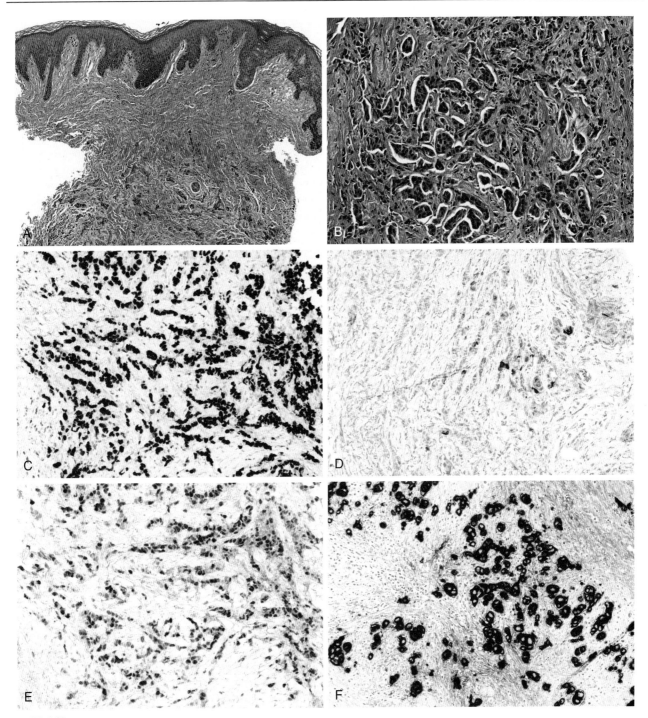

FIG. 1.32

Metastatic mammary adenocarcinoma to the anus. Adenocarcinoma is tubules and linear chains are seen undermining squamous mucosa of the anus **(A)**. The tumor cells are low cuboidal with mild to moderate cytologic atypia **(B)**. The tumor cells are positive for GATA3 **(C)**, mammaglobin **(D)**, ER **(E)**, and CK7 **(F)**.

Prognosis and Therapy

Adenocarcinomas of the anal canal are staged according to the TNM classification scheme for anal cancers in which the pT stage is determined by tumor size. The prognosis of anal canal adenocarcinoma is worse than that of anal squamous cell carcinoma and outcomes are largely dependent on pathologic TNM staging. Optimal or standardized therapeutic approaches to anal canal adenocarcinoma management are not well established. Most recommend radical surgical resection coupled with other preoperative or postoperative chemoradiotherapy.

LOW-GRADE MESENCHYMAL TUMORS

GASTROINTESTINAL STROMAL TUMOR

DDX: leiomyoma, schwannoma, inflammatory fibroid polyp, plexiform angiomyxoid myofibroblastic tumor

Clinical Features

Gastrointestinal stromal tumors (GISTs) are the most common mesenchymal neoplasms to involve the GI tract. They may occur in any part of the GI tract, most commonly in the stomach (60%), followed by jejunum and ileum (30%), duodenum (4%–5%), rectum (4%), colon and appendix (1%–2%), and distal esophagus (<1%). Rarely, GISTs may be found in extra-intestinal locations, but typically near GI organs, such as omentum and mesentery. Patients with GISTs may present with occult GI bleed, vague abdominal pain or discomfort, and rarely with an acute abdomen. Up to one fifth of patients with clinically identified GISTs present asymptomatically, with the lesions incidentally identified as submucosal lesions on endoscopic studies, or as mass lesions on imaging studies performed for other purposes.

Surveillance, epidemiology, and end results program-based studies estimate an incidence of 0.68 per 100,000 with a median age of 64 years at diagnosis. While autopsy series have found incidental, sub-centimeter GISTs in up to a third of cases, molecular studies have highlighted a series of alterations that may be responsible for progression from benign/incidental lesions to tumors that grow to clinically impactful size or harbor malignant/metastatic potential.

Pathologic Features

GROSS FINDINGS

GISTs are typically discrete, well-circumscribed lesions that are based in the muscularis propria. In some cases, the lesion may appear predominantly situated in the submucosa or perimuscular soft tissue but tethered to the muscularis propria. The overlying mucosa may be normal or show evidence of erosion or injury secondary to direct extension of tumor, or indirectly as a general result of mass effect.

MICROSCOPIC FINDINGS

GISTs may exhibit a broad histologic spectrum, with some patterns more common in certain anatomical locations. For example, GISTs of the colon and rectum are almost universally spindle cell in morphology. Overall, GISTs are typically cytologically bland, and the majority are of spindle cell type (~70%) with abundant amphophilic or eosinophilic cytoplasm and elongated nuclei (Fig. 1.33A–D). In some cases, the nuclei may be in an arrangement imparting a palisading appearance. Paranuclear vacuoles may also be seen. Epithelioid GISTs account for approximately 20% of cases, where tumor cells are round or plasmacytoid. The majority of the remaining GISTs are of mixed type, with separate components exhibiting spindle cell and epithelioid

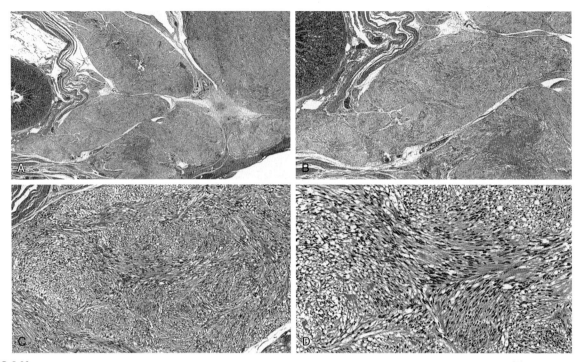

FIG. 1.33
Spindle cell gastrointestinal stromal tumor. The mass can be seen underlying gastric oxyntic mucosa. On high magnification, the lesion is composed of bland spindle cells and paranuclear vacuoles can be seen in this case **(A–D)**.

morphology. In the stomach, approximately 40% of GISTs will be epithelioid-type or contain an epithelioid component. While the majority of cases are cytologically bland, a minority of cases exhibit significant cytologic atypia, including nuclear pleomorphism and other overt features of malignancy. Rare cases of GISTs that develop a dedifferentiated/sarcomatous component have also been identified. Dedifferentiated components may lose expression of CD117 and DOG1 by IHC.

In 2006, Miettinen and Lasota found that tumor site, size, and mitotic activity were all independent prognostic factors and developed a prognostic model predicting the risk of recurrent disease that remains a staple in College of American Pathologists (CAP) reporting protocols for these tumors.

Ancillary Studies

GISTs are positive for KIT (CD117) in approximately 95% of cases and DOG1 in greater than 99% of cases. KIT and DOG1 positivities are usually strong and diffuse, although some cases may exhibit only focal KIT positivity. Although typically cytoplasmic, a variety of KIT staining patterns has been described, including perinuclear dot-like and membranous. However, these differing staining patterns have not clearly been associated with certain mutation types. The majority of KIT-negative, DOG1-positive GISTs are gastric or extra-intestinal in origin and

demonstrate PDGFRA mutations. Having said that, there is not a clear relationship between KIT expression on immunostain and KIT mutational status. That is, some cases of CD117-negative GISTs are found to have an activating KIT mutation, and conversely, some GISTs that are strongly positive for CD117 are KIT wild type on mutational testing.

IHC may also be used to identify cases of succinate dehydrogenase (SDH)-deficient GISTs, which account for approximately 8% of cases. SDH-deficient GISTs demonstrate aberrant loss of SDHB on immunostain. While some SDH-deficient GISTs are sporadic, they also account for the majority of GISTs seen in pediatric patients, as well as syndromic GISTs associated with Carney triad and Carney-Stratakis syndrome. SDH-deficient GISTs are usually in the stomach, may be associated with a plexiform or nodular growth pattern, are often associated with nodal or visceral metastasis, and are less likely to respond to imatinib. The majority of SDH-deficient GISTs are epithelioid or mixed type (Fig. 1.34A–D). Genetic counseling is recommended for all patients with SDH-deficient GISTs.

Increasingly, molecular studies examining KIT and PDGFRA, as well as SDH A/B/C/D, BRAF and NF1, are being performed in GISTs. Identifying a mutation in these genes may be confirmatory of a GIST diagnosis in cases where there was clinical uncertainty, such as cases of CD117-negative GISTs or tumors in unusual locations. In addition, hotspot analysis looking at mutations within particular exons of KIT and PDGFRA may have implications on treatment response.

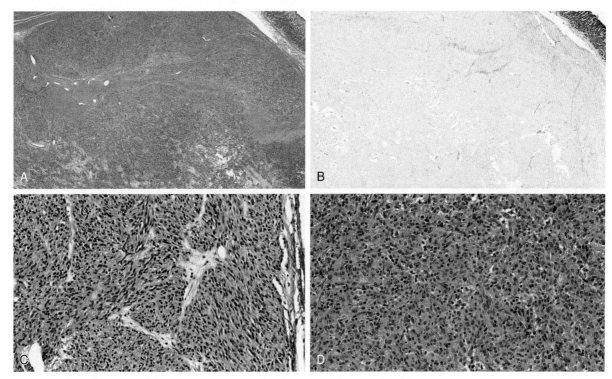

FIG. 1.34

Succinate dehydrogenase (SDH)-deficient gastrointestinal stromal tumor (GIST). A multilobulated architecture can be appreciated on low magnification **(A)** of this SDH-deficient GIST. SDH-B immunostain **(B)** confirms loss of expression in lesional cells and retained expression in the overlying mucosa. The tumor contains both spindle cell **(C)** and epithelioid **(D)** components.

Differential Diagnosis

GIST VERSUS LEIOMYOMA

Leiomyomas of the GI tract are bland, spindle tumors much like the majority of GISTs. Cytologically, the cytoplasm in leiomyomas is usually more densely eosinophilic and may contain eosinophilic globules. The nuclei in leiomyomas often appear cigar shaped (Fig. 1.35A and B). Grossly, leiomyomas also form firm, well-circumscribed nodules that may appear centered in the submucosa. However, leiomyomas typically arise in the muscularis mucosae. Immunohistochemical stains are often performed, particularly in biopsies, to differentiate between these entities. Leiomyomas are positive for SMA and desmin, but negative for CD117 and DOG1. Having said that, CD117 stain may highlight scattered mast cells or entrapped interstitial cells of Cajal. This staining may be robust and lead to concern for a GIST. In addition, SMA and desmin expression, typically weak and/or focal, may be seen in approximately 30% and 5% of GISTs, respectively. As such, it is often helpful to perform these stains as a panel in order to avoid over-interpretation of any one stain.

GIST VERSUS SCHWANNOMA

Schwannomas are benign tumors arising from the Schwann cells of peripheral nerves. The vast majority of

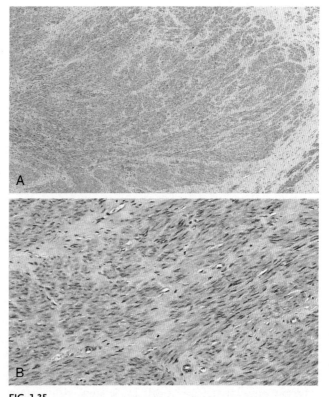

FIG. 1.35

Leiomyoma. Sequential images highlight a bland spindle cell neoplasm **(A)** with cigar-shaped nuclei and densely eosinophilic cytoplasm **(B)**.

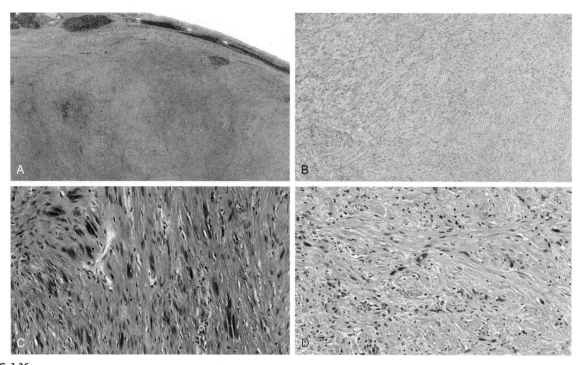

FIG. 1.36

Gastrointestinal schwannoma. These tumors classically exhibit a lymphoid cuff **(A)**. On intermediate magnification, a vaguely fascicular arrangement can be seen **(B)**. On high magnification, focal areas of nuclear atypia **(C)** may be seen, as well as intracytoplasmic vacuoles **(D)**.

GI schwannomas occur in the stomach, particularly the antrum. But overall, gastric schwannomas are much less common than GISTs. Grossly, schwannomas are typically based within the muscularis propria and extend into the submucosa. Larger lesions may be associated with mucosal ulceration. These lesions are characteristically well circumscribed but not encapsulated. Histologically, schwannomas are predominantly composed of bland spindle cells that are uniform, although focal nuclear atypia is common. In the GI tract, schwannomas classically exhibit a dense lymphoid cuff at the periphery (Fig. 1.36A). The nuclei may have a wavy appearance, and intranuclear inclusions may be seen. The spindle cells may form fascicles or whirls, and nuclear palisading can be seen (Fig. 1.36B–D). Having said that, these features are less commonly a feature of GI tract schwannomas compared with counterparts in the peripheral soft tissues. GI schwannomas are also less likely to have associated hyalinized vessels, Verocay bodies, or exhibit degenerative changes and are not associated with NF2 gene mutations. Mitotic figures are rare. Immunophenotypically, schwannomas show strong and diffuse staining for S100, but are negative for CD117, DOG1, and SMA.

GIST VERSUS INFLAMMATORY FIBROID POLYP

Inflammatory fibroid polyps (IFPs) are benign mesenchymal tumors that, like GISTs, can be found anywhere along the GI tract but are most commonly seen in the stomach or small bowel. The majority of these lesions

harbor activating PDGFRA mutations, suggestive of a neoplasm. IFPs typically arise in the submucosa and are histologically characterized by a spindle proliferation with bland, round to oval nuclei, with scant to moderate eosinophilic cytoplasm (Fig. 1.37A and B). The spindle cells often surround and accentuate vessels in a concentric fashion (Fig. 1.37C). The associated stroma may appear edematous, myxoid, or hyalinized, and contain a mixed inflammatory infiltrate with a predominance of eosinophils (Fig. 1.38D). Often, the predominance of eosinophils is the initial clue to the diagnosis. The spindle cells are often positive for CD34 but are negative for CD117 and DOG1.

GIST VERSUS PLEXIFORM ANGIOMYXOID MYOFIBROBLASTIC TUMOR

Plexiform angiomyxoid myofibroblastic tumors (PAMTs), previously called plexiform fibromyxomas, are rare tumors most commonly located in the gastric antrum or pylorus. These benign mesenchymal neoplasms are also primarily situated within the submucosa and muscularis propria, and exhibit a plexiform or nodular pattern of growth. PAMTs are another entry in this category of cytologically bland spindle cell proliferations. PAMTs have variable cellularity, and the accompanying stroma is typically myxoid, with some case cases also showing a fibrillary stroma (Fig. 1.38A–D). Immunohistochemically, the spindle cells are typically positive for SMA, but negative for CD117, DOG1, and CD34.

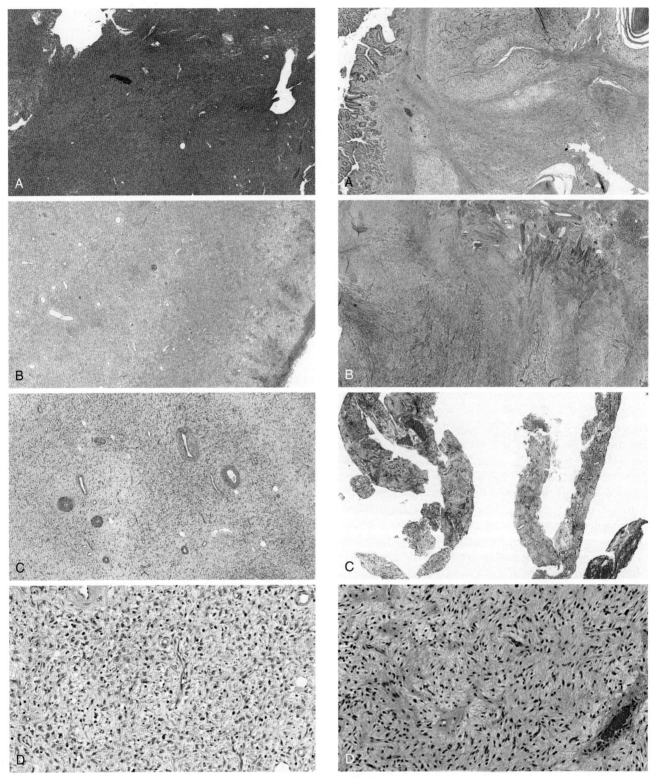

FIG. 1.37

Inflammatory fibroid polyp. These tumors may have variable cellularity **(A, B)**. Scattered, aberrant vessels are present, which may have thickened muscular walls and be accentuated by surrounding lesional spindle cells **(C)**. The associated inflammatory infiltrate is classically eosinophil rich **(D)**.

FIG. 1.38

Plexiform angiomyxoid myofibroblastic tumors. On low magnification, these tumors exhibit a multinodular architecture and a myxoid stroma **(A, B)**. On biopsy, this myxoid stroma may be the predominant finding **(C)**. Bland spindle cells, sometimes surrounded by a fibrillary stroma, without significant atypia is typical **(D)**.

GASTROINTESTINAL STROMAL TUMOR – DISEASE FACT SHEET

Definition
▶▶ Most common mesenchymal neoplasm of the GI tract, characterized by differentiation towards the interstitial cells of Cajal

Incidence and Location
▶▶ Relatively uncommon, with an incidence estimated at 0.68 per 100,000
▶▶ May occur at any site within the GI tract, most commonly occurring in the stomach (60%) followed by the small bowel (30%)

Sex and Age Distribution
▶▶ Sporadic GISTs may occur at any age, with a peak incidence in the sixth decade of life
▶▶ Slight male predominance
▶▶ Syndromic GISTs may occur in the pediatric population

Clinical Features
▶▶ Most common clinical presentation is vague abdominal pain

Endoscopic Features
▶▶ Submucosal or mural-based mass lesion

Prognosis and Therapy
▶▶ Prognosis is related to three main parameters: mitotic activity, tumor size, and tumor site
▶▶ Mutation status predicts response to imatinib, with *KIT* exon 11 mutations having the highest rate of response and *PDGFRA* exon 18 mutations demonstrating primary resistance

GASTROINTESTINAL STROMAL TUMOR – PATHOLOGIC FEATURES

Gross Findings
▶▶ Discrete, well-circumscribed mass lesion
▶▶ Usually mural based, typically in the muscularis propria
▶▶ Overlying mucosa may be unaffected or show evidence of injury secondary to the mass lesion or to direct extension of tumor

Microscopic Findings
▶▶ Three main tumor cell morphologies: spindled (70%), epithelioid (20%), or mixed (10%)
▶▶ GISTs are generally cytologically bland, regardless of morphology
▶▶ Spindle cells typically have elongated nuclei, paranuclear vacuoles, and abundant amphophilic cytoplasm
▶▶ Epithelioid type have round to plasmacytoid tumor cells
▶▶ In a minority of cases, cytologic atypia including nuclear pleomorphism may be identified

Pathologic Differential Diagnoses
▶▶ Leiomyoma
▶▶ Schwannoma
▶▶ Inflammatory fibroid polyp
▶▶ Plexiform angiomyxoid myofibroblastic tumor

SUGGESTED READINGS

Reflux Esophagitis

Delshad SD, Almario CV, Chey WD, Spiegel BMR. Prevalence of gastroesophageal reflux disease and proton pump inhibitor-refractory symptoms. *Gastroenterology*. 2020;158:1250-1261.

Fiocca R, Mastracci L, Riddell R, et al. Development of consensus guidelines for the histologic recognition of microscopic esophagitis in patients with gastroesophageal reflux disease: the Esohisto project. *Hum Pathol*. 2010;41:223-231.

Katzka DA, Kahrilas PJ. Advances in the diagnosis and management of gastroesophageal reflux disease. *BMJ*. 2020;371:m786.

Pascarenco OD, Boeriu A, Mocan S, et al. Barrett's esophagus and intestinal metaplasia of gastric cardia: prevalence, clinical, endoscopic, and histologic features. *J Gastrointestin Liv Dis*. 2014;23:19-25.

Irani MZ, Talley NJ, Ronkainen J, et al. Neutrophils, eosinophils, and intraepithelial lymphocytes in the squamous esophagus in subjects with and without gastroesophageal reflux symptoms. *Hum Pathol*. 2021;115:112-122.

Eosinophilic Esophagitis

Cohen MS, Kaufman AB, Palazzo JP, et al. An audit of endoscopic complications in adult eosinophilic esophagitis. *Clin Gastroenterol Hepatol*. 2007;5:1149-1153.

Dellon ES, Jensen ET, Martin CF, Shaheen NJ, Kappelman MD. Prevalence of eosinophilic esophagitis in the United States. *Clin Gastroenterol Hepatol*. 2014;12:589-596.

Dellon ES, Liacouras CA, Molina-Infante J, et al. Updated international consensus diagnostic criteria for eosinophilic esophagitis: proceedings of the AGREE conference. *Gastroenterology*. 2018;155:1022-1033.

Furuta GT, Liacouras CA, Collins MH, et al. Eosinophilic esophagitis in children and adults: a systematic review and consensus recommendations for diagnosis and treatment. *Gastroenterology*. 2007;133:1342-1363.

Kim HP, Dellon ES. An evolving approach to the diagnosis of eosinophilic esophagitis. *Gastroenterol Hepatol*. 2014;14:358-366.

Mansoor E, Cooper GS. The 2010-2015 Prevalence of eosinophilic esophagitis in the USA: a population-based study. *Dig Dis Sci*. 2016;61:2928-2934.

Okimoto E, Ishimura N, Ishihara S. Clinical characteristics and treatment outcomes of patients with eosinophilic esophagitis and eosinophilic gastroenteritis. *Digestion*. 2021;102:33-40.

Veerappan GR, Perry JL, Duncan TJ, et al. Prevalence of eosinophilic esophagitis in an adult population undergoing upper endoscopy: a prospective study. *Clin Gastroenterol Hepatol*. 2009;7:420-426, e426.e1–e2.

Lymphocytic Esophagitis

Rubio CA, Sjodahl K, Lagergren J. Lymphocytic esophagitis: a histologic subset of chronic esophagitis. *Am J Surg Pathol*. 2006;125:432-437.

Habbal M, Scaffidi MA, Rumman A, et al. Clinical, endoscopic, and histologic characteristics of lymphocytic esophagitis: a systematic review. *Esophagus*. 2019;16:123-132.

Purdy JK, Appelman HD, Golembeski CP, McKenna BJ. Lymphocytic esophagitis: a chronic or recurring pattern of esophagitis resembling allergic contact dermatitis. *Am J Clin Pathol*. 2008;130:508-513.

Pittman ME, Hissong E, Phillip KO, Yantiss RO. Lymphocyte-predominant esophagitis: a distinct and likely immune-mediated disorder encompassing lymphocytic and lichenoid esophagitis. *Am J Surg Pathol*. 2020;44:198-205.

Lichen Planus

Chryssostalis A, Gaudric M, Terris B, et al. Esophageal lichen planus: a series of eight cases including a patient with esophageal verrucous carcinoma. A case series. *Endoscopy.* 2008;40:764-768.

Dickens CM, Heseltine D, Walton S, et al. The oesophagus in lichen planus: an endoscopic study. *BMJ.* 1990;300:84.

Kern JS, Technau-Hafsi K, Schwacha H, et al. Esophageal involvement is frequent in lichen planus: study in 32 patients with suggestion of clinicopathologic diagnostic criteria and therapeutic implications. *Eur J Gastroenterol Hepatol.* 2016;28:1374-1382.

Peta Fox LP, Lightdale CJ, Grossman ME. Lichen planus of the esophagus: what dermatologists need to know. *J Am Acad Dermatol.* 2011;65:175-183.

Quispel R, van Boxel OS, Schipper ME, et al. High prevalence of esophageal involvement in lichen planus: a study using magnification chromoendoscopy. *Endoscopy.* 2009;41:187-193.

Squamous Dysplasia

Dry SM, Lewin KJ. Esophageal squamous dysplasia. *Semin Diagn Pathol.* 2002;19:2–11.

Shimizu M, Ban S, Odze RD. Squamous dysplasia and other precursor lesions related to esophageal squamous cell carcinoma. *Gastroenterol Clin North Am.* 2007;36:797–811.

Taylor PR, Abnet CC, Dawsey SM. Squamous dysplasia – the precursor lesion for esophageal squamous cell carcinoma. *Cancer Epidemiol Biomarkers Prev.* 2013;22:540-552.

Shekitka KM, Helwig EB. Deceptive bizarre stromal cells in polyps and ulcers of the gastrointestinal tract. *Cancer.* 1991;67:2111–2117.

Gastric Hyperplastic Polyp

Joao M, Areia M, Alves S, et al. Gastric hyperplastic polyps: a benign entity? Analysis of recurrence and neoplastic transformation in a cohort study. *GE Port J Gastroenterol.* 2021;28:328-335.

Waldum H, Fossmark R. Gastritis, gastric polyps and gastric cancer. *Int J Mol Sci.* 2021;22:6548.

Gonzalez-Obeso E, Fujita H, Deshpande V, et al. Gastric hyperplastic polyps: a heterogeneous clinicopathologic group including a distinct subset best categorized as mucosal prolapse polyp. *Am J Surg Pathol.* 2011;35:670-677.

Morais DJ, Yamanaka A, Zeitune JM, et al. Gastric polyps: a retrospective analysis of 26,000 digestive endoscopies. *Arq Gastroenterol.* 2007;44:14–17.

Zea-Iriarte WL, Sekine I, Itsuno M, et al. Carcinoma in gastric hyperplastic polyps. A phenotypic study. *Dig Dis Sci.* 1996;41:377-386.

Fundic Gland Polyp

Gao W, Huang Y, Lu S, Li C. The clinicopathological characteristics of gastric polyps and the relationship between fundic gland polyps, *Helicobacter pylori* infection, and proton pump inhibitors. *Ann Palliat Med.* 2021;10:2108-2114.

Orr CE, Beneck D, Jessurun J, et al. High interobserver variability and frequent overdiagnosis of dysplasia in fundic gland polyps can be improved by detecting atypia on the surface epithelium and an abrupt transition to non-neoplastic cells. *Histopathology.* 2022;80:314-321.

Carmack SW, Genta RM, Schuler CM, et al. The current spectrum of gastric polyps: a 1-year national study of over 120,000 patients. *Am J Gastroenterol.* 2009;104:1524-1532.

Sekine S, Shibata T, Yamauchi Y, et al. Beta-catenin mutations in sporadic fundic gland polyps. *Virchows Arch.* 2002;440:381-386.

Shaib WL, Nammour JP, Gill J, et al. Management of gastric polyps: an endoscopy-based approach. *Clin Gastroenterol Hepatol.* 2013;11:1374-1384.

Sonnenberg A, Genta RM. Prevalence of benign gastric polyps in a large pathology database. *Dig Liver Dis.* 2015;47:164-169.

Pyloric Gland Adenoma

Vieth M, Montgomery EA. Some observations on pyloric gland adenoma: an uncommon and long ignored entity! *J Clin Pathol.* 2014;67:882-890.

Pezhouh MK, Park JY. Gastric pyloric gland adenoma. *Arch Pathol Lab Med.* 2015;139:823-826.

Chlumska A, Waloschek T, Mukensnabl P, et al. Pyloric gland adenoma: a histologic, immunohistochemical and molecular genetic study of 23 cases. *Cesk Patol.* 2015;51:137-140.

Chen ZM, Scudiere JR, Abraham SC, et al. Pyloric gland adenoma: an entity distinct from gastric foveolar type adenoma. *Am J Surg Pathol.* 2009;33:186-193.

Choi WT, Brown I, Ushiku T, et al. Gastric pyloric gland adenoma: a multicenter clinicopathologic study of 67 cases. *Histopathology.* 2018;72:1007-1014.

Gastric Adenoma

Abraham SC, Montgomery EA, Singh VK, et al. Gastric adenomas: intestinal-type and gastric-type adenomas differ in the risk of adenocarcinoma and presence of background mucosal pathology. *Am J Surg Pathol.* 2002;26:1276-1285.

Lim CH, Cho YK, Kim SW, et al. The chronological sequence of somatic mutations in early gastric carcinogenesis inferred from multiregion sequencing of gastric adenomas. *Oncotarget.* 2016;7:39758.

Nakamura S, Matsumoto T, Kobori Y, et al. Impact of *Helicobacter pylori* infection and mucosal atrophy on gastric lesions in patients with familial adenpomatous polyposis. *Gut.* 2002;51:485-489.

Park DY, Srivastava A, Kim GH, et al. Adenomatous and foveolar gastric dysplasia: distinct patterns of mucin expression and background intestinal metaplasia. *Am J Surg Pathol.* 2008;32:524-533.

Hamartomatous/Syndromic Polyp

Vyas M, Yang X, Zhang X. Gastric hamartomatous polyps – review and update. *Clin Med Insights Gastroenterol.* 2016;9:3-10.

Giardiello FM, Brensinger JD, Tersmette AC, et al. Very high risk of cancer in familial Peutz-Jeghers syndrome. *Gastroenterology.* 2000;119:1447-1453.

Lam-Himlin D, Park JY, Cornisch TC, et al. Morphologic characterization of syndromic gastric polyps. *Am J Surg Pathol.* 2010;34:1656-1662.

Entuis MM, Keller JJ, Westerman AM, et al. Molecular genetic alterations in hamartomatous polyps and carcinomas of patients with Peutz-Jeghers syndrome. *J Clin Pathol.* 2001;54:126-131.

Cronkhite Jr LW, Canada WJ. Generalized gastrointestinal polyposis; an unusual syndrome of polyposis, pigmentation, alopecia and onychotrophia. *N Engl J Med.* 1955;252:1011-1015.

Intra-Ampullary Papillary-Tubular Neoplasms

Nappo G, Gentile D, Galvanin J, et al. Trans-duodenal ampullectomy for ampullary neoplasms: early and long-tern outcomes in 36 consecutive patients. *Surg Endosc.* 2020;34:4358-4368.

Ohike N, Kim GE, Tajiri T, et al. Intra-ampullary papillary-tubular neoplasm (IAPN): characterization of tumoral intraepithelial neoplasia occurring within the ampulla: a clinicopathologic analysis of 82 cases. *Am J Surg Pathol.* 2010;34:1731-1748.

Han S, Jang KT, Choi DW, et al. Prognostic impact of intra-ampullary papillary-tubular neoplasm versus flat dysplasia as precursor lesions of ampullary adenocarcinoma. *Dig Surg.* 2020;37:505-514.

Invasive Ampullary Adenocarcinoma

Xue Y, Reid MD, Balci S, et al. Immunohistochemical classification of ampullary carcinomas: critical reappraisal fails to confirm prognostic relevance for recently proposed panels, and highlights MUC5AC as a strong prognosticator. *Am J Surg Pathol.* 2017;41:865-876.

Han S, Jang KT, Choi DW, et al. Prognostic impact of intra-ampullary papillary-tubular neoplasm versus flat dysplasia as precursor lesions of ampullary adenocarcinoma. *Dig Surg.* 2020;37:505-514.

Moekotte AL, van Roessel S, Malleo G, et al. Development and external validation of a prediction model for survival in patients with resected ampullary adenocarcinoma. *Eur J Surg Oncol.* 2020;46:1717-1726.

Reid MD, Balci S, Ohike N, et al. Ampullary carcinoma is often of mixed or hybrid histologic type: an analysis of reproducibility and clinical relevance of classification as pancreatobiliary versus intestinal in 232 cases. *Mod Pathol.* 2016;29:1575-1585.

Adsay V, Ohike N, Tajiri T, et al. Ampullary region carcinomas: definition and site specific classification with delineation of four clinicopathologically and prognostically distinct subsets in an analysis of 249 cases. *Am J Surg Pathol.* 2012;36:1592-1608.

Adenoma of Ampullary Duodenum

Yamamoto Y, Nemoto T, Okubo Y, et al. Comparison between the location and the histomorphological/immunohistochemical characteristics of noninvasive neoplasms of the ampulla of Vater. *Hum Pathol.* 2014;45:1910-1917.

Onkendi EO, Naik ND, Rosedahl JK, et al. Adenomas of the ampulla of Vater: a comparison of outcomes of operative and endoscopic resections. *J Gastrointest Surg.* 2014;18:1588-1596.

Poorly Differentiated Neuroendocrine Carcinoma

Nassar H, Albores-Saavedra J, Klimstra DS. High-grade neuroendocrine carcinoma of the ampulla of Vater: a clinicopathologic and immunohistochemical analysis of 14 cases. *Am J Surg Pathol.* 2005;29:588-594.

Zamboni G, Franzin G, Bonetti F, et al. Small-cell neuroendocrine carcinoma of the ampullary region. A clinicopathologic, immunohistochemical, and ultrastructural study of three cases. *Am J Surg Pathol.* 1990;14:703-713.

Huang Z, Xiao WD, Li Y, et al. Mixed adenoneuroendocrine carcinoma of the ampulla: Two case reports. *World J Gastroenterol.* 2015;21: 2254-2259.

Cavazza A, Gallo M, Valcavi R, et al. Large cell neuroendocrine carcinoma of the ampulla of Vater. *Arch Pathol Lab Med.* 2003;127:221-223.

Appendiceal Mucinous Neoplasm

Valasek MA, Pai RK. An update on the diagnosis, grading, and staging of appendiceal mucinous neoplasms. *Adv Anat Pathol.* 2018;25:38-60.

Carr NJ, Cecil TD, Mohamed F, et al. A consensus for classification and pathologic reporting of pseudomyxoma peritonei and associated appendiceal neoplasia: the results of the Peritoneal Surface Oncology Group International (PSOGI) Modified Delphi Process. *Am J Surg Pathol.* 2016;40:14-26.

Carr NJ, Bibeau F, Bradley RF, et al. The histopathological classification, diagnosis and differential diagnosis of mucinous appendiceal neoplasms, appendiceal adenocarcinomas and pseudomyxoma peritonei. *Histopathology.* 2017;71:847-858.

Liao X, Vavinskaya V, Sun K, et al. Mutation profile of high-grade appendiceal mucinous neoplasm. *Histopathology.* 2020;76:461-469.

Koc C, Akbulut S, Akatli AN, et al. Nomenclature of appendiceal mucinous lesions according to the 2019 WHO Classification of Tumors of the Digestive System. *Turk J Gastroenterol.* 2020;31:649-657.

Retention Cyst

Morano WF, Gleeson EM, Sullivan SH, et al. Clinicopathological features and management of appendiceal mucoceles: a systematic review. *Am Surg.* 2018;84:273-281.

Singh MP. A general overview of mucocele of appendix. *J Family Med Prim Care.* 2020;31:5867-5871.

Kang DW, Kim BH, Kim JM, et al. Standardization of the pathologic diagnosis of appendiceal mucinous neoplasms. *J Pathol Transl Med.* 2021;55:247-264.

Ruptured Appendiceal Diverticulum

Abdullgaffar B. Diverticulosis and diverticulitis of the appendix. *Int J Surg Pathol.* 2009;17:231-237.

Lim CSH, Cheah SY, Kwok AMF, Ravindran P, Chan DL. Systematic review and meta-analysis of the association between diverticulosis of the appendix and neoplasia. *ANZ J Surg.* 2020;90:1871-1877.

Biyani DK, Benbow EW, Watson AJ. Diverticula of the appendix. *Colorectal Dis.* 2006;8:812-813.

Serrated Polyp

Ahadi M, Sokolova A, Brown I, Chou A, Gill AJ. The 2019 World Health Organization Classification of appendiceal, colorectal and anal canal tumours: an update and critical assessment. *Pathology.* 2021;53:454-461.

Pai RK, Hartman DJ, Gonzalo DH, et al. Serrated lesions of the appendix frequently harbor KRAS mutations and not BRAF mutations indicating a distinctly different serrated neoplastic pathway in the appendix. *Hum Pathol.* 2014;45:227-235.

Carr NJ. Updates in appendix pathology: the precarious cutting edge. *Surg Pathol Clin.* 2020;13:469-484.

Lu Y, Qi C, Xu H, Jin M. Differential diagnosis of appendiceal serrated lesions and polyps and low-grade appendiceal mucinous neoplasm: analysis of 88 cases. *J Cancer Res Clin Oncol.* 2022;148:1761-1769.

Munari G, Businello G, Mattiolo P, et al. Molecular profiling of appendiceal serrated lesions, polyps and mucinous neoplasms: a single-centre experience. *J Cancer Res Clin Oncol.* 2021;147:1897-1904.

Endometriosis with Intestinal Metaplasia

Vyas M, Wong S, Zhang X. Intestinal metaplasia of appendiceal endometriosis is not uncommon and may mimic appendiceal mucinous neoplasm. *Pathol Res Pract.* 2017;213:39-44.

Misdraji J, Lauwers GY, Irving JA, Batts KP, Young RH. Appendiceal or cecal endometriosis with intestinal metaplasia: a potential mimic of appendiceal mucinous neoplasms. *Am J Surg Pathol.* 2014;38: 698-705.

Crohn's Disease

Bergeron V, Vienne A, Sokol H, Seksik P, Nion-Larmurier I, Ruskone-Fourmestraux A, Svrcek M, Beaugerie L, Cosnes J. Risk factors for neoplasia in inflammatory bowel disease patients with pancolitis. *Am J Gastroenterol.* 2010;105(11):2405-2411. doi:10.1038/ajg.2010.248. Epub 2010 Jun 15. PMID: 20551939.

Friedman S, Rubin PH, Bodian C, Harpaz N, Present DH. Screening and surveillance colonoscopy in chronic Crohn's colitis: results of a surveillance program spanning 25 years. *Clin Gastroenterol Hepatol.* 2008;6(9):993-998; quiz 953-954. doi:10.1016/j.cgh.2008.03.019. Epub 2008 Jun 27. PMID: 18585966.

Gajendran M, Loganathan P, Catinella AP, Hashash JG. A comprehensive review and update on Crohn's disease. *Dis Mon.* 2018;64:20-57.

Kleer CG, Appelman HD. Surgical pathology of Crohn's disease. *Surg Clin North Am.* 2001;81:13-30.

Pai RK, Jairath V. What is the role of histopathology in the evaluation of disease activity in Crohn's disease? *Best Pract Res Clin Gastroenterol.* 2019;38-39:101601.

Ulcerative Colitis

Battat R, Duijvestein M, Guizzetti L, et al. Histologic healing rates of medical therapies for ulcerative colitis: a systematic review and meta-analysis of randomized controlled trials. *Am J Gastroenterol.* 2019; 114:733-745.

Battat R, Vande Casteele N, Pai RK, et al. Evaluating the optimum number of biopsies to assess histologic inflammation in ulcerative colitis: a retrospective cohort study. *Aliment Pharmacol Ther.* 2020; 52:1574-1582.

Joo M, Odze RD. Rectal sparing and skip lesions in ulcerative colitis: a comparative study of endoscopic and histologic findings in patients who underwent proctocolectomy. *Am J Surg Pathol.* 2010;34:689-696.

Robert ME, Skacel M, Ullman T, et al. Patterns of colonic involvement at initial presentation in ulcerative colitis: a retrospective study of 46 newly diagnosed cases. *Am J Clin Pathol.* 2004;122:94-99.

Kim B, Barnett JL, Kleer CG, Appelman HD. Endoscopic and histological patchiness in treated ulcerative colitis. *Am J Gastroenterol.* 1999;94: 3258-3262.

Infectious Colitis

Surawicz CM, Haggitt RC, Husseman M, et al. Mucosal biopsy diagnosis of colitis: acute self-limited colitis and idiopathic inflammatory bowel disease. *Gastroenterology.* 1994;107:755-763.

Lamps LW. Infectious diseases of the lower gastrointestinal tract. *Surg Pathol Clin.* 2010;3:297-326.

Lamps LW. Infective disorders of the gastrointestinal tract. *Histopathology.* 2007;50:55-63.

Drug/Medication-Induced Colitis

Elsayed AG, Srivastava R, Pacioles T, Limjoco T, Tirona MT. Ischemic colitis associated with paclitaxel and carboplatin combination. *Case Rep Oncol.* 2017;10:689-693.

Ambesh P, Siddiqui S, Obiagwu C, et al. Pseudoephedrine associated ischemic colitis. *Am J Ther.* 2018;25:e604-e606.

Bellaguarda E, Hanauer S. Checkpoint inhibitor-induced colitis. *Am J Gastroenterol.* 2020;115:202-210.

Ischemic Colitis

Danakas AM, Fazili BG, Huber AR. Mass-forming ischemic colitis: a potential mimicker of malignancy. *Case Rep Pathol.* 2019;17:8927872.

Patil DT, Odze RD. Biopsy diagnosis of colitis: an algorithmic approach. *Virchows Arch.* 2018;472:67-80.

Jessurun J. The differential diagnosis of acute colitis: clues to a specific diagnosis. *Surg Pathol Clin.* 2017;10:863-885.

Yantiss RK, Cui I, Panarelli NC, Jessurun J. Idiopathic myointeimal hyperplasia of mesenteric veins: an uncommon cause of ischemic colitis with distinct mucosal features. *Am J Surg Pathol.* 2017;41:1657-1665.

Diverticular Disease–Associated Colitis

Haddad FG, El Bitar S, Al Moussawi H, Chang Q, Deeb L. Diverticular disease-associated colitis: what do we know? A review of the liverature. *Cureus.* 2018;10:e2224.

Mulhall AM, Mahid SS, Petras RE, Galandiuk S. Diverticular disease associated with inflammatory bowel disease-like colitis: a systematic review. *Dis Colon Rectum.* 2009;52:1072-1079.

Sessile Serrated Lesion

Bleijenberg A, Klotz D, Loberg M, et al. Implications of different guidelines for surveillance after serrated polyp resection in United States of America and Europe. *Endopscopy.* 2019;51:750-758.

Kim JH, Kang GH. Evolving pathologic concepts of serrated lesions of the colorectum. *J Pathol Transl Med.* 2020;54:276-289.

Liu C, Walker NI, Leggett BA, Whitehall VLJ, Bettington ML, Rosty C. Sessile serrated adenomas with dysplasia: morphological patterns and correlations with MLH1 immunohistochemistry. *Mod Pathol.* 2017;30:1728-1738.

Melson J, Ma K, Arshad S, et al. Presence of small sessile serrated polyps increases rate of advanced neoplasia upon surveillance compared with isolated low-risk tubular adenomas. *Gastrointest Endosc.* 2016;84:307-314.

Hyperplastic Polyp

Hamoudah T, Ma K, Esteban M, et al. Patients with small and diminutive proximal hyperplastic polyps have higher rates of synchronous advanced neoplasia compared with patients without serrated lesions. *Gastrointest Endosc.* 2018;87:1518-1526.

Hazewinkel Y, de Wijkerslooth TR, Stoop EM, et al. Prevalence of serrated polyps and association with synchronous advanced neoplasia in screening colonoscopy. *Endoscopy.* 2014;46:219-224.

Traditional Serrated Adenoma

McCarthy AJ, Serra S, Chetty R. Traditional serrated adenoma: an overview of pathology and emphasis on molecular pathogenesis. *BMJ Open Gastroenterol.* 2019;6:e000317.

Anal Gland Adenocarcinoma

Mori M, Koda K, Hirano A, et al. Early anal gland adenocarcinoma with a characteristic submucosal tumor-like appearance: a case report. *World J Surg Oncol.* 2018;16:148.

Fistula-Associated Anal Adenocarcinoma

Yang BL, Shao WJ, Sun GD, Chen YQ, Huang JC. Perianal mucinous adenocarcinoma arising from chronic anorectal fistulae: a review from a single institution. *Int J Colorectal Dis.* 2009;24:1001-1006.

HPV-Associated Anal Adenocarcinoma

Voltaggio L, McCluggage WG, Iding JS, et al. A novel group of HPV-related adenocarcinomas of the lower anogenital tract (vagina, vulva, and anorectum) in women and men resembling HPV-related endocervical adenocarcinoma. *Mod Pathol.* 2020;33:944-952.

Koulos J, Symmans F, Chumas J, Nuovo G. Human papillomavirus detection in adenocarcinoma of the anus. *Mod Pathol.* 1991;4:58-61.

Mucosal Anal Adenocarcinoma

Anwar S, Welbourn H, Hill J, Sebag-Montefiore D. Adenocarcinoma of the anal canal – a systematic review. *Colorectal Dis.* 2013;15:1481-1488.

Shridhar R, Shibata D, Chan E, Thomas CR. Anal canal: current standards in care and recent changes in practice. *CA Cancer J Clin.* 2015;65:139-162.

Metastatic Adenocarcinoma to Anal Canal

Wakatsuki K, Oeda Y, Isono T, et al. Adenocarcinoma of the rectosigmoid colon seeing into pre-existing anal fistula. *Hepatogastroenterology.* 2008;55:952-955.

Dulskas A, Cereska V, Zurauskas E, Stratilatovas E, Jankevicius F. Prostate cancer solitary metastasis to anal canal: case report and review of the literature. *BMC Cancer.* 2019;19:374.

Gastrointestinal Stromal Tumor

Schaefer IM, Marino-Enriquez A, Fletcher JA. What is new in gastrointestinal stromal tumor? *Adv Anat Pathol.* 2017;24:259-267.

Yamamoto H, Oda Y. Gastrointestinal stromal tumor: recent advances in pathology and genetics. *Pathol Int.* 2015;65:9-18.

Miettinen M, Lasota J. Gastrointestinal stromal tumors: pathology and prognosis at different sites. *Semin Diagn Pathol.* 2006;23:70-83.

Hirota S. Differential diagnosis of gastrointestinal stromal tumor by histopathology and immunohistochemistry. *Transl Gastroenterol Hepatol.* 2018;3:27.

Leiomyoma

Virani N, Pang J, Lew M. Cytologic and immunohistochemical evaluation of low-grade spindle cell lesions of the gastrointestinal tract. *Arch Pathol Lab Med.* 2016;140:1038-1044.

Deshpande A, Nelson D, Corless CL, Deshpande V, O'Brien MJ. Leiomyoma of the gastrointestinal tract with interstitial cells of Cajal: a mimic of gastrointestinal stromal tumor. *Am J Surg Pathol.* 2014;38:72-77.

Schwannoma

Khan AA, Schizas AM, Cresswell AB, Kjan MK, Khawaja HT. Digestive tract schwannoma. *Dig Surg.* 2006;23:265-269.

Lin CS, Hsu HS, Tsai CH, Li WY, Huang MH. Gastric schwannoma. *J Chin Med Assoc.* 2004;67:583-586.

Inflammatory Fibroid Polyp

Garmpis N, Damaskos C, Garmpi A, et al. Inflammatory fibrous polyp of the gastrointestinal tract: a systematic review for a benign tumor. *In Vivo.* 2021;35:81-93.

Wang J, Tian X, Ning BF, et al. Clinical characteristics and prognosis of inflammatory fibrous polyp in the gastrointestinal tract: a series of nine cases and a literature review. *J Dig Dis.* 2020;21:737-740.

Plexiform Angiomyxoid Myofibroblastic Tumor

Takahashi Y, Suzuki M, Fukusato T. Plexiform angiomyxoid myofibroblastic tumor of the stomach. *World J Gastroenterol.* 2010;16:2835-2840.

Ma S, Wang J, Lu Z, Shi C, Yang D, Lin J. Plexiform fibromyxoma: a clinicopathological and immunohistochemical analysis of two cases with a literature review. *J Int Med Res.* 2021;49:3000605211027878.

Miettinen M, Makhlouf HR, Sobin LH, Lasota J. Plexiform fibromyxoma: a distinctive benign gastric antral neoplasm not to be confused with a myxoid GIST. *Am J Surg Pathol.* 2009;33:1624-1632.

Rau TT, Hartmann A, Dietmaier W, et al. Plexiform angiomyxoid myofibroblastic tumour: differential diagnosis of gastrointestinal stromal tumour in the stomach. *J Clin Pathol.* 2008;61:1136-1137.

2 Gynecologic Tract

Omonigho Aisagbonhi • Fadi W. Abdul-Karim • Oluwole Fadare

CLASSIC (USUAL-TYPE/HPV-ASSOCIATED) VULVAR INTRAEPITHELIAL NEOPLASIA

DIFFERENTIAL DIAGNOSES: DIFFERENTIATED (HPV-INDEPENDENT) VULVAR INTRAEPITHELIAL NEOPLASIA, INVASIVE SQUAMOUS CELL CARCINOMA OF THE VULVA, AND PAGET DISEASE

Clinical Features

The term vulvar intraepithelial neoplasia (VIN) describes non-invasive squamous lesions of the vulva, of which two major types exist—classic/usual-type VIN and differentiated/simplex-type VIN (DVIN). Usual-type/classic VIN typically occurs in reproductive age (premenopausal) women, whereas simplex-type/DVIN predominates in elderly (postmenopausal) women. Classic/usual-type VIN is caused by human papillomavirus (HPV) infection and is more common in smokers and people with HIV. It is further graded into low-grade squamous intraepithelial lesion (LSIL; VIN 1) and high-grade squamous intraepithelial lesion/HSIL (VIN 2 and 3). While LSIL is the preferred terminology for squamous lesions with low-grade dysplasia, other terminologies that may be encountered include condyloma (used when lesions have papillary appearance), mild dysplasia, and koilocytic atypia. Other terms used to describe high-grade classic/usual-type VIN include Bowen disease, bowenoid dysplasia, and bowenoid papulosis (if clinically multifocal and pigmented).

Pathologic Features

GROSS FINDINGS

LSIL (VIN 1) typically appears as a pale macule, papule, or hyperkeratotic lesion on clinical gross examination. HSIL (VIN 2 and VIN 3) typically appear as conspicuous white or erythematous macules, papules, or nodules on clinical gross examination.

MICROSCOPIC FINDINGS

Histologic sections of LSIL show epithelial thickening with dysplastic changes, including hypercellularity, nuclear enlargement with increased nuclear-to-cytoplasmic ratio, hyperchromasia, and increased mitosis, limited to the lower third of the epithelium. The lower third of the epithelium shows decreased cytoplasmic maturation, but normal maturation is seen in the middle to upper third. Superficial koilocytes with hyperchromatic, occasionally bi- or multinucleated, nuclei, and cytoplasmic halos are characteristic (Fig. 2.1A). Both low- and high-risk HPV types are associated with LSIL (VIN 1).

Histologic sections of HSIL show epithelial thickening with dysplastic changes, including hypercellularity, nuclear enlargement with irregular nuclear membranes, increased nuclear-to-cytoplasmic ratio, hyperchromasia, and increased mitosis (occasionally with atypical mitotic figures), involving the middle to upper two thirds of the epithelium. A lack of maturation is noted, with cells appearing more basal-/parabasal-like (Fig. 2.1B). Lesions are characterized as moderate dysplasia (VIN 2) when dysplastic changes involve the lower two thirds of the epithelium, and severe dysplasia (VIN 3) when full-thickness dysplastic changes are noted. Koilocytes may occasionally be present.

Ancillary Studies

Immunohistochemical stain with p16 can be useful in evaluating HPV-associated VIN. HPV infections in LSIL are typically episomal; thus, immunohistochemical stain for p16 is often negative (i.e., either completely negative or weak/patchy staining) but may occasionally be positive (with block-type staining limited to the basal layer). HSIL is typically associated with high-risk HPV types that have integrated into host genome and induced expression of viral E6 and E7 proteins that in turn inactivate the p53-mediated DNA damage response pathway and the pRb-mediated cell cycle, respectively. The inactivation of pRb leads to the upregulation of p16, which can be detected by immunohistochemical stains. HSIL shows strong, diffuse block-positive staining for p16. HSIL (VIN 2) may show some evidence of

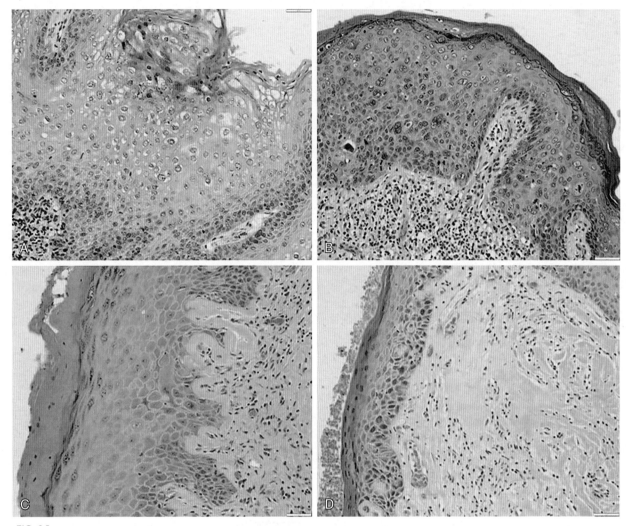

FIG. 2.1

Histology of vulva intraepithelial neoplasia. **A,** Low-grade squamous intraepithelial lesion shows epithelial maturation (the basal nuclei are palisaded and distinguishable from the cells of the superficial layers which have more abundant cytoplasm) and koilocytosis. **B,** High-grade squamous intraepithelial lesion shows lack of maturation for most of the epithelium; mitotic figures are not restricted to the base but are present in the middle and upper epithelial layers. **C,** Differentiated vulvar intraepithelial neoplasia (DVIN) can be subtle; elongated rete ridges and premature keratinization are clues. **D,** Another case of DVIN with basal keratinocyte atypia.

maturation with more abundant cytoplasm, occasionally with koilocytic change. Thus, distinguishing HSIL (VIN2) from LSIL may be a diagnostic challenge. Fortunately, immunohistochemical stain for p16 is useful (and recommended) in such cases. HSIL shows block-positive staining for p16 with extension to the middle third of the epithelium or higher, while p16 is often negative in LSIL (Fig. 2.2).

Differential Diagnosis

DIFFERENTIATED VULVAR INTRAEPITHELIAL NEOPLASIA

Differentiated vulvar intraepithelial neoplasia (DVIN) is HPV-independent and frequently arises in a background of vulvar dermatoses, particularly lichen sclerosus and lichen planus. The simplex type/DVIN is considered high grade. A substantial number of cases of DVIN are associated with *TP53* mutations. Three less common types of HPV-independent vulvar squamous intraepithelial neoplasms termed differentiated exophytic vulvar intraepithelial lesion (DEVIL), vulvar acanthosis with altered differentiation (VAAD), and basaloid DVIN have been described. Like DVIN, DEVIL and VAAD are HPV-independent. Mutations in *PIK3CA* have been described in DEVIL. *HRAS* mutations were found to be common in VAAD.

DVIN lesions are typically observed in areas of lichen sclerosus or lichen planus and may be associated with pruritus, pain, and burning. They typically appear erythematous or white, may have a rough irregular surface, and may be associated with hyperkeratosis or ulceration. DVIN lesions tend to be more clinically/grossly subtle than those observed in classic VIN. As a result, a

LSIL   HSIL   DVIN

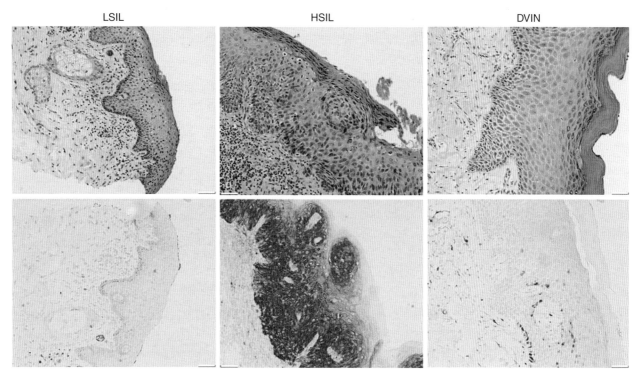

FIG. 2.2

p16 immunohistochemical staining pattern in low-grade squamous intraepithelial lesion (LSIL), high-grade squamous intraepithelial lesion (HSIL), and differentiated vulvar intraepithelial neoplasia (DVIN). p16 is negative in LSIL *(left panel)*, diffusely positive in HSIL *(middle panel)*, and negative in DVIN *(right panel)*.

high degree of clinical suspicion is warranted in patients with a history of lichen sclerosus or lichen planus.

Histologic sections may likewise be subtle due to the highly differentiated nature of the lesion. Sections of DVIN show epidermal thickening with hyper and/or parakeratosis and elongated rete ridges. The keratinocytes typically appear enlarged with large nuclei, prominent nucleoli, and abundant eosinophilic cytoplasm. The granular layer may be inconspicuous. Key diagnostic clues include premature keratinization (keratinocytes with abundant pink cytoplasm are abnormally located in the basal third of the epidermis), dyskeratosis of individual keratinocytes, and basal keratinocyte atypia (including karyomegaly, nuclear hyperchromasia, macronucleoli, and atypical mitosis). Given the association of DVIN with *TP53* mutations, mutant p53 immunohistochemical staining patterns are frequently present and the p53 immunohistochemical stain can be a diagnostic adjunct. Patterns of p53 staining that have been found to correlate with *TP53* mutations include the following: strong nuclear staining in consecutive basal tumor cells; diffuse strong nuclear staining in basal and parabasal layers; complete absence of staining in the setting of a positive internal control; diffuse cytoplasmic staining in the setting of a positive internal control.

Both DVIN and HSIL show acanthosis and significant keratinocyte atypia. In contrast to HSIL, which shows a loss of maturation, DVIN shows increased (abnormal) maturation, with superficial-type keratinizing cells being present in the basal third of the epidermis (Fig. 2.1C). The keratinocyte atypia in DVIN is typically restricted to the basal layer of the epidermis, while that of HSIL is more diffuse involving the middle third and upper layers. There, however, can be morphologic overlap, and in such cases, taking clinical features into account (i.e., patient's age, presence/history of lichen sclerosus or other dermatoses, sexual history, HIV status, or any history of abnormal cervical PAP smears) may be informative. Additionally, because DVIN is HPV-independent, and HSIL is HPV-associated, immunohistochemical staining for p16 (and/or direct HPV detection tests) is useful (see Fig. 2.2); p53 immunohistochemical stain may also be of use, if correctly interpreted (Fig. 2.3). Features useful in distinguishing usual-type VIN from DVIN are summarized in Table 2.1.

DVIN versus squamous hyperplasia: Both DVIN and benign hyperplastic squamous epithelium show acanthosis (i.e., epithelial thickening) and some degree of hyperkeratosis. However, benign squamous hyperplasia displays normal epidermal maturation (with preserved granular layer); it does not show abnormal keratinization and lacks the significant basal keratinocyte atypia that is characteristic of DVIN.

DVIN versus hypertrophic lichen planus: Like DVIN, lichen planus is often associated with acanthosis and hyperkeratosis and may even have individual dyskeratotic keratinocytes. However, the lesions may be distinguished based on preserved epidermal maturation

Lichen sclerosus	HSIL	DVIN with adjacent invasive SCC

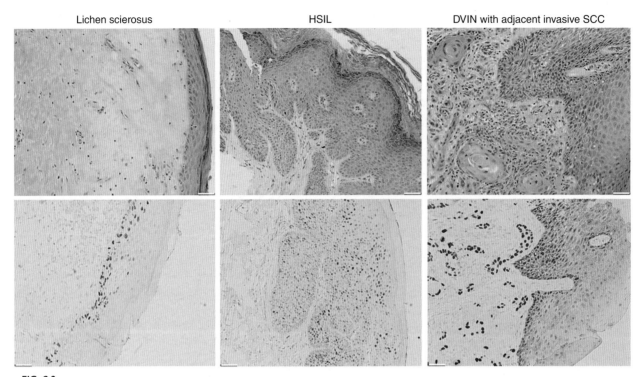

FIG. 2.3

p53 immunohistochemical stain in lichen sclerosus *(left panel)* versus high-grade squamous intraepithelial lesion (HSIL; *middle panel*) versus differentiated vulvar intraepithelial neoplasia (DVIN) with adjacent SCC *(right panel)*. Note p53 can be tricky to interpret—pay attention to basal layer. Confluent or near-confluent basal layer staining with suprabasal extension, as seen in the DVIN panel, is needed to be considered positive. Wild-type pattern can vary. In this case, the lichen sclerosus shows patchy staining and is negative, whereas the HSIL lacks staining in the basal layer and is therefore negative. *SCC*, Squamous cell carcinoma.

TABLE 2.1

Features Useful in Distinguishing Classic (HPV-associated) and Differentiated (HPV-independent) VIN

	CLASSIC (HPV-ASSOCIATED) VIN		Differentiated (HPV-independent) VIN
	LSIL	HSIL	
Epidemiology	Reproductive age	Reproductive age	Elderly (postmenopausal)
Etiology	Both high- and low-risk HPV	High-risk HPV	Chronic inflammation (lichen sclerosus, lichen planus) with resultant **Tp53**, PIK3CA, HRAS mutations
Histology	Intraepithelial lesion with dysplastic changes in the basal third of squamous epithelium associated with koilocytic change	Intraepithelial lesion with dysplastic changes and increased mitosis in the middle to upper third of squamous epithelium	Intraepithelial lesion with abnormal keratinization occurring in the middle to lower third of the squamous epithelium and associated with basal keratinocyte atypia
IHC	p16 typically negative (may occasionally be positive with staining limited to the basal third of the epithelium)	p16 shows strong diffuse block positivity involving the middle to upper third of the epithelium	p16 negative Mutant expression pattern of p53 (can either be p53 positive in basal and suprabasal cells or completely negative [null pattern])
Prognosis	Good: self-limited infection	30%–50% risk of invasive (typically basaloid/warty/non-keratinizing) squamous cell carcinoma over a 30-year period	Poor: >80% risk of concurrent or subsequent invasive squamous cell carcinoma within 2 years
Treatment	Only if symptomatic, treat like condyloma	Wide excision with clear margins	Wide excision with clear margins; also treat underlying lichen sclerosus or lichen planus

HPV, Human papillomavirus; *HSIL,* high-grade squamous intraepithelial lesion; *IHC,* immunohistochemistry; *LSIL,* low-grade squamous intraepithelial lesion; *VIN,* vulvar intraepithelial neoplasia.

with accentuation of the granular layer (wedge-shaped hypergranulosis) observed in lichen planus. In addition, lichen planus is typically associated with a lichenoid inflammatory infiltrate and clefting at the dermoepidermal junction. Lichen planus also lacks the significant basal keratinocyte atypia that is characteristic of DVIN.

DVIN versus lichen sclerosus: Early lichen sclerosus may show psoriasiform epidermal hyperplasia (i.e., elongated rete ridges) similar to DVIN. Lichen sclerosus, however, typically has associated dermal fibrosis (or homogenization in advanced lesions), lichenoid inflammatory infiltrate, and normal epidermal maturation. Lichen sclerosus also lacks the significant basal atypia that is characteristic of DVIN.

DVIN versus other HPV-independent VIN: The other types of HPV-independent VIN are only just beginning to be recognized. Watkins et al. coined the term differentiated exophytic vulvar intraepithelial lesion (DEVIL) to describe exophytic vulva lesions with prominent acanthosis or verruciform hyperplasia that lack the histomorphologic features of HPV-associated HSIL and also lack sufficient basal atypia to warrant a diagnosis of DVIN. In their study, DEVILs lacked *TP53* mutations but were associated with *PIK3CA* and *ARID2* mutations, supporting their categorization as a distinct entity from DVIN. Vulvar acanthosis with altered differentiation (VAAD) was described by Nascimento et al. as an intraepithelial squamous proliferation that displayed marked acanthosis with variable verruciform architecture, loss of granular cell layer with superficial epithelial cell pallor, and multilayered parakeratosis. Both VAAD and DEVIL are distinguished from DVIN by their lack of significant basal keratinocyte atypia. However, there is significant morphologic overlap between DEVIL and VAAD and establishing whether VAAD and DEVIL are distinct entities from each other requires more extensive studies. Ordi et al. described an unusual type of HPV-independent VIN that displayed architectural distortion with a homogenous population of basaloid keratinocytes, mimicking HSIL. All cases were HPV-negative by PCR and p16-negative by immunohistochemistry. In general, due to the varying morphologies and subtleties of HPV-independent vulvar squamous cancer precursors, it is prudent to be wary of acanthotic, hyperkeratotic (or even basaloid) lesions in postmenopausal women, especially those with a history of lichen sclerosus or lichen planus. Ancillary immunohistochemical stains with p16 and p53 may be of value.

INVASIVE SQUAMOUS CELL CARCINOMA OF THE VULVA

When HSIL extends into adnexal structures, distinction from invasive squamous cell carcinoma can be difficult, especially on tangential sections. Obtaining deeper sections may be helpful in such cases. Other clues that may help in distinguishing HSIL from invasive carcinoma include paying attention to the spatial orientation of the nests on low-power microscopic evaluation—the nests in HSIL tend to be rounded/organized—and noticing the preserved basement membrane of HSIL on higher power. Invasive squamous cell carcinoma is also typically associated with a desmoplastic stromal reaction that is not seen in HSIL.

A diagnosis of superficially invasive squamous cell carcinoma of the vulva (AJCC pT1a tumor) is rendered if all of the following conditions are met: (1) the tumor is 2 cm or less in size, (2) the tumor is confined to the vulva or perineum, and (3) the depth of invasion is less than or equal to 1 mm. The depth of invasion is measured from the base of epithelial-stromal junction of the adjacent most superficial dermal papilla to the deepest point of stromal invasion. Superficially invasive tumors have low risk of lymph node metastasis and are thus managed by wide local excision (simple partial vulvectomy) without the need for lymph node dissection. Additional surgery (radical vulvectomy with sentinel lymph node biopsy or inguinofemoral lymph node dissection) may be required if a tumor is discovered to have larger size and/or >1 mm of stromal invasion after initial partial vulvectomy.

PAGET DISEASE OF THE VULVA

Paget disease is an intraepithelial adenocarcinoma characterized by apocrine/eccrine large cells with abundant cytoplasm (Paget cells). Occasionally, HSIL can display a nested pattern that morphologically mimics Paget disease. Immunohistochemical stains are helpful in distinguishing HSIL from Paget. In contrast to HSIL, Paget cells stain positive for GCDFP-15 (an apocrine marker), CEA, CAM5.2, HER2/neu, and androgen receptors. Paget cells are also mostly negative for p40 and CK5/6. Given that Paget disease is a glandular neoplasm, mucin special stains also tend to be positive in Paget (but negative in HSIL).

Prognosis and Therapy

LSIL (VIN 1): LSILs are associated with transient (self-limited) episomal HPV infections and have a very low (in any) risk of progression to invasive cancer. Therefore, vulvar LSILs need not be treated, unless symptomatic. Symptomatic lesions are managed like condylomas.

HSIL (VIN2/3): HSILs are associated with persistent HPV infections secondary to the integration of viral DNA into the host genome. The invasive squamous cell carcinomas that arise in HSILs tend to have basaloid morphology, though keratinizing squamous cell carcinomas also occur. The 30-year risk of progression of untreated HSIL to invasive cancer is 30% to 50%. In addition, there is a potential for associated occult invasive cancer in HSIL. Therefore, the recommended treatment for HSIL is wide local excision with 0.5 to 1.0 cm gross margin clearance. When surgery is not possible, or occult invasion is not a concern, laser ablation and medical therapy with topical imiquimod are acceptable treatment options.

DVIN: DVINs are strongly associated with invasive cancer, with a risk of malignant progression estimated to be as high as 85%. The invasive squamous cell carcinomas that arise in DVINs tend to be keratinizing, though basaloid carcinomas occasionally occur. Due to the strong association with invasive cancer, lesions diagnosed as DVIN on biopsy require complete surgical excision with clear margins. DVINs are also associated with vulvar dermatoses; treatment of vulvar dermatoses, especially lichen sclerosus, reduces the risk of cancer.

VULVAR INTRAEPITHELIAL NEOPLASIA – DISEASE FACT SHEET

Definition
- Non-invasive vulvar neoplasms of two types:
  - HPV-associated (aka squamous intraepithelial lesions/classic or usual-type VIN)
  - HPV-independent (aka differentiated VIN)

Epidemiology
- HPV-associated squamous intraepithelial lesions typically occur in reproductive age women.
- Differentiated/HPV-independent VIN typically occur in elderly, postmenopausal women.

Clinical Features
- HPV-associated squamous intraepithelial lesions are often asymptomatic, though patients may present with pruritus and/or visible lesions (white, erythematous or pigmented macules, papules, or plaques).
- Patients with DVIN may be asymptomatic or present with long history of itching and burning related to pre-existing lichen sclerosus or lichen planus.

Prognosis and Therapy
- HSILs carry a 30%–50% risk of progressing into invasive squamous cell carcinoma over 30 years. HSILs are treated by wide local excision; topical imiquimod and laser ablation are also therapeutic options.
- DVINs carry a strong (as high as 85%) risk of progression into invasive squamous cell carcinoma over short period of time. DVINs are treated by complete surgical excisions with clear margins.

HPV-ASSOCIATED (CLASSIC/USUAL-TYPE) VIN – PATHOLOGIC FEATURES

Gross Findings
- May appear as white, erythematous or pigmented macules, papules, plaques, or nodules

Microscopic Findings
- LSILs show lack of maturation at the basal third of the squamous epithelium and are typically associated with superficial koilocytosis.
- HSILs show lack of maturation extending to the upper two thirds of the squamous epithelium; mitotic figures are often easily identified in the upper two thirds of the epithelium.

Pathologic Differential Diagnoses
- Invasive squamous cell carcinoma
- Differentiated VIN

INVASIVE SQUAMOUS CELL CARCINOMA OF THE UTERINE CERVIX

DIFFERENTIAL DIAGNOSIS: SQUAMOUS INTRAEPITHELIAL LESIONS

Clinical Features

Almost all invasive cervical squamous cell carcinomas are caused by high-risk HPV infection. The median age of invasive cervical squamous cell carcinoma diagnosis is 51 years. Patients may be asymptomatic or present with abnormal vaginal bleeding, discharge, and/or pain.

Pathologic Features

GROSS FINDINGS

Gross findings vary depending on the size of the carcinoma—varying from erythematous, raised lesions to exophytic or endophytic masses with necrosis.

MICROSCOPIC FINDINGS

Morphologic types: There are various morphologic types of invasive squamous cell carcinoma, such as non-keratinizing (also called usual-type), keratinizing, basaloid, verrucous, papillary, warty, squamotransitional, and lymphoepithelioma-like; HPV has been identified in all described morphologic types. Except for verrucous carcinoma, a well-differentiated tumor with a bulbous pushing (rather than infiltrative) invasive front, which does not metastasize but has a tendency for local recurrence if incompletely excised, squamous cell carcinoma morphologic type has little effect on prognosis once grade and stage have been taken into account. Nevertheless, papillary squamous cell carcinoma and lymphoepithelial-like carcinoma are variants worth noting. Papillary squamous cell carcinoma is superficially exophytic with papillae/connective tissue stroma covered by HSIL-like epithelium but is often associated with an underlying stromal invasive carcinoma, often usual-type. This variant is worth noting because it can be underdiagnosed as HSIL on superficial biopsies. Lymphoepithelial-like carcinoma is composed of poorly defined islands of undifferentiated-appearing squamous cells (i.e., lack keratinization and intercellular bridges) in a background of a dense lymphocytic infiltrate. This variant is worth noting because the associated dense lymphocytic infiltrate may mask the presence of the underlying malignant epithelial cells, which can be highlighted by pancytokeratin, p40, and p16 immunohistochemical stains.

Occasionally a tumor may be composed of clearly distinguishable glandular and squamous carcinoma components—a mixture of a definite adenocarcinoma and squamous cell carcinoma. Such tumors are termed adenosquamous carcinomas. Adenosquamous carcinomas are typically HPV-associated and stage for stage appear to have similar prognosis and behavior to cervical squamous cell carcinoma. Of note, scattered mucin-producing cells may be seen in poorly differentiated squamous cell carcinoma, but their presence is insufficient to render a diagnosis of adenosquamous carcinoma. A diagnosis of adenosquamous carcinoma is rendered when a tumor contains well-developed recognizable glands in addition to a squamous cell carcinoma component.

Grading: The 2014 WHO mentions criteria for grading cervical squamous cell carcinoma that include extent of squamous differentiation, nuclear pleomorphism, size of nucleoli, mitotic frequency, and necrosis; however, details on how to implement such criteria are lacking.

A three-tiered grading system based on tumor budding activity and tumor nest size (TBNS) has been proposed for cervical squamous cell carcinoma. The TBNS system assigns a score from 1 to 3 based on tumor budding activity per 10 high-power fields (HPF): score 1, no budding; score 2: <15 budding foci; score 3, ≥15 budding foci. A score from 1 to 4 is assigned for the smallest cell nest size within the tumor: score 1, > 15 cells; score 2, 5–15 cells; score 3, 2–4 cells; score 4, single-cell invasion. The grade is then assigned based on the total score: grade 1, score 2–3; grade 2, score 4–5; and grade 3, score 6–7. The TBNS system has been found to be a significant prognostic indicator. The system likely assesses a tumor's dispersion propensity, that is, level of epithelial to mesenchymal transition and metastatic potential.

Ancillary Studies

In rare cases of very poorly differentiated carcinomas, immunohistochemical stains confirming squamous differentiation: p40, p63, CK5/6 may be useful, in addition to p16 immunohistochemical stain and HPV testing.

Differential Diagnosis

SQUAMOUS INTRAEPITHELIAL LESIONS

Squamous intraepithelial lesions of the uterine cervix are non-invasive HPV-associated neoplasms. LSILs as associated with transient HPV infections, episomal infections that end up being cleared. The episomal phase of infection is associated with morphologic features, such as koilocytosis, that define LSIL.

In immunocompromised people, those who smoke, those infected with particularly virulent high-risk HPV strains such as HPV types 16 and 18, and those with other less understood risk factors, high-risk HPV infections may persist, allowing for viral integration into the host genome and progression to HSIL. Untreated HSIL has a 30% to 50% risk of progressing into invasive squamous cell carcinoma over 30 years.

HSIL may occasionally extend into endocervical glands; extensive glandular involvement by HSIL may be confused with invasive squamous cell carcinoma. Helpful distinguishing features include smooth rounded contours with intact basement membrane in HSIL versus irregular angulated contours in invasive carcinoma. Stromal desmoplasia, detached small tumor nests, and single isolated cells within the stroma are features of invasive carcinoma (Fig. 2.4D). A diagnosis of superficially invasive squamous cell carcinoma is rendered if all of the following conditions are met: (1) the tumor has been completely excised, (2) the tumor is not grossly visible, (3) the depth of invasion is less than or equal to 3 mm, and (4) the horizontal spread is less than or equal to 7 mm. The depth of invasion is measured from the base of epithelium involved by HSIL to the deepest point of stromal invasion by carcinoma. After complete cone excision or loop electrosurgical excision procedure (LEEP), tumors diagnosed as superficially invasive squamous cell carcinomas that lack lymphovascular invasion may be managed by observation to spare fertility, if surgical margin clearance is 3 mm or greater. Some histologic features useful in distinguishing invasive squamous cell carcinoma from HSIL are presented in Table 2.2.

LSIL versus HSIL: LSIL shows cell maturation and often has associated koilocytic change, whereas cell maturation is often lost in HSIL (i.e., the basal epithelium is not easily distinguished from the superficial epithelium) (Fig. 2.4). However, in flat or tangentially sectioned epithelium or in cases of CIN 2 where some surface maturation occurs, it may be difficult to distinguish LSIL from HSIL. A diagnosis of HSIL should be rendered in the presence of extreme basal/parabasal nuclear atypia, atypical mitosis, and mitosis higher than the basal third of the epithelium. A combination of p16 and Ki67 immunohistochemical stains may be useful in challenging cases. HSIL shows strong and diffuse p16 positivity and Ki67 activity higher than the basal epithelium, while LSIL is p16 negative or if

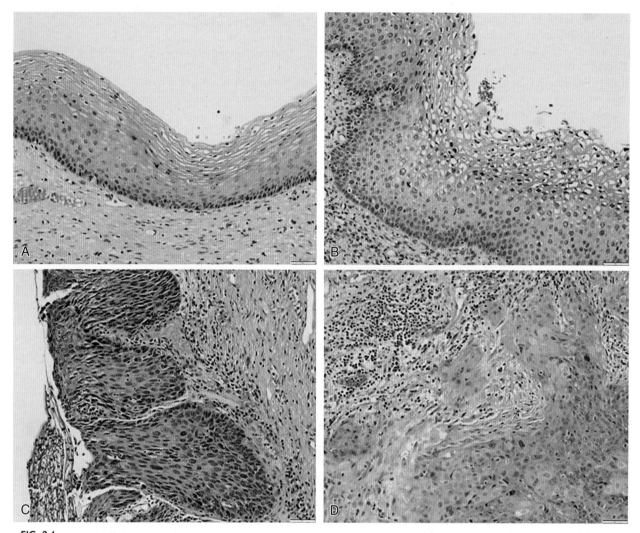

FIG. 2.4

Histology of normal cervix in contrast to low-grade squamous intraepithelial lesion (LSIL), high-grade squamous intraepithelial lesion (HSIL), and squamous cell carcinoma (SCC). **A,** Normal cervix shows maturation of the epithelium with increasing keratinization from basal to superficial epithelium; note the small size of superficial nuclei. **B,** LSIL shows maturation of the epithelium but with superficial koilocytes displaying nuclear enlargement and hyperchromasia along with cytoplasmic clearing. **C,** HSIL lacks epithelial maturation and mitotic figures are not restricted to the base, but the basement membrane is preserved. **D,** Invasive SCC lacks a basement membrane and shows stromal desmoplasia; small tumor nests detached from the main invasive front may also be noted.

TABLE 2.2

Histologic Features Helpful in Distinguishing Invasive Squamous Cell Carcinoma from High-Grade Squamous Intraepithelial Lesion

Invasive Squamous Cell Carcinoma	High-Grade Squamous Intraepithelial Lesion
Invades stroma	Limited to the epithelium
Angulated nests, single isolated cells, or expansile solid sheets within the stroma	Smooth; defined epithelial-stromal junction with intact basement membrane
Stromal desmoplasia	No desmoplasia
Lymphovascular invasion may be present	No lymphovascular invasion

positive, has staining limited to the basal third of the epithelium. In addition, Ki67 is limited to the epithelial base in LSIL. Of note, the immunohistochemical stain results need to be interpreted in conjunction with morphologic findings. Immunohistochemistry is not recommended in cases that are clearly LSIL or HSIL based on morphology. A diagnosis of LSIL should not be changed to HSIL based solely on immunohistochemical staining results.

Benign, reactive, atrophic, and metaplastic squamous epithelium versus HPV-related squamous intraepithelial lesions: The cytoplasmic clearing in mature glycogenated squamous epithelium and perinuclear clearing in squamous epithelium reacting to infections like trichomoniasis may mimic LSIL. LSIL, however, is characterized by nuclear enlargement, hyperchromasia, and membrane irregularities that distinguish it from benign and reactive processes. Squamous metaplasia and atrophy may show a lack of maturation that mimics HSIL. However, the cellular uniformity, smooth nuclear contours, and lack of mitosis and presence of small nucleoli distinguish squamous metaplasia from HSIL. Atrophy similarly has cellular uniformity, smooth nuclear contours, and lack of mitosis, whereas HSIL often shows enlarged irregular hyperchromatic nuclei that lack appreciable nucleoli in addition to the presence of mitotic figures higher than the basal third of the epithelium. A combination of p16 and Ki67 immunohistochemical stains is useful in challenging cases. HSIL shows strong and diffuse p16 positivity and Ki67 activity higher than the basal epithelium, while squamous metaplasia and atrophy are p16 negative (focal reactivity is considered negative) and have Ki67 limited to the epithelial base.

Prognosis and Therapy

The prognosis and treatment of cervical squamous cell carcinomas are stage-dependent. Localized tumors have an approximately 92% 5-year survival rate which drops to 17% in advanced stage (stage IV) cancers. Treatment modalities range from fertility-sparing LEEP or cone excisions in superficially invasive (AJCC pT1a1) squamous cell carcinomas to radical hysterectomy with lymphadenectomy and/or chemoradiation in more advanced stages.

INVASIVE SQUAMOUS CELL CARCINOMA OF THE UTERINE CERVIX – DISEASE FACT SHEET

Definition
- ▸▸ Squamous tumor with infiltrative, pushing, or exophytic invasion

Epidemiology
- ▸▸ Fourth most frequent cancer in women
- ▸▸ Median age at diagnosis: 51 years
- ▸▸ Almost all (approximately 95%) are high-risk HPV-associated

Clinical Features
- ▸▸ Range from asymptomatic to abnormal vaginal bleeding, discharge, and pelvic pain
- ▸▸ Colposcopy may show erythematous raised lesions in early stages; advanced stage cancers are usually apparent as palpable and/or visible masses on routine clinical exam.

Prognosis and Therapy
- ▸▸ Depend on stage

INVASIVE SQUAMOUS CELL CARCINOMA OF THE UTERINE CERVIX – PATHOLOGIC FEATURES

Gross Findings
- ▸▸ Range from erythematous raised lesions and/or ulcers in early cancers to exophytic or endophytic masses with necrosis in more progressed cancers

Microscopic Findings
- ▸▸ Tumor may invade stroma as sheets, nests, cords or single cells. Exophytic growth with fibrovascular cores may be present in papillary squamous cell carcinoma.
- ▸▸ Stromal desmoplasia often present
- ▸▸ Various histomorphologic patterns: keratinizing, basaloid, warty, papillary, verrucous, and lymphoepithelial

Pathologic Differential Diagnosis
- ▸▸ Squamous intraepithelial lesions

HPV-ASSOCIATED ENDOCERVICAL ADENOCARCINOMAS

DIFFERENTIAL DIAGNOSIS: HPV-INDEPENDENT (NON–HPV-ASSOCIATED) ENDOCERVICAL ADENOCARCINOMAS

General Information

In 2018, the International Endocervical Adenocarcinoma Criteria and Classification (IECC) was introduced to link morphologic features of endocervical adenocarcinomas to their etiology. Based on these criteria, endocervical adenocarcinomas can be classified into two major categories: human papillomavirus–associated (HPVA) endocervical adenocarcinomas and adenocarcinomas unassociated with HPV (i.e., non–HPV-associated adenocarcinomas [NHPVA]).

Clinical Features

On average, patients with HPVA endocervical adenocarcinomas are aged 40 to 42 years. Patients may be asymptomatic, with cancer detected on screening cytology, or may present with abnormal vaginal bleeding and/or mass.

Pathologic Features

GROSS FINDINGS

HPVA endocervical adenocarcinomas grossly appear as ulcers and/or exophytic or endophytic masses in the endocervix.

MICROSCOPIC FINDINGS

HPVA endocervical adenocarcinomas are invasive tumors morphologically defined by easily detected apical mitosis and apoptosis (i.e., mitosis and apoptosis can be identified at scanning to low-power [4–10×] magnification) and are

often diffusely p16 positive by immunohistochemistry (Fig. 2.5). They encompass different morphologic types: usual type, villoglandular, mucinous (intestinal type), mucinous (signet ring cell type), and invasive stratified mucin producing.

Usual type is the most common type of endocervical adenocarcinoma, accounting for approximately 75% of all endocervical adenocarcinomas. It is relatively mucin-poor; intracytoplasmic mucin is present in less than 50% of the cells. Usual-type endocervical adenocarcinomas can be further classified into prognostic groups based on the pattern of stromal invasion. Pattern A tumors carry an excellent prognosis; all studied tumors have been stage I at diagnosis and have not been associated with lymph node metastasis or recurrence. Pattern A tumors are characterized by well-formed glands with preserved lobular architecture and a lack of stromal reaction (i.e., stromal desmoplasia is absent). Single detached cells,

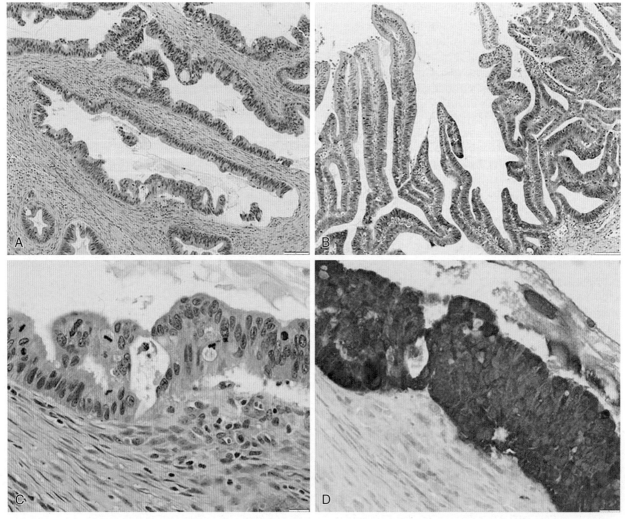

FIG. 2.5

Human papillomavirus–associated endocervical adenocarcinoma. Mitotic and apoptotic figures are easily appreciated at low power. **A,** Usual type. **B,** Villoglandular. **C,** High power showing apical mitosis. **D,** p16 immunohistochemical stain is positive (diffuse strong staining).

detached tumor clusters, solid growth, and lympho-vascular invasion must be absent for tumors to be categorized as pattern A. Pattern C tumors display diffuse destructive stromal invasion with desmoplasia, solid growth, and lymphovascular invasion. Extravasated mucin with admixed tumor cells, band-like lymphocytic infiltrate, papillary and/or micropapillary architecture, and confluent glands may be present. Pattern C tumors often present at stage II or higher and are associated with lymph node metastasis (22.5% of the studies cases), recurrences (19.7% of cases), and death from disease. Pattern B tumors are associated with limited (<5 mm; one 4× field) destructive stromal invasion in a background of pattern A. Lymphovascular invasion may be present, but solid growth must be absent. Most patients with pattern B tumors were stage I at diagnosis; less than 5% had lymph node metastasis. Assigning a pattern to usual-type endocervical adenocarcinomas should only be done in a completely excised specimen. Data suggest that regardless of size or depth of stromal invasion, pattern A tumors can be managed with localized complete surgical excision (e.g., cone or LEEP with negative margins) without the need for more radical surgery. Pattern B tumors can be managed with localized complete resection and sentinel node excision to determine the need for adjuvant therapy, while radical surgery may be necessary in pattern C tumors.

Other histologic types of HPVA endocervical adenocarcinoma include: *Villoglandular* carcinomas which display distinct exophytic long slender papillae. Villoglandular adenocarcinomas typically occur in a younger age group (median age, 34 years) than usual-type adenocarcinomas (median age, 42 years). *Mucinous* carcinomas comprise cells with intracytoplasmic mucin making up >50% of the tumor population. The mucinous cells may be goblet cells (intestinal type) or signet ring cells (signet ring cell type). *Invasive stratified mucin-producing intraepithelial lesion (iSMILE)* is characterized by invasive nests of stratified columnar cells with peripheral palisading and variable amounts of intracytoplasmic mucin. At least one study suggests that iSMILE may be more aggressive than usual-type endocervical adenocarcinoma.

Precursor glandular lesions for HPVA endocervical adenocarcinomas include adenocarcinoma *in situ* (AIS), HPVA, and SMILE. HSIL is occasionally identified as a precursor in HPVA endocervical adenocarcinomas.

Ancillary Studies

Immunohistochemical staining showing strong, diffuse p16 expression is a useful ancillary test as a molecular studies for high-risk HPV.

Differential Diagnosis

HPV-INDEPENDENT ENDOCERVICAL ADENOCARCINOMAS (NHPVA ADENOCARCINOMAS)

NHPVA endocervical adenocarcinomas are invasive adenocarcinomas with various etiologies unrelated to HPV infection. They encompass different morphologic types, the most common being gastric-type adenocarcinomas, including minimal deviation adenocarcinoma/adenoma malignum. STK11 mutations, gains in chromosome 3p, and loss of 1p have been described in gastric-type adenocarcinomas. Lobular endocervical glandular hyperplasia is a potential precursor lesion for gastric-type adenocarcinomas. Other NHPVA morphologic types of endocervical adenocarcinomas are rare and include: endometrioid (thought to arise from endometriosis), clear cell, serous, and mesonephric.

NHPVA endocervical adenocarcinomas tend to present as larger tumors (median tumor size, 38 mm) and in older women (median age, 55 years) compared with HPVA endocervical adenocarcinomas (median tumor size, 21 mm; median patient age, 42 years). The gastric-type endocervical adenocarcinomas have a significantly worse prognosis than HPVA adenocarcinomas, being more frequently associated with distant metastasis.

In contrast to usual type adenocarcinoma and other HPV-associated subtypes, the NHPVA adenocarcinoma subtypes do NOT have easily identifiable apical mitosis or apoptosis. Mitotic and apoptotic figures may be present but require high-power diligent evaluation to identify. If readily identifiable apical mitotic or apoptotic figures are found even focally, p16 immunohistochemical stain and testing for high-risk HPV types is recommended to avoid misclassifying HPVA adenocarcinomas as one of the NHPVA subtypes. The NHPVA subtypes include:

1. *Gastric type:* contains cells with abundant clear, foamy, or pale eosinophilic cytoplasm with distinct cytoplasmic borders and basally located nuclei similar to gastric pyloric glands (Fig. 2.6). Adenoma malignum (minimal deviation adenocarcinoma) is part of the spectrum of gastric-type adenocarcinoma. Gastric-type adenocarcinomas carry a worse prognosis than usual-type adenocarcinoma, being more frequently associated with deep stromal invasion, higher pathologic stage at presentation, and lower disease-free survival (30% 5-year disease-free survival in gastric type versus 74% in usual type).

2. *Endometrioid:* lacks readily identifiable apical mitosis and apoptosis and has classic endometrioid features—glands lined by columnar cells with pseudostratified nuclei that demonstrate no more than moderate atypia. Squamous metaplasia and/or endometriosis may be present. Of note, in the IECC study, a number of cancers that were initially called endometrioid adenocarcinomas were reclassified as usual-type adenocarcinoma. It is important to exclude

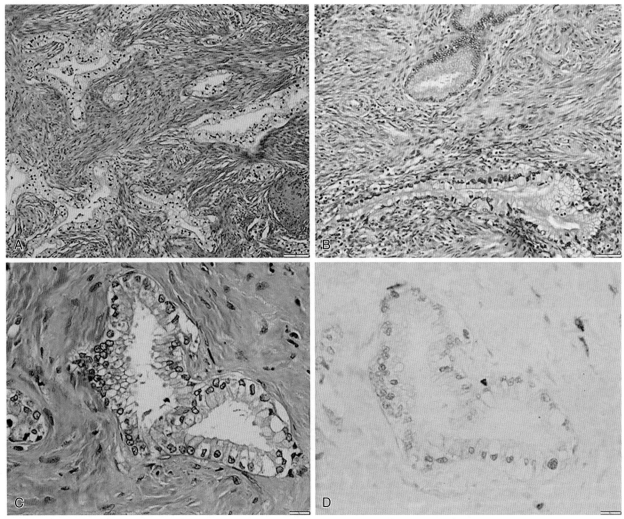

FIG. 2.6

Non–human papillomavirus-associated endocervical adenocarcinoma. Gastric type is the most common. Mitotic and apoptotic figures are NOT easily appreciated at low power. **A,** Low power. **B,** Medium power. Gastric-type adenocarcinoma (bottom gland) has pale/eosinophilic cytoplasm in comparison with the bluish/basophilic tinge of normal endocervical glands (top gland). **C,** High power showing tumor cells with pale cytoplasm and sharp cytoplasmic boundaries. **D,** p16 immunohistochemical stain is negative (patchy weak reactivity).

HPVA usual-type adenocarcinoma by performing p16 immunohistochemical stain and/or HPV testing before classifying an endocervical adenocarcinoma as endometrioid.

3. *Serous:* resemble their endometrial and tubo-ovarian counterparts, being composed of cells with high-grade nuclei displaying slit-like glands, papillary, and/or micropapillary architecture. Endocervical serous carcinomas are exceedingly rare and should only be diagnosed after HPV testing has been performed to exclude HPVA serous-like usual-type adenocarcinomas. In addition, direct extension from the endometrium and drop metastasis from the endometrium, tubes, and ovaries need to be excluded before a diagnosis of primary endocervical serous adenocarcinoma is rendered.

4. *Clear cell:* composed of clear or eosinophilic hobnail cells displaying solid, papillary, and/or tubulocystic architecture. Endocervical clear cell adenocarcinomas

are rare and are associated with *in utero* diethylstilbestrol (DES) exposure. Sporadic tumors rarely occur.

5. *Mesonephric:* arises from mesonephric remnants, typically in the lateral to posterior cervical wall. Mesonephric carcinomas show a variety of architectural growth patterns (ductal, tubular, retiform, cord-like, papillary, solid, spindle, among others) but have characteristic luminal eosinophilic colloid-like material. Mesonephric carcinomas are pancytokeratin positive and are often also positive for calretinin, PAX-8, and TTF1. They may be p16 immunoreactive focally but are HPV negative. Key features distinguishing HPVA endocervical adenocarcinomas from NHPVA carcinomas are summarized in Table 2.3.

HPVA in situ lesions versus NHPVA in situ lesions (lobular endocervical glandular hyperplasia): HPVA *in situ* lesions include AIS and SMILE. *AIS, HPVA:* shows cytologic atypia with nuclear enlargement, crowding, pseudostratification and hyperchromasia, cytoplasmic

TABLE 2.3

Features Distinguishing HPV-associated Endocervical Adenocarcinomas from Non-HPV-associated Adenocarcinomas

	HPV-associated Endocervical Adenocarcinomas	HPV-independent Endocervical Adenocarcinomas
Etiology	High-risk HPV	Not HPV-related; various etiologies, e.g., STK11 mutation in gastric-type, *in utero* DES exposure in clear cell
Histology	Easily identifiable apical mitosis and apoptosis at scanning to low power (4–10×) magnification	Apical mitosis and apoptosis are NOT easily identified
IHC/molecular	Diffusely p16 positive; high-risk HPV detected	p16 negative; HPV negative
Morphologic types	Usual type: mucin-poor; median patient age 42 years. Important to note pattern of invasion (see text) Villoglandular: exophytic slender papillae; younger patients, median 34 years Mucinous: >50% of tumor cells contain intracytoplasmic mucin; may be intestinal or signet ring iSMILE: stratified columnar cells with peripheral palisading and intracytoplasmic mucin	**Gastric type:** tumor cells resemble gastric pyloric glands, i.e., have basally located nuclei and abundant clear, foamy, or pale eosinophilic cytoplasm with distinct cytoplasmic borders **Endometrioid:** columnar cells with pseudostratified nuclei; squamous metaplasia and/or endometriosis may be present **Serous:** slit-like/gaping glands, papillary and/or micropapillary architecture and high-grade nuclei with ≥3:1 variation in nuclei size and prominent nucleoli **Clear cell:** clear or eosinophilic hobnail cells with solid, papillary and/or tubulocystic architecture **Mesonephric:** characteristic luminal eosinophilic colloid-like material; displays variety of growth patterns
Prognosis	Usual type: depends on pattern of invasion and stage; on average, 74% 5-year disease free survival	**Poor:** more frequently associated with higher stage and distant metastasis; gastric type has 30% 5-year disease-free survival

HPV, Human papillomavirus; *IHC,* immunohistochemistry.

mucin depletion, and easily recognizable apical mitosis and apoptosis; however, normal lobular endocervical architecture is preserved. Intestinal metaplasia may occasionally be present. *SMILE:* shows cytologic atypia with nuclear hyperchromasia and easily recognizable apical mitosis and apoptosis but is characterized by stratified epithelium with mucin-containing cells (either present as discrete vacuoles or cytoplasmic clearing) being present in all cell layers. Both AIS and SMILE show strong and diffuse p16 immunoreactivity and are always associated with high-risk HPV, most commonly types 16 and/or 18. Strong diffuse p16 immunoreactivity and high Ki67 mitotic index are useful features helpful in distinguishing AIS and SMILE from benign mimics such as tubal metaplasia. The presence of cilia and absence of apical mitosis and apoptosis are morphologic features present in tubal metaplasia that are helpful in distinguishing it from AIS and SMILE. *Lobular endocervical glandular hyperplasia:* is a lobular proliferation of endocervical glands displaying pyloric-type epithelium. Lobular endocervical glandular hyperplasia often shows small- to moderate-sized glands surrounding a larger gland. The glands are often benign-appearing and limited to the inner half of the cervical stroma. The cells express pyloric-type mucins, MUC6, and HIK1083. Gains of chromosome 3p and loss of 1p have been identified in some cases of lobular endocervical glandular hyperplasia. Lobular endocervical glandular hyperplasia is a precursor to gastric-type adenocarcinomas. Patients

with Peutz-Jeghers syndrome (*STK11* mutations) are susceptible to lobular endocervical glandular hyperplasia and gastric-type adenocarcinomas. Lobular endocervical glandular hyperplasia is distinguished from AIS by the lack of easily identifiable apical mitosis and apoptosis. In addition, lobular endocervical glandular hyperplasia is NOT associated with HPV and as such is p16 negative and without detectable high-risk HPV.

AIS versus invasive endocervical adenocarcinoma: Distinguishing AIS from pattern A invasion in usual-type HPVA endocervical adenocarcinoma can be difficult (and may not be of much clinical significance) as both do not elicit a stromal response. However, increased glandular density with small confluent or cribriform glands and the presence of deep glands suggests an invasive over an *in situ* process. AIS is distinguished from other patterns of invasion in usual-type adenocarcinoma and other subtypes of endocervical adenocarcinoma by the presence of stromal desmoplasia, lymphovascular invasion, solid cell nests and/or individual malignant cells, or small incomplete malignant glands within the stroma.

Usual-type endocervical adenocarcinoma versus endocervical involvement by endometrial adenocarcinoma: Distinguishing endometrial from endocervical adenocarcinoma on biopsy has important implications for treatment—type and extent of surgery (e.g., total versus radical hysterectomy) and/or chemoradiation options. The distinction can be diagnostically challenging if based solely on morphologic findings. Nevertheless, morphologic clues include readily identifiable apical mitotic and apoptotic figures in HPVA endocervical adenocarcinoma. Clinical and gross pathologic evaluations such as location of the mass are also important clues. Immunohistochemical stains and molecular testing for high-risk HPV infection are helpful adjuncts. Usual-type endocervical adenocarcinoma stains strongly and diffusely positive for p16 and is often estrogen receptor (ER) and progesterone receptor (PR) negative (or only focally positive) and vimentin negative, while endometrial adenocarcinomas (particularly International Federation of Gynecology and Obstetrics [FIGO] grades I and II) are p16 negative, ER and PR positive and vimentin positive. As p16 is a cell cycle protein that can be activated in high-grade tumors independently of HPV status, testing for high-risk HPV may be required in high-grade tumors as FIGO grade III endometrial adenocarcinomas can be p16 positive.

Prognosis and Therapy

Prognosis and treatment are predominantly dictated by stage. Survival in early invasive (stage 1A1) HPVA endocervical adenocarcinomas is 93% but drops to 3% in stage IV disease. Early invasive tumors can be treated with LEEP or cone excisions, whereas more advanced disease may require radical hysterectomy with lymphadenectomy and/or chemoradiation. Other factors that influence prognosis of endocervical adenocarcinomas include pattern of invasion (pattern A conferring better prognosis than B or C) and HPV status (HPVA endocervical adenocarcinomas have better prognosis than NHPVA endocervical adenocarcinomas).

ENDOCERVICAL ADENOCARCINOMA – DISEASE FACT SHEET

Definition
▸▸ Glandular tumor with stromal invasion and/or exophytic expansile growth of two etiologic categories:
  ▸▸ HPVA (usual-type, villoglandular, mucinous, and iSMILE).
  ▸▸ NHPVA (gastric-type, clear cell, mesonephric, endometrioid)

Epidemiology
▸▸ HPVA endocervical adenocarcinomas typically occur in reproductive age women (average age, 42 years).
▸▸ NHPVA endocervical adenocarcinomas occur over a wide age range from reproductive age to postmenopausal women (average age, 50–55 years).

Clinical Features
▸▸ HPVA endocervical adenocarcinomas may be discovered incidentally at routine cervical PAP screenings or due to symptoms of abnormal uterine bleeding and/or mass.
▸▸ NHPVA endocervical adenocarcinomas are often discovered due to symptoms of uterine bleeding, pain, and/or discharge.

Prognosis and Therapy
▸▸ HPVA endocervical adenocarcinomas: stage-dependent prognosis and treatment
▸▸ NHPVA endocervical adenocarcinomas: poor prognosis; often presents at advanced stage, requiring radical hysterectomy with lymphadenectomy and/or chemoradiation

---

HPVA ENDOCERVICAL ADENOCARCINOMA – PATHOLOGIC FEATURES

Gross Findings
▸▸ Endocervical mass and/or ulcer

Microscopic Findings
▸▸ Invasive carcinoma with easily identified apical mitotic figures
▸▸ May be mucin-depleted (usual type), composed of >50% cells with intracytoplasmic mucin (mucinous) or exophytic with papillary growth (villoglandular)
▸▸ Diffusely p16 positive
▸▸ High-risk HPV detected on molecular studies

Pathologic Differential Diagnoses
▸▸ NHPVA endocervical adenocarcinoma
▸▸ Endometrial adenocarcinoma involving the cervix

ENDOMETRIAL ENDOMETRIOID ADENOCARCINOMA

DIFFERENTIAL DIAGNOSES: ENDOMETRIAL HYPERPLASIA, SEROUS CARCINOMA, CLEAR CELL CARCINOMA, NEUROENDOCRINE CARCINOMA, AND UNDIFFERENTIATED CARCINOMA

Clinical Features

Endometrioid adenocarcinomas are the most common malignancies of the uterine corpus. Patients are typically postmenopausal (average age, 63 years). Reproductive age patients typically present with abnormal uterine bleeding, while older patients present with postmenopausal bleeding.

Endometrial carcinomas are typically classified into type I (low-grade endometrioid types) and type II (high-grade non-endometrioid types such as serous, clear cell, neuroendocrine, and undifferentiated) carcinomas. Risk factors for type I carcinomas include factors associated with hyperestrogenism such as obesity, nulliparity, early menarche, polycystic ovarian syndrome, and estrogen-secreting ovarian neoplasms. Genetic associations include Lynch syndrome (microsatellite instability) and Cowden syndrome (PTEN mutations). Type I carcinomas often arise in a background of atypical hyperplasia. Type II carcinomas are typically aggressive high-grade tumors with risk factors that include smoking and p53 mutations. ARID1A loss has been described in clear carcinoma. Type II tumors typically arise in a background of endometrial atrophy. Mixed carcinomas comprise two or more different histological types of endometrial carcinoma, with at least one of which being a type II carcinoma. For a diagnosis of mixed carcinoma to be rendered, the second component has to comprise at least 5% of the tumor.

Pathologic Features

GROSS FINDINGS

Endometrial endometrioid adenocarcinomas typically appear as nodules, exophytic, or infiltrative masses in the uterine corpus or lower uterine segment.

MICROSCOPIC FINDINGS

Endometrioid adenocarcinoma typically displays glandular growth pattern with glands lined by stratified columnar cells. Foci of squamous differentiation, mucinous differentiation, secretory change, and ciliated cells may be present. Solid growth pattern may be present, and endometrioid adenocarcinomas are graded based on the amount of solid growth present. Tumors with solid growth comprising 5% or less of the total tumor are grade 1, tumors with 6% to 50% solid growth are grade 2, and those with >50% solid growth are grade 3. Mitosis and necrosis may be present in endometrioid adenocarcinomas as well as severe nuclear atypia (i.e., pleomorphic nuclei with prominent nucleoli; grade 3 nuclei). Tumors with severe nuclear atypia involving greater than 50% of the nuclei are upgraded by one grade; for example, an otherwise grade 1 endometrioid tumor, composed of 95% glands, should be upgraded to grade 2 if the nuclei of cells lining the glands display pleomorphism and prominent nucleoli.

Ancillary Studies

Grade 1 to 2 endometrial endometrioid adenocarcinomas typically stain diffusely positive for PAX-8, ER, and PR. They are typically p16 negative and p53 wild-type.

Differential Diagnosis

ENDOMETRIAL HYPERPLASIA

The term "hyperplasia" as applied to the endometrium encompasses two somewhat related processes: "hyperplasia

without atypia" and "atypical hyperplasia/endometrioid intraepithelial neoplasia" (AH/EIN). Hyperplasia without atypia results from prolonged, unopposed, or suboptimally opposed estrogen exposure. Accordingly, epidemiologic associations include obesity, diabetes, and polycystic ovarian syndrome, among others. The changes are proliferative and diffusely present within the endometrium. Alternatively, AH/EIN is a clonal alteration that results in an initially localized cytologic atypia, and which is associated with a substantially increased risk of carcinoma concurrent with, and subsequent to its diagnosis in a sampling specimen. AH/EIN is frequently seen in a background of hyperplasia without atypia, which suggests that unopposed estrogen exposure may be involved in the clonal selection process that eventuates in the development of AH/EIN. The clinicopathologic features of hyperplasia without atypia and AH/EIN are compared in Table 2.4.

Hyperplasia without atypia versus disordered proliferative endometrium: The term "disordered proliferative endometrium" (DPE) is applied to mitotically active, proliferative-type glands that are devoid of cytologic atypia, but which display scattered gland dilatations (microcysts). Associated glands in the background may display tubular or slightly irregular architecture. Tubal metaplasia is frequent. The changes of DPE are essentially those seen in hyperplasia without atypia but in a more localized form. DPE is frequently found in women with anovulatory cycles and is a manifestation of unopposed estrogen stimulation. It also frequently regresses without treatment.

Hyperplasia without atypia versus AH/EIN: General differences between these two diagnostic categories are outlined in Table 2.3. Although AH/EIN may be seen in a background of hyperplasia without atypia, the distinction is of ample clinical significance given the marked differences between them in their rates of concurrent or subsequent carcinoma, and accordingly, management approaches. The key diagnostic feature that helps in their distinction is the presence of cytologic demarcation in AH/EIN and the lack thereof in hyperplasia without atypia (Fig. 2.7). The cytologic features of the crowded glands in a putative focus of AH/EIN should be compared with those of the background glands. If AH/EIN is present in an endometrial polyp, their features should be compared with those of the background glands within the polyp. The presence of metaplastic alterations may complicate the determination of cytologic demarcation, but every attempt should be made to compare the focus to the background endometrium. Ancillary immunohistochemical studies may also be helpful: The concurrent loss of PTEN, BAF-250a (ARID1A), and PAX2 expression is substantially more likely to be encountered in AH/EIN than in hyperplasia without atypia.

AH/EIN versus FIGO grade 1 endometrioid adenocarcinoma: The distinction between AH/EIN and grade I

TABLE 2.4

Useful Features to Distinguish Hyperplasia without Atypia From Atypical Hyperplasia/Endometrioid Intraepithelial Neoplasia (AH/EIN)

	Hyperplasia Without Atypia (Fig. 2.7A and B)	AH/EIN (Fig. 2.7C and D)
Associations	Long term, unopposed or suboptimally opposed hyperestrogenism	Long term, unopposed or suboptimally opposed hyperestrogenism
Mean prevalence of concurrent endometrial cancer	Unknown	32.6%
Mean risk of progression to cancer	2.3%	13%
Mean age at diagnosis (years)	48	53
Presenting symptoms	Vaginal bleeding	Vaginal bleeding
Gross features	Variable; mostly diffusely thickened or polypoid endometrium	Variable; mostly diffusely thickened or polypoid endometrium
Microscopic features	Irregularly distributed and shaped glands; glands are frequently cystic; remodeled glands, vascular thrombi, and stromal microinfarcts may be present. Glands often show tubal metaplasia.	Crowded glands that display cytologic demarcation from background, frequently due to nuclear atypia (nuclear pleomorphism, rounding, enlargement), and/or nucleolomegaly

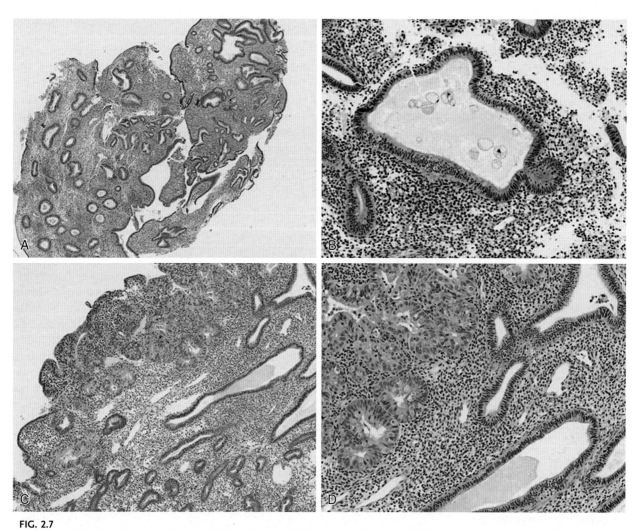

FIG. 2.7

Hyperplasia. **(A, B)** Hyperplasia without atypia: irregularly distributed and shaped glands; glands are frequently cystic and show tubal metaplasia. **(C, D)** Atypical hyperplasia/endometrioid intraepithelial neoplasia. Crowded glands with cytological atypia *(upper left)*, the latter manifested by cytologic demarcation from the background glands *(lower right)*, which in this case show hyperplasia without atypia.

endometrioid carcinoma may be difficult. In general, the following features are exclusively seen in carcinoma: Extensive glandular or confluent patterns (i.e., back to back glands, generally exceeding 3 contiguous mm); papillary architectures associated with any other architectural complexity; solid pattern; and cribriform pattern. Features that favor carcinoma include significant cytologic atypia beyond what is typically seen in AH/EIN (including macronucleoli) and a desmoplastic stromal response. Features that may be seen in either category include abundant mitoses, necrosis, and neutrophilic aggregates. If the distinction cannot be readily made in a biopsy, a descriptive diagnosis that acknowledges both possibilities should be rendered.

ENDOMETRIAL SEROUS CARCINOMA

Endometrial serous carcinomas are the prototypical type II tumor with aggressive behavior. Endometrial serous carcinomas can metastasize to extra-uterine sites even in the absence of demonstrable myometrial invasion. Serous carcinomas typically display papillary, glandular, or solid architecture with diffuse nuclear pleomorphism and frequent mitosis. Therefore, if one considers upgrading an endometrioid adenocarcinoma because of nuclear atypia, a serous carcinoma should first be excluded, as serous carcinomas can form well-defined glands that mimic endometrioid adenocarcinoma. Immunohistochemical stains are crucial in such settings. An initial limited panel composed of p53, p16, PR, and PTEN is helpful. Most endometrial serous carcinomas (80%–90%) display mutant pattern of p53 immunohistochemical staining, that is, may be diffusely positive ($\geq$75% of nuclei) or completely negative (null pattern) while endometrioid carcinomas are typically p53 wild-type. Likewise, serous carcinomas typically show diffuse strong positive staining with p16, while endometrioid adenocarcinomas are typically p16 negative or have patchy weak expression. Endometrioid adenocarcinomas typically are strongly and diffusely PR positive and typically show PTEN loss, while serous carcinomas show patchy PR expression and have retained PTEN. Once endometrioid histology is confirmed, immunohistochemical stain for mismatch repair proteins (MLH1, PMS2, MSH2, and MSH6) is important to exclude Lynch syndrome, an autosomal-dominant heritable cause of endometrial carcinoma that is associated with an increased risk of colon cancer.

ENDOMETRIAL CLEAR CELL CARCINOMA

Clear cell carcinoma comprises polygonal or hobnail cells with high-grade nuclear atypia (at least focally) and clear or eosinophilic cytoplasm, displaying papillary, tubulocystic, and/or solid growth patterns. Clear cell carcinomas are typically diffusely napsin-A positive, ER and PR negative, and p53 wild-type.

ENDOMETRIAL NEUROENDOCRINE CARCINOMA

Endometrial neuroendocrine carcinomas may be morphologically small cell neuroendocrine carcinomas or large cell neuroendocrine carcinomas. Small cell neuroendocrine carcinomas are characterized by loosely cohesive cells with scant cytoplasm, nuclear molding, frequent mitosis, apoptosis, and necrosis. Large cell neuroendocrine carcinomas comprise polygonal cells with prominent nucleoli and moderate to abundant cytoplasm displaying neuroendocrine growth patterns, that is, organoid nests, trabeculae growth, rosette-like formations, cords, and/or peripheral palisading. Neuroendocrine carcinomas stain positive for CD56, synaptophysin, and chromogranin.

UNDIFFERENTIATED CARCINOMA

Undifferentiated endometrial carcinomas typically form large polypoid partially necrotic endometrial masses and occur in postmenopausal women. Histologic sections show discohesive small to intermediate monomorphic cells displaying diffuse growth pattern. A differential diagnosis of lymphoma, plasmacytoma, and high-grade sarcoma is often entertained as no well-formed glands, or neuroendocrine growth features such as trabeculae, cords, or organoid nests are appreciable. Classification as a carcinoma is often based on immunohistochemical stains showing EMA positivity (at least focally); cytokeratins may be negative. A diagnosis of dedifferentiated carcinoma is rendered when a component of FIGO grade 1 or grade 2 endometrioid adenocarcinoma is present in an otherwise monomorphic undifferentiated carcinoma.

Features useful in distinguishing endometrioid adenocarcinoma from the various type II tumors are summarized in Table 2.5.

Prognosis and Therapy

The prognosis of endometrial adenocarcinoma depends on stage (i.e., depth of myometrial invasion, cervical stroma involvement, and extent of extra-uterine spread). Molecular sub-classification of endometrial adenocarcinomas into four classes: POLE-ultramutated, MMR-deficient, p53-mutant, and no specific molecular profile (NSMP) are used for prognostication; POLE-ultramutated endometrial carcinomas carry excellent prognosis, MMR-deficient and NSMP carcinomas carry intermediate prognosis, and p53-mutant carcinomas carry poor prognosis. Treatment depends on clinical stage. Patients with tumors limited to the uterus on clinical exam are typically treated with total abdominal hysterectomy, bilateral salpingo-oophorectomies, and surgical staging, with need for adjuvant therapy dictated by the final

TABLE 2.5

Features Helpful in Distinguishing Endometrial Endometrioid Adenocarcinoma (Type I Carcinoma) From Type II Endometrial Carcinomas

	Endometrioid Adenocarcinoma	Serous Carcinoma	Clear Cell Carcinoma	Neuroendocrine Carcinoma	Undifferentiated Carcinoma
Risk factors	Hyperestrogenism Lynch syndrome	Smoking; history of breast cancer and/or tamoxifen use	Smoking	Non-specific	Possibly Lynch syndrome
Histology	Stratified columnar epithelial cells form crowded (back-to-back) glands with acinar, papillary or solid architecture. Grade 1: well-defined glands (<5% solid growth); grade 2: 6%–50% solid growth; grade 3: >50% solid growth. Typically lacks significant nuclear pleomorphism and prominent nucleoli; if present even focally, first exclude serous carcinoma. Once serous carcinoma is excluded, upgrade tumor by one grade if pleomorphism in >50% of nuclei.	Epithelial cells with marked nuclear pleomorphism, high nuclear-to-cytoplasmic ratio and prominent nucleoli grow in papillary, glandular and/or solid patterns. Mitotic figures are numerous.	Polygonal or hobnail cells with clear or eosinophilic cytoplasm and high-grade nuclear atypia (at least focally) grow in papillary, solid and/or tubulocystic patterns. Hyaline bodies may be present.	Small cell neuroendocrine carcinoma: diffuse, trabecular, nested or rosette-like growth of cells with high nuclear-to-cytoplasmic ratio, nuclear molding, numerous mitosis and apoptosis, often with necrosis. Large cell neuroendocrine carcinoma: large polygonal cells with prominent nucleoli grow in organoid nests, trabeculae, rosette-like formations, or cords with peripheral palisading.	Monomorphic small to intermediate sized discohesive cells grow diffusely (in sheets). No obvious gland formation, papillae, organoid nests or trabeculae; resembles lymphoma or high-grade sarcoma.
Genetics and/or IHC	*PTEN* mutation/ inactivation in >50% of tumors (PTEN loss by IHC); *ARID1A* mutation in 40% of low-grade tumors (ARID1A loss by IHC); MSI-high in 35% (loss of MLH1, MSH2, MSH6, or PMS2 by IHC). *TP53* mutations in 30% of grade 3 tumors (diffuse or null p53 by IHC). Other mutations: *PIK3CA* (30%), *POLE* (10%). Other IHC: diffuse positive ER and PR.	*TP53* mutations in 80%–90% (diffuse or null p53 by IHC). Other mutations: *PIK3CA* (24%–40%), *FBXW7* (20%–30%), *PPP2R1A* (18%–28%). Other helpful IHC: diffuse positive p16.	Useful IHC: Positive for Napsin-A and HNF-1B in most cases; often ER and PR negative, and p53 wild type. Loss of ARID1A by IHC may also be observed.	Useful IHC: positive for synaptophysin, chromogranin, and CD56.	Useful IHC: strong positive EMA (at least focally); ER, PR negative. Microsatellite instability high in 50%.
Prognosis	Depends on stage (predicted by depth of myometrial invasion and presence of lymphovascular invasion), grade and patient age; worse with increase.	Poor: often associated with extra-uterine spread. However, occasional cases confined to the endometrium have good prognosis.	Poor: 5-year survival < 50%, regardless of stage.	Poor	Poor; highly aggressive

pathologic stage. Patients whose clinical exams reveal more advanced tumors may be treated with external beam radiation therapy, brachytherapy, and/or systemic chemotherapy.

ENDOMETRIAL ENDOMETRIOID ADENOCARCINOMA – DISEASE FACT SHEET

Definition
▶▶ Malignant glandular tumor displaying various growth patterns—glandular, papillary, or solid—and endometrioid (i.e., varying mix of columnar, secretory, mucinous, ciliated and/or squamous) cytologic features.

Epidemiology
▶▶ Most common malignancy of the uterine corpus
▶▶ Typically occurs in postmenopausal women

Clinical Features
▶ Patients typically have risk factors associated with hyperestrogenism.
▶ Patients typically present with abnormal uterine/postmenopausal bleeding.

Prognosis and Therapy
▶▶ Prognosis depends on stage, grade, and molecular sub-class.
▶▶ Treatment depends on stage.

ENDOMETRIAL ENDOMETRIOID ADENOCARCINOMA – PATHOLOGIC FEATURES

Gross Findings
▶▶ Nodule or mass in the uterine corpus or lower uterine segment.

Microscopic Findings
▶▶ Confluent glandular, papillary, and/or solid growth in varying amounts.
▶▶ Component cells display columnar, secretory, ciliated, mucinous, ciliated, and/or squamous differentiation.
▶▶ Stromal desmoplasia and myometrial invasion may be present.
▶▶ Lymphovascular invasion may be present.

Pathologic Differential Diagnoses
▶▶ Atypical hyperplasia
▶▶ Type II carcinomas

LEIOMYOMA OF THE UTERUS

DIFFERENTIAL DIAGNOSES: LEIOMYOSARCOMA AND ENDOMETRIAL STROMAL SARCOMA

Clinical Features

Leiomyomas are benign mesenchymal tumors that display smooth muscle differentiation. Most patients with leiomyoma are in the fourth to sixth decade of life. Most are asymptomatic, but a significant subset present with vaginal bleeding or pelvic pain. Patients with hereditary leiomyomatosis and renal cell carcinoma (HLRCC) generally present at an earlier age. The most common molecular alterations in leiomyomas include *MED12* mutations, *COL4A5* and *COL4A6* deletions, *HMGA2* and *HMGA1* rearrangements, and FH mutations.

Pathologic Features

GROSS FINDINGS

Grossly, leiomyomas are frequently multiple and may be situated intramurally, subserosally, or submucosally. They vary in size from microscopic to >30 cm, are rounded, unencapsulated, and frequently display a tan-white, whorled cut surface.

MICROSCOPIC FINDINGS

Morphologic variants include conventional (spindle cell) leiomyoma, cellular leiomyoma, mitotically active leiomyoma, hydropic leiomyoma, myxoid leiomyoma, dissecting leiomyoma, leiomyoma with bizarre nuclei, apoplectic leiomyoma, lipoleiomyoma, epithelioid leiomyoma, diffuse leiomyomatosis, and fumarate hydratase (FH)–deficient leiomyoma.

The most common variant of leiomyoma, spindle cell leiomyoma (i.e., leiomyoma with spindled morphology), is comprised of spindle cells with eosinophilic cytoplasm, cigar-shaped, and pale nuclei that are arranged in fascicles (Fig. 2.8A). Mitotic figures are uncommon (<5 MF/10 HPF), unless directly adjacent to an area of necrosis, where mitotic activity may be higher. The necrosis seen in leiomyoma is of the infarct type, characterized by a zone of generalized death of tumor cells and vessels, often accompanied by hemorrhage, and bordering the viable areas by foci of granulation-like tissue or hyalinization (Fig. 2.8B).

Morphologic variations for spindle cell leiomyomas include diffuse hyalinization, an abundance of vessels, nuclear palisading that result in a schwannoma-like appearance, tumor cell nesting, or cording. Other variants or unusual growth patterns are briefly described below.

Leiomyoma with bizarre nuclei show large nuclei with bizarrely shaped, hyperchromatic, often multilobulated nuclei, but are devoid of tumor cell necrosis or an increased mitotic index (Fig. 2.8C). Atypical cells are often distributed in a background of otherwise typical or cellular leiomyoma.

Highly cellular leiomyomas show a level of cellularity that is comparable to endometrial stromal tumors, but display areas of spindling, peripheral clefting, and thick-walled vessels, and are devoid of tumor cell necrosis or increased mitotic index (Fig. 2.8D).

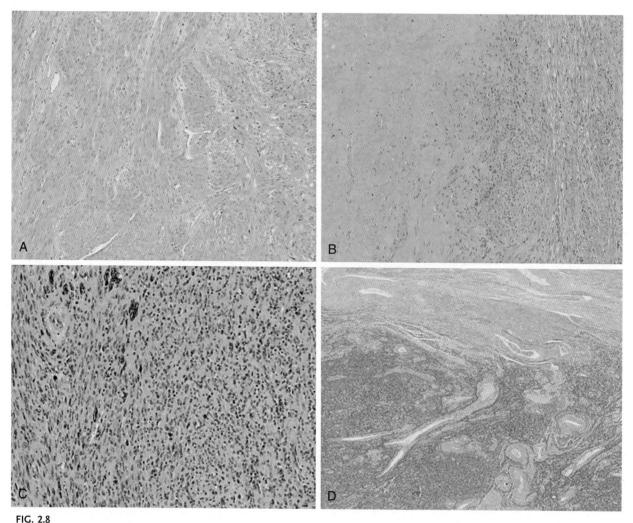

FIG. 2.8

Leiomyoma and selected variants. **A,** Conventional spindle cell leiomyoma composed of spindle cells with eosinophilic cytoplasm and cigar-shaped, pale nuclei that are arranged in fascicles. **B,** Conventional spindle cell leiomyoma with an area of infarct-type necrosis. There is a zone of granulation-like tissue between the viable areas *(right field)* and non-viable areas *(left field)*. **C,** Leiomyoma with bizarre nuclei. Bizarre nuclei scattered in a background of less atypical nuclei. **D,** Highly cellular leiomyoma; note the thick-walled vessels.

Cellular leiomyoma show more cellularity than the background myometrium but are similarly devoid of tumor cell necrosis, a high mitotic index, or cytologic atypia.

FH-deficient leiomyoma shows alveolar pattern edema, staghorn vasculature, scattered bizarre nuclei, eosinophilic cytoplasmic inclusions, and eosinophilic macronucleoli that may be surrounded by perinuclear halos. These changes are not specific but may be part of diagnostic trigger to initiate further testing for germline FH mutations.

Epithelioid leiomyomas show round or polygonal cells with abundant cytoplasm, should have less than 2 MF/10 HPF, and should be devoid of necrosis and severe cytologic atypia. A diagnosis of epithelioid leiomyosarcoma is rendered in a tumor that shows epithelioid appearance (i.e., round to polygonal cells with abundant cytoplasm) in >50% of the tumor, severe cytologic atypia, tumor cell necrosis, and/or ≥5 MF/10 HPF.

Mitotically active leiomyomas are otherwise similar to conventional spindle cell leiomyomas in morphology and behavior but have a mitotic index of 6 to 14 MF/10 HPF.

Myxoid leiomyomas are well-circumscribed and are comprised of cells that are separated by myxoid Alcian blue–positive acid-mucin stroma. Myxoid leiomyomas are devoid of cytologic atypia and should have very low mitotic activity (<2 MF/10 HPF). In contrast, myxoid leiomyosarcomas show infiltrative growth in a background of myxoid stroma and have ≥2 mitosis/10 HPF.

Hydropic leiomyomas are characterized by the accumulation of watery fluid between tumor cells, often accompanied by large areas of hyalinization, and prominent thick-walled vessels.

Leiomyoma with vascular invasion describes an unusual scenario in which an otherwise typical leiomyoma is seen within an intravascular space. This finding has no known clinical significance.

Dissecting leiomyoma has nests or groups of leiomyoma cells that are seen to infiltrate or dissect in the myometrium, hence its name. The most frequent variant of dissecting leiomyoma is the cotyledonoid variant, wherein a large, exophytic, placenta-like mass is seen extending from the uterine wall into the broad ligament or parametrial soft tissue. The component cells lack tumor cell necrosis, cytologic atypia, and increased mitotic activity.

Diffuse leiomyomatosis is characterized by numerous hypercellular nodules of otherwise typical bland smooth muscle cells diffusely involving the myometrium.

Intravenous leiomyomatosis shows intravenous smooth muscle outside of the confines of a leiomyoma. They frequently involve the ovarian veins and may extend all the way into the inferior vena cava. Recurrences are not infrequent.

Benign metastasizing leiomyoma is a scenario in which a well-characterized benign smooth muscle tumor is synchronously or subsequently associated with extra-uterine nodules of morphologically similar tumor.

Ancillary Studies

Leiomyomas are typically positive for muscle markers like desmin, SMA, and h-caldesmon as well as ER, PR, and WT-1 (nuclear). Of note, CD10 (a marker typically associated with endometrial stroma) is positive in up to 40% of leiomyomas.

Differential Diagnosis

LEIOMYOSARCOMA

This section centers primarily on the distinction of spindle cell leiomyoma from spindle cell leiomyosarcoma, which represent the vast majority, that is, >75% of uterine sarcomas. Leiomyosarcomas are clinically aggressive, with a median survival of approximately 20 months. The key diagnostic features are tumor cell/coagulative necrosis, mitotic index ≥10 MF/10 HPF and diffuse moderate to severe cytologic atypia. The presence of at least any two of the aforementioned features in a uterine smooth muscle tumor defines it as malignant, although most tumors display all three. Cytologic atypia must be discernible at scanning magnification (10×). Mitotic figures must be carefully counted to exclude inflammatory cells, apoptotic bodies, or tumor cells. The necrosis must be of the tumor cell or coagulative type, which is characterized by an abrupt transition between viable tumor cells and necrotic areas. This is in contrast to the aforementioned infarct-type necrosis that is typical of leiomyomas. Table 2.6 outlines the key clinicopathologic differences between these two tumors.

Leiomyoma with bizarre nuclei and FH-deficient leiomyoma versus leiomyosarcoma: The nuclei atypia in leiomyomas with bizarre nuclei and FH-deficient leiomyomas may sometimes result in a differential consideration of leiomyosarcoma. Both FH-deficient leiomyomas and leiomyomas with bizarre nuclei are distinguished from leiomyosarcoma by their lack of tumor cell

TABLE 2.6

Features Useful in Distinguishing Spindle Cell Leiomyoma from Spindle Cell Leiomyosarcoma

	Leiomyoma	Leiomyosarcoma
Proportion of all uterine smooth muscle tumors	>95%	<5%
Most common patient age group at presentation	Fourth to sixth decades	Fourth to seventh decades
Clinical presentation	Asymptomatic; non-specific pelvic pain or vaginal bleeding	Non-specific
Gross features	Frequently multiple; intramural, subserosal, or submucosal. Rounded, unencapsulated, well-circumscribed. Frequently displays a tan-white, whorled cut surface.	Mostly solitary and intramural. Average size of 10 cm. Well-circumscribed or infiltrative. Cut surface soft and fleshy with areas of degeneration.
Cytologic atypia (severe pleomorphism, uniform nuclear enlargement, diffuse hyperchromasia)	Moderate to severe, diffuse atypia absent at scanning magnification (10×)	Moderate to severe, diffuse atypia easily discernible at scanning magnification (10×)
Tumor cell/coagulative necrosis (abrupt transition between viable tumor cells and necrotic areas)	Absent	Present
Infarct type necrosis (granulation-like or fibrous tissue between viable and non-viable areas; viable areas often display hemorrhage, mummified tumor cells, and vessels)	May be present	May be present
Mitotic index	<5 MF/10 HPF	≥10 MF/10 HPF

necrosis and relatively low mitotic index ($<$10 MF/10 HPF). FH loss by immunohistochemical stain distinguishes FH-deficient leiomyoma from leiomyoma with bizarre nuclei.

Smooth muscle tumor of uncertain malignant potential versus spindle cell leiomyoma and leiomyosarcoma: Smooth muscle tumor of uncertain malignant potential (STUMP) is a diagnostic term for those tumors whose aberrations exceed what are allowable for leiomyoma or variants, but which are nonetheless insufficient for a diagnosis of malignancy. The STUMP discussed in this section pertains only to conventional (spindle cell) STUMP, as the diagnostic criteria for myxoid and epithelioid STUMP are different. Tumors diagnosed as STUMP have been reported to recur in 7% to 28% of cases. The patients are younger than patients diagnosed with leiomyosarcoma. Grossly, the tumors are mostly similar to leiomyomas, although areas of infiltration have rarely been reported, and may be associated with adverse outcome. A STUMP should be diagnosed only after extensive attempts have been made to definitively characterize the lesion. Spindle cell smooth muscle tumors that may be classified as STUMP include tumors with $>$15 MF/10 HPF, but which are devoid of tumor cell/coagulative necrosis or diffuse severe cytologic atypia; tumors with 6 to 9 MF/10 HPF and diffuse atypia but no tumor cell/coagulative necrosis; tumors in which the type or presence of necrosis is uncertain; or tumors with diffuse severe atypia in which the mitotic count is uncertain.

ENDOMETRIAL STROMAL SARCOMA

There are two histologic variants of endometrial stromal sarcomas: low-grade endometrial stromal sarcoma (LGESS) and high-grade endometrial stromal sarcoma (HGESS). LGESS comprises cells resembling proliferative-phase endometrium but displays permeative (tongue-like) myometrial infiltration and/or lymphovascular invasion. Spiral arterioles are common. Mitotic activity is often low (usually $<$5 MF/10 HPF) and cytologic atypia is minimal. LGESS is often associated with *JAZF1*, *SUZ12(JJAZ1)*, and *PHF1* rearrangements. HGESS displays high-grade round cell morphology, frequent mitosis ($>$10 MF/10 HPF), apoptosis, necrosis, and lymphovascular invasion and is often associated with *YWHAE* and *BCOR* rearrangements. LGESS may occasionally transform into HGESS. LGESS may have focal smooth muscle differentiation and thus enter into the differential diagnostic consideration with spindle cell leiomyosarcoma. Distinguishing morphologic clues common in LGESS include the presence of spiral arterioles and the tongue-like infiltrative growth pattern. Helpful immunohistochemical stains include CD10, desmin, and caldesmon—LGESS stains strongly and diffusely positive for CD10, but only focally positive for desmin and caldesmon (in foci of smooth muscle

differentiation), while spindle cell leiomyosarcomas often stain diffusely positive for desmin and caldesmon with only focal CD10 immunoreactivity. The round cell morphology of HGESS may occasionally lead to diagnostic confusion with epithelioid leiomyosarcoma. Helpful immunohistochemical stains include cyclin D1, desmin, and caldesmon. HGESS is often diffusely cyclin D1 positive ($>$70% nuclei) and negative to only focally positive for desmin and caldesmon, while epithelioid leiomyosarcomas are often cyclin D1 negative but strongly desmin and caldesmon positive.

Prognosis and Therapy

Leiomyomas are benign; symptomatic patients are treated surgically with either myomectomy or hysterectomy. Patients with FH-deficient leiomyomas should be referred for genetic counseling to exclude HLRCC. Leiomyosarcomas carry a poor prognosis even with early stage disease due to high recurrence rates. The 5-year overall survival rate ranges from 15% to 25%. Treatment is mainly surgical with hysterectomy and resection of metastasis.

LEIOMYOMA OF THE UTERUS– DISEASE FACT SHEET

Definition
▶▶ Benign mesenchymal neoplasm with smooth muscle differentiation

Epidemiology
▶▶ Most common uterine tumor
▶▶ Affects reproductive age and postmenopausal women
▶▶ More common among women of African descent

Clinical Features
▶▶ Typically asymptomatic but may be associated with menorrhagia and pelvic pain; large tumors may present with symptoms attributable to abdominopelvic mass effect.

Prognosis and Therapy
▶▶ Benign; symptomatic cases are treated with surgical excision

LEIOMYOMA OF THE UTERUS – PATHOLOGIC FEATURES

Gross Findings
▶▶ Typically multiple, well-circumscribed whorled bulging firm white to tan nodules and/or masses.
▶▶ Large tumors may have infarction and edema and cystic degenerative changes.

Microscopic Findings
▶▶ Well-demarcated borders.
▶▶ Multiple morphologic variants: conventional (spindle cell) leiomyoma, cellular leiomyoma, mitotically active leiomyoma,

hydropic leiomyoma, myxoid leiomyoma, dissecting leiomyoma, leiomyoma with bizarre nuclei, apoplectic leiomyoma, lipoleiomyoma, epithelioid leiomyoma, diffuse leiomyomatosis, and FH-deficient leiomyoma
▸▸ Spindle cell leiomyoma is the most common—comprises spindle cells with fascicular arrangement
▸▸ Low mitotic index (<5 MF/10 HPF)

Pathologic Differential Diagnosis
▸▸ Leiomyosarcoma
▸▸ Endometrial stromal tumors

HIGH-GRADE SEROUS CARCINOMA OF THE FALLOPIAN TUBE

DIFFERENTIAL DIAGNOSES: SEROUS TUBAL INTRAEPITHELIAL CARCINOMA, SEROUS TUBAL INTRAEPITHELIAL LESION, AND P53 SIGNATURE

Clinical Features

High-grade serous carcinomas typically occur in post-menopausal patients (average age, 65 years) but can occur in younger, reproductive age patients, particularly those with germline mutations in genes such as *BRCA1* and *BRCA2*. Patients with high-grade serous carcinomas typically present with stage III to IV disease and symptoms related to abdominopelvic mass, such as bloating, increased abdominal girth, and change in bowel habits. Serum CA-125 levels are often elevated.

Data support the concept that the fallopian tube is the origin of most extra-uterine high-grade serous carcinomas. Studies have revealed the existence of precursor lesions in the fallopian tube, most commonly in the distal portion/fimbriated end and as such, it is advisable to thoroughly examine excised fallopian tubes using the sectioning and extensively examining the fimbriated end/SEE-FIM protocol, particularly in high-risk patients, such as those with *BRCA* mutations. Precursor lesions range from p53 signatures to serous tubal intraepithelial lesions (STILs) and serous tubal intraepithelial carcinomas (STICs).

Pathologic Features

GROSS FINDINGS

High-grade serous carcinomas are typically bilateral masses with varying amount of solid and cystic components. Papillary excrescences are often present. Early stage disease may be unilateral.

MICROSCOPIC FINDINGS

High-grade serous carcinoma shows stromal invasion, papillary, glandular, and/or solid growth patterns and high-grade nuclear atypia with nuclear pleomorphism (>3 times size variation) and prominent nucleoli; mitosis, apoptosis, and necrosis are often present (Fig. 2.9D). Psammoma bodies may be present.

Ancillary Studies

High-grade serous carcinomas typically stain positive for PAX-8, WT-1, and ER. Most (80%–95%) are associated with *TP53* mutations and show mutant pattern immunohistochemical stain with p53—either strong diffuse staining in at least 70% to 80% of the cells or null pattern. Most tumors show diffuse p16 expression.

Differential Diagnoses

Stromal invasion differentiates high-grade serous carcinoma from STIC. STICs are defined as stretches of tubal epithelium that show evidence of p53 mutation and marked intra-mucosal atypia including loss of cilia, nuclear enlargement, increased N:C ratio, loss of polarity, detached papillary clusters, intraepithelial fractures, and/or marked cytologic atypia (Fig. 2.9C). The Ki67 proliferation index is often increased compared with the background tubal epithelium. Genetic counseling (and testing for BRCA mutation) should be considered for women in whom STICs are detected incidentally.

STILs are defined as stretches of tubal epithelium that show evidence of p53 mutation and morphologic changes that include loss of cilia and epithelial atypia (such as nuclear enlargement and increased N:C ratio) but with preservation of cell polarity (Fig. 2.9A and B). There is variable increase in the Ki67 proliferation index in STIL compared with the background tubal epithelium.

Evidence of *TP53* mutations accompanied by only subtle morphologic changes in the fallopian tube characterize p53 signature. Fallopian tubes with p53 signatures show small stretches of non-ciliated epithelium that display mutant-pattern p53 immunohistochemical stain (i.e., stain either strongly positive or completely negative [null pattern] in comparison with the background tubal epithelium). Apart from the loss of cilia, there is often no significant morphologic difference between the stretch of tubal epithelium with p53 signature and the background tubal epithelium. p53 signatures are found in approximately 30% to 50% of fallopian tubes from women, regardless of their BRCA mutation status, and are considered early (latent) events in the carcinogenesis of high-grade serous carcinomas.

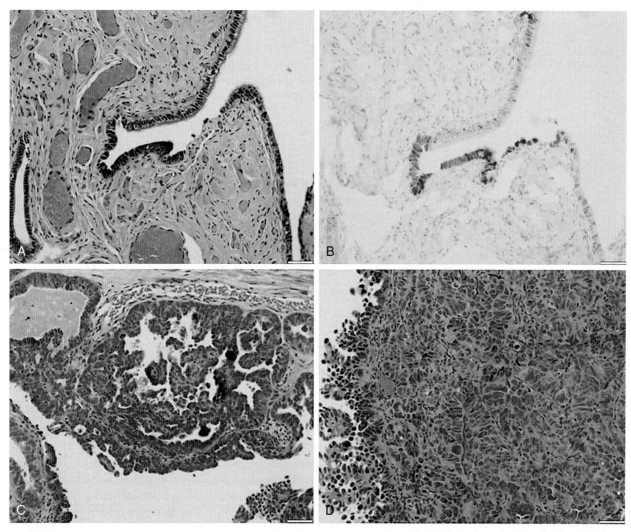

FIG. 2.9
Fallopian tube serous neoplasia. **A,** Serous tubal intraepithelial lesion (STIL) shows loss of cilia and nuclear enlargement but with preserved polarity; note normal background ciliated tubal epithelium. **B,** p53 is mutated within the STIL focus; note wild-type pattern in the background. **C,** Serous tubal intraepithelial carcinoma shows loss of cell polarity, marked cytologic atypia, and detached papillary clusters but is confined to the lumen. **D,** Invasive serous carcinoma shows stromal invasion by cells with high-grade cytologic atypia.

Features useful in distinguishing serous carcinomas from STICs, STILs, and p53 signatures are presented in Table 2.7.

Prognosis and Therapy

The prognosis of high-grade serous carcinoma depends on the stage and degree of tumor debulking—optimally debulked stage 1 disease carries a >80% 5-year survival rate, while the 5-year survival rate for stage III–IV tumors ranges from 15% to 20%. Approximately 5% of STICs progress to high-grade serous carcinoma. Incidental discovery of isolated STIC should prompt consideration for genetic counseling and testing for *BRCA* mutation. STILs and p53 signatures are considered latent/early

phases of serous carcinogenesis without significantly increased risk for recurrence or subsequent high-grade serous carcinoma.

HIGH-GRADE SEROUS CARCINOMA– DISEASE FACT SHEET

Definition

▸▸ Malignant epithelial neoplasm with serous differentiation, i.e., papillary, glandular, and/or solid growth and high-grade nuclear atypia; typically stains positive for WT-1 and PAX-8.
▸▸ Most are *TP53* mutated and show mutant pattern immunohistochemical staining with p53 antibody.

Epidemiology

▸▸ Typically occurs in postmenopausal women (average age, 65 years)
▸▸ May occur during reproductive age in women with familial predisposition such as BRCA mutations

TABLE 2.7

Summary of Features Useful in Distinguishing High-grade Serous Carcinoma From Serous Tubal Intraepithelial Carcinoma (STIC), Serous Tubal Intraepithelial Lesion (STIL), and p53 Signature

	High-grade Serous Carcinoma	STIC	STIL	p53 Signature
Morphology	Diffuse nuclear pleomorphism, prominent nucleoli, stromal invasion. p53 mutation.	No stromal invasion but lack of cilia, marked nuclear atypia/pleomorphism, prominent nucleoli, and loss of cell polarity. p53 mutation.	Lack of cilia and presence of nuclear atypia but preserved cell polarity. p53 mutation.	Lack of cilia but otherwise relatively normal appearing tubal epithelium. p53 mutation.
Prognosis	Depends on stage and degree of tumor debulking	Approximately 5% risk of progression to high-grade serous carcinoma	Minimal risk of progression to high-grade serous carcinoma	No significant risk of progression to high-grade serous carcinoma

Clinical Features

▸▸ Most patients present with stage III or IV disease.
▸▸ Abdominopelvic mass symptoms, bloating, and changes in bowel/bladder habits may be reported.
▸▸ Serum CA-125 is often elevated.

Prognosis and Therapy

▸▸ Tumor debulking, combined with adjuvant and/or neoadjuvant platinum-based chemotherapy is the main treatment modality.
▸▸ Median 5-year survival rates range from 15% to 55%, depending on tumor stage and degree of debulking.

HIGH-GRADE SEROUS CARCINOMA – PATHOLOGIC FEATURES

Gross Findings

▸▸ Typically bilateral masses with varying amount of solid and cystic components, and papillary excrescences

Microscopic Findings

▸▸ Solid, papillary, glandular, and/or cribriform architecture
▸▸ High-grade cytology with marked nuclear pleomorphism (>3:1 nuclear size variation), prominent nucleoli, mitosis, apoptosis, and necrosis

Pathologic Differential Diagnosis

▸▸ Serous tubal intraepithelial carcinoma

SEROUS BORDERLINE TUMOR OF THE OVARY

DIFFERENTIAL DIAGNOSES: BENIGN SEROUS CYSTADENOMA, LOW-GRADE SEROUS CARCINOMA, AND HIGH-GRADE SEROUS CARCINOMA

Clinical Features

Serous borderline tumors are non-invasive proliferative epithelial neoplasms with branching papillae and low-grade nuclear cytologic features. Serous borderline tumors occur over a wide age range, principally affecting reproductive age and perimenopausal women (average age, 45 years). Patients typically present with symptoms attributable to mass or masses confined to the ovary/ovaries.

Pathologic Features

GROSS FINDINGS

Serous borderline tumors are typically solid and/or cystic with varying amounts of intra-cystic and/or surface papillary excrescences. Solid areas/papillary excrescences should grossly comprise >10% of the tumor volume.

MICROSCOPIC FINDINGS

Histologic sections typically show hierarchical branching papillae lined by (often ciliated) cuboidal or columnar epithelial cells with minimal nuclear atypia. Serous borderline tumors may contain foci, measuring <5 mm, of confluent growth and/or stromal invasion by rounded cells with abundant eosinophilic cytoplasm may be present, and if present, such tumors are termed serous borderline tumor with microinvasion. Of note, the rounded cells with abundant eosinophilic cytoplasm are thought to be senescent based on their lack of expression of ER, PR, and WT-1, decreased Ki67 labeling and increased staining with apoptotic marker, M30, in comparison to columnar/cuboidal tumor cells. Their senescent nature may explain why serous borderline tumors with microinvasion and/or lymph node involvement by eosinophilic cells have similar outcome to borderline tumors lacking these features. Pelvic lymph nodes containing eosinophilic cells are thus not classified as metastasis, though the presence of such cells should be documented.

The micropapillary variant of serous borderline tumor is architecturally characterized by long slender micropapillae (usually five times taller than wide) emanating from large papillary cores; cribriform growth may be present in some tumors. Cytologically, the component cells are uniform (often non-ciliated) cuboidal to polygonal cells with high nuclear-to-cytoplasmic ratio and prominent small nucleoli. Of note, otherwise typical serous borderline tumors may contain focal micropapillary growth pattern; if such foci measure less than 5 mm, the tumors are classified as serous borderline tumors with focal micropapillary features.

Ancillary Studies

Serous borderline tumors typically stain positive for PAX-8, WT-1, and ER. Mutations in *KRAS* and *BRAF* have been identified in serous borderline tumors.

Differential Diagnosis

BENIGN SEROUS CYSTADENOMA

Grossly, benign serous tumors have smooth outer surfaces and smooth inner lining and contain clear watery (serous) fluid. Cystadenomas are entirely cystic, while cystadenofibromas may contain solid uniform fibrotic areas. On histologic sections, benign serous tumors are comprised of cysts lined by a single layer of fallopian tube-like ciliated cuboidal to columnar epithelium. Focal epithelial proliferation comprised of branching papillae of <10% of the epithelial volume may be present and if present, such tumors are termed serous cystadenoma/cystadenofibroma with focal epithelial proliferation. In contrast, serous borderline tumors typically have papillary excrescences grossly comprising >10% of the tumor volume and histologic sections show hierarchical branching papillae (Fig. 2.10).

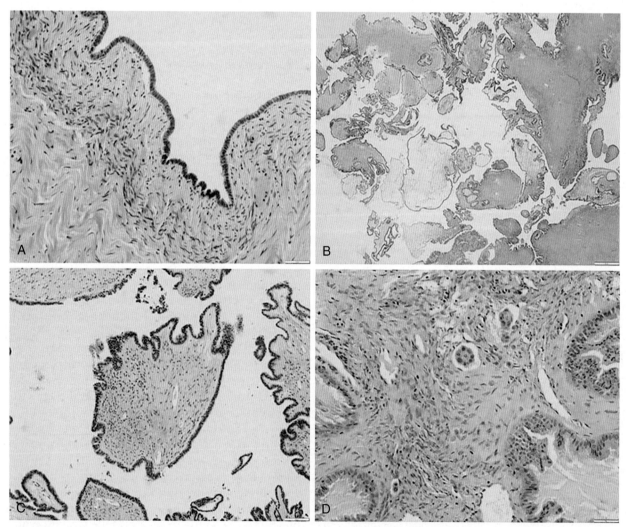

FIG. 2.10

Benign versus borderline serous tumors. **A,** Benign serous cystadenoma shows cyst lined by ciliated epithelium without hierarchal branching. **(B, C)** Borderline serous tumor shows hierarchal branching papillae in the cyst lumen; there is no stromal invasion. **D,** Borderline serous tumor with microinvasion shows rounded eosinophilic cells within the stroma.

LOW-GRADE SEROUS CARCINOMA

Low-grade serous carcinomas are invasive carcinomas with low-grade cytologic atypia. On histologic sections, low-grade serous carcinomas display stromal invasion by uniform cuboidal or polygonal cells with high nuclear-to-cytoplasmic ratio and prominent small nucleoli. The cells may invade stroma as single cells, small nests, micropapillae, macropapillae with surrounding clear space, or a combination of patterns. Psammoma bodies are often present and may be numerous. Low-grade serous carcinomas are distinguished from serous borderline tumors by the presence of stromal, lymph node, and/or peritoneal involvement by columnar or cuboidal cells with uniform nuclei, small nucleoli, and high nuclear-to-cytoplasmic ratio exhibiting micropapillary, cribriform, or solid growth pattern and/or destructive invasion with associated desmoplastic response. Low-grade serous carcinomas display similar *KRAS* and *BRAF* mutations as serous borderline tumors. Immunohistochemical staining patterns are likewise similar in serous borderline tumors and low-grade serous carcinomas; both are p53 wild-type and p16 negative but pancytokeratin, WT-1, and PAX-8 positive with high levels of ER and PR expression. Attention to morphology—mainly detection of solid growth and/or stromal invasion—is therefore key in distinguishing borderline serous tumor from low-grade serous carcinoma (Fig. 2.11).

HIGH-GRADE SEROUS CARCINOMA

High-grade serous carcinoma is distinguished from serous borderline tumor and low-grade serous carcinoma by the presence of high-grade nuclear cytologic atypia (Fig. 2.12). The nuclei in high-grade serous carcinoma are pleomorphic with greater than 3:1 size variation; nucleoli are prominent; mitotic figures are numerous; apoptosis, necrosis, and psammoma calcifications may be readily identifiable. High-grade serous carcinomas may display papillary, solid, or slit-like glandular

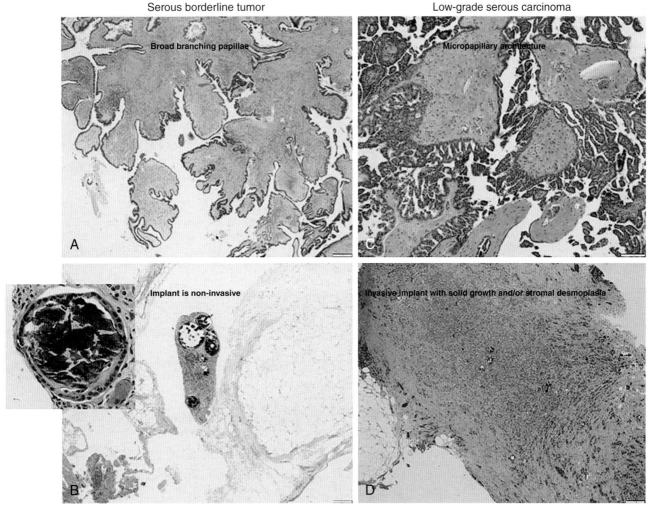

Serous borderline tumor

Low-grade serous carcinoma

Broad branching papillae

Micropapillary architecture

A

C

Implant is non-invasive

Invasive implant with solid growth and/or stromal desmoplasia

B

D

FIG. 2.11

Serous borderline tumor versus low-grade serous carcinoma. **A,** Serous borderline tumor shows hierarchal branching papillae in the cyst lumen; there is no stromal invasion. **B,** Implants of serous borderline tumors are non-invasive: limited to the peritoneal surface without stromal desmoplasia. Low-grade serous carcinoma shows micropapillary architecture **(C)**, solid growth, and/or destructive stromal invasion **(D)**.

Low-grade serous carcinoma   High-grade serous carcinoma

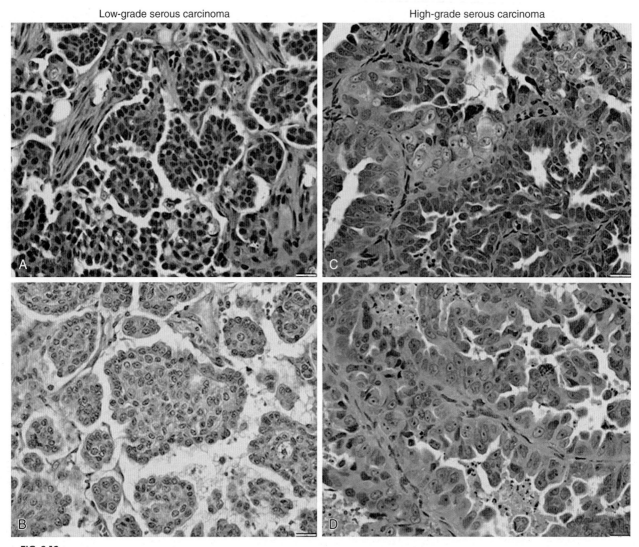

FIG. 2.12

Low-grade serous carcinoma versus high-grade serous carcinoma. **(A, B)** Nuclear features distinguish low-grade from high-grade serous carcinomas. Low-grade serous carcinoma shows relatively uniform, occasionally grooved nuclei with visible small nucleoli. **(C, D)** High-grade serous
carcinoma shows nuclear pleomorphism, apoptosis, necrosis, mitosis. and prominent nucleoli.

architecture. *BRCA*-related high-grade serous carcinomas may display solid, pseudoendometrioid and transitional carcinoma-like (SET) foci. Of note, serous tumors
with high-grade nuclear cytology are classified as high-
grade serous carcinomas irrespective of the presence or
absence of stromal invasion. Like serous borderline
tumors and low-grade serous carcinomas, high-grade
serous carcinomas stain positive for pancytokeratin,
WT-1, and PAX-8. However, high-grade serous carcinomas are distinguished by a high frequency of *TP53*
mutations. They thereby display p53 immunohistochemical staining patterns that correspond with *TP53*
mutation. High-grade serous tumors may either stain
strongly and diffusely positive (>70% of the tumor)
for p53, correlating with missense *TP53* mutation, or
display complete absence of p53 staining, correlating
with nonsense *TP53* mutation. Diffuse staining for p16

is also frequently observed in high-grade serous carcinomas in contrast to low-grade tumors.

Features useful in distinguishing serous borderline
tumors from low-grade and high-grade serous carcinomas are summarized in Table 2.8.

Prognosis and Therapy

Serous borderline tumors generally carry good prognosis
and are treated by complete surgical excision. Occasionally (in about 5% of patients), serous borderline tumors
recur as low-grade serous carcinomas. Risk factors for
recurrence include micropapillary/cribriform architecture, bilaterality, surface involvement, and incomplete
surgical excision.

TABLE 2.8

Summary of Features Useful in Distinguishing Borderline Serous Tumors From Low-grade and High-grade Serous Carcinomas

	Serous Borderline Tumor	Low-grade Serous Carcinoma	High-grade Serous Carcinoma
Histology in the ovary	Architecture: hierarchal branching papillae. Cytology: ciliated cuboidal or columnar cells; may have polygonal hobnail cells with eosinophilic cytoplasm but lacks significant nuclear pleomorphism.	Architecture: non-hierarchal branching slender micropapillae, occasionally with cribriform architecture **and** stromal invasion by single cells, small nests of cells, micropapillae, or macropapillae. Psammoma bodies may be prominent. Cytology: cuboidal to polygonal, typically non-ciliated cells with high nuclear to cytoplasmic ratio and uniform nuclei with small prominent nucleoli. Lacks significant nuclear pleomorphism. Mitosis ≤12 MF/10 HPF.	Architecture: solid, papillary, or glandular (slit-like or cribriform) growth patterns. Psammoma bodies may be present. Cytology: high-grade pleomorphic nuclei with >3:1 variation in nuclear size, prominent nucleoli, frequent mitosis, apoptosis, and often necrosis. Mitosis >12 MF/10 HPF.
Histology in the peritoneum, if involved	Implants are non-invasive: • easily shelled out during surgery. • limited to the peritoneal surface or in peritoneal invaginations of serous cells surrounded by a cyst with mesothelial cell (calretinin-positive) rim without stromal response. • desmoplastic implants have glands, small nests or single eosinophilic cells within granulation tissue-like stroma. The stroma predominates.	Implants are invasive; display any of: • destructive invasion of the underlying normal tissue associated with a desmoplastic response. • solid growth/epithelial dominant growth.	Implants are not applicable; tumors with high-grade nuclear cytology are designated high-grade serous carcinomas regardless of whether or not they invade the stroma at ovarian or extra-ovarian sites.
Genetics	*BRAF* and *KRAS* mutations	*BRAF* and *KRAS* mutations	*TP53*, *BRCA1*, and *BRCA2* mutations; prominent DNA copy number changes
Immunohistochemistry	p53 wild type; p16 negative (i.e., not diffuse)	p53 wild type; p16 negative (i.e., not diffuse)	Mutant pattern p53: either diffusely positive (>60%) or completely negative (null pattern) Diffusely p16 positive
Prognosis	Good	Depends on stage and completeness of surgical resection.	Aggressive: even low stage tumors require adjuvant chemotherapy.

SEROUS BORDERLINE TUMOR– DISEASE FACT SHEET

Definition
▶▶ Non-invasive proliferative epithelial neoplasms with branching papillae and low-grade nuclear cytologic features

Epidemiology
▶▶ Typically occurs in reproductive age and perimenopausal women (average age, 45 years)

Clinical Features
▶▶ Patients present with ovarian mass-related symptoms

Prognosis and Therapy
▶▶ Prognosis is generally good.
▶▶ Treated by complete surgical resection
▶▶ Risk of recurrence in patients with micropapillary variant, bilateral tumors, surface involvement, and incomplete surgical excision

SEROUS BORDERLINE TUMOR – PATHOLOGIC FEATURES

Gross Findings
▶▶ Solid and/or cystic mass with varying amounts of intra-cystic and/or surface papillary excrescences

Microscopic Findings
▶▶ Classic: Non-invasive with hierarchal branching papillae
▶▶ Micropapillary variant: Non-invasive with "Medusa head" appearance—slender micropapillae that emanate directly from large papillae
▶▶ Low-grade nuclear cytology: uniform cells with small nucleoli; lacks significant pleomorphism

Pathologic Differential Diagnosis
▶▶ Low-grade serous carcinoma
▶▶ High-grade serous carcinoma

MUCINOUS BORDERLINE TUMOR OF THE OVARY

DIFFERENTIAL DIAGNOSES: BENIGN MUCINOUS CYSTADENOMA, OVARIAN MUCINOUS ADENOCARCINOMA, MUCINOUS ADENOCARCINOMA METASTATIC TO THE OVARY, AND OVARIAN ENDOMETRIOID ADENOCARCINOMA

Clinical Features

Mucinous borderline tumors are non-invasive proliferative neoplasms with gastrointestinal-type epithelium displaying architectural complexity (i.e., epithelial stratification, tufting, and/or slender papillae). Mucinous borderline tumors occur over a wide age range—from pediatric to postmenopausal patients (average age, 45 years). Patients present with symptoms attributable to a unilateral ovarian mass.

Pathologic Features

GROSS FINDINGS

Mucinous borderline tumors are typically large unilateral ovarian masses with smooth outer surface (average size, 20 cm). Cross-sections typically reveal multilocular cysts containing thick mucinous fluid. The presence of solid nodules grossly is a worrisome feature and solid areas need to be thoroughly sampled (2 sections per cm) to exclude invasive carcinoma.

MICROSCOPIC FINDINGS

Histologic sections of mucinous borderline tumors reveal cysts lined by gastrointestinal epithelium displaying epithelial stratification, tufting, and/or slender papillae. Nuclear enlargement and pseudostratification may be present, but high-grade nuclear features (defined by marked nuclear enlargement, nuclear hyperchromasia, and large prominent nucleoli involving the full thickness of the epithelium, i.e., similar to high-grade dysplasia in gastrointestinal adenomas) are absent in borderline tumors. Mucinous borderline tumors showing high-grade atypia without evidence of stromal invasion are termed mucinous borderline tumor with intraepithelial carcinoma. Mucinous borderline tumors with foci, measuring <5 mm, of confluent growth and/or stromal invasion by single cells or glands with mild to moderate cytologic atypia (with nuclei that are not much different from the background non-invasive borderline component) are termed mucinous borderline tumor with microinvasion. However, if the invasive cells in the

<5-mm foci display high-grade nuclear features, the tumors are termed microinvasive carcinoma. Of note, if the stromal invasion is of the destructive pattern (i.e., infiltrative glands associated with desmoplasia), the tumors should be classified as mucinous carcinomas even if the invasive focus is <5 mm, as such tumors are associated with worse prognosis. A note about the small size of the focus may be warranted.

Ancillary Studies

Immunohistochemical stains are only occasionally useful when evaluating mucinous tumors—attention to gross and histologic morphology is more useful in distinguishing mucinous tumors from other ovarian tumors such as serous and endometrioid tumors. Attention to clinical history is more useful in distinguishing primary ovarian mucinous tumors from metastasis to the ovary. Nevertheless, ovarian mucinous tumors typically stain diffusely positive for CK7, variable positive for PAX-8, CK20, CDX2, and SATB2 and are often negative for p16, WT-1, napsin-A, ER, and PR. Immunohistochemical stain with p53 may reveal either wild-type or mutant pattern.

BENIGN MUCINOUS CYSTADENOMA/ CYSTADENOFIBROMA

Benign mucinous tumors may be entirely cystic (mucinous cystadenomas) or may have fibromatous stroma (mucinous cystadenofibromas). Grossly, benign mucinous tumors have smooth outer surfaces and smooth inner lining and contain thick mucoid fluid. Cystadenomas usually present as unilateral cysts, while cystadenofibromas may contain solid uniform spongy/fibrotic areas. On histologic sections of benign mucinous tumors, the lining epithelial cells display basally located nuclei with abundant apical mucin, absent to minimal stratification, and absent to minimal nuclear atypia. Focal epithelial proliferation comprised of stratification or papillae of <10% of the epithelial volume may be present and if present, such tumors are termed mucinous cystadenoma/cystadenofibroma with focal epithelial proliferation. Mucinous borderline tumors may be difficult to reliably distinguish from benign mucinous cystadenofibromas grossly. Histologic features that distinguish mucinous borderline tumors from benign cystadenomas include epithelial stratification, tufting, and villous/slender papillae in mucinous borderline tumors. KRAS mutations are present in both benign mucinous cystadenomas and mucinous borderline tumors.

MUCINOUS ADENOCARCINOMA

Like mucinous borderline tumors, mucinous adenocarcinomas are typically large smooth-surfaced unilateral solid and cystic masses with mucinous cyst contents.

However, necrosis may be grossly present in carcinomas. On histologic sections, mucinous adenocarcinoma is distinguished from mucinous borderline tumor by the presence of stromal invasion and/or high-grade cytologic atypia. Importantly, histologic sections of mucinous carcinomas characteristically show a spectrum of epithelial changes ranging from benign mucinous cystadenoma-like areas to borderline-like areas and areas of frank carcinoma showing either high-grade cytologic atypia and/or stromal invasion. Therefore, careful sampling, specifically targeting solid areas, is important during intraoperative pathologic assessment. At least 2 sections per cm of tumor should be evaluated prior to final pathology sign out. Two patterns of stromal invasion may be present in mucinous carcinoma. The expansile pattern of invasion, characterized by back-to-back confluent glands with little to no intervening stroma, is more common and carries a relatively good prognosis. The destructive pattern of stromal invasion, characterized by infiltrating glands eliciting a desmoplastic stromal response, tends to follow a more aggressive course regardless of the size of the invasive focus. Hence, it is important that the type of stromal invasion is mentioned in the pathology report. Like benign and borderline mucinous tumors, mucinous carcinomas are associated with *KRAS* mutations. *HER2* amplification has also been described.

Features useful in distinguishing benign, borderline, and malignant ovarian mucinous tumors are summarized in Table 2.9 and Fig. 2.13. Of note, distinguishing low-grade mucinous carcinomas with expansile pattern invasion from mucinous borderline tumors can be difficult and subjective. Fortunately, both tumors carry similar prognosis. The more easily recognized destructive pattern of stromal invasion portends an adverse prognosis in mucinous carcinomas.

MUCINOUS ADENOCARCINOMA METASTATIC TO THE OVARY

Just like primary ovarian mucinous carcinoma often displays a full spectrum of differentiation from benign-appearing areas to borderline-like areas and areas with frank invasive carcinoma, mucinous carcinomas metastatic to the ovary likewise can display this full differentiation spectrum. Hence, histologic findings alone are insufficient to distinguish primary mucinous carcinoma from metastasis to the ovary. Gross features and clinical history provide the most helpful clues in distinguishing primary ovarian mucinous tumors from metastasis. Features to suggest metastasis include clinical history of mucinous neoplasm or adenocarcinoma at other site (typically gastrointestinal tract or uterine cervix), involvement of bilateral ovaries, the presence of ovarian surface nodules, and the presence of extra-ovarian disease/mucinous ascites. Unilaterality and large tumor size favor primary ovarian origin. An algorithm, whereby tumors ≥13 cm were considered primary to the ovary unless they displayed surface nodules or bilaterality, and tumors <13 cm were considered metastatic unless they were

	TABLE 2.9		
	Features Useful in Distinguishing Benign From Borderline and Malignant Mucinous Tumors		
	Mucinous Cystadenoma	Mucinous Borderline Tumor (MBT)	Mucinous Adenocarcinoma
Gross features	Smooth outer surface; interior may contain smooth-walled unilocular or multiloculated cysts (cystadenoma) or smooth-walled cysts admixed with uniformly solid/spongy fibrous areas (cystadenofibroma).	Smooth outer surface; interior often contains multiloculated cysts; solid nodules may be present.	Smooth outer surface; interior may contain unilocular or multiloculated cysts; solid nodules are often present and should be well-sampled. Necrosis and hemorrhage may be present.
Histology	Lined by non-stratified columnar mucinous epithelium with basally located nuclei with no to minimal cytologic atypia. Focal epithelial stratification and low-grade nuclear atypia comprising <10% of the tumor may be present.	Lined by stratified columnar mucinous epithelium often with papillary tufts reminiscent of intestinal polyps and adenomas, comprising >10% of the tumor. MBT with microinvasion: foci of confluent growth or stromal invasion by cells with low to moderate nuclear atypia measuring < 5 mm.	Displays stromal invasion. Invasion may be expansile pattern, i.e., back-to-back glands with minimal intervening stroma (requires invasive focus >5 mm to be called mucinous adenocarcinoma) or destructive/infiltrative with stromal desmoplasia (classified as mucinous adenocarcinoma regardless of the size of invasive focus). Cytologic grade varies from low to high.
Prognosis	Benign; excellent prognosis.	Excellent prognosis with complete surgical excision.	Carcinomas with expansile pattern of invasion are often stage I and have excellent prognosis. Carcinomas with destructive pattern of stromal invasion have worse prognosis. Prognosis with extra-ovarian disease is poor.

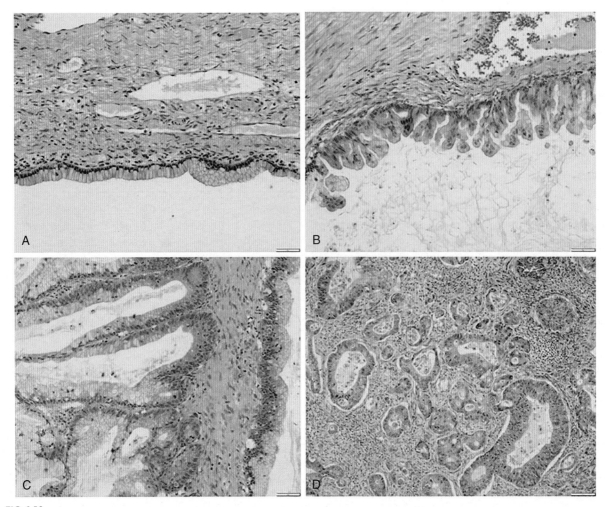

FIG. 2.13
Benign versus borderline versus malignant mucinous tumors. **A,** Benign mucinous cystadenoma shows cyst lined by mucinous epithelium with basally located nuclei. **(B)** Borderline mucinous tumor shows stratified epithelium; there is no stromal invasion. **(C, D)** Mucinous adenocarcinoma shows a range of epithelial differentiation and stromal invasion.

unilateral, correctly classified 94% of metastatic tumors and 98% of primary ovarian tumors in one study. Though not entirely specific, histologic features more commonly identified in metastasis include infiltrative pattern of stromal invasion and vascular invasion. Immunohistochemical stains, particularly PAX-8 and SATB2, may occasionally be helpful in distinguishing primary ovarian mucinous carcinoma from gastrointestinal metastasis, as 30% to 50% of primary ovarian mucinous tumors express PAX-8, while SATB2 expression is more common in gastrointestinal tumors. Most treatment guidelines recommend routine appendectomies in cases in which mucinous borderline tumors or mucinous adenocarcinomas are diagnosed intraoperatively in order to exclude metastasis to the ovary from an appendiceal primary.

ENDOMETRIOID ADENOCARCINOMA

Ovarian endometrioid adenocarcinoma displays infiltrative and/or back-to-back endometrioid glands and typically arises in a background of endometriosis or endometrioid adenofibroma. Endometrioid adenocarcinomas typically display a spectrum of cytoplasmic changes including secretory, squamous, ciliated, sex cord-like, and mucinous differentiation. When mucinous differentiation is present in an endometrioid adenocarcinoma, the differential with ovarian mucinous tumors arises. The findings of background endometriosis and/or endometrioid adenofibroma combined with the presence of squamous differentiation are helpful clues that favor endometrioid adenocarcinoma. Immunohistochemical stains that may be of aid include PR and vimentin for which endometrioid adenocarcinomas are often positive, while mucinous tumors are often negative.

Prognosis and Therapy

Most patients with mucinous borderline tumors and ovarian mucinous adenocarcinomas present with stage I disease, confined to the ovary. As such, both borderline and malignant mucinous tumors generally carry good prognosis. Patients with mucinous borderline tumors are often cured by unilateral salpingo-oophorectomy. The prognosis of mucinous adenocarcinoma is stage-dependent, with 5-year survival rates of 91% for stage I, 76% for stage II, and 17% for stage III/IV disease.

MUCINOUS BORDERLINE TUMOR– DISEASE FACT SHEET

Definition
▸▸ Non-invasive proliferative epithelial neoplasm with gastrointestinal epithelium and architectural complexity

Epidemiology
▸▸ Occurs over a wide age range—from pediatric to postmenopausal (average age, 45 years).

Clinical Features
▸▸ Patients present with ovarian mass–related symptoms.

Prognosis and Therapy
▸▸ Prognosis is generally excellent.
▸▸ Often cured by unilateral salpingo-oophorectomy

MUCINOUS BORDERLINE TUMOR – PATHOLOGIC FEATURES

Gross Findings
▸▸ Large smooth-surfaced ovarian mass with internal multilocular cysts containing thick mucin.

Microscopic Findings
▸▸ Gastric and/or intestinal-type mucinous epithelium
▸▸ Architectural complexity: stratification, tufting, villous, and/or slender papillae.
▸▸ No invasion or high-grade cytology

Pathologic Differential Diagnosis
▸▸ Mucinous cystadenoma
▸▸ Mucinous adenocarcinoma
▸▸ Endometrioid adenocarcinoma
▸▸ Metastasis from extra-ovarian sites

OVARIAN FIBROMA

DIFFERENTIAL DIAGNOSES: FIBROSARCOMA, THECOMA, AND STEROID CELL TUMOR

Clinical Features

Sex cord stromal tumors represent approximately 8% of all primary ovarian neoplasms. Clinically, sex cord

stromal tumors may be hormonally silent or may present with estrogenizing hormonal manifestations (such as precocious pseudo-puberty and dysfunctional uterine bleeding secondary to endometrial hyperplasia/carcinoma), or androgenizing/virilizing hormonal manifestations (such as hypertrophied clitoris, hirsutism, male-pattern baldness, increased testosterone levels, and amenorrhea or dysfunctional uterine bleeding secondary to endometrial inactivity). The hormonally silent tumors tend to be grossly white (or tan), while the hormonally active tumors are characterized by a vibrant yellow color (at least focally) (Fig. 2.14). The tumors that are generally hormonally inactive include fibroma, luteinized thecoma associated with sclerosing peritonitis, sclerosing stromal tumor, and signet ring stromal tumor. The tumors commonly associated with estrogenizing symptoms include thecoma, Sertoli cell tumor, granulosa cell tumor (both adult and juvenile types), and sex cord tumor with annular tubules (SCTAT). The tumors usually associated with androgenizing symptoms include Leydig cell tumor, steroid cell tumor, and Sertoli-Leydig cell tumor.

Fibromas are the most common sex cord stromal tumors, representing 70% of ovarian sex cord stromal tumors and 4% of all ovarian neoplasms. Fibromas typically occur in middle-age women (i.e., women > 40 years old; average age, 48 years) and are typically unilateral, hormonally inactive, and asymptomatic. Symptomatic cases are often secondary to mass effect. Rarely (1% of the time), fibromas are associated with Meigs syndrome (i.e., concurrent ascites and pleural effusion) or ascites alone. In patients with Gorlin syndrome (also known as nevoid basal cell carcinoma syndrome), fibromas tend to be bilateral, calcified, and present at a younger age (including childhood).

Pathologic Features

GROSS FINDINGS

Typical gross features of fibromas include smooth surface with circumscribed firm white to tan homogenous cut section (see Fig. 2.14).

MICROSCOPIC FINDINGS

On histologic sections, fibromas are composed of benign-appearing cells with ovoid to fusiform bland nuclei and scant cytoplasm. Fibromas may contain collagen bands or hyaline plaques. Mitotic figures are typically rare. However, occasional fibromas may have increased cellularity (cellular fibromas) and/or greater than 4, but <19 MF/10 HPF (mitotically active cellular fibromas). Fibromas may occasionally have areas of hemorrhage and infarct-type necrosis secondary to torsion.

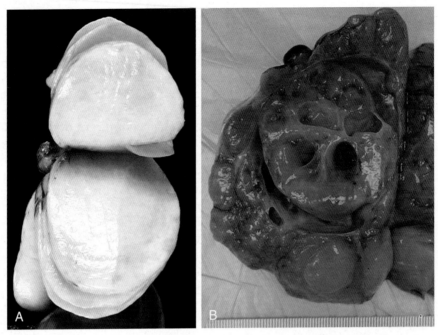

FIG. 2.14

Gross appearance of sex cord stromal tumors. Sex cord stromal tumors are typically solid masses (or may be solid and cystic, but only rarely entirely cystic). Hormonally inactive sex cord stromal tumors, such as fibroma **(A)**, are typically white. Hormonally active sex cord stromal tumors, such as juvenile granulosa cell tumor **(B)**, are typically vibrant yellow.

Ancillary Studies

Fibromas are typically immunoreactive for smooth muscle actin and tend to be focally positive for inhibin, calretinin, WT-1, and other sex cord markers.

Differential Diagnosis

FIBROSARCOMA

Patients with fibrosarcomas typically present at an older age (average age, 58 years) than those with fibromas. Histologically, fibrosarcomas display moderate to marked cytologic atypia, necrosis, and frequent mitosis, including atypical mitotic figures. The absence of significant nuclear atypia is an important feature for distinguishing mitotically active cellular fibromas from fibrosarcomas. Helpful clues to distinguish fibromas from fibrosarcomas are summarized in Table 2.10.

THECOMA

Thecomas account for 1% (or less) of all ovarian tumors, are typically unilateral, and occur in postmeno-pausal women (average age, 59 years). Hormonal manifestations are common and often estrogenic (e.g., vaginal bleeding, thickened endometrial stripe, increased risk of concurrent endometrial cancer in about 20% of cases). Thecomas containing lutein cells

may be androgenic. Thecomas are typically grossly cir-cumscribed solid yellow tumors with lobulated cut surface but may occasionally be cystic. Their sizes range from <1 to 15 cm, but are typically 5 to 10 cm. Histo-logic sections of thecomas (Fig. 2.15A) show cells that resemble the normal ovarian theca interna, that is, uniform cells with oval to round nuclei and pale grey-ish-pink cytoplasm with ill-defined borders. There may be an alternating spindle cell (fibromatous) background separated by collagen. Hyaline plaques and lutein cells (i.e., cells with round nuclei, prominent nucleoli, and abundant eosinophilic or clear cytoplasm) may be present. Stromal calcification may be seen in thecomas from younger patients. Bizarre degenerative nuclei may rarely be present, but significant mitotic activity is absent. Thecomas may have a prominent fibromatous back-ground and hence be difficult to distinguish from fibro-mas. Clinical presentation and gross features are key to distinguishing thecoma from fibroma. Fibromas are typically hormonally inactive and grossly white, while thecomas typically present with hormonal manifesta-tions and are grossly yellow. If information about the clinical and gross features is somehow unavailable, the diagnosis of fibrothecoma may be rendered in histo-logically ambiguous cases. Thecomas are strongly im-munoreactive for sex cord stromal markers.

STEROID CELL TUMOR

Steroid cell tumors are hormone-secreting tumors comprised entirely of cells that resemble lutein cells,

TABLE 2.10

Features Useful in Distinguishing Fibromas From Fibrosarcomas

	Fibroma	Fibrosarcoma
Epidemiology and clinical	• Most common ovarian stromal tumor. • Typically presents in perimenopausal women (average age, 48 years). • Typically asymptomatic, but if symptomatic, presents with mass-related symptoms.	• Rare. • Typically presents in postmenopausal women (average age, 58 years). • Typically presents with mass-related symptoms.
Gross	• Typically unilateral uniform, smooth white ovarian masses.	• Typically large solid unilateral ovarian masses with hemorrhage and necrosis.
Histology	• **Bland** spindle cells with varying amounts of collagenous background. • Mitosis may be present in mitotically active cellular fibromas (4–19 MF/10 HPF).	• **Cytologically atypical** densely hypercellular spindle cells with disordered fascicles; nuclei display moderate to severe atypia/pleomorphism. • Mitotic figures are typically numerous (>19 MF/10 HPF); abnormal mitosis may be present; necrosis may be present.
Prognosis	Benign	Aggressive malignancy: 50% of patients die within 2 years of diagnosis.

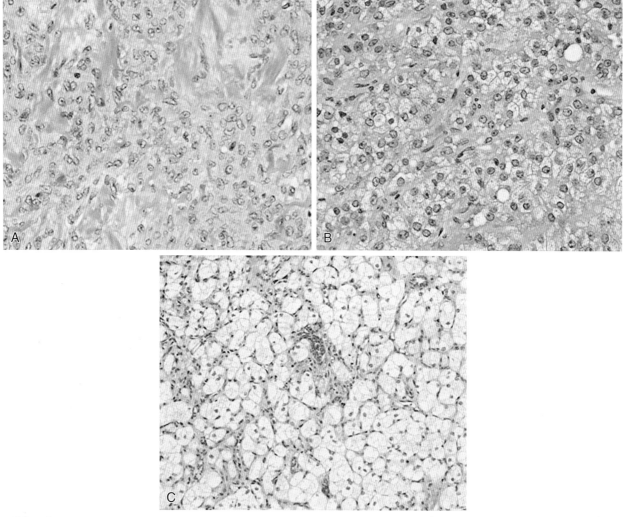

FIG. 2.15

Thecoma versus steroid cell tumor. Both thecomas and steroid cell tumors have abundant cytoplasm. **A,** Thecomas have oval to spindled nuclei and indistinct cytoplasmic boundaries. **(B, C)** Steroid cell tumors tend to have round nuclei and abundant lipid-rich cytoplasm with well-defined cytoplasmic boundaries. Clinically, thecomas are typically estrogenic, while patients with steroid cell tumors often present with androgenic symptoms.

Leydig cells, or adrenal cortical cells. Steroid cell tumors are epithelioid (i.e., tend to have centrally placed round nuclei and abundant eosinophilic or clear cytoplasm and well-defined cytoplasmic borders). Because thecomas also tend to have abundant cytoplasm, the differential diagnosis with steroid cell tumor arises. Helpful clinical features include the type of hormonal manifestations—thecomas are typically estrogenic, while steroid cell tumors are typically androgenic. Histologic clues to the differential include the presence of a spindle cell component (fibromatous background) in thecomas. Thecomas also tend to have ill-defined cytoplasmic boundaries, while steroid cell tumors have well-defined cytoplasmic borders (Fig. 2.15). Immunohistochemical stains are not helpful as both tumors stain positive for sex cord stromal markers.

Prognosis and therapy

Fibromas, like most sex cord stromal tumors, are benign and cured by complete surgical excision (oophorectomies). The malignant sex cord stromal tumors include fibrosarcoma and granulosa cell tumor (both adult and juvenile types). Steroid cell tumor is malignant 30% to 40% of the time, particularly tumors with size >7 cm, mitotic count >2 MF/10 HPF, necrosis, hemorrhage, and significant nuclear atypia. SCTAT typically occurs in patients with Peutz-Jehgers syndrome and has a benign course in those patients. However, sporadic cases of SC-TAT have low-grade malignant potential.

OVARIAN FIBROMA – DISEASE FACT SHEET

Definition
▸▸ Benign stromal tumor comprised of bland spindle cells (resembles normal ovarian stroma, but may be collagenous).

Epidemiology
▸▸ Most common ovarian sex cord stromal tumor
▸▸ Occurs at any age, but most common in perimenopausal women (average age, 48 years)

Clinical Features
▸▸ Most patients are asymptomatic, but when symptomatic, patients present with ovarian mass–related symptoms

Prognosis and Therapy
▸▸ Benign
▸▸ Recurrence risk: cellular fibromas; ovarian rupture

OVARIAN FIBROMA – PATHOLOGIC FEATURES

Gross Findings
▸▸ Typically unilateral firm, white smooth-surfaced ovarian mass with uniform cut surface. May occasionally have cystic degeneration.

▸▸ May occasionally be bilateral and calcified (in patients with Gorlin syndrome).

Microscopic Findings
▸▸ Bland spindle cells within variably collagenous stroma
▸▸ Occasionally increased cellularity and mitotic activity occur in mitotically active cellular fibromas
▸▸ No significant nuclear atypia

Pathologic Differential Diagnosis
▸▸ Fibrosarcoma
▸▸ Thecoma

ADULT GRANULOSA CELL TUMOR

DIFFERENTIAL DIAGNOSES: THECOMA, JUVENILE GRANULOSA CELL TUMOR, SERTOLI-LEYDIG CELL TUMOR, AND CARCINOMA (PRIMARY OR METASTATIC)

Clinical Features

Adult granulosa cell tumors are the second most common sex cord stromal tumors, accounting for 2% to 3% of all primary ovarian tumors. They occur from the first to tenth decade (median age, 50 years). Patients with adult granulosa cell tumors commonly present with estrogenic manifestations (i.e., postmenopausal bleeding, menometrorrhagia, or isosexual pseudoprecocity). Concurrent endometrial hyperplasia is present approximately 50% of the time and endometrial carcinoma in about 10% of cases. Hence, endometrial sampling is necessary in patients with granulosa cell tumors. Serum inhibin levels may be elevated.

Pathologic Features

GROSS FINDINGS

Adult granulosa cell tumors are typically unilateral, yellow and red, hemorrhagic, mixed solid and cystic masses (Fig. 2.16A). The tumors may, however, occasionally be entirely solid or, rarely, entirely cystic.

MICROSCOPIC FINDINGS

On histologic sections, adult granulosa cell tumors show a variety of growth patterns (Fig. 2.16B–D)—diffuse (most common), insular, microfollicular (with Call-Exner bodies), macrofollicular, trabecular, pseudopapillary, and watered silk (least common). Mixed growth patterns are typically present in the same tumor. However, on rare occasions, tumors may be

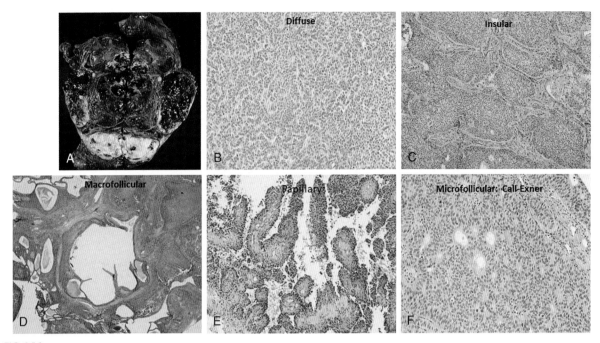

FIG. 2.16

Adult granulosa cell tumor. **A,** The tumors are typically yellow and red hemorrhagic solid and cystic masses; may have regions of necrosis. Histologic sections typically show a variety of growth patterns. **B,** Diffuse. **C,** Insular. **D,** Macrofollicular. **E,** Papillary. **F,** Microfollicular (microfollicles are also called Call-Exner bodies). A prominent fibromatous or thecomatous background may be present (not shown).

homogenous. The component cells are granulosa cells with round to oval angulated or grooved nuclei and scant cytoplasm that may occasionally be luteinized. The nuclei of the granulosa cells may occasionally appear less mature with scant cytoplasm reminiscent of small blue cell tumors. The background stroma in granulosa cell tumors is typically fibromatous or thecomatous. Variable mitotic activity may be present, though significant nuclear atypia is rare. On rare occasions, granulosa cell tumors may have bizarre nuclei, heterologous mucinous epithelium, or hepatoid differentiation. Adult granulosa cell tumors may have a minor component of juvenile granulosa cell tumor.

Ancillary Studies

Adult granulosa cell tumors stain strongly positive for sex cord stromal markers—calretinin, inhibin, SF1, WT-1. *FOXL2* is mutated in most adult granulosa cell tumors and tumors stain positive with FOXL2 by immunohistochemistry.

Differential Diagnosis

THECOMA

The differential diagnosis with thecoma arises because both thecoma and granulosa cell tumor may present as unilateral grossly yellow ovarian masses associated with estrogenizing clinical symptoms. In addition, on histologic sections, adult granulosa cell tumors may occasionally display diffuse growth and/or more abundant (luteinized) cytoplasm, making it difficult to distinguish from thecoma. Furthermore, both tumors stain positive for sex cord markers (calretinin, inhibin, etc.) and though *FOXL2* mutations are very common in granulosa cell tumors, they may also be seen in 12.5% to 21% of thecomas. Thorough sampling for more typical granulosa cell features (i.e., morphologic variety, epithelial differentiation, and nuclear grooves) may be helpful. Otherwise, reticulin stain is the most useful in distinguishing the entities. Reticulin surrounds individual cells in thecoma and nests of cells in granulosa cell tumor (Fig. 2.17).

JUVENILE GRANULOSA CELL TUMOR

Juvenile granulosa cell tumors occur over a wide age range, but most tumors (97%) occur in patients younger than 30 years old. Juvenile granulosa tumors are typically estrogenizing. Children present with isosexual pseudoprecocity, premenopausal adults present with menstrual irregularities, and postmenopausal women present with postmenopausal bleeding. Other presenting symptoms include those associated with the presence of an abdominopelvic mass such as abdominal distension or pain. Like adult granulosa cell tumors, juvenile granulosa cell tumors are typically unilateral solid and cystic yellow ovarian masses, occasionally

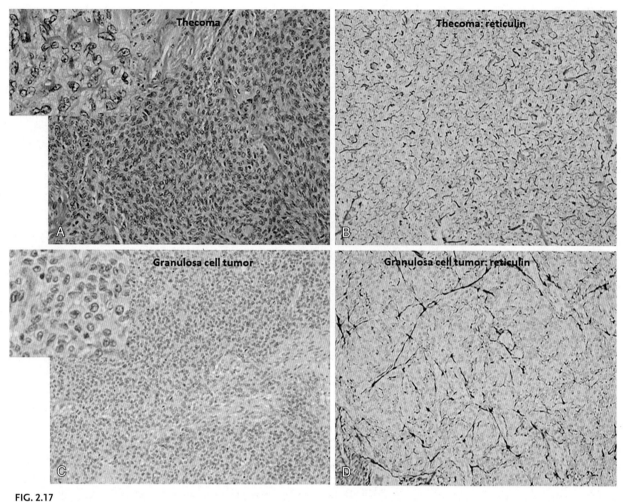

FIG. 2.17

Thecoma versus granulosa cell tumor. **A,** Occasionally nuclear grooves reminiscent of granulosa cell tumor may be present in thecomas (inset). **B,** Reticulin surrounds individual cells in thecomas. This helps distinguish thecoma from granulosa cell tumor with diffuse growth pattern **(C, D).**

with foci of hemorrhage and necrosis. Tumors may rarely be entirely solid or entirely cystic. Histologic sections (Fig. 2.18) show nodular or diffuse growth of granulosa cells in a myxoid or edematous background, punctuated by follicles of varying shapes and sizes. The follicles may contain eosinophilic or basophilic secretions. The component cells have round to oval nuclei with tiny nucleoli and moderate to abundant eosinophilic cytoplasm (Fig. 2.19). Nuclear grooves are rare. There is variable cytologic atypia, and mitotic activity may be frequent. Atypical mitotic figures may be present. Juvenile granulosa cell tumors generally have less conspicuous stroma than adult granulosa cell tumors but may occasionally have prominent fibromatous or sclerotic stroma and may have frequent luteinized cells. Morphologic features of juvenile granulosa cell tumors that typically distinguish them from adult granulosa cell tumors include nodular growth pattern, myxoid background, more varied irregular-sized and shaped follicles, and component cells that lack nuclear grooves but tend to have more pronounced mitotic activity, bizarre nuclei, and more abundant "luteinized"

cytoplasm. Juvenile granulosa cell tumors may have a component of adult granulosa cell tumor, but the tumor is classified based on the predominant histology.

Juvenile granulosa cell tumor versus yolk sac tumor: Yolk sac tumor is a malignant germ cell tumor that occurs in children and young adults (average age, 19 years). Like sex cord stromal tumors, endocrine manifestations may be observed in yolk sac tumor but is rare. Morphologic overlap between yolk sac tumor and juvenile granulosa cell tumor includes myxoid background, microcystic (follicle-like) architecture, and brisk mitosis. The following features of yolk sac tumor help establish its diagnosis: pronounced nuclear atypia, the presence of Schiller-Duval bodies, association with other germ cell components, positive staining for CDX-2, AFP, and SALL4, and absent inhibin expression. Clinically, patients with yolk sac tumors present with markedly elevated serum AFP, whereas those with juvenile granulosa cell tumor may present with elevated serum inhibin (in addition to endocrine manifestations).

Juvenile granulosa cell tumor versus small cell carcinoma, hypercalcemic type: Small cell carcinoma,

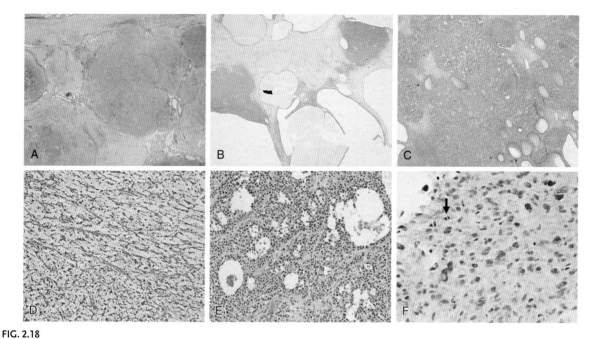

FIG. 2.18

Juvenile granulosa cell tumor. Histologic sections typically show: nodular growth, **(A)** follicles and follicle-like spaces of various sizes containing eosinophilic secretions, **(B)** or basophilic secretions **(C)**. Myxoid background, occasionally with sieve-like spaces **(D)**. Microcystic spaces may also be present, **(E)**. Component cells may be round with high nuclear-to-cytoplasmic ratio **(E)** or may have more abundant luteinized cytoplasm **(F)**; note mitotic figure *(arrow)*.

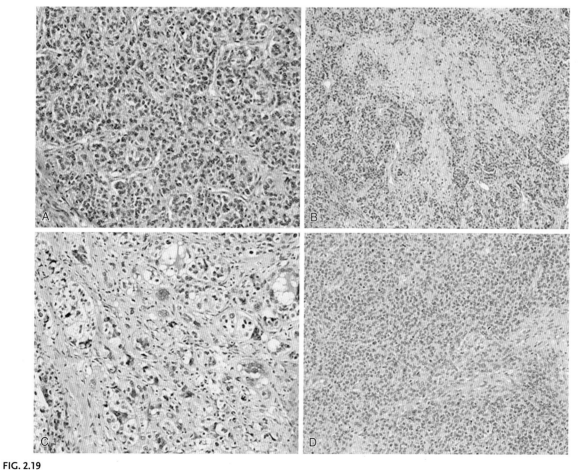

FIG. 2.19

Juvenile granulosa cell tumor. Cytologic features. The component cells typically have round nuclei with small nucleoli and moderate amount of cytoplasm **(A)**. Occasionally, the cells appear small with scant amount of cytoplasm; seen here in a myxoid background **(B)**. Regions of cytologic atypia may be present **(C)**. Occasionally, adult granulosa-like grooved nuclei may be present focally **(D)**.

hypercalcemic type is a rare, undifferentiated, highly aggressive neoplasm that occurs in young women (average age, 23 years) and is often associated with a paraneoplastic hypercalcemia. Like juvenile granulosa cell tumor, small cell carcinoma, hypercalcemic type has follicle-like spaces and brisk mitotic activity. Distinguishing features of small cell carcinoma, hypercalcemic type include more striking mitotic activity, more varied architecture to the follicle-like spaces (versus better-defined follicles of juvenile granulosa cell tumor), more diffuse/sheet-like growth pattern (versus nodular growth pattern of juvenile granulosa cell tumor), lack of reactivity for inhibin, and extra-ovarian spread at the time of diagnosis.

Juvenile granulosa cell tumor versus microcystic stromal tumor: Microcystic stromal tumor is a benign ovarian tumor that is characterized by a distinctive microcystic appearance. It has been described in women aged 26 to 63 years (average age, 45 years). Like juvenile granulosa cell tumor, microcystic stromal tumor contains cysts/follicle-like spaces and may have nodular

growth pattern and myxoid background. Immunohistochemical stains are key to distinguishing the tumors. Microcystic stromal tumors are positive for CD10, have nuclear immunoreactivity to beta-catenin (due to *CTNNB1* mutations), and are negative for inhibin and calretinin (Fig. 2.20). Juvenile granulosa cell tumors and microcystic stromal tumors are distinguished from metastatic carcinomas by epithelial membrane antigen (EMA) immunohistochemical stain—both juvenile granulosa cell tumor and microcystic stromal tumor are EMA negative, while carcinomas metastatic to the ovary (including signet ring carcinomas/Krukenberg tumors) are generally EMA positive.

SERTOLI-LEYDIG CELL TUMOR

Sertoli-Leydig cell tumors are rare and represent <0.5% of all ovarian neoplasms. They have been reported over a wide age range (1–84 years) but are more common in young patients (average age, 25 years). Patients with

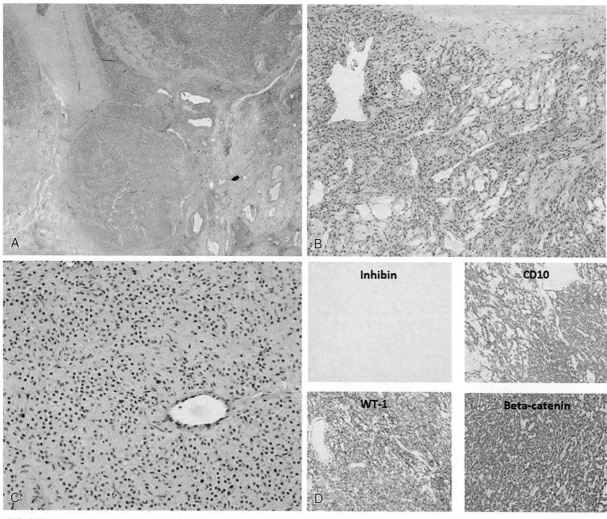

FIG. 2.20

Microcystic stromal tumor. Like juvenile granulosa cell tumor, microcystic stromal tumor may have nodular growth pattern **(A)**, microcystic spaces in myxoid background **(B)**, and luteinized cells **(C)**. **D,** Immunohistochemical stains were key to reaching the correct diagnosis. Microcystic stromal tumors are inhibin negative, CD10 and WT-1 positive, and show nuclear beta-catenin.

Sertoli-Leydig cell tumors present with androgenic manifestations 40% to 60% of the time. On rare occasions, Sertoli-Leydig cell tumors may be estrogenizing or result in elevated AFP (though not as marked an elevation as that seen in yolk sac tumor). Sertoli-Leydig cell tumors are typically unilateral solid and cystic yellow masses; occasionally, particularly in poorly differentiated tumors, areas of hemorrhage and necrosis may be present. Sertoli-Leydig cell tumors are assigned into three prognostically significant grade categories based on the degree of tubular differentiation of the Sertoli component and the quantity of primitive gonadal stroma.

1. Well-differentiated Sertoli-Leydig cell tumors (Fig. 2.21): Sertoli cells form open or closed tubules and are separated into lobules by fibromatous stroma containing Leydig cells. There is minimal cytologic atypia and low mitotic rate.

2. Moderately differentiated Sertoli-Leydig cell tumors (Fig. 2.22): Sertoli cells are arranged diffusely or form poorly developed tubules, nests, cords, or thyroid follicle-like microcysts and are separated by hypocellular edematous stroma. Leydig cells may be admixed with the Sertoli cells or present in the stroma. Mitotic figures may be seen (average, 5 MF/10 HPF).

3. Poorly differentiated Sertoli-Leydig cell tumors (Figs. 2.23 and 2.24): Sarcomatoid stroma predominates. Mitotic rate is variable but usually high (up to 20 MF/10 HPF). Poorly formed Sertoli tubules may be focally present, aiding the diagnosis. Leydig cells are rare or absent.

Heterologous elements may be present in moderately and poorly differentiated Sertoli-Leydig cell tumors. The most common heterologous element is mucinous epithelium of gastrointestinal type. The heterologous mucinous

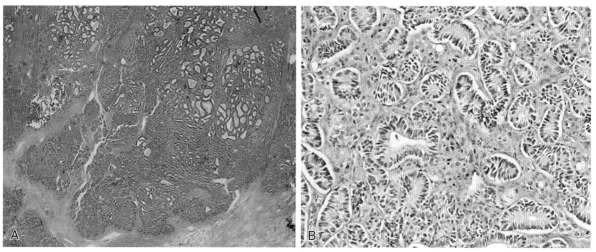

FIG. 2.21
Well-differentiated Sertoli-Leydig cell tumor. **A,** Sertoli cells form tubules separated into lobules by fibromatous stroma. **B,** Numerous Leydig cells are present in the stroma.

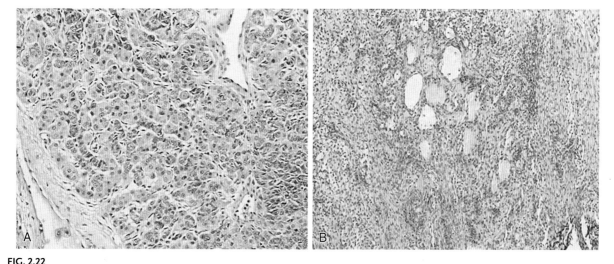

FIG. 2.22
Moderately differentiated Sertoli-Leydig cell tumor. **A,** Sertoli cells form ill-defined tubules/cords with admixed Leydig cells. **B,** Foci of thyroid follicle-like microcysts may be present in a background of edematous stroma.

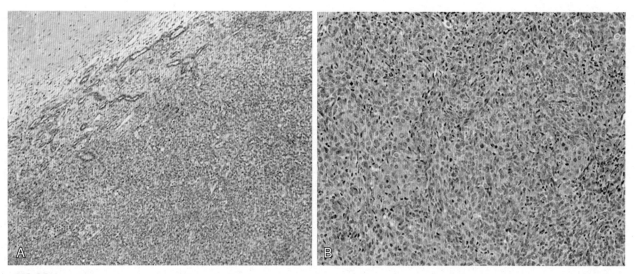

FIG. 2.23

Poorly differentiated Sertoli-Leydig cell tumor. **A,** Sarcomatoid stroma predominates; however, tubules may be present focally aiding the diagnosis. **B,** Leydig cells may rarely also be present and are a helpful diagnostic aid when observed.

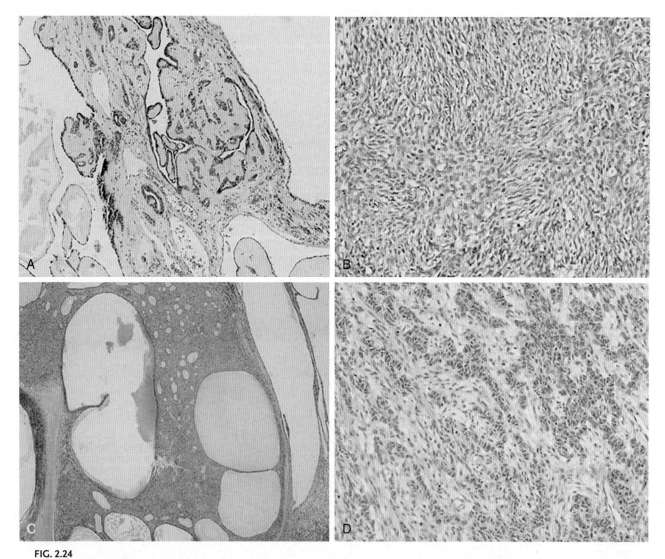

FIG. 2.24

Poorly differentiated Sertoli-Leydig cell tumor. Other histologic features that may be observed include: **A,** Retiform regions. **B,** Diffuse growth of primitive-appearing mesenchyme. Focal granulosa cell–like areas with macrocysts/follicles **(C)** or trabeculae **(D)**.

epithelium is typically benign but may be borderline or malignant. Other heterologous elements encountered in Sertoli-Leydig cell tumors include carcinoid tumor, heterologous mesenchyme (commonly cartilage and skeletal muscle), hepatic differentiation, and neuroblastoma. Moderately and poorly differentiated Sertoli-Leydig cell tumors may occasionally display areas of anastomosing slit-like spaces resembling rete testis. When the retiform pattern is substantial, the term retiform Sertoli-Leydig cell tumor is used. Sertoli-Leydig cell tumors may have a granulosa cell tumor component, but the tumor is classified based on the predominant histology. It is recommended that the term gynandroblastoma (or sex cord stromal tumor of mixed types) be reserved for those tumors where significant, large discrete foci (perhaps 40%–50%) of a neoplasm represents one variant of sex cord stromal tumor and the other sizable component represents another.

The microfollicular and trabecular patterns of adult granulosa cell tumor may mimic the tubules of well-to-moderately differentiated Sertoli-Leydig cell tumor. Sertoli-Leydig cell tumor is distinguished by the presence of Leydig cells. Adult granulosa cell tumors also have grooved nuclei and, upon thorough sampling, often show a diversity of growth patterns. Clinically, granulosa cell tumors tend to be estrogenizing in contrast to typically androgenizing Sertoli-Leydig cell tumors. Poorly differentiated Sertoli-Leydig cell tumors are distinguished from fibrosarcomas by the clinical features (Sertoli-Leydig cell tumors occur in younger reproductive age group and often have associated androgenizing hormonal manifestations, while fibrosarcomas occur in postmenopausal women and are often hormonally silent) and the findings of Leydig cells and/or better-differentiated areas resembling typical Sertoli-Leydig cell tumor on thorough histologic evaluation.

Sertoli-Leydig cell tumor versus gonadoblastoma: Gonadoblastoma is a rare tumor comprising a mixture of sex cord cells and germ cells that occurs predominantly in patients with Swyer syndrome (i.e., patients with 46 XY karyotype but who are phenotypically females due to *SRY* mutations that lead to gonadal dysgenesis). Gonadoblastoma can be viewed as an *in situ* form of malignant germ cell tumor. Histologic sections of gonadoblastoma show nests formed by sex cord-type cells surrounding primitive germ cells, separated by fibrous stroma that may contain lutein or Leydig cells (Fig. 2.25). Due to the presence of stromal Leydig cells, the differential diagnosis with Sertoli-Leydig cell tumor may arise. Distinguishing features of gonadoblastoma include bilaterality and the presence of germ cells, which can be highlighted by SALL4 immunohistochemical stain.

CARCINOMA (PRIMARY OR METASTATIC)

Adult granulosa cell tumors have striking epithelial differentiation, that is, form cohesive clusters/nests raising a morphologic differential diagnosis of various primary ovarian carcinomas or carcinomas metastatic to the ovary. For example, adult granulosa cell tumors with insular, trabecular, and microfollicular patterns may resemble endometrioid adenocarcinoma, adult granulosa cell tumors with papillary growth pattern may resemble serous or transitional cell carcinoma, and adult granulosa cell tumors with watered silk pattern may resemble metastatic breast carcinoma. Likewise, Sertoli-Leydig cell tumors form tubules that may mimic ovarian endometrioid adenocarcinomas. Helpful morphologic clues present in carcinomas but not observed in granulosa or Sertoli-Leydig cell tumors include stromal desmoplasia, which, though not always present in ovarian carcinomas, is a helpful clue when present, cytoplasmic mucin, squamous differentiation (in endometrioid carcinoma), and high-grade cytologic atypia and/or necrosis (serous/transitional cell carcinoma). Other useful background clues include concurrent endometriosis or adenofibroma in endometrioid adenocarcinomas (Fig. 2.26). Useful immunohistochemical stains include EMA (positive in carcinomas, but negative in most sex cord stromal tumors) and sex cord stromal markers (FOXL2, inhibin, etc.), which are positive in sex cord stromal tumors but negative in primary ovarian carcinomas. The clinical history of malignancy at other site, presence of bilateral masses, and involvement of the ovarian surface are noteworthy features in cases of metastasis to the ovary.

Prognosis and Therapy

Adult granulosa cell tumors are initially treated with surgical resection and complete staging. Prognosis is stage-dependent. Most patients present with stage I disease have good prognosis with 10-year survival rates at 90% to 95%. Late recurrences (up to 20 years postop) do occur. Recurrence risk is associated with stage (patients with extra-ovarian spread at initial presentation are at increased risk of recurrence) and tumor rupture. Adjuvant chemotherapy and/or radiation may be needed for stage II–IV disease.

The malignant potential of Sertoli-Leydig cell tumors depends on the grade of the tumor. Well-differentiated Sertoli-Leydig cell tumors are benign, while poorly differentiated tumors are generally malignant; the moderately differentiated tumors behave in a malignant fashion about 10% of the time. Sertoli-Leydig cell tumors are associated with *Dicer1* mutations; patients with germline *Dicer1* mutations may have a syndrome: Sertoli-Leydig cell tumors, pleuropulmonary blastomas, multinodular goiters, cervical embryonal rhabdomyosarcomas—testing for germline *Dicer1* mutation is recommended in patients diagnosed with Sertoli-Leydig cell tumors.

Useful diagnostic features of select ovarian sex cord stromal tumors are summarized in Table 2.11.

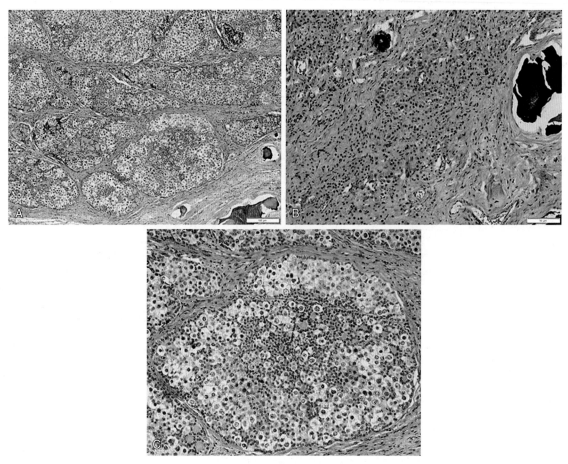

FIG. 2.25

Gonadoblastoma. Like Sertoli-Leydig cell tumor, gonadoblastoma may be separated into lobules by fibromatous stroma **(A)** and contain stromal Leydig cells **(B)**. The germ cell component of gonadoblastoma is appreciated (cells with clear cytoplasm) on high power **(C)**.

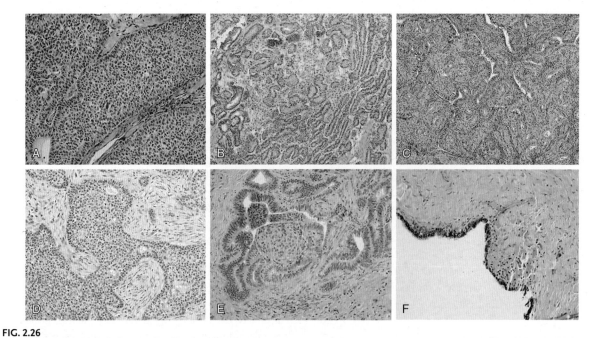

FIG. 2.26

Sex cord stromal tumor versus primary ovarian carcinoma or metastasis to the ovary. Adult granulosa cell tumors may show striking epithelial differentiation **(A)**, while both Sertoli-Leydig cell tumor **(B)** and endometrioid adenocarcinoma **(C)** form tubules. Note lack of stromal desmoplasia in adult granulosa cell tumor **(A)** in contrast to carcinoma **(D)**. Note presence of Leydig cells in Sertoli-Leydig cell tumor **(B)**. Helpful clues in endometrioid adenocarcinoma include background adenofibroma with squamous morules **(E)** and background endometriosis **(F)**.

TABLE 2.11

Summary of Characteristics of Select Ovarian Sex Cord Stromal Tumors

	Fibroma	Thecoma	Adult Granulosa Cell Tumor	Juvenile Granulosa Cell Tumor	Sertoli-Leydig Cell Tumor
Clinical	Most common sex cord stromal tumor. Typically unilateral and in patients aged > 40 years. Typically **lacks endocrine manifestations.**	Typically unilateral; postmenopausal women (avg. 59 years) Often **estrogenic;** concurrent endometrial cancer in 20% of cases.	Second most common sex cord stromal tumor. Typically unilateral and occurs over a wide age range (avg. 53 year). **Estrogenic;** concurrent endometrial cancer in 10%. Serum inhibin may be elevated.	Typically in patients aged <30 years; (avg. 15 years). Typically unilateral. Estrogenic; (isosexual pseudoprecocity in prepubescent; menometrorrhagia or postmenopausal bleeding in older). Serum inhibin may be elevated.	Rare (<0.5% of ovarian neoplasms). Typically unilateral; wide age range (1–84 years) but more common in young patients (avg. 25 years). **Androgenic** (40%–60% of patients).
Pathology	**Gross:** white to tan; well-circumscribed; smooth surface Microscopic: resembles ovarian stroma, i.e., composed of bland spindle cells; may have collagen bands or hyaline plaques; may be mitotically active (4–19 MF/10 HPF); may have diffuse calcification (Gorlin syndrome); may have minor sex cord elements (<10% of the neoplasm). Reticulin surrounds individual cells.	**Gross:** typically solid, yellow lobulated cut surface Microscopic: cells resemble the theca interna—uniform oval to round nuclei and pale grayish-pink cytoplasm with ill-defined borders; alternating with spindle cells (fibromatous background); separated by collagen; Reticulin surrounds individual cells.	**Gross:** typically solid/cystic; solid areas usually yellow; cystic areas may be hemorrhagic or necrotic Microscopic: variety of growth patterns—diffuse, insular, microfollicular (Call-Exner bodies), macrofollicular (larger follicles), trabecular, pseudopapillary, watered silk (less common). May be homogenous but often mixed patterns in the same tumor. Component cells resemble normal ovarian granulosa cells: round to oval angulated/grooved nuclei, scant cytoplasm; occasionally may be luteinized. Variable mitotic activity; rarely nuclear atypia. Fibromatous or thecomatous background stroma common. Reticulin surrounds aggregates of tumor cells.	**Gross:** similar to adult granulosa cell tumor: solid/cystic yellow; +/−hemorrhage/necrosis. Microscopic: nodular or diffuse growth; myxoid or edematous background; punctuated by follicles (or follicle-like spaces) of varying shapes and sizes. Follicles may contain eosinophilic or basophilic secretions. Cytology: round to oval nuclei; tiny nucleoli, abundant eosinophilic cytoplasm; nuclear grooves are rare. Variable cytologic atypia and mitotic activity; atypical mitosis may be present. Generally less conspicuous stroma than AGCT, but may occasionally have prominent fibromatous or sclerotic stroma. May have frequent luteinized cells. Reticulin surrounds aggregates of tumor cells.	**Gross features:** solid/cystic yellow; +/−hemorrhage/necrosis (especially poorly differentiated) Microscopic: well-differentiated; Sertoli cells form tubules (may be open or closed); minimal cytologic atypia; low mitotic rate; separated into lobules by fibromatous stroma containing Leydig cells—may occur singly or in clusters. Moderately differentiated: lobulated growth pattern with cellular regions (contain Sertoli cells arranged diffusely or forming poorly developed tubules, nests, or cords; may occasionally form thyroid follicle-like microcysts) separated by hypocellular edematous stroma; Leydig cells may be admixed with the Sertoli cells or be present in the periphery or in the stroma. **Poorly differentiated:** diffuse sarcomatous growth; may be difficult to make a diagnosis of SLCT, but minor component of moderately differentiated areas helps. Heterologous elements may be present.

Continued

TABLE 2.11

Summary of Characteristics of Select Ovarian Sex Cord Stromal Tumors—cont'd

	Fibroma	Thecoma	Adult Granulosa Cell Tumor	Juvenile Granulosa Cell Tumor	Sertoli-Leydig Cell Tumor
Molecular	Gorlin syndrome a/w PTCH mutations LOH at 9q22.3 LOH at 19p13.3 (STK11) Trisomy/ Tetrasomy 12.	FOXL2 mutations in 12.5%–21% of cases.	FOXL2 (402 C to G) point mutation; Trisomy 12, 14; Monosomy 16, 22; del 16q; TERT promoter mutations → more aggressive behavior.	Trisomy 12 Generally lack FOXL2 mutations Associated with Ollier disease Maffucci syndrome	*Dicer1* mutations;
Prognosis	Benign—cured by oophorectomy	Benign—cured by oophorectomy	Malignant. Late recurrences (5–20 years after initial treatment). Unfavorable factors: advanced stage; large size; bilaterality; rupture.	Malignant. Stage-dependent. Recurrences within 3 years; Recurrence risk: rupture, positive peritoneal cytology, extra-ovarian spread.	Depends on grade adverse outcomes: grade, mesenchymal heterologous elements, rupture, stage.

ADULT GRANULOSA CELL TUMOR– DISEASE FACT SHEET

Definition
▶▶ Low-grade malignant sex cord tumor composed of granulosa cells, often displaying a variety of growth patterns

Epidemiology
▶▶ Second most common ovarian sex cord stromal tumor (most common ovarian sex cord tumor)
▶▶ Occurs at any age, but most common in perimenopausal women (median age, 50 years)

Clinical Features
▶▶ Most patients present with estrogenizing hormonal manifestations—e.g., precocious pseudopuberty and abnormal uterine bleeding.
▶▶ Serum β−inhibin levels may be elevated.

Prognosis and Therapy
▶▶ Treated by surgical resection and staging
▶▶ Stage-dependent prognosis

ADULT GRANULOSA CELL TUMOR – PATHOLOGIC FEATURES

Gross Findings
▶▶ Typically yellow solid and cystic masses with foci of necrosis and hemorrhage

Microscopic Findings
▶▶ Variety of growth patterns—diffuse, insular, macrofollicular, papillary, microfollicular with Call-Exner bodies
▶▶ Often has fibromatous or thecomatous background stroma
▶▶ Component cells are often grooved

Pathologic Differential Diagnosis
▶▶ Fibroma/thecoma
▶▶ Juvenile granulosa cell tumor
▶▶ Sertoli-Leydig cell tumor
▶▶ Carcinoma (primary or metastatic)

OVARIAN MATURE TERATOMA

DIFFERENTIAL DIAGNOSES: IMMATURE TERATOMA AND MONODERMAL TERATOMAS

Clinical Features

Germ cell tumors are a heterogeneous group of neoplasms that arise from the primordial germ cell and can occur anywhere along the midline axis of migration of primordial germ cells to the gonadal ridge; hence, germ cell tumors are found in both gonadal (ovaries/testes) and extragonadal sites (e.g., mediastinum, abdominopelvic cavity, sacrum, vagina, and vulva). Ovarian germ cell tumors account for 30% to 50% of all ovarian neoplasms. Germ cell tumors are the most common ovarian neoplasms in children, adolescents, and young adults.

Mature teratomas, composed of mature tissue derived from two or three germ cell layers, are by far the most common ovarian germ cell tumors accounting for 80% to 95% of all ovarian germ cell tumors. Both mature and immature teratomas may be associated with N-methyl-D-aspartate (NMDA) receptor encephalitis, a potentially fatal paraneoplastic encephalitis, characterized by psychiatric symptoms, seizures, and autonomic dysfunction as a result of antibodies to NMDA receptors produced by some teratomas. Patients often recover after a combination of teratoma resection and immunosuppression.

Pathologic Features

GROSS FINDINGS

Mature teratomas may be cystic (mature cystic teratoma) or solid (mature solid teratoma). The mature cystic teratomas are far more common. The cysts often contain varying amounts of sebaceous material and hair. Adipose tissue, teeth, and bone may occasionally be grossly apparent.

Microscopic Findings

Histologic sections of mature teratomas show mature tissue derived from two to three germ cell layers—most commonly ectoderm-derived tissues such as skin and mature neuroectoderm. Mesoderm derivatives such as adipose tissue and bone are commonly also present. Endoderm derivatives such as gastrointestinal tract, respiratory tract, and thyroid may also be present (Fig. 2.27).

Ancillary Studies

Not useful.

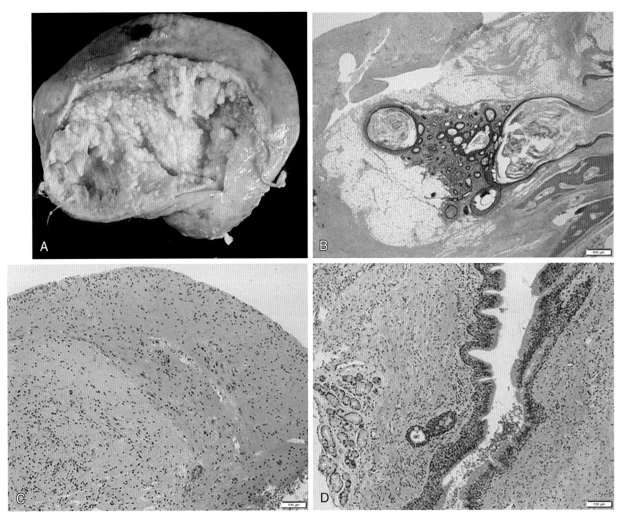

FIG. 2.27

Mature teratoma. **A,** Gross. Mature teratomas are typically unilocular cystic masses containing sebaceous material and hair. Teeth may also be present. **B,** Sections of mature teratomas show mature tissue derived from two to three germ cell layers, such as ectoderm-derived epidermis and brain tissue and mesoderm-derived adipose tissue and bone. **C,** Mature brain tissue, medium power. **D,** Endoderm-derived tissue such as respiratory epithelium may also be present.

Differential Diagnosis

IMMATURE TERATOMA

Immature teratomas most often occur in children and young adults (median age, 18 years). Patients with immature teratomas present with symptoms associated with an abdominopelvic mass. AFP may be elevated, though not to the extent observed in yolk sac tumor.

Immature teratomas are typically large solid masses with fleshy cut sections grossly (Fig. 2.28). On histologic sections, immature teratomas are defined by the presence of immature neuroepithelium (Fig. 2.29) and are graded by the amount of immature neuroepithelium present. Low-grade (grade 1) tumors contain rare foci (<1 low-power [4×]) field) of immature neuroepithelium, whereas high-grade tumors contain 1 to 3 low-power fields (grade 2) or > 3 low-power fields (grade 3) of immature neuroepithelium in any slide. Variations of mature teratomas that should be distinguished from immature teratoma include:

Mature solid teratoma versus immature teratoma: Both mature solid teratoma and immature teratoma are grossly solid masses. However, histologic sections of mature solid teratoma reveal only mature tissues without any immature neuroepithelium. Thorough sampling of mature solid teratomas is necessary to exclude the diagnosis of immature teratoma.

Mature teratoma with differentiated neural tissue versus immature teratoma (Fig. 2.30): Fully differentiated cellular neural tissue such as granular layer of cerebellum and ependymal rests in mature teratomas should not be misdiagnosed as immature teratoma. Truly immature neural elements that warrant a diagnosis of immature teratoma show vesicular chromatin, apoptosis, and mitosis. Differentiated neural tissue tends to be organized and lacks apoptosis and mitosis.

Mature cystic teratoma with microscopic foci of immature neuroepithelium versus immature teratoma: An otherwise grossly typical mature cystic teratoma/dermoid cyst may rarely contain microscopic foci of immature neuroepithelium. Because mature cystic teratomas, even with microscopic foci of immature neuroepithelium, have good prognosis, the presence of immature neuroepithelium in an otherwise grossly typical dermoid cyst is insufficient to warrant a diagnosis of immature teratoma. Such cases are diagnosed as mature teratoma with microscopic foci of neuroepithelium.

Features useful in distinguishing mature from immature teratomas are presented in Table 2.12.

MONODERMAL TERATOMAS

Monodermal teratomas, composed predominantly of one tissue type, include struma ovarii (thyroid tissue), carcinoid tumors (may be insular, trabecular, strumal [i.e., mixture of carcinoid and thyroid tissue], or mucinous/goblet cell), sebaceous tumors, and neuroectodermal-type tumors. The prognosis of monodermal teratomas depends on the component tissue type. Struma ovarii is typically benign (though a small subset of patients with thyroid-type carcinomas has poor outcomes). Stage I insular, trabecular, and strumal carcinoids have excellent prognosis (100% 5-year survival); patients with stage III–IV tumors fare worse (33% 5-year survival). Mucinous/goblet cell carcinoids may be aggressive, especially if associated with carcinomatous component. Sebaceous tumors composed of histologically benign sebaceous components have benign outcome, whereas sebaceous carcinomas may be clinically malignant.

Neuroectodermal-type tumors are divided into the differentiated group (ependymoma, astrocytoma, and oligodendroglioma), primitive group (primitive

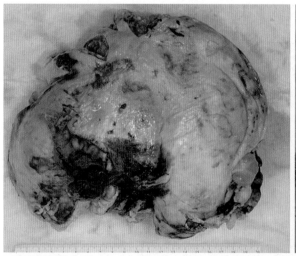
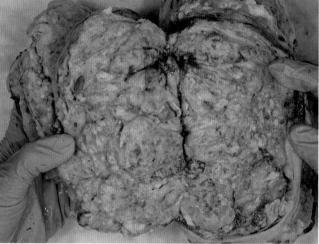

FIG. 2.28

Immature teratoma. Immature teratomas are typically large solid masses with fleshy (and sometimes fatty) cut surfaces.

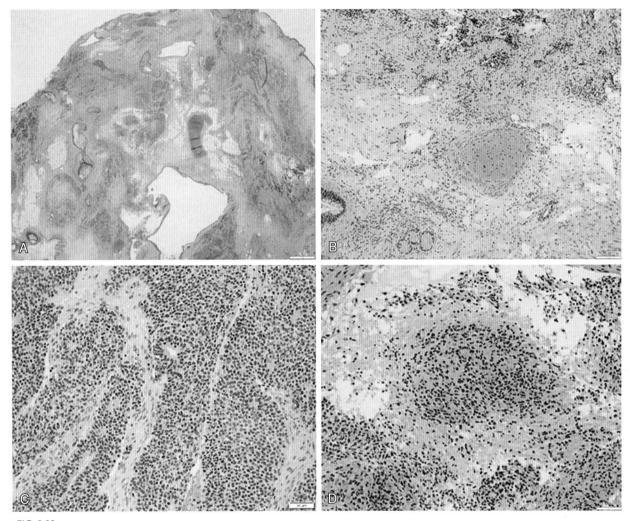

FIG. 2.29

Histologic sections of immature teratoma. **A,** Ectodermal, mesodermal, and endodermal derivatives are observed (2×). Immature cartilage may be present **(B)**. It is the presence of immature neuroepithelium that defines immature teratoma—primitive neuroepithelial tubules **(C),** cellular atypical neuroglia **(D)**.

neuroectodermal tumors [PNETs], neuroblastoma, medulloblastoma, embryonal tumor with multilayered rosettes, and medulloepithelioma), and anaplastic group (glioblastoma). The neuroectodermal-type tumors are generally malignant, with their prognosis being stage-dependent. The primitive and anaplastic group tumors are more aggressive than the differentiated group tumors.

Immature teratoma versus PNET and other monodermal neuroectodermal-type tumors: High-grade immature teratomas may contain abundant mitotically active neuroepithelium raising the differential of malignant neuroectodermal tumors. The malignant neuroectodermal tumors are distinguished by confluent growth and effacement of the pre-existing architecture of the underlying teratoma, that is, a significant proportion of a single tumor displays immature neuroectodermal tissue without the admixture of other ectoderm-, mesoderm-, or endoderm-derived tissue types.

Prognosis and Therapy

Mature teratomas are benign and have excellent prognosis. On rare occasions, somatic-type malignancies may arise from mature teratomas. Somatic-type carcinomas that arise are most commonly squamous cell carcinomas, but adenocarcinomas may also be found. Other somatic-type malignancies, including melanoma and various sarcomas, may also arise in mature teratomas but are uncommon. The prognosis of immature teratomas depends on stage and grade.

Mixed germ cell tumors account for around 8% to 10% of ovarian germ cell tumors. As the presence of yolk sac tumor, embryonal carcinoma, and/or choriocarcinoma warrants adjuvant chemotherapy in even stage I tumors, thorough sampling of all germ cell tumors (at least one section per centimeter), including additional sections of areas that appear different, is

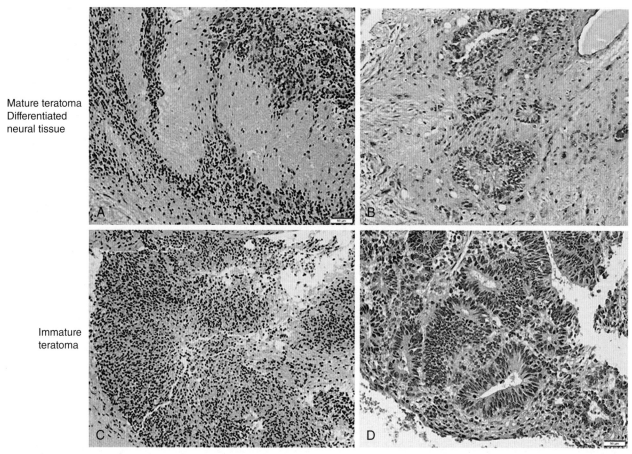

Mature teratoma
Differentiated
neural tissue

Immature
teratoma

FIG. 2.30

Mature teratoma with differentiated neural tissue versus immature teratoma. Differentiated neural tissue of mature teratoma such as cerebellum (**A**; note organization with molecular layer, Purkinje cell layer, and granular layer) and ependymal rests (**B**) should not be mistaken for immature teratoma, which shows disorganized cellular neuroglia (**C**) and neuroepithelial tubules/rosettes with frequent mitosis (**D**).

TABLE 2.12

Mature Versus Immature Teratoma

	Mature Teratoma	Immature Teratoma
Epidemiology/clinical presentation	Wide age range, typically reproductive age. Patients present with mass symptoms. Rarely, NMDA receptor encephalitis.	Mostly children and young adults (average age, 18 years). Patients present with mass symptoms; AFP may be mildly elevated. Rarely, NMDA receptor encephalitis.
Gross features	Typically cystic; typically contains sebaceous material and hair.	Typically solid with fleshy cut surface; may have hemorrhage and necrosis.
Histology	Composed of mature tissue from two or three germ layers—typically ectoderm predominant. May have cellular mature neural tissue (e.g., cerebellar granular layer) that should not be confused for immature teratoma. A microscopic focus of immature neuroepithelium in an otherwise grossly typical mature cystic teratoma/dermoid cyst should be diagnosed as mature cystic teratoma with microscopic foci of neuroepithelium and not as immature teratoma.	Defined by the presence of immature neuroepithelium that is mitotically active and has notable apoptosis. Graded based on the amount of immature neuroepithelium present.
Treatment	May be treated by cystectomy or unilateral oophorectomy.	Low-grade stage I tumors are treated by surgery and observation, while high-grade/stage II or higher tumors are treated with surgery and adjuvant chemotherapy.
Prognosis	Good: benign.	Depends on the grade and stage.

important in order to identify or exclude other components. The percentages of the various germ cell components should be reported.

MATURE TERATOMA – DISEASE FACT SHEET

Definition
▸▸ Benign germ cell tumor composed of mature tissues derived from two to three germ cell layers—ectoderm, mesoderm, and/or endoderm

Epidemiology
▸▸ Most common ovarian germ cell tumor
▸▸ Occurs in all age groups—most commonly reproductive age

Clinical Features
▸▸ Most patients present with symptoms attributable to ovarian mass.
▸▸ Rarely, patients present with anti-NMDA receptor encephalitis.

Prognosis and Therapy
▸▸ Treated by surgical resection
▸▸ Benign; good prognosis
▸▸ Rare cases are associated with somatic-type malignancies and have poor outcomes.

MATURE TERATOMA – PATHOLOGIC FEATURES

Gross Findings
▸▸ Typically cystic masses with varying amounts of sebaceous material and hair

Microscopic Findings
▸▸ Varying components of mature ectoderm-, mesoderm-, and endoderm-derived tissues.

Pathologic Differential Diagnosis
▸▸ Immature teratoma
▸▸ Monodermal teratomas

DYSGERMINOMA

DIFFERENTIAL DIAGNOSES: EMBRYONAL CARCINOMA, YOLK SAC TUMOR, AND LYMPHOMA

Clinical Features

Dysgerminomas are the most common malignant germ cell tumors and typically occur in children and young women (average age, 22 years). Patients with dysgerminomas typically present with abdominopelvic mass symptoms and elevated lactate dehydrogenase (LDH). Occasionally, β-HCG may be elevated and accompanied

with estrogenic hormonal manifestations. Rarely, paraneoplastic hypercalcemia may be observed.

Pathologic Features

GROSS FINDINGS

Dysgerminomas are typically solid masses with lobulated tan/light brown cut surface. Necrosis, hemorrhage, and/or cystic degeneration may occasionally be present. Foci of calcification suggest the possibility of an underlying gonadoblastoma. Dysgerminomas should be thoroughly sampled to exclude other germ cell components that may alter the type of adjuvant therapy.

MICROSCOPIC FINDINGS

Histologic sections of dysgerminomas show sheets of polygonal cells with abundant granular eosinophilic or clear cytoplasm with distinct cell membranes, separated by lymphocyte-rich fibrous septa (Fig. 2.31). Epithelioid histiocytes and sarcoid-like granulomas may be present. β-HCG-producing syncytiotrophoblastic giant cells may also occasionally be observed. Smears from fine-needle aspiration of dysgerminomas show uniform cells with round to oval nuclei, granular chromatin, and prominent nucleoli in a tigroid background, composed of stripped glycogen-rich cytoplasm. A second population comprising lymphocytes and/or granulomas is typically observed.

Ancillary Studies

Dysgerminomas stain positive for SALL4, OCT3/4, and c-Kit (CD117).

Differential Diagnosis

EMBRYONAL CARCINOMA

Embryonal carcinoma is a rare aggressive malignant germ cell neoplasm that, like dysgerminoma, occurs in children and young women and may be associated with elevated β-HCG. Similar to dysgerminoma, histologic sections may show sheets/diffuse growth of polygonal cells with abundant cytoplasm and distinct cytoplasmic boundaries, occasionally with interspersed syncytiotrophoblasts. Embryonal carcinomas are distinguished from dysgerminomas by their more extreme cytologic atypia—embryonal carcinomas have pleomorphic nuclei, abundant mitotic figures, apoptosis, and a dirty, necrotic background. Embryonal carcinomas also lack the lymphocyte-rich fibrous stroma that

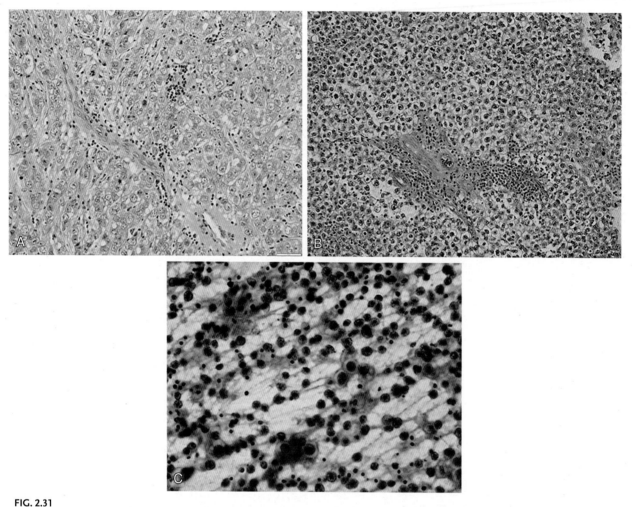

FIG. 2.31

Dysgerminoma. Ovarian dysgerminomas **(A)** are morphologically identical to seminomas **(B)**. Sections show cells with squared-off nuclei, prominent nucleoli, and clear cytoplasm with distinct cell borders; fibrous septate-containing lymphocytes are notable. Smears show cells with clear cytoplasm and distinct cell borders in a tigroid background containing lymphocytes **(C)**.

is characteristic of dysgerminomas. CD30 and c-KIT are useful immunohistochemical stains; embryonal carcinomas are CD30 positive and cKIT negative, whereas dysgerminomas are cKIT positive and CD30 negative (Fig. 2.32). Embryonal carcinomas stain diffusely positive for cytokeratins (vs. limited cytokeratin positivity in dysgerminomas).

YOLK SAC TUMOR

Yolk sac tumors are rapidly growing highly malignant germ cell tumors composed of cells that exhibit differentiation into endodermal structures, namely yolk sac (reticular/microcystic/cribriform/tubular patterns), allantois (polyvesicular pattern), primitive gut (glandular pattern), liver (hepatoid pattern), and mesenchyme (mesenchymal overgrowth). Yolk sac tumors occur in childhood and adolescence (average age, 19 years) and are almost as common as dysgerminomas in females younger than 20 years old. Patients with yolk sac tumors typically present with abdominopelvic mass

symptoms and markedly elevated AFP (>1000 ng/mL). CA-125 may also be elevated. Up to one third of patients present with extra-ovarian spread. Yolk sac tumors are typically large solid and cystic masses with friable fleshy cut surface, frequently containing areas of hemorrhage and necrosis. There may be gross evidence of other germ cell components—most often mature cystic teratoma and/or dysgerminoma. Histologic sections (Fig. 2.33) show primitive cells with clear to eosinophilic cytoplasm and large hyperchromatic nuclei with brisk mitotic activity growing in various patterns, including reticular, microcystic, pseudopapillary, solid, polyvesicular, glandular, and hepatoid. Typically, a combination of two or more patterns co-exists. Schiller-Duval bodies (central blood vessels surrounded by loose stroma and an outer mantle of cuboidal to columnar neoplastic cells) are pathognomonic but only occur in ~30% of cases. Hyaline globules are common. Due to the significantly worse prognosis of yolk sac tumors, it is important to distinguish the solid pattern yolk sac tumors from dysgerminomas. Helpful histologic

Dysgerminoma   Embryonal carcinoma

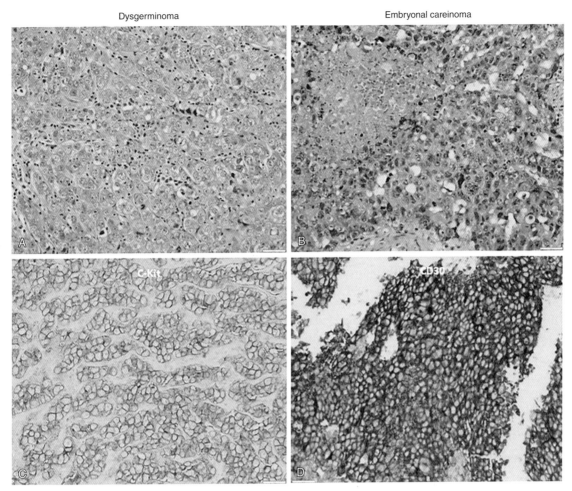

FIG. 2.32

Dysgerminoma versus embryonal carcinoma. **A,** Dysgerminoma contains stromal lymphocytes. **B,** Embryonal carcinoma has more pleomorphic cells with notable necrosis, apoptosis, and frequent mitosis. Dysgerminomas stain positive for c-Kit **(C)**, while embryonal carcinomas stain positive for CD30 **(D).**

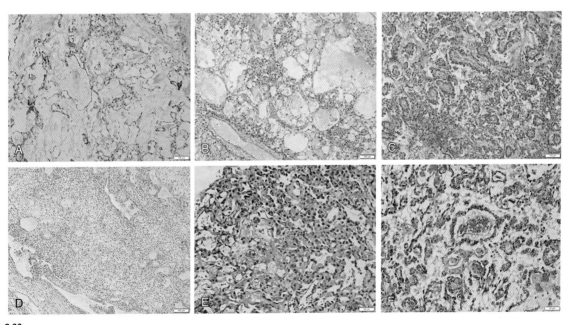

FIG. 2.33

Yolk sac tumor. Yolk sac tumors typically display a variety of growth patterns including reticular **(A),** microcystic **(B)** and papillary **(C)**. Mesenchymal overgrowth **(D)** and hyaline globules **(E)** may be present. Schiller-Duval bodies **(F)** are pathognomonic (when present).

clues include the presence of lymphoid-rich stroma in dysgerminomas and the presence of hyaline globules and Schiller-Duval bodies in yolk sac tumors. In addition, well-sampled yolk sac tumors would typically display other more characteristic growth patterns, at least focally. Dysgerminomas stain positive for OCT3/4, whereas yolk sac tumors stain positive for CDX-2, AFP, and glypican 3.

Features useful in distinguishing the non-teratomatous malignant germ cell tumors—dysgerminoma, embryonal carcinoma, yolk sac tumor, and choriocarcinoma—are presented in Table 2.13.

Yolk sac tumor versus clear cell carcinoma: Both yolk sac tumor and clear cell carcinoma have growth patterns that include papillary, tubular, cystic, and solid architectures. Furthermore, both tumors are composed of cells with clear cytoplasm, and the fibrovascular cores of clear cell carcinoma may mimic yolk sac's Schiller-Duval bodies (Fig. 2.34). However, clear cell carcinoma typically occurs in older women (average age, 55 years), is frequently associated with

background endometrioisis or adenofibroma, and often shows characteristic hobnailing. Helpful immunohistochemical stains include EMA (positive in clear cell carcinomas but negative in yolk sac tumors) and SALL4 (positive in yolk sac tumors but negative in clear cell carcinomas).

LYMPHOMA

Ovarian lymphomas may have lobulated solid tan appearance, grossly similar to dysgerminomas. However, bilaterality and gross fallopian tube involvement are more commonly observed in lymphomas. Smears and/or touch preps are very helpful in distinguishing the neoplasms during intraoperative consultation. Lymphomas lack the tigroid background and second population of epithelioid cells with eosinophilic or clear cytoplasm and distinct cell borders characteristically observed in dysgerminomas. Lymphomas may stain positive for Oct4 and SALL4; therefore, careful attention to gross and histologic features in addition

---

TABLE 2.13

Distinguishing Features of Non-teratomatous Malignant Germ Cell Tumors

	Dysgerminoma	Embryonal Carcinoma	Yolk Sac Tumor	Choriocarcinoma
Epidemiology	Most common malignant germ cell tumor; occurs in children and young adults (average age, 22 years).	Rare. Occurs in children and young adults (average age, 15 years).	Common malignant germ cell tumor; occurs in children and young adults (average age, 19 years).	Rare. Typically occurs in children and young adults. Rare cases in postmenopausal women.
Clinical/serum findings	Elevated LDH; may have elevated beta-HCG (if syncytiotrophoblasts are present).	Often have elevated beta-HCG as syncytiotrophoblasts are often present. LDH may also be elevated.	Often have markedly elevated AFP (>1000 ng/mL). **If AFP is elevated clinically, sample tumor thoroughly to identify yolk sac component if not initially identified.**	Elevated beta-HCG (range from hundreds to >2 million mIU/mL).
Histology	Typically diffuse growth of polygonal cells with abundant eosinophilic to clear glycogen-rich cytoplasm and distinct cell boundaries separated by lymphoid stroma. Oct3/4 and c-KIT/CD117 positive. CD30 and AFP negative.	Typically diffuse growth of highly pleomorphic cells with vesicular nuclei, prominent nucleoli, and abundant cytoplasm with distinct boundaries. Numerous mitosis and apoptosis. Necrosis may be present. Syncytiotrophoblasts are common. No lymphoid stroma. CD30 and cytokeratin positive; c-KIT and AFP negative.	Typically displays variety of growth patterns—reticular most common, but can have solid growth mimicking dysgerminoma/embryonal carcinoma. Distinguished by the presence of Schiller-Duval bodies and hyaline globules. CDX-2, AFP, and glypican 3 positive; Oct3/4 and CD30 negative.	Cytotrophoblasts (round polygonal mononuclear cells with prominent nucleoli) in sheets/nests draped by syncytiotrophoblasts (multinucleated large cells with abundant cytoplasm). Extensive hemorrhage; vascular invasion is common. **Chorionic villi are typically absent (if present, exclude molar gestation).**
Treatment	Stage I—surgery and observation. Stage II or higher—surgery and adjuvant chemotherapy.	Surgery and adjuvant chemotherapy; BEP is typically used for malignant germ cell tumors.	Surgery and adjuvant chemotherapy.	Surgery and adjuvant chemotherapy
Prognosis	Good; chemo and radiation sensitive; >90% survival.	Aggressive tumors, but are chemosensitive.	Good with advent of cisplatin-based chemotherapies.	Aggressive—frequent lymphatic and hematogenous spread.

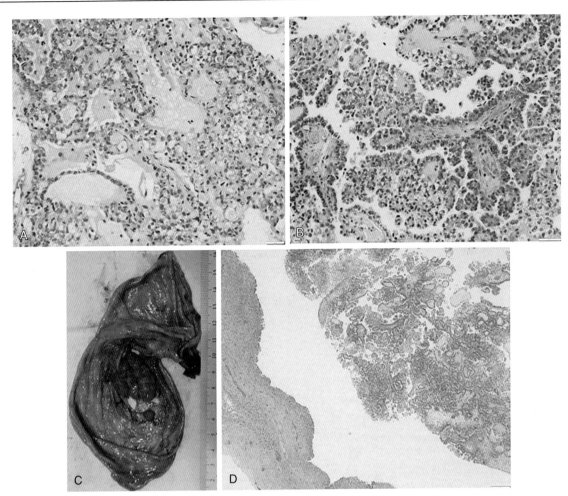

FIG. 2.34
Ovarian clear cell carcinoma. Like yolk sac tumors, ovarian clear cell carcinomas may have microcystic **(A)** and papillary growth patterns; fibrovascular cores in papillae may even mimic Schiller-Duval bodies **(B)**. However, In contrast to yolk sac tumors, clear cell carcinomas typically arise in a background of endometriosis/endometriotic cyst; gross **(C)**, low-power histology **(D)**. Clinically, clear cell carcinomas occur in older women.

to a panel of antibodies is necessary in distinguishing dysgerminomas from lymphomas. A PAS/diastase stain to highlight glycogen in dysgerminomas may be useful.

Prognosis and Therapy

Dysgerminomas generally carry good prognosis—the 10-year progression-free survival rate is >90%. Most patients have stage I disease at presentation and are treated with surgical resection and staging without need for adjuvant therapy. In contrast, patients with any stage of embryonal carcinoma, yolk sac tumor, or choriocarcinoma, or any of these components as part of a mixed germ cell tumor, require adjuvant chemotherapy. Patients with higher stage dysgerminomas also require adjuvant chemotherapy.

DYSGERMINOMA – DISEASE FACT SHEET

Definition
▶▶ Malignant germ cell tumor composed of polygonal cells with granular or clear cytoplasm, separated by lymphocyte-rich fibrous septae

Epidemiology
▶▶ Most common malignant ovarian germ cell tumor
▶▶ Occurs predominantly in children and young reproductive age women (average age, 22 years)

Clinical Features
▶▶ Most patients present with symptoms attributable to ovarian mass.
▶▶ Serum LDH is often elevated.

Prognosis and Therapy
▶▶ Treated by surgical resection and complete staging
▶▶ Generally good for stage I disease; most patients present with stage I disease

---

DYSGERMINOMA – PATHOLOGIC FEATURES

Gross Findings

▸▸ Typically large solid/fleshy tan or cream lobulated masses; hemorrhage and/or necrosis may be present

Microscopic Findings

▸▸ Typically sheets of polygonal cells with abundant clear or granular eosinophilic cytoplasm separated by fibrous septa containing lymphocytes
▸▸ The polygonal cells often display distinct cell membranes.
▸▸ Scattered syncytiotrophoblasts and granulomas may be present.

Pathologic Differential Diagnosis

▸▸ Embryonal carcinoma
▸▸ Yolk sac tumor, solid pattern
▸▸ Lymphoma

SUGGESTED READINGS

Vulvar Intraepithelial Neoplasia

Crum CP, Herrington CS, McCluggage WG, et al. Epithelial tumors. Tumors of the vulva. In: Kurman RJ, Carcangiu ML, Herrington CS, Young RH, eds. *World Health Organization Classification of Tumors of Female Reproductive Organs.* Lyon: IARC; 2014:232-234.

Darragh TM, Colgan TJ, Cox T, et al. The lower anogenital squamous terminology standardization project for HPV-associated lesions. *Arch Pathol Lab Med.* 2012;136:1266-1297.

Pinto AP, Miron A, Yassin Y, et al. Differentiated vulvar intraepithelial neoplasia contains Tp53 mutations and is genetically linked to vulvar squamous cell carcinoma. *Mod Pathol.* 2010;23:404-412.

Choschzick M, Hantaredja W, Tennstedt P, et al. Role of TP53 mutations in vulvar carcinomas. *Int J Gynecol Pathol.* 2011;30:497-504.

Watkins JC, Howitt BE, Horowitz NS, et al. Differentiated exophytic vulvar intraepithelial lesions are genetically distinct from keratinizing squamous cell carcinomas and contain mutations in PIK3CA. *Mod Pathol.* 2017;30:448-458.

Nascimento AF, Granter SR, Cviko A, et al. Vulvar acanthosis with altered differentiation. A precursor to verrucous carcinoma? *Am J Surg Pathol.* 2004;28:638-643.

Ordi J, Alejo M, Fuste V, et al. HPV-negative vulvar intraepithelial neoplasia with basaloid histologic pattern; an unrecognized variant of simplex (differentiated) VIN. *Am J Surg Pathol.* 2009;33:1659-1665.

Nooij LS, Ter Haar NT, Ruano D, et al. Genomic characterization of vulvar (pre)cancers identities distinct molecular subtypes with prognostic significance. *Clin Cancer Res.* 2017;23:6781-6789.

Kortekaas KE, Solleveld-Westerink N, Tessier-Cloutier B, et al. Performance of the pattern-based interpretation of p53 immunohistochemistry as a surrogate for TP53 mutations in vulvar squamous cell carcinoma. *Histopathology.* 2020;77(1):92-99.

Abu-Rustum N, Yashar CM, Bradley K, et al. *NCCN Clinical Practice Guidelines in Oncology: Vulvar Cancer (Squamous Cell Carcinoma).* Available at: https://www.nccn.org/professionals/physician_gls/pdf/vulvar.pdf.

Goje O, Reutter J, Lawson H, Stockdale C. Committee opinion No. 675: management of vulvar intraepithelial neoplasia. American college of obstetricians and gynecologists; American society for colposcopy and cervical pathology. *Obstet Gynecol.* 2016;128:e178-e182.

Invasive Squamous Cell Carcinoma of the Uterine Cervix

Saco A, Carriho C, Focchi GRA, et al. Squamous cell carcinoma, HPV-associated of the uterine cervix. Chapter 8, tumors of the uterine cervix. In: WHO Classification of Tumors Editorial Board, ed. *Female Genital Tumors. WHO Classification of Tumors Series.* 5th ed. Lyon (France): IARC; 2020:336-349.

Wilbur DC, Colgan TJ, Frenczy AS, et al. Glandular tumors and precursors. Tumors of the uterine cervix. In: Kurman RJ, Carcangiu ML, Herrington CS, Young RH, eds. *World Health Organization Classification of Tumors of Female Reproductive Organs.* Lyon: IARC; 2014:183-194.

Jesinghaus M, Strehl J, Boxberg M, et al. Introducing a novel highly prognostic grading scheme based on tumor budding and cell nest size for squamous cell carcinoma of the uterine cervix. *J Pathol Clin Res.* 2018;4:93-102.

Zare SY, Aisagbonhi O, Hasteh F, Fadare O. Independent validation of tumor budding activity and cell nest size as determinants of patient outcome in squamous cell carcinoma of the uterine cervix. *Am J Surg Pathol.* 2020;44:1151-1160.

Abu-Rustum NR, Yashar CM, Bradley K, et al. *NCCN Practice Guidelines in Oncology: Cervical Cancer.* 2020. Available at: https://www.nccn.org/professionals/physician_gls/pdf/cervical.pdf.

Siegel RL, Miller KD, Jemal A. Cancer statistics, 2020. *CA Cancer J Clin.* 2020;70:7-30.

HPV-Associated Endocervical Adenocarcinomas

Stolnicu S, Barsan I, Hoang L, et al. International Endocervical Adenocarcinoma Criteria and Classification (IECC): a new pathogenetic classification for invasive adenocarcinomas of the endocervix. *Am J Surg Pathol.* 2018;42:214-226.

Parra-Herran C, Alvarado-Cabrero I, Hoang LN, et al. Adenocarcinoma, HPV-associated, of the uterine cervix. Tumors of the uterine cervix. In: WHO Classification of Tumors Editorial Board, ed. *Female Genital Tumors. WHO Classification of Tumors Series.* 5th ed. Lyon (France): IARC; 2020:336-371.

Diaz De Vivar A, Roma AA, Park KJ, et al. Invasive endocervical adenocarcinoma: proposal for a new pattern-based classification system with significant clinical implications: a multi-institutional study. *Int J Gynecol Pathol.* 2013;32:592-601.

Roma AA, Diaz De Vivar A, Park KJ, et al. Invasive endocervical adenocarcinoma: a new pattern-based classification system with important clinical significance. *Am J Surg Pathol.* 2015;39:667-672.

Park KJ, Roma AA. Pattern based classification of endocervical adenocarcinoma: a review. *Pathology.* 2018;50:134-140.

Roma AA, Fadare O. The pattern is the issue: recent advances in adenocarcinoma of the uterine cervix. *Virchows Archiv.* 2018;472:897-905.

Horn LC, Handzel R, Borte G, et al. Invasive stratified mucin-producing carcinoma (i-SMILE) of the uterine cervix: report of a case series and review of the literature indicating poor prognostic subtype of cervical adenocarcinoma. *J Cancer Res Clin Oncol.* 2019;145:2573-2582.

Kuragaki C, Enomoto T, Ueno Y, et al. Mutations in the STK11 gene characterize minimal deviation adenocarcinoma of the uterine cervix. *Lab Invest.* 2003;83:35-45.

Endometrial Endometrioid Adenocarcinoma

Bosse T, Davidson B, Euscher ED, et al. Endometrioid carcinoma of the uterine corpus. Tumors of the uterine corpus. In: WHO Classification of Tumors Editorial Board, ed. *Female Genital Tumors. WHO Classification of Tumors Series.* 5th ed. Lyon (France): IARC; 2020:252-255.

Weigand KC, Lee AF, Al-Agha OM, et al. Loss of BAF250a (ARID1A) is frequent in high-grade endometrial carcinomas. *J Pathol.* 2011;224:328-333.

Mutter GL, Zaino RJ, Baak JP, Bentley RC, Robboy SJ. Benign endometrial hyperplasia sequence and endometrial intraepithelial neoplasia. *Int J Gynecol Pathol.* 2007;26(2):103-114.

Doherty MT, Sanni OB, Coleman HG, et al. Concurrent and future risk of endometrial cancer in women with endometrial hyperplasia: a systematic review and meta-analysis. *PLoS One.* 2020;15(4):e0232231.

Baak JP, Mutter GL, Robboy S, et al. The molecular genetics and morphometry-based endometrial intraepithelial neoplasia classification system predicts disease progression in endometrial hyperplasia more accurately than the 1994 World Health Organization classification system. *Cancer.* 2005;103(11):2304-2312. doi:10.1002/cncr.21058.

Kasper HG, Crum CP. The utility of immunohistochemistry in the differential diagnosis of gynecologic disorders. *Arch Pathol Lab Med.* 2015;139:39-54.

McAlpine J, Leon-Castillo A, Bosse T. The rise of a novel classification system for endometrial carcinoma; integration of molecular subclasses. *J Pathol.* 2018;244:538-549.

Abu-Rustum NR, Yashar CM, Bradley K, et al. *NCCN Practice Guidelines in Oncology: Uterine Neoplasms*. 2020. Available at: https://www.nccn.org/professionals/physician_gls/pdf/uterine.pdf.

Leiomyoma of the Uterus

Oliva E, Young RH, Amin MB, et al. An immunohistochemical analysis of endometrial stromal and smooth muscle tumors of the uterus: a study of 54 cases emphasizing the importance of using a panel because of overlap in immunoreactivity for individual antibodies. *Am J Surg Pathol.* 2002;26:403-412.

Bell SW, Kempson RL, Hendrickson MR. Problematic uterine smooth muscle neoplasms. A clinicopathologic study of 213 cases. *Am J Surg Pathol.* 1994;18:535-558.

Ip PP, Cheung AN, Clement PB. Uterine smooth muscle tumors of uncertain malignant potential (STUMP): a clinicopathologic analysis of 16 cases. *Am J Surg Pathol.* 2009;33:992-1005.

Gupta M, Laury AL, Nucci MR, et al. Predictors of adverse outcome in uterine smooth muscle tumours of uncertain malignant potential (STUMP): a clinicopathological analysis of 22 cases with a proposal for the inclusion of additional histological parameters. *Histopathology.* 2018;73(2):284-298.

Oliva E, Carcangiu ML, Carinelli SG, et al. Mesenchymal tumors. Tumors of the uterine corpus. In: Kurman RJ, Carcangiu ML, Herrington CS, Young RH, eds. *World Health Organization Classification of Tumors of Female Reproductive Organs.* Lyon: IARC; 2014:142-144.

Lewis N, Soslow RA, Delair DF, et al. ZCH7B-BCOR high-grade endometria stromal sarcomas: a report of 17 cases of a newly defined entity. *Mod Pathol.* 2018;4:674-684.

Aisagbonhi O, Harrison B, Zhao L, et al. YWHAE rearrangement in a purely conventional low-grade endometrial stromal sarcoma that transformed over time to high-grade sarcoma: importance of molecular testing. *Int J Gynecol Pathol.* 2018;5:441-447.

Zou Y, Turashvili G, Soslow RA, et al. High-grade transformation of low-grade endometrial stromal sarcomas lacking YWHAE and BCOR genetic abnormalities. *Mod Pathol.* 2020;9:1861-1870.

Lin JF, Slomovitz BM. Uterine sarcoma. *Curr Oncol Rep.* 2008;10:512-518.

Longacre TA, Lim D, Parra-Herran C. Uterine leiomyosarcoma. Tumors of the uterine corpus. In: WHO Classification of Tumors Editorial Board, ed. *Female Genital Tumors. WHO Classification of Tumors Series.* 5th ed. Lyon (France): IARC; 2020:283-285.

High-Grade Serous Carcinoma of the Fallopian Tube

Meserve EEK, Brouwer J, Crum CP. Serous tubal intraepithelial neoplasia: the concept and its application. *Mod Pathol.* 2017; 30:710-721.

Longacre TA, Wells M. Serous tumors. Tumors of the ovary. In: Kurman RJ, Carcangiu ML, Herrington CS, Young RH, eds. *World Health Organization Classification of Tumors of Female Reproductive Organs.* Lyon: IARC; 2014:15-16.

Zweemer RP, van Diest PJ, Verheijen RH, et al. Molecular evidence linking primary cancer of the fallopian tube to BRCA1 germline mutations. *Gynecol Oncol.* 2000;76:45-50.

Medeiros F, Muto MG, Lee Y, et al. The tubal fimbria is a preferred site for early adenocarcinoma in women with familial ovarian cancer syndrome. *Am J Surg Pathol.* 2006;30:230-236.

Gilks CB, Irving J, Köbel M, et al. Incidental nonuterine high-grade serous carcinomas arise in the fallopian tube in most cases: further evidence for the tubal origin of high-grade serous carcinomas. *Am J Surg Pathol.* 2015;39:357-364.

Morrison JC, Blanco Jr LZ, Vang R, Ronnett BM. Incidental serous tubal intraepithelial carcinoma and early invasive serous carcinoma in the nonprophylactic setting: analysis of a case series. *Am J Surg Pathol.* 2015;39:442-453.

Lee Y, Miron A, Drapkin R, et al. A candidate precursor to serous carcinoma that originates in the distal fallopian tube. *J Pathol.* 2007;211:26-35. [Published erratum appears in: *J Pathol.* 2007;213:116].

Serous Borderline Tumor of the Ovary

Maniar KP, Wang Y, Visvanathan K, et al. Evaluation of microinvasion and lymph node involvement in ovarian serous borderline/atypical proliferative serous tumors: a morphologic and Immunohistochemical analysis of 37 cases. *Am J Surg Pathol.* 2014;38:743-755.

Ho CL, Kurman RJ, Dehari R, et al. Mutations of BRAF and KRAS precede the development of ovarian serous borderline tumors. *Cancer Res.* 2004;64:6915-6918.

Young RH. Ovarian tumors: a survey of selected advances of note during the life of this journal. *Hum Pathol.* 2020;95:169-206.

Vang R, Davidson B, Kong CS, et al. Serous borderline tumor of the ovary. Chapter 1, tumors of the ovary. In: WHO Classification of Tumors Editorial Board, ed. *Female Genital Tumors. WHO Classification of Tumors Series.* 5th ed. Lyon (France): IARC; 2020:38-42.

Mucinous Borderline Tumor of the Ovary

Young RH. Ovarian tumors: a survey of selected advances of note during the life of this journal. *Hum Pathol.* 2020;95:169-206.

Garrett AP, Lee KR, Colitti CR, et al. K-ras mutation may be an early event in mucinous ovarian tumorigenesis. *Int J Gynecol Pathol.* 2001;20:244-251.

Anglesio MS, Kommoss S, Tolcher MC, et al. Molecular characterization of mucinous ovarian tumors supports a stratified treatment approach with HER2 targeting in 19% of carcinomas. *J Pathol.* 2013;229:111-120.

Hu J, Khalifa RD, Roma AA, Fadare O. The pathologic distinction of primary and metastatic mucinous tumors involving the ovary: a re-evaluation of algorithms based on gross features. *Ann Diagn Pathol.* 2018;37:1-6.

Aldaoud N, Erashdi M, Alkhatib S, et al. The utility of PAX8 and SATB2 immunohistochemical stains in distinguishing ovarian mucinous neoplasms from colonic and appendiceal mucinous neoplasms. *BMC Res Notes.* 2019;12:770.

Armstrong DK, Alvarez RD, Bakkum-Gamez JN, et al. *NCCN Clinical Practice Guidelines in Oncology: Ovarian Cancer, Including Fallopian Tube Cancer and Primary Peritoneal Cancer.* 2019. Available at: https://www.nccn.org/professionals/physician_gls/pdf/ovarian.pdf.

Peres LC, Cushing-Haugen KL, Kobel M, et al. Invasive epithelial ovarian cancer survival by histotype and disease stage. *J Natl Cancer Inst.* 2019;111:60-68.

Ovarian Fibroma and Adult Granulosa Cell Tumor

Young RH, Clement PB, Scully RE. Calcified thecomas in young women. A report of four cases. *Int J Gynecol Pathol.* 1988;7:343-350.

Deavers M, Oliva E, Nucci M. Sex cord-stromal tumors of the ovary. In: Nucci MR, Oliva E, eds. *Gynecologic Pathology, A Volume in the Series Foundations in Diagnostic Pathology.* Elsevier; 2009:445-500.

Kim MS, Hur SY, Yoo NJ, Lee SH. Mutational analysis of FOXL2 codon 134 in granulosa cell tumor of ovary and other human cancers. *J Pathol.* 2010;221:147-152.

Shah SP, Kobel M, Senz J, et al. Mutation of FOXL2 in granulosa cell tumors of the ovary. *N Engl J Med.* 2009;360:2719-2729.

Stall JN, Young RH. Granulosa cell tumors of the ovary with prominent thecoma-like foci: a report of 16 cases emphasizing the ongoing utility of the reticulin stain in the modern era. *Int J Gynecol Pathol.* 2019;38:143-150.

Gui T, Cao D, Shen D, et al. A clinicopathological analysis of 40 cases of ovarian Sertoli-Leydig cell tumors. *Gynecol Oncol.* 2012;127:384-389.

Young RH. Ovarian sex cord–stromal tumors: reflections on a 40-year experience with a fascinating group of tumors, including comments on the seminal observations of Robert E. Scully, MD. *Arch Pathol Lab Med.* 2018;142:1459-1484.

Irving JA, Young RH. Microcystic stromal tumor of the ovary: report of 16 cases of a hitherto uncharacterized distinctive ovarian neoplasm. *Am J Surg Pathol.* 2009;33:367-375.

Ovarian Mature Teratoma and Dysgerminoma

Euscher ED. Germ cell tumors of the female genital tract. *Surg Pathol.* 2019;12:621-649.

Prat J, Cao D, Carinelli SG, et al. Germ cell tumors. Tumors of the ovary. In: Kurman RJ, Carcangiu ML, Herrington CS, Young RH, eds. *World Health Organization Classification of Tumors of Female Reproductive Organs.* Lyon: IARC; 2014:57-66.

Dalmau J, Tuzun E, Wu H, et al. Paraneoplastic anti-N-methyl-D-asparate receptor encephalitis associated with ovarian teratoma. *Ann Neurol.* 2007;61:25-36.

Wei S, Baloch ZW, LiVolsi V. Pathology of struma ovarii: a report of 96 cases. *Endocr Pathol.* 2015;26:342-348.

Davis KP, Hartmann LK, Keeney GL, Shapiro H. Primary ovarian carcinoid tumors. *Gynecol Oncol.* 1996;61:259-265.

Baker PM, Oliva E, Young RH, et al. Ovarian mucinous carcinoids including some with a carcinomatous component: a report of 17 cases. *Am J Surg Pathol.* 2001;25:557-568.

Chumas JC, Scully RE. Sebaceous tumors arising in ovarian dermoid cysts. *Int J Gynecol Pathol.* 1991;10:356-363.

Morovic A, Damjanov I. Neuroectodermal ovarian tumors: a brief overview. *Histol Histopathol.* 2008;23:765-771.

Kleinman GM, Young RH, Scully RE. Primary neuroectodermal tumors of the ovary. A report of 25 cases. *Am J Surg Pathol.* 1993;17:764-778.

Al Wazzan A, Popowich S, Dean E, et al. Malignant transformation of mature cystic teratoma of the ovary: a 30-year experience of a single tertiary care center. *Eur J Gynaecol Oncol.* 2016;37:809-813.

Armstrong DK, Alvarez RD, Bakkum-Gamez JN, et al. *NCCN Clinical Practice Guidelines in Oncology: Ovarian Cancer, Including Fallopian Tube Cancer and Primary Peritoneal Cancer.* 2019. Available at: https://www.nccn.org/professionals/physician_gls/pdf/ovarian.pdf.

Osman H, Cheng L, Ulbright TM, Idrees MT. The utility of CDX-2, GATA-3 and DOG-1 in the diagnosis of testicular neoplasms: an immunohistochemical study of 109 cases. *Hum Pathol.* 2016; 48:18-24.

3

Neuropathology

Richard A. Prayson

GLIOSIS VERSUS GLIOMA

Clinical Features

One of the most challenging differential diagnostic issues in surgical neuropathology is distinguishing between gliosis or reactive astrocytosis and an infiltrating low-grade glioma. Patients with low-grade gliomas may present at any age, although the peak is in the third through fifth decades of life. Often, patients present with signs or symptoms related to their tumor. Presentation is often tied to the location of the neoplasm. Most commonly, gliomas present with focal neural deficits (cranial nerve, sensory motor, or visual), seizures, or symptoms related to increased intracranial pressure (headaches, nausea/vomiting, and papilledema). Gliosis is not in and of itself a pathology, it develops secondary to some other pathology. It stands to reason that some degree of gliosis is expected in proximity to a low-grade glioma. Most low-grade infiltrative gliomas (fibrillary astrocytomas and oligodendrogliomas) arise in the cerebral hemispheres and are white matter based. They may also arise in the cerebellum, brain stem, and spinal cord. By nature, they are infiltrative lesions. On imaging studies, low-grade gliomas are usually nonenhancing, ill-defined masses best visualized on T2-weighted or fluid-attenuated inversion recovery (FLAIR) magnetic resonance imaging (MRI). The tumors often extend beyond what is apparent on imaging studies and so marginating these lesions on excised tissues is a fruitless activity. Because of their infiltrative nature, they may cross midline structures, such as the corpus callosum, and infiltrate tissue on the contralateral side, so-called "butterfly gliomas."

Pathologic Features

GROSS FINDINGS

Reliable detection of gliosis or infiltrating low-grade gliomas grossly is not possible. In some cases, low-grade gliomas, as they involve the overlying cortex, may cause blurring of the gray–white interface grossly. Sometimes, a subtle discoloration of the parenchyma or cystic change may be evident. Gliosis, if prominent, may give the tissue an increased firmness.

MICROSCOPIC FINDINGS

In gliosis, hypertrophic astrocytes are marked by increased eosinophilic cytoplasm, stellate cytoplasmic processes, and an eccentrically placed nucleus (Fig. 3.1A and B). The nuclei may be enlarged and are generally oval or kidney bean shaped. Occasionally, binucleate cells may be seen. The hypertrophic or reactive astrocytes are usually evenly distributed. In contrast, gemistocytes are usually unevenly distributed and present in greater numbers, usually in the context of an astrocytoma. Gemistocytes have shorter and thinner cytoplasmic processes, best seen on a glial fibrillary acidic protein (GFAP) stain. Morphologically, the subtle differences between a reactive astrocyte and gemistocyte may not be evident on a hematoxylin and eosin–stained tissue section. In some cases, other changes including Rosenthal fibers and eosinophilic granular bodies may develop in association with the gliosis. One needs to be cautious about not assuming that these findings are exclusively seen in gliosis or in a tumor; they may be also encountered in other processes such as Alexander's disease.

Table 3.1 summarizes characteristic features of glioma versus low-grade glioma. Low-grade gliomas morphologically are marked by tumor cells with high nuclear-to-cytoplasmic ratios (Fig. 3.1C). Astrocytoma nuclei are typically enlarged compared with normal astrocytes and are marked by irregular nuclear contours (nuclear pleomorphism). Nuclear chromatin may be more clumped and irregular in distribution. Nuclei also tend to be more hyperchromatic. Oligodendroglioma nuclei tend to more rounded and monomorphic and less hyperchromatic than astrocytoma nuclei (Fig. 3.1D). Other morphologic features which, if present are more indicative of a tumor than gliosis include the presence of mitotic figures, calcification, and microcytic changes. These findings are not present in all tumors but, when seen, are more indicative of a glioma than gliosis. One needs to be careful not to confuse freeze artifact changes, seen frequently at the time of frozen section intraoperative consultation, with true microcytic change. Satellitosis is a fairly common occurrence at the infiltrating edge of a glioma. Tumor cells have

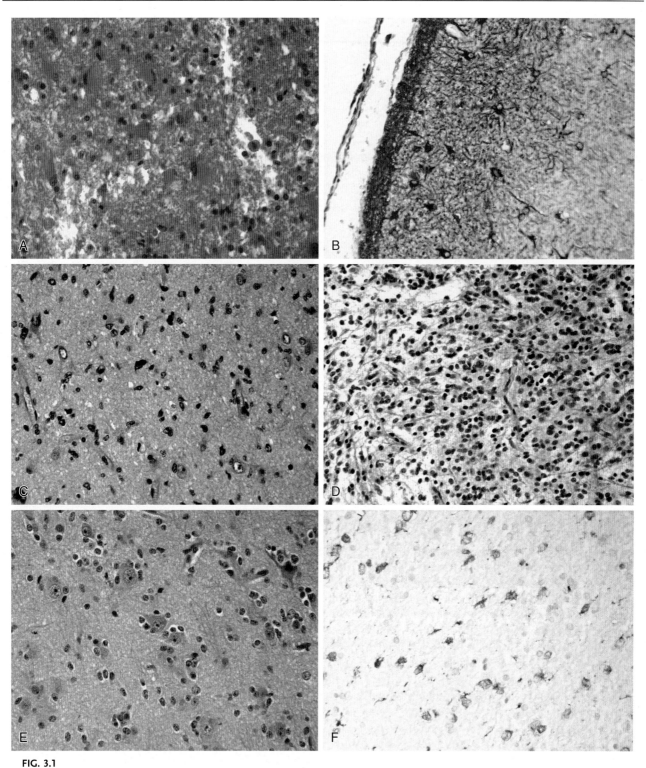

FIG. 3.1

A, Reactive astrocytes marked by abundant eosinophilic cytoplasm and eccentric nuclei (hematoxylin and eosin [H&E], original magnification 400×). **B,** Reactive astrocytes highlighted on a GFAP immunostain showing multiple cytoplasmic processes (original magnification 400×). **C,** Diffuse astrocytoma (grade 2) marked by tumor cells with a high nuclear-to-cytoplasmic ratio, irregular nuclear contours, and hyperchromasia (H&E, original magnification 400×). **D,** Oligodendroglioma (grade 2) characterized by more rounded cell nuclei and scant cytoplasm (H&E, original magnification 400×). **E,** Oligodendroglioma (grade 2) with satellitosis of tumor cells around neurons in the cortex and capillaries (H&E, original magnification 400×). **F,** Diffuse astrocytoma (grade 2) staining with antibody to IDH-1 (R132H) consistent with a mutant status (original magnification 400×).

TABLE 3.1

Gliosis Versus Low-grade Glioma

	Gliosis	Low-grade Glioma
Age	Any	Peak third to fifth decades, but can occur at any age
Location	Gray or white matter	White > gray matter
Gross	Firm	Obscure gray–white interface
Atypia	Prominent eosinophilic cytoplasm with long tapered process	High nuclear-to-cytoplasmic ratio, nuclear pleomorphism, and hyperchromasia
Mitosis	Absent	May be present
Microcystic change	Absent	May be present
Calcification	Absent	May be present
Satellitosis	Absent	May be present
IDH-1 stain	Negative	May be positive
p53 stain	Minimal	May be diffusely positive
ATRX stain	Diffuse staining	May show loss of staining

a tendency to satellite around preexisting structures like blood vessels and neurons (Fig. 3.1E). Reactive astrocytes typically do not satellite around other structures. The term secondary structure of Scherer has been used to describe this phenomenon in astrocytomas.

Ancillary Studies

At times, distinction of gliosis from an infiltrating low-grade glioma may be impossible based on morphology alone. There are certain immunomarkers that may be helpful in some of these cases. Probably the single most useful marker is isocitrate dehydrogenase-1 (IDH-1). The antibody stain will never stain reactive processes including gliosis. Most oligodendrogliomas and many fibrillary astrocytomas will stain positively with the antibody, indicating the presence of a mutation (Fig. 3.1F). Therefore, a positive staining result is useful in the differential diagnosis; a negative stain is not helpful. The p53 staining, if diffusely present, is indicative of a tumor. Rare positive staining is not helpful and can be seen in both. ATRX loss of staining is seen in a subset of astrocytomas (not oligodendrogliomas) and not gliosis. Low rates of cell proliferation, as evidenced by Ki-67 or MIB-1 staining, can be seen in both processes; a high labeling index is more likely indicative of a tumor.

Prognosis and Therapy

Gliosis is a benign condition and is generally not the target of surgery and does not require further treatment. Prognosis and treatment of infiltrating gliomas will be addressed later in this chapter. Both World Health Organization (WHO) grade 2 oligodendrogliomas and astrocytomas will progress over time to higher-grade tumors. Use of adjuvant treatment is dependent on tumor type and a variety of other factors including location of tumor, symptomatology, imaging appearance, age of patient, baseline health, and overall prognosis.

RADIATION CHANGE VERSUS RECURRENT/RESIDUAL GLIOMA

Clinical Features

Radiation therapy is one of the commonly employed treatment modalities for many brain tumors, including high-grade gliomas. The techniques employed in delivering the radiation and the doses used depend on a variety of factors including age and location of tumor, tumor type and grade, and the extent of the tumor. The goal is to kill tumor cells, cause chromosomal damage to cancer cells, and disrupt tumor growth (cell proliferation), while minimizing damage to the adjacent non-tumoral tissue. Unfortunately, there are adverse effects associated with the administration of radiation to the brain and pathologic changes that may be seen. These patients are often followed with serial imaging studies. Changes on imaging studies are sometimes difficult to interpret with certainty. The scenario that may result in tissue being taken and sent for evaluation centers around the question of whether or not changes seen on imaging represent tumor necrosis (beneficial effects of radiation) or whether the changes seen are secondary to the radiation in surrounding tissue and there has been relatively little effect on the tumor.

A variety of factors impact the extent of damage sustained by the brain from radiation; these include the total dose administered, how the dose is administered (fractionation) and time intervals in administration, beam energy and composition, other drugs or chemotherapeutic agents being simultaneously used, location, and the patient's condition and age. In general, smaller tumors respond better than larger tumors. Tissue in some parts of the brain, such as the brain stem, is more sensitive than frontal or parietal lobe cortex. Pediatric and geriatric brains are more sensitive to the effects of radiation than other age groups.

Pathologic Features

GROSS FINDINGS

Grossly, the findings associated with radiotherapy may include findings of cerebral edema in the acute stages. Changes of demyelination may be evident due to damage of oligodendroglial cells, typically in weeks 2 to 12 after administration. Delayed effects, which may occur anywhere from months to years after the radiation was administered, may result in grossly evident necrosis. Another long-term risk of radiation treatment, often years later, is the development of a secondary neoplasm; these tumors most commonly include meningiomas, sarcomas, and gliomas.

MICROSCOPIC FINDINGS

As previously described, changes of edema may be seen histologically. Blood vessels often show a hyalinized thickening of the vessel walls accompanied by varying degrees of perivascular fibrosis (Fig. 3.2A). Some of these thickened vessels are accompanied by variable numbers of benign lymphocytes. Endothelial cells lining the vessels show reactive changes. Vascular thrombosis may sometimes be seen. Adjacent parenchyma shows gliosis and microglial cell proliferation. Foci of coagulative necrosis, sometimes accompanied by prominent numbers of macrophages, may be seen (Fig. 3.2B). Areas of increased collagen deposition and granulation tissue may be present. Dystrophic calcification may also be evident. Foci of petechial hemorrhages may be noted. Direct injury to oligodendrocytes may result in changes of demyelination (myelin loss, gliosis, white matter macrophages, and perivascular chronic inflammation).

Radiation may also manifest with evidence of cytologic atypia, which is what most commonly can cause confusion with an astrocytoma (Fig. 3.2C). The classic scenario encountered in surgical neuropathology is the patient with a known astrocytoma who has been irradiated and the

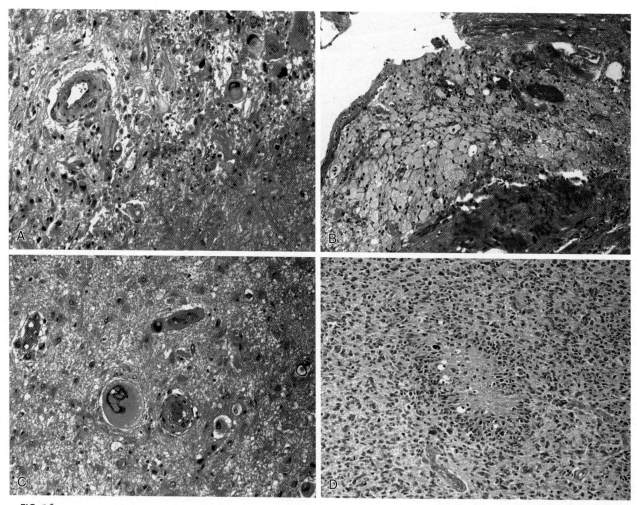

FIG. 3.2

A, Radiation changes in a residual glioblastoma marked by vascular wall thickening and necrosis (hematoxylin and eosin [H&E], original magnification 200×). **B,** Focal radiation necrosis associated with increased number of macrophages (H&E, original magnification 200×). **C,** Large, bizarre appearing cells represent radiation atypia in a residual astrocytoma (H&E, original magnification 200×). **D,** Necrosis rimmed by a pseudopalisade of tumor cells represents intrinsic tumor (glioblastoma) necrosis, not radiation necrosis (H&E, original magnification 200×).

TABLE 3.2

Radiation Change Versus Recurrent/Residual Glioma

	Radiation Change	Recurrent/ Residual Glioma
Edema	Present	Present
Reactive astrocytes	Present	Present
Blood vessels	Hyalinized	Vascular proliferation (high grade)
Atypia	Radiation atypia	Tumor cell atypia (high nuclear-to-cytoplasmic ratio cells)
Perinecrotic pseudopalisading	Absent	Maybe present
Non-perinecrotic pseudopalisading	Present	Maybe present
Macrophages	Frequently present	Usually absent
Calcification in necrosis	Maybe present	Usually absent
Demyelination	Maybe present	Absent
Mitoses	Absent	Often present (especially in high-grade tumors)

question is whether the post radiation findings are secondary to the treatment or whether the tumor has continued to grow and persist despite the treatment. Comparison of radiation changes to recurrent/residual astrocytoma is summarized in Table 3.2. Radiation atypia may be quite pronounced and manifest as bizarre-appearing cells with multinucleation and cytoplasmic vacuolization. Features more typically characteristic of a fibrillary astrocytoma rather than radiation change include cells marked by a high nuclear-to-cytoplasmic ratio, mitotic activity, vascular proliferative changes, and perinecrotic pseudopalisading by tumor cells (Fig. 3.2D). Necrosis accompanied by macrophages and/or calcifications is much more typical of radionecrosis than tumor necrosis.

Ancillary Studies

Ancillary immunostains that may be helpful in selected cases in the differential diagnosis include markers typically encountered in low-grade gliomas. IDH-1 (R132H) staining is present in most oligodendrogliomas and in a subset of astrocytoma; it is not a feature of radiation changes. Loss of ATRX staining, indicating a mutation, may be seen in a subset of astrocytomas but is not a feature of radiation changes. Widespread p53 immunoreactivity, likewise, may be encountered in a subset of astrocytomas but is not a feature of radiation.

Prognosis and Therapy

As previously mentioned, the question usually comes down to whether or not there is recurrent or residual tumor in the setting of prior radiation and changes on imaging. In most cases of infiltrating gliomas, if there is enough viable tissue to assess, there is likely to be some infiltrating tumor cells present; the challenge lies in how discernible they are. The follow-up question is whether the tumor has upgraded, particularly if one is dealing with a low-grade or anaplastic astrocytoma. Necrosis, a feature diagnostic of glioblastoma, may be present but due to the radiation. Unless there is a pseudopalisading of tumor cells around the necrotic focus, it is difficult to be absolutely certain that the necrosis seen in this setting is intrinsic tumor necrosis and therefore using necrosis as a grading parameter needs to be done with caution. True vascular proliferation is a feature of glioblastoma and not radiation (which gives one vascular sclerosis) and can be used as a grading parameter.

Radiation does predispose one to the development of secondary neoplasms. These usually transpire several years after administration of the radiation. A variety of tumors have been described as arising in this setting; most commonly these include meningiomas, sarcomas, and gliomas.

FIBRILLARY ASTROCYTOMA VERSUS OLIGODENDROGLIOMA

Clinical Features

Fibrillary astrocytomas are the most common primary tumors of the central nervous system (CNS). Glioblastoma is the most frequent malignant tumor, accounting for about 15% of all intracranial tumors and almost half of all primary malignant tumors of the brain. Oligodendrogliomas are much less frequently encountered, comprising about 1.7% of all primary brain tumors. Both tumors are most frequently encountered in adults with peak incidences of the low-grade tumors in the third to fifth decades of life; higher-grade tumors more commonly present in an older age group. Tumors arise in the lobes of the brain; low-grade fibrillary astrocytomas and low-grade oligodendrogliomas both arise most commonly in the frontal lobes. Clinical presentation is dependent on the location of the tumors but most commonly includes seizures, headaches, and signs related to increased intracranial pressure, focal neurologic deficits, and cognitive or mental changes.

On computed tomography (CT) imaging, grade 2 astrocytomas and oligodendrogliomas appear as ill-defined, homogeneous masses of low density. Calcifications and cystic changes may be present in some tumors. MRI studies show hypodensity on T1-weighted images and hyperintensity on T2-weighted images. Glioblastoma, or high-grade astrocytomas, are classically ring-enhancing lesions.

Pathologic Features

GROSS FINDINGS

Both fibrillary astrocytomas and oligodendrogliomas are infiltrative lesions. They typically arise in the white matter and infiltrate into the overlying cortex, grossly obscuring the gray–white interface, causing an enlargement and distortion of invaded areas. The classic "butterfly glioma" is marked by infiltration by tumor of commissural structures with involvement of the contralateral brain parenchyma. The gross appearances of these tumors may be altered by cystic change, microcalcifications, or hemorrhage. High-grade tumors may demonstrate areas of necrosis. Rarely, tumors may extend to involve the overlying leptomeninges.

MICROSCOPIC FINDINGS

Table 3.3 compares and contrasts features of fibrillary astrocytomas versus oligodendrogliomas. Fibrillary astrocytomas are graded by the WHO into diffuse astrocytomas (WHO grade 2), anaplastic astrocytomas (WHO grade 3), and glioblastomas (WHO grade 4). All tumors are marked by a proliferation of atypical appearing astrocytes, characterized by nuclear enlargement, nuclear pleomorphism, and nuclear hyperchromasia. Grade 2 tumors are characterized by mild hypercellularity and rare mitotic figures (Fig. 3.3A). Grade 3 tumors are more cellular than grade 2 tumors and mitotic activity is more readily discernible (Fig. 3.3B). The hallmarks of a grade 4 tumor are vascular proliferation (a proliferation of cells that normally comprise blood vessel walls) and necrosis (Figs. 3.2D and 3.3C). Perineuronal or perivascular satellitosis by tumor cells is a common finding at the infiltrating margin of the tumor.

Oligodendrogliomas are stratified into low-grade (WHO grade 2) and anaplastic (WHO grade 3) lesions. Oligodendroglioma tumor cells, in contrast to astrocytoma cells, are generally more monomorphic in appearance. They are typically rounded with scant cytoplasm (Fig. 3.1D). Pericellular clearing (fried egg appearance) is an artifact of delayed formalin fixation and a common finding in oligodendrogliomas (Fig. 3.3D). Due to the paucity of cytoplasm and cytoplasmic processes, the vasculature of the tumor is readily discernible (chicken wire or arcuate capillary vascular pattern). The parameters used for grading astrocytomas are the same for oligodendrogliomas; the thresholds for assigning grades are different. Grade 3 oligodendrogliomas are typically more cellular than grade 2 tumors and are characterized by prominent mitotic activity (at least 4 or 5 mitotic

	Fibrillary Astrocytoma	Oligodendroglioma
Infiltration	Present	Present
Perineuronal satellitosis	May be present	May be present
Nuclear pleomorphism	Present	Less prominent
Nuclear hyperchromasia	Present	Less prominent
Pericellular clearing	Less common	More common (related to delayed formalin fixation)
Arcuate capillary vasculature	Absent	Present
Calcification	Occasionally	Frequently
Gemistocytic-like cells	Occasionally, larger size	Occasionally, smaller size
Vascular proliferation	Frequent in WHO grade 4	Frequent in WHO grade 3
Necrosis	Frequent in WHO grade 4	Frequent in WHO grade 3
Mitoses	Increased with higher grade	Increased with higher grade
IDH mutation	Sometimes present	Always present
p53 mutation	Sometimes present	Absent
ATRX mutation	Sometimes present	Absent
Chromosome 1p/19q co-deletion	Almost always absent	Always present
EGFR amplification	Sometimes present	Absent

TABLE 3.3
Fibrillary Astrocytoma Versus Oligodendroglioma

figures [MFs] per 10 high-power fields [HPFs]), often accompanied by vascular proliferation or necrosis (Fig. 3.3E). Calcifications are more commonly encountered in oligodendrogliomas. Similar to astrocytomas, tumor cells may be seen satelliting around preexisting structures or aggregating under the pial surface (Fig. 3.1E). In contrast to the larger gemistocytic astrocytes sometimes encountered in fibrillary astrocytomas, marked by oval- to kidney bean–shaped nuclei and abundant eosinophilic cytoplasm with short processes on GFAP staining, oligodendrogliomas sometimes have minigemistocytes, marked by more rounded nuclei and overall smaller size.

Ancillary Studies

Both tumor types may demonstrate GFAP and S-100 protein positivity; GFAP positivity is often more pronounced in astrocytomas given the more abundant cytoplasm filled

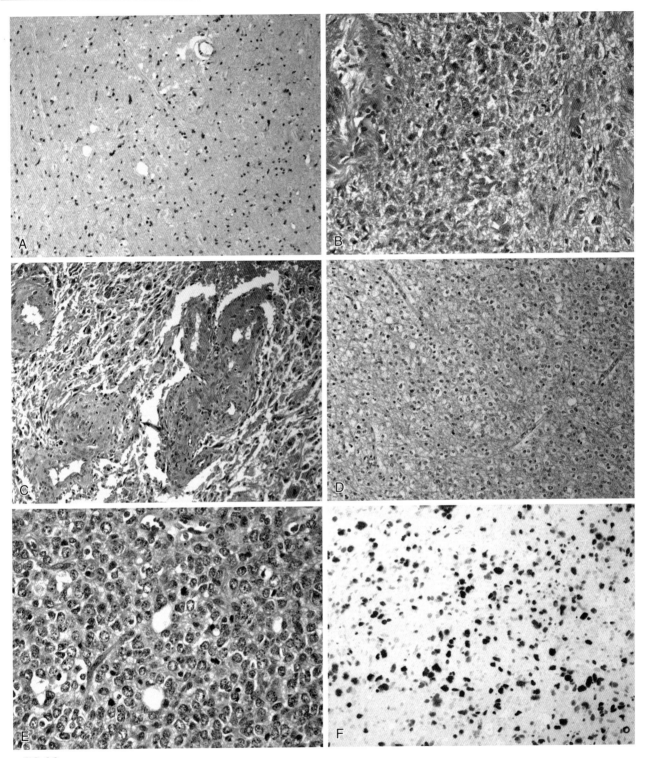

FIG. 3.3

A, Frozen section of a diffuse astrocytomas (grade 2) marked by mild hypercellularity and atypical appearing tumor cells (hematoxylin and eosin [H&E], original magnification 200×). **B,** Anaplastic astrocytoma (grade 3) characterized by increased cellularity (as compared with grade 2 tumors) and identifiable mitotic activity (H&E, original magnification 400×). **C,** Glioblastoma (grade 4) marked by vascular proliferative changes (H&E, original magnification 200×). **D,** Oligodendroglioma (grade 2) with tumor cells showing pericellular clearing ("fried egg appearance"), an artifact of delayed formalin fixation (H&E, original magnification 200×). **E,** Anaplastic oligodendroglioma (grade 3) marked by prominent cellularity and 3 mitotic figures in a single high-power field (H&E, original magnification 400×). **F,** An anaplastic astrocytoma showing prominent p53 immunostaining (>50%) (original magnification 200×).

Continued

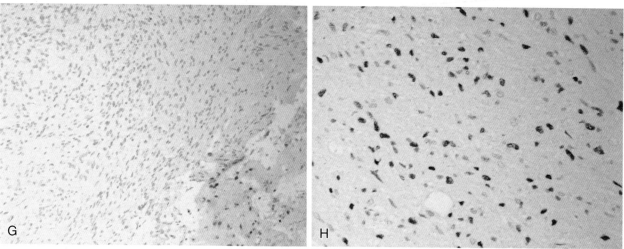

FIG. 3.3, cont'd

G, An anaplastic astrocytoma marked by loss of ATRX staining (original magnification 200×). **H,** Diffuse midline gliomas (grade 4) are characterized by an astrocytoma phenotype and evidence of H3K27M immunostaining, seen here (original magnification 400×).

with intermediate molecular weight filaments. Olig 2 staining may be seen in both tumor types. Non-specific cross-immunoreactivity with certain keratin markers, such as cytokeratins AE1/3 may be seen in some astrocytomas.

Oligodendrogliomas, as of the 2021 WHO Classification of Tumours of the Central Nervous System, require demonstrated evidence of a IDH mutation and codeletion on chromosomes 1p and 19q. IDH mutation may also be encountered in a subset of fibrillary astrocytomas (Fig. 3.1F). Codeletion on chromosomes 1p and 19q is a very rare occurrence in fibrillary astrocytomas and when present are smaller deletions compared with the near full arm deletions that mark oligodendrogliomas. Markers that are seen in a subset of fibrillary astrocytomas but are absent in oligodendrogliomas include p53 mutation (in excess of 30%–40% immunostaining) (Fig. 3.3F), ATRX mutation (loss of staining on immunohistochemistry; Fig. 3.3G), and epidermal growth factor receptor (EGFR) overexpression or amplification by fluorescent *in situ* hybridization (FISH) testing.

A rare, particularly aggressive neoplasm, diffuse midline glioma (WHO grade 4) arises in the brainstem and midline areas and can look like any grade of astrocytoma. The tumor is defined by an H3K27M alteration (Fig. 3.3H).

Prognosis and Therapy

Grade for grade, oligodendrogliomas have a better prognosis than their astrocytomas counterparts. IDH-mutant astrocytomas do significantly better than IDH wild-type tumors. Astrocytomas with a genotype of 7q gain and 10q loss, TERT promotor mutation or EGFR gene amplification have a poorer outcome. Most patients with glioblastoma die within 15 to 18 months after diagnosis. MGMT promotor methylation is associated with

chemoresponsiveness in astrocytomas. Most tumors are treated with radiation with or without chemotherapy. Oligodendrogliomas are typically chemoresponsive (PCV [procarbazine, lomustine, and vincristine] and temozolomide). Often, radiation is used to treat oligodendrogliomas as well. Mean survival for high-grade oligodendrogliomas is 3 to 4 years.

PILOCYTIC ASTROCYTOMA VERSUS FIBRILLARY ASTROCYTOMA

Clinical Features

Pilocytic astrocytomas are low-grade tumors (WHO grade 1) that most commonly present in children. They typically arise in the cerebellum (juvenile cerebellar astrocytoma), adjacent to the third ventricle, optic nerve, brain stem, and thalamus. Classic signs and symptoms are dependent on the location of the tumor. There is a well-known association of this variant with neurofibromatosis type I, especially optic nerve tumors. On imaging, the classic appearance of the tumor (about two third of cases) is that of a cystic neoplasm with enhancing mural nodule; this is very distinct from the appearance of the majority of fibrillary astrocytomas. The remaining cases are either cystic with a central non-enhancing zone or a solid mass.

Pathologic Features

GROSS FINDINGS

Most tumors are soft, gray, well-circumscribed masses with a cystic component. Tumors may show calcification

TABLE 3.4

Pilocytic Astrocytoma Versus Fibrillary Astrocytoma

	Pilocytic Astrocytoma	Fibrillary Astrocytoma
Age	Children, young adults	Adults
Location	Cerebellum, third ventricle region, brain stem	Frontal > parietal > temporal > occipital lobe
Imaging/gross	Cystic with enhancing mural nodule, circumscribed	Ill-defined, infiltrative, higher-grade tumors with enhancement
Biphasic appearance	Often	Rare
Nuclear pleomorphism	Mild to marked	Mild to marked
Mitosis	Rare	More common
Vascular proliferation	Present	In high-grade tumors
Necrosis	Absent	In high-grade tumors
Eosinophilic granular bodies	Present	Absent
Rosenthal fibers	Present	Absent
Hyalinized blood vessels	Sometimes present	Absent
Malignant progression	Rare	Frequent
Ki-67/MIB-1	Low index	Low to high indices
IDH mutation	Absent	Sometimes present
p53 mutation	Absent	Sometimes present
ATRX mutation	Absent	Sometimes present
BRAF alterations	Sometimes present	Generally absent

or evidence of hemosiderin deposition. Optic nerve tumors often involve the subarachnoid space circumferentially around the nerve.

MICROSCOPIC FINDINGS

Table 3.4 compares pilocytic astrocytoma with fibrillary astrocytoma. The classic appearance of pilocytic astrocytoma is that of a biphasic neoplasm: compact areas marked by spindled or piloid cells arranged against a fibrillary background juxtaposed with looser areas with a microcystic background (Fig. 3.4A and B). Nuclear pleomorphisms and cellularity may range from mild to marked, potentially causing confusion with an anaplastic astrocytoma. The presence of vacuolar proliferative changes can potentially cause the tumor to be confused with a glioblastoma. Hyalinized blood vessels, similar to what is seen in radiation, are also not uncommon in pilocytic astrocytoma (Fig. 3.4C). In contrast to high-grade fibrillary astrocytoma, mitotic figures and necrosis are not common. Two histologic features which are distinctively characteristic of pilocytic astrocytoma and not fibrillary astrocytoma are Rosenthal fibers (Fig. 3.4D) and eosinophilic granular bodies (Fig. 3.4E). Both of these features can be encountered in other low-grade glial and glioneuronal tumors (gangliogliomas and pleomorphic xanthoastrocytomas [PXAs]) and may be seen in gliosis.

Ancillary Studies

The most common genetic abnormality encountered in pilocytic astrocytoma is a 7q34 duplication, resulting in a KIAA1549-BRAF fusion gene. MAPK pathway alterations including NF1 mutations, BRAF-V600E mutations, and KRAS mutations may also be encountered. ATRX, p53, and IDH mutations, which may be encountered in a subset of fibrillary astrocytomas, are not typically seen in pilocytic astrocytomas. Cell proliferation markers, such as Ki-67 and MIB-1, show low labeling indices in pilocytic astrocytomas and have overlapping index ranges with grade 2 fibrillary astrocytomas.

Prognosis and Therapy

Most tumors are amenable to surgical resection due to their circumscription and do not require adjuvant therapy. In contrast to most grade 2 diffuse astrocytomas that will eventually progress to a higher-grade tumor, malignant progression is a very rare occurrence in pilocytic astrocytomas. The rare pilomyxoid variant of pilocytic astrocytoma has a high frequency of local recurrence and may seed the cerebrospinal fluid. This variant is characterized by a perivascular orientation of

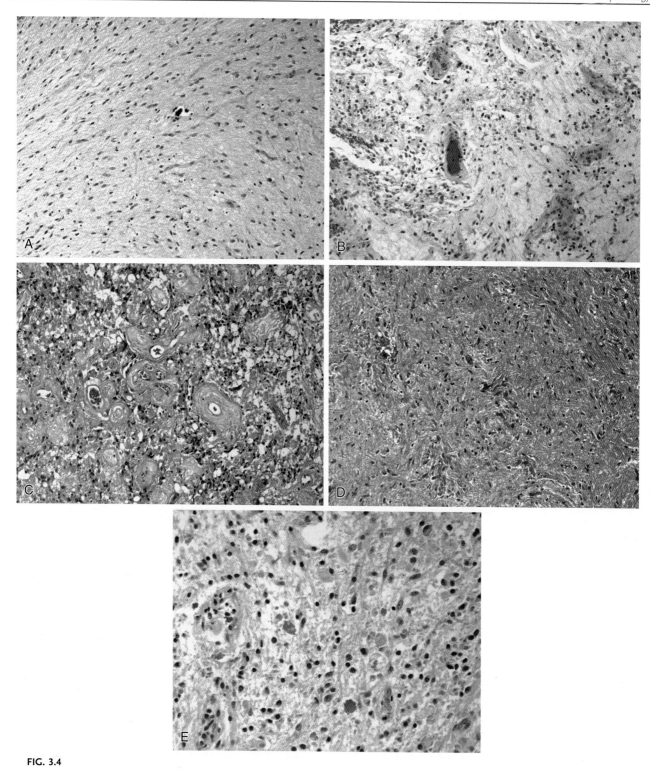

FIG. 3.4

A, Pilocytic astrocytoma (grade 1) showing a more compact area composed of spindled "piloid" cells with focal calcification (hematoxylin and eosin [H&E], original magnification 200×). **B,** Pilocytic astrocytoma showing microcystic changes (H&E, original magnification 200×). **C,** Focal perivascular sclerosis in a pilocytic astrocytoma (H&E, original magnification 200×). **D,** Brightly eosinophilic Rosenthal fibers are encountered in most (but not all) pilocytic astrocytomas (H&E, original magnification 200×). **E,** Eosinophilic granular bodies are also encountered in a majority (but not all) of pilocytic astrocytomas (H&E, original magnification 400×).

small, bipolar cells around blood vessels and mostly arise in children in the third ventricular and hypothalamic regions.

GEMISTOCYTIC ASTROCYTOMA VERSUS SUBEPENDYMAL GIANT CELL ASTROCYTOMA

Clinical Features

Subependymal giant cell astrocytoma (SEGA) comprises large, eosinophilic cells similar to gemistocytic astrocytoma cells (a variant of fibrillary astrocytoma). SEGA, however, is a distinctive tumor. They arise within the lateral ventricle around the foramen of Monro and present with signs and symptoms related to increased intracranial pressure. Most arise in the first two decades of life. The incidence of SEGA in patients with tuberous sclerosis is 5% to 15%. On imaging, they appear as a solid, sometimes partially calcified mass, contrast enhancing on MRI studies.

Pathologic Features

GROSS FINDINGS

They are typically located in the walls of the lateral ventricles and are sharply demarcated, multinodular lesions in contrast to the infiltrative gemistocytic astrocytomas. SEGAs may be focally cystic, hemorrhagic, calcified, and rarely necrotic.

MICROSCOPIC FINDINGS

Table 3.5 compares SEGA with the gemistocytic astrocytoma. As already mentioned, SEGAs are marked by large, plump cells with abundant eosinophilic cytoplasm and arranged in sheets, fascicles, or nests (Fig. 3.5A and B). The cells are larger than those typically seen in a gemistocytic astrocytoma. Areas resembling a more typical fibrillary astrocytoma with high nuclear-to-cytoplasmic ratio tumor cells are not present. Nuclear pseudoinclusions may be present in some SEGAs. Nuclear pleomorphism may be prominent in some cases and may be accompanied by multinucleated cells. Hyalinized blood vessels with perivascular T lymphocytes are common (Fig. 3.5C). Scattered mast cells are present in SEGAs. Mitotic figures, a feature of higher-grade gemistocytic astrocytomas, are not typical of SEGA. Occasionally, vascular proliferative changes and necrosis may be seen in a SEGA, but these features do not indicate that the tumor is higher grade as they do with a gemistocytic astrocytoma (Fig. 3.5D). SEGAs are considered WHO grade 1 neoplasms.

TABLE 3.5

Gemistocytic Astrocytoma Versus Subependymal Giant Cell Astrocytoma

	Gemistocytic Astrocytoma	Subependymal Giant Cell Astrocytoma
Age	Adults	Young
Location	Lobar	Lateral ventricle/foramen of Monro region
Gross	Infiltrative	Circumscribed
Large eosinophilic cells	Yes (smaller)	Yes (larger)
Spindle cell component	Sometimes	Sometimes
Cytoplastic processes (GFAP)	Circumferentially radiating	Polar
Nuclear pseudoinclusions	Absent	Present
Mast cells	Absent	Present
Lymphocytes	Generally absent	Present
Mitosis	Rare to common	Rare
Vascular proliferation	Common in high grade	Rare
Necrosis	Common in high grade	Rare (autoinfarct)
Malignant progression	Frequent	Very rare
Association	None	Tuberous sclerosis
IDH mutation	Sometimes	Absent
p53 mutation	Sometimes	Absent
ATRX mutation	Sometimes	Absent

Ancillary Studies

On GFAP staining, cytoplasmic processes are polar in their arrangement in a SEGA compared with gemistocytic astrocytes, which demonstrate circumferentially radiating cytoplasmic processes. Similar to other astrocytic tumors, SEGAs are S-100 protein positive. Some SEGAs may demonstrate immunoreactivity with neuronal markers such as synaptophysin and NeuN, staining patterns not seen in gemistocytic astrocytomas. IDH, p53, and ATRX abnormalities observed in a subset of gemistocytic astrocytomas are not features of SEGA. Cell proliferation labeling indices are low in SEGA but in an overlapping range with low-grade gemistocytic astrocytoma.

Prognosis and Therapy

SEGAs are considered low-grade lesions and have an excellent prognosis after gross total resection. Incompletely

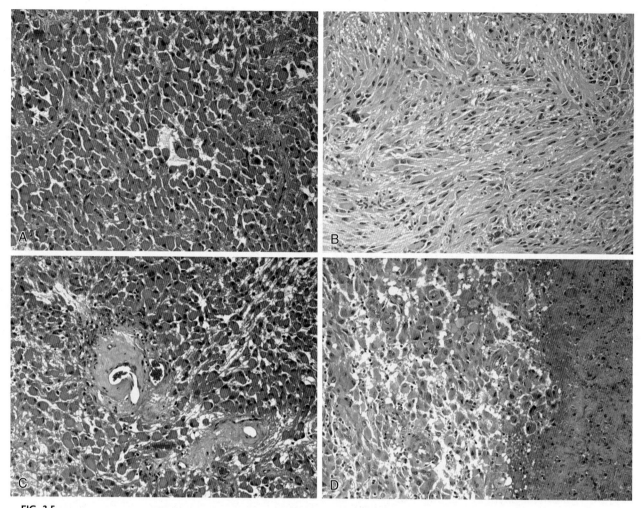

FIG. 3.5

A, Subependymal giant cell astrocytoma (grade 1) marked by a sheet-like proliferation of large, rounded cells with abundant eosinophilic cytoplasm (hematoxylin and eosin [H&E], original magnification 200×). **B,** Some subependymal giant cell astrocytomas may show areas in which the tumor cells are more spindled and arranged in fascicles (H&E, original magnification 200×). **C,** Perivascular sclerosis and perivascular lymphocytes may be encountered in some subependymal giant cell astrocytomas (H&E, original magnification 200×). **D,** An astrocytoma with gemistocytes and necrosis, consistent with a glioblastoma (grade 4) (H&E, original magnification 200×).

resected tumors may recur. In young patients with tuberous sclerosis, regular surveillance by MRI every 1–3 years is recommended until age 25 years. Malignant progression, a common occurrence with low-grade gemistocytic astrocytomas, is very rare in SEGAs.

PLEOMORPHIC XANTHOASTROCYTOMA VERSUS GANGLIOGLIOMA

Clinical Features

PXA (WHO grade 2) is rare astrocytic neoplasm that arises primarily in children and young adults. Tumors are located in the superficial cortex and meninges, most commonly in the temporal lobe. Given the usual location of the tumor, the vast majority of PXAs present with epilepsy.

On MRI, PXAs are either hypointense or isointense to gray matter on T1-weighted images and hyperintense or show mixed signal intensity on T2-weighted images.

Gangliogliomas are low-grade (WHO grade 1) glioneuronal tumors which similarly arise in young patients, most commonly in the temporal lobe as well. It is the most common neoplasm to be associated with pharmacoresistant epilepsy. On imaging, the tumors are typically intracortical and circumscribed and often have a cystic component to them. Contrast enhancement is variable and may be negligible to prominent.

Pathologic Features

GROSS FINDINGS

PXAs are usually superficially situated, fairly circumscribed, and extend sometimes to involve the overlying leptomeninges. Often, they have a cystic component with mural nodule. Higher-grade tumors may contain areas of necrosis. Gangliogliomas are grossly circumscribed masses which may be either solid or cystic. Calcifications may be evident in a subset of gangliogliomas.

MICROSCOPIC FINDINGS

Table 3.6 compares and contrasts PXAs with gangliogliomas. Microscopically, PXAs are marked by prominent cellularity and often comprise a mixture of large, frequently multinucleated giant astrocytes, spindled cells, and cells which may show lipidized cytoplasmic changes (Fig. 3.6A). Intranuclear inclusions are commonly seen. Vascular proliferative changes are fairly commonly encountered but do not necessarily portend a worse outcome. Other features that are somewhat more unique to PXA in addition to the lipidized astrocytes are the presence of perivascular lymphocytes and plasma cells, eosinophilic granular bodies, Rosenthal fibers, and the presence of increased reticulin deposition, not only around blood vessels but also in between tumor cells (Fig. 3.6B and C). Rare anaplastic PXAs

(WHO grade 3) are marked additionally by increased mitotic activity and necrosis.

Gangliogliomas are characterized by a biphasic appearance; areas of the tumor resemble a glioma (usually low grade) and other foci contain atypical appearing neuronal or ganglionic cells (Fig. 3.6D). Both components are usually not uniformly distributed throughout the neoplasm and extensive tissue sampling of the lesion is recommended in order to identify both components of the neoplasm (Fig. 3.6E). The degree of pleomorphism that characterizes PXA is not seen in most gangliogliomas. Xanthomatous change in astrocytes, increased pericellular reticulin, and vascular proliferative changes are not features of ganglioglioma. Prominent mitotic activity and necrosis are not typical features of gangliogliomas but may be encountered in rare cases of anaplastic ganglioglioma (WHO grade 3). Perivascular chronic inflammatory cells, Rosenthal fibers, and eosinophilic granular bodies are variably encountered, similar to PXA. Calcifications are more commonly seen in gangliogliomas (Fig. 3.6F). Many gangliogliomas are accompanied by adjacent focal cortical dysplasia (cortical architectural disorganization) warranting a designation of type IIIb focal cortical dysplasia, according to the International League Against Epilepsy (ILAE) classification of focal cortical dysplasia (Fig. 3.6G); this finding has been also described in a minority of PXAs.

Ancillary Studies

Both tumors typically demonstrate focal areas of GFAP and S-100 protein immunoreactivity. The neuronal cell component of ganglioglioma will stain with neural markers including MAP2, neurofilaments, synaptophysin, and NeuN. Interestingly, most PXAs contain a second population of cells that also stain with neural markers. BRAF alterations may be seen in a subset of both tumors. IDH, ATRX, and p53 mutations, all features of a subset of fibrillary astrocytomas, are not a feature of either of these tumors.

Prognosis and Therapy

PXAs generally do well. About 70% of patients have recurrence-free survival at 5 years. Extent of resection is most important in predicting recurrence. Anaplastic tumors have poorer outcomes than the lower-grade tumors and overall poorer 5-year survival and higher 5-year recurrence rates. Gangliogliomas have much better outcomes than PXAs. Control of epilepsy in patients with ganglioglioma is often related to excision of the adjacent focal cortical dysplasia (the actual cause of seizures in these patients).

TABLE 3.6

Pleomorphic Xanthoastrocytoma Versus Ganglioglioma

	Pleomorphic Xanthoastrocytoma	Ganglioglioma
Age	Pediatric	Pediatric
Location	Temporal and parietal lobes	Temporal lobe most common
Gross	Superficial, circumscribed	Circumscribed
Nuclear pleomorphism	Prominent	Mild to prominent
Xanthomatous changes	Often present	Absent
Mitoses	Variable, prominent in anaplastic tumors	Rare, prominent in anaplastic tumors
Vascular proliferation	Present	Absent
Necrosis	Generally absent except in anaplastic tumors	Absent
Perivascular lymphocytes	Common	Variable
Rosenthal fibers	May be present	May be present
Eosinophilic granular bodies	Often present	Often present
Pericellular reticulin	Present	Generally absent
Neuronal component	Sometimes present	Present
BRAF alterations	Sometimes	Sometimes

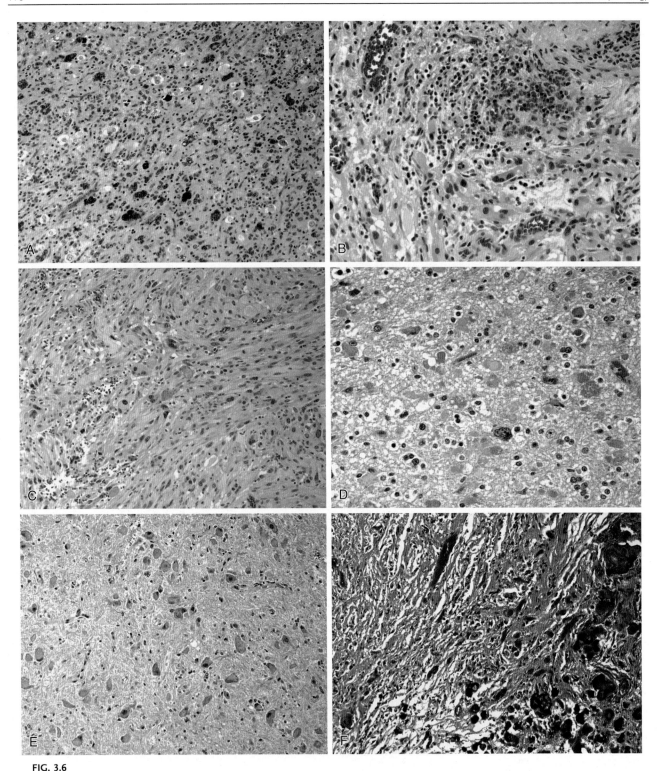

FIG. 3.6

A, Pleomorphic xanthoastrocytoma (grade 2) marked by prominent variation in nuclear size, multinucleated giant tumor cells and occasional cells with lipidized cytoplasm (xanthoastrocytes) (hematoxylin and eosin [H&E], original magnification 200×). **B,** Perivascular lymphocytes may be encountered in pleomorphic xanthoastrocytoma (H&E, original magnification 400×). **C,** Eosinophilic granular bodies may also be seen in some pleomorphic xanthoastrocytomas (H&E, original magnification 200×). **D,** Gangliogliomas (grade 1) are marked by a proliferation of atypical appearing glial cells with an associated atypical ganglion cell component. This tumor also shows some eosinophilic granular bodies (original magnification 400×). **E,** The two components of the ganglioglioma may not be evenly distributed throughout the tumor; this area shows a predominantly ganglion cell component (H&E, original magnification 200×). **F,** Calcifications may be focally present in some gangliogliomas (H&E, original magnification 200×).

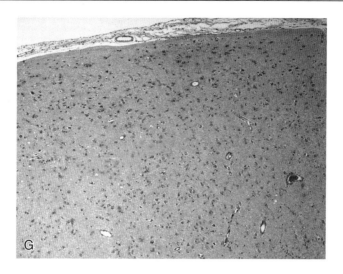

FIG. 3.6, cont'd

G, An area of cortical architectural disorganization (focal cortical dysplasia) adjacent to a ganglioglioma; the two pathologies are commonly coexistent (H&E, original magnification 100×).

DYSEMBRYOPLASTIC NEUROEPITHELIAL TUMOR VERSUS CENTRAL NEUROCYTOMA VERSUS OLIGODENDROGLIOMA

Clinical Features

Two tumors which can microscopically resemble oligodendroglioma and run the risk of being confused with an oligodendroglioma are the dysembryoplastic neuroepithelial tumor (DNT) and central neurocytoma. Both of these tumors have unique characteristics that allow for distinction from oligodendroglioma and both lack the molecular signature (IDH mutation and chromosome 1p/19q codeletion) that are part of the definition of an oligodendroglioma.

DNTs are low-grade glioneuronal neoplasms (WHO grade 1) which classically present in pediatric patients and in young adults, most commonly in the temporal lobe, with a history of pharmacoresistant epilepsy. Less commonly, they can be encountered in other locations such as the frontal lobe (second most common site), basal ganglia, brain stem, and cerebellum. On imaging, they are generally cortical based and on MRI appear as T2-hyperintense, multiple or single pseudocysts.

Central neurocytomas are WHO grade 2 neural neoplasms that arise in the lateral ventricles and in the region of the foramen of Monro. Most patients present in the third and fourth decades of life. Symptoms are related to increased intracranial pressure caused by the tumor. On imaging, central neurocytomas appear as T1-isointense masses with a soap-bubble multicystic appearance on T2-weighted images.

Pathologic Features

GROSS FINDINGS

Grossly, DNT can range in size from a few millimeters to several centimeters. They are typically circumscribed, cortical based, frequently multinodular masses. In the area of the tumor, the surface of the brain often looks blistered due to microcystic changes. Central neurocytomas appear as somewhat circumscribed, gray, friable masses. Foci of calcification and hemorrhage may be apparent grossly. Rare cases of extraventricular neurocytoma and cases of neurocytomas with fat tissue (liponeurocytomas) have been described.

MICROSCOPIC FINDINGS

Table 3.7 compares the salient features of DNTs and central neurocytomas with oligodendrogliomas. Microscopically, DNTs resemble multinodular oligodendrogliomas (Fig. 3.7A). Most of the nodules are cortical based. Tumor cells are generally rounded with scant cytoplasm. Intermixed with the rounded cells is a second population of benign neuronal cells (Fig. 3.7B). Often, the tumor has a microcystic background and neuronal cells can be seen "floating" in the cystic spaces. Pericellular clearing, calcifications, and an arcuate capillary pattern, similar to what is commonly seen in oligodendroglioma, may be encountered in DNTs as well. Rarely, minigemistocytes may be present in some of the nodules (Fig. 3.7C). Vascular proliferative changes, perineuronal satellitosis, prominent mitotic activity, and necrosis are not seen. Similar to gangliogliomas, most DNTs are accompanied by adjacent focal cortical dysplasia.

TABLE 3.7

Dysembryoplastic Neuroepithelial Tumor Versus Central Neurocytoma Versus Oligodendroglioma

	Dysembryoplastic Neuroepithelial Tumor	Central Neurocytoma	Oligodendroglioma
Age	Pediatric, young adult	Adult	Adult
Location	Temporal lobe most common	Lateral ventricle	Frontal lobe most common
Gross	Circumscribed, cortical based	Circumscribed	Infiltrative, white matter based
Microcystic	Often	Rare	Sometimes
Perineuronal satellitosis	Absent	Absent	May be present
Minigemistocytes	Rare	Absent	Sometimes
Floating neurons	Present	Absent	Absent
Calcifications	Rare	Rare	Frequent
Vascular proliferation	Absent	Absent	Frequent in WHO grade 3
Mitoses	Usually absent	Occasionally seen	Frequent in WHO grade 3
Necrosis	Absent	Absent	Frequent in WHO grade 3
Associated focal cortical dysplasia	Present	Absent	Absent
GFAP	Astrocytic cells	Absent	Usually weakly positive
Synaptophysin/NeuN	Scattered positive cells	Diffusely positive	Negative
IDH mutation	Absent	Absent	Present
Chromosomes 1p/19q co-deletion	Absent	Absent	Present

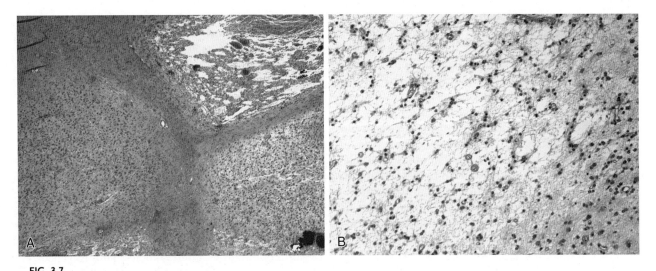

FIG. 3.7

A, Dysembryoplastic neuroepithelial tumors (grade 1) are typically marked by a multinodular architectural pattern with most nodules situated primarily in the cortex (hematoxylin and eosin [H&E], original magnification 40×). **B,** Dysembryoplastic neuroepithelial tumors are composed of rounded cells intermixed with normal-appearing neuronal cells, often arranged against a microcystic background (H&E, original magnification 200×).

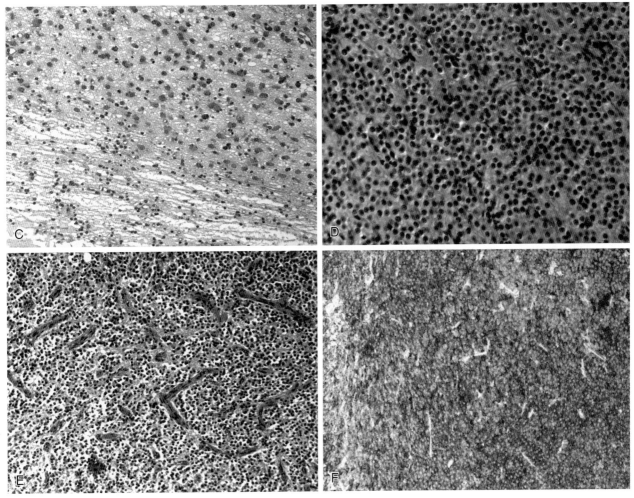

FIG. 3.7, cont'd

C, Occasionally, minigemistocytic cells may be encountered in a dysembryoplastic neuroepithelial tumor (H&E, original magnification 200×). **D,** Central neurocytomas (grade 2) are composed of rounded cells with scant cytoplasm and a "salt-and-pepper" nuclear chromatin pattern (H&E, original magnification 400×). **E,** Similar to oligodendrogliomas, an arcuate capillary vascular pattern is readily discernible in most central neurocytomas (H&E, original magnification 200×). **F,** Diffuse positivity with synaptophysin antibody is observed in central neurocytomas (original magnification 200×).

Central neurocytomas, likewise, are marked by a proliferation of cells with scant cytoplasm and rounded nuclei; nuclei tend to have a salt-and-pepper chromatin pattern (Fig. 3.7D). Areas of the tumor may have a more fibrillary appearance. A prominent arcuate capillary vascular pattern is often seen (Fig. 3.7E). Microcalcifications may be present. Perineuronal satellitosis and minigemistocytes are not typical findings. Occasional cases may show Homer Wright–like pseudorosettes and/or ganglion cells. Prominent mitotic activity, vascular proliferative changes, and necrosis are also not frequent findings in grade 2 central neurocytomas. Rare cases of so-called central neurocytomas with anaplastic features may show prominent mitotic activity, elevated Ki-67 or MIB-1 labeling indices (often greater than 3%), necrosis, or vascular proliferation.

Ancillary Studies

Both DNTs and central neurocytomas do not demonstrate the molecular features of oligodendrogliomas—IDH mutation and 1p/19q codeletions. GFAP immunoreactivity may be seen in the minigemistocytic component, if present, of DNT. The neuronal component of DNT as well as neurocytomas stains with a variety of neural markers including synaptophysin, NeuN, MAP2, and class III beta-tubulin (Fig. 3.7F).

Prognosis and Therapy

Given their relative circumscription, DNTs are amenable to gross total resection. Recurrences are rare. Similar to gangliogliomas, the epilepsy symptoms are often due to the coexistent focal cortical dysplasia. Malignant transformation is also a very rare occurrence. Most central neurocytomas behave in a benign fashion; extent of surgical resection is the best predictor of outcome. Postoperative radiotherapy is recommended by some for subtotally resected tumors.

EPENDYMOMA VERSUS SUBEPENDYMOMA VERSUS MYXOPAPILLARY EPENDYMOMA

Clinical Features

Ependymomas comprise about 6% to 7% of all tumors of the CNS. Ependymomas, similar to oligodendrogliomas, are grouped by the WHO into low-grade (grade 2) and anaplastic (grade 3) lesions. They are more commonly encountered in children; they are the third most common primary CNS tumor of childhood (first two being pilocytic astrocytoma and medulloblastoma). These tumors are derived from ependymal cells and so most of them arise in the ventricular system or central canal of the spinal cord. About 60% of them arise in the posterior fossa region, 30% in the supratentorial compartment, and the rest in the spinal cord and in other rare sites (e.g., ovaries, broad ligaments, and mediastinum/lung). Their clinical presentation is related to signs and symptoms secondary to increased intracranial pressure or mass effect. Spinal cord tumors may present with back pain or focal sensory and/or motor deficits. There is an association of ependymomas with neurofibromatosis type II. Spinal cord tumors are associated with syringomyelia. On MRI studies, these circumscribed tumors may show focal enhancement. Cystic changes, hemorrhage, and calcifications may be variably present.

Subependymomas, WHO grade 1, are benign, slow-growing lesions that may arise at any age but are most common in middle-aged and elderly individuals and more common in men. They arise within the ventricular system, most commonly growing in the fourth ventricle; occasional cases have been documented in the spinal cord. Similar to ordinary ependymoma, clinical presentation usually manifests as symptoms related to increased intracranial pressure. Spinal cord tumors present with motor or sensory deficits. On imaging, subependymomas present as circumscribed masses which range from hypointense to hyperintense on T1- and T2-weighted MRI studies.

Myxopapillary ependymomas are also WHO grade 2 neoplasms that arise almost exclusively in the region of the conus medullaris, cauda equina, and filum terminale and present with back pain. They typically present in young adults and are more commonly encountered in males. On imaging, they are circumscribed, enhancing masses.

Pathologic Features

GROSS FINDINGS

Ependymomas are well-circumscribed, intraventricular masses that are soft and gray-tan colored. They may be calcified. High-grade tumors may show areas of necrosis. Similarly, both subependymomas and myxopapillary ependymomas are circumscribed. Both of these tumors may also demonstrate calcifications and areas of hemorrhage.

MICROSCOPIC FINDINGS

Table 3.8 summarizes and compares features of ependymomas with subependymomas and myxopapillary ependymomas. Histologically, ependymomas are characterized by the presence of either true rosettes (ependymal cells arranged around a space or lumen; Fig. 3.8A) or pseudorosettes (ependymal cells arranged around a blood vessel; Fig. 3.8B). Tumor cell nuclei are typically uniform in appearance (although some pleomorphism may be evident in some tumors) with slight elongation of nuclei. Some tumors have a more epithelial appearance (Fig. 3.8A) and microvilli may be evident in those cases. Other less commonly encountered subtypes include papillary, clear cell (Fig. 3.8C), tanycytic (spindled cells; Fig. 3.8D), and melanotic. Anaplastic tumors are variably marked by increased mitotic activity, vascular proliferative changes, and/or necrosis (Fig. 3.8E). Ultrastructurally, ependymomas demonstrate microvilli, cilia, and ciliary body attachments (blepharoplasts).

Subependymomas have a variable hypercellularity pattern best seen at low magnification—clusters of cells with intervening hypocellular zones ("islands of blue in a sea of pink"; Fig. 3.8F). Microcystic areas are frequent. Rarely, mitotic figures may be encountered. Occasionally, nuclear pleomorphism may be encountered. Rosettes or pseudorosettes are not a feature of subependymoma, although rare cases of composite tumors which have mixed patterns of ependymoma and subependymoma have been documented. Rarely, the tumor may autoinfarct focally and result in focal necrosis. Vascular proliferative changes are not a feature of subependymoma.

Myxopapillary ependymoma classically has a pseudopapillary architecture marked by blood vessels surrounded by variable amounts of mucin material which in turn is surrounded by tumor cells (Fig. 3.8G). Rosettes and pseudorosettes are not seen in these tumors. In areas, the tumor may grow in a more solid pattern. Tumor cells contain variable amounts of eosinophilic cytoplasm and elongated nuclei with small nucleoli. Focally prominent nuclear pleomorphism

TABLE 3.8
Ependymoma Versus Subependymoma Versus Myxopapillary Ependymoma

	Ependymoma	Subependymoma	Myxopapillary Ependymoma
Age	Pediatric	Adult	Young adult
Location	Ventricles and spinal cord	Ventricles	Filum terminale and lower spinal cord
Gross	Circumscribed	Circumscribed	Circumscribed
True rosettes	Present	Absent	Absent
Perivascular pseudorosettes	Present	Absent	Absent
Papillary architecture	Rare	Absent	Often
Mucoid stroma (mucin positive)	Absent	Absent	Present
Microcystic change	Rare	Common	Rare
Nuclear pleomorphism	Variable	Variable	Variable
Vascular hyalinization	Rare	Rare	More common
Mitoses	Variable, more in high-grade tumors	Rare	Rare
Necrosis	High-grade tumors	Rare	Rare
Vascular proliferation	High-grade tumors	Absent	Absent

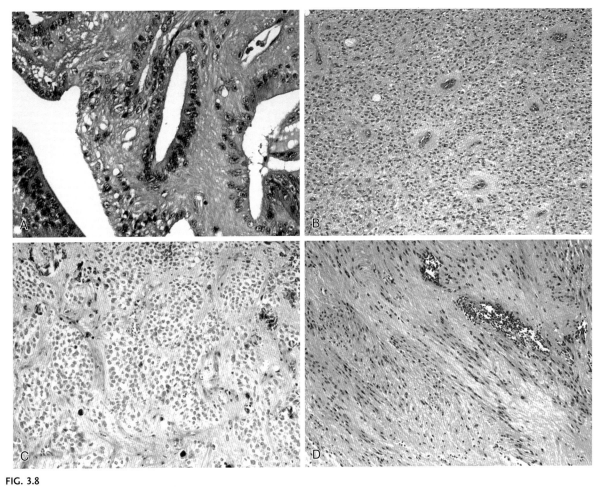

FIG. 3.8

A, An ependymoma (grade 2) marked by true ependymal rosette—tumor cells arranged around a space (hematoxylin and eosin [H&E], original magnification 400×). **B,** An ependymoma marked by perivascular pseudorosettes, characterized by blood vessels rimmed by cytoplasmic processes and tumor cell nuclei (original magnification 200×). **C,** An ependymoma demonstrating focal clear cell change with mild nuclear pleomorphism and calcifications (H&E, original magnification 200×). **D,** Tanycytic ependymomas are marked by cells with an elongated, spindled appearance (H&E, original magnification 200×).

Continued

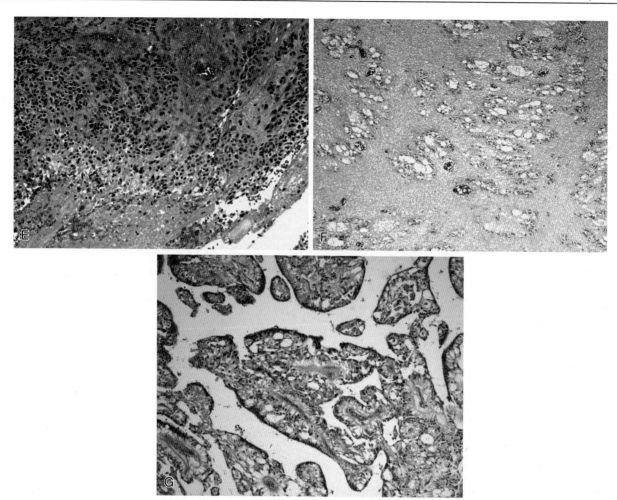

FIG. 3.8, cont'd

E, An anaplastic ependymoma (grade 3) marked by focal necrosis and vascular proliferative changes (H&E, original magnification 200×). **F,** Subependymomas (grade 1) are marked by loose arrangements of tumor cell nuclei with intervening hypocellular zones. Microcystic changes are commonly present (H&E, original magnification 100×). **G,** Myxopapillary ependymomas (grade 2) are characterized by blood vessels surrounded by variable amounts of mucin material, which is surrounded by tumor cells. An overall papillary architecture pattern is seen in some tumors (H&E, original magnification 100×).

may be evident. Mitotic figures, vascular proliferative changes, and necrosis are not typical. Vascular sclerosis, hemorrhage, and hemosiderin deposition may be present in some tumors.

Ancillary Studies

Ependymomas stain with antibodies to GFAP, S-100 protein, vimentin, and EMA. Olig 2 immunostaining is usually sparse as compared with other gliomas. Focally, cytokeratin immunostaining may be present. Myxopapillary ependymomas stain similarly with the aforementioned antibodies. Subependymomas are usually not EMA positive.

Ependymomas arising in the spinal cord and arising in the setting of neurofibromatosis type 2 frequently harbor chromosome 22 abnormalities. NF2 gene involvement is involved in the pathogenesis of ependymomas. Fusion genes RELA and YAP1 are commonly seen in supratentorial ependymomas.

Prognosis and Therapy

Adults with ependymomas do significantly better than children with ependymomas. Extent of surgical resection is the most reliable predictor of outcome in ependymomas, irrespective of tumor grade. Supratentorial tumors fare better than posterior fossa neoplasms. Spinal tumors do better than tumors in the brain. Metastases are a bad prognostic sign. Ependymomas which are RELA fusion positive typically fare worse. Treatment usually involves surgical resection accompanied by radiation and/or chemotherapy. Subependymomas have an excellent prognosis and are generally curable with gross total resection. Incompletely resected myxopapillary ependymomas may develop late recurrence or they may rarely metastasize; most do very well with surgical resection. Adjuvant radiotherapy may improve progression-free survival in incompletely resected tumors.

MENINGIOMA VERSUS SCHWANNOMA VERSUS SOLITARY FIBROUS TUMOR

Clinical Features

Meningiomas are the most commonly encountered primary non-glial tumors of the brain. They arise most commonly in older adults (median age, 65 years), and there is a marked female predilection for the development of meningioma. They are well known to be associated with neurofibromatosis type II and arise with increased frequency in patients who have received prior radiation to the head (post radiation–induced neoplasm). Increased risk has also been associated with breast cancer, use of endogenous/exogenous hormones, smoking, and increased body mass index. The vast majority of cases arise in the intracranial, spinal, or orbital regions; less commonly, tumors may arise in the ventricles, epidural region or in other locations in the body (e.g., ear, lung, skin). They are generally slow-growing, circumscribed tumors which produce signs and symptoms secondary to compression of adjacent structures. On MRI studies, they appear as isodense, contrast-enhancing, dural-based tumors. Calcifications in the form of psammoma bodies or sometimes osseous metaplasia may be seen. The perimeter of the tumor may show a dural tail. Cystic changes may sometimes be evident. Peritumoral edema may be present adjacent to certain subtypes and in higher-grade tumors. Tumors may invade into adjacent structures (skull and soft tissues); higher-grade tumors may show evidence of brain invasion. Some tumors may grow in a flattened configuration (meningioma en plaque).

Schwannomas are low-grade tumors (WHO grade 1) derived from the myelin-producing Schwann cells of the peripheral nervous system. Most arise outside the CNS. Intracranial tumors can arise from any of the cranial nerves (most commonly involving the eighth cranial nerve in the cerebellopontine angle region). They also arise fairly commonly from the spinal nerve roots. Most arise as solitary masses; about 4% of them arise in the setting of neurofibromatosis type II and a subset may arise in the setting of schwannomatosis. Bilateral cranial nerve VIII schwannomas are diagnostic of neurofibromatosis type II. The peak incidence is in patients in the fourth to sixth decades, and there appears to be no strong sex predilection overall. Cranial nerve VIII tumors present with symptoms of hearing loss, tinnitus, and vertigo. Spinal tumors present with radicular pain and signs of nerve root or cord compression. On imaging, schwannomas are well-circumscribed, variably enhancing masses. Vestibular tumors may demonstrate an ice cream cone appearance with a tapered interosseous component widening out as it exits the internal auditory canal. Evidence of adjacent bone erosion may be seen in some tumors.

Solitary fibrous tumor (SFT) are mesenchymal tumors marked by a prominent vascular pattern. They run the gamut from low-grade neoplasms (WHO grade 1) to high-grade tumors (WHO grade 3). They are typically dural-based, generally circumscribed lesions which arise most commonly in the fourth and fifth decades of life, slightly more frequently in males. Symptoms are dependent on location of the mass. On MRI, they are isointense on T1-weighted images and hyperintense or show mixed intensity on T2-weighted studies.

Pathologic Features

GROSS FINDINGS

Meningiomas, grossly, are rubbery or firm, circumscribed, sometimes lobulated tumors that are frequently dural based. They may be associated with hyperostosis of the adjacent skull. As previously mentioned, they may grow in a flat, en-plaque fashion in some cases. The gross appearance may vary depending on the subtype of tumor (e.g., metaplastic, angiomatous, psammomatous, and microcystic). Schwannomas are rounded, circumscribed, light tan, often encapsulated masses. They may demonstrate cystic areas, yellow patches with increased macrophages, or hemorrhagic foci. SFTs are usually well-circumscribed, white (more collagenized tumors) to brown masses. Areas with a hemorrhagic or myxoid appearance may be seen. High-grade tumors may show areas of necrosis.

MICROSCOPIC FINDINGS

Table 3.9 compares and contrasts features of meningioma, schwannoma, and SFT. Meningiomas come in a variety of histologic subtypes. The fibrous variant (WHO grade 1) is the one that most resembles a schwannoma or spindled SFT. The tumor cells are elongated and arranged in fascicles with variable amounts of intermixed collagen and hyalinized blood vessels (Fig. 3.9A). Elongated cell nuclei tend to have more rounded ends versus the more tapered ends of schwannoma nuclei. Psammoma bodies may be variably present. Focal areas of these tumors may contain cells with more oval nuclei, arranged in a syncytial-like growth pattern (meningothelial type; Fig. 3.9B). In these areas, intranuclear pseudoinclusions representing cytoplasmic invaginations into the nuclei may be present (Fig. 3.9C). Tumors with mixed pattern are often referred to as transitional meningiomas.

TABLE 3.9

Meningoma Versus Schwannoma Versus Solitary Fibrous Tumor/Hemangiopericytoma

	Meningioma	Schwannoma	Solitary Fibrous Tumor
Age	Adult	Adult	Adult
Sex prediction	Female > male	None	None
Association	Neurofibromatosis II breast cancer, prior radiation	Neurofibromatosis II	None
Location	Dural based, rarely intraventricular	Associated with peripheral nerve	Most dural based
Gross	Circumscribed	Circumscribed	Most circumscribed
Spindled cells	Some (fibrous variant)	Present	Present
Psammoma bodies	Often	Generally absent	Absent
Biphasic	Absent	Often	Absent
Verocay bodies	Absent	Absent	Present
Intranuclear pseudoinclusions	Often	Absent	Absent
Staghorn vessels	Absent	Absent	Present
Hyalinized blood vessels	Often	Often	Rare
Mitoses	In grade 2 and 3 tumors	Generally rare	Sometimes (higher grade)
EMA	Positive	Negative	Negative
Progesterone receptor	Positive	Negative	Negative
SSRT 2a	Positive	Negative	Negative
Stat 6	Negative	Negative	Positive
S-100 protein	May be totally positive	Positive	Negative

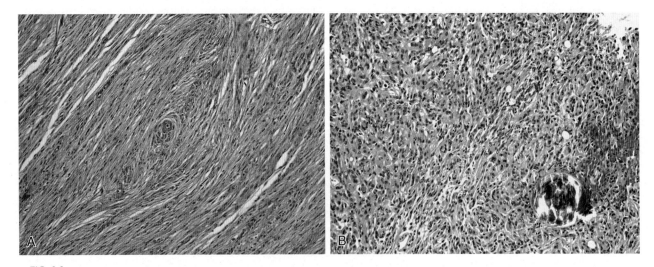

FIG. 3.9

A, Fibrous meningioma (grade 1) marked by a proliferation of bland spindled cells with rounded nuclear ends (hematoxylin and eosin [H&E], original magnification 200×). **B,** Meningothelial or syncytial meningioma pattern characterized by more rounded cells. Psammomas bodies may be seen in any of the meningioma subtypes (H&E, original magnification 200×).

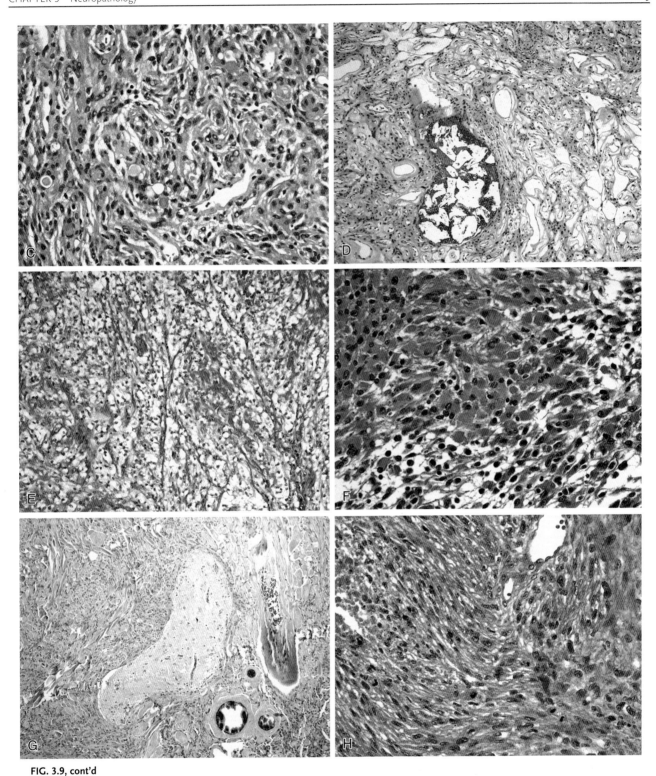

FIG. 3.9, cont'd

C, A secretory meningioma (with eosinophilic amorphous protein collections) (grade 1) with intranuclear pseudoinclusions representing cytoplasmic invaginations which are a common cytologic feature of meningioma (H&E, original magnification 400×). **D,** Angiomatous meningioma (grade 1) with microcystic changes and evidence of embolization within a blood vessel in the tumor (H&E, original magnification 100×). **E,** A clear cell meningioma (grade 2) characterized by tumor cells with glycogen-rich clear cytoplasm (H&E, original magnification 200×). **F,** Rhabdoid meningioma (grade 3) marked by tumor cells with cytoplasmic inclusions and eccentrically placed nuclei (H&E, original magnification 400×). **G,** Brain-invasive meningiomas are more aggressive behaving tumors (grade 2) (H&E, original magnification 100×). **H,** An anaplastic meningioma (grade 3) marked by multiple mitotic figures in a single high-power field and focal necrosis (H&E, original magnification 400×).

Continued

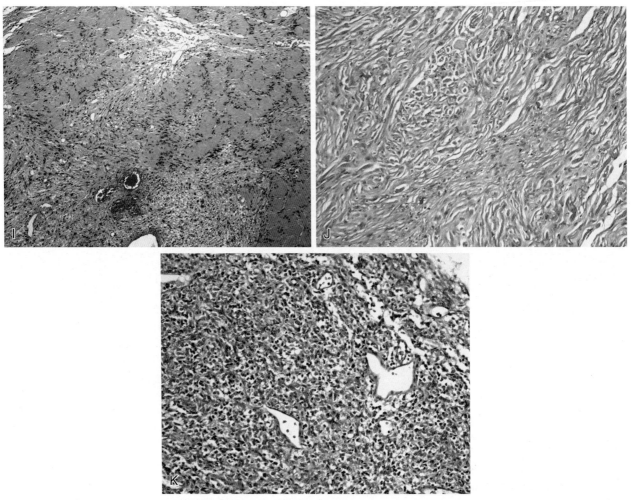

FIG. 3.9, cont'd

I, Schwannoma (grade 1) marked by compact Antoni A pattern with Verocay bodies and a looser Antoni B pattern (H&E, original magnification 100×). **J,** Low-grade solitary fibrous tumor (grade 1) marked by bland, often spindled cells with increased collagen between individual tumors cell (H&E, original magnification 200×). **K,** Grade 2 solitary fibrous tumor characterized by a staghorn vascular pattern and more prominent cellularity (H&E, original magnification 200×).

A host of other meningioma subtypes are well documented. Most of these do not morphologically resemble schwannomas or SFT. Other grade 1 variants include psammomatous, angiomatous (Fig. 3.9D), microcystic, secretory, metaplastic, and lymphoplasmacytic-rich types. Clear cell (Fig. 3.9E) and chordoid variants represent grade 2 lesions; rhabdoid (Fig. 3.9F) and papillary variants are grade 3 tumors. Brain invasion warrants a grade 2 designation (Fig. 3.9G). Tumors with ≥4 MF/10 HPF are also grade 2 neoplasms, and ≥20 MF/10 HPF defines grade 3 tumors. High-grade SFT (WHO grade 2 or 3) tumors may resemble atypical meningiomas (WHO grade 2), marked by the presence of three or more worrisome features (disordered architecture or sheeting, small cell change, hypercellularity, prominent nucleoli, and necrosis). Tumors with overly malignant cytology are also designated as grade 3 meningiomas and can also be confused with high-grade SFT (Fig. 3.9H).

Schwannomas classically are marked by a proliferation of spindled cells. Tumors demonstrate areas in which cells are more compactly arranged (Antoni A) juxtaposed with areas marked by microcystic change (Antoni B; Fig. 3.9I). In any given tumor, one or the other pattern may predominate. The Antoni A pattern most resembles the fibrous meningioma. Hyalinized blood vessels and perivascular whorling may be seen in both tumors. Nuclear palisading (Verocay bodies) is a distinctive feature of some schwannomas (see Fig. 3.9I). Schwannomas may show areas of nuclear pleomorphism (degenerative or ancient change), cystic change, hemosiderin deposition, or increased lipid-rich macrophages. Most schwannomas, except the rare psammomatous melanotic schwannoma, do not contain psammoma bodies.

SFTs are marked by a staghorn vascular pattern. Low-grade tumors often are marked by spindle-shaped cells arranged in a patternless manner with increased collagen deposition between individual cells (Fig. 3.9J). Parameters used for grading include necrosis and elevated mitotic counts. Tumors with ≥ 5 MF/10 HPF are considered grade 3 (Fig. 3.9K).

Ancillary Studies

Most meningiomas demonstrate EMA immunostaining and the majority show progesterone receptor immunoreactivity. Somatostatin receptor 2A (SSTR 2A) immunostaining is expressed in the majority of tumors, including high-grade tumors. Focal S-100 protein immunostaining may be encountered in a minority of cases. In contrast, schwannomas demonstrate diffuse strong immunostaining with S-100 protein antibody and do not stain with the other aforementioned meningioma markers. SOX-10 staining is also commonly encountered in schwannomas. STAT-6 and CD34 staining are features of SFT and are not seen in meningiomas. The typical immunomarkers of meningioma do not stain SFT.

Prognosis and Therapy

Most meningiomas are curable by gross total resection. If tumor is left behind after surgery, regrowth can occur (sooner in higher-grade tumors than in grade 1 neoplasms). Grade 2 and 3 tumors are more likely to recur in a shorter period of time and are more likely to metastasize (grade 3). High-grade tumors may require adjuvant radiation therapy following surgery. Schwannomas are curable by surgical resection. Only rarely do they recur, if incompletely excised, and only rare cases undergo malignant degeneration. Recurrences are commonly encountered (30%–40% of cases) with cellular and plexiform schwannomas. Low-grade SFT lesions are considered benign and curable by surgical resection. Higher-grade tumors are more likely to recur and develop extracranial metastases (particularly to lung, liver, and bone). Adjuvant radiotherapy is often employed in the postoperative management of high-grade SFT.

HEMANGIOBLASTOMA VERSUS METASTATIC CLEAR CELL RENAL CARCINOMA

Clinical Features

Hemangioblastomas are low-grade (WHO grade 1) neoplasms that arise in adults in the cerebellum, brain stem, and spinal cord. About 30% of cases are associated

with von Hippel-Lindau disease. As its name suggests, it is a vascular tumor which is marked by stromal cells with clear cytoplasm. The main differential diagnostic consideration is with a metastatic clear cell renal cell carcinoma, especially in the setting of von Hippel-Lindau disease, where patients are also prone to develop renal cell carcinoma. Hemangioblastomas show no sex predilection. On imaging, the tumor is a cystic neoplasm with a gadolinium-enhancing mural nodule on MRI study. Spinal cord tumors may be associated with a syrinx. Intracranial tumors often present with symptoms related to impaired cerebrospinal fluid flow, causing increased intracranial pressure. Dysmetria and ataxia may also be seen in cerebellar tumors. Spinal tumors can present with pain, hypesthesia, and incontinence. About 5% of cases are associated with secondary polycythemia vera due to erythropoietin production by the tumor.

Metastatic renal cell carcinoma typically presents in older adults, although patients with von Hippel-Lindau disease may develop a renal cell carcinoma at a much younger age. Metastases are more likely multifocal, circumscribed masses with lesions developing anywhere in the brain, brain stem, or spinal cord. Symptoms will depend on the location of the tumor. Overall, tumors most likely to metastasize to the brain originate from the lung, breast, skin (melanoma), kidney, and gastrointestinal tract.

Pathologic Features

GROSS FINDINGS

Hemangioblastomas present as well-circumscribed, partially cystic (about 60%), highly vascularized tumors. Tumors rich in lipid content may have a more yellow appearance. Metastatic renal cell carcinoma may also appear as a grossly circumscribed lesion which can be highly vascularized as well and may show evidence of hemorrhage. Necrosis may be evident in some cases. Multifocality is not uncommon. A cyst with mural nodule configuration would be unusual in a renal cell carcinoma metastasis.

MICROSCOPIC FINDINGS

Table 3.10 compares and contrasts features of hemangioblastoma with metastatic renal cell carcinoma. Hemangioblastomas are marked by a proliferation of stromal cells with abundant clear vacuolated (lipid-filled) cytoplasm, intermixed with a prominent vasculature (Fig. 3.10A). Clear cell renal cell carcinoma cells are glycogen rich. In the reticular variant of hemangioblastoma, the stromal cells are uniformly distributed within the vascular network. The cellular variant is characterized by clustering of the stromal cells (Fig. 3.10B); this latter variant more closely resembles the typical

TABLE 3.10

Hemangioblastoma Versus Metastatic Renal Carcinoma (Clear Cell)

	Hemangioblastoma	Metastatic Clear Cell Carcinoma
Age	Young adults	Older adults
Location	Most cerebellum	Anywhere in the brain and spinal cord
Association	von Hippel-Lindau	von Hippel-Lindau (renal cell)
Gross	Cystic with mural nodule	Solid, often multiple
Intracellular lipid	Present	Absent
Intracellular glycogen	Absent	Present
Hypervascularity	Present	Present
Necrosis	Generally absent	May be present
Mitoses	Rare	Common
Reticulin staining	Around individual cells	Delineates cell nests
EMA	Negative	Positive
Inhibin	Positive	Negative
PAX8	Negative	Positive

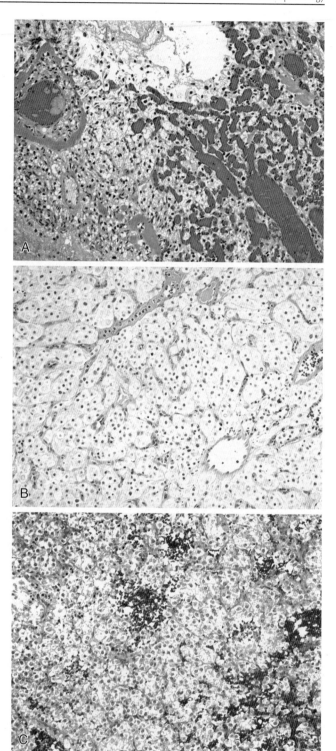

FIG. 3.10

A, Hemangioblastoma (grade 1) characterized by a prominent vasculature with intervening rounded stromal cells with clear or lightly eosinophilic cytoplasm (hematoxylin and eosin [H&E], original magnification 200×). **B,** A cellular variant of hemangioblastoma with stromal cells arranged in nests or clusters, more reminiscent of a renal cell carcinoma (H&E, original magnification 200×). **C,** Metastatic renal cell carcinoma marked by tumor cells arranged in clusters and accompanied by hemorrhage. When in doubt, an inhibin stain in combination with renal cell carcinoma markers such as PAX8 can be used to sort out the differential (H&E, original magnification 200×).

growth pattern of a metastatic renal cell carcinoma (Fig. 3.10C). Prominent mitotic activity and necrosis, features not uncommon in metastases, are unusual in hemangioblastoma. Occasional tumors may show increased numbers of mast cells or extramedullary hematopoiesis. The tissue surrounding the tumor is gliotic and may show prominent numbers of Rosenthal fibers. Consequently, care should be taken not to misinterpret this gliosis with a pilocytic astrocytoma (which can also present on imaging as a cystic tumor with an enhancing mural nodule).

Ancillary Studies

Most hemangioblastomas show at least focal areas in which individual cells are invested by reticulin. In most renal cell carcinoma metastases, reticulin outlines nests or clusters of tumor cells. The stromal cells have been described to stain with a variety of markers including vimentin, S-100 protein, neuron-specific enolase, ezrin, aquaporin-1, and brachyury. Markers that stain hemangioblastoma and not renal cell carcinomas are inhibin and D2-40. EMA and renal cell carcinoma markers such as CD10 and PAX8 generally do not stain hemangioblastomas.

Prognosis and Therapy

Hemangioblastomas have an excellent prognosis, if completely resected. In the setting of von Hippel-Lindau disease, patients are at risk of developing multiple lesions over time. Individual metastases can be resected, but prognosis is ultimately related to patient age, number of brain lesions, extent of disease outside the brain, and Karnofsky performance score.

MEDULLOBLASTOMA VERSUS ATYPICAL TERATOID/RHABDOID TUMOR

Clinical Features

Medulloblastomas are high-grade (WHO grade 4) embryonal neuroepithelial tumors that arise in the cerebellum, predominantly in children (median age, 9 years). It is the most common malignant tumor and the second most common tumor of childhood (pilocytic astrocytoma being the most common), accounting for 25% in intracranial neoplasms in children. A similar percentage of medulloblastomas arise in adults. There appears to be a slight male predominance (especially in patients over the age of 3 years). Presentation typically manifests with signs of increased intracranial pressure (headaches, nausea/vomiting, and ataxia). They have a propensity to seed the cerebrospinal fluid and spread in that fashion. On imaging, they appear as solid, contrast-enhancing masses with associated edema.

Atypical teratoid/rhabdoid tumors (AT/RTs) are malignant embryonal neoplasms (WHO grade 4) that also arise primarily in children and arise in a broader distribution (in both supratentorial and infratentorial compartments). They account for about 1% to 2% of pediatric brain tumors and most arise in the first 3 years of life. There is a slight male predominance. Clinical presentation varies depending on the site of origin and may include lethargy, vomiting, failure to thrive, cranial nerve palsies, headaches, or hemiplegia. Like medulloblastoma, the tumor tends to seed the cerebrospinal fluid pathway. They appear as isodense or hyperintense masses on FLAIR images and show restricted diffusion. Like medulloblastomas, tumors that are cystic or focally necrotic may show areas of heterogenous signal intensity.

Pathologic Features

GROSS FINDINGS

Both tumors present as variably soft, predominantly pink-gray, solid, and often focally necrotic masses.

Those with mesenchymal tissue or intratumoral desmoplasia may be firmer in consistency and have a more tan-white appearance.

MICROSCOPIC FINDINGS

Table 3.11 compares and contrasts medulloblastoma with AT/RT. The typical appearance of a medulloblastoma is that of a sheet of small, relatively rounded cells with hyperchromatic nuclei and scant cytoplasm (Fig. 3.11A). Mitotic figures, apoptotic cells, and foci of geographic necrosis are common (Fig. 3.11B). Occasional tumors may demonstrate Homer Wright pseudorosettes, marked by a rim of nuclei surrounding a neuritic fibrillary core (Fig. 3.11C). A variety of morphologic variants of medulloblastoma have been described in the literature: classic, desmoplastic (Fig. 3.11D), nodular/excessive nodularity, large cell, and anaplastic (Fig. 3.11E) types. Additionally, some tumors may show evidence of myogenic or melanotic differentiation or may have an epithelioid appearance.

AT/RTs are heterogeneous lesions. A subset of tumor cells have a rhabdoid appearance, characterized by abundant eosinophilic cytoplasm and eccentric nuclei with vesicular chromatin and prominent nucleoli (Fig. 3.11F). Eosinophilic globular cytoplasmic inclusions, comprising aggregates of intermediate molecular weight filaments, are a hallmark of these cells. These

TABLE 3.11
Medulloblastoma Versus Atypical Teratoid/Rhabdoid Tumor

	Medulloblastoma	Atypical Teratoid/ Rhabdoid Tumor
Age	Pediatric	Pediatric
Location	Cerebellum	Infratentorial > supratentorial
Gross	Variably soft, focally necrotic	Variably soft, focally necrotic
Small, "blue" cells	Present	Present
Spindle cells	Occasional	Occasional
Rhabdoid morphology	Absent	Present
Synaptophysin	Positive	Positive
EMA	Negative	Positive
Smooth muscle actin	Negative	Positive
GFAP	Variably positive	Variably positive
INI1	Retained	Loss
Keratin	Negative	Variably positive
WNT – activated	Some (10%)	None
SHH – activated	Some (30%)	None
p53 mutated	Some	None

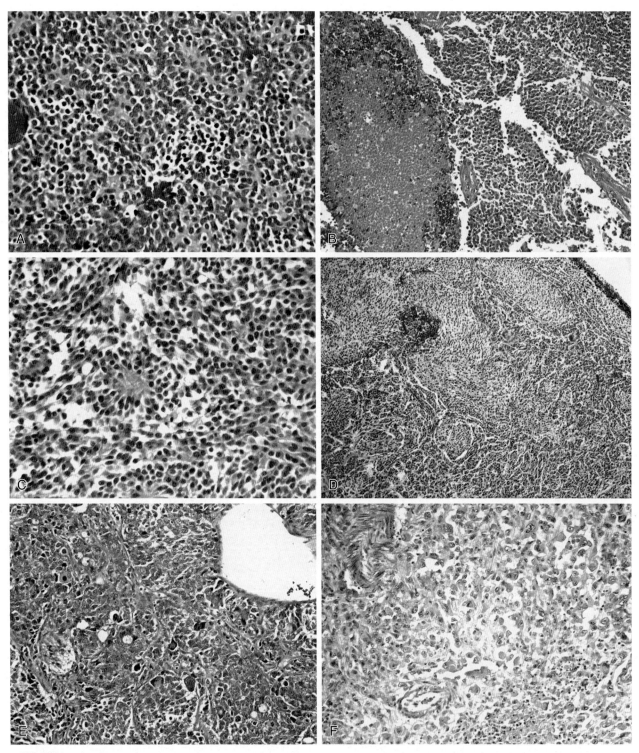

FIG. 3.11

A, Medulloblastoma (grade 4) marked by a proliferation of small cells with scant cytoplasm (hematoxylin and eosin [H&E], original magnification 400×). **B,** Medulloblastoma frequently contain foci of necrosis (H&E, original magnification 200×). **C,** Occasional medulloblastomas demonstrate Homer Wright pseudorosettes (H&E, original magnification 400×). **D,** Desmoplastic medulloblastomas have a nodular architectural pattern with some nodules marked by a looser arrangement of cells (H&E, original magnification 100×). **E,** An anaplastic medulloblastoma characterized by large atypical appearing tumor cells (H&E, original magnification 200×). **F,** An atypical teratoid/rhabdoid tumor (grade 4) with focal necrosis and a population of tumor cells with eccentric nuclei and abundant eosinophilic cytoplasm, composed of intermediate molecular weight filaments (H&E, original magnification 200×).

tumors may also be composed of cells with mesenchymal (spindled), epithelial, and embryonal (resembling medulloblastoma) features. Areas of the tumor may demonstrate a mucopolysaccharide-rich background. Similar to medulloblastoma, easily identifiable mitotic figures, apoptotic bodies, geographic necrosis, and hemorrhage are commonly seen.

Ancillary Studies

Medulloblastoma typically demonstrates diffuse positive immunoreactivity to markers of neuronal differentiation (synaptophysin, NeuN, class III beta-tubulin). Focally, areas of GFAP immunoreactivity may be observed. In tumors with myogenic differentiation, desmin or myogenin immunostaining may be present but not smooth muscle actin. Melanotic differentiation may be confirmed with HMB45 and melan-A immunoreactivity. INI-1 staining is retained in medulloblastoma.

In the 2021 WHO classification schema, a genetically defined system was presented for medulloblastomas. Tumors are generally grouped into four main categories: WNT-activated, SHH-activated, and non-WNT/non-SHH tumors (divided into group 3 and group 4 lesions). The WNT-activated group usually has classic morphology, APC gene with germline mutation, and frequent CTNNB1, DDX3X, and TP53 mutations. The SHH-activated group is divided into those tumors marked by TP53 mutations (often large cell and anaplastic morphology) and those that do not harbor a TP53 mutation (often desmoplastic or nodular morphology). The latter group may demonstrate mutations in PTCH 1, SMO, SUFU, or TERT promoter. The group 3 non-WNT/non-SHH tumors are marked by MYC amplification and the group 4 tumors by MYCN amplification. None of these alterations seen in medulloblastomas are typically encountered in AT/RT.

The rhabdoid cells of AT/RT stain with a variety of markers including smooth muscle actin, EMA, vimentin, GFAP, synaptophysin, cytokeratin, and neurofilament protein. Loss of nuclear staining with INI-1 (SMARCB1 protein) antibody is a hallmark of AT/RT.

Prognosis and Therapy

Medulloblastomas are generally associated with a variable prognosis and are prone to disseminate via cerebrospinal fluid seeding. Tumors with excessive nodularity and desmoplastic/nodular tumors tend to have a better prognosis; large cell and anaplastic tumors tend to have a worse prognosis. Treatment includes surgery (gross total resection, if possible), craniospinal radiation, and adjuvant chemotherapy. The overall 5-year

survival rate is in the 60% to 80% range. WNT-activated tumors generally have a better prognosis than SHH-activated, TP53-mutated tumors. AT/RTs are notoriously aggressive tumors with a median survival rate of 17 months. Tumors are similarly treated with surgical resection, radiation, and intensive chemotherapy.

LYMPHOMA VERSUS VASCULITIS

Clinical Features

Primary CNS lymphomas account for about 2% to 3% of all brain tumors. Most cases arise in people in the fifth to seventh decades of life with a slight male predominance. Immunocompromised patients or post-transplant lesions (post-transplant lymphoproliferative disorders) may present at a younger age and the tumor may be associated with viral infections (e.g., Epstein-Barr virus [EBV]). The majority of tumors arise in the supratentorial compartment (frontal lobe most commonly) and 60% to 70% of patients present with a single lesion. Leptomeninges may be involved (more commonly seen in secondary involvement of the CNS by lymphoma or leukemia). Symptoms can be varied depending on tumor location but most commonly include psychomotor slowing, cognitive impairment, and focal neurologic deficits. On imaging, lesions appear hypointense on T1-weighted images and hyperintense to isointense on T2 images. Peritumoral edema, more common with high-grade gliomas and metastases, is generally not prominent in lymphoma.

Primary angiitis of the CNS is a relatively rare disorder similarly marked by angiocentric inflammation. Patients commonly present with headaches, stroke-like events, or myelopathy (in the case of spinal cord involvement). Males are more likely to be affected and peak incidence is in the fifth and sixth decades of life. Imaging findings are relatively non-specific and therefore a biopsy is often needed to confirm a clinical impression. Vessels in more superficial locations (meninges and cortex) are more likely to be involved than white matter vessels. Secondary involvement of the CNS by systemic vasculitis may also be encountered. Threshold for biopsying a suspected patient may be dependent on a variety of clinical and serological factors and index of suspicion.

Pathologic Features

GROSS FINDINGS

Lymphoma may present as a single or multiple lesions. Often, they are periventricular in location. Tissue can be firm, friable, granular, hemorrhagic, and focally necrotic. Demarcation from the adjacent tissue is variable. Vasculitis is not grossly evident. Secondary consequences of vasculitis, such as infarct or hemorrhage, may be grossly evident if present.

MICROSCOPIC FINDINGS

Table 3.12 compares and contrasts features of lymphoma with those of vasculitis. Lymphoma is marked by a proliferation of atypical appearing lymphoid cells (Fig. 3.12A). These are often highly cellular tumors and the tumor cells preferentially arrange themselves in an angiocentric fashion (Fig. 3.12B). At times, the tumor growth may result in a sheet-like arrangement of cells, which conjures up differential diagnostic considerations of high-grade oligodendroglioma or a small cell astrocytoma. Areas of necrosis and prominent mitotic activity may be present. Most tumors represent diffuse large B-cell lymphomas, although less commonly, other lymphoma types (low-grade B-cell lymphomas, T-cell lymphoma, NK/T-cell lymphomas, anaplastic large cell lymphoma, extranodal marginal zone lymphoma-MALT lymphoma, and intravascular lymphoma (Fig. 3.12C) may be encountered. Tumors that have been treated recently with steroids prior to surgery may demonstrate extensive tumor necrosis, making diagnosis a challenge.

In vasculitis, blood vessels are marked by infiltration of blood vessel walls by inflammatory cells (Fig. 3.12D). In some cases, multinucleated giant cells or fibrinoid necrosis of vessel walls may be evident (Fig. 3.12E). Atypical cells, such as one sees with lymphoma, are not part of the vasculitis pathology. A number of processes may manifest with a vasculitic pattern of injury (e.g., infection, autoimmune encephalitis, drugs); so ultimately, the diagnosis is one of exclusion.

Ancillary Studies

The atypical cells of diffuse large B-cell lymphoma will be highlighted by B-cell lymphoid markers such as CD20, CD19, and CD79a. Evidence of EBV infection may indicate that the patient is immunocompromised. Most tumors are marked by a second population of benign-appearing T lymphocytes (CD3 positive) that represent tumor infiltrating lymphocytes. In occasional cases, the number of benign T lymphocytes may predominate and obscure the malignant cells. Gene rearrangement studies can be used to demonstrate monoclonality, but care should be taken in how one uses this information (i.e., not everything that is monoclonal is lymphoma). In addition to lymphoid cells, vasculitis may show other inflammatory cells in the vessel wall (neutrophils, plasma cells, macrophages, eosinophils). Stains for microorganisms may be useful in evaluating for potential infection. A subset of cases appear to be associated with varicella zoster infection. Occasional cases may be accompanied by amyloid deposition and evaluation for amyloid (Congo red, thioflavin S, beta-amyloid) should be undertaken.

Prognosis and Therapy

The prognosis of diffuse large B-cell lymphoma of the CNS is generally poor, even with treatment, which may include a variety of chemotherapy agents, such as steroids and methotrexate, and radiation. Older patients (over the age of 65 years) do much worse. Immunosuppressive therapy is traditionally employed to treat primary CNS vasculitis with variable results.

TABLE 3.12

Lymphoma Versus Vasculitis

	Lymphoma	Vasculitis
Age	Older patients	Adults
Location	Supratentorial, frontal lobe most common	Meninges and cortex > white matter
Associations	Acquired immunodeficiency syndrome, post-transplantation	Sometimes associated with systemic vasculitis
Atypical cells	Present, most common type: diffuse large B-cell lymphoma (CD20 and CD79a positive)	Absent, generally more T cells (CD3 positive) than B cells
Fibrinoid necrosis of vessel walls	Absent	Occasionally present
EBV association	Sometimes	Absent
VZV association	Absent	Sometimes

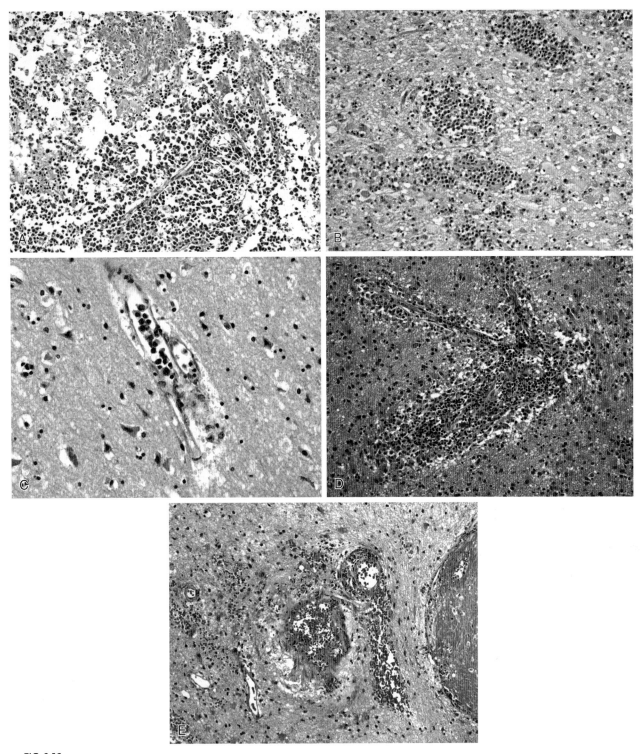

FIG. 3.12

A, Primary CNS lymphoma with focal necrosis and marked by a proliferation of atypical lymphoid cells (usually diffuse large B-cell lymphomas) (hematoxylin and eosin [H&E], original magnification 400×). **B,** Primary CNS lymphomas often grow in an angiocentric pattern (H&E, original magnification 200×). **C,** Intravascular lymphoma or angiocentric lymphoma is marked by a proliferation of lymphoid cells confined to vascular lumina (H&E, original magnification 400×). **D,** Non-necrotizing vasculitis characterized by infiltration of blood vessel walls by benign appearing chronic inflammatory cells (H&E, original magnification 200×). **E,** Fibrinoid necrosis of blood vessel walls in a necrotizing vasculitis (H&E, original magnification 200×).

DEMYELINATING DISEASE VERSUS INFARCT

Clinical Features

Multiple sclerosis (MS) is the prototypical demyelinating disease. The most common presenting form of MS arises in young adults, preferentially women, and follows a remitting and relapsing clinical course. Populations living in temperate climates are at higher risk of developing disease. MS primarily targets the white matter and classically presents with multifocal white matter lesions (plaques). Classically, lesions are periventricularly situated and neural parenchyma at any level of the CNS may be involved. Occasional patients may have only a few attacks and stabilize for extended periods of time. Occasional patients present with a single lesion (acute tumefactive MS); often, these lesions are targeted for biopsy since they can resemble a tumor on imaging. Marburg type of MS is a monophasic, sometimes rapidly progressive disease. Imaging studies are not pathognomonic for MS. Plaques appear as areas of hyperintensity on T2-weighted MRI images and "black holes" on T1-weighted images. Tumefactive MS has a distinctive horseshoe or C-shaped appearance of partial rim enhancement, which contrasts with the circumferential ring of enhancement encountered more typically in tumors and abscesses. Other less commonly encountered demyelinating lesions, such as necrotizing hemorrhagic leukoencephalitis or progressive multifocal leukoencephalopathy (PML) due to papovavirus infection, may also be targets for biopsy on occasion because of their unusual presentations or to establish a definitive diagnosis.

Infarcts (stroke) represent areas of geographic necrosis most commonly due to atherosclerotic disease, vascular thrombosis, or embolization of blood vessels. Risk factors for the development of infarct include hypertension, diabetes, smoking, positive family history, truncal obesity, and hyperlipidemia. The risk increases with increasing age. Signs and symptoms relate to multiple factors including size and location of the infarct, duration of reduced blood flow, collateral circulation status, and the vulnerability of cells in the region affected. So-called watershed infarcts are due to diffuse or global anoxic damage in arterial border zones corresponding to end artery regions of supply between main arteries. CT imaging may show no changes in the first few hours but usually within 6 to 8 hours, the area of necrosis will become hypodense. Older lesions often demonstrate evidence of cavitary change. Infarcts are not typically a routine target for biopsy but rarely may be biopsied because of an atypical appearance on imaging. Evidence of infarct is also frequently seen adjacent to other pathologies such as vasculitis, infections, immune-mediated diseases, vascular malformations, or following radiation.

Pathologic Features

GROSS FINDINGS

Plaques usually appear as irregularly shaped and variably sized areas of gray in the white matter. Infarcts undergo changes as the lesions age. Initially, there is a blurring of the gray–white interface and swelling due to edema in the involved area. Vascular congestion, which may or may not be accompanied by hemorrhage, may develop. The lesions are more commonly situated, at least partially, in the gray matter (in contrast to MS plaques). The tissue is soft and over time may cavitate (usually after a few months have passed). The subpial region of the cortex is often relatively spared.

MICROSCOPIC FINDINGS

Table 3.13 compares and contrasts features of demyelinating disease and infarct. Both pathologies are marked by the presence of macrophages and associated reactive astrocytes. In MS, the macrophages are situated in the white matter and are filled with myelin material; reactive astrocytes are intermixed within the macrophages in the plaque (Fig. 3.13A). Perivascular chronic inflammation, consisting primarily of benign-appearing T lymphocytes, is common (Fig. 3.13B). The lesions are typically sharply demarcated from the adjacent uninvolved parenchyma (Fig. 3.13C). Occasional lesions may be marked by Creutzfeldt cells. Viral inclusions within oligodendrocytes in the background of a demyelinating lesion in an immunocompromised individual should raise the possibility of PML due to papovavirus infection (Fig. 3.13D and E). Small areas of infarction and hemorrhage may be encountered in acute hemorrhagic leukoencephalitis, a rare usually monophasic and rapidly progressive disorder (Fig. 3.13F).

Infarcts undergo an evolution of change as the lesion ages. Within the first 24 hours, edema develops around the perimeter of the lesion. Neurons may undergo ischemic changes where the nucleus condenses and the cell body shrinks, and cell cytoplasm becomes hypereosinophilic (red and dead appearance; Fig. 3.13G). Reactive endothelial changes, sometimes accompanied by small number of neutrophils, may be evident. Vascular congestion and sometimes evidence of hemorrhage may be seen. Macrophages move in as early as 24 to 36 hours out, peak at 3 to 5 days, and stick around for months afterward (Fig. 3.13H). Reactive astrocytes become evident at about 7 to 10 days around the perimeter of the infarct (defines subacute infarct). Cavitary changes (defines remote infarct) may become evident 6 to 8 weeks out (Fig. 3.13I). Perivascular lymphocytes are not as prominently noted in

TABLE 3.13
Demyelinating Disease Versus Infarct

	Demyelinating Disease	Infarct
Age	Younger adults most common	Older adults most common
Location	White matter	Cortex > white matter
Macrophages	Present	Present
Reactive astrocytes	Present, intermixed in the lesion	Present, at edge of the lesion, 7 or more days out
Perivascular lymphocytes	Present	Usually absent
Viral inclusions	Present in progressive multifocal leukoencephalopathy	Absent
Hemorrhage	Rarely with acute hemorrhage leukoencephalitis	Often
Necrosis	Absent	Present
Myelin stain	Loss	Loss if white matter affected
Neurofilament stain	Relative preservation	Loss

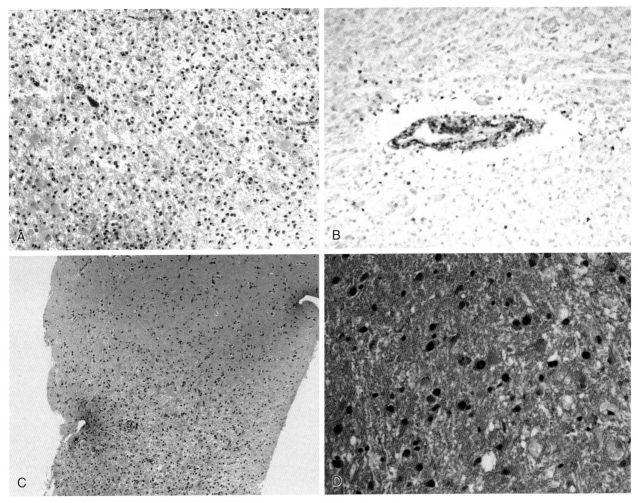

FIG. 3.13

A, Multiple sclerosis plaque or area of demyelination marked by increased numbers of white matter macrophages and intermixed reactive astrocytes (hematoxylin and eosin [H&E], original magnification 200×). **B,** CD3 immunostain highlighting perivascular T lymphocytes in multiple sclerosis (original magnification 200×). **C,** There is typically a sharp demarcation between areas of demyelination in multiple sclerosis and the surrounding, uninvolved parenchyma (H&E, original magnification 100×). **D,** Progressive multifocal leukoencephalopathy is a papovavirus infection which can manifest as intranuclear inclusions within oligodendrocytes in the background of demyelination (H&E, original magnification 400×).

Continued

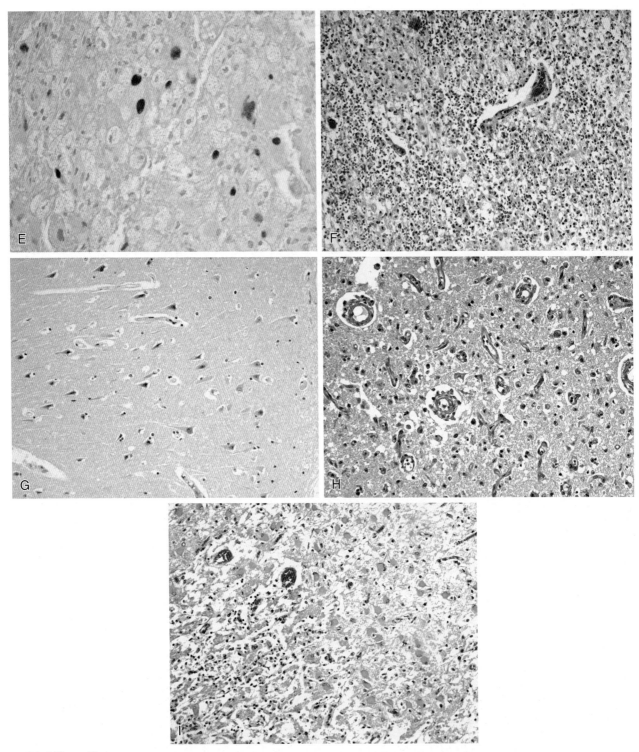

FIG. 3.13, cont'd

E, Polyoma virus antibody staining affected nuclei in progressive multifocal leukoencephalopathy (original magnification 400×). **F,** Acute hemorrhagic leukoencephalitis often shows areas of hemorrhage in the background of demyelinating disease (H&E, original magnification 200×). **G,** Ischemic neurons are marked by cell shrinkage and hypereosinophilia (H&E, original magnification 200×). **H,** An area of acute infarct marked by reactive vascular endothelial changes and increased macrophages (H&E, original magnification 200×). **I,** Remote infarct with early cavitary change and adjacent reactive astrocytes around the perimeter (H&E, original magnification 200×).

most infarcts, unless the etiology is related to an inflammatory process such as vasculitis or infection.

Ancillary Studies

Special stains can sometimes help in sorting out the two processes, particularly in infarcts that are primarily white matter based. Both processes will show decreased myelin staining. In demyelinating lesions, there is a relative preservation of axons and so there is some retention of neurofilament staining or silver staining (Bodian or Bielschowsky). This is in contrast to infarcts where neurofilament staining is generally absent in the dead tissue.

Prognosis and Therapy

As mentioned previously, most patients with MS experience a remitting and relapsing clinical course. In some cases, the course is fulminant and in others, relatively asymptomatic. There are a host of drugs that can be used to help in the management of MS such as steroids, type I beta interferons, and natalizumab. Protocols for the immediate administration of thrombolytic agents have been effective in improving survival and reducing morbidity in strokes. Stroke prevention for at-risk patients may include a regimen of aspirin or antiplatelet agents as well as strategies to treat risk factors such as diabetes and hypertension.

ARTERIOVENOUS MALFORMATION VERSUS CAVERNOUS ANGIOMA

Clinical Features

The vascular malformations are a group of disorders marked by an abnormal proliferation of blood vessels. Four major types are recognized: arteriovenous (AVM), cavernous angioma (CA) (cavernoma), venous angioma, and capillary telangiectasia. Because of the risk of hemorrhage and size of the lesions causing focal neural deficits or seizures, AVMs and CAs are the ones that most commonly require surgical intervention, and features of these two lesions are outlined in Table 3.14. The other two malformations are usually asymptomatic and are incidental findings on imaging or at autopsy. AVMs most commonly arise within the vascular territory of the middle cerebral artery. Angiographic examination is usually diagnostic; however, some cases may be angiographically "occult" due to thrombosis of the arterial

TABLE 3.14
Arteriovenous Malformation Versus Cavernous Angioma

	Arteriovenous Malformation	Cavernous Angioma
Abnormal arteries	Present	Absent
Intervening parenchyma	Present	Absent
Gliosis	Present	Present
Calcification	Sometimes	Sometimes
Hemosiderin	Sometimes	Sometimes
Multiple	Rare	More common
Familial	Rare	More common

feeding vessels. CAs are not as reliably discernible on angiographic studies. Cases of familial CAs are documented, especially among people of Hispanic-American heritage; these cases have been associated with mutations on the KRIT1, CCM2, and PDCD10 genes. Multiple CAs are commonly seen in familial cases.

Pathologic Features

GROSS FINDINGS

The classic appearance of an AVM is that of a wedge-shaped malformation with the base of the wedge situated near the surface of the brain. Intervening brain parenchyma is seen between the blood vessels comprising the malformation. CAs are often more deep-seated, well-circumscribed, irregularly shaped (mulberry appearance) lesions; no discernible intervening brain parenchyma is observed.

MICROSCOPIC FINDINGS

As its name suggests, AVMs comprise an admixture of arteries and veins with intervening brain parenchyma (Fig. 3.14A). The intervening parenchyma frequently shows reactive changes including gliosis, calcification, osseous metaplasia, hemosiderin deposition, and sometimes evidence of ischemic injury (Fig. 3.14B). Since hemodynamics in AVMs is not normal, pathology of the vessel walls themselves is commonly observed including atherosclerosis, fibrosis, and thrombosis (Fig. 3.14C). Sometimes, amyloid deposition may be seen in elderly patients. Evidence of embolization (if employed preoperatively) may be observed within vessels and make infarct in the region more likely.

CAs are characterized by a back-to-back arrangement of venous vessels without intervening brain parenchyma (Fig. 3.14D). Again, the vessels frequently

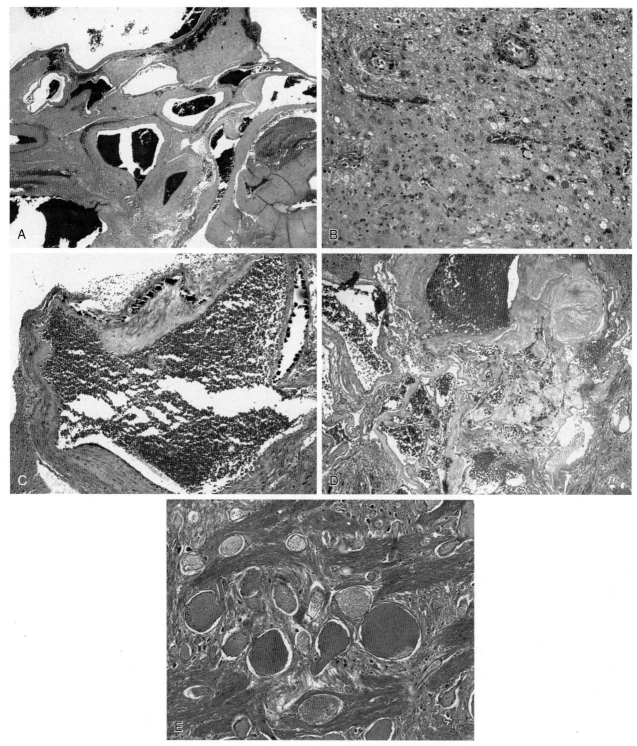

FIG. 3.14

A, An arteriovenous malformation marked by a mixture of arteries and veins with intervening brain parenchyma (hematoxylin and eosin [H&E], original magnification 40×). **B,** Parenchyma adjacent to an arteriovenous malformation with gliosis, macrophages, hemosiderin, and eosinophilic granular bodies (H&E, original magnification 200×). **C,** Blood vessels in an arteriovenous malformation often show atherosclerotic changes with calcification in vessel walls (H&E, original magnification 100×). **D,** Cavernous angioma characterized by venous blood vessels arranged in a back-to-back configuration (H&E, original magnification 100×). **E,** Venous angioma in the pons, marked by venous blood vessels with intervening brain parenchyma (Luxol fast blue, original magnification 100×).

show thickened walls due to atherosclerotic changes and occasional evidence of thrombosis. The adjacent parenchyma may show reactive changes including gliosis, Rosenthal fibers, calcification, and hemosiderin deposition.

Venous angiomas are marked by venous vessels with intervening brain parenchyma (Fig. 3.14E). Capillary telangiectasias comprise capillary-sized vessels with intervening brain parenchyma.

Ancillary Studies

Elastic or Movat stains can be useful in highlighting the internal elastic lamina and media in arterial vessels, if present in the malformation.

Prognosis and Therapy

About two third of patients with AVMs experience a clinically significant bleed and have a mortality rate of 10%. Treatment options include surgical resection, embolization, and radiosurgery. Superficially located AVMs generally have an overall better prognosis than deep-seated malformations. CAs are usually managed surgically, if symptomatic; embolization is usually not employed and radiosurgery is less frequently utilized.

MENINGITIS VERSUS ENCEPHALITIS/ CEREBRITIS VERSUS ABSCESS

Clinical Features

There are a variety of patterns of injury that may be associated with infections of the CNS. Inflammation confined to the leptomeninges is referred to as meningitis or leptomeningitis. Cerebrospinal fluid may have a cloudy appearance and contain inflammatory cells and abnormal glucose and protein levels. Certain bacterial organisms may be more commonly encountered at certain ages in community-acquired infections (first month of life: group B *Streptococcus*, *Escherichia coli*, and *Listeria*; childhood: *Neisseria meningitidis*; adults: *Streptococcus pneumoniae*). Empyema refers to a collection of purulent material on the surface of the brain. Inflammation within the substance of the brain itself is referred to as encephalitis or cerebritis. A localized suppurative process represents an abscess. Other patterns of injury may be secondary to infection and are less commonly encountered, such as demyelination in the setting of Papova virus infection in PML.

Infections may arise at any age in both immunocompetent and more commonly in immunocompromised individuals. Processes may be focal or diffuse in distribution. Signs and symptoms are very much dependent on the pattern of injury and type and distribution of infection. On imaging, meningitis causes leptomeningeal enhancement on MRI studies. Encephalitis may be undetectable on CT imaging and may be variably discernible on MRI studies, depending on the pattern of injury. An abscess can present as a ring-enhancing lesion on imaging and may mimic a glioblastoma.

Pathologic Features

GROSS FINDINGS

Meningitis may be characterized by clouding of the meninges with associated cerebral edema and vascular congestion. Many cases may appear grossly normal in appearance and the diagnosis requires microscopic examination to make. Encephalitis/cerebritis may run the gamut of a normal-appearing brain grossly to hemorrhagic and necrotizing brain tissue with organisms such as herpes or ameba. An abscess often is grossly somewhat circumscribed in appearance. Early on, it may have a purulent appearance. As the lesion organizes, it forms a firmer wall around the centrally necrotic/purulent portion. In certain infections (e.g., cysticercosis), the organism at the center of the organizing process may serve as a nidus for eventual calcification.

MICROSCOPIC FINDINGS

Most cases of bacterial meningitis are preferentially located in the region of the basal cistern and Sylvian fissure, due to the effect of gravity. Histologically, bacterial meningitis is marked by predominantly acute inflammatory cells (neutrophils) and smaller numbers of plasma cells, lymphocytes, and macrophages (Fig. 3.15A and B). The inflammatory infiltrate may extend along the Virchow-Robin spaces. Edema, vascular congestion, and sometimes infarct and hemorrhage (due to blood vessel damage) may be evident in the underlying parenchyma. With healing or treatment, the inflammatory infiltrate may become predominantly chronic and the development of granulation tissue and fibrosis may be seen. Viral meningitis tends to most commonly start with a chronic inflammatory cell infiltrate. Fungal organisms (and mycobacterial infections) may be associated with granulomatous inflammation (Fig. 3.15C).

Table 3.15 compares and contrasts features of granulomatous infection in the setting of an infection versus sarcoidosis. When granulomas are encountered, whether it be in meningitis or in the wall of an abscess, the differential diagnosis should include certain infectious agents (fungal and mycobacteria), sarcoidosis, foreign

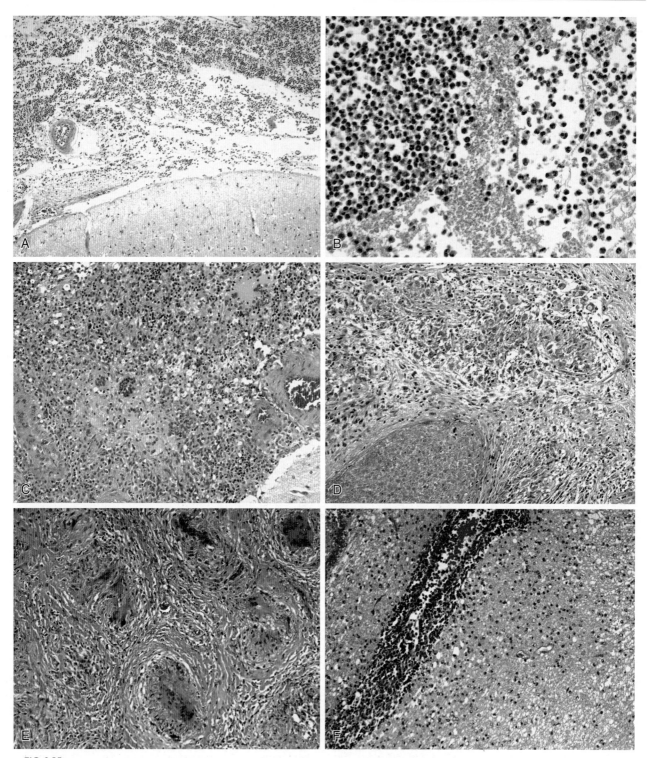

FIG. 3.15

A, Marked inflammation in the meninges (leptomeningitis) (hematoxylin and eosin [H&E], original magnification 100×). **B,** Bacterial meningitis is often marked by increased neutrophils (H&E, original magnification 400×). **C,** Cryptococcal meningitis with increased chronic inflammatory cells, scattered multinucleated giant cells, and reactive fibroblasts (H&E, original magnification 200×). **D,** Necrotizing granulomatous inflammation in the setting of tuberculosis (H&E, original magnification 200×). **E,** Sarcoidosis involving the dura, characterized by non-necrotizing granulomas with multinucleated giant cells (H&E, original magnification 200×). **F,** Herpes encephalitis with a focus on non-necrotizing vasculitis (original magnification 200×).

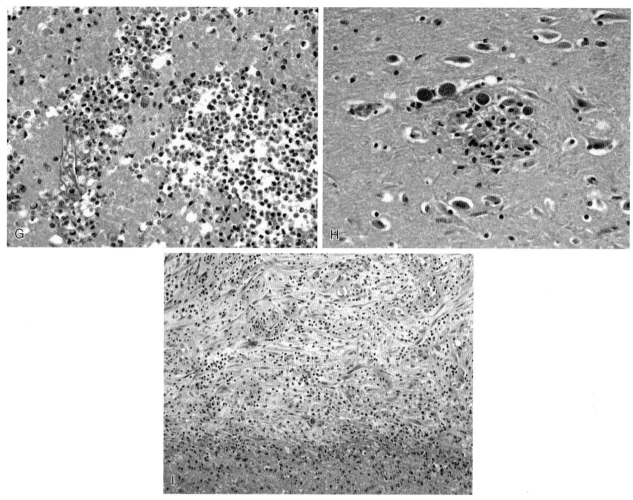

FIG. 3.15, cont'd

G, Naegleria encephalitis marked by a mixed acute and chronic inflammatory infiltrate and amebic organisms (H&E, original magnification 400×). **H,** Toxoplasmosis cysts associated with a microglial nodule (H&E, original magnification 400×). **I,** The wall of an organizing abscess characterized by a mixture of acute and chronic inflammatory cells and reactive fibroblasts (H&E, original magnification 200×).

TABLE 3.15		
Sarcoid Versus Infectious Granulomas		
	Sarcoid	Infectious Granulomas
Age	Younger adults	Any
Multisystem disease	Usually	Often
Base of brain involvement	Usually	Usually
Meningeal disease	Often	Sometimes (meningitis)
Parenchymal disease	Less frequent	Sometimes (abscess)
Caseous necrosis	Usually absent	Often present
Vasculitic pattern of injury	Often	Sometimes
AFB/FITE stains	Negative	Variably positive (culture or in molecular testing for infection is more definitive)

body reaction (in the setting of prior surgery or trauma), and rare other conditions such as idiopathic hypertrophic pachymeningitis or granulomatous vasculitis. Both processes may be multisystem disease and both often target the base of the brain. Both may involve the meninges or parenchyma. The association of necrosis is more commonly encountered with an infectious etiology than sarcoid (exceptions exist in both camps, however; Fig. 3.15D and E). Both may be associated with a vasculitic pattern of injury. Distinction often relies on culture or identifying organisms by microscopic examination and/or staining. In both sarcoid and infections associated with granulomas, biopsies may be done when the clinical picture is unclear or the presentation is unusual.

Encephalitis and cerebritis are marked by inflammation within the brain parenchyma (Fig. 3.15F and G). It may or may not be accompanied by overlying meningitis. The inflammation may be acute and/or chronic, depending on the cause. Bacterial infections, in general, tend to show a predominance of neutrophils and viral infections show more chronic inflammatory cells; however, there are exceptions on both sides. Microglial cell proliferation or aggregates (nodules) may be encountered, especially with certain viral and rarely parasitic organisms (Fig. 3.15H). One should look for evidence of viral inclusions or organisms. Certain organisms (such as herpes, aspergillus, and mucormycetes) may be associated with a hemorrhagic component. In some cases, necrosis may also be evident.

An abscess often starts as a focus of purulent material (collection of neutrophils). It may be accompanied by a variable amount of necrosis or granulomatous inflammation. The surrounding tissue usually transitions to a more chronic inflammatory cell infiltrate with adjacent gliosis (Fig. 3.15I). Fibroblastic proliferation and neovascularization proceeds around the perimeter as the abscess is organizing.

Ancillary Studies

Special stains for microorganisms (Gram, Gomori methenamine silver, Ziehl-Neelsen, PAS) can be useful sometimes in making a quick diagnosis. With many organisms, culture remains a gold standard for diagnosis and in suspected infectious cases, some tissue removed at the time of surgery should be directed to the Microbiology laboratory. Antibody stains exist which target certain organisms; these can be particularly helpful in identifying certain common viral organisms. Molecular studies and polymerase chain reaction testing may be employed to help increase the yield in identifying certain difficult-to-identify organisms in more timely fashion.

Prognosis and Therapy

Targeted treatment usually is optimally predicated on identifying the organism. When infection is suspected, but an organism cannot be identified, preemptive treatment is often employed. Prognosis is dependent on a variety of factors including the extent of disease, immune status, organism or organisms involved, effectiveness of existing treatments, and baseline overall health of the patient being treated.

SUGGESTED READINGS

General Text References

Burger PC, Scheithauer BW. *Tumors of the Central Nervous System. AFIP Atlas of Tumor Pathology Series 4*. Washington, DC: AFIP; 2007.
Gray F, Duyckaerts C, de Girolami U. *Manual of Basic Neuropathology*. 6th ed. Oxford University Press; 2019.
Perry A, Brat DJ, eds. *Practical Surgical Neuropathology. A Diagnostic Approach*. 2nd ed. Philadelphia, PA: Elsevier; 2018.
Prayson RA. *Neuropathology. Foundations in Diagnostic Pathology Series*. 2nd ed. Philadelphia, PA: Elsevier Saunders; 2012.
WHO Classification of Tumours Editorial Board. *Central Nervous System Tumours*. 5th ed. Lyon: International Agency for Research on Cancer; 2021.
Yachnis A, Rivera-Zengotita ML. *Neuropathology. High-Yield Pathology*. Philadelphia, PA: Elsevier Saunders; 2014.

Gliosis Versus Glioma

Brandner S, von Deimling A. Diagnostic, prognostic and predictive relevance of molecular markers in gliomas. *Neuropathol Appl Neurobiol*. 2015;41(6):694-720.
Carmelo-Piragua S, Jansen M, Ganguly A, et al. Mutant IDH1-specific immunohistochemistry distinguishes diffuse astrocytoma from astrocytosis. *Acta Neuropathol*. 2010;119(4):509-511.
Kleinschmidt-DeMasters BK, Prayson R. An algorithmic approach to the brain biopsy – part 1. *Arch Pathol Lab Med*. 2006;130:1630-1638.
Schittenhelm J, Mittelbronn M, Nguyen TD, et al. WT1 expression distinguishes astrocytic tumor cells from normal and reactive astrocytes. *Brain Pathol*. 2008;18(3):344-353.
Takami H, Yoshida A, Fukushima S, et al. Revisiting TP53 mutations and immunohistochemistry – A comparative study in 157 diffuse gliomas. *Brain Pathol*. 2015;25(3):256-265.

Radiation Change Versus Recurrent/Residual Glioma

Burger PC, Mahley Jr MS, Dudka L, et al. The morphologic effects of radiation administered therapeutically for intracranial gliomas: a postmortem study of 25 cases. *Cancer*. 1979;44:1256-1272.
Kleinschmidt-DeMasters BK, Kang JS, Lillehei KO. The burden of radiation-induced central nervous system tumors: a single institutions' experience. *J Neuropathol Exp Neurol*. 2006;65:204-216.
Perry A, Schmidt RE. Cancer therapy-associated CNS neuropathology: an update and review of the literature. *Acta Neuropathol*. 2006;111:197-212.

Fibrillary Astrocytoma Versus Oligodendroglioma

Cancer Genome Atlas Research Network, Brat DJ, Verhaak RG, et al. Comprehensive, integrative genomic analysis of diffuse lower-grade gliomas. *N Engl J Med*. 2015;372(26):2481-2498.
Capper D, Zentgraf H, Balss J, et al. Monoclonal antibody specific for ISH1 R132H mutations. *Acta Neuropathol*. 2009;118(5):599-601.
Kannan K, Inagaki A, Silber J, et al. Whole-exome sequencing identifies ATRX mutations as a key molecular determinant in lower-grade gliomas. *Oncotarget*. 2012;3(10):1194-1203.
Eckel-Passow JE, Lachance DH, Molinaro AM, et al. Glioma groups based on 1p/19q, IDH, and TERT promoter mutations in tumors. *N Engl J Med*. 2015;372(26):2499-2508.
Jiao Y, Killela PJ, Reitman ZJ, et al. Frequent ATRX, CIC, FUBP1, and IDH mutations refine the classification of malignant gliomas. *Oncotarget*. 2012;3(7):709-722.
Leeper HE, Caron AA, Decker PA, et al. IDH mutation, 1p19q codeletion and ATRX loss in WHO grade II gliomas. *Oncotarget*. 2015;6(30):30295-30305.
Olar A, Wani KM, Alfaro-Munoz KD, et al. IDH mutations status and role of WHO grade and mitotic index in overall survival in grade II-III diffuse gliomas. *Acta Neuropathol*. 2015;129:585-596.
Ostrom QT, de Blank PM, Kruchko C, et al. Alex's Lemonade Stand Foundation infant and childhood primary brain and central nervous system tumors diagnosed in the United States in 2007-2011. *Neuro Oncol*. 2015;16(suppl 10):x1-x36.
Wesseling P, van den Bent M, Perry A. Oligodendroglioma: pathology, molecular mechanisms and markers. *Acta Neuropathol*. 2015;129(6):809-827.

Pilocytic Astrocytoma Versus Fibrillary Astrocytoma

Colin C, Padovani L, Chappé C, et al. Outcome analysis of childhood pilocytic astrocytomas: a retrospective study of 148 cases at a single institution. *Neuropathol Appl Neurobiol*. 2013;39(6):693-705.
Collins VP, Jones DT, Giannini C. Pilocytic astrocytoma: pathology, molecular mechanisms and markers. *Acta Neuropathol*. 2015;129:775-788.

Marko NF, Weil RJ. The molecular biology of WHO grade I astrocytomas. *Neuro Oncol*. 2012;14(12):1424-1431.

Packer RJ, Pfister S, Bouffet E, et al. Pediatric low-grade gliomas: implications of the biologic era. *Neuro Oncol*. 2017;19(6):750-761.

Schindler G, Capper D, Meyer J, et al. Analysis of BRAF V600E mutations in 1,320 nervous system tumors reveals high mutation frequencies in pleomorphic xanthoastrocytoma, ganglioglioma and extra-cerebellar pilocytic astrocytoma. *Acta Neuropathol*. 2011;121(3):397-405.

Gemistocytic Astrocytoma Versus Subependymal Giant Cell Astrocytoma

Goh S, Butler W, Thiele EA. Subependymal giant cell tumors in tuberous sclerosis complex. *Neurology*. 2004;63(8):1457-1461.

Krouwer HG, Davis RL, Silver P, et al. Gemistocytic astrocytomas: a reappraisal. *J Neurosurg*. 1991;74(3):399-406.

Roth J, Roach ES, Bartels U, et al. Subependymal giant cell astrocytoma: diagnosis, screening, and treatment. Recommendations from the International Tuberous Sclerosis Complex Consensus Conference 2012. *Pediatr Neurol*. 2013;49:439-444.

Watanabe K, Peraud A, Gratas C, et al. p53 and PTEN gene mutations in gemistocytic astrocytomas. *Acta Neuropathol*. 1998;95(6):559-564.

Pleomorphic Xanthoastrocytoma Versus Ganglioglioma

Giannini C, Scheithauer BW, Burger PC, et al. Pleomorphic xanthoastrocytoma: what do we really know about it? *Cancer*. 1999;85:2033-2045.

Giannini C, Scheithauer BW, Lopes MB, et al. Immunophenotype of pleomorphic xanthoastrocytoma. *Am J Surg Pathol*. 2002;26(4):479-485.

Ida CM, Rodriguez FJ, Burger PC, et al. Pleomorphic xanthoastrocytoma: natural history and long-term follow-up. *Brain Pathol*. 2015;25:575-586.

Powell SZ, Yachnis AT, Rorke LB, et al. Divergent differentiation in pleomorphic xanthoastrocytoma. Evidence for a neuronal element and possible relationship to ganglion cell tumors. *Am J Surg Pathol*. 1996;20(1):80-85.

Prayson RA, Khajavi K, Comair YG, et al. Cortical architectural abnormality and MIB1 immunoreactivity in gangliogliomas: a study of 60 patients with intracranial tumors. *J Neuropathol Exp Neurol*. 1995; 54(4):513-520.

Dysembryoplastic Neuroepithelial Tumor Versus Central Neurocytoma versus Oligodendroglioma

Daumas-Duport C, Scheithauer BW, Chodkiewicz JP, et al. Dysembryoplastic neuroepithelial tumour: a surgically curable tumour of young patients with intractable partial seizures. Report of thirty-nine cases. *Neurosurgery*. 1988;23:545-556.

Figarella Branger D, Pellissier JF, Daumas-Duport C, et al. Central neurocytomas. Critical evaluation of a small-cell neuronal tumour. *Am J Surg Pathol*. 1992;16:97-109.

Honavar M, Janota I, Polkey CE. Histological heterogeneity of dysembryoplastic neuroepithelial tumour: identification and differential diagnosis in a series of 74 cases. *Histopathology*. 1993;34:342-356.

Patel DM, Schmidt RF, Liu JK. Update on the diagnosis, pathogenesis, and treatment strategies for central neurocytoma. *J Clin Neurosci*. 2013;20(9):1193-1199.

Schild SE, Scheithauer BW, Haddock MG, et al. Central neurocytomas. *Cancer*. 1997;79:790-795.

Thom M, Toma A, An S, et al. One hundred and one dysembryoplastic neuroepithelial tumors: an adult epilepsy series with immunohistochemical, molecular genetic, and clinical correlations and a review of the literature. *J Neuropathol Exp Neurol*. 2011;70(10):859-878.

Ependymoma Versus Subependymoma Versus Myxopapillary Ependymoma

Akyurek S, Chang EL, Yu TK, et al. Spinal myxopapillary ependymoma outcomes in patients treated with surgery and radiotherapy at M.D. Anderson Cancer Center. *J Neurooncol*. 2006;80:177-183.

Bi Z, Ren X, Zhang J, et al. Clinical, radiological, and pathological features in 43 cases of intracranial subependymoma. *J Neursurg*. 2015;122:49-60.

Ellison D, Kocak M, Figarella-Branger D, et al. Histopathological grading of pediatric ependymoma: reproducibility and clinical relevance in European trial cohorts. *J Negat Results Biomed*. 2011;10:7.

Pajtler KW, Witt H, Sill M, et al. Molecular classification of ependymal tumors across all CNS compartments, histopathological grades, and age groups. *Cancer Cell*. 2015;27:728-743.

Reni M, Gatta G, Mazza E, et al. Ependymoma. *Crit Rev Oncol Hematol*. 2007;63:81-89.

Sonneland PR, Scheithauer BW, Onofrio BM. Myxopapillary ependymoma. A classification and immunohistochemical study 77 cases. *Cancer*. 1985; 56:883-893.

Meningioma Versus Schwannoma Versus Solitary Fibrous Tumor/Hemangiopericytoma

Matthies C, Samii M. Management of 1000 vestibular schwannomas (acoustic neuromas): clinical presentation. *Neurosurgery*. 1997; 40(1):1-9.

Menke JR, Raleigh DR, Gown AM, et al. Somatostatin receptor 2 alpha is a more sensitive diagnostic marker of meningioma than epithelial membrane antigen. *Acta Neuropathol*. 2015;130:441-443.

Perry A, Scheithauer BW, Stafford SL, et al. "Malignancy" in meningiomas: clinicopathologic study of 116 patients with grading implications. *Cancer*. 1999;85:2046-2056.

Rogers CL, Perry A, Pugh S, et al. Pathology concordance levels for meningioma classification and grading in NRG Oncology RTOG Trial 0539. *Neuro Oncol*. 2016;18:565-574.

Schweizer L, Koelsche C, Sahm F, et al. Meningeal hemangiopericytoma and solitary fibrous tumors carry the NAB2-STAT6 fusion and can be diagnosed by nuclear expression of STAT6 protein. *Acta Neuropathol*. 2013;125:651-658.

Sobel RA. Vestibular (acoustic) schwannomas: histologic features in neurofibromatosis 2 and in unilateral cases. *J Neuropathol Exp Neurol*. 1993;52(2):106-113.

Wolfsberger S, Doostkam S, Boecher-Schwarz HG, et al. Progesterone-receptor index in meningiomas: correlation with clinico-pathological parameters and review of the literature. *Neurosurg Rev*. 2004;27: 238-245.

Yalcin CE, Tihan T. Solitary fibrous tumor/hemangiopericytoma dichotomy revisited: a restless family of neoplasms in the CNS. *Adv Anat Pathol*. 2016;23:104-111.

Hemangioblastoma Versus Metastatic Carcinoma

Hasselblatt M, Jeibmann A, Gerss J, et al. Cellular and reticular variants of haemangioblastoma revisited: a clinicopathologic study of 88 cases. *Neuropathol Appl Neurobiol*. 2005;31:618-622.

Polydorides AD, Rosenblum MK, Edgar MA. Metastatic renal cell carcinoma to hemangioblastoma in von Hippel-Lindau disease. *Arch Pathol Lab Med*. 2007;131:641-645.

Shehata BM, Stockwell CA, Castellano-Sanchez AA, et al. Von Hippel-Lindau (VHL) disease: an update on the clinico-pathologic and genetic aspects. *Adv Anat Pathol*. 2008;15:165-171.

Medulloblastoma Versus Atypical Teratoid/Rhabdoid Tumor

Eberhart CG. Molecular diagnostics in embryonal brain tumors. *Brain Pathol*. 2011;21:96-104.

Massimino M, Biassoni V, Gandola L, et al. Childhood medulloblastoma. *Crit Rev Oncol Hematol*. 2016;105:35-51.

Perry A, Fuller CE, Judkins AR, et al. INI1 expression is retained in composite rhabdoid tumors, including rhabdoid meningiomas. *Mod Pathol*. 2005;18:951-958.

Reddy AT. Atypical teratoid/rhabdoid tumors of the central nervous system. *J Neurooncol*. 2005;75:309-313.

Taylor MD, Northcott PA, Korshunov A, et al. Molecular subgroups of medulloblastoma: the current consensus. *Acta Neuropathol*. 2012;123:465-472.

Lymphoma Versus Vasculitis

Carnevale J, Rubenstein JL. The challenge of primary central nervous system lymphoma. *Hematol Oncol Clin North Am*. 2016;30(6):1293-1316.

Giannini C, Salvarani C, Hunder G, et al. Primary central nervous system vasculitis: pathology and mechanisms. *Acta Neuropathol*. 2012;123(6):759-772.

Gilden D, Nagel MA. Varicella zoster virus and giant cell arteritis. *Curr Opin Infect Dis*. 2016;29:275-279.

Hoang-Xuan K, Bessell E, Bromberg J, et al. Diagnosis and treatment of primary CNS lymphoma in immunocompetent patients: guidelines from the European Association for Neuro-Oncology. *Lancet Oncol*. 2015;16(7):e322-e332.

Swerdlow SH, Campo E, Pileri SA, et al. The 2016 revision of the World Health Organization classification of lymphoid neoplasms. *Blood.* 2016;127:2375-2390.

Demyelinating Disease Versus Infarct

Frohman EM, Racke MK, Raine CS. Multiple sclerosis – the plaque and its pathogenesis. *N Engl J Med.* 2006;354:942-955.

Ginsberg MD. Adventures in the pathophysiology of brain ischemia: penumbra, gene expression, neuroprotection. *Stroke.* 2003;34:214-223.

Lammie GA. Hypertensive cerebral small vessel disease and stroke. *Brain Pathol.* 2002;12:358-370.

Love S. Demyelinating diseases. *J Clin Pathol.* 2006;59:1151-1159.

Ludwin SK. The pathogenesis of multiple sclerosis: relating human pathology to experimental studies. *J Neuropathol Exp Pathol.* 2006; 65:305-318.

Arteriovenous Malformation Versus Cavernous Angioma

Frischer JM. Cerebral cavernous malformations congruency of histopathological features with the current clinical definition. *J Neurol Neurosurg Psychiatry.* 2008;79:783-788.

Hanjani SA. The genetics of cerebrovascular malformations. *J Stroke Cerebrovasc Dis.* 2002;11:279-287.

Jahan R, Murayama Y, Gobin YP, et al. Embolization of arteriovenous malformations with Onyx: clinicopathological experience in 23 patients. *Neurosurgery.* 2001;48:984-995.

Labauge P, Denier C, Bergametti F, et al. Genetics of cavernous angiomas. *Lancet Neurol.* 2007;6:237-244.

McCormick WF. Vascular malformations ("angiomas") of the brain, with special reference to those occurring in the posterior fossa. *J Neurosurg.* 1968;28:241-251.

Moriarity JL. The natural history of cavernous malformations: a prospective study of 68 patients. *Neurosurgery.* 1999;44:1166-1171.

Meningitis Versus Encephalitis/Cerebritis Versus Abscess

Hofman P, Lucas S, Jouvion G, et al. Pathology of infectious diseases: what does the future hold? *Virchows Arch.* 2018;470(5):483-492.

Hoitsma E, Faber CG, Drent M, et al. Neurosarcoidosis: a clinical dilemma. *Lancet Neurol.* 2004;3(7):397-407.

Stern BJ. Neurological complications of sarcoidosis. *Curr Opin Neurol.* 2004;17(3):311-316.

Strickland-Marmol LB, Fessler RG, Rojiani AM. Necrotizing sarcoid granulomatosis mimicking an intracranial neoplasm: clinicopathologic features and review of the literature. *Mod Pathol.* 2000;13(8):909-913.

Thigpen MC, Whitney CG, Messonnier NE, et al. Bacterial meningitis in the United States, 1998-2007. *N Engl J Med.* 2011;364(21):2016-2025.

4

Hepatobiliary and Pancreas

Daniel E. Roberts • Clifton G. Fulmer

LIVER

HEPATOCELLULAR TUMORS

FOCAL NODULAR HYPERPLASIA

DDX: Hepatocellular adenoma, well-differentiated hepatocellular carcinoma, regenerative nodule

Clinical Features

Focal nodular hyperplasia (FNH) is the most common benign hepatocellular tumor and is thought to represent a localized, regenerative proliferation of hepatocytes in an area of abnormal blood flow. While it most often affects women between 20 and 50 years, FNH can occur in either sex and in all age groups. Lesions are usually solitary, ranging in size from subcentimeter masses to more than 10 cm across, and the background liver is not cirrhotic.

FNH has been associated with vascular malformations or hemangiomas in 20% to 30% of cases. Most are discovered incidentally on imaging, and FNH-like areas may also arise adjacent to other hepatic tumors due to localized vascular changes secondary to mass effect. Molecular studies have shown that the hepatocellular component is polyclonal. Consequently, FNH is termed a lesion rather than a neoplasm, and it carries no risk of malignant transformation.

Pathologic Features

GROSS FINDINGS

Classically, FNH appears as a single well-circumscribed, tan-white, nodular mass. Most are less than 5 cm, but they can grow larger. The characteristic feature is a central stellate scar that radiates through the lesion and imparts a grossly nodular appearance.

MICROSCOPIC FINDINGS

FNH contains hyperplastic nodules of benign hepatocytes separated by fibrous bands radiating from a central scar-like area (Fig. 4.1A). Ductular reaction spreads alongside the periphery of these fibrous septae (Fig. 4.1B), but the lesion itself does not contain true portal tracts. Instead, the fibrous areas may contain thick-walled dystrophic arteries with medial hypertrophy and intimal fibrosis, and variable amounts of lymphocyte-predominant inflammation are present.

Within the hepatocellular nodules, the trabecular width is largely normal (i.e., 1 or 2 cells across), but focal areas may show mild regenerative changes manifesting as patchy plate widening or slight architectural disarray. Hepatocytes can sometimes exhibit cytoplasmic swelling or Mallory hyaline accumulation around fibrous septae.

Ancillary Studies

Immunohistochemistry (IHC) for glutamine synthetase (GS) highlights a characteristic "geographic" or "map-like" staining pattern within the lesion that manifests as broad, interconnecting channels of cytoplasmic labeling (Fig. 4.2). This differs from the pattern of GS expression in normal liver, which is restricted to a thin rim of hepatocytes around central veins.

Prognosis and Therapy

FNH is a benign lesion with no significant risk of malignant transformation, rupture, or hemorrhage. As such, surgery is not always indicated, and prognosis is excellent.

Differential Diagnosis

The primary differential diagnosis for FNH is hepatocellular adenoma (HCA), as both are mass lesions that arise in noncirrhotic livers. The presence of fibrous bands containing large dystrophic vessels and lined by prominent ductular reaction is characteristic of FNH. "Map-like" GS expression is not seen in HCA and is diagnostic of FNH. Between the characteristic

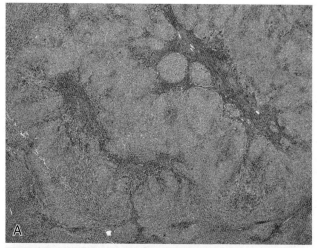

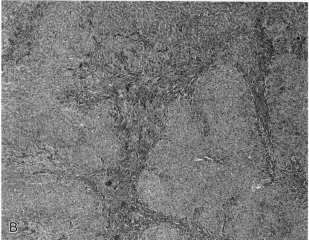

FIG. 4.1

Focal nodular hyperplasia. **A,** Bands of fibrosis radiate from a larger central scar and impart a nodular appearance at low power. **B,** Prominent ductular reaction is seen along the fibrous bands.

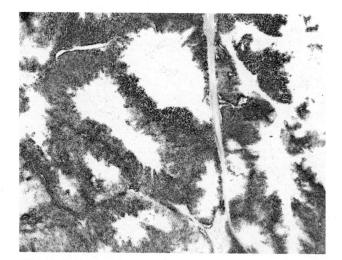

FIG. 4.2

Focal nodular hyperplasia. Immunohistochemistry for glutamine synthetase demonstrates a characteristic geographic or map-like pattern of staining at low power.

morphologic features and GS expression pattern, this diagnosis is usually straightforward on resection specimens.

However, this differential is more often encountered on small biopsy samples, which may not show distinct morphologic features or a well-developed geographic staining pattern with GS. The presence of fibrosis, ductular reaction, and thick-walled vessels may suggest a diagnosis of FNH in such cases, but these features are often not well-developed, and focal scarring or ductular reaction can also be present in adenomas. For truly inconclusive biopsies, our practice is to exclude β-catenin activation by IHC (see Hepatocellular Adenoma section) and diagnose these as well-differentiated hepatocellular lesions.

FNH is not diagnosed in cirrhotic livers. However, if the presence of cirrhosis is unknown, the differential diagnosis may include regenerative nodules of cirrhosis or even a well-differentiated hepatocellular carcinoma (HCC). Regenerative nodules will contain portal tract components that are absent in FNH. If considering a diagnosis of HCC, reticulin staining in FNH will show a preserved framework and normal hepatic plate thickness, while HCC will feature abnormally widened hepatic plates, a disrupted reticulin framework, and/or increased cytologic atypia on hematoxylin and eosin (H&E) staining.

FOCAL NODULAR HYPERPLASIA – DISEASE FACT SHEET

Definition

▸▸ Non-neoplastic proliferation of hepatocytes due to alterations in hepatic blood flow

Incidence and Location

▸▸ More common in women
▸▸ Occurs in noncirrhotic livers
▸▸ Often found incidentally

Age Distribution

▸▸ Most often between 20 and 50 years of age

Clinical Features

▸▸ Usually solitary, but can be multiple in up to 20% of cases
▸▸ FNH-like areas can appear adjacent to other mass lesions due to locally altered blood flow
▸▸ Typically asymptomatic, but rarely can present with abdominal pain

Radiologic Features

▸▸ Prominent central scar
▸▸ Hypodense lesion on CT with arterial enhancement

Prognosis and Therapy

▸▸ Observation if asymptomatic
▸▸ Resection if symptomatic
▸▸ No risk of malignant transformation or significant hemorrhage

---

FOCAL NODULAR HYPERPLASIA – PATHOLOGIC FEATURES

Gross Findings

▸▸ Well-circumscribed, often solitary, nodular lesion, typically under 5 cm

▸▸ Most characteristic feature is a central stellate scar

Microscopic Findings

▸▸ Bands of irregular fibrosis with ductular reaction impart a nodular appearance

▸▸ Large vessels present with thick walls and intimal fibrosis within central scar

▸▸ Hepatocytes appear normal

▸▸ Map-like staining pattern with GS

Pathologic Differential Diagnoses

▸▸ Hepatocellular adenoma

▸▸ Regenerative nodule

▸▸ Well-differentiated hepatocellular carcinoma

HEPATOCELLULAR ADENOMA

DDX: focal nodular hyperplasia, well-differentiated hepatocellular carcinoma, normal liver

Clinical Features

HCA is a clonal proliferation of benign hepatocytes that arises in noncirrhotic livers and accounts for approximately 10% of benign hepatocellular tumors. Three major subtypes are recognized, each with specific clinical, molecular, and morphologic characteristics: (1) inflammatory adenoma, (2) hepatocyte nuclear factor 1α (HNF1α)–inactivated adenoma, and (3) β-catenin–activated adenoma. The overwhelming majority of cases are seen in women of reproductive age (20–40 years), and the association between adenomas and oral contraceptive use, as well as observations of rapid tumor growth during pregnancy, suggest that sex hormones promote HCA proliferation. HCAs have also been reported in association with exogenous androgen administration, and this particular risk factor has shown an increased association with the β-catenin–activated subtype. Any adenoma greater than 5 cm is at risk of hemorrhage, but inflammatory adenomas have an increased bleeding risk at any size.

Inflammatory adenomas are defined by stimulation of signal transducer and activator of transcription 3 (STAT3), a major inflammatory response pathway component. STAT3 promotion is caused by an activating mutation in one of several pathway constituents (*IL6ST, FRK, STAT3, GNAS, JAK1*) and these tumors are characterized by overexpression of STAT3 targets such as serum amyloid A (SAA) and C-reactive protein (CRP).

HNF1α-inactivated adenomas are characterized by loss of HNF1α function, a transcription factor involved in hepatocellular differentiation. Consequently, these lesions lack expression for downstream HNF1α targets, such as liver fatty acid binding protein (LFABP).

β-catenin–activated adenomas are defined by activation of the Wnt/β-catenin pathway, either by mutation of *CTNNB1* directly or a β-catenin suppressor gene such as *APC*. While malignant transformation can be seen in any adenoma, it is far more common in β-catenin–activated adenomas harboring mutations in exon 3 of *CTNNB1*.

Pathologic Features

GROSS FINDINGS

HCA typically appears as a well-circumscribed tan-brown mass in a non-cirrhotic liver, usually lacking a fibrous capsule. HCA is most often a solitary lesion, although multiple can occur synchronously, and the presence of 10 or more adenomas is referred to as *adenomatosis*. The prototypical HCA measures between 5 and 15 cm in greatest dimension and may show foci of gross discoloration due to bile excess, hemorrhage, or necrosis.

MICROSCOPIC FINDINGS

HCAs are well-differentiated hepatocellular neoplasms characterized by normal-appearing hepatocytes with minimal cytologic atypia, arranged in trabeculae of normal thickness (1–2 cells wide). Adenomas may either blend seamlessly with the background parenchyma or compress the adjacent liver and produce a thin fibrous rim. They are identified by their lack of normal portal structures and scattered small arterioles without paired bile ducts (Fig. 4.3).

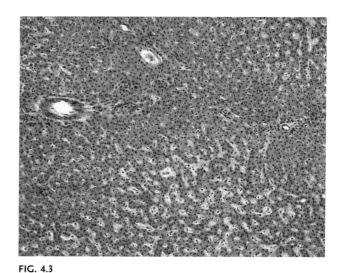

FIG. 4.3

Hepatocellular adenoma. Typical appearance of an adenoma, with scattered unpaired arterioles in a background of normal hepatocytes arranged in trabecular plates of normal width (1–2 across).

The hepatocytes in HCAs harbor minimal cytologic atypia, with relatively monomorphic nuclei, eosinophilic cytoplasm, and a nucleus-to-cytoplasm (N/C) ratio comparable with the background liver. Focally, HCAs can show mildly increased cytologic atypia as well as regenerative architectural changes that manifest as occasionally thickened or disordered cell plates. However, these changes are mild and localized. Adenomas may contain a variable amount of steatosis and sinusoidal changes, but certain morphologic features are more commonly seen in certain HCA subtypes.

Inflammatory adenomas often contain foci of lymphocytic inflammation and areas of dilated sinusoidal spaces, which are often prominent and filled with blood (Fig. 4.4A), explaining their increased association with spontaneous hemorrhage if left untreated. Focal ductular reaction can be seen more often in this subtype.

HNF1α-inactivated adenomas are classically associated with bland steatosis (Fig. 4.5A), which may or may not be present in the background liver. Notably, HNF1α-inactivated adenomas do not contain features of steatohepatitis such as Mallory hyaline or pericellular fibrosis.

β-catenin–activated adenomas lack any characteristic morphologic features on H&E, and hepatocytes vary from cytoarchitecturally unremarkable to mildly atypical. This diagnosis is principally made by IHC or molecular testing, and β-catenin activation can overlap with other phenotypically distinct adenoma subtypes.

Rarely, some adenomas may show features that are suspicious for, but not diagnostic of, well-differentiated HCC, such as very focal reticulin loss or increased cytologic atypia. These lesions have been called atypical adenomas and definitive diagnosis may only be possible on resection specimens.

Ancillary Studies

Despite certain characteristic morphologic features, the adenoma subtypes show considerable histologic

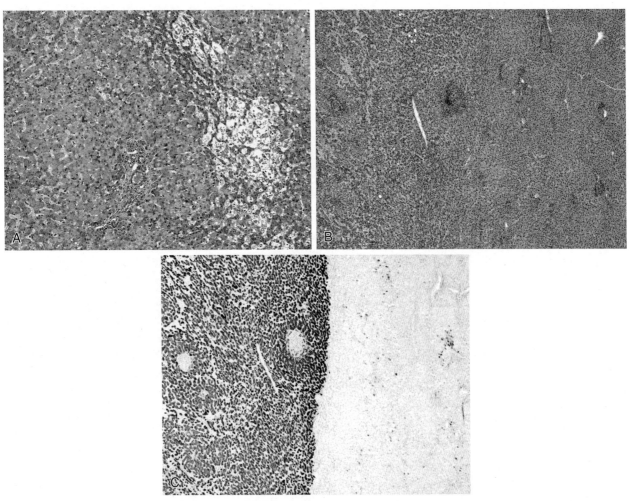

FIG. 4.4

Hepatocellular adenoma, inflammatory type. **A,** In addition to unpaired arterioles, inflammatory adenomas often show patchy sinusoidal dilatation with congestion and chronic inflammation. Compared with the background liver parenchyma (**B** and **C,** right), inflammatory adenomas often demonstrate increased staining for CRP (**B** and **C,** left) and SAA.

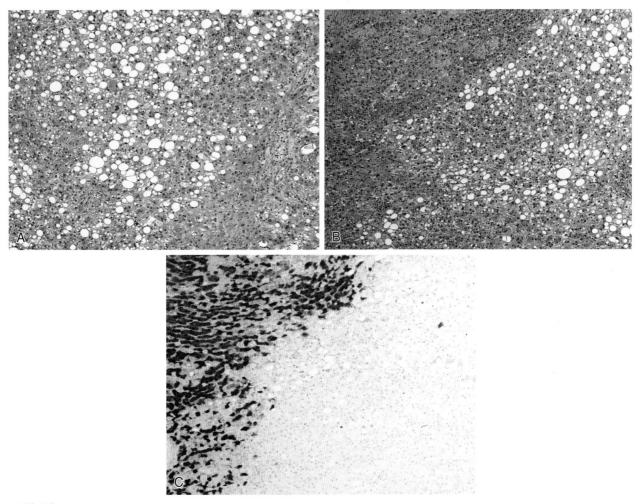

FIG. 4.5

Hepatocellular adenoma, HFN1α-inactivated type. **A,** These adenomas often contain bland macrosteatosis. The interface between the adenoma and background liver (**B**) highlights the characteristic loss of LFABP expression (**C,** right), which is preserved in the background liver (**C,** left).

overlap and are best distinguished using either IHC or molecular testing. Adenoma markers are typically ordered as a panel, and consist of β-catenin, GS, LFABP, CRP, and SAA. The characteristic staining pattern of each subtype is summarized below.

HCA Subtype	β-Catenin	Glutamine Synthetase	LFABP	CRP	SAA
β-Catenin activated	Nuclear localization	Diffuse expression	+/−	+/−	+/−
Inflammatory	−	Variable	+	+	+
HNF1α inactivated	−	Variable	−	+/−	+/−

In clinical practice, the presence of β-catenin activation is critical to identify because this confers an increased risk of malignant transformation. Normal liver typically shows membranous expression of β-catenin on IHC, but *CTNNB1* mutation in adenomas manifests as focal nuclear staining. While this pattern is diagnostic of β-catenin activation, it has a low sensitivity in practice due to focality of staining.

GS is an extremely useful surrogate marker, as studies have correlated diffuse expression of GS with β-catenin mutation status. Diffuse GS expression is defined as moderate-to-strong staining in more than half of tumor cells without a map-like distribution, and this is further subdivided into two groups. A pattern of *diffuse, homogenous* GS expression is defined as staining in more than 90% of tumor cells (Fig. 4.6A) and is highly correlated with β-catenin activation, often involving deletions in exon 3 of *CTNNB1*. The *diffuse, heterogenous* pattern is defined as expression in 50% to 90% of tumor cells (Fig. 4.6B), and this immunophenotype shows a weaker

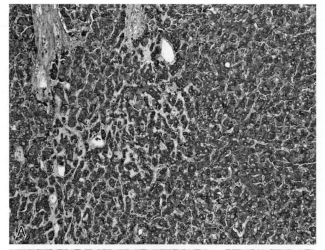

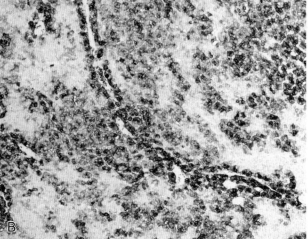

FIG. 4.6

Hepatocellular adenoma, β-catenin–activated type. These adenomas are morphologically variable but characterized by diffuse glutamine synthetase expression, which is a sensitive marker for β-catenin activation. **A,** Diffuse, homogenous expression is defined by staining of >90% of tumor cells and is strongly linked to β-catenin activation. **B,** Diffuse heterogenous expression describes adenomas in which 50% to 90% of the tumor express GS and shows a weaker correlation with β-catenin activation.

correlation with β-catenin activation. However, either pattern of diffuse GS labeling is considered a high-risk feature. In small biopsies, however, the pattern of expression may appear abnormal yet cannot be reliably characterized. In these cases, molecular testing may be prudent.

Inflammatory adenomas are characterized by increased CRP and/or SAA expression (Fig. 4.4B and C). Both markers are nonspecific acute-phase reactants that may be variably expressed in the liver depending on physical state, and diagnosis is most reliable when expression patterns in the adenoma can be compared to the background liver. Diagnostic confidence increases when both CRP and SAA are positive, although SAA often demonstrates a weak cytoplasmic staining profile that is less sensitive (but more specific) than CRP.

HNF1α-inactivated adenomas will show loss of LFABP (Fig. 4.5B and C), a marker normally expressed at variable levels in all hepatocytes.

In some cases, especially biopsy specimens, the diagnosis of adenoma will be clear, but tumor cells are negative for β-catenin, GS, CRP, SAA, and they retain LFABP expression. These lesions are termed unclassified HCAs.

Prognosis and Therapy

The most common complication of HCA is massive hemorrhage into the peritoneal cavity. Inflammatory adenomas have an increased association with bleeding, but any adenoma greater than 5 cm is at heightened risk of hemorrhage and is usually resected for this reason. HCAs are premalignant lesions, and the published rate of transformation ranges from 3% to 12%.

Differential Diagnosis

The diagnosis of a well-differentiated hepatocellular tumor requires two steps. The first step is identifying lesional tissue by the absence of normal portal structures. This is usually straightforward but can be challenging in biopsies that only contain minimal tissue and/or heavy fragmentation. IHC can be helpful in this situation, as lesional areas of the liver often exhibit abnormal endothelialization of the sinusoidal spaces that manifests by expanded CD34 expression. Normal liver sinusoids should be negative for CD34 apart from focal periportal expression, but hepatocellular lesions such as adenomas, FNH, and HCC typically show more diffuse CD34 staining that can be helpful in identifying lesional tissue in small or disrupted biopsies.

The second step is classifying the tumor, and the differential diagnosis changes depending on the status of the background liver. In a non-cirrhotic liver, the most common hepatocellular lesions are HCA and FNH. Well-differentiated HCC can also arise in non-cirrhotic livers and may recapitulate the bland cytomorphology and largely intact architecture seen in HCA.

Both HCA and FNH are composed of bland hepatocytes without cytologic atypia. The hepatic plate architecture may show focal regenerative changes in either lesion, but the reticulin framework remains intact. FNH characteristically shows a central scar with radiating bands of fibrosis and accompanying ductular reaction that yields a nodular structure. Conversely, the typical HCA lacks a central scar, nodular fibrosis, and ductular reaction. Instead, HCA contains small, thin-walled, unpaired arterioles in the lobule without corresponding veins and ducts. These morphologic features can show some degree of overlap, but the diagnosis is usually clear on large resection specimens.

In practice, however, this diagnosis is usually rendered on needle core biopsies, where features may not be well-developed and the diagnosis can be challenging. In these cases, IHC for GS is essential. GS expression in normal liver highlights only a thin rim of perivenular hepatocytes in zone 3, but this pattern changes in lesional tissue. FNH demonstrates a characteristic "map-like" staining pattern. In contrast, HCA can exhibit multiple staining patterns: entirely negative, diffusely positive with either a homogenous or heterogenous distribution, or indeterminate expression that is neither map-like nor indicative of definite β-catenin mutation. The combination of morphologic features and GS expression pattern is usually sufficient to separate FNH from HCA.

The diagnosis of HCC primarily relies on H&E features and reticulin integrity, and all adenoma subtypes harbor risk of malignant transformation (Fig. 4.7). In this differential, the status of the reticulin framework is essential to diagnosis. Adenomas exhibit an intact reticulin network, while well-differentiated HCC will show at least focal disruption. However, the presence of fat can complicate reticulin evaluation, as macrosteatosis disrupts the framework and causes reticulin fragmentation even in non-neoplastic tissue. Given that steatosis can be seen in adenomas, especially the HNF1α-inactivated subtype, the reticulin framework may not always be easily evaluated. In problematic cases, glypian-3 IHC may help distinguish these entities. Adenomas are negative for this marker, but HCC may be positive (see Hepatocellular Carcinoma section). In addition, features of steatohepatitis within a tumor, such as ballooning degeneration, Mallory hyaline, and pericellular fibrosis, are indicative of the steatohepatitic variant of HCC and should not be mistaken for an adenoma, which only contain bland steatosis.

Importantly, adenomas should only be subtyped after a diagnosis of HCA is rendered, as the stains involved in subtyping are not diagnostically helpful and provide no additional insight without a clear diagnosis of HCA. For instance, while LFABP expression is lost in HNF1α-inactivated adenomas, its expression may also be absent in HCC.

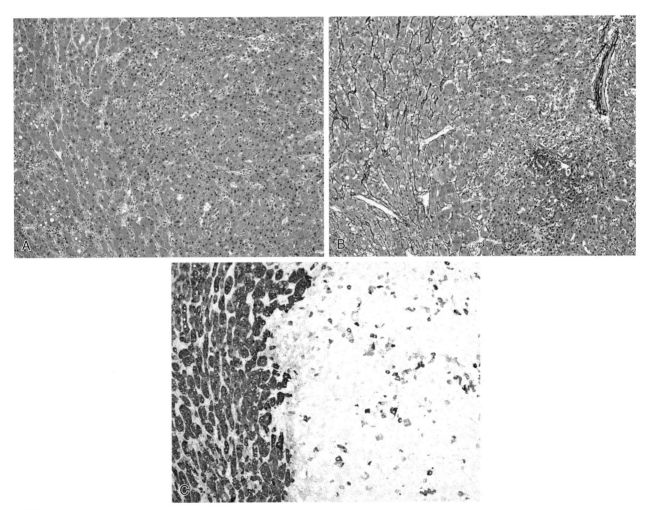

FIG. 4.7

Malignant transformation within inflammatory-type hepatocellular adenoma. H&E staining **(A)** demonstrates the transition from relatively normal-appearing hepatocytes arranged in thin trabeculae to a more disordered arrangement of hepatocytes with increased cytoarchitectural atypia and profound loss of reticulin framework **(B)**. CRP immunohistochemistry is diffusely positive in the adenoma **(C)** and is increased compared with the background parenchyma.

HEPATOCELLULAR ADENOMA – DISEASE FACT SHEET

Definition
►► Clonal proliferation of benign hepatocytes

Incidence and Location
►► Account for 10% of benign hepatocellular tumors
►► Mostly occur in women, rare in men
►► Can be seen in children with glycogen storage disease

Age Distribution
►► 20–40 years

Clinical Features
►► Most patients have history of oral contraceptive use
►► Also associated with exogenous androgen use (β-catenin mutant subtype)
►► Presents incidentally or with right upper quadrant pain
►► Usually solitary, but can be multiple (adenomatosis if > 10 lesions)

Radiologic Features
►► Vascular lesion with irregular enhancement on CT
►► Well-defined mass on MRI, low signal on T1-weighted images

Prognosis and Therapy
►► Overall malignant transformation rate ranges from 3% to 12%
►► β-catenin–activated subtype has increased risk of malignant transformation
►► Large size (>5 cm) and inflammatory subtype are risk factors for clinically significant hemorrhage

HEPATOCELLULAR ADENOMA – PATHOLOGIC FEATURES

Gross Findings
►► Circumscribed, usually non-encapsulated tumors
►► Arise in non-cirrhotic livers
►► May be hemorrhagic

Microscopic Findings
►► Identified by lack of portal tracts and thin-walled arterioles within tumor
►► Benign hepatocytes without appreciable atypia
►► No thickened hepatic plates or loss of reticulin
►► Divided into four subtypes:
  ►► Inflammatory subtype: scattered lymphocytic inflammation, dilated sinusoidal spaces with or without congestion, may have focal ductular reaction. Positive for CRP and SAA.
  ►► HNF1α-inactivated subtype: usually contains bland steatosis. Shows loss of LFABP.
  ►► β-catenin–activated subtype: no distinct morphology. Shows nuclear β-catenin staining and/or diffuse GS expression.
  ►► Unclassified subtype: does not fit any specific morphologic pattern or immunophenotype

Pathologic Differential Diagnoses
►► Focal nodular hyperplasia
►► Well-differentiated hepatocellular carcinoma
►► Normal liver

HEPATOCELLULAR CARCINOMA

DDX: hepatocellular adenoma, regenerative nodule, cholangiocarcinoma, neuroendocrine tumor

Clinical Features

HCC is the most common primary liver cancer in adults, accounting for more than 75% of malignant hepatic tumors. It represents a complex and heterogenous cancer linked to behavioral factors, environmental exposures, genetic disorders, and chronic liver disease. Approximately 60% to 90% of HCC arises in cirrhotic livers, and the presenting symptoms typically reflect the patient's underlying liver disease: upper abdominal pain, weight loss, jaundice, ascites, and hemorrhage from esophageal varices, among others.

Cirrhosis of any cause is a major risk factor for HCC. As the primary agent of chronic hepatitis worldwide, hepatitis B and hepatitis C infections can be attributed to most cases of HCC globally. The mechanism of carcinogenesis is believed to be a combination of direct genomic changes due to viral insertion, oncogenic viral proteins, and a continuous cycle of injury and regeneration over many years. In addition to viral infection, exposure to aflatoxin, a fungal toxin produced by the *Aspergillus* family, is another significant risk factor due to relatively high rates of food contamination in certain parts of the world. Iron accumulation has been associated with HCC as well, and this seems to hold true whether iron overload is secondary to hereditary hemochromatosis or merely a consequence of cirrhosis.

Several other risk factors are not directly carcinogenic but do represent leading causes of cirrhosis and are therefore indirectly associated with HCC development. Alcohol consumption and metabolic syndrome (diabetes, obesity, etc.) represent some of the most common risk factors for cirrhosis in the United States and Europe, and the annual risk of developing HCC once cirrhotic is estimated at 3%. In addition to hereditary hemochromatosis, other inherited metabolic disorders, such as α1-antitrypsin deficiency, show a stronger association with HCC development beyond the risk conferred by cirrhosis alone.

Rates of incidence and mortality show a striking geographic diversity. While HCC represents the third leading cause of cancer mortality worldwide, HCC is far more common in Southeastern Asia and sub-Saharan Africa than in the United States and Europe. This is believed to largely reflect the geographic distribution of viral hepatitis and aflatoxin contamination, both of which are significant risk factors.

In areas with a lower incidence of HCC, such as the United States and Europe, most tumors occur between

60 and 70 years of age. In higher-incidence regions like sub-Saharan Africa, peak incidence is seen in the 20s and 30s. Regardless of the geographic region, HCC arises more often in men with a ratio between 2:1 and 5:1.

Most HCC is diagnosed radiographically by CT or MRI. Criteria proposed by the American Association for the Study of Liver Diseases state that tumors larger than 1 cm in a cirrhotic background do not require biopsy confirmation, so long as characteristic imaging features are present. A standardized system of reporting HCC risk has been developed, termed Liver Imaging Reporting and Data Systems (LI-RADS), which summarizes imaging findings into five categories ranging from definitely benign (LR-1) to definitely malignant (LR-5).

In addition to imaging modalities, serum alpha fetoprotein (AFP) is a helpful biomarker used to track the development of HCC. Although its sensitivity is somewhat limited, measuring the serum AFP level can be a useful screen in patients at high risk for developing HCC, and for monitoring recurrence in patients who have undergone treatment.

Pathologic Features

GROSS FINDINGS

Macroscopically, HCC can present as a single mass (with or without adjacent satellite nodules), multiple distinct masses, or rarely as the so-called "cirrhosis-like" pattern with diffuse and innumerable tumor nodules that mimic cirrhosis. HCC within a cirrhotic background is usually well-demarcated and wreathed by a dense fibrous capsule due to atrophy and fibrosis of the surrounding parenchyma, secondary to mass effect. HCC arising in a non-cirrhotic liver may instead appear diffusely infiltrative, with ill-defined borders. Most HCC are soft masses that bulge outward from their cut surface. Exceptions to this include fibrolamellar or scirrhous variants, which appear firm and densely fibrous. Tumor size is quite variable, ranging from around 1 cm to larger than 30 cm. HCC is typically tan, yellow, or green if bile-stained. Necrosis can be seen, either from a large tumor outgrowing its blood supply or secondary to preoperative treatment. Involvement of the portal or hepatic vein is not uncommon in advanced disease.

MICROSCOPIC FINDINGS

The microscopic appearance of HCC is quite variable, and any given tumor may contain multiple clonal populations exhibiting different morphologic phenotypes. Four primary architectural patterns have been described and correlated with tumor behavior. The most common growth pattern is *trabecular*, which recapitulates the

normal arrangement of hepatic plates, but with expansion to more than 3 cells in width (Fig. 4.8A). These trabeculae remain separated by modified sinusoidal spaces and do not contain intervening stroma. Often, the bile canaliculi can dilate to form vague acinar or *pseudoglandular* structures, which may contain bile plugs or central debris (Fig. 4.8B). The *solid* growth pattern is associated with more aggressive HCC and is characterized by obliteration of the normal sinusoidal channels to form a sheet-like tumor mass (Fig. 4.9A). *Macrotrabecular* growth is another architectural pattern associated with more aggressive tumor behavior and is defined as widely expanded trabecular plates greater than 6 cells thick (Fig. 4.9B). In general, the trabecular and pseudoglandular patterns are the most common tumor architecture, while solid and macrotrabecular patterns are considered evidence of poorer differentiation and have been associated with more aggressive tumor behavior. Other specialized growth patterns include fibrolamellar, steatohepatitic, scirrhous, sarcomatoid, and lymphoepithelioma-like, which are described later.

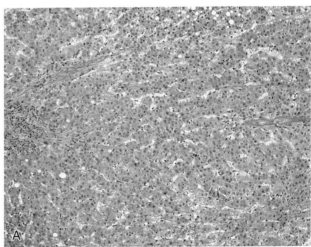
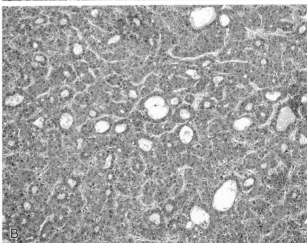

FIG. 4.8

Hepatocellular carcinoma (HCC). The most common architectural patterns in HCC are trabecular **(A)** and pseudoglandular **(B)**, which are often intermixed. Trabeculae thickness averages to 3–6 cells wide, and pseudoglands may contain either bile plugs or debris.

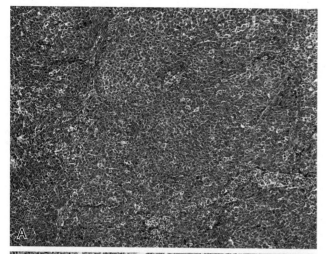

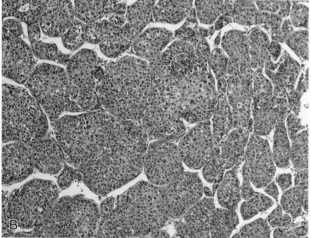

FIG. 4.9

Hepatocellular carcinoma. Several architectural patterns have been correlated with more aggressive tumor behavior. **A,** The solid pattern is characterized by sheets of hepatocytes with obliteration of the normal sinusoidal spaces. **B,** Macrotrabecular architecture is defined by widened trabeculae that average more than 6 cells across.

Cytologically, a well-differentiated HCC resembles non-neoplastic hepatocytes, with abundant granular, eosinophilic cytoplasm and round-to-ovoid nuclei without significant pleomorphism. There may be a slightly increased N/C ratio compared with the background liver. Macronucleoli, mitotic activity, and nuclear hyperchromasia are variably present. As HCC becomes more poorly differentiated, its overall appearance becomes less hepatoid. This manifests as a shift from eosinophilic to more amphophilic or basophilic cytoplasm, an increase in the N/C ratio toward and beyond a 1:1 proportion, and prominent nuclear pleomorphism. Additional non-specific histologic changes can be seen occasionally, including clear cell features and multinucleated giant cells. The presence of bile or Mallory hyaline can be helpful evidence of hepatocellular derivation. While a few studies have delineated specific cytoarchitectural criteria for assigning HCC tumor grade, current WHO guidelines advocate for a synthesis

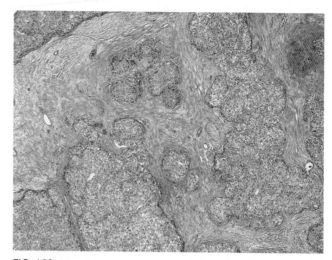

FIG. 4.10

The scirrhous variant of hepatocellular carcinoma shows infiltrative tumor nests separated by abundant fibrous stroma.

of cytologic and architectural features along the aforementioned spectrum.

Special staining for reticulin is a tremendously helpful way to assess the hepatic plate architecture, and it may be diagnostically critical in well-differentiated tumors. In most HCC, the reticulin framework is at least focally fragmented or lost, and this architectural disruption may not always be apparent on H&E sections. Some very well-differentiated HCC will retain an intact reticulin framework, but the stain can also help confirm diffuse expansion of the hepatic plates, bizarre architecture, and in some tumors, the reticulin framework may show an abnormal encasement of single cells or small clusters of cells in a way that is not typical of benign lesions. In fatty lesions, however, reticulin staining becomes unreliable, as disruption of the normal framework typically occurs secondary to steatosis.

Several distinct histologic variants of HCC are described below, and awareness of these variants is important to prevent misdiagnosis.

Scirrhous hepatocellular carcinoma describes a subset of HCC that contains nests of tumor set within prominent fibrotic stroma that comprises a significant proportion of the total tumor mass (Fig. 4.10). Scirrhous HCC tends to occur in subcapsular areas, and some reports indicate a higher rate of K7 and K19 expression compared with typical HCC, although most will also express arginase and glyican-3. The scirrhous variant is associated with worse outcome than traditional HCC.

Fibrolamellar hepatocellular carcinoma is a rare tumor distinct from other forms of HCC. It occurs in young adults without cirrhosis and is characterized by a somatic deletion that yields a characteristic DNAJB1-PRKACA fusion transcript, which can be detected by RT-PCR and FISH assays. Histologically, the fibrolamellar variant shows parallel bands of collagen-rich fibrosis infiltrating and separating tumor nests (Fig. 4.11A). The

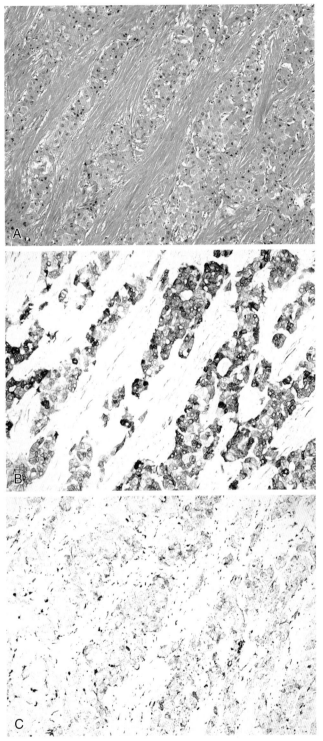

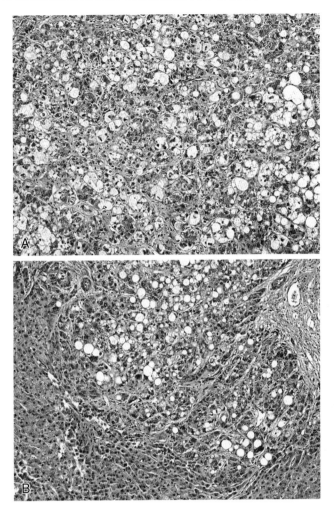

FIG. 4.12

The steatohepatitic variant of hepatocellular carcinoma recapitulates the ballooning degeneration, Mallory hyaline, and pericellular fibrosis characteristic of steatohepatitis (**A**), but shows striking cytologic atypia when compared with background hepatocytes (**B**).

FIG. 4.11

The fibrolamellar variant of hepatocellular carcinoma is characterized by large polygonal cells with brightly eosinophilic cytoplasm and dense intratumoral fibrosis (**A**). Unlike the scirrhous variant, tumor cells are positive for CK7 (**B**) and CD68 (**C**), and molecular testing can confirm the characteristic *DNAJB1-PRKACA* gene fusion.

tumor cells are large and polygonal, with abundant eosinophilic cytoplasm that often contain subtle cytoplasmic inclusions known as "pale bodies." Tumor nuclei are rounded and contain a single prominent macronucleoli. Hepatocellular markers are positive, but

this HCC variant differs in that it is nearly always positive for K7 and CD68 as well (Fig. 4.11B and C). While early studies suggested a favorable outcome compared with traditional HCC, recent evidence has shown that outcomes are in fact similar, and that fibrolamellar HCC is an aggressive tumor with a greater propensity for early nodal spread.

Steatohepatitic hepatocellular carcinoma is a relatively common variant of HCC that recapitulates the prototypical features of steatohepatitis within HCC, including steatosis, ballooning degeneration, prominent Mallory hyaline inclusion, and pericellular fibrosis (Fig. 4.12). This form of HCC can occur even in the absence of background steatohepatitis or any associated risk factors. Outcome is similar to typical HCC.

Lymphocyte-rich hepatocellular carcinoma is a rare HCC variant characterized by a prominent lymphoid infiltrate (Fig. 4.13). Some cases can superficially resemble a nasopharyngeal carcinoma, but Epstein-Barr virus

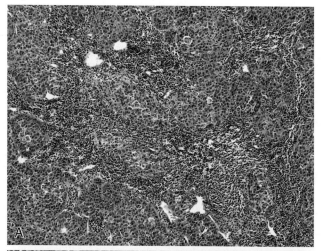

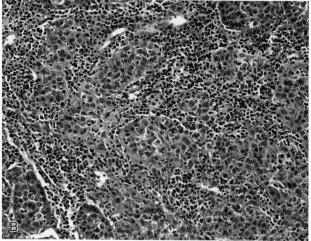

FIG. 4.13

The lymphocyte-rich variant of hepatocellular carcinoma is a rare subtype that may be mistaken for lymphoma. (**A**) 100x. (**B**) 200x.

testing is nearly always negative. The hepatocellular component is usually well-to-moderately differentiated. Tumors with a more poorly differentiated hepatocellular component alongside a dense lymphoinflammatory infiltrate have been called *lymphoepithelioma-like hepatocellular carcinoma.*

Sarcomatoid hepatocellular carcinoma describes a very rare HCC subtype that features sarcoma-like foci, often alongside more classical HCC. The sarcomatous component consists of malignant spindle and epithelioid cells that often express keratins, but rarely stain for hepatocellular markers. Heterologous elements may be present. Sarcomatoid changes can be seen following chemotherapy or embolization. In the absence of a recognizable HCC component, this diagnosis can be extremely difficult, and these tumors have a worse prognosis than typical forms of HCC.

Combined hepatocellular-cholangiocarcinoma (CHC) is defined as a tumor containing unequivocal and mixed elements of both HCC and cholangiocarcinoma. This entity is discussed in the cholangiocarcinoma section.

Ancillary Studies

Several immunohistochemical markers are available to confirm hepatocellular origin, although most do not distinguish benign from malignant hepatocytes. Arginase and HepPar1 are both highly sensitive and specific hepatocyte markers. Both tend to be quite useful in confirming hepatocellular lineage in well-to-moderately differentiated HCC, but they tend to exhibit less reliable staining in poorly differentiated HCC. Glypican-3 shows the opposite pattern, with increased utility in poorly differentiated HCC and less reliable staining in more well-differentiated tumors (Fig. 4.14). Glypican-3 also differs from the other two markers in that it is not specific to the liver. However, it is also not expressed in benign hepatocellular lesions like FNH and HCA. Albumin *in situ* hybridization is a new and fairly specific marker of hepatic origin that is positive in liver tumors of either hepatocytic or cholangiocytic derivation, but this marker is not widely available at present.

Less useful markers include polyclonal carcinoembryonic antigen (CEA), which demonstrates a characteristic canalicular staining pattern in normal and neoplastic hepatocytes. However, this stain is unreliable in more poorly differentiated HCC, and the distinction between canalicular and membranous staining can sometimes be challenging to interpret. CD10 and villin are similar stains with similar drawbacks. AFP is an oncofetal protein expressed in hepatocellular and germ cell tumors, but its use as a marker of HCC is limited by poor sensitivity.

In general, keratin expression profiles are not useful in HCC. Most will stain with K8, K18, and CAM5.2. A minority of tumors will also express K7 and/or K19, which some research has associated with a less favorable prognosis.

Prognosis and Therapy

Overall, the median survival after diagnosis lies between 10 and 18 months, and the primary prognostic determinant is tumor resectability. Surgical resection is the only cure, and liver transplantation may be offered to patients who meet certain radiographic criteria regarding tumor size and extent (e.g., Milan criteria and others). Successful surgical resection or transplantation has a 5-year survival up to 80%, although more than half of patients do experience tumor recurrence. Imaging guided ablation and transarterial embolization are other common treatment modalities, used as definitive therapy for small lesions or as bridging therapy in patients awaiting resection or transplantation.

Favorable prognostic factors include well-to-moderate tumor differentiation, low serum AFP, absence of

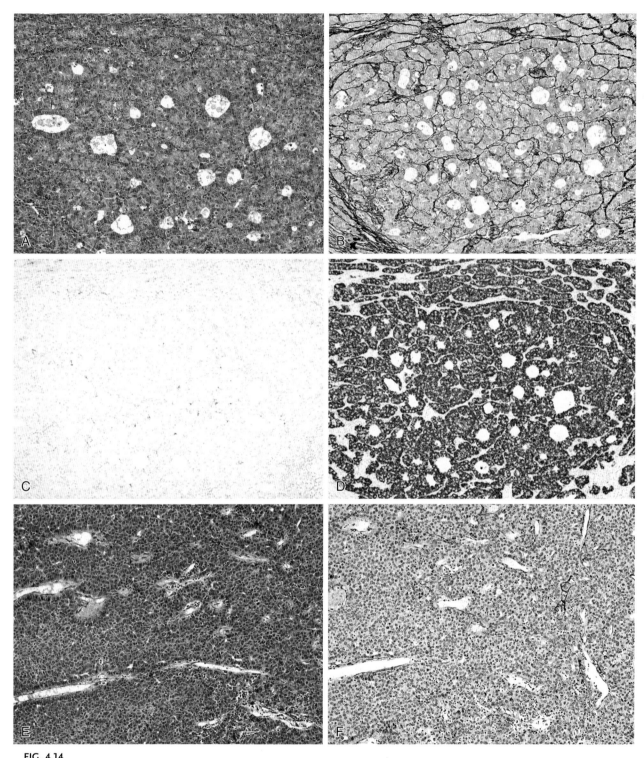

FIG. 4.14

Immunohistochemistry often shows differential sensitivity in well-differentiated and poorly differentiated hepatocellular carcinoma (HCC). In well-differentiated HCC (**A,** H&E; **B,** reticulin), glypican-3 is typically a poor marker (**C**), but arginase and HepPar1 (**D**) frequently show diffuse expression. However, in poorly differentiated HCC (**E,** H&E; **F,** reticulin), glypican-3 may be extremely helpful

Continued

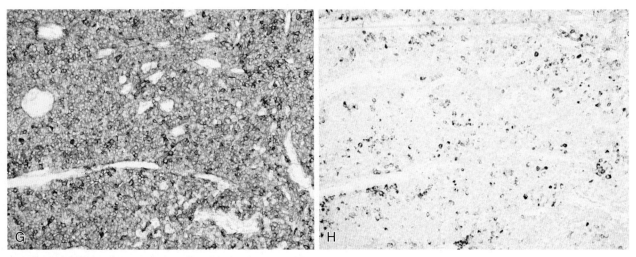

FIG. 4.14, cont'd

(**G**), while arginase and HepPar1 (**H**) are less reliable than in more well-differentiated HCC.

vascular invasion, patient age less than 50 years, female sex, and lack of background cirrhosis.

Differential Diagnosis

The differential diagnosis of HCC is broad and varies with morphology. In most cases of well-differentiated HCC, the tumor will retain a clearly hepatoid appearance and the main considerations will include other hepatocellular lesions, notably HCA. If the background liver is cirrhotic, a diagnosis of HCA is highly unlikely, but HCC also arises *de novo* in non-cirrhotic livers and through malignant transformation of an existing adenoma. In these situations, the distinction is primarily based on H&E evaluation. Both lesions lack portal structures and may contain unpaired arterioles, but the hepatocytes of HCA are generally bland, without notable cytologic atypia or mitotic activity. Well-differentiated HCC can pose a diagnostic challenge, as cytologic features may be similarly bland, so demonstration of reticulin framework disruption/loss is often critical to making this diagnosis. IHC is of marginal utility. Markers of hepatocellular differentiation (arginase, HepPar1) will be positive in both. However, glypican-3 is not expressed in adenomas and can potentially help distinguish these two entities. In practice, however, glypican-3 is less frequently positive in well-differentiated HCC, so morphologic features and reticulin integrity are often more diagnostically useful.

Moderately differentiated HCC is not typically confused with benign hepatocellular tumors due to more obvious cytoarchitectural atypia, but poorly differentiated HCC may not appear overtly hepatoid and can resemble other cancers. HCC with clear cell features can mimic clear cell renal cell carcinoma (RCC) or adrenocortical carcinoma. IHC for hepatocellular markers, PAX8, inhibin, and calretinin will distinguish these entities. Epithelioid-predominant angiomyolipoma (AML) can appear hepatoid, but these lack expression of hepatocellular markers and instead label with HMB-45 and smooth muscle actin (SMA). Epithelioid gastrointestinal stromal tumors can also mimic HCC, but these tumors show diffuse expression of CD117 and/or DOG-1 without labeling by hepatocellular markers. Neuroendocrine tumors commonly metastasize to the liver and can resemble a poorly differentiated HCC with a high N/C ratio; some even exhibit clear cell features, which can complicate the H&E interpretation. However, these strongly express neuroendocrine markers (synaptophysin, chromogranin, insulinoma-associated protein 1 [INSM1]) and are negative for arginase and HepPar1.

Cholangiocarcinoma can sometimes appear as hepatoid tumor nests, and the pseudoglandular structures of HCC may mimic an adenocarcinoma. The presence of intraluminal mucin supports a diagnosis of cholangiocarcinoma (or metastatic adenocarcinoma), and strong K7, K19, and MOC-31 expression is characteristic of cholangiocarcinoma. While some HCCs will also express these keratin markers, MOC-31 staining is not typically seen in HCC, and cholangiocarcinoma lacks arginase and HepPar1 labeling. Importantly, the diagnosis of CHC can only be made in the context of two separate morphologic patterns and not solely on the basis of a biphasic immunophenotype (see Cholangiocarcinoma section).

Finally, tumor growth patterns typically differ between HCC, cholangiocarcinoma, and metastatic tumors. While HCC often exhibits a pushing border, cholangiocarcinoma and metastatic lesions are generally more infiltrative and accompanied by a densely fibrous or desmoplastic stroma. However, certain forms of HCC are also embedded within dense background fibrosis, such as the fibrolamellar and scirrhous variants, and immunophenotype can be helpful if the morphology is unclear.

HEPATOCELLULAR CARCINOMA – DISEASE FACT SHEET

Definition
▶▶ Most common malignant primary liver tumor
▶▶ Carcinoma derived from hepatocytes

Incidence and Location
▶▶ Incidence varies widely with the geographic distribution of viral hepatitis and aflatoxin
▶▶ Southeast Asia and sub-Saharan Africa have highest incidence and mortality

Age Distribution
▶▶ Age of incidence varies geographically
▶▶ In the United States and Europe, mean age is 60–70 years
▶▶ In Southeast Asia and sub-Saharan Africa, mean age is 20–40 years

Clinical Features
▶▶ Most arise in cirrhotic livers (70%–90%)
▶▶ Cirrhosis of any cause is a risk factor and confers worse prognosis
▶▶ Additional risk factors include HBV, HCV, aflatoxin, metabolic disorders

Radiologic Features
▶▶ LI-RADS criteria used to confer risk of malignancy
▶▶ In cirrhotic livers with imaging characteristics of HCC, no biopsy is indicated

Prognosis and Therapy
▶▶ Only cure is surgical resection or transplantation
▶▶ Survival measured in months if left untreated, but 5-year survival up to 80% if successfully resected
▶▶ Embolization or ablation therapies used to treat small tumors or as bridging therapy in larger tumors before surgery

---

HEPATOCELLULAR CARCINOMA – PATHOLOGIC FEATURES

Gross Findings
▶▶ Soft tumor of varying size, may contain hemorrhage or necrosis
▶▶ May be encapsulated or have infiltrative edges
▶▶ Rare "cirrhosis-like" pattern shows diffuse small nodules of HCC

Microscopic Findings
▶▶ Characterized by expanded hepatic plates, fragmented or abnormal reticulin staining
▶▶ Bile sometimes seen in well-differentiated HCC
▶▶ Well-differentiated features include: trabecular or pseudoglandular architecture, eosinophilic cytoplasm, low N/C ratio, minimal nuclear pleomorphism
▶▶ Poorly differentiated features include: solid or macrotrabecular architecture, amphophilic/basophilic cytoplasm, increased N/C ratio, prominent nuclear pleomorphism
▶▶ Notable variants: fibrolamellar, scirrhous, steatohepatitic, sarcomatoid, lymphocyte-rich

---

Pathologic Differential Diagnoses
▶▶ Hepatocellular adenoma
▶▶ Regenerative nodule
▶▶ Cholangiocarcinoma
▶▶ Neuroendocrine tumor
▶▶ Renal cell carcinoma
▶▶ Adrenocortical carcinoma

HEPATOBLASTOMA

DDX: hepatocellular carcinoma, pediatric small round blue cell tumors, germ cell tumor, normal liver

Clinical Features

Hepatoblastoma is the most common liver tumor in children. Most occur before age 5, and the majority of patients are male. Presenting symptoms typically include abdominal swelling with occasional pain, weight loss, nausea, vomiting, and/or jaundice. Low birth weight confers a higher risk of developing hepatoblastoma, although the mechanism behind this is unclear. Most patients will have a markedly elevated serum AFP level.

Approximately 5% of patients also report concurrent congenital anomalies, and hepatoblastoma is associated with various disorders such as familial adenomatous polyposis, Li-Fraumeni syndrome, Beckwith-Wiedemann syndrome, trisomy 18, and others. Studies have shown mutations in the Wnt/β-catenin signal transduction pathway in more than 80% of hepatoblastomas, and *CTNNB1* is mutated in more than half.

Pathologic Features

GROSS FINDINGS

Most hepatoblastomas present as a single, well-circumscribed mass that can grow over 20 cm, but they are occasionally multifocal. The background liver parenchyma is normal. The tumor's macroscopic appearance depends on its histologic makeup, but a purely epithelial hepatoblastoma will appear as a soft, tan-white mass. In tumors with a prominent mesenchymal component, cystic degeneration with possible necrosis, hemorrhage, and/or calcification can be seen.

MICROSCOPIC FINDINGS

Hepatoblastoma mimics the histologic appearance of the embryonal liver. Broadly, these tumors are categorized as either purely epithelial (70% of all hepatoblastomas) or mixed epithelial and mesenchymal patterns (30%). The epithelial pattern is divided into several histologic subtypes.

The *fetal pattern* is the most common epithelial subtype, seen alone or in combination with other patterns in the vast majority of hepatoblastomas. Fetal morphology is characterized by thin trabeculae or sheets of polygonal cells that resemble immature hepatocytes, with round nuclei, prominent nucleoli, and variably distributed eosinophilic and clear cytoplasm that imparts a distinctive alternating "light and dark" appearance at low magnification (Fig. 4.15). Extramedullary hematopoiesis is often seen. In most cases, the fetal pattern exhibits a low proliferative rate, but occasional examples of high mitotic activity are seen (defined as >2 mitoses [MF] per 10 high-power fields [HPFs]).

The *embryonal pattern* is seen in about 30% of tumors and is nearly always admixed with fetal morphology.

This pattern is defined by sheets or clusters of small, hyperchromatic cells with a high N/C ratio, prominent nucleoli, and more brisk mitotic activity than the fetal form (Fig. 4.16). Extramedullary hematopoiesis is typically more prominent than in the fetal pattern.

The *pleomorphic pattern* is uncommon and often resembles adult HCC more so than the primitive morphology seen in other hepatoblastomas subtypes (Fig. 4.17A). This pattern exhibits more pronounced nuclear atypia than the previous growth patterns.

The *macrotrabecular pattern* is a rare architectural variant defined by the presence of prominently widened trabeculae (>10 cells in thickness) and can be composed of cells showing either fetal or embryonal morphology (Fig. 4.17B). This appearance can also be mistaken for HCC but is usually mixed with other, more common hepatoblastoma patterns.

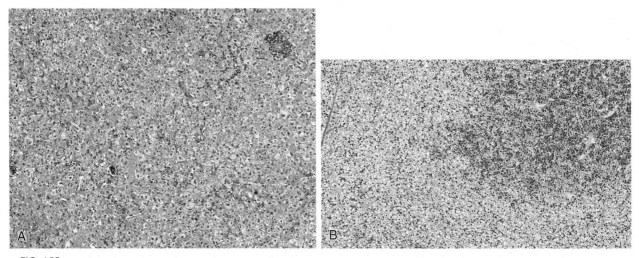

FIG. 4.15
Hepatoblastoma, fetal pattern. **(A)** Tumor cells resemble immature hepatocytes, arranged in thin trabeculae or sheets with extramedullary hematopoiesis. **(B)** Variably eosinophilic cytoplasm imparts an alternating light and dark appearance at low power. (Photos provided by Dr. Soo-Jin Cho, University of California, San Francisco.)

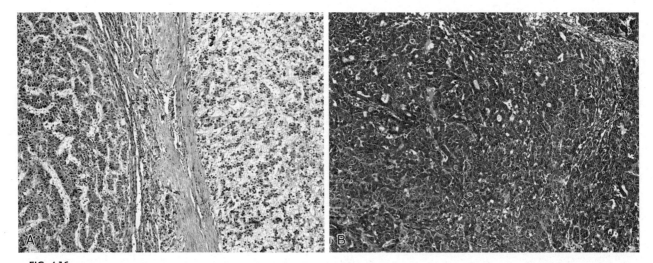

FIG. 4.16
Hepatoblastoma, embryonal pattern. Compared with the fetal pattern **(A,** right), the embryonal morphology **(A,** left) consists of smaller, hyperchromatic tumor cells, characterized by a higher nucleus-to-cytoplasm ratio **(B)**.

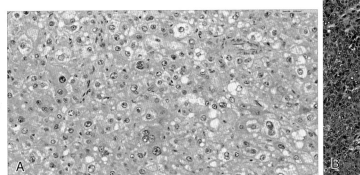
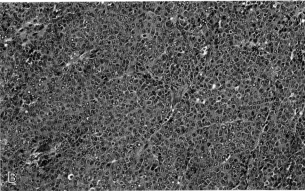

FIG. 4.17

Hepatoblastoma, pleomorphic and macrotrabecular patterns. Both patterns are uncommon variants that may resemble adult hepatocellular carcinoma. The pleomorphic pattern (**A**) exhibits more pronounced nuclear size variance than fetal or embryonal patterns, and the macrotrabecular pattern (**B**) features prominently widened trabeculae often seen in more poorly differentiated hepatocellular carcinomas. As with other rare hepatoblastoma subtypes, however, these are often admixed with more recognizable forms. (Photos provided by Dr. Soo-Jin Cho, University of California, San Francisco.)

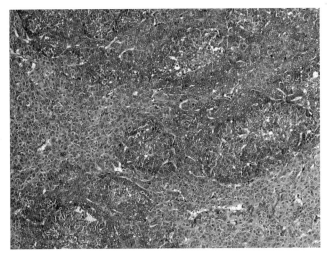

FIG. 4.18

Hepatoblastoma, small undifferentiated pattern. This variant is rarely seen and describes a tumor with aggregates of "small round blue cells" that shares a non-specific and undifferentiated morphology with several other pediatric tumors. The presence of intermixed fetal morphology helps with diagnosis in this case.

Another uncommon morphology is the *cholangioblastic pattern*, which contains scattered duct-like structures within loose stroma that superficially resembles ductular reaction. However, the degree of cytologic atypia is usually more pronounced than in reactive ductules, and while ductular reaction might be expected at the periphery of the tumor, this morphologic variant is more often seen toward the central portion of the mass.

The *small cell undifferentiated pattern* is rarely seen and describes a tumor with clusters or sheets of "small round blue cells" that share a non-specific and undifferentiated morphology with a number of other pediatric tumors (Fig. 4.18). Mitotic activity can be brisk or inconspicuous. Occasional rhabdoid morphology can be seen, characterized by eccentric nuclei and eosinophilic globules within the cytoplasm.

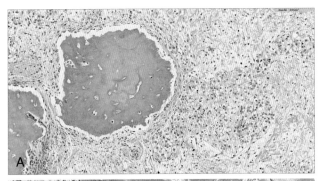
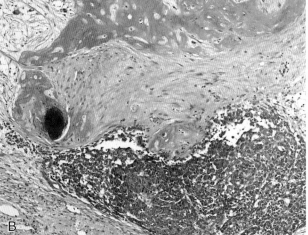

FIG. 4.19

Hepatoblastoma, mixed epithelial-mesenchymal pattern. About 30% of hepatoblastomas contain a mixture of epithelial subtypes such as fetal (**A**) or embryonal (**B**) with various mesenchymal components, commonly osteoid. (Photos provided by Dr. Soo-Jin Cho, University of California, San Francisco.)

Approximately 30% of hepatoblastomas are classified as *epithelial-mesenchymal pattern* and contain a mixture of the aforementioned epithelial subtypes with various mesenchymal components such as osteoid, fibrous tissue, and/or hyaline cartilage (Fig. 4.19). These mesenchymal areas are often positive for keratin markers and are therefore believed to represent metaplastic changes. Some mixed hepatoblastomas also exhibit *teratoid* features and include heterologous elements such as neuroectodermal, squamous, and intestinal structures.

Ancillary Studies

The immunophenotype varies based on histologic pattern, but nuclear and/or cytoplasmic β-catenin expression is typical of most hepatoblastomas, excepting small cell undifferentiated and well-differentiated fetal patterns, which can show variable β-catenin patterns. In very well-differentiated fetal patterns, membranous expression is more common.

In addition, the fetal patten of hepatoblastoma shows keratin positivity, labeling by hepatocellular markers (arginase, HepPar1), glypican-3 staining, and diffuse expression of GS. The embryonal immunophenotype is similar, but its expression of hepatocellular markers and GS is less reliable.

The small cell undifferentiated pattern exhibits variable nuclear and cytoplasmic expression of β-catenin. but is typically negative for hepatocellular markers and GS. Glypican-3 and keratin expression may be focally present. A subset of small cell undifferentiated hepatoblastomas show loss of INI1 and behave similar to malignant rhabdoid tumors.

Prognosis and Therapy

Surgery is the primary treatment for hepatoblastoma, and complete resection is the only cure. The most important prognostic factor is the tumor stage at the time of resection. Approximately 20% are metastatic at diagnosis. In most unresectable disease, however, chemotherapy can reduce the tumor burden prior to definitive surgery, and liver transplantation can be offered to many patients who remain unresectable after chemotherapy. The overall survival rate is 80%, with early-stage disease approaching 100% and falling to 40% once metastatic. Macrotrabecular and small cell undifferentiated patterns are associated with worse outcomes.

Differential Diagnosis

The differential diagnosis of hepatoblastoma depends on the tumor's predominant morphologic subtype. Hepatoblastoma with a purely fetal pattern can resemble the normal developing liver with extramedullary hematopoiesis. However, the low-power appearance of alternating light and dark zones is not typical of developing liver, and hepatoblastoma will lack both normal portal zones and central veins. IHC can also help distinguish these entities, as normal liver will not express glypican-3 or show diffuse GS, and it exhibits only membranous expression of β-catenin.

Pleomorphic and macrotrabecular areas can be mistaken for HCC. Although HCC rarely affects this age group, the cytologic features, immunophenotype, and serum AFP levels do exhibit considerable overlap and may prove a diagnostic challenge in some cases. The presence of other hepatoblastoma components, such as fetal, embryonal, or mesenchymal patterns, can be extremely helpful in excluding HCC. In addition, the presence or absence of chronic disease in the background liver may be diagnostically useful, as the former would strongly favor HCC.

The small cell undifferentiated pattern resembles any number of morphologically similar pediatric tumors such as Wilms tumor, neuroblastoma, rhabdomyosarcoma, Ewing sarcoma, and lymphoma. As before, the presence of other hepatoblastoma patterns is diagnostically helpful, but these are not always seen. In their absence, clinicoradiographic correlation and immunophenotype are critical, and the lack of a renal or adrenal mass argues against both Wilms tumor and neuroblastoma. In addition, the small cell undifferentiated pattern of hepatoblastoma will often show nuclear β-catenin localization while lacking expression for WT-1, neuroendocrine or lymphoid markers, desmin, and CD99.

Germ cell tumors enter the differential if a teratoid component is present. These are often focal, and the hepatocellular component of a teratoma usually resembles more mature liver as opposed to the fetal or embryonal patterns seen in hepatoblastoma. Glypican-3 is not diagnostically useful in this scenario, but the presence of nuclear β-catenin supports hepatoblastoma.

HEPATOBLASTOMA – DISEASE FACT SHEET

Definition
▸▸ Most common malignant liver tumor in children
▸▸ Composed of fetal and/or embryonal liver

Incidence and Location
▸▸ Rare disease (approximately 1 per 1 million children)
▸▸ Slight male predominance

Age Distribution
▸▸ Peak incidence in first 2 years, almost never seen beyond age 5

Clinical Features
▸▸ Associated with very low birth weight
▸▸ Most often presents with abdominal swelling noticed by parents
▸▸ 5% of patients also have congenital anomalies
▸▸ Associated with congenital disorders such as familial adenomatous polyposis, Li-Fraumeni syndrome, Beckwith-Wiedemann syndrome, trisomy 18, and others

Radiologic Features

▸▸ Usually a solid mass

▸▸ Calcifications present in more than 50% of cases

Prognosis and Therapy

▸▸ Prognosis determined by tumor stage at resection

▸▸ Surgical excision is only cure, preoperative chemotherapy often used to reduce tumor stage

▸▸ Small cell undifferentiated and macrotrabecular patterns have worse outcome

HEPATOBLASTOMA – PATHOLOGIC FEATURES

Gross Findings

▸▸ Typically a single, well-defined mass in a normal liver

▸▸ Epithelial tumors are usually tan-white and solid

▸▸ Mixed tumors have heterogenous appearance

Microscopic Findings

▸▸ Divided into distinct subtypes:

  ▸▸ Fetal pattern: sheets of uniform cells resembling hepatocytes, have characteristic "light and dark" appearance on low power

  ▸▸ Embryonal pattern: cells are smaller and show higher N/C ratio

  ▸▸ Pleomorphic pattern: fetal or embryonal morphology with prominent cytologic atypia

  ▸▸ Macrotrabecular pattern: fetal or embryonal cells arranged in expanded sheets at least 10 cells wide

  ▸▸ Cholangioblastic pattern: resembles ductular reaction, but cells are more atypical and located within lesion

  ▸▸ Small cell undifferentiated pattern: sheets of small round blue cells resembling several other childhood tumors

  ▸▸ Mixed epithelial-mesenchymal pattern: contains fetal and/or embryonal components admixed with primitive mesenchymal elements like osteoid, fibrous tissue, cartilage

  ▸▸ Teratoid pattern: a mixed epithelial-mesenchymal pattern that also contains heterologous elements such as neuroectodermal and intestinal derivatives

Pathologic Differential Diagnoses

▸▸ Hepatocellular carcinoma

▸▸ Pediatric small round blue cell tumors

▸▸ Germ cell tumor

▸▸ Normal liver

BILIARY TUMORS

BILE DUCT HAMARTOMA

DDX: bile duct adenoma, well-differentiated cholangiocarcinoma

Clinical Features

Bile duct hamartoma (also known as von Meyenburg complex) is an asymptomatic, subcentimeter liver lesion considered a type of ductal plate malformation. While they often arise sporadically, bile duct hamartomas have a strong association with adult polycystic disease, congenital hepatic fibrosis, and other entities on the ductal plate malformation spectrum. These lesions are found near portal areas and are frequently multiple. Bile duct hamartomas are benign and carry no risk of malignant transformation.

Pathologic Features

GROSS FINDINGS

When seen, bile duct hamartomas present as white nodules less than 5 mm in diameter dispersed throughout the liver parenchyma. Small hamartomas may not be grossly visible.

MICROSCOPIC FINDINGS

These lesions are found directly adjacent to portal areas and consist of dilated, often branching and irregularly shaped bile ductules embedded in a dense fibrous stroma (Fig. 4.20). These dilated spaces are lined by a layer of monomorphic cuboidal epithelium without appreciable atypia, and lumen frequently contain inspissated bile or proteinaceous debris. They do not contain mucin.

Differential Diagnosis

The primary differential diagnosis for bile duct hamartomas includes other benign biliary proliferations such as a bile duct adenoma or, occasionally, even

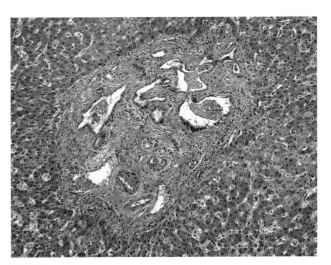

FIG. 4.20

Bile duct hamartoma. Lesions are found near portal tracts and are characterized by dilated, irregularly shaped bile ductules within dense fibrous stroma. The lumen often contains bile or proteinaceous debris, but not mucin.

well-differentiated cholangiocarcinoma. Bile duct adenomas are generally located in subcapsular areas of the liver, while hamartomas are dispersed throughout the hepatic parenchyma. The glands of a bile duct adenoma are smaller and more uniform in size compared with a bile duct hamartoma, and they lack intraluminal bile.

Well-differentiated cholangiocarcinoma is typically much larger than a bile duct hamartoma and is unlikely to be mistaken for one in most scenarios, although biopsy specimens can mask the overall size, and radiographic correlation is not always immediately available. Features that favor cholangiocarcinoma include significant variation in gland shape and spacing, desmoplastic stromal response, cribriform gland architecture, and notable cytologic atypia that manifests as nuclear pleomorphism, irregular membrane contours, and/or an increased N/C ratio. If needed, IHC for Ki-67 and p53 can often help separate benign from malignant biliary lesions. Benign lesions such as bile duct hamartoma will not show a Ki-67 proliferation index greater than 10%, and p53 will exhibit a wild-type expression pattern.

BILE DUCT HAMARTOMA – DISEASE FACT SHEET

Definition
▸▸ Common ductal plate malformation seen near portal tracts

Incidence and Location
▸▸ Often sampled incidentally at surgery or found at autopsy
▸▸ No geographic predilection

Age Distribution
▸▸ Seen in all ages

Clinical Features
▸▸ Asymptomatic
▸▸ If numerous, may suggest genetic ductal plate disease

Prognosis and Therapy
▸▸ Benign lesion with excellent prognosis
▸▸ No treatment indicated

BILE DUCT HAMARTOMA – PATHOLOGIC FEATURES

Gross Findings
▸▸ Often inapparent
▸▸ Small, subcentimeter white nodule
▸▸ May be single or multiple, spread throughout liver

Microscopic Findings
▸▸ Located immediately adjacent to portal tracts
▸▸ Consist of dilated, branching ductules set in dense fibrous stroma
▸▸ Dilated ductules often contain bile or pink proteinaceous material without mucin
▸▸ Low Ki-67 proliferation rate and wild-type p53 pattern

Pathologic Differential Diagnoses
▸▸ Bile duct adenoma
▸▸ Well-differentiated cholangiocarcinoma

BILE DUCT ADENOMA

DDX: bile duct hamartoma (von Meyenburg complex), cholangiocarcinoma, metastatic adenocarcinoma

Clinical Features

Bile duct adenomas were once thought to arise as a proliferative response to localized trauma or injury, but molecular studies now suggest that at least a subset represent true neoplasms. They are asymptomatic, often discovered incidentally, and typically located in subcapsular areas. Their distribution makes them grossly visible during abdominal surgery, where these lesions may be biopsied over concern for metastatic cancer. Bile duct adenomas may be found in both cirrhotic and noncirrhotic livers.

Pathologic Features

GROSS FINDINGS

Bile duct adenomas are usually well-demarcated, firm, tan-white lesions located beneath the capsular surface. Most are less than 1 cm, and they can be multiple.

MICROSCOPIC FINDINGS

Lesions are well-circumscribed, composed of small tubules with relatively uniform features and spacing, and are lined by a single layer of monomorphic cuboidal cells (Fig. 4.21). Tubular dilatation is not typical, and intraluminal bile is not seen. The background stroma is variable, ranging from loosely fibrous to prominently hyalinized. Accompanying inflammation is occasionally present. The glandular epithelium typically lacks mitotic activity or atypia. Normal portal zones can be seen within a bile duct adenoma, often located near the periphery.

Differential Diagnosis

The differential diagnosis contains both benign and malignant glandular lesions. Bile duct adenomas do

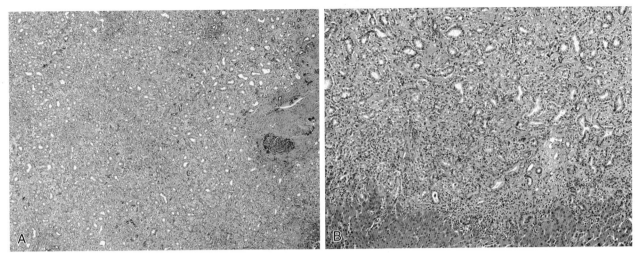

FIG. 4.21
Bile duct adenoma consists of small tubules with relatively uniform cytology and gland spacing set within fibrous stroma. **(A)** 40×. **(B)** 100×.

not feature the cystically dilated tubules with inspissated bile that characterize bile duct hamartomas, and they are not associated with polycystic diseases of the liver or kidney.

Clinically, bile duct adenomas are often sampled over concern for a primary or metastatic cancer. The circumscription of the lesion and presence of portal structures within bile duct adenomas can help distinguish these lesions from invasive adenocarcinoma. The cytomorphology also differs. Bile duct adenomas typically exhibit more uniform tubular size and spacing than a typical adenocarcinoma, with smooth rather than angular gland contours. There should not be significant mitotic activity or nuclear pleomorphism, although some well-differentiated pancreatobiliary adenocarcinomas can closely mimic this bland appearance and complicate diagnosis, especially on small biopsy specimens.

For difficult cases, IHC may be helpful. Benign biliary lesions such as a bile duct adenoma or hamartoma will exhibit a low Ki-67 proliferation index (less than 10%) and a wild-type pattern of p53 expression, whereas adenocarcinoma typically shows a higher proliferation rate and/or aberrant p53 expression (Fig. 4.22).

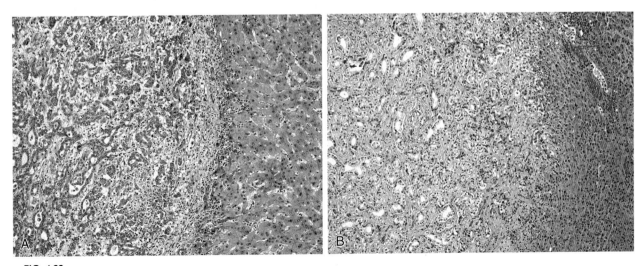

FIG. 4.22
Compared with cholangiocarcinoma **(A)**, a bile duct adenoma **(B)** contains less cytologic atypia and mitotic activity. These entities can often be distinguished by Ki-67 index, which is generally high in cholangiocarcinoma

Continued

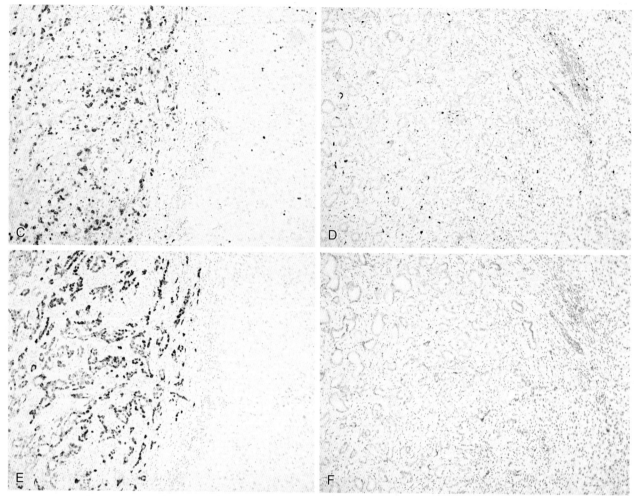

FIG. 4.22, cont'd

(**C**) but always less than 10% in adenomas (**D**). In addition, p53 is often aberrant in cholangiocarcinoma (**E**) but shows wild-type expression in adenomas (**F**).

BILE DUCT ADENOMA – DISEASE FACT SHEET

Definition
▸▸ Benign lesion composed of uniform tubular structures

Incidence and Location
▸▸ Typically located immediately beneath liver capsule

Age Distribution
▸▸ All ages

Clinical Features
▸▸ Incidentally discovered, often during abdominal surgery or autopsy

Prognosis and Therapy
▸▸ Excellent prognosis, no treatment indicated

BILE DUCT ADENOMA – PATHOLOGIC FEATURES

Gross Findings
▸▸ Small subcapsular lesion, usually less than 1 cm
▸▸ Usually solitary, but can be multiple

Microscopic Findings
▸▸ Small, uniform tubules within variably fibrous background
▸▸ Lacks notable mitotic activity or atypia
▸▸ Low Ki-67 proliferation rate and wild-type p53 pattern

Pathologic Differential Diagnoses
▸▸ Bile duct hamartoma (von Meyenburg complex)
▸▸ Cholangiocarcinoma
▸▸ Metastatic adenocarcinoma

CHOLANGIOCARCINOMA

DDX: benign biliary proliferations/neoplasms, metastatic adenocarcinoma, hepatocellular carcinoma

Clinical Features

Cholangiocarcinoma is a form of adenocarcinoma arising from bile duct epithelium, and it is further subclassified based on location. Intrahepatic cholangiocarcinoma (ICC) arises from the biliary system within the liver. Extrahepatic cholangiocarcinoma arises from biliary epithelium outside the liver and is divided into perihilar and distal bile duct cholangiocarcinoma, depending on whether the tumor origin is proximal or distal to the insertion of the cystic duct. While histologically similar, the molecular features of these subtypes cluster into somewhat distinct groups.

The majority of this discussion will focus on ICC, which accounts for approximately 15% of primary liver cancers. ICC exhibits tremendous geographic variability, as it is strongly associated with parasitic biliary infections endemic to certain parts of Southeast Asia (e.g., liver flukes such as *Clonorchis, Opisthorchis,* and *Schistosoma*). In the United States, roughly 40% of cholangiocarcinoma is intrahepatic, 10% is hilar, and the remaining half arises in the distal biliary tree. These tumors show a slight male preponderance, and mostly affect people between 50 and 70 years of age. Patients with extrahepatic cholangiocarcinoma may present early with symptoms of biliary obstruction, but the majority of patients with ICC are asymptomatic until advanced disease.

Cholangiocarcinoma is classically associated with primary sclerosing cholangitis (PSC) and has been linked to several other conditions that also induce a chronic inflammatory state within the biliary tract, such as the aforementioned biliary parasites and hepatolithiasis. Congenital biliary malformations such as Caroli disease have been associated with an increased risk of ICC, and cirrhosis also acts as an independent risk factor.

Pathologic Features

GROSS FINDINGS

Cholangiocarcinoma typically appears as a firm, tan-white mass. Although cirrhosis is a risk factor, ICC most often arises in non-cirrhotic livers. Hilar and extrahepatic cholangiocarcinoma show a similar gross appearance, but both are often accompanied by global discoloration of the liver secondary to obstructive jaundice.

The macroscopic growth behavior of ICC has been separated into three basic patterns. *Mass-forming* tumors are solid lesions within the liver parenchyma. *Periductal* tumors infiltrate along the portal zones and lead to bile duct strictures. Lastly, *intraductal* tumors exhibit papillary or polypoid growth within a dilated bile duct. These macroscopic growth patterns are significant when determining resectability.

MICROSCOPIC FINDINGS

Cholangiocarcinoma usually forms invasive glands, but solid nests, cords, and papillary structures are not uncommon architectural patterns. The tumor is often set in a backdrop of abundant fibrous or desmoplastic stroma, containing at least focal mucin within glandular elements. Perineural invasion is common, and ICC has a tendency for intravascular spread within the liver and to regional lymph nodes.

ICC has been subdivided into small duct and large duct variants, with the small duct pattern usually showing mass-forming growth at the periphery of the liver, and the large duct variant typically located near the hilum and exhibiting an infiltrative periductal growth. *Small duct* ICC resembles benign bile ducts, lined by cuboidal cells with ovoid nuclei and scant cytoplasm, growing in well-defined tubules or small anastomosing glands (Fig. 4.23A and B). In contrast, *large duct* ICC is characterized by large infiltrating glands lined by columnar epithelium (Fig. 4.23C and D). Uncommon and distinct morphologic subtypes of cholangiocarcinoma include mucinous, clear cell, signet ring, adenosquamous, mucoepidermoid, lymphoepithelioma-like, and sarcomatoid variants.

A rare subset of primary liver cancer exhibits a biphasic morphology that merges hepatocellular and cholangiocytic elements, due in part to its origin from progenitor cells in the bile ductules that contain the potential for differentiation along either lineage. This CHC contains visually distinct patterns of hepatocellular and cholangiocytic differentiation on H&E, which also demonstrate a corresponding biphasic immunophenotype (Fig. 4.24A).

Ancillary Studies

IHC is of limited utility for cholangiocarcinoma. Most will stain for K7, K19, MOC-31, and show variable K20 expression, an immunoprofile that is frequently shared by pancreatic and upper gastrointestinal cancers as well. ICC is negative for hepatocellular markers (HepPar1 and arginase) but can express the colorectal tissue marker CDX2 in up to 50% of cases.

As mentioned earlier, CHC exhibits a biphasic morphology and immunophenotype, with areas of hepatoid differentiation that stain for arginase and/or HepPar1 alongside an adenocarcinoma showing an immunoprofile consistent with cholangiocarcinoma (Fig. 4.24B and C). Importantly, a differential immunophenotype alone is insufficient to diagnose CHC; visualizing two distinct morphologic elements is necessary.

Prognosis and Therapy

The overall prognosis for cholangiocarcinoma is heavily tied to the extent of disease at the time of

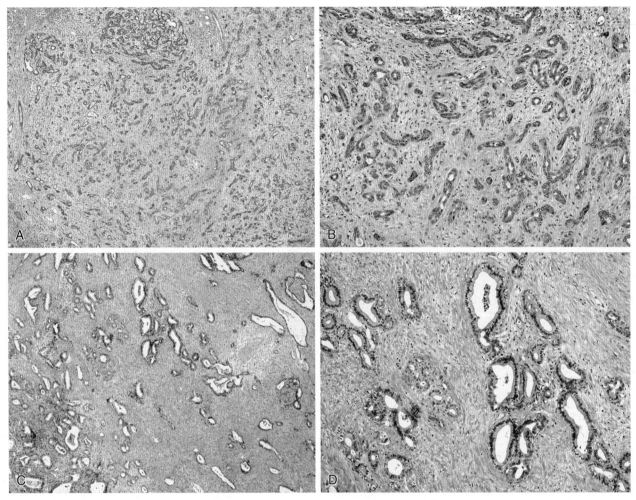

FIG. 4.23
Cholangiocarcinoma. The small duct variant (**A, B**) shows well-defined or anastomosing tubules lined by cuboidal cells, while the large duct variant (**C, D**) contains larger, more dilated glands lined by columnar epithelium.

resection. As many patients present with advanced, unresectable tumors, the usual prognosis for cholangiocarcinoma is poor, with a median survival of 6 months. For resectable tumors, the most important prognostic factors are margin status and nodal involvement. The 5-year survival for ICC with lymph node metastasis is less than 10%, but node-negative disease with clear surgical margins increases the 5-year survival to approximately 40%.

Differential Diagnosis

The two primary considerations in the differential diagnosis of ICC are benign biliary proliferations and other primary or metastatic cancers. Small duct ICC can mimic the features of benign tumors such as a bile duct adenoma. Resection specimens permit assessment of the lesion edge, which can be quite helpful—bile duct

adenomas have a well-circumscribed, smooth border, while cholangiocarcinomas often exhibit an irregular and infiltrative margin. However, small biopsy specimens can be problematic to interpret, since the presence or absence of an infiltrative border often cannot be assessed. Further complicating this differential, both benign and malignant bile duct lesions may contain a densely fibrous or hyalinized background.

In difficult biopsies, borders and gland cytoarchitecture are the most helpful features. Small duct ICC and bile duct adenomas are both comprised of small glands or tubules, but the invasive glands of ICC more often show angular contours and complex, anastomosing growth, whereas the glands comprising adenomas are smooth and exhibit more separation. Bile duct adenomas should not contain more than rare mitotic figures, and the cuboidal lining cells should not harbor any significant atypia. Features such as nuclear pleomorphism and irregular nuclear contours favor ICC. If the diagnosis remains unclear,

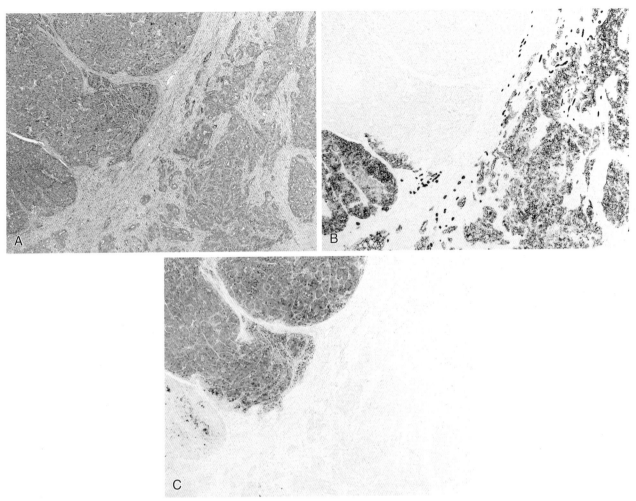

FIG. 4.24

Combined hepatocellular-cholangiocarcinoma. **A,** This biphasic tumor contains two distinct morphologic patterns that resemble intermixed elements of hepatocellular carcinoma and adenocarcinoma. Immunohistochemistry for CK19 (**B**) will highlight the cholangiocarcinoma component, while arginase (**C**) will only stain the areas of hepatocellular carcinoma.

IHC can help separate benign from malignant biliary lesions. Benign lesions do not show a Ki-67 proliferation index greater than 10% or aberrant p53 expression. However, not all malignant tumors will show the opposite immunophenotype, so correlation with morphology is needed.

The other challenge lies in distinguishing ICC from metastatic adenocarcinoma or other primary liver tumors. Where appropriate, common tumors that metastasize to the liver can be excluded with an immunohistochemical panel that includes markers of colorectal, pulmonary, breast, gynecologic, and/or prostatic origin. Metastatic adenocarcinomas from the upper gastrointestinal tract and pancreas represent a particular challenge, as these tumors have overlapping immunophenotypes with strong K7 positivity and variable expression of CDX2. Albumin *in situ* hybridization is a useful marker of hepatic origin (labeling both HCC and ICC) and therefore has

utility in separating ICC from metastatic adenocarcinomas. In cases of a non-specific immunophenotype, however, correlation with clinical and imaging findings is critical.

Epithelioid hemangioendothelioma (EHE) contains a prominent desmoplastic stroma that can mimic poorly differentiated ICC at low power, and the presence of intracellular lumen can be confused with vague gland formation. However, EHE lacks mucin and stains readily with vascular markers (ERG, CD31, CD34) as well as the fusion-specific CAMTA1.

In addition, ICC with a solid-predominant growth pattern and minimal/absent gland formation could be confused with HCC exhibiting compact architecture. Likewise, HCC with abundant pseudoglandular architecture may mimic a CHC. In both cases, immunohistochemical distinction is usually straightforward, as hepatocellular markers (HepPar1, arginase) will be negative in ICC and MOC-31 is almost never expressed in HCC.

MESENCHYMAL TUMORS

ANGIOMYOLIPOMA

DDX:
- Myomatous AML: hepatocellular adenoma, hepatocellular carcinoma, melanoma
- Lipomatous AML: focal fatty change, steatotic liver neoplasm (such as HNF1α-inactivated subtype of hepatocellular adenoma)
- Angiomatous AML: hemangioma, vascular malformation

Clinical Features

AMLs are rare tumors of the liver that arise from the perivascular epithelioid cell and have historically been grouped among the "PEComa" family. Most are found in non-cirrhotic livers. The majority of hepatic angiolipomas are sporadic and only 5% to 10% occur in patients with tuberous sclerosis (unlike AMLs arising in the kidney). Most cases are clinically silent and only detected incidentally when the patient is imaged for other reasons, but large tumors can present with abdominal pain.

Pathologic Features

GROSS FINDINGS

AMLs are typically solitary, circumscribed, non-encapsulated lesions. Their size shows tremendous variance, ranging from a few millimeters to well over 30 cm. Their gross appearance depends on the microscopic composition of the tumor. Lipomatous areas will be yellow and soft, while the angiomatous component is grossly hemorrhagic, and myomatous regions will be solid, firm, and tan-white.

MICROSCOPIC FINDINGS

AML is a triphasic tumor composed of three elements: epithelioid or spindled myoid cells, blood vessels, and adipose tissue. They have a variable histologic appearance due to the relative proportion of their component elements, and tumors featuring a single primary component have been termed angiomatous, myomatous, or lipomatous AMLs. The smooth muscle element of these tumors originates from vascular walls and can appear spindled or epithelioid with varying degrees of pleomorphism and cellularity. The vascular component consists of tortuous, thick-walled arterial spaces and/or thin-walled venous channels. The fatty elements are generally composed of mature adipose tissue, either scattered as individual cells throughout the tumor or coalesced into large sheets. Scattered lipoblasts may also be present.

Mixed AMLs will demonstrate all three components clearly, and these tumors are typically not a diagnostic challenge. However, hepatic AMLs frequently present with a single predominant element that can complicate diagnosis. In particular, hepatic AMLs often feature a prominent epithelioid myoid cell element with only scattered blood vessels and a minimal fat (Fig. 4.25A). These epithelioid cells are rounded or polygonal, with ovoid nuclei, prominent nucleoli, and eosinophilic cytoplasm that sometimes condenses around the nucleus after fixation, which may mimic swollen hepatocytes. Although mitotic activity is not pronounced, these cells can show a surprising degree of cytologic atypia. A myomatous AML with a prominent spindle cell component will be variably cellular, and myoid cells will also contain ovoid nuclei with eosinophilic cytoplasm, although their spindled histologic appearance is more obviously mesenchymal.

Ancillary Studies

The different elements of AML stain with various markers, but all components are negative for keratins. The epithelioid or spindled myoid component stains with

HMB-45, Melan-A, SMA, and caldesmon. Any vascular component will express endothelial markers (CD31, CD34, ERG), mature adipocytes labeled with S-100, and scattered lipoblasts stain with either S-100 or HMB-45.

Prognosis and Therapy

Hepatic AMLs are benign lesions that can be managed by observation or, if needed, surgical resection. Malignant angiomyolipomas in the liver have been reported but are extremely rare.

Differential Diagnosis

AMLs with a single prominent component can be diagnostically challenging. Most problematic are epithelioid myomatous tumors, which can exhibit a remarkably

FIG. 4.25
Hepatic angiomyolipomas with a prominent epithelioid component can look hepatoid (**A**). These can be easily misdiagnosed as hepatocellular carcinoma. However, immunohistochemistry for arginase will be negative (**B**), and melanomyoid markers like HMB-45 (**C**) will stain the epithelioid component.

hepatoid morphology, with polygonal cells containing abundant eosinophilic cytoplasm and well-demarcated cell borders. These kinds of AML can easily mimic HCAs or, if even mild cytologic atypia is present, well-differentiated HCC. Furthermore, reticulin staining on AML will highlight a poorly developed or obliterated framework, which may reinforce a mistaken diagnosis of HCC. A hepatoid neoplasm in a non-cirrhotic liver with a vaguely mesenchymal appearance and/or reticulin loss out of proportion to the degree of cytologic atypia should raise suspicion for AML, and staining for hepatocellular derivation may be prudent. Arginase and HepPar1 will be negative in AML (Fig. 4.25B), while myomelanocytic markers like HMB-45 and SMA will be diffusely positive (Fig. 4.25C). This distinction can be especially challenging in biopsy specimens, where IHC is often crucial to avoiding misdiagnosis.

Myomatous AML with a mixture of epithelioid and spindled cells can also mimic metastatic melanoma, further complicated by their overlapping immunophenotype. However, melanoma typically shows a greater degree of cytologic atypia. While melanocytic markers like HMB-45 are positive in both entities, melanoma will not co-express smooth muscle markers, and SOX10 is negative in AML.

If the tumor exhibits a vascular predominance, it may be mistaken for a hemangioma or vascular malformation. If the dominant element is fatty, these can be misinterpreted as focal fatty change or a hepatocellular lesion with prominent steatosis (such as the HNF1α-inactivated subtype of HCA). In either case, immunohistochemical staining should label associated myoid cells and confirm the diagnosis of AML.

ANGIOMYOLIPOMA – DISEASE FACT SHEET

Definition
▸▸ Benign tumor composed of myoid cells, blood vessels, and fat

Incidence and Location
▸▸ Rare tumors with no geographic predilection

Age Distribution
▸▸ More common in females
▸▸ Average age between 30 and 50 years

Clinical Features
▸▸ Most AMLs are asymptomatic and detected incidentally
▸▸ Larger lesions may present with abdominal pain

Radiologic Features
▸▸ Heterogenous and circumscribed mass on imaging
▸▸ Radiographic differential frequently includes hepatocellular lesions if tumor fat content is low

Prognosis and Therapy
▸▸ Excellent prognosis
▸▸ Patients are either observed or undergo surgical resection

---

ANGIOMYOLIPOMA – PATHOLOGIC FEATURES

Gross Findings
▸▸ Well-circumscribed lesion, size can vary tremendously
▸▸ Some combination of fatty, hemorrhagic, and tan-white solid areas, depending on tumor composition
▸▸ Non-cirrhotic background liver

Microscopic Findings
▸▸ Triphasic tumor with a varying proportion of three cell types: epithelioid/spindled myoid cells, blood vessels, and adipose tissue
▸▸ Myomatous AML is common in the liver
▸▸ Fatty component is often inconspicuous in hepatic AML

Pathologic Differential Diagnoses
▸▸ Myomatous AML: hepatocellular adenoma, hepatocellular carcinoma, melanoma
▸▸ Lipomatous AML: focal fatty change, steatotic liver neoplasm (HNF1α-inactivated subtype of hepatocellular adenoma)
▸▸ Angiomatous AML: hemangioma, vascular malformation

EPITHELIOID HEMANGIOENDOTHELIOMA

DDX: adenocarcinoma (including cholangiocarcinoma), angiosarcoma, bland fibrosis

Clinical Features

EHE is a rare, malignant vascular tumor that can arise in multiple sites, including the liver. It affects adults and is seen more often in women than in men. Hepatic EHE tends to cause venous occlusion, and involvement of the hepatic vein can result in sinusoidal obstruction or Budd-Chiari syndrome. Although this is a vascular tumor, its dense stroma protects from rupture and hemorrhage, so risk of significant bleeding is minimal.

A distinct chromosomal translocation has been identified in more than 90% of EHEs, which results in a *WWTR1-CAMTA1* fusion. A small subset (fewer than 5%) also contains the *YAP-TFE3* gene fusion.

Pathologic Features

GROSS FINDINGS

EHE is typically multifocal at the time of resection, usually involves both lobes, and individual masses vary in size from a few millimeters to more than 10 cm. The cut surface is firm, tan-white, and sometimes gritty due to dystrophic calcifications.

MICROSCOPIC FINDINGS

These tumors typically exhibit prominent fibromyxoid stroma and relative paucicellularity at the center of the lesion. Cellularity increases toward the periphery of the tumor, imparting a zonal appearance at low power. At the leading front, EHE grows through sinusoidal spaces and characteristically entraps normal hepatic structures such as portal zones and hepatocyte clusters (Fig. 4.26A). Within the tumor's fibromyxoid stroma are a mixture of spindled dendritic cells and rounded epithelioid cells, the latter containing vacuoles that represent intracellular capillary-type lumina ("blister cells"). These can mimic signet ring cells, but the intracellular channels occasionally contain red blood cells and lack mucin (Fig. 4.26B). Toward the center of the lesion, the tumor appears more solid, stroma-rich, and sometimes calcified. Obliteration of portal and central veins is a common finding.

Ancillary Studies

All cases of EHE are positive for at least one endothelial marker (CD31, CD34, ERG). If available, IHC for CAMTA1 is essentially diagnostic for EHE (Fig. 4.26B and C), and molecular testing can be performed to detect the characteristic fusion products. Notably, EHE can sometimes show anomalous keratin expression.

Prognosis and Therapy

EHE tends to behave in a low-grade manner compared with other malignant vascular tumors such as angiosarcoma. It grows relatively slowly, and the 5-year survival is approximately 50%.

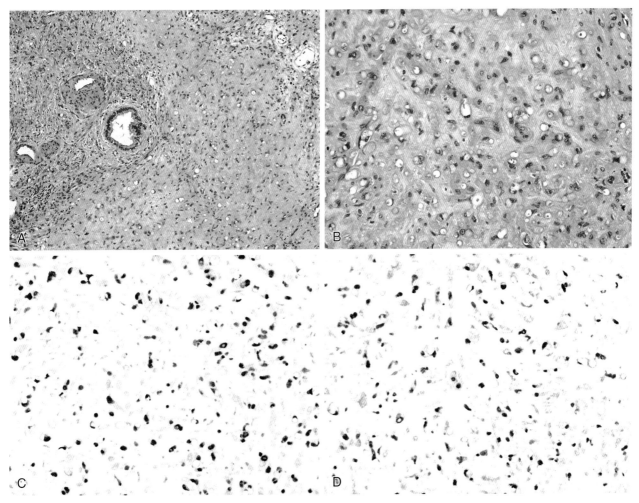

FIG. 4.26
Epithelioid hemangioendothelioma tends to entrap native liver structures such as hepatocytes or portal zones (**A**) and is characterized by "blister cells," epithelioid tumor cells with intracellular capillary lumen that may contain red blood cells (**B**). There is no mucin. Immunohistochemistry for ERG (**C**) and CAMTA1 (**D**) are strongly positive in tumor cells.

Differential Diagnosis

The primary differential diagnosis for hepatic EHE includes adenocarcinoma, angiosarcoma, or a benign sclerosing process. The prominent myxoid-type stroma and presence of epithelioid elements can resemble the desmoplastic response of adenocarcinoma, and the blister cell morphology can especially resemble signet ring cells or abortive gland structures. However, the intracellular vacuoles of EHE blister cells will occasionally contain erythrocytes and lack mucin. EHE will also express vascular endothelial markers and the vast majority will also label with CAMTA1 IHC, both of which will be negative in adenocarcinoma. Be wary of focal keratin staining, as EHE can occasionally be positive, and atrophic hepatic structures may be entrapped within the tumor.

Angiosarcoma shows an overlapping immunophenotype, with variable keratin expression and strong labeling by vascular markers such as ERG, but the morphologic distinction is straightforward. Angiosarcomas tend to be larger and more hemorrhagic than EHE. They demonstrate a significantly higher degree of nuclear atypia and show prominent mitotic activity. The characteristic fibromyxoid stroma and calcifications of EHE are not shared by angiosarcoma, and the latter tumor has a notably more destructive growth pattern, without entrapment and preservation of hepatic structures.

In small biopsies, it can be challenging to distinguish EHE from areas of bland fibrosis, such as a sclerosed hemangioma or parenchymal extinction adjacent to an unsampled mass lesion. These areas of bland fibrosis tend to be more hypocellular than EHE. They may contain small, normal capillaries within the fibrous background, which will label with endothelial markers. However, the characteristic "blister cells" of EHE will be absent, and no atypical dendritic cells are seen. If available, IHC for CAMTA1 can be very helpful in these situations.

EPITHELIOID HEMANGIOENDOTHELIOMA – DISEASE FACT SHEET

Definition
▸▸ Rare, low-grade malignant endothelial neoplasm

Incidence and Location
▸▸ Slightly more prevalent in women

Age Distribution
▸▸ Mean age of diagnosis is 40 years

Clinical Features
▸▸ Patients present with non-specific symptoms
▸▸ 90% are characterized by *WWTR1-CAMTA1* fusion
▸▸ Can present with elevated alkaline phosphatase level
▸▸ Diagnosis made incidentally in about 50% of cases

Radiologic Features
▸▸ Usually appear as multiple liver masses

Prognosis and Therapy
▸▸ Prognosis is variable
▸▸ 5-year survival is approximately 50%

EPITHELIOID HEMANGIOENDOTHELIOMA – PATHOLOGIC FEATURES

Gross Findings
▸▸ Usually multiple
▸▸ Firm, tan-white cut surface
▸▸ Can have gritty texture if calcified

Microscopic Findings
▸▸ Zonal pattern at low power, with increased cellularity in peripheral areas
▸▸ Entraps hepatic structures at periphery, tends to occlude veins
▸▸ Prominent fibromyxoid stroma
▸▸ Contains spindled dendritic cells and epithelioid "blister cells"
▸▸ Only mild cytologic atypia

Pathologic Differential Diagnoses
▸▸ Adenocarcinoma (including cholangiocarcinoma)
▸▸ Angiosarcoma
▸▸ Bland fibrosis

PANCREAS

NON-NEOPLASTIC DISEASE

A diverse array of inflammatory disorders, developmental variants, and non-neoplastic mass-forming lesions can affect the pancreas and Vaterian system. Familiarity with these entities is essential, as they have the potential to be mistaken for neoplastic processes, both clinically and histologically. Careful review of laboratory and imaging studies, as well as discussion with the clinical team, may be invaluable in arriving at the correct diagnosis and ultimately informing safe and appropriate patient care.

CHRONIC PANCREATITIS

DDX: pancreatic ductal adenocarcinoma, autoimmune pancreatitis, well-differentiated pancreatic neuroendocrine tumor

Clinical Features

Chronic pancreatitis (CP) is a fibroinflammatory process that leads to the irreversible loss of the acinar, and ultimately endocrine, parenchymal tissue. Although initially considered to be distinct entities, it is now thought that CP exists on a continuum with and develops following multiple episodes of acute pancreatitis (discussed later). In the United States and other Western countries, alcohol abuse is by far the most common cause of CP, though the development of this disease appears to be multifactorial with contributions from numerous other environmental and genetic factors.

Classically, CP presents in the fourth or fifth decades of life with epigastric abdominal pain. Loss of acinar cell mass ultimately results in exocrine insufficiency leading to malabsorption, steatorrhea, and nutritional deficiencies. Perhaps not surprisingly, islet cell destruction also occurs over time and leads to endocrine failure and the development of diabetes mellitus in most patients with longstanding CP.

Pathologic Features

GROSS FINDINGS

CP is typically not a surgical disease. However, it may occasionally present as a mass-forming lesion on imaging studies leading to surgical resection. In these situations, gross examination may reveal a firm, tan-white mass that is essentially indistinguishable from a pancreatic ductal adenocarcinoma (PDAC) (Fig. 4.27). In the absence of tumefactive lesions, the pancreas is typically shrunken and fibrotic, lacking the well-defined lobular architecture of the normal gland. Cystic structures, representing either intrapancreatic retention cysts or pseudocysts, may also be identified after the pancreas is sectioned and are occasionally prominent. The cut surface of the gland typically has a gritty texture resulting from calcification of the obliterated parenchyma. Larger calculi may also be embedded within the ductal system, leading to obstruction and upstream dilation. These pancreatic calcifications and calculi may also be

seen on cross-sectional imaging studies, though they are not present in all instances.

MICROSCOPIC FINDINGS

CP is characterized by atrophy of the acinar parenchyma with expansion of the normally inconspicuous interlobular connective tissue by broad swaths of dense fibrosis. This expanded interlobular fibrous tissue is relatively paucicellular, containing fibroblasts and myofibroblasts in addition to a modest, lymphocyte-predominant inflammatory infiltrate (Fig. 4.28A). Over time and with increasing parenchymal atrophy, intralobular fibrosis develops, further distorting and obscuring the normal lobular architecture of the gland. Calcifications are frequently identified within this fibrous stroma, as well as the peripancreatic adipose tissue.

Relative to the acinar parenchyma, the islets of Langerhans are relatively preserved early in the course of CP. The residual islets may appear particularly prominent in

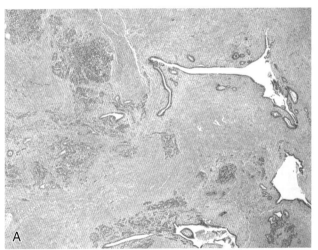

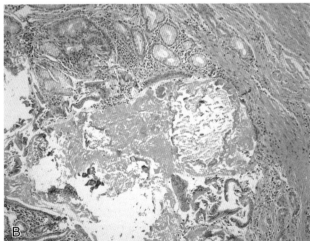

FIG. 4.28
Chronic pancreatitis. **A,** There is atrophy of the acinar parenchyma with expansion of the interlobular connective tissue by dense fibrosis. **B,** Dilated pancreatic duct with proteinaceous material, cellular debris, and calcifications.

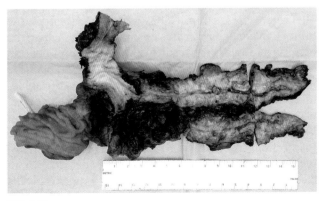

FIG. 4.27
Total pancreatectomy bisected through main pancreatic duct and demonstrating atrophy of the normal lobular architecture with calculi embedded within the ductal system.

a background of expansile fibrosis with the loss of acinar cell mass and have been mistaken for neuroendocrine neoplasms (discussed later). Pancreatic ducts are frequently dilated in CP. Classically, impaction of the ductal system with dense concretions or calculi has been associated with alcohol abuse, though this finding is not entirely specific and proteinaceous plugs may also be found in individuals with cystic fibrosis–related pancreatitis (Fig. 4.28B).

Ancillary Studies

Ancillary immunohistochemical and molecular diagnostic studies have limited utility in the diagnosis of CP with classic histologic features.

Differential Diagnosis

Distinguishing well- and moderately differentiated PDACs from CP can be extremely challenging, particularly in small biopsy fragments and at the time of intraoperative consultation with frozen sections. The challenging nature of this diagnosis is compounded by the fact that adenocarcinoma and CP may coexist in the same pancreas; carcinomas frequently obstruct the ductal system leading to upstream parenchymal atrophy and fibrosis that is indistinguishable from CP developing in other settings.

Architectural cues are invaluable in the assessment of pancreatic lesions. In contrast to ductal adenocarcinoma, the normal lobular architecture of the pancreas is typically retained in CP, even in the setting of extensive parenchymal atrophy and fibrosis. Ducts restricted to residual or atrophic lobules are generally non-neoplastic, while small ducts infiltrating interlobular septae and peripancreatic adipose tissue are highly suggestive of a neoplastic process regardless of the degree of cytologic atypia. Similarly, glands adjacent to muscular arteries, infiltrating nerve sheaths, or within lymphovascular spaces are not seen in the setting of CP and should be considered to be essentially pathognomonic for malignancy (Fig. 4.29). Incomplete glands and glands with luminal necrosis are also highly suggestive of a neoplastic process.

Cytologic assessment is also essential in distinguishing benign reactive glands in the setting of CP from an infiltrating ductal adenocarcinoma, particularly in fine-needle aspirates and fine-needle biopsies where architectural features may be obscured or absent. Significant nuclear pleomorphism and anisonucleosis with greater than 4:1 variation in nuclear size, particularly within a single gland, is often cited as a feature of malignancy that distinguishes ductal adenocarcinoma from reactive glands in the setting of CP (Fig. 4.30). Similarly, significant nuclear membrane and chromatin abnormalities are generally associated with carcinoma rather than reactive atypia, though these subtle findings are best appreciated on cytologic preparations (Table 4.1).

Although immunohistochemical studies are not needed in most instances, and are not possible at the time of intraoperative consultation, several markers may be useful in rare situations when distinguishing benign, reactive pancreatic ducts from an infiltrative process is challenging based upon H&E-stained sections alone. The transcription factor *SMAD4* has been reported to be lost in approximately 60% of PDACs and shows retained nuclear expression in CP. Preserved reactivity for *SMAD4*, therefore, does nothing to exclude a malignant process. Some groups have suggested that strong nuclear reactivity for the tumor suppressor gene *TP53* favors malignancy, though expression is not universal in adenocarcinomas. Similarly, the Ki-67 proliferative index is generally elevated in PDAC, but may also be increased in the benign, reactive glands of CP, again limiting the utility of this immunohistochemical stain somewhat. In general, given the less-than-ideal performance characteristics of the currently available immunohistochemical studies, ancillary tests should be used judiciously and interpreted after careful review of the H&E-stained tissue sections in the context of the clinical picture.

Significant atrophy of the acinar parenchyma early in the course of CP with relative preservation of the islets of Langerhans may lead to the pseudohypertrophy of the endocrine population. Occasionally, the residual islets may cluster and be so prominent as to mimic a pancreatic neuroendocrine microadenoma or, if greater than 0.5 cm, a well-differentiated pancreatic neuroendocrine tumor (WDNET). The distinction is typically relatively straightforward on H&E-stained sections from resection specimens, where neuroendocrine tumors are mass-forming lesions while pseudohypertrophic islets of Langerhans tend to be distributed throughout the gland in a background of CP. The lobular architecture is also typically maintained in cases of pseudohypertrophy, whereas it is completely absent in neuroendocrine tumors. In challenging cases or small biopsies where the preserved lobular architecture may be difficult to appreciate, immunohistochemical stains for the islet peptides insulin, glucagon, pancreatic polypeptide, and somatostatin can be employed in order to exclude a neoplastic process. Immunostains for glucagon and insulin will highlight the normal spatial distribution of alpha and beta cells in pseudohypertrophic islets of Langerhans, with significantly less prominent, singly dispersed pancreatic polypeptide and somatostatin producing cells (Fig. 4.31). In contrast, neuroendocrine tumors lack this spatial organization and generally show either diffuse reactivity for glucagon, or lack expression for insulin and glucagon altogether.

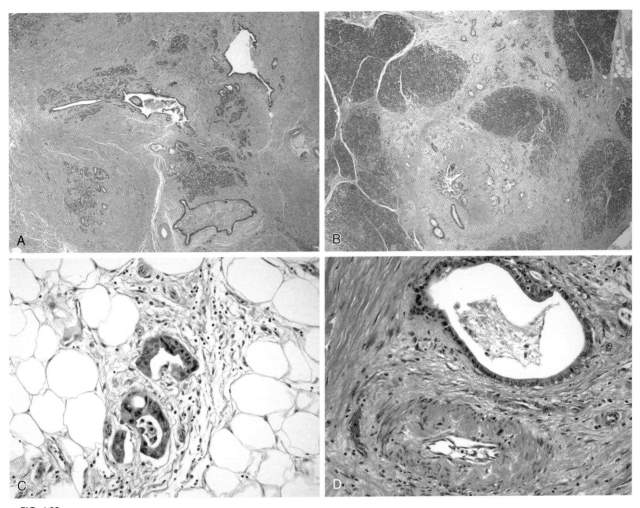

FIG. 4.29

Chronic pancreatitis versus pancreatic ductal adenocarcinoma. **A,** Despite the atrophy of the acinar parenchyma and increase in fibrous tissue, the normal lobular architecture is still identifiable in the setting of chronic pancreatitis. **B,** In contrast, neoplastic glands infiltrate between normal and atrophic lobules in pancreatic ductal adenocarcinoma. **C,** Glands infiltrating peripancreatic adipose tissue is not a feature of chronic pancreatitis but is frequently encountered in invasive adenocarcinoma. **D,** Non-neoplastic glands do not abut muscular arteries.

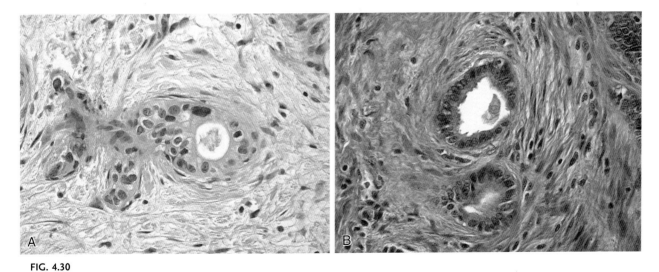

FIG. 4.30

Pancreatic ductal adenocarcinoma versus chronic pancreatitis. **A,** Infiltrating malignant glands of pancreatic ductal adenocarcinoma show significant nuclear pleomorphism with marked variation of nuclear size within a single gland. **B,** In contrast, the benign glands of chronic pancreatitis contain cells with relatively uniform nuclei and maintained polarity.

TABLE 4.1
Chronic Pancreatitis Versus Pancreatic Ductal Adenocarcinoma

	Chronic Pancreatitis	Pancreatic Ductal Adenocarcinoma
Preserved lobular architecture	Yes	No
Glands infiltrating fibrous septae	No	Yes
Glands in adipose tissue	No	Yes
Glands adjacent to muscular arteries	No	Yes
Glands infiltrating nerve sheaths	No	Yes
Glands in lymphovascular spaces	No	Yes
Incomplete glands and glands with luminal necrosis	No	Yes
Nuclear variation >4:1	No	Yes
Nuclear pleomorphism	No	Yes
Chromatin irregularities	No	Yes
Nuclear membrane irregularities	No	Yes

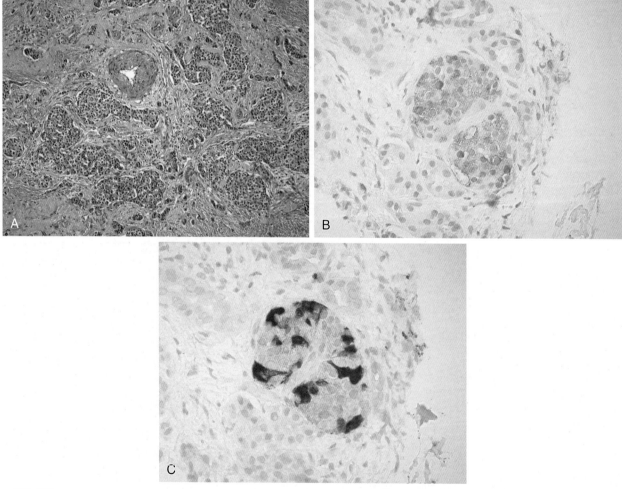

FIG. 4.31

A, Chronic pancreatitis with atrophy and loss of acinar parenchyma can lead to pseudohypertrophy of islets of Langerhans and lead to diagnostic confusion with well-differentiated pancreatic neuroendocrine tumors. **B,** Immunohistochemical stains for insulin and glucagon **(C)** demonstrate normal distribution and spatial arrangements of peptide-producing endocrine cells and support a non-neoplastic process.

Autoimmune pancreatitis (AIP) may occasionally enter the differential diagnosis for CP and is discussed in more detail below. Briefly, type 1 AIP (also referred to as lymphoplasmacytic sclerosing pancreatitis) is an immune-mediated process characterized by dense, plasma cell–rich inflammatory infiltrate, cellular storiform-type fibrosis, obliterative phlebitis, and increased IgG4-positive plasma cells. In contrast to type 1 AIP, the inflammatory infiltrate seen in CP is significantly less robust and is predominantly lymphocytic. Swirling, duct-centric fibrosis is generally not a feature of CP, which tends to be relatively paucicellular, nor is obliterative venulitis or arteritis. Perhaps most importantly, as type 1 AIP is an IgG4-related disease, patients tend to have an elevated serum IgG4. Although occasional IgG4-positive plasma cells may be encountered in CP, they are generally sparse and fall far short of the threshold of 50 IgG4-positive plasma cells per HPF needed to suggest a diagnosis of type 1 AIP.

Prognosis and Therapy

The prognosis for patients with CP is poor with up 80% of patients exhibiting chronic abdominal pain and nearly half developing diabetes and exocrine insufficiency which require medical support. Abstinence from alcohol and tobacco should be encouraged and pain control is generally achievable with oral analgesics, though endoscopic drainage procedures or surgical resection with celiac plexus blockade may be offered in patients refractory to medical therapy. Despite advances in management, the median survival for patients with CP is only 15 to 20 years after initial diagnosis.

CHRONIC PANCREATITIS – DISEASE FACT SHEET

Definition
▶▶ Fibroinflammatory disorder of the pancreas characterized by parenchymal loss with associated exocrine insufficiency and endocrine failure

Incidence and Location
▶▶ Common with annual incidence of 5–8 per 100,000 adults in the United States

Sex and Age Distribution
▶▶ Two thirds of patients are men
▶▶ Alcohol-related chronic pancreatitis presents between 40 and 60 years
▶▶ Chronic pancreatitis related to genetic mutations presents between 10 and 40 years

Clinical Features
▶▶ Exocrine insufficiency with malabsorption and steatorrhea
▶▶ Endocrine failure leading to diabetes mellitus

Radiologic Features
▶▶ Pancreatic calcifications and/or marked ductal changes on CT
▶▶ Magnetic resonance cholangiopancreatography demonstrates main pancreatic duct dilation or irregularity, dilation of the side branches, and strictures

Prognosis and Therapy
▶▶ Poor long-term survival
▶▶ Supportive care with enzyme replacement, management of endocrine insufficiency, and pain control

---

CHRONIC PANCREATITIS – PATHOLOGIC FEATURES

Gross Findings
▶▶ Firm, shrunken gland with loss of normal lobular architecture
▶▶ Gritty cut surface
▶▶ Pancreatic and peripancreatic cysts and ductal dilation

Microscopic Findings
▶▶ Paucicellular interlobular and intralobular fibrosis
▶▶ Early atrophy of acinar parenchyma with relative preservation of islets of Langerhans
▶▶ Mild, patchy, lymphocyte-predominant inflammatory infiltrate
▶▶ Proteinaceous ductal concretions and calculi

Pathologic Differential Diagnoses
▶▶ Pancreatic ductal adenocarcinoma
▶▶ Well-differentiated pancreatic neuroendocrine tumor
▶▶ Autoimmune pancreatitis

AUTOIMMUNE PANCREATITIS

DDX: chronic pancreatitis, pancreatic ductal adenocarcinoma

Clinical Features

AIP is uncommon relative to CP. Although the incidence and prevalence of this disorder is difficult to estimate, reports from South Korea and Japan suggest a prevalence of approximately 5% in patients with idiopathic pancreatitis. AIP is an umbrella term used to describe at least two distinct entities: type 1 AIP and type 2 AIP. Type 1 AIP is a prototypical IgG4-related disease and tends to affect primarily elderly men. Classical symptoms of CP, namely abdominal pain, weight loss, and steatorrhea, are uncommon in patients with type 1 AIP. Rather, the vast majority of patients present with either painless jaundice or cholangitis, prompting workup with cross-sectional imaging studies that frequently demonstrate an inflammatory mass within the pancreatic head or body. At presentation, bilateral swelling of the parotid, submandibular, and lacrimal glands are also frequently identified, and AIP may be associated with other autoimmune disease including lymphocytic thyroiditis, Sjögren disease, and retroperitoneal fibrosis.

In contrast, type 2 AIP occurs in a slightly younger population and affects men and women in roughly equal proportions. Obstructive jaundice is not a universal feature of type 2 AIP and there is considerable overlap with symptoms of CP and, occasionally, acute pancreatitis. There is less of an association with elevated serum IgG4 levels and other systemic autoimmune diseases, though a minority of patients with type 2 AIP may have concomitant ulcerative colitis, or less frequently, Crohn disease.

Pathologic Features

GROSS FINDINGS

Resections are occasionally performed because of a clinical and radiographic concern for a neoplastic process. The pancreas is typically firm and fibrotic with a homogenous tan-white cut surface. Occasionally, a distinct, infiltrative-appearing, tan-white mass lesion may be identified that is indistinguishable from typical ductal adenocarcinoma at gross inspection (Fig. 4.32). More often, however, no such lesion is identified macroscopically necessitating the submission of the entire gland for histology in order to exclude carcinoma. Careful dissection and inspection of the ductal system may reveal long or multiple strictures without significant upstream dilation, which correlates with features described in endoscopic retrograde pancreatography and magnetic resonance cholangiopancreatography (MRCP).

MICROSCOPIC FINDINGS

Type 1 AIP has several features in common with other IgG4-related diseases. It is characterized by a dense, periductal, lymphoplasmacytic inflammation (Fig. 4.33A). While plasma cells are typically the most conspicuous component of the infiltrate, eosinophils and T lymphocytes are also abundant, and mature lymphoid follicles with germinal centers are not uncommon. Though classically the inflammatory infiltrate is centered on the medium-sized pancreatic duct branches, it may also extend into the peripancreatic adipose tissue and lymph nodes and may also involve the intrapancreatic portion of the distal common bile duct. Inflammation of veins, and less commonly arteries, is also characteristic of type 1 AIP, but is difficult to identify and may be unsampled in small biopsies. Obliterative venulitis, that is inflamed veins with complete or near-complete lumenal obliteration, should be present in larger tissue samples, and are best seen adjacent to muscular arteries away from the denser aspects of the fibroinflammatory process (Fig. 4.33B). The fibrosis that develops in the setting of type 1 AIP is typically duct-centric, swirling, and cellular with conspicuous fibroblasts in addition to the previously described lymphoplasmacytic inflammatory infiltrate (Fig. 4.33C).

In contrast to type 1 AIP, type 2 AIP is not an IgG4-related disease. While duct-centric and stromal lymphocytes and plasma cells are typically seen in type 2 AIP, the characteristic histologic features of this entity are microabscesses and a robust neutrophilic inflammatory infiltrate involving the duct epithelium and lobular parenchyma (Fig. 4.34). The larger ducts may be ulcerated with residual ductal epithelial cells showing marked epithelial atypia. A moderate degree of duct-centric fibrosis may be present in type 2 AIP, though it

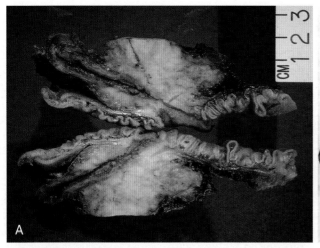
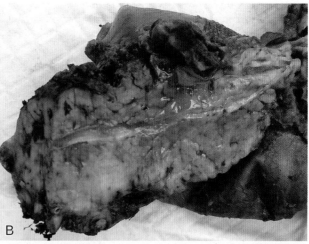

FIG. 4.32

Utoimmune pancreatitis versus pancreatic ductal adenocarcinoma. **A,** Autoimmune pancreatitis can present as an infiltrative-appearing, firm, tan-white mass that is grossly indistinguishable from carcinoma. **B,** Pancreatic ductal adenocarcinoma showing similar gross features to autoimmune pancreatitis.

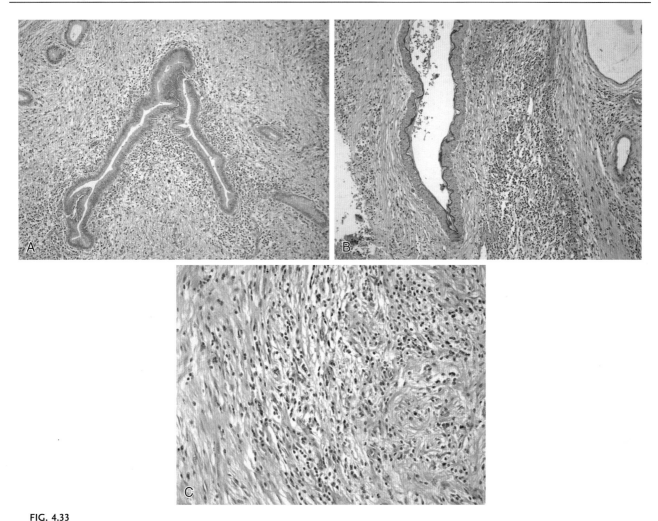

FIG. 4.33

Type 1 autoimmune pancreatitis. **A,** Characterized by dense, periductal lymphoplasmacytic inflammation. **B,** Movat stain demonstrating large muscular artery with adjacent obliterative venulitis. **C,** Swirling, cellular, duct centric pattern of fibrosis.

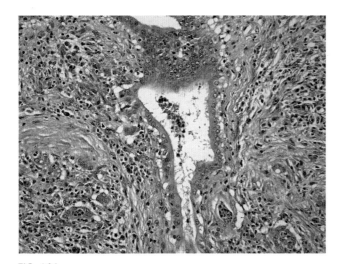

FIG. 4.34

Type 2 autoimmune pancreatitis with microabscesses and neutrophils infiltrating the duct epithelium and acinar parenchyma.

is typically not storiform or as cellular as that seen in type 1 AIP.

Ancillary Studies

Although elevated serum IgG4 levels are characteristic of type 1 AIP, the performance characteristics of this laboratory test are less than ideal and levels may also be elevated in patients with pancreatic cancer and pancreatitis, though typically only mildly. Immunohistochemical stains for IgG4 may be used to demonstrate an increase in the IgG4-producing plasma cells. In small biopsies, greater than 10 IgG4-positive plasma cells per HPF with a ratio of IgG4/IgG-positive cells of over 40% is generally regarded as an appropriate cutoff to support a diagnosis of type 1 AIP. Conversely, in resection specimens, the criteria is more stringent, with greater than 50 IgG4-positive plasma cells per HPF required to maintain specificity.

Differential Diagnosis

In contrast to type 1 AIP, a dense, duct-centric lympho-plasmacytic inflammatory infiltrate is not typically seen in the setting of CP. Instead, lymphocytes tend to be the dominant inflammatory cell present in CP and are generally sparse. The character of the fibrosis is also dramatically different and is swirling or storiform and cellular in type 1 AIP, but dense, sclerotic, and paucicellular with focal calcifications in the setting of CP (Fig. 4.35). The fibrosis of CP is also generally interlobular, at least initially, while it may show periductal accentuation in type 1 AIP. Obliterative venulitis is also not characteristic of CP and is fairly specific for type 1 AIP in the proper context.

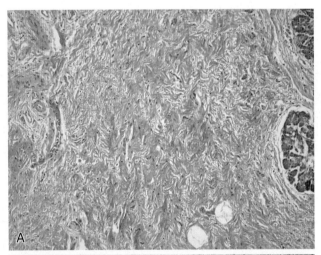

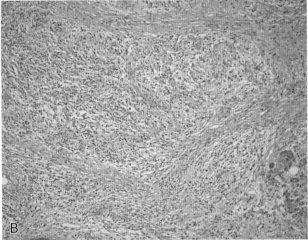

FIG. 4.35

Chronic pancreatitis versus autoimmune pancreatitis. **A,** The fibrosis of chronic pancreatitis is dense, sclerotic, and relatively paucicellular. **B,** In contrast, the fibrosis of autoimmune pancreatitis type 1 is cellular and swirling with periductal accentuation.

The distinction between CP and AIP is generally not a diagnostic challenge in resection specimens where there is ample tissue to evaluate for the characteristic triad of dense lymphoplasmacytic inflammation, obliterative venulitis, and storiform fibrosis, particularly when laboratory studies evaluating serum IgG4 levels have already been performed. Immunohistochemical studies demonstrating greater than 50 IgG4-positive plasma cells per HPF, preferably in multiple HPFs, support a diagnosis of type 1 AIP, whereas their absence or lower levels of positivity suggest an alternate diagnosis.

The distinction between type 2 AIP and CP is extremely challenging given the significant degree of overlap both in demographic and histologic features between these two entities and may not always be possible. While periductal inflammation may be seen in association with CP, it is generally less well-developed than that seen in type 2 AIP. Granulocytic epithelial lesions, or microabscesses and the infiltration of the ductal epithelium and lobular parenchyma by neutrophils, are a characteristic histologic feature of type 2 AIP, but active ductal inflammation may also be a component of CP, particularly if the pancreatic ducts have been manipulated, such as with stenting or pancreatography. Neutrophilic lobular inflammation is more characteristic of type 2 AIP than is lobular atrophy, and, while common in CP, the presence of pseudocysts, dilated ducts, and calculi are unusual in this entity.

Distinguishing AIP from PDAC is not a trivial undertaking, particularly in cases that present as a mass lesion where the pre-test probably for a malignant process is high. In resection material, the triad of duct-centric plasma cell–rich inflammation, storiform fibrosis, and obliterative phlebitis are usually obvious in cases of type 1 AIP. Pancreatic ducts may show reactive-type atypia, but maintain an orderly lobular distribution with no haphazardly arranged or destructive glands infiltrating between lobules or into the peripancreatic adipose tissue. Care should be taken not to rely exclusively on the presence of a plasma cell–rich inflammation for the diagnosis of type 1 AIP, as otherwise typical PDACs may have a prominent lymphoplasmacytic inflammatory that includes IgG4-positive plasma cells. Identifying greater than 50 IgG4-positive plasma per HPF across multiple HPFs appears to increase the specificity for the diagnosis of type 1 AIP. The fact that a minority of patients with pancreatic cancer have significantly elevated serum IgG4 levels may also cause diagnostic confusion, but should not dissuade the pathologist from rendering a diagnosis of adenocarcinoma in the presence of an obviously infiltrative process.

Fine-needle aspirates and biopsies assisted by endoscopic ultrasound are increasingly employed to sample solid pancreatic lesions and pose diagnostic challenges that are not encountered in H&E-stained resection material. Architectural features are often heavily distorted or completely absent from these limited specimens. The stroma of AIP is generally denser and more sclerotic than the cellular desmoplastic reaction associated with carcinoma, though this distinction is somewhat subjective and not always possible. Identifying greater than 10 IgG4-positive plasma cells per HPF in small biopsies generally supports a diagnosis of type 1 AIP and should trigger further workup for IgG4-related disease. An isolated increase in IgG4-positive plasma cells should, however, be interpreted with caution as it does not exclude the presence of a parallel malignant process.

Rarely, the orderly lobular distribution of benign pancreatic ducts is obvious in biopsy cores. However, cytology becomes extremely important when these architectural cues are not present for evaluation. Cytologic feature of ductal malignancy are discussed more extensively above but include nuclear pleomorphism, membrane irregularities, and atypical chromatin distribution and staining quality. Generally, the degree of atypia seen in the setting of PDAC is more pronounced than that seen in reactive processes like AIP. However, atypia may be widespread and pronounced following duct manipulation and with significant inflammation such as that seen in type 2 AIP where there are exuberant neutrophilic infiltrates in the pancreatic ducts. As in other organ systems, extreme caution should be taken to avoid the over interpretation of reactive atypia as neoplasia in the setting of a robust inflammatory infiltrate. In challenging cases, the use of immunohistochemical markers may be of some utility in distinguishing neoplastic from reactive processes. SMAD4 staining is lost in approximately 60% of PDACs and retained in benign pancreatic epithelium. In general, one should have a low threshold for ordering deeper tissue sections, as examining additional tissue levels frequently assists in rendering a definitive diagnosis.

AUTOIMMUNE PANCREATITIS – DISEASE FACT SHEET

Definition
▶▶ Autoimmune, frequently mass-forming variant of chronic pancreatitis that is prototypical IgG4-related disease

Incidence and Location
▶▶ Type 1 autoimmune pancreatitis is rare in the United States, but annual incidence of 1.4 per 100,000 population in Japan
▶▶ The incidence of type 2 autoimmune pancreatitis is unknown, but this entity is distinctly uncommon in Japan and is reported more frequently in Europe and the United States

Sex and Age Distribution
▶▶ Patients with type 1 autoimmune pancreatitis are generally elderly and male
▶▶ Type 2 autoimmune pancreatitis has no sex bias and generally presents in the fifth and sixth decades of life

Clinical Features
▶▶ Obstructive jaundice related to pancreatic mass lesion
▶▶ Submandibular gland swelling

▶▶ Elevated serum IgG4 levels with associated stigmata of IgG4-related disease at other sites
▶▶ Type 2 autoimmune pancreatitis associated with inflammatory bowel disease and may present with features indistinguishable from acute pancreatitis

Radiologic Features
▶▶ Focal form of disease may present as mass lesion indistinguishable from pancreatic ductal adenocarcinoma
▶▶ Diffuse, "sausage-shaped" enlargement with long main pancreatic duct strictures

Prognosis and Therapy
▶▶ Relapses common for type 1 autoimmune pancreatitis but do not occur for type 2 disease
▶▶ Excellent response to steroids and immunomodulators

AUTOIMMUNE PANCREATITIS – PATHOLOGIC FEATURES

Gross Findings
▶▶ Focal form with mass-forming lesions that are fibrotic, tan-white, and virtually indistinguishable from pancreatic ductal adenocarcinoma
▶▶ In diffuse form of disease, gland is either enlarged or shrunken and fibrotic
▶▶ Main pancreatic duct strictures with no discrete mass lesion

Microscopic Findings
▶▶ Type 1 autoimmune pancreatitis with duct-centric lymphoplasmacytic inflammation, storiform fibrosis, obliterative phlebitis, and increased IgG4-positive plasma cells
▶▶ Type 2 autoimmune pancreatitis with granulocytic epithelial lesions, and neutrophils infiltrating ducts and acinar parenchyma

Pathologic Differential Diagnoses
▶▶ Chronic pancreatitis
▶▶ Pancreatic ductal adenocarcinoma

PARADUODENAL PANCREATITIS ("GROOVE PANCREATITIS")

DDX: adenocarcinoma of the pancreas, duodenum, and ampulla, gangliocytic paraganglioma

Clinical Features

Paraduodenal pancreatitis is a variant of CP centered on the minor papilla and associated duct system that involves the second portion of the duodenum, superior aspect of the pancreas, and distal common bile duct. There is significant overlap with regard to demographics and presumptive risk factors between paraduodenal pancreatitis and CP, with the disease primarily affecting men in their fifth and sixth decades of life who abuse alcohol.

Clinically, most patients develop severe upper abdominal pain and postprandial vomiting, and upper endoscopy and gastric emptying studies frequently demonstrate duodenal stenosis and impaired motility, respectively.

Cross-sectional imaging studies frequently show thickening of the duodenum with associated cysts, both within the duodenal wall and the adjacent pancreatic parenchyma. Other cases appear more solid and infiltrative, compressing the distal common bile duct and main pancreatic ducts and mimicking a periampullary or pancreatic head carcinomas.

Pathologic Features

GROSS FINDINGS

Paraduodenal pancreatitis is centered in the duodenal wall at the minor papilla, approximately 2 cm proximal to the ampulla of Vater. The duodenal wall in this area is thickened and fibrotic. Scarring of the wall and adjacent tissues leads to distortion of the normal duodenal mucosal folds, occasionally with associated ulceration. Sieve-like cystic changes are seen in the muscular wall of the duodenum and extend into the paraduodenal pancreas in the "groove region" adjacent to the distal common bile duct. Larger cysts may also develop and compress the distal common bile duct leading to biliary obstruction. Scarring of the paraduodenal pancreas distorts the normal soft, tan lobular parenchyma, which is replaced by homogenous, dense, sclerotic tissue that is similar to that seen in forms of CP (Fig. 4.36).

MICROSCOPIC FINDINGS

Within the duodenal wall near the minor papilla, there is an exuberant adenomyomatous proliferation of whorling smooth muscle cells with embedded, cystically dilated pancreatic ducts that are lined by cuboidal to low-columnar biliary-type epithelium. Mucinous plugs and, rarely, calcified concretions similar to that seen in the setting of alcoholic pancreatitis are encountered in the dilated ducts which may rupture. Larger cysts may lack an identifiable epithelial lining and instead resemble pseudocysts that are lined by granulation tissue and contain inflammatory debris (Fig. 4.37A). Inflammation is generally lymphoplasmacytic and, as a rule, relatively sparse. Dense fibrosis develops in the duodenal wall, replacing the submucosa and muscularis propria, and extends into the paraduodenal pancreas where it is accompanied by acinar atrophy. Some cases exhibit prominent Brunner gland hyperplasia, which may contribute to the mucosal thickening seen at the time of endoscopy and may be the only diagnostic clue to the presence of paraduodenal pancreatitis in superficial mucosal biopsies (Fig. 4.37B).

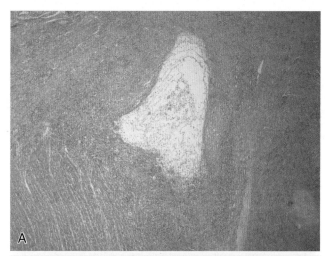
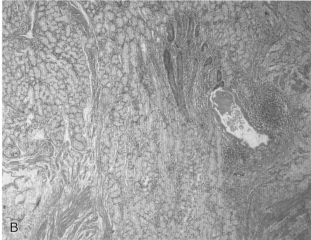

FIG. 4.37
Paraduodenal pancreatitis. **A,** Large paraduodenal cyst lined by granulation tissue and containing inflammatory debris. **B,** Brunner gland hyperplasia with whorling smooth muscle and cystically dilated pancreatic duct containing inspissated proteinaceous material.

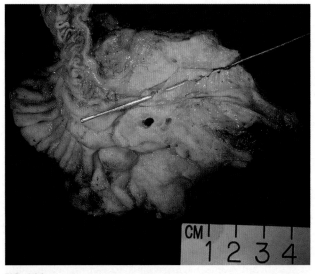

FIG. 4.36
Paraduodenal pancreatitis with fibrous thickening of the duodenal wall and associated cystic changes in the groove region adjacent to the intrapancreatic portion of the common bile duct.

Ancillary Studies

Ancillary studies have very limited utility in the diagnosis of paraduodenal pancreatitis. Careful gross examination of the specimen to document the relationship of the lesion with the minor papilla is essential. Correlation with endoscopic and cross-sectional imaging studies is potentially helpful, but extensive tissue sampling for histology may be required to exclude a neoplastic process in many instances.

Differential Diagnosis

From a clinical and radiologic standpoint, paraduodenal pancreatitis frequently mimics infiltrating neoplasms of the pancreatic head, ampulla, and periampullary duodenum. Endoscopically, the lumen of the duodenum is typically narrowed and distorted. Mucosal-based lesions are typically not a feature of paraduodenal pancreatitis. However, the duodenal folds may be thickened or nodular as a result of scarring and Brunner gland hyperplasia, potentially mimicking adenomatous polyps to the endoscopist. These superficial mucosal biopsies may only show non-specific Brunner gland or adenomyomatous hyperplasia. Discussion with the endoscopist might reveal that the lumenal narrowing of the duodenum appeared to be via extrinsic compression rather than by intrinsic stenosis via a mucosal-based mass lesion. In general, however, a definitive diagnosis of paraduodenal pancreatitis is not possible based upon histologic examination of superficial mucosal biopsies, requiring instead correlation with endoscopic and imaging findings. Excluding the presence of dysplasia and carcinoma in biopsy material is generally sufficient to trigger further workup on the part of the clinical team.

The presence of a mass-forming lesion within or adjacent to the pancreatic head may result in surgical resection in the absence of a definitive tissue diagnosis of adenocarcinoma, particularly if other stigmata of a neoplastic process such as biliary obstruction are also present. Careful gross dissection of the specimen is essential and universally demonstrates involvement of the duodenal wall at the level of the minor papilla. Trabeculation and sieve-like cysts are nearly always seen in the duodenal wall and adjacent paraduodenal pancreas in this location and should be documented. Though infiltrative appearing fibrosis involving the paraduodenal pancreas and duodenum is very characteristic of paraduodenal pancreatitis and may mimic some features of an invasive carcinoma, the presence of a discrete mass lesion centered within the pancreatic head and obstructing the pancreatic duct is not and should raise suspicion for a neoplastic process.

Definitive diagnosis of paraduodenal pancreatitis requires extensive tissue sampling and histologic examination. Fibrous tissue replaces the muscular wall of the duodenum and extends into the paraduodenal pancreas leading to atrophy of the acinar parenchyma. In contrast to the relatively paucicellular fibrosis of paraduodenal pancreatitis, the desmoplastic stroma of ductal adenocarcinoma is far more cellular and contains infiltrating neoplastic glands and single carcinoma cells. The presence of cysts in the pancreatic head may evoke the possibility of a side branch intraductal papillary mucinous neoplasm (IPMN) on gross examination. However, the contents of the cysts in paraduodenal pancreatitis are thin rather than mucinous, and histologic examination reveals bland biliary-type epithelium lacking appreciable atypia and mucin.

Gangliocytic paragangliomas are rare neoplasms that involve the duodenal wall in the vicinity of the ampulla of Vater. In contrast to paraduodenal paragangliomas which lead to diffuse scarring and distortion of the duodenum with associated extrinsic compression, gangliocytic paragangliomas generally form submucosal nodules. Histologically, the lesions are quite distinct from one another. Gangliocytic paragangliomas are composed of a triphasic proliferation of epithelioid neuroendocrine cells, ganglion cells, and spindle cells. The epithelioid proliferation of neuroendocrine cells is perhaps most conspicuous and forms nests and trabeculae that resemble WDNETs. Large, individual ganglion cells with ample granular cytoplasm and large round nuclei with prominent central nucleoli are scattered throughout the lesion (Fig. 4.38). The spindle component is bland and composed of elongated cells with wavy, tapered nuclei with darkly staining but uniform chromatin that resemble Schwann cells. Although the spindled proliferation of myoid cells seen in paraduodenal pancreatitis may

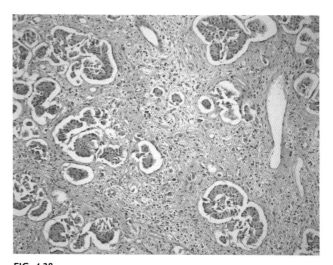

FIG. 4.38

Gangliocytic paraganglioma. Triphasic proliferation composed of nests of epithelioid neuroendocrine cells, singly dispersed and clustered ganglion cells, and bland spindle cells that resemble Schwann cells.

occasionally be evocative of a mesenchymal neoplasm, smooth muscle differentiation is usually obvious from a histologic and immunohistochemical perspective, and this component of the larger lesion is typically readily distinguishable from the Schwannian component of gangliocytic paraganglioma.

- ▶▶ Chronic inflammatory infiltrate composed primarily of lymphocytes set in a fibrotic stroma that involves both muscular duodenal wall and pancreas
- ▶▶ Adenomyomatous proliferation of smooth muscle cells and myofibroblasts
- ▶▶ Marked Brunner gland hyperplasia

Pathologic Differential Diagnoses
- ▶▶ Pancreatic ductal adenocarcinoma
- ▶▶ Gangliocytic paraganglioma

PARADUODENAL PANCREATITIS – DISEASE FACT SHEET

Definition
- ▶▶ Chronic inflammatory disorder involving the duodenal wall at the level of the minor papilla and paraduodenal pancreas in the groove region

Incidence and Location
- ▶▶ Rare entity defined by pseudotumoral inflammatory process involving the peripapillary duodenum and groove region of the pancreas

Sex and Age Distribution
- ▶▶ Similar sex and age distribution to chronic pancreatitis
- ▶▶ Primarily affects men in the fifth and sixth decades of life
- ▶▶ Strong association with history of alcohol abuse

Clinical Features
- ▶▶ Presents with abdominal pain and weight loss
- ▶▶ Disordered gastric emptying and duodenal stenosis may lead to vomiting
- ▶▶ Obstruction of the common bile duct may occur leading to jaundice

Radiologic Features
- ▶▶ Cystic changes in the peripancreatic duodenal wall
- ▶▶ Tumefactive lesions obstructing the distal common bile duct and pancreatic ducts frequently misdiagnosed as carcinoma

Prognosis and Therapy
- ▶▶ Non-neoplastic lesion with excellent prognosis
- ▶▶ May be resected if clinical concern for malignancy is high, or for intractable symptoms related to obstruction

PARADUODENAL PANCREATITIS – PATHOLOGIC FEATURES

Gross Findings
- ▶▶ Centered in the duodenal wall and paraduodenal pancreas at the level of the minor papilla
- ▶▶ Characterized by trabeculation/variable-sized cysts containing clear, non-mucinous fluid or granular necrotic debris
- ▶▶ Thickening of the duodenal wall with associated scarring leads to distortion of the mucosal folds
- ▶▶ Scarring of the paraduodenal pancreas with homogenous, tan-white fibrous tissue effaces the normal tan-yellow architecture of the pancreas and may mimic a mass lesion

Microscopic Findings
- ▶▶ Cysts in the duodenal wall and paraduodenal soft tissue/pancreas that are lined by bland biliary-type epithelium or granulation tissue

LYMPHOEPITHELIAL CYST

DDX: squamoid cyst, dermoid cyst, mucinous cystic neoplasm

Clinical Features

Lymphoepithelial cysts of the pancreas is extremely rare, comprising less than 0.5% of pancreatic cysts and with approximately 150 cases currently reported in the world literature. These lesions are more frequently detected in older adults (mean age 55) but have reported in individuals as young as 20 years. The majority (80%) of individuals with lymphoepithelial cysts are men. In contrast to lymphoepithelial cysts of the salivary glands, there does not appear to be an association with HIV infection or Sjögren disease. Patients may present with non-specific gastrointestinal symptoms including nausea, vomiting, and abdominal pain, but most lesions are incidentally detected with cross-sectional imaging studies performed for another indication.

Pathologic Features

GROSS FINDINGS

Lymphoepithelial cysts are typically well demarcated from the surrounding pancreatic parenchyma and average approximately 4 cm, though much larger lesions have also been reported. Although lymphoepithelial cysts may be located within the pancreatic parenchyma, they are frequently peripancreatic and may be either unilocular or multilocular. The lesion typically has rounded, spherical contours and cut section reveals a thin-walled cyst with cheesy, yellow-brown keratinaceous debris. Thick serous fluid may also be encountered, but the presence of obvious mucin is not a feature of lymphoepithelial cysts and should suggest another diagnosis.

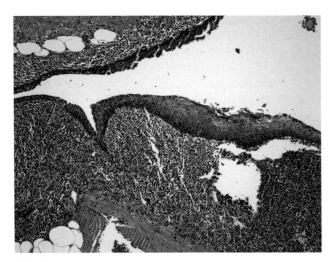

FIG. 4.39
Lymphoepithelial cyst. These lesions are composed of mature keratinizing squamous epithelium with a granular cell layer that sits on a dense band of lymphocytes.

MICROSCOPIC FINDINGS

Lymphoepithelial cysts are lined by mature keratinizing squamous epithelium with a granular cell layer that sits directly on a dense band of bland lymphocytes with scattered lymphoid follicles that generally resembles nodal tissue (Fig. 4.39). The cyst typically contains abundant intraluminal keratin debris. Small foci of sebaceous differentiation are occasionally encountered, but true skin appendages and mesenchymal elements are universally absent. Similarly, minute foci of mucinous epithelium and occasional goblet cells may be seen in a minority of otherwise typical lymphoepithelial cysts that are predominantly lined by squamous epithelium.

Ancillary Studies

Although lymphoepithelial cysts cannot be reliably distinguished from other pancreatic cysts based upon cross-sectional imaging studies alone, endoscopic ultrasound with fine-needle aspiration (EUS-FNA) has emerged as an increasingly important modality for the preoperative assessment of cystic pancreatic lesions and may facilitate conservative treatment of these benign lesions. Evaluation of lymphoepithelial cysts by a cytopathologist may reveal squamous fragments, keratin debris, and intact squamous epithelial cells. These specific features are, however, not present in all cases and the presence of mildly atypical mucinous glandular epithelium may lead to the erroneous characterization of the lesion as a mucinous cyst, or suspicious for malignancy. Unfortunately, chemical analysis of fluid aspirated from lymphoepithelial cysts has been shown to be of limited utility, as CEA levels are frequently elevated in these lesions, potentially contributing to their mischaracterization as mucinous cysts preoperatively.

Differential Diagnosis

In contrast to the mature, keratinizing squamous epithelium that lines lymphoepithelial cysts, squamoid cysts are lined by non-keratinizing squamous epithelium that lacks a granular cell layer. While lymphoepithelial cysts contain cheesy keratinaceous debris, squamoid cysts contain a thinner serous fluid. The subepithelial lymphoid layer is typically prominent in lymphoepithelial cysts, whereas squamoid cysts lack this lymphoid stroma.

Lymphoepithelial cysts are primarily lined by a mature, keratinizing squamous epithelium. Sebaceous and mucinous metaplasia are present in only a minority of otherwise typical lymphoepithelial cysts and are at most focal. In contrast, in addition to sebaceous elements, dermoid cysts typically contain true skin adnexal structures such as hair follicles and sweat glands, as well as mesenchymal elements like cartilage. The presence of more extensive mucinous epithelium, or of respiratory-type epithelium, further supports a diagnosis of dermoid cyst.

Mucinous pancreatic cysts may occasionally enter the differential diagnosis based upon imaging features or cytologic evaluation of a lymphoepithelial cyst. Though occasionally present focally, mucinous epithelium is not a common finding in lymphoepithelial cysts, which are lined by a mature keratinizing squamous epithelium. Mildly atypical mucinous epithelium is rarely sampled during EUS-FNA, but distinguishing a mucinous cyst from a lymphoepithelial cyst is rarely a diagnostic challenge in resection specimens. In addition to their more complex papillary architecture (in the case of IPMNs) and extensive mucin-producing glandular epithelium, mucinous cysts lack the dense subepithelial lymphoid stroma that is characteristic of lymphoepithelial cysts.

Caution is advised regarding the use of ancillary studies to distinguish lymphoepithelial cysts from mucinous cysts in the preoperative setting. Fresh aspirates from cystic pancreatic lesions are frequently sent for chemical analysis for CEA and amylase to aid in the diagnosis of mucinous cysts and pseudocysts, respectively. Unfortunately, despite the near complete absence of mucin-producing epithelium, CEA levels are frequently elevated, often to high levels, in lymphoepithelial cysts, which may triage the patient to surgical resection in the setting of a presumed mucinous cyst. Correlation with cytologic evaluation is essential in order to prevent overtreatment of these benign lesions.

SQUAMOID CYST

DDX: lymphoepithelial cyst, dermoid cyst

Clinical Features

Squamoid cysts of the pancreas are extremely rare lesions that were first described in 2007. In general,

squamoid cysts of the pancreas are small, averaging only 1.5 cm in greatest extent, and are detected most frequently with cross-sectional imaging performed during the evaluation of an unrelated condition. Squamoid cysts of the pancreas are generally identified in older adults (mean age, 63 years). In contrast to lymphoepithelial cysts, they are found with approximately equal frequency in men and women.

Pathologic Features

GROSS FINDINGS

Squamoid cysts of the pancreas are generally unilocular, well-circumscribed lesions most frequently detected in the pancreatic head. The wall of the cyst is thin and fibrotic with a smooth inner surface lacking papillary excrescences and mural nodules. The cyst contents are generally thin and serous with suspended aggregates of flaky, off-white material.

MICROSCOPIC FINDINGS

Squamoid cysts of the pancreas are lined by squamous epithelium that is either flat and attenuated or stratified, but lacking a granular cell layer and keratinization (Fig. 4.40). Mucinous cyst-lining cells are not characteristic, nor is cytologic atypia. The cyst wall is thin and paucicellular without associated dense lymphoid tissue or ovarian stroma. Careful microscopic examination may reveal continuity with the pancreatic ductal system, and the lumen of the cyst frequently contains proteinaceous concretions. Microcysts with similar histologic

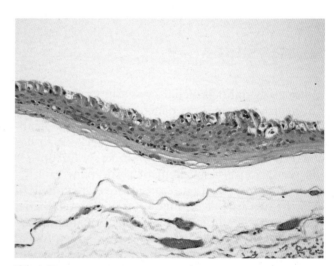

FIG. 4.40

Squamoid cyst. The walls of squamoid cysts are thin and paucicellular. Careful gross and microscopic examination may demonstrate continuity with the ductal system. The cysts are lined by a simple, non-keratinizing squamous epithelium with no adnexal structures, lymphoid tissue, or cytologic atypia.

features may occasionally be encountered in pancreata resected for other reasons.

Ancillary Studies

Ancillary studies have limited diagnostic utility in the diagnosis of squamoid cysts of the pancreas. As discussed previously, incidentally detected pancreatic cysts may be investigated further with EUS-FNA, with a portion of fresh cyst aspirates triaged for chemical or molecular analysis. CEA and CA19-9 levels are generally lower in squamoid cysts of the pancreas than they are in mucinous pancreatic cysts, though experience is limited with these rare tumors and the results of these ancillary studies should be interpreted in conjunction with imaging studies and conventional cytology.

Differential Diagnosis

From a demographic perspective, lymphoepithelial cysts are far more common in men than in women, whereas squamoid cysts of the pancreas have no such sex predilection. Squamoid cysts of the pancreas are continuous with the pancreatic ductal system and acini and are therefore universally intrapancreatic. In contrast, while lymphoepithelial cysts can also be found anywhere in the pancreas, it is not uncommon to find these lesions in the peripancreatic soft tissue. On histologic exam, squamoid cysts are lined by attenuated or stratified squamous epithelium that lacks a granular cell layer and is non-keratinizing. This is in stark contrast to the mature keratinizing epithelium of lymphoepithelial cysts which is responsible for the lamellated keratin debris that fill these lesions. Finally, the wall of squamoid cysts is thin and fibrous, lacking the obvious subepithelial lymphoid tissue of lymphoepithelial cysts.

Squamoid cysts of the pancreas are lined by a simple non-keratinizing squamous epithelium and are frequently in continuity with the ductal system. In contrast, while dermoid cysts also contain squamous epithelium, other epithelial components (such as respiratory-type) are also frequently encountered, as are sebaceous glands, skin adnexal structures, and mesenchymal elements.

SQUAMOID CYST – DISEASE FACT SHEET

Definition
▸▸ Benign pancreatic cyst in continuity with pancreatic ducts and lined by simple non-keratinizing squamous epithelium

Incidence and Location
▸▸ Extremely rare
▸▸ Predominantly located in pancreatic head

Sex and Age Distribution
▸▸ No sex predilection
▸▸ Older adults in the seventh decade of life

Clinical Features
▸▸ Generally asymptomatic and detected incidentally

Radiologic Features
▸▸ Unilocular cyst with no internal septations, mural nodules, or communication with the main pancreatic duct

Prognosis and Therapy
▸▸ Benign lesion with excellent prognosis
▸▸ Managed conservatively with resection reserved for large or symptomatic lesions

---

SQUAMOID CYST – PATHOLOGIC FEATURES

Gross Findings
▸▸ Unilocular cyst with thin fibrotic wall and smooth inner surface
▸▸ No papillary excrescences or mural nodules
▸▸ Thin serous fluid with suspended, flaky concretions
▸▸ Normal background pancreas

Microscopic Findings
▸▸ Cyst lined by attenuated or stratified squamous epithelium
▸▸ No granular cell layer or keratinization
▸▸ Cyst wall thin and fibrotic
▸▸ Occasionally, microscopic continuity with pancreatic ductal system

Pathologic Differential Diagnoses
▸▸ Lymphoepithelial cyst
▸▸ Dermoid cyst

INTRAPANCREATIC ACCESSORY SPLEEN

DDX: well-differentiated pancreatic neuroendocrine tumor

Clinical Features

Accessory spleens are relatively common and are identified in 10% to 30% of individuals in some autopsy series. While the majority of accessory spleens are identified adjacent to the splenic hilum, approximately 17% are found within the tail of the pancreas. This accessory splenic tissue is typically small (less than 3 cm) and discovered incidentally in otherwise asymptomatic patients who have cross-sectional imaging studies performed for another indication.

Pathologic Features

GROSS FINDINGS

Intrapancreatic accessory spleens are well-circumscribed, rounded masses with a beefy-red cut surface that is grossly indistinguishable from normal splenic tissue. The accessory spleen is typically encapsulated and situated within the soft, tan, lobular parenchyma of the normal pancreatic tail.

MICROSCOPIC FINDINGS

Intrapancreatic accessory spleen is histologically indistinguishable from native splenic tissue. The red pulp is composed of reticular cords of connective tissue with macrophages and other inflammatory cells separating vascular sinuses that are filled with circulating blood and lined by specialized endothelial cells. The white pulp comprises a minority of the splenic mass and is made up of periarteriolar lymphoid sheaths and B-lymphocyte–rich follicles (Fig. 4.41). Germinal centers are generally not present in the white pulp of adult spleens.

Ancillary Studies

Cross-sectional imaging studies are valuable in the preoperative diagnosis of these benign lesions. Triple-phase contrast CT may show similar attenuation in the intrapancreatic accessory spleen to the native splenic tissue, which is typically higher than that seen in adjacent pancreatic parenchyma. Diffusion-weighted magnetic resonance imaging is another useful modality that differentiates intrapancreatic accessory spleen from small solid neoplasms of the pancreatic tail with good performance characteristics.

Differential Diagnosis

Despite advances in preoperative cross-sectional imaging, there is significant overlap in the radiographic characteristics of solid lesions of the pancreatic tail, which may lead to resection of an intrapancreatic accessory spleen. Both intrapancreatic accessory spleen and WDNETs tend to be well-circumscribed lesions firmly situated within the pancreatic parenchyma. Gross examination of intrapancreatic accessory spleen universally reveals a beefy-red cut surface that is characteristic of all splenic tissue. WDNETs have a more diverse gross appearance, but typically have a homogeneous soft, tan-yellow cut surface. Cystic degeneration of WDNETs is also not infrequently encountered.

The histologic distinction between intrapancreatic accessory spleen and WDNETs is typically not a diagnostic challenge. Intrapancreatic accessory spleen shows cords of stromal and inflammatory cells and vascular sinuses, in addition to mature lymphoid tissue. While a variety of architectural patterns have been described for WDNETs, they tend to be composed of cohesive epithelioid cells with amphophilic to clear cytoplasm and relatively uniform, round to ovoid nuclei with granular stippled chromatin. Immunohistochemical stains for synaptophysin, chromogranin, and INSM1 can be used to demonstrate neuroendocrine differentiation in these tumors and will be absent in intrapancreatic accessory spleen.

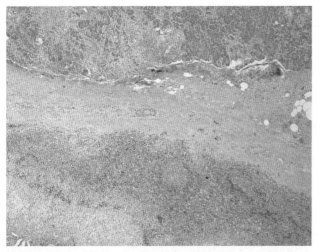

FIG. 4.41

Intrapancreatic accessory spleen. Histologically indistinguishable from native spleen with cords of red pulp and B-lymphocyte–rich follicles.

INTRAPANCREATIC ACCESSORY SPLEEN – DISEASE FACT SHEET

Definition
▶▶ Ectopic splenic tissue located within the pancreatic tail

Incidence and Location
▶▶ Relatively common in general population
▶▶ Accessory splenic tissue frequently identified near splenic hilum and within pancreatic tail

Sex and Age Distribution
▶▶ Slight male predilection (55% in one study)
▶▶ Wide age distribution with median of 52 years

Clinical Features
▶▶ Generally asymptomatic and detected incidentally

Radiologic Features
▶▶ Solid pancreatic tail lesion with imaging characteristics similar to native spleen

Prognosis and Therapy
▶▶ Benign lesion with excellent prognosis

INTRAPANCREATIC ACCESSORY SPLEEN – PATHOLOGIC FEATURES

Gross Findings

▸▸ Solid pancreatic tail tumor generally smaller than 3 cm
▸▸ Well circumscribed with fibrous capsule and beefy-red cut surface

---

Microscopic Findings

▸▸ Histologically indistinguishable from native spleen
▸▸ Red pulp with cords and stromal and inflammatory cells, and vascular sinuses lined by specialized endothelial cells
▸▸ White pulp composed of perivascular lymphoid cuffs and well-formed lymphoid follicles without germinal centers

---

Pathologic Differential Diagnoses

▸▸ Well-differentiated neuroendocrine tumor

EXOCRINE NEOPLASMS

Neoplasms of the exocrine pancreas are by far the most common malignant processes involving the organ and include carcinomas related to the ductal system and associated precursor cells. Tumors of the endocrine pancreas and cystic neoplasms are considered separately.

PANCREATIC DUCTAL ADENOCARCINOMA AND VARIANTS

DDX: chronic pancreatitis, autoimmune pancreatitis, adenocarcinoma of the distal common bile duct

Clinical Features

PDAC is the most common pancreatic neoplasm, with nearly 500,000 new cases diagnosed worldwide in 2018. Despite advances in early diagnosis and therapeutics, the incidence of PDAC appears to be increasing, particularly in high-income countries with aging populations, and the overall 5-year survival is considerably less than 10%. With few exceptions, PDAC is a disease of the elderly, primarily affecting individuals older than 55 years with a slight male predilection. Smoking tobacco products is a well-established risk factor, as is hereditary pancreatitis caused by gain of function mutations in the trypsinogen gene (*PRSS1*).

Classically, PDAC presents with painless jaundice resulting from the obstruction of the intrapancreatic portion of the distal common bile duct in tumors involving the pancreatic head. Non-specific abdominal pain and weight loss are also frequent clinical findings. New-onset pancreatogenic, or type 3c diabetes mellitus, also appears to be associated with underlying PDAC, particularly in individuals older than 50 years.

Pathologic Features

GROSS FINDINGS

The majority of PDACs occur in the pancreatic head, but can also develop in the pancreatic body and tail. Palpation of the resected gland may reveal a poorly defined, rock-like mass in the gland. On cut section, ductal adenocarcinomas form solid, poorly defined, gritty, white, infiltrative lesion. Frequently, the carcinoma obstructs the main pancreatic duct, which may make it impossible to probe the duct system to the ampulla of Vater. Careful gross dissection of the pancreas by bisecting the gland through the main pancreatic duct may help to demonstrate its relationship with the tumor (Fig. 4.42). Obstruction of the pancreatic duct frequently leads to atrophy and fibrosis of the upstream pancreatic parenchyma, which may make it difficult to distinguish the infiltrating neoplasm from the background of CP.

MICROSCOPIC FINDINGS

Conventional PDAC is characterized by a proliferation of infiltrative, malignant glands centered within the pancreatic parenchyma. Well-differentiated ductal adenocarcinomas are composed of tubular glands made up of slightly atypical cuboidal to columnar cells with basally oriented, hyperchromatic, ovoid nuclei and abundant pale-eosinophilic or foamy mucinous cytoplasm. It may be challenging to distinguish well-differentiated ductal adenocarcinomas from benign reactive pancreatic ductal

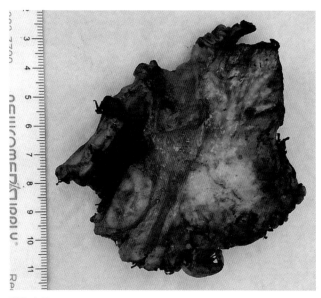

FIG. 4.42

Pancreatic ductal adenocarcinoma. Bisecting the pancreatic head through the distal common bile duct and pancreatic duct reveals a stellate, firm, infiltrative lesion. The lesion obliterates the pancreatic duct and infiltrates the intrapancreatic portion of the distal common bile duct and peripancreatic adipose tissue.

epithelium based upon cytologic features alone, though these very well-differentiated neoplastic glands are typically admixed with a population showing more convincing cellular and architectural atypia. Well-differentiated PDACs, however, universally exhibit a haphazard, infiltrative pattern of growth that is set in a cellular, desmoplastic stroma and is best appreciated on low power (Fig. 4.43A). This haphazard growth pattern does not respect the normal lobular architecture of the gland and infiltrates between acini and into the peripancreatic adipose tissue. In the absence of cytologic atypia, other features of malignancy in well-differentiated ductal adenocarcinomas include the presence of lymphovascular or perineural invasion, as well as the juxtaposition of neoplastic glands with muscular arteries (Fig. 4.43B).

Moderately and poorly differentiated PDACs exhibit increasing levels of cytologic and architectural atypia. The infiltrating glands of moderately differentiated carcinomas frequently have angulated contours with

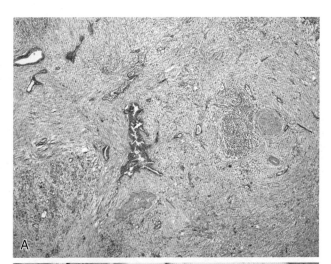

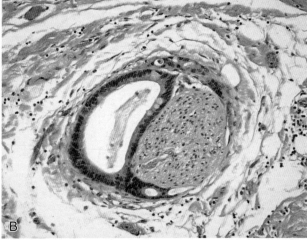

FIG. 4.43

Well-differentiated pancreatic ductal adenocarcinoma. **A,** Low-power examination of pancreatic ductal adenocarcinomas reveals a haphazard pattern of growth that does not respect normal lobular architecture. **B,** Perineural invasion, even in the absence of significant cytologic atypia, is a feature of a malignant process.

incomplete lumina, or form complex branching or cribriform structures (Fig. 4.44A). There is typically significant nuclear pleomorphism, with marked variation in nuclear size, irregular nuclear membrane contours, and hyperchromatic, clumpy chromatin (Fig. 4.44B). Mitotic figures, including atypical forms, are usually conspicuous, as are foci of luminal necrosis (Fig. 4.44C). Single infiltrating carcinoma cells, including occasional pleomorphic tumor cells, may be encountered, particularly at the interface of the tumor with the surrounding non-neoplastic pancreatic parenchyma.

Poorly differentiated ductal adenocarcinomas are composed of sheets and single infiltrating pleomorphic tumor cells with only minimal gland formation. Tumor giant cells are frequently encountered, as are foci of sarcomatoid or squamous differentiation (Fig. 4.44D). The expansile, destructive pattern of growth that obscures an intraductal component, coupled with the lack of significant mucin production and desmoplasia, may make it challenging to identify these poorly differentiated carcinomas as ductal in origin.

The large duct morphologic pattern of PDAC is frequently diagnostically challenging, particularly in small fine-needle biopsies where it is difficult to appreciate architectural cues. In contrast to the small, angulated, atypical infiltrating ducts that are characteristic of typical PDAC, the neoplastic ducts seen in the large duct variant measure between 0.5 mm and 1 cm in diameter and are lined by relatively bland cells with columnar epithelial cells that have cytoplasmic mucin, a prominent apical brush border-like zone, and minimal nuclear atypia. Intraluminal papillary growth may also be encountered but is not as well-developed as that seen in IPMNs. The large neoplastic glands are typically dilated and somewhat angular or jagged, and often contain luminal neutrophils or necrotic debris (Fig. 4.45A). Close inspection of the periglandular stroma may reveal a cellular desmoplastic stromal response that should be distinguished from the ovarian-like stroma of mucinous cystic neoplasms (MCNs), but more frequently has a myxoid quality. Regardless of these somewhat subtle histologic features, the malignant nature of the large duct variant of PDAC is frequently betrayed by the haphazard arrangement and infiltrative nature of the glands seen on low-power inspection.

Foci of squamous differentiation are occasionally seen in typical PDACs. Rarely, more extensive squamous differentiation (greater than 30% of the tumor mass) in an otherwise typical PDAC is encountered and the tumor can be classified as adenosquamous carcinoma. Adenosquamous carcinomas may be large but well circumscribed and frequently exhibit prominent cystic degeneration or tumor necrosis on gross examination. The squamous component of adenosquamous carcinoma is indistinguishable from squamous cell carcinoma arising in other sites and is characterized by clusters and solid sheets of polygonal epithelioid cells

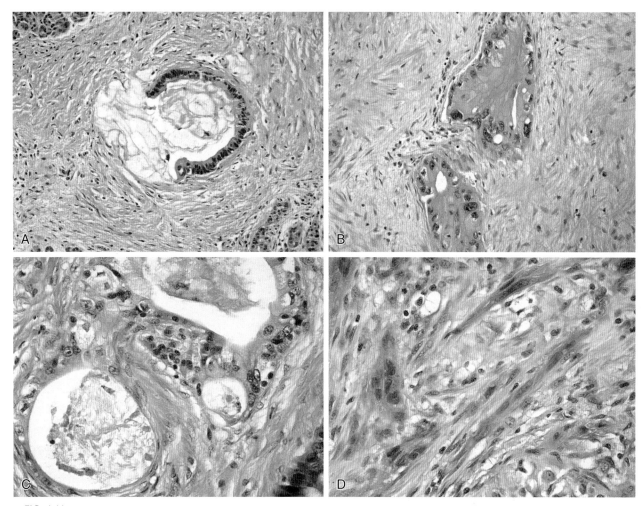

FIG. 4.44

Pancreatic ductal adenocarcinoma. **A,** Angulated, infiltrative glands with incomplete lumina are characteristic of pancreatic ductal adenocarcinoma. **B,** Moderately differentiated pancreatic ductal adenocarcinomas show significant nuclear membrane irregularities and marked nuclear pleomorphism and irregularly distributed, hyperchromatic chromatin. **C,** Many neoplastic glands exhibit luminal necrosis. **D,** Poorly differentiated pancreatic ductal adenocarcinomas exhibit foci with sarcomatoid of squamous transformation.

with dense eosinophilic cytoplasm and large, hyperchromatic nuclei. Close inspection may reveal intercellular desmosomal bridges. The neoplastic squamous cells may exhibit a whorling pattern of growth with the formation of keratin pearls, or alternatively, more subtle, abrupt, single cell keratinization (Fig. 4.45B). As with squamous cell carcinomas at other sites, the squamous component of adenosquamous carcinoma is typically immunoreactive for p40, p63, and CK5/6.

Hepatoid carcinoma is a rare histologic subtype of pancreatic ductal carcinoma that exhibits morphologic and immunohistochemical features of hepatocellular differentiation in the majority of the tumor. Like primary HCCs, pancreatic hepatoid carcinomas exhibit a solid or trabecular pattern of growth and are made up of polygonal cells with abundant, granular eosinophilic cytoplasm and large central nuclei with clumpy or vesicular chromatin and often prominent nucleoli (Fig. 4.45C). Hepatoid carcinomas produce AFP and are immunoreactive for HepPar-1 and arginase-1, though

these markers are not entirely specific for this entity, and non-hepatoid neoplasms, including acinar cell carcinoma, may also express AFP. *In situ* hybridization studies for albumin is a more specific marker for hepatocellular differentiation in hepatoid carcinomas but does not distinguish this entity from true HCC or ICC.

Colloid carcinomas (formerly mucinous non-cystic adenocarcinoma) are unique neoplasms that arise in association with intestinal-type IPMNs and are associated with significantly better 5-year survival than conventional PDAC. Greater than 80% of the tumor mass is composed of mucinous epithelial cells arranged in strips, clusters, and tubules floating in pools of mucin that dissect through the stromal tissue (Fig. 4.45D). Signet ring cells are not uncommonly encountered within the mucin pools but are, as a rule, only a minor component. The epithelial component of colloid carcinomas exhibit immunohistochemical evidence of intestinal differentiation and express CK20, CDX2, and the intestinal mucin MUC2.

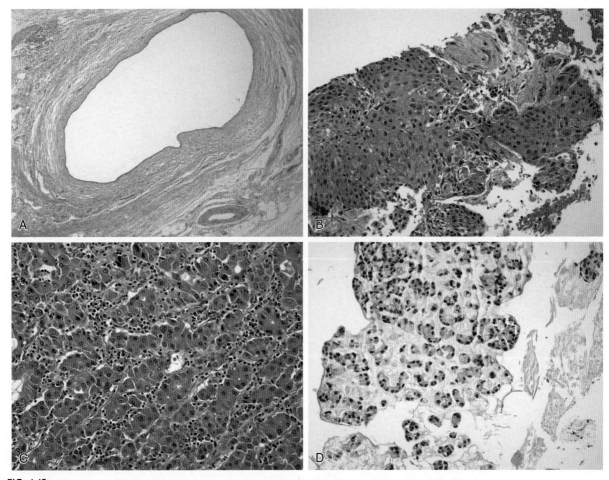

FIG. 4.45

Histologic subtypes of pancreatic ductal adenocarcinoma. **A,** The large duct morphologic pattern is characterized by infiltrative glands that measure greater than 0.5 mm in greatest extent and exhibit relatively bland cytologic features. **B,** Squamous differentiation is focally present in many pancreatic ductal adenocarcinomas but is more extensive in a minority of cases. Cells with squamous differentiation are polygonal with ample eosinophilic cytoplasm and show foci of abrupt keratinization. **C,** Hepatoid carcinoma is rare and resembles hepatocellular carcinoma, exhibiting a solid or trabecular pattern of growth. **D,** Colloid carcinoma shows abundant mucin with embedded strips and clusters of mucinous epithelial cells.

Undifferentiated carcinomas of the pancreas are malignant epithelial neoplasms that show no histologic evidence of lineage-specific differentiation. The anaplastic variant of undifferentiated carcinoma displays a sheet-like growth of poorly cohesive tumor giant cells with eosinophilic cytoplasm, pleomorphic nuclei, bizarre mitotic figures, and, often, emperipolesis of inflammatory cells. The sarcomatoid variant of undifferentiated carcinoma is composed of at least 80% atypical spindle cells and may contain heterologous mesenchymal elements, while carcinosarcomas of the pancreas show a biphasic growth pattern where gland-forming epithelial elements coexist with sarcomatoid spindle or anaplastic tumor giant cells.

Ancillary Studies

Ancillary immunohistochemical stains and molecular studies have limited utility in the daily practice of pancreatic surgical pathology. PDACs lack a defining immunophenotype, but generally express CK7 and CK19, with a smaller proportion coexpressing CK20. A notable exception to this is colloid carcinomas which, as previously discussed, show intestinal differentiation and express CK20, CDX2, and MUC2, as well as neuroendocrine markers like synaptophysin.

Approximately 60% of PDACs lose expression of *SMAD4*, a component of the TGF-beta signaling cascade. Loss of nuclear SMAD4 immunoreactivity supports a diagnosis of PDAC, but preserved nuclear staining does not exclude malignancy. Similarly, alterations in *TP53* are frequently identified in PDACs. Immunohistochemical staining demonstrating either abnormal nuclear accumulation of TP53 or, alternatively, complete loss may also support a diagnosis of adenocarcinoma. In general, these ancillary immunohistochemical studies should be used judiciously with great caution and interpreted in the context of conventional morphologic assessment and the clinical scenario. When interpreting small fine-needle biopsies, requesting additional H&E-stained tissue sections be cut from the paraffin block allows additional diagnostic material to be reviewed and may facilitate the delivery of a definitive diagnosis when one was not previously available.

Differential Diagnosis

There is considerable histologic overlap between the benign, reactive glands seen in the setting of pancreatitis and the neoplastic glands of well- and moderately differentiated PDACs. Extensive fibrosis and atrophy of the acinar units is characteristic of CP. Extensive parenchymal loss leaves angulated, slightly atypical ductules embedded in loose fibrous stroma that formerly supported the acinar structures and can be quite concerning for a malignant process. However, low-power inspection of the pancreas in the setting of CP reveals a preserved lobular orientation which are large central ducts entering atrophic but well-circumscribed lobules that lack significant acinar cell mass and are now populated by reactive ductules. In contrast, PDACs lack this lobular orientation and atypical glands infiltrate the dense interlobular fibrous stroma. Invasion of the duodenal wall or peripancreatic adipose tissue is also highly specific for malignancy, as naked glands embedded within fat are never seen outside the setting of carcinoma regardless of the degree of cytologic atypia present in the infiltrating glands. Other architectural clues that are very specific for a diagnosis of PDAC include the presence of perineural and lymphovascular invasion, as well as the close apposition of glands with thick-walled muscular arteries.

In fine-needles biopsies, architectural assessment may be difficult, making familiarity with the cytologic features of PDAC essential for surgical pathologists. Nuclear pleomorphism, that is variability in size, shape, and staining quality, is highly characteristic of PDAC. Anisonucleosis of 4:1 or more within a single gland or cluster of cells is a feature of malignancy, as are irregularities in the contours of the nuclear membrane or distribution of chromatin. Irregular nuclear spacing and polarity in sheets of ductal cells, conferring the so-called drunken honeycomb appearance, may be particularly helpful in identifying well-differentiated PDACs where the cytologic atypia is subtle (Fig. 4.46). PDAC cells may also acquire dense eosinophilic cytoplasm or, alternatively, abundant, lacy, finely vacuolated or bubbly appearing cytoplasm.

The distinction between PDAC and type 1 AIP was discussed extensively earlier. Extreme caution should be utilized when evaluating small fine-needles biopsies or fine-needle aspirates so as not to over interpret reactive ductular atypia in the setting of AIP for carcinoma. Conversely, increased IgG4-positive plasma cells can

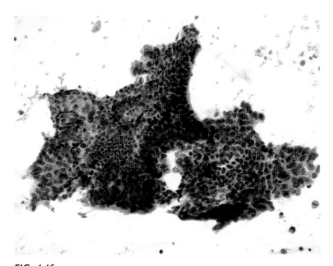

FIG. 4.46

Pancreatic ductal adenocarcinoma. Sheets of malignant pancreatic ductal cells exhibit uneven nuclear spacing and anisonucleosis imparting a "drunken honeycomb" appearance (Conventional smear, Papanicolaou stain). (Photo provided by Dr. Jordan Reynolds, The Cleveland Clinic.)

sometimes be seen in otherwise typical PDACs and should not be overinterpreted to suggest IgG4-related disease. In general, an interdisciplinary approach should be employed for difficult cases with close communication with cytopathologists, radiologists, endoscopists, and surgical colleagues which can help to avoid diagnostic pitfalls and potentially devastating outcomes.

Adenocarcinomas of the distal common bile duct are challenging to distinguish from PDACs. The distinction, however, is potentially important and may have prognostic and therapeutic implications for the patient. Carcinomas originating in the intrapancreatic portion of the distal common bile duct are also staged differently than PDACs according to the eighth edition of the AJCC cancer staging manual. Both tumor types are composed of infiltrating glands made up of cuboidal to low columnar pancreatobiliary-type cells with eosinophilic to pale finely vacuolated cytoplasm and large, irregular, hyperchromatic nuclei making distinction based upon histologic features alone difficult, though carcinomas originating in the distal common bile duct more frequently displayed a smaller tubular pattern and abundant intraglandular neutrophil-rich debris.

Careful gross dissection of the pancreatic head through the common bile duct and main pancreatic duct is essential and may demonstrate a circumferential, constrictive thickening of the wall of the distal common bile duct, rather than a mass centered within the pancreatic parenchyma and associated with the ductal system. Low-power histologic examination of the common bile duct frequently shows a band-like circumferential ductal lesion that may also infiltrate the pancreatic parenchyma and peripancreatic structures. Unfortunately, the vast majority of typical PDACs infiltrate the intrapancreatic common bile duct, complicating microscopic assessment, and highlight the need for careful gross inspection of the tumor to identify the epicenter prior to submitting sections of histology.

PANCREATIC DUCTAL ADENOCARCINOMA – DISEASE FACT SHEET

Definition
▶▶ Infiltrating epithelial neoplasm of the exocrine pancreas with ductal differentiation

Incidence and Location
▶▶ Most common pancreatic neoplasm
▶▶ 6.2 cases per 100,000 person-years in high-income countries
▶▶ Can involve any portion of pancreas, but most commonly pancreatic head

Sex and Age Distribution
▶▶ Slight male predilection
▶▶ Elderly individuals with mean age of 70 years in the United States

Clinical Features
▶▶ Painless jaundice
▶▶ Weight loss
▶▶ Epigastric abdominal pain
▶▶ Diabetes mellitus type 3c

Radiologic Features
▶▶ Solid pancreatic mass with infiltrative borders and associated abrupt pancreatic duct obstruction
▶▶ Double-duct sign with dilation of both main pancreatic duct and distal common bile duct

Prognosis and Therapy
▶▶ Poor prognosis with dismal 5-year survival (approximately 8%)
▶▶ Surgical resection (pancreaticoduodenectomy, distal pancreatectomy) for minority of patients with resectable disease
▶▶ Chemotherapy and radiation

PANCREATIC DUCTAL ADENOCARCINOMA – PATHOLOGIC FEATURES

Gross Findings
▶▶ Poorly defined rock-like mass
▶▶ Gritty, gray-white infiltrative lesion with irregular borders
▶▶ May be associated with pancreatic ductal system
▶▶ Upstream dilation of main pancreatic duct with obstruction and associated atrophy/fibrosis of non-neoplastic pancreatic parenchyma

Microscopic Findings
▶▶ Infiltrative malignant glands with haphazard arrangement that does not respect the normal lobular architecture of pancreas
▶▶ Cuboidal to low columnar biliary-type cells with eosinophilic or finely vacuolated foamy cytoplasm
▶▶ Nuclear anisonucleosis with variation of greater than 4:1 within a single gland or group
▶▶ Pleomorphic nuclei with irregular nuclear membranes and clumpy irregularly distributed chromatin
▶▶ Mitotic activity common with frequent atypical forms
▶▶ Incomplete, angulated glands
▶▶ Glands with luminal necrosis
▶▶ Infiltration of peripancreatic adipose tissue

▶▶ Lymphovascular and perineural invasion
▶▶ Juxtaposition with muscular arteries
▶▶ Variant patterns with large ducts, squamous or hepatoid differentiation, abundant extracellular mucin, and anaplastic or sarcomatoid features

Pathologic Differential Diagnoses
▶▶ Chronic pancreatitis, autoimmune pancreatitis, adenocarcinoma of the distal common bile duct

---

ACINAR CELL CARCINOMA

DDX: pancreatoblastoma, well-differentiated pancreatic neuroendocrine tumor, solid pseudopapillary neoplasm

Clinical Features

Acinar cell carcinoma is a rare malignant neoplasm of the exocrine pancreas that accounts for less than 2% of pancreatic neoplasms in adults and approximately 15% of pediatric tumors. In contrast to PDACs, acinar cell carcinomas rarely present with obstructive jaundice. Instead, the majority of patients with acinar cell carcinoma present with non-specific gastrointestinal symptoms related to mass-effect or metastatic spread to other sites like the liver. As acinar cell carcinomas, by definition, show acinar differentiation, production of lipase by the tumor can lead to a syndrome of widespread subcutaneous fat necrosis and polyarthralgia in a minority of patients with metastatic disease.

Patients with acinar cell carcinoma tend to be slightly younger than those with PDAC, averaging 60 years, although it affects individuals over a wide age range. Men are affected by acinar cell carcinoma twice a frequently as women. Acinar cell carcinoma is an aggressive neoplasm with a 5-year survival of 25%.

In contrast to PDACs, variants in *KRAS* and *TP53* are uncommon in acinar cell carcinoma. Alterations in the APC/β-catenin pathway are found in a subset of acinar cell carcinomas, typically through gene loss or promoter hypermethylation, and 23% harbor *SND1-BRAF* fusions that potentially confer sensitivity to treatment with MEK inhibitors. It is also clear now that a significant subset of acinar cell carcinomas are microsatellite unstable, which has important therapeutic implications in the era of immune checkpoint inhibitors.

Pathologic Features

GROSS FINDINGS

Acinar cell carcinomas are large, well-circumscribed neoplasms that can be found at anywhere within the pancreas. They are often at least partially encapsulated and have a fleshy, pink-tan cut surface that is soft and friable. In larger tumors, areas of hemorrhage, cystic degeneration, and necrosis are not uncommon. Infiltration of adjacent structures, including the stomach, duodenum, spleen, kidneys, and large blood vessels, is frequently encountered.

MICROSCOPIC FINDINGS

Acinar cell carcinoma is a cellular neoplasm lacking a prominent stromal component. The neoplastic cells grow in nests, sheets, and trabeculae. The formation of acini or small glands with dilated lumina are also frequently encountered. The epithelioid cells have a moderate amount of finely granular eosinophilic cytoplasm and characteristic uniform, basally oriented nuclei with a prominent central nucleolus (Fig. 4.47A). Uncommon variants include acinar cell carcinomas showing oncocytic features, that is polygonal cells with dense, hypereosinophilic, granular cytoplasm, or those abundant cytoplasmic clearing or sarcomatoid features.

Ancillary Studies

Immunohistochemical studies are essential for the accurate diagnosis of acinar cell carcinoma. The expression of the neuroendocrine markers synaptophysin and chromogranin is detected in approximately 33% of acinar cell carcinomas and can lead to diagnostic confusion with WDNETs for which prognosis and therapy are quite different. Immunohistochemical stains targeting the exocrine digestive enzymes trypsin and chymotrypsin, as well as a monoclonal antibody directed against

the carboxy-terminal portion of BCL10 which reacts with pancreatic carboxyl ester lipase, appear to be exquisitely sensitive and specific as markers for acinar cell carcinoma (Fig. 4.47B).

Differential Diagnosis

Distinguishing acinar cell carcinoma from WDNETs can be challenging, particularly in small fine-needle biopsy specimens, as both are cellular neoplasms composed of medium-sized epithelioid cells. Both tumors can show a predominantly solid growth pattern. Densely hyalinized, amyloid-like stroma may be seen in WDNETs, while the stromal component of acinar cell carcinomas is decidedly less prominent. Acinar structures with small lumina may be identifiable in acinar cell carcinomas and are typically not a feature of WDNETs, though some may form pseudoglandular structures. Cytologically, acinar cell carcinomas tend to have granular eosinophilic cytoplasm and round, relatively uniform nuclei with prominent nucleoli. This is in contrast to the evenly distributed, coarsely granular salt-and-pepper chromatin of WDNETs.

Immunohistochemical studies are indispensable for distinguishing between acinar cell carcinomas and WDNETs. While a significant proportion of acinar cell carcinomas show reactivity for neuroendocrine markers, markers of acinar differentiation, namely antibodies to trypsin, chymotrypsin, and some clones of BCL10 are highly sensitive and specific for this entity. There should be a low threshold for employing the use of immunohistochemical markers if acinar cell carcinoma enters the differential diagnosis of a solid, cellular pancreatic lesion, as treatment modalities and patient prognosis differ significantly from WDNETs.

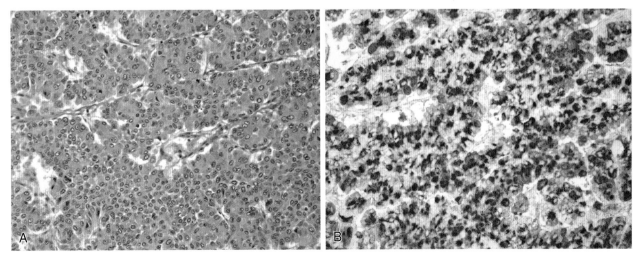

FIG. 4.47

Acinar cell carcinoma. **A,** Solid neoplasm composed of nests, sheets, and trabeculae of epithelioid cells with granular eosinophilic or amphophilic cytoplasm. Acinar structures may be prominent in some foci. Nuclei are basally oriented, round, and basally oriented. Prominent central nucleoli are usually identifiable. **B,** Strong, diffuse reactivity for chymotrypsin is characteristic.

Pancreatoblastoma is a rare neoplasm and the most frequent pancreatic neoplasm occurring in children. Like acinar cell carcinoma, pancreatoblastomas are typically large, solid tumors. There is significant histologic overlap between acinar cell carcinoma and pancreatoblastoma, with both composed of lobules of epithelioid neoplastic cells with granular eosinophilic cytoplasm and round, regular nuclei with prominent nucleoli. The neoplastic cells may be arranged in acinar units, solid sheets, and trabecular structures. Discrete acini with small lumina are generally identifiable in both tumor types, and both show reactivity for markers of acinar differentiation.

The presence of discrete squamoid nests composed of whorled epithelioid to plump spindled cells with eosinophilic cytoplasm and ovoid nuclei is the principle feature distinguishing pancreatoblastoma from acinar cell carcinoma. The squamoid nests are immunoreactive for EMA and show nuclear labeling for β-catenin but may not be present in small biopsies or fine-needle aspiration specimens.

Solid pseudopapillary neoplasms primarily affect young women, whereas acinar cell carcinoma is a disease of older adults. Both tumors can grow to reach a large size and have both solid areas and foci with hemorrhagic necrosis and cystic degeneration. Solid areas of solid pseudopapillary tumors are composed of hyalinized or myxoid fibrovascular cords set in a sea of poorly cohesive neoplastic cells with eosinophilic to clear vacuolated cytoplasm and ovoid nuclei with finely granular chromatin and prominent grooves indenting the nuclear membrane. In some areas, neoplastic cells cling to the fibrovascular cords, lending a pseudopapillary appearance to the neoplasm. In contrast to acinar cell carcinoma, prominent, discrete nucleoli are not a feature of solid pseudopapillary neoplasms. The cytoplasm is also less abundant and granular than that of acinar cell carcinomas and may contain prominent eosinophilic, PAS/D-positive hyaline globules.

A panel of immunostains can help to distinguish solid pseudopapillary neoplasms from acinar cell carcinomas in difficult cases. Solid pseudopapillary tumors show variable reactivity for keratins and synaptophysin, raising other diagnostic pitfalls, but always show nuclear labeling for β-catenin, as well as reactivity for the progesterone receptor and CD10. Markers of acinar differentiation, namely trypsin, chymotrypsin, and BCL10, are not expressed in solid pseudopapillary neoplasms.

ACINAR CELL CARCINOMA – DISEASE FACT SHEET

Definition
▸▸ Infiltrating epithelial neoplasm of the exocrine pancreas with acinar differentiation

---

Incidence and Location
▸▸ Rare carcinoma accounting for less than 2% of all pancreatic malignancies
▸▸ 15% of pancreatic neoplasms in children
▸▸ Any portion of pancreas

Sex and Age Distribution
▸▸ Male-to-female ratio of 2:1
▸▸ Primarily disease of elderly (median age, 60 years) but with wide age distribution (including children)

Clinical Features
▸▸ Weight loss
▸▸ Abdominal pain
▸▸ Metastatic fat necrosis and polyarthralgia
▸▸ Jaundice rare relative for pancreatic ductal adenocarcinoma

Radiologic Features
▸▸ Large, well-marginated, round to oval tumor
▸▸ Homogeneously enhancing and hypovascular

Prognosis and Therapy
▸▸ Aggressive neoplasm with median survival of 19 months and 5-year survival of approximately 25%
▸▸ Resection and chemotherapy
▸▸ MEK inhibitors in tumors with *SND1-BRAF* fusions

ACINAR CELL CARCINOMA – PATHOLOGIC FEATURES

Gross Findings
▸▸ Large, well-circumscribed, soft mass (average 10 cm)
▸▸ Flesh, homogenous pink-tan cut surface
▸▸ Hemorrhage and foci of necrosis not uncommon
▸▸ Rare cystic transformation

Microscopic Findings
▸▸ Cellular neoplasm with scant fibrous stroma
▸▸ Lobular growth pattern with nests, sheets, and trabeculae composed of neoplastic cells
▸▸ Acini with lumina frequently encountered
▸▸ Medium-sized epithelioid cells with granular eosinophilic cytoplasm
▸▸ Basally oriented round nuclei with prominent nucleoli
▸▸ Variants with oncocytic change, cytoplasmic clearing, or spindle cells

Immunohistochemistry
▸▸ Positive for trypsin, chymotrypsin, BCL10 (clone 331.3)
▸▸ Positive for cytokeratins (CK AE1/AE3, Cam5.2)
▸▸ Up to 33% express neuroendocrine markers

Pathologic Differential Diagnoses
▸▸ Well-differentiated pancreatic neuroendocrine tumor
▸▸ Pancreatoblastoma
▸▸ Solid pseudopapillary neoplasm

PANCREATOBLASTOMA

DDX: acinar cell carcinoma

Clinical Features

Pancreatoblastoma is a malignant epithelial neoplasm of the pancreas with acinar differentiation and is the most common pancreatic neoplasm in children with a quarter of cases presenting in the first 10 years of life (median age, 5 years). Though considerably less common, both young adults and the elderly may also be affected by pancreatoblastoma (range, 18–78 years). Most reported cases are sporadic, occurring outside the setting of a known genetic syndrome. However, there is a strong association of pancreatoblastoma, including congenital cases, with Beckwith-Wiedemann syndrome. Biallelic inactivation of *APC* in the setting of familial adenomatous polyposis, as well as *RASSF1a* promoter methylation have also been reported in some instances.

Non-specific abdominal pain, weight loss, and nausea are common presenting complaints in adults, while jaundice is distinctly uncommon relative to the incidence seen with PDAC. A palpable abdominal mass is identified in approximately 20% of adults with pancreatoblastoma, and is frequently encountered in children with this tumor.

Although tumors may reach a large size, pancreatoblastoma is a fairly indolent pancreatic neoplasm, particularly in children who tend to have localized disease. The 5-year survival is approximately 65% in patients with resectable disease, though local recurrence is not an uncommon occurrence. Metastasis to the liver, regional lymph nodes, and lung is detected in approximately half of all adults with pancreatoblastoma and significantly worsens the overall prognosis.

Pathologic Features

GROSS FINDINGS

Pancreatoblastomas are large (mean 10 cm), well-circumscribed, solid tumors that may be partially encapsulated and have a lobular, soft, fleshy, whitish-yellow cut surface with only scant fibrous stroma. Foci of hemorrhage, necrosis, and cystic degeneration may also be encountered.

MICROSCOPIC FINDINGS

Highly cellular lobules of neoplastic cells are separated by thin fibrous bands which impart a geographic appearance to the tumor. Occasionally, more extensive fine fibrous septations create a micronodular architecture that is reminiscent of lymphoid follicles. The neoplastic cells are arranged in solid sheets, broad trabeculae, and acinar structures. Most show acinar differentiation and have granular eosinophilic cytoplasm and round eccentric nuclei with a prominent central nucleolus.

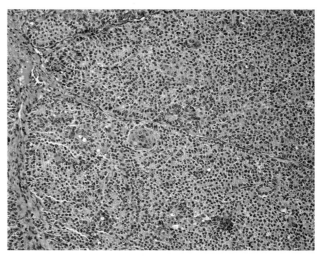

FIG. 4.48

Pancreatoblastoma. Solid neoplasm composed of acinar structures, trabeculae, and solid sheets of epithelioid cells with granular cytoplasm and round basally oriented nuclei. Squamoid nests composed of whorling epithelioid and plump spindle cells with nuclear clearing differentiate pancreatoblastoma from acinar cell carcinoma. Abrupt keratinization may be encountered. (Photo provided by Dr. Meredith Pittman, Maimonides Medical Center.)

Interspersed amongst the acinar component are squamoid nests which are the defining feature of pancreatoblastoma (Fig. 4.48). These structures are composed of whorling epithelioid and plump spindle cells with eosinophilic to clear cytoplasm and ovoid nuclei with occasional nuclear clearing that are well defined from the background acinar population. Keratinization may be present in some squamoid nests but is not a necessary feature.

In addition to the squamoid nests and acinar component, isolated single cells and small nests of neuroendocrine cells may also be identified in a pancreatoblastoma, as can true mucin-producing glands and primitive, small blue, undifferentiated round cells. While the stromal component of pancreatoblastoma is often inconspicuous, some cases show increased stromal cellularity with sarcomatous atypia and, rarely heterologous neoplastic mesenchymal elements.

Ancillary Studies

Pancreatoblastomas show multiple lines of differentiation which can be demonstrated with immunohistochemical studies. Like acinar cell carcinoma, the acinar component of pancreatoblastoma is immunoreactive for several cytokeratins, as well as for markers of acinar differentiation like trypsin, chymotrypsin, and BCL10. Foci of neuroendocrine cells can be demonstrated with immunohistochemical stains for synaptophysin and chromogranin A. The squamoid nests are immunoreactive for EMA and show nuclear labeling with β-catenin.

Differential Diagnosis

There is significant overlap with the gross and histologic features of pancreatoblastoma and acinar cell carcinoma. Both are large, solid neoplasms composed primarily of acinar cells with granular eosinophilic cytoplasm and eccentric round nuclei with single prominent nucleoli. In contrast to acinar cell carcinoma, pancreatoblastoma is far more common in the pediatric population and, by definition, shows multiple lines of differentiation. The identification of discrete squamoid elements, with or without mesenchymal, glandular, and neuroendocrine elements, is necessary to distinguish pancreatoblastoma from acinar cell carcinoma. This may be particularly challenging in small biopsy specimens and fine-needle aspirations, though the preparation of cell blocks may aid in the identification of squamoid nests and facilitate immunohistochemical studies to exclude other entities in the differential diagnosis like neuroendocrine tumors and neuroendocrine carcinomas.

PANCREATOBLASTOMA – DISEASE FACT SHEET

Definition
▸▸ Pancreatic exocrine neoplasm showing multiple lines of differentiation including acinar and squamous

Incidence and Location
▸▸ Extremely rare neoplasm (0.5% of all pancreatic exocrine tumors)
▸▸ No predilection for particular pancreatic site

Sex and Age Distribution
▸▸ Most common pancreatic neoplasm of children (median age, 4 years)
▸▸ Congenital cases reported
▸▸ Rarely presents in adults with wide age range (range, 18–78 years)
▸▸ No sex predominance

Clinical Features
▸▸ Weight loss
▸▸ Abdominal pain
▸▸ Palpable abdominal mass
▸▸ Cushing syndrome secondary to tumor secretion of ACTH

Radiologic Features
▸▸ Large, well-marginated, round to oval tumor
▸▸ Large size may displace adjacent organs, distorting internal anatomy and making identifying pancreas as primary site challenging

Prognosis and Therapy
▸▸ Surgical resection associated with 5-year survival of 65%
▸▸ Recurrence no uncommon
▸▸ More aggressive disease in adults with frequent metastasis and worse survival
▸▸ Platinum-based chemotherapy and radiotherapy frequently employed

---

PANCREATOBLASTOMA – PATHOLOGIC FEATURES

Gross Findings
▸▸ Large, well-circumscribed, solid mass (average 10 cm)
▸▸ Frequently at least partially encapsulated
▸▸ Flesh, soft, whitish-yellow cut surface
▸▸ Lobular arrangement with scant fibrous stroma
▸▸ Foci of hemorrhage, necrosis, and cystic degeneration

Microscopic Findings
▸▸ Lobules composed primarily of neoplastic cells with acinar differentiation
▸▸ Interspersed squamoid nests composed of whorling epithelioid and plump spindle cells, with or without keratinization
▸▸ Neuroendocrine and glandular components frequently encountered
▸▸ Stroma may be cellular/sarcomatoid with occasional malignant heterologous mesenchymal elements

Immunohistochemistry
▸▸ Acinar component immunoreactive for trypsin, chymotrypsin, BCL10
▸▸ Squamoid nests immunoreactive for EMA and shows nuclear labeling for β-catenin
▸▸ Neuroendocrine component immunoreactive for synaptophysin and chromogranin A

Pathologic Differential Diagnoses
▸▸ Acinar cell carcinoma

UNDIFFERENTIATED CARCINOMA WITH OSTEOCLAST-LIKE GIANT CELLS

DDX: undifferentiated carcinoma

Clinical Features

Undifferentiated carcinoma with osteoclast-like giant cells (UC-OGC) is a variant of PDAC with distinct histologic features and a less aggressive clinical course than anaplastic, sarcomatoid, and typical PDACs. UC-OGCs are rare, representing approximately 1% of pancreatic carcinomas. There is a slight female predominance to these tumors and they affect adults over a wide age range, though it is generally a disease of older adults (mean, 58 years). Clinical behavior is somewhat unpredictable, though UC-OGCs appear to have a better prognosis than conventional PDACs with a 5-year survival rate of 59.1% and a median survival of 7.7 years.

Pathologic Features

GROSS FINDINGS

UC-OGCs are large tumor (mean, 5.3 cm) and can be found throughout the pancreas and biliary tree, though about a third are localized to the pancreatic body and tail. The cut surface is frequently soft and hemorrhagic and may show extensive necrosis. Cyst formation is identified in many UC-OGCs, with a third of tumors showing prominent intraductal and intracystic polypoid growth.

MICROSCOPIC FINDINGS

UC-OGCs are composed of three distinct populations. Osteoclast-like multinucleated giant cells are histologically identical to those seen in bone and have abundant dense eosinophilic cytoplasm and multiple centrally clustered, relatively uniform nuclei lacking significant atypia. The osteoclast-like giant cell component of these tumors may be prominent or only focal but tend to be clustered in distinct nodules in areas of necrosis and hemorrhage. In addition to osteoclast-like giant cells, numerous mononuclear histiocytes are also present within the tumor but may be inconspicuous on H&E-stained sections.

In contrast to the osteoclast-like giant cell and histiocytic components of UC-OGCs, which are reactive in nature and generally quite prominent, the neoplastic component of these tumors may be harder to appreciate on H&E-stained sections. These mononuclear histiocyte-like sarcomatoid carcinoma cells are typically round to oval and epithelioid, or plump and somewhat spindled, and display some degree of nuclear atypia, especially compared with the non-neoplastic background histiocytes and osteoclast-like giant cells. In addition to these histiocyte-like sarcomatoid carcinoma cells, obviously malignant pleomorphic giant carcinoma cells with anaplastic hyperchromatic nuclei can be identified in some cases (Fig. 4.49).

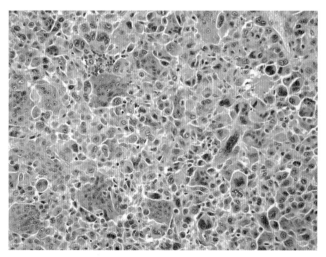

FIG. 4.49

Undifferentiated carcinoma with osteoclast-like giant cells. Characterized by three distinct cell populations including osteoclast-like giant cells with abundant eosinophilic cytoplasm and multiple nuclei, background mononuclear histiocytes, and neoplastic histiocyte-like sarcomatoid cells, some of which show marked nuclear atypia.

Interestingly, component of typical PDAC is identified in approximately 75% of UC-OGCs. An association with MCNs and IPMNs has been identified in a minority of cases.

Ancillary Studies

The histologic features of UC-OGCs are distinct obviating the need for ancillary studies in routine clinical practice. Not surprisingly, both the osteoclast-like giant cells and reactive histiocytic component of these tumors are reactive for CD68. The neoplastic histiocytic sarcomatoid carcinoma cells and pleomorphic giant carcinoma cells occasionally show focal, weak staining for CK AE1/AE3 and Cam5.2, while foci containing typical PDAC are reactive for keratins.

Sequencing studies performed on UC-OGCs have identified similar variants in *KRAS* and *TP53* to those detected in typical PDACs. As such, abnormal expression of p53 can be detected by immunohistochemical stains in the neoplastic component of these tumors.

Differential Diagnosis

Other undifferentiated pancreatic carcinomas may occasionally enter the differential for UC-OGCs. While large, highly atypical tumor cells are seen in both anaplastic undifferentiated carcinoma and UC-OGCs, these pleomorphic bizarre-appearing cells are significantly less abundant in the latter. Furthermore, the neoplastic cells in UC-OGC are admixed with non-neoplastic histiocytes and obviously benign osteoclast-like giant cells.

Osteoid may be identified at least focally in about a third of UC-OGCs, which may result in carcinosarcoma entering the differential diagnosis. In contrast to the malignant heterologous sarcomatoid elements seen in carcinosarcoma, the osteoid seen in UC-OGCs is reactive in nature and associated with foci of metaplastic bone. Overgrowth of osteoid in an osteosarcomatous pattern with associated malignant osteoclasts is not a feature of UC-OGCs.

UNDIFFERENTIATED CARCINOMA WITH OSTEOCLAST-LIKE GIANT CELLS – DISEASE FACT SHEET

Definition
▸▸ Undifferentiated variant of pancreatic ductal adenocarcinoma containing numerous osteoclast-like giant cells and non-neoplastic histiocytic inflammation

Incidence and Location
▸▸ Rare neoplasm
▸▸ Develop at any site within the pancreas
▸▸ Rarely reported in bile ducts and other sites

Continued

UNDIFFERENTIATED CARCINOMA WITH OSTEOCLAST-LIKE GIANT CELLS – DISEASE FACT SHEET—cont'd

Sex and Age Distribution
▸▸ Generally disease of older adults (mean age, 58 years)
▸▸ Slight female predominance

Clinical Features
▸▸ Abdominal and back pain
▸▸ Unintentional weight loss
▸▸ Nausea

Radiologic Features
▸▸ Large mass with delayed enhancement
▸▸ Occasional intraductal/intracystic growth
▸▸ Rarely predominantly cystic

Prognosis and Therapy
▸▸ Unpredictable clinical course
▸▸ Potentially aggressive but better prognosis than conventional pancreatic ductal adenocarcinoma (5-year survival rate of 59.1%)
▸▸ Surgical resection

UNDIFFERENTIATED CARCINOMA WITH OSTEOCLAST-LIKE GIANT CELLS – PATHOLOGIC FEATURES

Gross Findings
▸▸ Large mass (mean, 5.3 cm) found anywhere in pancreas
▸▸ Cut surface lobulated, soft, and hemorrhagic
▸▸ Extensive necrosis not uncommon
▸▸ Rarely intraductal or intracystic polypoid growth

Microscopic Findings
▸▸ Multiphasic tumor
▸▸ Prominent osteoclast-like giant cells with abundant dense eosinophilic cytoplasm and multiple uniform nuclei without atypia
▸▸ Reactive background non-neoplastic histiocytes
▸▸ Histiocyte-like sarcomatoid carcinoma cells epithelioid or plump and spindled with obvious nuclear atypia
▸▸ Pleomorphic giant carcinoma cells with bizarre anaplastic nuclei
▸▸ Often associated with component of conventional pancreatic ductal adenocarcinoma
▸▸ Reactive bone and osteoid seen in 30% of cases

Immunohistochemistry
▸▸ Reactive histiocytic component and osteoclast-like giant cells immunoreactive for CD68
▸▸ Neoplastic histiocyte-like sarcomatoid and pleomorphic giant carcinoma cells with occasional weak keratin expression
▸▸ High Ki-67 proliferative index and abnormal p53 expression in neoplastic component

Pathologic Differential Diagnoses
▸▸ Undifferentiated carcinoma

ENDOCRINE NEOPLASMS

Pancreatic neuroendocrine neoplasms are a class of pancreatic tumors with distinct histologic and clinical features that display immunohistochemical and ultrastructural evidence of neuroendocrine differentiation.

Though considerably less common than conventional PDACs, pancreatic neuroendocrine neoplasms are the second most common malignant neoplasm of the pancreas. These neoplasms are diverse with respect to both histologic appearance, presentation and symptomatology, and clinical course. Broadly, pancreatic neuroendocrine tumors can be classified as either WDNETs or poorly differentiated neuroendocrine carcinomas (PDNEC), which resemble small and large cell neuroendocrine carcinomas of other sites.

WELL-DIFFERENTIATED PANCREATIC NEUROENDOCRINE TUMOR

DDX: pancreatic neuroendocrine microadenoma, acinar cell carcinoma, solid pseudopapillary neoplasm

Clinical Features

WDNETs have been reported over a wide age range, but most commonly adults (mean age, 55 years). Although most WDNETs are sporadic, they may also develop in the setting of underlying genetic disorders such as multiple endocrine neoplasia, type 1 (100% of patients), von Hippel-Lindau (VHL) syndrome (11%–17% of patients), and, less commonly, tuberous sclerosis.

Historically, most WDNETs were functional, that is, associated with a clinical syndrome related to the production of peptide hormones and biogenic amines. Insulin-producing WDNETs (insulinomas) are the most commonly encountered syndromic neuroendocrine tumor, accounting for up to 20% of all resected neoplasms. Patients with insulinomas frequently present with profound hypoglycemia (frequently less than 40 mg/dL) with associated neuroglycopenic and autonomic symptoms, or even hypoglycemic coma. Although multiple insulinomas are seen in a subset of patients, most exhibit a benign clinical course with only 10% of patients developing metastatic disease.

Gastrin-producing WDNETs (gastrinomas) are the second most common neuroendocrine tumor and account for less than 8% of all cases, with an estimated incidence of 0.5 to 3 cases per million per year worldwide. Excessive, inappropriate gastrin production leads to gastric enterochromaffin-like cell hyperplasia and gastric acid hypersecretion which results in severe gastroesophageal reflux disease and duodenal as well as distal intestinal ulcers. In contrast to insulinomas, most gastrinomas exhibit an aggressive clinical course with over 60% of cases presenting with metastatic nodal disease.

Other functional WDNETs are considerably less common and include, in descending order of frequency, vasoactive intestinal peptide tumors (VIPomas), glucagonomas, somatostatinomas, ACTH-producing tumors, and the extremely rare serotonin-producing neuroendocrine tumors, which resemble classical midgut carcinoid tumors. The clinical syndrome associated with each of these neoplasms is, not surprisingly, related to the peptide hormones and biogenic amines that they produce. For example, high plasma levels (greater than pmol/L) of circulating VIP produce a syndrome of severe secretory diarrhea with associated hypokalemia, achlorhydria, and acidosis, while elevated glucagon levels cause the glucagonoma syndrome with a characteristic symmetric skin rash (necrolytic migratory erythema) involving the buttocks, perineum, and limbs, as well as diabetes mellitus, weight loss, anemia, and venous thrombosis.

In contrast to functional WDNETs, non-functioning neuroendocrine tumors are not associated with a clinical syndrome related to the production of peptide hormones or biogenic amines. In the era of widespread, high-quality cross-sectional imaging studies, the detection of non-functioning WDNETs has increased and now account for up to 80% of all neuroendocrine tumors. Incidental small non-functioning tumors are occasionally encountered in the tail of the pancreas as rounded, well-circumscribed and enhancing masses. Tumors involving the head of the pancreas may lead to biliary obstruction causing jaundice and abdominal pain. Unfortunately, over half of patients with non-functioning WDNETs present with metastatic disease to the regional lymph nodes and liver. Modern functional imaging studies using gallium-68 DOTA peptides (i.e., [68]GA-DOTATATE) are increasingly being employed and increase the sensitivity of detection of metastatic disease relative to older technologies which may alter clinical management, particularly with regard to surgical debulking of metastatic disease and liver-directed procedures.

Pathologic Features

GROSS FINDINGS

WDNETs are well-circumscribed, soft, fleshy lesions with homogeneous yellow-brown to pink cut surfaces. Some tumors have more abundant fibrous tissue or cystic areas, which may be prominent and are degenerative in nature. Tumor necrosis is generally not a feature of WDNETs. Non-functioning pancreatic neuroendocrine tumors average 2 to 5 cm in greatest extent and are more commonly encountered in the head of the pancreas. This is in contrast to functional neuroendocrine tumors, particularly insulin-producing tumors, which tend to be smaller but may still grow to form large masses.

MICROSCOPIC FINDINGS

WDNETs exhibit a diverse array of cytologic features and architectural growth patterns. Generally, the

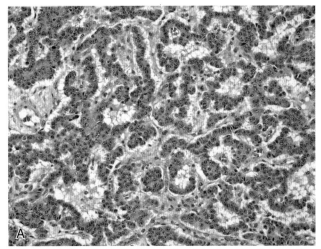
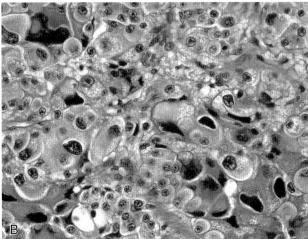

FIG. 4.50

Well-differentiated pancreatic neuroendocrine tumor. **A,** Well-differentiated neuroendocrine tumors exhibit a diverse array of cytologic features and growth patterns. Generally, they are composed of epithelioid cells with round, regular nuclei that have a characteristic coarsely granular "salt-and-pepper" chromatin. **B,** Some well-differentiated neuroendocrine tumors show variable, though sometimes striking nuclear pleomorphism.

neoplastic cells of WDNETs are epithelioid and round or cuboidal and have a moderate amount of finely granular eosinophilic cytoplasm and round to ovoid, regular nuclei with the characteristic granular, coarsely stippled "salt-and-pepper" chromatin (Fig. 4.50A). Other histologic variants include tumors that exhibit variable nuclear pleomorphism (Fig. 4.50B), extensive foamy cytoplasm with clear cell change, rhabdoid features, or an oncocytic phenotype. Aside from the association of clear cell change with VHL syndrome, these histologic patterns have minimal prognostic significance, though tumors with extensive stromal fibrosis and oncocytic features may exhibit a more aggressive clinical course.

The neoplastic cells of WDNETs assume a variety of architectural patterns of growth. Solid or organoid patterns of growth are common, as are trabecular structures, ribbons, nests, and acinar or pseudoglandular structures (Fig. 4.51). Most tumors are highly cellular

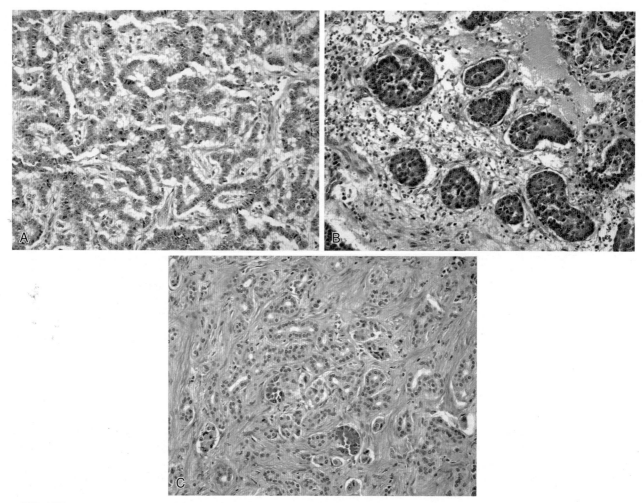

FIG. 4.51
Well-differentiated pancreatic neuroendocrine tumor. These neoplasms exhibit a diverse array of growth patterns, including within the same tumor, including: **A,** gyriform or trabecular, **B,** organoid and nested, **C,** pseudoglandular.

with minimal intervening stroma, though tumors with thick fibrous septae, extensive hyalinized stroma, or even amyloid deposition are frequently encountered. Calcifications, including psammomatous calcifications in somatostatinomas, are seen in some cases.

Pancreatic microadenomas are common incidental findings composed of nests and trabeculae of neuroendocrine cells with granular eosinophilic cytoplasm and round or ovoid nuclei with stippled chromatin that are histologically indistinguishable from WDNETs but measure less than 0.5 cm in diameter. They are typically of no clinical significance and detected at the time of autopsy or during the histologic examination of pancreata resected for another reason.

Ancillary Studies

WDNETs are generally immunoreactive for the neuroendocrine markers synaptophysin, chromogranin A,

and INSM1, at least focally. There are, unfortunately, no specific immunohistochemical markers that can reliably differentiate WDNETs from neuroendocrine tumors arising in other sites. The immunohistochemical stains that recognize the transcription factors ISL1 and PAX8 appear to label pancreatic neuroendocrine tumors preferentially, but also recognize tumors originating in other sites.

Occasionally, particularly in the setting of a pseudoglandular pattern of growth, WDNETs may be mistaken for conventional PDAC. While immunohistochemical markers such as synaptophysin and INSM1 will demonstrate neuroendocrine differentiation in the former, care must be taken not to rely too heavily on immunohistochemical studies to differentiate pancreatic neuroendocrine tumors from ductal adenocarcinomas. For example, over half of all WDNETs express CK7 and CK19, and nearly all are reactive for MOC-31.

In 2011, genetic studies have revealed alterations in the chromatin remodeling genes *ATRX* and *DAXX*. Genetic variants impacting this pathway result in loss of

TABLE 4.2

Grading Well-Differentiated Pancreatic
Neuroendocrine Tumors

	Mitoses per 2 mm²	Ki-67 Proliferative Index
Low grade (G1)	<2	<3%
Intermediate grade (G2)	2–20	3%–20%
High grade (G3)	>20	>20%

immunohistochemical staining for ATRX or DAXX in over 40% of WDNETs.

The accurate assessment of mitotic activity and the estimated Ki-67 proliferative index is critical for the grading and risk stratification of WDNETs. Low-grade (G1) WDNETs exhibit < 2 MF/2 mm² and a Ki-67 proliferative index of < 3%, while intermediate grade (G2) tumors have between 2 and 20 MF/2 mm² and a Ki-67 proliferative index of between 3% and 20%. The most recent 2019 WHO classification of digestive system tumors (fifth edition) creates a novel category of high-grade (G3) WDNETs, which show the typical histologic features of WDNETs and lack genetic abnormalities in *TP53* and *RB1* but exhibit >20 MF/2 mm² and have a Ki-67 proliferative index of >20% (Table 4.2). While high-grade (G3) WDNETs have a proliferative index of >20%, it rarely exceeds 55%. This is in stark contrast to PDNECs (discussed later) which have a markedly elevated proliferative index, frequently exhibit genetic variant in *TP53* and *RB1*, and have histologic features reminiscent of pulmonary small cell and large cell neuroendocrine carcinoma.

Occasionally, there will be discordance between the assigned grade with respect to the formal mitotic count and the estimated Ki-67 proliferative index. In these situations, the higher grade should be assigned to the tumor.

Differential Diagnosis

Neuroendocrine microadenomas are distinguished from WDNETs on the basis of size, with microadenomas measuring less than 5 mm. Microadenomas are, otherwise, indistinguishable from WDNETs and are composed of relatively uniform, medium-sized cells with round to ovoid nuclei with coarsely stippled neuroendocrine-type chromatin that are arranged in nests, cords, and thick trabeculae. Microadenomas are nearly always discovered incidentally in specimens that were resected from another indication.

By definition, neuroendocrine microadenomas are non-functioning. Neuroendocrine proliferations smaller than 5 mm but associated with a clinical syndrome should be considered to be WDNETs and graded and staged appropriately. The distinction between pancreatic neuroendocrine microadenoma and WDNETs is potentially clinically important because, despite rare case reports of nodal metastasis, microadenomas nearly always behave in a benign fashion while even low-grade WDNETs have significant malignant potential.

This distinction between WDNETs and acinar cell carcinoma is potentially challenging, particularly on small fine-needle biopsies and in cytologic preparation, but is of great clinical significance. While the formation of acinar structures is seen in some WDNETs, this architectural pattern is typically not as prominent or diffuse as that seen in acinar cell carcinomas. There are several important cytologic clues that can assist in the differentiation of these neoplasms from one another. While the cytoplasm of WDNETs may be eosinophilic and finely granular, it is typically more abundant and coarser in acinar cell carcinomas, and PAS/D special stains highlight cytoplasmic zymogen granules. The nuclei of acinar cell carcinoma cells are also typically eccentric and basally oriented and often contain prominent conspicuous nucleoli. This contrasts starkly with the round, regular, centrally located nuclei with smooth contours and coarsely granular "salt-and-pepper" chromatin that are characteristic of WDNETs.

In particularly challenging cases, a limited panel of immunohistochemical stains can greatly assist in the proper classification of these neoplasms. The expression of neuroendocrine markers, particularly synaptophysin, is characteristic of WDNETs and is typically strong and diffuse. Up to a third of acinar cell carcinomas, however, also express neuroendocrine markers which can potentially lead to diagnostic confusion. There should be a low threshold for employing immunohistochemical stains for trypsin, chymotrypsin, and certain clones of BCL10 which support acinar differentiation and are highly specific for the diagnosis of acinar cell carcinoma.

WDNETs share some histologic features with solid pseudopapillary neoplasms. Both tumors may show solid and cystic areas on cross-sectional imaging studies and at the time of gross examination. Histologically, both neoplasms are composed of epithelioid cells with somewhat granular eosinophilic cytoplasm. Cells with clear vacuolated cytoplasm are also seen in some solid pseudopapillary neoplasms. Occasional intensely eosinophilic hyaline globules may be encountered within the cytoplasm of solid pseudopapillary neoplasms, which are not typically seen in WDNETs. In contrast with the diverse architectural patterns of growth seen in WDNETs, solid pseudopapillary neoplasms exhibit a predominantly solid pattern of growth with poorly cohesive epithelioid cells seemingly falling apart and clinging to myxoid fibrovascular stalks and imparting a pseudopapillary appearance to the tumor. There are also significant differences in the nuclear features of these two neoplasms. While WDNETs have round to ovoid nuclei with smooth, regular contours and coarsely granular chromatin, the nuclei of solid pseudopapillary neoplasms have prominent linear grooves.

Immunohistochemical stains may also aid in the distinction of WDNETs from solid pseudopapillary neoplasms. Focal positive expression for synaptophysin may be seen in some solid pseudopapillary neoplasms but is never as strong and diffuse as that seen in WDNETs. In contrast, abnormal nuclear accumulation of β-catenin with associated loss of membranous E-cadherin expression is seen in nearly all solid pseudopapillary neoplasms, as is nuclear reactivity for the progesterone receptor and cyclin D1.

WELL-DIFFERENTIATED PANCREATIC NEUROENDOCRINE TUMOR – DISEASE FACT SHEET

Definition
▶▶ Malignant pancreatic neoplasm with evidence of neuroendocrine differentiation and frequently clinical syndromes associated with the elaboration of peptide hormones

Incidence and Location
▶▶ Relatively rare neoplasm accounting for less than 5% of pancreatic tumors
▶▶ Can be found at any location within the pancreas

Sex and Age Distribution
▶▶ No substantial sex differences
▶▶ Wide age range with highest incidence between 30 and 60 years

Clinical Features
▶▶ Functioning or syndromic neuroendocrine tumors produce symptoms related to the specific peptide hormone elaborated by neoplastic cells (i.e., insulin, gastrin, glucagon, VIP)
▶▶ Pancreatic head tumors may cause biliary obstruction
▶▶ Large proportion of patients with non-functioning neuroendocrine tumors present with sequelae of metastatic disease (frequently liver and regional lymph nodes)
▶▶ Strong association with MEN, type 1 and VHL syndrome

Radiologic Features
▶▶ Well-demarcated pancreatic mass
▶▶ Functional imaging studies using gallium-68 DOTA peptides are exquisitely sensitive and specific

Prognosis and Therapy
▶▶ Variable with neuroendocrine microadenomas typically incidentally discovered and behaving in a benign fashion and most larger non-functioning tumors presenting with hepatic or nodal metastasis
▶▶ Elevated proliferative index associated with more aggressive phenotype
▶▶ Mutated *DAXX* or *ATRX* associated with worse prognosis
▶▶ Surgical resection and tumor debulking
▶▶ Clinical course may be prolonged even in setting of metastatic disease (10-year survival 36%)

WELL-DIFFERENTIATED PANCREATIC NEUROENDOCRINE TUMOR – PATHOLOGIC FEATURES

Gross Findings
▶▶ Well-circumscribed, soft, flesh lesions
▶▶ Homogenous yellow-brown to pink cut surface
▶▶ Cystic degeneration not uncommon

Microscopic Findings
▶▶ Variable architecture with tumors showing solid, nested, trabecular, gyriform, or pseudoglandular patterns of growth
▶▶ Stroma variable ranging from richly vascular and inconspicuous to densely hyalinized
▶▶ Epithelioid cells with granular eosinophilic cytoplasm and regular round to ovoid nuclei with smooth contours and stippled "salt-and-pepper" chromatin
▶▶ Occasional pleomorphic nuclei clinically insignificant
▶▶ Mitotic figures identifiably but rare

Immunohistochemistry
▶▶ Strong, diffuse immunoreactivity for synaptophysin, chromogranin A, and INSM1
▶▶ Subset show loss of reactivity for ATRX or DAXX
▶▶ Variable Ki-67 proliferative index; required for grading

Pathologic Differential Diagnoses
▶▶ Pancreatic neuroendocrine microadenoma
▶▶ Acinar cell carcinoma
▶▶ Solid pseudopapillary neoplasm

POORLY DIFFERENTIATED NEUROENDOCRINE TUMOR

DDX: lymphoma, acinar cell carcinoma, high-grade well-differentiated pancreatic neuroendocrine tumor (G3)

Clinical Features

PDNECs are extremely rare neoplasms, accounting for less than 1% of all primary pancreatic tumors. Like ductal adenocarcinoma, PDNEC is primarily a disease of older adults (mean, 59 years), though it has been reported in individual as young as 21 years in one series. The majority of these tumors arise in the head of the pancreas, resulting in back pain and obstructive jaundice developing as the most common presenting symptoms. In contrast to functioning WDNETs, the elaboration of peptide hormones and amine neurotransmitters is not a feature of PDNECs.

Like PDNECs arising in other sites, the prognosis for these pancreatic tumors is dismal with a median survival of only 11 months. Over 80% of patients with PDNECs have metastatic disease at the time of initial presentation.

There are significant differences in between the genetic drivers of WDNETs and PDNECs. While mutations in *DAXX* or *ATRX* are seen in 44% of WDNETs, alterations in these genes are not a feature of PDNEC. Instead, *TP53* mutations and inactivation of *RB1* are seen in variable proportions of small and large cell neuroendocrine carcinomas several sites and support a diagnosis of PDNEC in the pancreas.

Pathologic Features

GROSS FINDINGS

More than half of PDNECs arise in the pancreatic head, though they have also been reported in the tail of the pancreas and, less frequently, the body. They form fairly large tumors, with a median size of 4 cm and have a fleshy tan-red to yellow, vaguely nodular or lobulated cut surface.

MICROSCOPIC FINDINGS

Similar to neuroendocrine carcinomas of other sites, PDNEC of the pancreas can show either large cell or small cell cytologic features. The large cell subtype is more common and displays variable patterns of growth, often within the same tumor, including solid, nested, trabecular, and pseudopapillary architecture. The neoplastic cells of large cell carcinoma are polygonal with ample amphophilic cytoplasm and large round nuclei with vesicular chromatin and prominent nucleoli.

In contrast, the small cell type of PDNEC is composed of sheets of medium-sized cells with scant cytoplasm and large, elongated nuclei with hyperchromatic, finely granular chromatin and inconspicuous nucleoli. Nuclear molding may be prominent. Numerous apoptotic bodies are frequently present, as are confluent foci of tumor necrosis (Fig. 4.52A). While numerous mitotic figures are present in both large and small cell types of neuroendocrine carcinoma, they are generally more abundant in the small cell type and average over 50 MF/10 HPF.

A subset of PDNECs (approximately 20% in one series) contained identifiable elements of ductal adenocarcinoma or acinar cell carcinoma. These non-neuroendocrine elements can either be sharply segregated from the neuroendocrine carcinoma or be admixed with it. If these non-neuroendocrine components account for greater than 30% of the tumor mass, the neoplasm can be classified as a mixed neuroendocrine–non-neuroendocrine carcinoma (MiNEC). The poorly differentiated neuroendocrine component of the neoplasm, however, typically dictates the clinical course and should drive treatment decisions.

Ancillary Studies

Although the morphologic features of PDNECs are somewhat distinct, demonstrating neuroendocrine differentiation with the aid of immunohistochemical stains may be essential to exclude other high-grade poorly differentiated neoplasms, including large cell lymphoma and melanoma. Synaptophysin is an extremely sensitive marker and labels nearly all PDNECs with a moderately strong intensity, though the distribution may be often be patchy. A panel-based approach including either chromogranin or INSM1 along with synaptophysin may be required to demonstrate neuroendocrine differentiation in rare neuroendocrine carcinomas with negative or equivocal synaptophysin reactivity, though this is usually not the case (Fig. 4.52B).

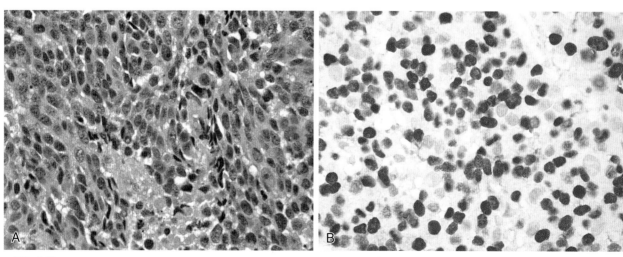

FIG. 4.52

Poorly differentiated neuroendocrine carcinoma. **A,** Small cell-type poorly differentiated neuroendocrine carcinomas are histologically similar to small cell carcinomas arising in other sites. They are characterized by a solid or sheet-like growth of medium-sized cells with scant cytoplasm and large nuclei with granular, hyperchromatic cytoplasm. Mitotic figures, including atypical forms are frequently encountered, as are foci of tumor necrosis. **B,** Strong nuclear reactivity for synaptophysin and INSM1 (pictured) supports neuroendocrine differentiation.

PDNECs of the pancreas have an extremely high proliferative rate, as evidenced by the high mitotic counts seen in both large cell and small cell types. This is, not surprisingly, supported by immunohistochemical stains for Ki-67 as well, where the large cell type of PDNEC has an average proliferative index of 66%, while the small cell types have a mean proliferative index of 75%. This high proliferative index can be useful diagnostically, particularly in distinguishing high-grade (G3) WDNETs that generally have a proliferative index of less than 55%, from PDNECs that frequently have a proliferative index greater than 55%. There are, however, exceptions to this generalization that necessitate further workup for more challenging cases.

As mutations in *TP53* and inactivation of the RB1/p16 pathway are frequently encountered in neuroendocrine carcinomas from several anatomic sites, but are not seen in WDNETs, immunohistochemical stains for p53 and Rb can be leveraged to support a diagnosis of PDNEC in ambiguous high-grade neuroendocrine neoplasms of the pancreas. An abnormal pattern of p53 staining or loss of nuclear Rb by neoplastic cells supports a diagnosis of PDNEC and should be employed in cases with challenging or ambiguous histologic features in order to accurately classify these tumors and direct appropriate therapy.

Differential Diagnosis

The presence of monotonous, poorly differentiated neoplastic cells with high N/C ratios may occasionally invoke the possibility of hematologic malignancy, particularly in small, often crushed fine-needle biopsies. Differentiating PDNEC from diffuse large B-cell lymphoma can be accomplished with a limited panel of immunohistochemical stains, since neuroendocrine carcinomas express synaptophysin and other markers of neuroendocrine differentiation at least focally, while large B-cell lymphomas express the B-lymphocyte markers CD19 and CD20, show light chain restriction, and lack reactivity for broad-spectrum cytokeratins.

Like PDNEC, acinar cell carcinomas frequently exhibit high-grade cytologic features with an elevated proliferative index and a sheet-like, monotonous pattern of growth. Adding to the potential diagnostic confusion, a significant proportion of acinar cell carcinomas express markers of neuroendocrine differentiation, though it is usually focal. PDNECs do not, however, express the acinar markers trypsin and chymotrypsin in their pure form. A minority of otherwise typical acinar cell carcinomas, however, show a morphologically and immunohistochemically distinct component of small cell- or large cell-type neuroendocrine carcinoma cells and are best categorized as mixed acinar-neuroendocrine carcinomas. These mixed acinar-neuroendocrine

carcinomas have similar driver mutations to acinar cell carcinomas and exhibit a comparable clinical course.

In some instances, it may be challenging to classify a high-grade neuroendocrine neoplasm showing increased mitotic activity and a proliferative index of greater than 20%. While the majority of PDNECs show a proliferative index of greater than 50%, there is substantial overlap in this metric with G3 WDNETs and it alone cannot be used to distinguish between these biologically distinct neoplasms. In resection material, careful histologic examination may reveal a minor component of conventional ductal adenocarcinoma which favors a diagnosis of PDNEC. Alternatively, immunohistochemical studies demonstrating loss of nuclear ATRX or DAXX is fairly specific for WDNETs, though it is not seen in all cases. Conversely, abnormal p53 expression including both strong, near universal nuclear reactivity or a null pattern is commonly seen in PDNECs, as is loss of Rb.

Correlation with clinical and radiologic studies is also indispensable and should be employed to accurately classify high-grade neuroendocrine neoplasms and direct appropriate therapy. Like other WDNETs, G3 WDNETS may be associated with clinical symptoms related to the elaboration of peptide hormones and biogenic amines, which is not a feature of neuroendocrine carcinoma. Similarly, elevated plasma chromogranin levels and positive DOTA peptide nuclear medicine scans are not seen in the setting of PDNEC. Instead, laboratory studies may show elevations of carcinoma markers like CEA, CA19.9, or CA125.

POORLY DIFFERENTIATED NEUROENDOCRINE TUMOR – DISEASE FACT SHEET

Definition
▶▶ Poorly differentiated carcinoma with neuroendocrine differentiation, an extremely high proliferative index, and genetic alterations in *TP53* and *RB1*

Incidence and Location
▶▶ Extremely rare (less than 1% of all primary pancreatic tumors)
▶▶ Majority arise in pancreatic head

Sex and Age Distribution
▶▶ Slight male preference
▶▶ Generally disease of older adults (mean, 59 years)
▶▶ Reported in individuals as young as 21 years

Clinical Features
▶▶ Abdominal and back pain, obstructive jaundice
▶▶ No clinical syndrome related to the elaboration of peptide hormones or biogenic amines
▶▶ Frequently associated with elevated plasma CEA and CA19.9

Radiologic Features
▶▶ Negative or very weak DOTA peptide scans

Prognosis and Therapy

▶▶ Majority with metastatic disease at time of initial presentation

▶▶ Extremely aggressive neoplasm with median survival of 11 months

▶▶ Platinum-based chemotherapy protocols with etoposide

POORLY DIFFERENTIATED NEUROENDOCRINE CARCINOMA – PATHOLOGIC FEATURES

Gross Findings

▶▶ Large tumors with flesh tan-red to yellow cut surface

▶▶ Vaguely nodular or lobulated

Microscopic Findings

▶▶ Histologically indistinguishable from neuroendocrine carcinomas of other sites

▶▶ Small cell-type morphology with sheets of medium-sized carcinoma cells with elongated, hyperchromatic nuclei and inconspicuous nucleoli

▶▶ Frequent nuclear molding and numerous mitotic figures

▶▶ Large cell type morphology with variable growth patterns and larger, polygonal carcinoma cells

▶▶ Large nuclei with vesicular chromatin and frequently prominent nucleoli

▶▶ Foci of tumor necrosis frequent

▶▶ Components of typical ductal adenocarcinoma or acinar carcinoma frequently encountered

Immunohistochemistry

▶▶ Display at least focal neuroendocrine differentiation with immunoreactivity for synaptophysin, INSM1, or chromogranin

▶▶ Abnormal p53 expression in subset of poorly differentiated neuroendocrine carcinomas

▶▶ Loss of Rb expression

▶▶ Preserved DAXX and ATRX expression

▶▶ Ki-67 proliferative index universally greater than 20% and nearly always greater than 50%

Pathologic Differential Diagnoses

▶▶ Large cell lymphoma

▶▶ Acinar cell carcinoma

▶▶ High-grade well-differentiated neuroendocrine tumor (G3)

CYSTIC NEOPLASMS

Cystic neoplasms of the pancreas are relatively common and frequently discovered incidentally with cross-sectional imaging of the abdomen performed for another indication. While some are essentially benign, others represent important precursor lesions to a subset of PDACs.

SEROUS CYSTIC NEOPLASM

DDX: mucinous pancreatic neoplasms, metastatic renal clear cell carcinoma

Clinical Features

Serous cystic neoplasms of the pancreas are relatively rare benign neoplasms that affect individuals over a wide age range (mean age, 60 years) with a strong predilection for women. Approximately 60% of patients are asymptomatic and the neoplasm is incidentally discovered during cross-sectional imaging performed for another reason. However, a minority of patients present with non-specific abdominal complaints like pain, nausea, vomiting, or weight loss.

On CT, serous cystic neoplasms are well circumscribed and typically centered in the pancreatic body or tail. In contrast to intraductal pancreatic mucinous neoplasms, there is no demonstrable continuity with the pancreatic ductal system. The more common microcystic variant of serous cystic neoplasms exhibits small microlobular cysts that are less than 20 mm in size and delicate septae which can also be seen on endoscopic ultrasound and impart a honeycomb appearance to the tumor. Approximately 20% of these neoplasms have a well-defined central scar with an associated sunburst pattern of calcification.

Serous cystic neoplasms are typically solitary lesions outside the setting of VHL syndrome where they are frequently multiple and may diffusely involve the entire pancreas. While there are rare reports of malignant serous cystadenocarcinomas, the vast majority of serous cystic neoplasms behave in a benign fashion and have an excellent prognosis. Given the potential morbidity and mortality associated with pancreatic surgery, resection is reserved for large, symptomatic lesion in good surgical candidates, as well as for lesions where there is uncertainty regarding the preoperative diagnosis and a mucinous neoplasm cannot be entirely excluded after endoscopic sampling. Small, asymptomatic lesions with biopsy-confirmed or classic radiographic features of serous cystic neoplasm can be safely observed with surveillance imaging.

Pathologic Features

GROSS FINDINGS

Benign serous cystadenomas are well-circumscribed, bosselated lesions that are typically unifocal in the sporadic setting but can grow to impressive dimensions (up to 25 cm). The microcystic variant of serous cystadenoma is encountered most frequently and cut sections show a sponge-like cut surface made up of numerous small cysts that contain a watery serous fluid (Fig. 4.53A). Extremely small cysts may impart a solid appearance to the tumor. Approximately 20% of microcystic serous cystadenomas show a prominent central stellate scar which is variably gritty and

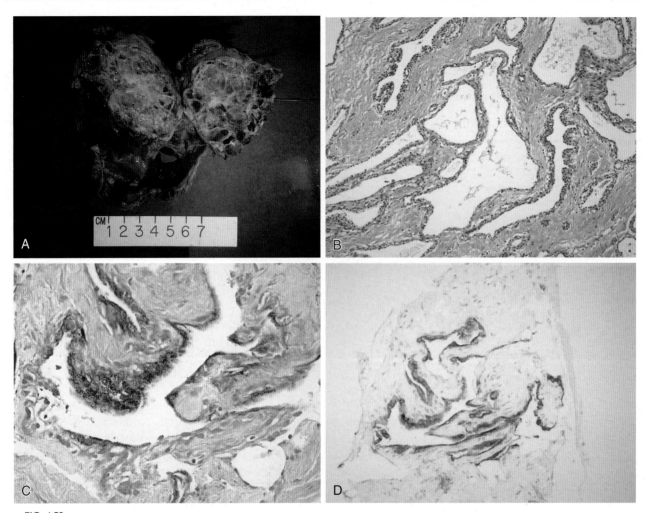

FIG. 4.53

Serous cystadenoma. **A,** Microcystic serous cystadenomas are well-circumscribed lesions that have a sponge-like cut surface. Numerous small cysts are filled with watery serous fluid. A prominent central scar is present in some instances. **B,** The cystic spaces are lined by flattened or cuboidal cells with round, regular nuclei with darkly staining uniform chromatin. **C,** The neoplastic cells are strongly reactive for PAS that is sensitive to diastase digestion. **D,** Most also show strong immunoreactivity for inhibin, though this marker is not specific for this neoplasm.

calcified. The oligocystic variant is considerably less common, representing less than 10% of serous neoplasms, and tends to be less well circumscribed than the microcystic variant with cysts greater than 1 cm.

MICROSCOPIC FINDINGS

Regardless of the gross classification, all serous cystadenomas are lined by a single layer of uniform cuboidal to flattened cells with clear to light eosinophilic cytoplasm, well-defined cell borders, and centrally placed, round, regular nuclei with dense homogenous chromatin (Fig. 4.53B). Pronounced mitotic activity and significant nuclear atypia are not characteristic.

Some cases may show tufting of the epithelium into the cystic spaces, or even blunt papillary projections, but large, complex papillary structures are not a feature of serous cystadenomas and should raise the possibility of a mucinous neoplasm. Embedded within the delicate fibrous tissue subjacent to the epithelial component of

this tumor is a fine network of conspicuous capillaries with plump endothelial cells. Normal components of the pancreatic parenchyma, including acinar structures and islets of Langerhans, may also be entrapped within the fibrous septae.

Cytologically, the neoplastic cells of the solid pancreatic serous neoplasms are indistinguishable from those that form cysts. Similarly, vanishingly rare serous cystadenocarcinomas may demonstrate an infiltrative pattern of growth into adjacent structures, in addition to lymphovascular invasion and metastasis, but show cytologic features that are identical to those seen in benign serous neoplasms.

Ancillary Studies

The striking clear cytoplasm of serous neoplasms is due to the presence of abundant cytoplasmic glycogen. As such, the neoplastic cells stain intensely with PAS but are sensitive for diastase digestion (Fig. 4.53C). Serous neoplasms of the pancreas express a wide array of cytokeratins, as well as EMA, inhibin, CA9, and GLUT1 (Fig. 4.53D). Care should be taken when interpreting the results of immunohistochemical stains, as clear cell morphology coupled with reactivity for CA9 may cause metastatic clear cell RCC to enter the differential diagnosis. Similarly, the clear cell variant of WDNETs, like serous neoplasms, frequently develop in the setting of VHL and also show reactivity for CA9 and inhibin, highlighting the need to interpret immunohistochemical studies in the context of the overall clinical picture.

Differential Diagnosis

Occasionally, there may be clinical and radiographic uncertainty with regard to the nature of a cystic pancreatic lesion necessitating fine-needle aspiration or biopsy. This is particularly challenging for oligocystic serous neoplasms, which may be mistaken for MCNs on cross-sectional imaging studies. Thick, neoplastic mucin is generally abundant and easily identified in conventional smears prepared from material aspirated from MCNs, while that derived from serous cystic neoplasms is thin, proteinaceous, and bloody. Biochemical and genetic studies can also help to differentiate serous neoplasms from mucinous neoplasms, as fluid CEA levels are typically low in serous neoplasms and *KRAS* and *GNAS* variants have not been reported in this tumor type.

Following resection, the distinction is generally less difficult. While small micropapillary tufts and simple papillary structures are occasionally encountered in serous cystic neoplasms, they are generally not as florid and complex as that seen in IPMNs. There are also obvious cytologic differences. While serous cystic neoplasms are composed of relatively uniform cuboidal cells with clear, glycogen-rich cytoplasm and round, regular nuclei, cytoplasmic and extracellular mucin is generally present, and frequently abundant, in pancreatic mucinous neoplasms. Similarly, cytologic and architectural atypia is not a feature of serous cystic neoplasms but is seen in mucinous pancreatic cysts and may be severe.

Clear cell RCC frequently metastasizes to the pancreas and may be extremely difficult to distinguish from a serous cystic neoplasm, particularly in the absence of radiographic information or if the clinical history is not known or provided. Both neoplasms are composed of epithelioid cells with clear cytoplasm and well-defined cell boarders. Cystic change is frequently encountered in clear cell RCC but is generally not as prominent as that seen in serous cystic neoplasms. Nuclear atypia is generally more pronounced in clear cell RCC, but these neoplasms are on occasion deceptively bland and lack obvious nucleoli (Fig. 4.54). Complicating matters

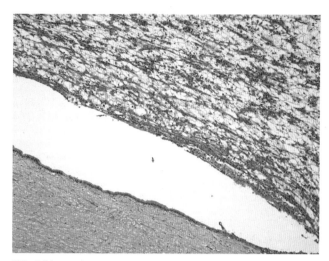

FIG. 4.54
Metastatic clear cell renal cell carcinoma may involve the pancreas and cause diagnostic confusion with other clear cell neoplasms, including serous cystadenoma and well-differentiated pancreatic neuroendocrine tumors with clear cell change.

further, as discussed previously, is the fact that serous cystic neoplasms, like many neoplasms with increased HIF1 activity, express CA9. Fortunately, reactivity for inhibin is not a feature of clear cell RCC and can be used to differentiate metastasis from a primary serous neoplasm.

SEROUS CYSTIC NEOPLASM – DISEASE FACT SHEET

Definition
▶▶ Epithelial neoplasm with frequent cyst formation composed of bland cuboidal cells with glycogen-rich cytoplasm

Incidence and Location
▶▶ Relatively rare neoplasm, frequently discovered incidentally
▶▶ Solitary lesions most frequent in the body or tail of pancreas
▶▶ VHL-associated lesions may be multiple or diffusely involve pancreas

Sex and Age Distribution
▶▶ Strong female predominance (approximately 3:1)
▶▶ Wide age distribution with mean age at presentation 60 years

Clinical Features
▶▶ Association with VHL syndrome
▶▶ Majority of patients are asymptomatic
▶▶ Minority with non-specific abdominal complaints related to mass effect including pain, nausea, vomiting, weight loss
▶▶ Palpable mass
▶▶ Biliary obstruction generally not a feature

Radiologic Features
▶▶ Well-defined, lobulated mass
▶▶ Microcystic variant with microlobular cysts less than 20 mm in size and delicate septae
▶▶ Occasional stellate central scar with sunburst calcifications
▶▶ Macro(oligo)cystic variant less well defined with larger cysts and absent central scar
▶▶ No communication with main pancreatic duct

Continued

SEROUS CYSTIC NEOPLASM – DISEASE FACT SHEET—cont'd

Prognosis and Therapy

▶▶ Excellent prognosis with only rare reports of malignant behavior/metastasis

▶▶ Small lesions can be safely followed

▶▶ Larger, symptomatic lesions treated with resection

SEROUS CYSTIC NEOPLASM – PATHOLOGIC FEATURES

Gross Findings

▶▶ Well-circumscribed, typically unifocal lesion with bosselated surface

▶▶ Microcystic variant with sponge-like cut surface made up of numerous small cysts and fine septae

▶▶ Watery serous fluid with no thick mucin

▶▶ Central stellate scar with gritty calcifications

▶▶ Oligocystic variant less well circumscribed with larger cysts

Microscopic Findings

▶▶ Cysts lined by single layer of uniform cuboidal to flattened cells with clear to light eosinophilic cytoplasm and well-defined cell borders

▶▶ Round, regular, centrally placed nuclei with dense, homogenous chromatin

▶▶ No significant mitotic activity or nuclear pleomorphism

▶▶ Occasional intracystic tufting and blunt papillary projections

▶▶ Fine subepithelial capillary network

▶▶ Very rare infiltration into adjacent structures

Immunohistochemistry

▶▶ Glycogen-rich cytoplasm stains strongly with PAS and sensitive to diastase digestion

▶▶ Immunoreactive for cytokeratins and EMA, along with inhibin, CA9, and GLUT1

Pathologic Differential Diagnoses

▶▶ Mucinous pancreatic neoplasms, metastatic clear cell renal cell carcinoma

---

MUCINOUS CYSTIC NEOPLASM

DDX: intraductal papillary mucinous neoplasm, oligocystic serous cystadenoma

Clinical Features

MCNs are cyst-forming, mucinous neoplasms with a characteristic "ovarian-type" stroma that account for approximately 8% of resected pancreatic cysts. With very rare exceptions, MCNs occur in women. Like most cystic pancreatic neoplasms, MCNs have been reported in individuals over a wide age range, but they are most commonly detected in women during the fifth decade of life (mean age at presentation, 48 years).

Some patients with MCNs present with non-specific abdominal complaints that can be attributed to mass effect, whereas a significant proportion of individuals are entirely asymptomatic and the lesion is discovered incidentally via cross-sectional imaging studies performed for another indication. In over 98% of cases, the neoplasm is present in the distal pancreatic body or tail, though they have rarely been reported in the pancreatic head as well. The lesion is typically solitary and well-defined with central and peripheral septations, occasional mural nodules, and no communication with the main pancreatic duct.

MCNs are established precursor lesions to a subset of PDAC. There appears to be a strong association with tumor size and risk of concomitant invasive adenocarcinoma. In one series, MCNs with foci of invasive adenocarcinoma averaged 9.4 cm, whereas those without an invasive component were significantly smaller at 5.4 cm. The presence of intracystic papillary mural nodules is also a well-defined risk factor for malignant progression and is detectable with high-quality cross-sectional imaging studies. However, it is important to note that invasive adenocarcinomas do develop in smaller MCNs and those without solid mural nodules, highlighting the difficulty in risk-stratifying these lesions preoperatively. Given that MCNs without an invasive component are cured with resection, and even small foci of invasive carcinoma are associated with significant mortality, all patients with these lesions should be referred for potential surgical intervention.

Pathologic Features

GROSS FINDINGS

MCNs form well-circumscribed cystic masses in the distal pancreas with thick, occasionally calcified fibrous capsules. Careful dissection will universally fail to demonstrate continuity of the lesion with the pancreatic ductal system, though fistula tracts may develop with the ducts and adjacent structures, including the stomach. These neoplasms can grow to impressive sizes, but average 6 cm in greatest extent. On cut section, MCNs are generally multilocular, composed of variably sized cysts containing thick, inspissated mucus and blood that are separated by internal septations.

Thickened septae, foci of nodular growth of stromal tissue, and true intracystic papillary excrescences are occasionally encountered and may be associated with foci of invasive carcinoma, particularly when these papillary nodules measure greater than 1 cm. Extensive sampling of these foci is absolutely required. However, complete submission of the entire cyst for histologic examination should be strongly considered in most instances since even small foci of septal invasion may be associated with a risk for disease progression and poor outcome.

MICROSCOPIC FINDINGS

The cysts of MCNs are predominantly lined by tall columnar cells with abundant apical neutral mucin, though cuboidal cells with no obvious cytoplasmic mucin are occasionally encountered as well, as are foci with intestinal-type epithelium and goblet cells. The degree of cytologic and architectural atypia in the lining epithelium is graded in a two-tiered system. The epithelium of MCNs with low-grade dysplasia is simple with minimal architectural complexity and only mild to moderate cytologic atypia (Fig. 4.55). Some loss of nuclear polarity is generally considered to be acceptable in MCNs with low-grade dysplasia. In contrast, high-grade dysplasia is characterized by marked cytologic atypia with large, hyperchromatic nuclei, prominent nucleoli, and loss of cellular polarity. Complex papillary and microcapillary structures that project into the cysts are also frequently seen in the setting of high-grade dysplasia. Careful histologic examination of these lesions is required as foci of invasive carcinoma are identified in up to 15% of MCNs. While carcinoma arising in a background of MCNs is typically conventional PDAC, rare variants including undifferentiated carcinomas and UC-OGCs have also been reported.

Regardless of the degree of dysplasia or the presence of concomitant invasive carcinoma, the defining feature of all MCNs is the presence of a distinctive hypercellular subepithelial "ovarian-type" stroma made up of plump, uniform spindle cells with sparse cytoplasm. This distinctive stroma may be atrophic and hyalinized in postmenopausal patients or in foci of invasive carcinoma. Conversely, this spindle population may be exuberant in some cases, overshadowing the mucinous component of the tumor, or contain clusters of luteinized epithelioid cells with clear to eosinophilic cytoplasm.

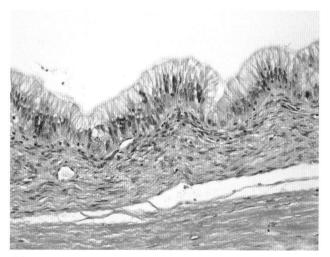

FIG. 4.55

Mucinous cystic neoplasm. Cysts are lined by tall columnar cells with abundant apical mucin. There is a distinctive subepithelial ovarian-type stroma composed of plump, uniform spindle cells. Lesions with low-grade dysplasia have a relatively simple epithelial lining, lacking complex papillary projections, and exhibit only mild to moderate cytologic atypia.

Ancillary Studies

The epithelium of MCNs express numerous cytokeratins, including CK7 and CK19, as well as MUC5AC, but generally not CK20 in the absence of significant intestinal differentiation. Conversely, MUC1 is not typically expressed in MCNs, but may be seen in foci of invasive carcinoma along with concomitant loss of SMAD4 expression.

The subepithelial ovarian-type stroma expresses SMA and desmin, as well as the progesterone receptor in most instances, which can assist in the accurate classification of these tumors in small biopsies or when the stromal component is atrophic and sparse.

EUS-FNA is useful in demonstrating the mucinous nature of MCNs but may not accurately classify these lesions if the stromal component is not adequately sampled. Similarly, biochemical studies performed on fresh cyst aspirates may reveal elevated CEA levels and again support the mucinous nature of these lesions. Molecular testing performed on these aspirates frequently demonstrate variants in *KRAS* and *TP53*, as well as *RNF43*, which do not distinguish MCNs from other mucinous pancreatic cysts. However, in contrast to IPMNs, alterations in *GNAS* are not a feature of MCNs and exclude this entity if detected in preoperative studies.

Differential Diagnosis

Differentiating MCNs from branch duct IPMNs is occasionally challenging, particularly if definite communication with the pancreatic ductal system cannot be demonstrated for the latter. In general, MCNs tend to occur in a slightly younger demographic, and nearly all patients are women. In contrast, IPMNs affect older individuals with a slight predilection for men. Furthermore, the vast majority of MCNs develop in the distal pancreatic body and tail, whereas IPMNs can be seen throughout the entire ductal system but are enriched in the pancreatic head.

There is significant overlap in the histologic features of MCNs and IPMNs, particularly with regard to the lining epithelium. The predominant cell type seen in MCNs is columnar with abundant apical neutral mucin, which is nearly indistinguishable from that seen in gastric-type IPMNs. Enteric-type epithelium with the formation of villi is generally not a feature of MCNs and strongly favors a diagnosis of intestinal-type IPMN, particularly if there is documented involvement of the main pancreatic duct. While papillary excrescences and large mural nodules are seen in a subset of cases, papillary structures are not frequent findings in MCNs but are typically florid and extensive in IPMNs.

Finally, the presence of distinctive ovarian-type stroma is highly specific for MCNs and is a required feature in order to render this diagnosis. It is important to remember that this ovarian-stroma may be thin and atrophic or hyalinized in postmenopausal patients, as well as in areas with high-grade dysplasia or carcinoma. Immunoreactivity for the progesterone receptor can assist with the identification of this stroma in challenging cases.

The radiographic differential diagnosis for cystic pancreatic tail lesions may include both MCNs and serous cystic neoplasms. This is particularly true for oligocystic serous cystadenomas which may lack the characteristic honeycomb appearance and central stellate scar seen in the more common microcystic variant of these tumors. The accurate preoperative classification of these tumors is, however, essential, given the significant differences in clinical management for mucinous and serous pancreatic neoplasms.

Sampling the contents of MCNs with EUS-FNA frequently yields obvious thick mucin, along with sheets of mucinous epithelium that can accurately classify these lesions as a neoplastic mucinous cyst, while aspirates from serous tumors are thin, proteinaceous, or bloody, and relatively paucicellular. Biochemical and molecular studies performed on cyst aspirates may also demonstrate an elevated CEA, as well as genetic variants in *KRAS*, *TP53*, and *RNF43* that are not features of serous neoplasms but fairly specific for neoplastic mucinous cysts of all types. Conversely, the detection of *VHL* variants supports a serous neoplasm.

MUCINOUS CYSTIC NEOPLASM – DISEASE FACT SHEET

Definition
▶▶ Mucinous neoplasm of the pancreas with distinctive ovarian-type stroma and absence of continuity with the ductal system

Incidence and Location
▶▶ Account for approximately 8% of resected pancreatic cysts
▶▶ Majority arise in the distal pancreatic body and pancreatic tail

Sex and Age Distribution
▶▶ Very strong predilection for women (greater than 98% of cases)
▶▶ Wide age range but most common in fifth decade of life (mean, 48 years)

Clinical Features
▶▶ Non-specific abdominal complaints
▶▶ Smaller lesions detected incidentally on cross-sectional imaging studies

Radiologic Features
▶▶ Solitary cystic lesions of the distal pancreas with septae
▶▶ No demonstrable communication with pancreatic ductal system
▶▶ Mural nodules and septal thickening high-risk features for associated malignancy

Prognosis and Therapy
▶▶ High risk of associated invasive carcinoma is larger lesions and those with mural nodules greater than 1 cm

▶▶ Given high risk of malignancy, resection standard of care in good surgical candidates
▶▶ Excellent prognosis if no associated invasive component
▶▶ Aggressive clinical course if associated with invasive carcinoma, particularly larger invasive carcinoma and those infiltrating beyond cyst wall

---

MUCINOUS CYSTIC NEOPLASM – PATHOLOGIC FEATURES

Gross Findings
▶▶ Well-circumscribed cystic mass in distal pancreas with thick fibrous capsule
▶▶ No true continuity with pancreatic ductal system but may fistulize with ducts and adjacent structures
▶▶ Average 6 cm in greatest extent
▶▶ Cut surfaces show multilocular cysts separated by internal septations of variable thickness
▶▶ Cysts contain tenacious neoplastic mucus
▶▶ Variable septal thickening and mural nodules

Microscopic Findings
▶▶ Cysts predominantly lined by tall columnar cells with apical neutral mucin that resemble gastric foveolar-type epithelium
▶▶ Smaller population of cuboidal pancreatobiliary-type cells
▶▶ Large amounts of enteric-type epithelium not characteristic but acceptable focally
▶▶ Low-grade lesions show relatively uniform cells with only mild to moderate atypia and an absence of complex papillary or cribriform architecture
▶▶ High-grade lesions show severe cytologic with loss of polarity, nuclear pleomorphism, and architectural complexity
▶▶ Distinctive hypercellular subepithelial ovarian-type stroma composed of spindle cells; may show hyalinization or patchy luteinization

Immunohistochemistry
▶▶ Mucinous epithelial cells express cytokeratins, including CK7 and CK19, but generally not CK20
▶▶ Reactive for MUC5AC
▶▶ Associated invasive component may express MUC1 and lose nuclear reactivity for SMAD4
▶▶ Ovarian-type stroma expresses SMA and desmin, and is at least focally reactive for the progesterone receptor in most instances

Pathologic Differential Diagnoses
▶▶ Intraductal papillary mucinous neoplasm, oligocystic serous cystadenoma

---

INTRADUCTAL PAPILLARY MUCINOUS NEOPLASM

DDX: intraductal tubulopapillary neoplasm, intraductal oncocytic papillary neoplasm

Clinical Features

IPMNs are mucin-producing epithelial neoplasms that arise within the pancreatic ductal system. They are fairly common neoplasms that are detected with increasing frequency in aging populations and are established precursor lesions to a subset of invasive ductal adenocarcinomas. Although some patients may present with abdominal pain, weight loss, or jaundice, many more IPMNs are detected incidentally on cross-sectional imaging studies performed for another indication. Endoscopic examination of the upper gastrointestinal tract may demonstrate mucin extrusion from a patulous ampulla of Vater, which is nearly pathognomonic for involvement of the main pancreatic duct.

Generally speaking, the intraductal neoplasms that are not associated with foci of invasive carcinoma have an excellent prognosis and are potentially cured with surgical resection alone. Approximately 23% of resected IPMNs, however, harbor invasive carcinoma or high-grade dysplasia, which follows a significantly more aggressive clinical course. In contrast to IPMNs confined to the pancreatic branch ducts, those involving the main pancreatic duct, or both branch ducts and the main pancreatic duct, are higher-risk lesions associated with an increased risk for progression to adenocarcinoma. Other high-risk features include large cyst size, or those that are increasing in size on serial imaging studies, as well as those associated with solid mural nodules or showing high-grade dysplasia on cytology.

Pathologic Features

GROSS FINDINGS

By definition, main-duct IPMNs involve the main pancreatic duct. Most involve the distal portion of the main pancreatic duct within the head of the pancreas, but can involve the entire length of the main pancreatic duct and extend into side-branch ducts as well. The ductal system is dilated and frequently filled with thick, tenacious mucin as well as soft, friable, mass-like papillary projections (Fig. 4.56). The ampulla of Vater may be soft and bulging as a result of the intraductal proliferation and may show the characteristic fish-mouth deformity.

Branch duct–type IPMNs do not directly involve the main pancreatic duct, though continuity may be demonstrable with careful gross examination and dissection. Branch duct–type IPMNs are most frequently encountered in the uncinate process but can develop anywhere in the pancreas. They form multilocular, grape-like cystic clusters filled with papillary excrescences and tenacious mucin.

MICROSCOPIC FINDINGS

All IPMNs are characterized by an intraductal proliferation of papillary structures lined by mucin-producing cuboidal to columnar epithelial cells. These neoplasms can be graded based upon the degree of architectural

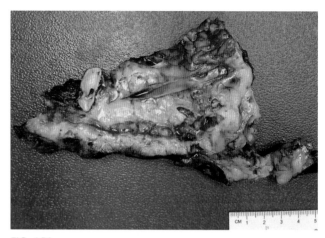

FIG. 4.56

Intraductal papillary mucinous neoplasm. The main pancreatic duct is diffusely dilated and contains thick, inspissated mucin. Branch ducts are similarly dilated in this case and contain friable, intracystic papillary projections.

complexity and cytologic atypia present. Low-grade IPMNs exhibit a flat to undulating pattern of growth with relatively simple papillary projections. The lining cells show mild to moderate atypia with nuclear enlargement and hyperchromasia, but no nuclear pleomorphism or loss of polarity. Nucleoli are generally inconspicuous and mitotic figures can be present but should not be abundant.

In contrast, high-grade IPMNs show more pronounced architectural complexity with branching papillary structures, cribriforming glands, and micropapillary tufts. Accompanying this increase in architectural complexity is higher grade cytology with marked variation in nuclear size, irregular nuclear contours and chromatin distribution, prominent nucleoli, and loss of polarity of neoplastic cells with respect to the basement membrane and adjacent cells. Brisk mitotic activity is frequently encountered in high-grade IPMNs, as are foci of tumor necrosis.

IPMNs can be further subtyped based upon the specific cytomorphologic features they display and mucin protein family they express. Gastric-type IPMNs are the most common subtype and are composed of epithelial cells that resemble gastric foveolar-type or endocervical-type epithelium. The have prominent apical neutral mucin caps and relatively regular, basally oriented, round to ovoid hyperchromatic nuclei (Fig. 4.57A). Gastric-type IPMNs typically lack significant architectural complexity. Simple papillae are commonly encountered, but many cysts lack such structures and exhibit undulating or even flat, attenuated surfaces. Most exhibit low-grade dysplasia.

Intestinal-type IPMNs frequently develop in the main pancreatic duct and resemble villous adenomas of the luminal gastrointestinal tract. The papillary structures of intestinal-type IPMNs are lined by crowded columnar cells with hyperchromatic pencillate nuclei and variable intracellular mucin that is typically less than that seen

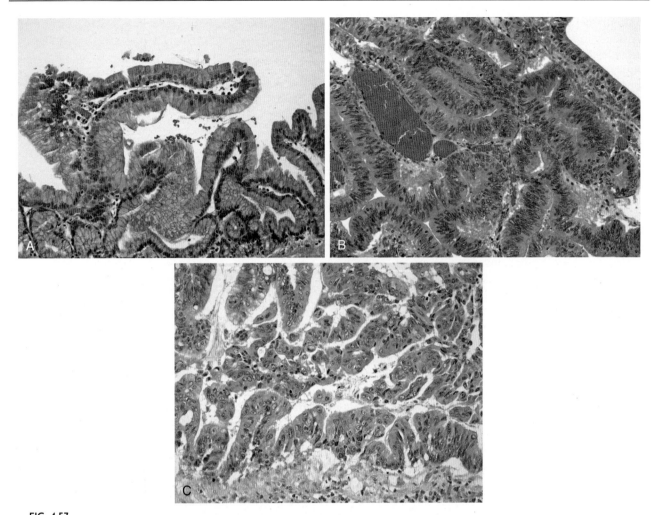

FIG. 4.57
Intraductal papillary mucinous neoplasm. **A,** Gastric-type intraductal papillary mucinous neoplasms lack significant architectural complexity and are lined by bland cells with abundant apical neutral mucin and basally oriented nuclei. **B,** Intestinal-type intraductal papillary mucinous neoplasms primarily develop in the main pancreatic duct and resemble villous adenomas of the luminal gastrointestinal tract. **C,** Pancreato-biliary-type intraductal papillary mucinous neoplasms exhibit a complex architectural pattern of growth and are composed of biliary-type cells with severe nuclear atypia.

in gastric-type neoplasms (Fig. 4.57B). Most show sufficient architectural complexity and cytologic atypia to warrant classification as high grade, though foci with less dramatic atypia and low-grade foveolar-type epithelium may also be encountered.

Pancreatobiliary-type IPMNs are the least common subtype and are universally high grade. They form complex branching papillary and tufting micropapillary structures that are lined by cuboidal and low columnar cells with amphophilic cytoplasm and pleomorphic nuclei with irregular contours and chromatin distribution, and variably prominent nucleoli (Fig. 4.57C). Cribriforming structures are frequently encountered, as are mitotic figures and foci of tumor necrosis.

A significant proportion of surgically resected IPMNs are associated with contiguous foci of invasive adenocarcinoma. Most carcinomas associated with IPMNs are typical gland-forming ductal adenocarcinomas. Approximately half of IPMN-associated carcinomas, however, are composed of large pools of paucicellular mucin containing strips and clusters of malignant epithelial cells and signet ring cells. These mucinous non-cystic, or colloid carcinomas, most frequently develop in association with intestinal-type IPMNs.

Ancillary Studies

Cystic neoplasms of the pancreas, particularly larger or growing lesions, or those associated with solid mural nodules, frequently undergo examination with EUS-FNA. Nearly all IPMNs contain detectable background mucin, which is frequently viscous or colloid-like. Clusters or sheets of columnar epithelial are detected in over 80% of IPMN aspirates, but the absence of an epithelial component does not exclude a neoplastic process.

The detection of high-grade cytologic atypia in pancreatic cyst aspirates may drive treatment decisions and result in patients being triaged to surgical resection. While the distinction between low-grade and high-grade dysplasia has historically been plagued by poor interobserver variability, the presence of large cells with increased N/C ratios, irregular nuclear membrane contours, and abnormal chromatin patterns, as well as the presence of background necrosis, appear to be associated with high-grade lesions.

Chemical analysis of fresh cyst aspirates may also assist in the accurate classification of cystic pancreatic neoplasms, particularly when combined with conventional cytologic studies. CEA levels greater than 192 ng/mL are fairly sensitive and specific for mucinous pancreatic cysts, while amylase levels less than 250 IU/L essentially exclude non-neoplastic pseudocysts. Similarly, next-generation sequencing studies can be performed on fresh cyst aspirates, as well as fixative-preserved genetic material, and may reveal alterations in *KRAS* and *GNAS* that support a mucinous etiology.

Like most epithelial pancreatobiliary neoplasms, IPMNs express broad-spectrum cytokeratins like CK AE1/AE3 and Cam5.2, as well as CK7 and CK19. Perhaps not surprisingly, intestinal-type IPMNs also express the intestinal transcription factor CDX2, as well as CK20. Specific mucin stains may also aid in the subtyping of IPMNs, as well as in differentiating these tumors from intraductal tubulopapillary neoplasms. Most IPMNs express MUC5AC. Pancreatobiliary-type IPMNs also express MUC1 and MUC6, while intestinal-type tumors lack expression of these markers but express the intestinal mucin MUC2. Gastric-type IPMNs lack expression of MUC1 and MUC2 but may express MUC6.

Differential Diagnosis

Intraductal tubulopapillary neoplasms are rare lesions with overlapping clinical and pathologic findings with IPMNs. They are more common in middle age individuals, though they have been reported over a wide range of ages, and are slightly more common in women. Patients may present with vague abdominal complaints, but these neoplasms are more commonly detected incidentally on cross-sectional imaging studies. On CT, intraductal tubulopapillary neoplasms show an irregularly dilated main pancreatic duct that is similar to that seen with main duct IPMNs, but lacking abundant low-attenuation mucin. Intraductal growth causes obstruction and accumulation of non-mucinous fluid in the distal pancreatic duct, leading to a "two-tone duct" or "cork-of-wine-bottle" signs on cholangiopancreatography.

In contrast to the predominantly papillary architecture seen in IPMNs, intraductal tubulopapillary neoplasms form cellular nodules that expand and fill the

ductal system with tubules and irregular cribriform glands (Fig. 4.58A). The nodules of intraductal growth are usually well circumscribed and separated from the adjacent pancreatic parenchyma by dense fibrosis. Cytologically, intraductal tubulopapillary neoplasms are composed of relatively uniform cuboidal cells with amphophilic cytoplasm and ovoid nuclei with coarse chromatin. Intracellular and luminal mucin is not typical, though amorphous acidophilic secretions may be seen in some cases. Brisk mitotic activity is usually present and, coupled with the architectural complexity of this intraductal proliferation, warrants a diagnosis of high-grade dysplasia by default.

Intraductal tubulopapillary neoplasms are associated with a component of invasive carcinoma in 70% of cases. The associated invasive carcinoma is usually a gland-forming typical ductal adenocarcinoma, but may

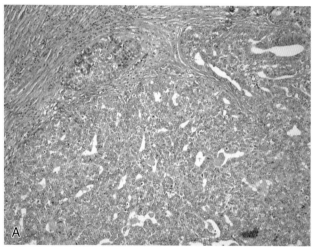

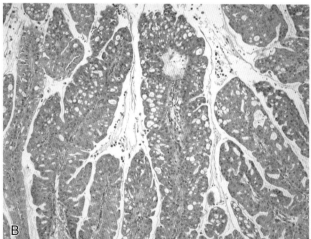

FIG. 4.58

A, Intraductal tubulopapillary neoplasms expand the pancreatic ductal system with obvious tubules and cribriform glands. Mitotic activity is usually identifiable and glands may contain acidophilic secretions rather than mucin. **B,** Intraductal oncocytic papillary neoplasms show papillary growth but may fuse into more solid sheets of neoplastic cells. The cells are polygonal and have granular eosinophilic cytoplasm. Intracytoplasmic lumina with mucin are conspicuous and impart an appearance of punched-out spaces.

be very focal and difficult to appreciate necessitating extensive or complete sampling for histologic evaluation. Generally, however, invasive carcinomas associated with intraductal tubulopapillary neoplasms have a significantly better prognosis that typical PDACs and those associated with IPMNs.

Given the relatively good prognosis associated with these tumors, the accurate distinction between intraductal tubulopapillary neoplasms and IPMNs is essential. Immunohistochemical stains for specific mucin glycoproteins may be helpful in some instances, as all IPMNs regardless of subtype express MUC5AC, while MUC5AC expression is extremely rare in intraductal tubulopapillary neoplasms. Molecular studies may also be useful in some instances. While most pancreatic epithelial neoplasms show alterations in *KRAS*, MAPK pathway alterations are not a feature of intraductal tubulopapillary neoplasms. Instead, alterations in chromatin remodeling genes, the PI3K pathway, and, rarely, *FGFR2* fusions are characteristic of these tumors.

Intraductal oncocytic papillary mucinous neoplasms are relatively rare intraductal proliferations that develop over a wide age range (mean age, 67 years) and have a slight predilection for women. While some patients present with abdominal pain, CP, or features of biliary obstruction, many, like other intraductal pancreatic neoplasms, are discovered incidentally on cross-sectional imaging.

There is, however, significant overlap between the imaging characteristics and gross pathologic features of intraductal tubulopapillary neoplasms with IPMNs, with both showing cystic transformation of a portion of the ductal system and associated mural nodules or friable papillary projections. Histologically, intraductal oncocytic papillary neoplasm exhibits a complex, arborizing pattern of papillary growth supported by fine fibrovascular cores. Cytologically, the papillary structures are lined by epithelioid cells with abundant granular eosinophilic cytoplasm and large, round nuclei with prominent nucleoli (Fig. 4.58B). Goblet cells may be present and do not imply intestinal differentiation in the setting of extensive background oncocytic transformation. Papillary structures may fuse and form solid sheets of neoplastic cells that frequently contain punched-out mucin-containing spaces. Up to a third of these tumors contain foci of invasive carcinoma. The invasive component is usually tubular in nature, but single infiltrating cells that retain the oncocytic features of the precursor lesion may also be present. Rarely, the invasive component may contain elements that resemble colloid carcinoma with abundant pools of extracellular mucin similar to that seen associated with intestinal-type IPMNs, though pure colloid carcinomas are not characteristic.

It may be challenging to differentiate intraductal oncocytic papillary neoplasms from pancreatobiliary-type IPMN. Both usually show sufficient cytologic atypia and architectural atypia to be classified as exhibiting high-grade dysplasia. Distinction may be important as

carcinomas associated with intraductal oncocytic papillary neoplasms are generally associated with an outstanding prognosis, and local recurrence can be treated with re-excision. The presence of abundant oncocytic cytoplasm and punched-out, mucin-containing intracellular lumina are fairly specific for intraductal oncocytic papillary neoplasm. Immunohistochemical stains for specific mucin glycoproteins are generally not helpful, though pancreatobiliary-type IPMNs are more consistently positive for MUC1 and show less intense MUC6 expression than intraductal oncocytic papillary neoplasms. Intraductal oncocytic papillary neoplasms show immunoreactivity for the hepatocellular marker HepPar1 but are negative for albumin by *in situ* hybridization. From a molecular standpoint, while most IPMNs, including pancreatobiliary-type tumors, exhibit genetic alterations in *KRAS*, *GNAS*, or *TP53* (particularly if there is high-grade dysplasia), intraductal oncocytic papillary neoplasm are generally believed to lack mutations in these genes, though exceptions have been reported.

INTRADUCTAL PAPILLARY MUCINOUS NEOPLASM – DISEASE FACT SHEET

Definition
▸▸ Intraductal mucin-producing neoplasm that involves main pancreatic duct and/or branch ducts

Incidence and Location
▸▸ Fairly common accounting for approximately 5% of all pancreatic neoplasms
▸▸ Can involve any portion of the ductal system, though most frequently identified in pancreatic head (up to 80%)
▸▸ May be multifocal

Sex and Age Distribution
▸▸ Strong male predilection for main duct–type intraductal papillary mucinous neoplasms in Japan and Korea
▸▸ Less pronounced sex disparity in the United States
▸▸ Increasing frequency with advancing age
▸▸ Mean age of 62–67 years

Clinical Features
▸▸ Epigastric abdominal pain
▸▸ Weight loss
▸▸ Jaundice
▸▸ Asymptomatic

Radiologic Features
▸▸ MRCP demonstrates segmental or diffuse dilation (greater than 5 mm) of the main pancreatic duct filled with low-density mucinous material (main duct type)
▸▸ Branch duct–type intraductal papillary mucinous neoplasm show cystic mass-like lesion resembling bunch of grapes
▸▸ Solid mural nodules concerning for malignant transformation

Prognosis and Therapy
▸▸ Surgical resection of large or growing intraductal papillary mucinous neoplasms, as well as those involving the main pancreatic duct, with solid mural components, or demonstrating high-grade cytology

▸▸ Low-grade intraductal papillary mucinous neoplasms cured with resection, though tumor recurrence/metachronous tumor development is common
▸▸ Prognosis significantly worse if associated with foci of invasive adenocarcinoma

---

INTRADUCTAL PAPILLARY MUCINOUS NEOPLASM – PATHOLOGIC FEATURES

Gross Findings

▸▸ Dilation of main pancreatic duct and/or branch ducts
▸▸ Main duct intraductal papillary mucinous neoplasms are frequently associated with patulous ampulla of Vater with fish-mouth appearance and extruding mucin
▸▸ Ductal system with thick, inspissated mucin
▸▸ Mass-like papillary projections project into dilated ductal system
▸▸ Firm mural nodules and infiltrative appearing periductal fibrous tissue suspicious for associated carcinoma

Microscopic Findings

▸▸ Complex papillary structures lined by mucin-producing cells
▸▸ Gastric-type lesions most common and lined by tall columnar cells with abundant apical neutral mucin caps
▸▸ Intestinal-type lesions typically involve main pancreatic duct and have enlarged, overlapping penicillate nuclei and less conspicuous cytoplasmic mucin; resembles villous adenoma
▸▸ Pancreatobiliary-type lesions have complex branching papillary structures lined by atypical cuboidal to low columnar cells with marked atypia
▸▸ Most intestinal and pancreatobiliary-type intraductal papillary mucinous neoplasms interpreted as having high-grade dysplasia

Immunohistochemistry

▸▸ Immunoreactive for CK7 and CK19
▸▸ All subtypes express the mucin glycoprotein MUC5AC
▸▸ Intestinal-type intraductal papillary mucinous neoplasms express MUC2, CK20, and CDX2
▸▸ Pancreatobiliary-type intraductal papillary mucinous neoplasms express MUC1 and MUC6

Pathologic Differential Diagnoses

▸▸ Intraductal tubulopapillary neoplasm
▸▸ Intraductal oncocytic papillary neoplasm

SUGGESTED READINGS

Focal Nodular Hyperplasia

Altavilla G, Guariso G. Focal nodular hyperplasia of the liver associated with portal vein agenesis: a morphological and immunohistochemical study of one case and review of the literature. *Adv Clin Path*. 1999; 3(4):139-145.

Bioulac-Sage P, Laumonier H, Rullier A, et al. Over-expression of glutamine synthetase in focal nodular hyperplasia: a novel easy diagnostic tool in surgical pathology. *Liver Int*. 2009;29(3):459-465.

Joseph NM, Ferrell LD, Jain D, et al. Diagnostic utility and limitations of glutamine synthetase and serum amyloid-associated protein immunohistochemistry in the distinction of focal nodular hyperplasia and inflammatory hepatocellular adenoma. *Mod Pathol*. 2014; 27(1):62-72.

Navarro AP, Gomez D, Lamb CM, Brooks A, Cameron IC. Focal nodular hyperplasia: a review of current indications for and outcomes of hepatic resection. *HPB (Oxford)*. 2014;16(6):503-511.

Nguyen BN, Fléjou JF, Terris B, Belghiti J, Degott C. Focal nodular hyperplasia of the liver: a comprehensive pathologic study of 305 lesions and recognition of new histologic forms. *Am J Surg Pathol*. 1999;23(12):1441-1454.

Paradis V, Laurent A, Flejou JF, Vidaud M, Bedossa P. Evidence for the polyclonal nature of focal nodular hyperplasia of the liver by the study of X-chromosome inactivation. *Hepatology*. 1997;26(4):891-895.

Hepatocellular Adenoma

Bioulac-Sage P, Rebouissou S, Thomas C, et al. Hepatocellular adenoma subtype classification using molecular markers and immunohistochemistry. *Hepatology*. 2007;46(3):740-748.

Bioulac-Sage P, Sempoux C, Balabaud C. Hepatocellular adenoma: classification, variants and clinical relevance. *Semin Diagn Pathol*. 2017;34(2):112-125.

Cho SJ, Ferrell LD, Gill RM. Expression of liver fatty acid binding protein in hepatocellular carcinoma. *Hum Pathol*. 2016;50:135-139.

Evason KJ, Grenert JP, Ferrell LD, Kakar S. Atypical hepatocellular adenoma-like neoplasms with β-catenin activation show cytogenetic alterations similar to well-differentiated hepatocellular carcinomas. *Hum Pathol*. 2013;44(5):750-758.

Hale G, Liu X, Hu J, et al. Correlation of exon 3 β-catenin mutations with glutamine synthetase staining patterns in hepatocellular adenoma and hepatocellular carcinoma. *Mod Pathol*. 2016;29(11):1370-1380.

Joseph NM, Umetsu SE, Shafizadeh N, Ferrell L, Kakar S. Genomic profiling of well-differentiated hepatocellular neoplasms with diffuse glutamine synthetase staining reveals similar genetics across the adenoma to carcinoma spectrum. *Mod Pathol*. 2019;32(11):1627-1636.

Kakar S, Grenert JP, Paradis V, Pote N, Jakate S, Ferrell LD. Hepatocellular carcinoma arising in adenoma: similar immunohistochemical and cytogenetic features in adenoma and hepatocellular carcinoma portions of the tumor. *Mod Pathol*. 2014;27(11):1499-1509.

Liu L, Shah SS, Naini BV, et al. Immunostains used to subtype hepatic adenomas do not distinguish hepatic adenomas from hepatocellular carcinomas. *Am J Surg Pathol*. 2016;40(8):1062-1069.

Nault JC, Bioulac-Sage P, Zucman-Rossi J. Hepatocellular benign tumors-from molecular classification to personalized clinical care. *Gastroenterology*. 2013;144(5):888-902.

Rebouissou S, Franconi A, Calderaro J, et al. Genotype-phenotype correlation of CTNNB1 mutations reveals different ß-catenin activity associated with liver tumor progression. *Hepatology*. 2016;64(6):2047-2061.

Zucman-Rossi J, Jeannot E, Nhieu JT, et al. Genotype-phenotype correlation in hepatocellular adenoma: new classification and relationship with HCC. *Hepatology*. 2006;43(3):515-524.

Hepatocellular Carcinoma

Calderaro J, Couchy G, Imbeaud S, et al. Histological subtypes of hepatocellular carcinoma are related to gene mutations and molecular tumour classification. *J Hepatol*. 2017;67(4):727-738.

Graham RP, Torbenson MS. Fibrolamellar carcinoma: a histologically unique tumor with unique molecular findings. *Semin Diagn Pathol*. 2017;34(2):146-152.

Honeyman JN, Simon EP, Robine N, et al. Detection of a recurrent DNAJB1-PRKACA chimeric transcript in fibrolamellar hepatocellular carcinoma. *Science*. 2014;343(6174):1010-1014.

Jakate S, Yabes A, Giusto D, et al. Diffuse cirrhosis-like hepatocellular carcinoma: a clinically and radiographically undetected variant mimicking cirrhosis. *Am J Surg Pathol*. 2010;34(7):935-941.

Jeon Y, Benedict M, Taddei T, Jain D, Zhang X. Macrotrabecular hepatocellular carcinoma: an aggressive subtype of hepatocellular carcinoma. *Am J Surg Pathol*. 2019;43(7):943-948.

Liu PH, Hsu CY, Hsia CY, et al. Prognosis of hepatocellular carcinoma: assessment of eleven staging systems. *J Hepatol*. 2016;64(3):601-608.

Krings G, Ramachandran R, Jain D, et al. Immunohistochemical pitfalls and the importance of glypican 3 and arginase in the diagnosis of scirrhous hepatocellular carcinoma. *Mod Pathol*. 2013;26(6):782-791.

Mazzaferro V, Regalia E, Doci R, et al. Liver transplantation for the treatment of small hepatocellular carcinomas in patients with cirrhosis. *N Engl J Med*. 1996;334(11):693-699.

Roberts DE, Kakar S, Mehta N, Gill RM. A point-based histologic scoring system for hepatocellular carcinoma can stratify risk of posttransplant tumor recurrence. *Am J Surg Pathol*. 2018;42(7):855-865.

Salomao M, Yu WM, Brown Jr RS, Emond JC, Lefkowitch JH. Steatohepatitic hepatocellular carcinoma (SH-HCC): a distinctive histological variant of HCC in hepatitis C virus-related cirrhosis with associated NAFLD/NASH. *Am J Surg Pathol*. 2010;34(11):1630-1636.

Ziol M, Poté N, Amaddeo G, et al. Macrotrabecular-massive hepatocellular carcinoma: a distinctive histological subtype with clinical relevance. *Hepatology.* 2018;68(1):103-112.

Hepatoblastoma

Adesina AM, Lopez-Terrada D, Wong KK, et al. Gene expression profiling reveals signatures characterizing histologic subtypes of hepatoblastoma and global deregulation in cell growth and survival pathways. *Hum Pathol.* 2009;40(6):843-853.

Czauderna P, Lopez-Terrada D, Hiyama E, Häberle B, Malogolowkin MH, Meyers RL. Hepatoblastoma state of the art: pathology, genetics, risk stratification, and chemotherapy. *Curr Opin Pediatr.* 2014;26(1):19-28.

López-Terrada D, Alaggio R, de Dávila MT, et al. Towards an international pediatric liver tumor consensus classification: proceedings of the Los Angeles COG liver tumors symposium. *Mod Pathol.* 2014;27(3):472-491.

Malogolowkin MH, Katzenstein HM, Meyers RL, et al. Complete surgical resection is curative for children with hepatoblastoma with pure fetal histology: a report from the Children's Oncology Group. *J Clin Oncol.* 2011;29(24):3301-3306.

Sharma D, Subbarao G, Saxena R. Hepatoblastoma. *Semin Diagn Pathol.* 2017;34(2):192-200.

Spector LG, Birch J. The epidemiology of hepatoblastoma. *Pediatr Blood Cancer.* 2012;59(5):776-779.

Sumazin P, Chen Y, Treviño LR, et al. Genomic analysis of hepatoblastoma identifies distinct molecular and prognostic subgroups. *Hepatology.* 2017;65(1):104-121.

Bile Duct Adenoma

Allaire GS, Rabin L, Ishak KG, Sesterhenn IA. Bile duct adenoma. A study of 152 cases. *Am J Surg Pathol.* 1988;12(9):708-715.

Bhathal PS, Hughes NR, Goodman ZD. The so-called bile duct adenoma is a peribiliary gland hamartoma. *Am J Surg Pathol.* 1996;20(7):858-864.

Pujals A, Bioulac-Sage P, Castain C, Charpy C, Zafrani ES, Calderaro J. BRAF V600E mutational status in bile duct adenomas and hamartomas. *Histopathology.* 2015;67(4):562-567.

Tsokos CG, Krings G, Yilmaz F, Ferrell LD, Gill RM. Proliferative index facilitates distinction between benign biliary lesions and intrahepatic cholangiocarcinoma. *Hum Pathol.* 2016;57:61-67.

Hornick JL, Lauwers GY, Odze RD. Immunohistochemistry can help distinguish metastatic pancreatic adenocarcinomas from bile duct adenomas and hamartomas of the liver. *Am J Surg Pathol.* 2005;29(3):381-389.

Biliary Hamartoma

Jain D, Ahrens W, Finkelstein S. Molecular evidence for the neoplastic potential of hepatic Von-Meyenburg complexes. *Appl Immunohistochem Mol Morphol.* 2010;18(2):166-171.

Jain D, Sarode VR, Abdul-Karim FW, Homer R, Robert ME. Evidence for the neoplastic transformation of Von-Meyenburg complexes. *Am J Surg Pathol.* 2000;24(8):1131-1139.

Raynaud P, Tate J, Callens C, et al. A classification of ductal plate malformations based on distinct pathogenic mechanisms of biliary dysmorphogenesis. *Hepatology.* 2011;53(6):1959-1966.

Song JS, Lee YJ, Kim KW, Huh J, Jang SJ, Yu E. Cholangiocarcinoma arising in von Meyenburg complexes: report of four cases. *Pathol Int.* 2008;58(8):503-512.

Torbenson MS. Hamartomas and malformations of the liver. *Semin Diagn Pathol.* 2019;36(1):39-47.

Cholangiocarcinoma

Aishima S, Oda Y. Pathogenesis and classification of intrahepatic cholangiocarcinoma: different characters of perihilar large duct type versus peripheral small duct type. *J Hepatobiliary Pancreat Sci.* 2015;22(2):94-100.

Bridgewater J, Galle PR, Khan SA, et al. Guidelines for the diagnosis and management of intrahepatic cholangiocarcinoma. *J Hepatol.* 2014;60(6):1268-1289.

Cardinale V, Semeraro R, Torrice A, et al. Intra-hepatic and extra-hepatic cholangiocarcinoma: new insight into epidemiology and risk factors. *World J Gastrointest Oncol.* 2010;2(11):407-416.

Hayashi A, Misumi K, Shibahara J, et al. Distinct clinicopathologic and genetic features of 2 histologic subtypes of intrahepatic cholangiocarcinoma. *Am J Surg Pathol.* 2016;40(8):1021-1030.

Krasinskas AM. Cholangiocarcinoma. *Surg Pathol Clin.* 2018;11(2):403-429.

Nakanuma Y, Sato Y, Ikeda H, et al. Intrahepatic cholangiocarcinoma with predominant "ductal plate malformation" pattern: a new subtype. *Am J Surg Pathol.* 2012;36(11):1629-1635.

Nasir A, Lehrke HD, Mounajjed T, et al. Albumin in situ hybridization can be positive in adenocarcinomas and other tumors from diverse sites. *Am J Clin Pathol.* 2019;152(2):190-199.

Shahid M, Mubeen A, Tse J, et al. Branched chain in situ hybridization for albumin as a marker of hepatocellular differentiation: evaluation of manual and automated in situ hybridization platforms. *Am J Surg Pathol.* 2015;39(1):25-34.

Sigel CS, Drill E, Zhou Y, et al. Intrahepatic cholangiocarcinomas have histologically and immunophenotypically distinct small and large duct patterns. *Am J Surg Pathol.* 2018;42(10):1334-1345.

Tsokos CG, Krings G, Yilmaz F, Ferrell LD, Gill RM. Proliferative index facilitates distinction between benign biliary lesions and intrahepatic cholangiocarcinoma. *Hum Pathol.* 2016;57:61-67.

Wang T, Drill E, Vakiani E, et al. Distinct histomorphological features are associated with IDH1 mutation in intrahepatic cholangiocarcinoma. *Hum Pathol.* 2019;91:19-25.

Angiomyolipoma

Jimbo N, Nishigami T, Noguchi M, et al. Hepatic angiomyolipomas may overexpress TFE3, but have no relevant genetic alterations. *Hum Pathol.* 2017;61:41-48.

Kamimura K, Nomoto M, Aoyagi Y. Hepatic angiomyolipoma: diagnostic findings and management. *Int J Hepatol.* 2012;2012:410781.

Kannangai R, Diehl AM, Sicklick J, Rojkind M, Thomas D, Torbenson M. Hepatic angiomyolipoma and hepatic stellate cells share a similar gene expression profile. *Hum Pathol.* 2005;36(4):341-347.

Klompenhouwer AJ, Verver D, Janki S, et al. Management of hepatic angiomyolipoma: a systematic review. *Liver Int.* 2017;37(9):1272-1280.

Petrolla AA, Xin W. Hepatic angiomyolipoma. *Arch Pathol Lab Med.* 2008;132(10):1679-1682.

Tsui WM, Colombari R, Portmann BC, et al. Hepatic angiomyolipoma: a clinicopathologic study of 30 cases and delineation of unusual morphologic variants. *Am J Surg Pathol.* 1999;23(1):34-48.

Xie L, Jessurun J, Manivel JC, Pambuccian SE. Hepatic epithelioid angiomyolipoma with trabecular growth pattern: a mimic of hepatocellular carcinoma on fine needle aspiration cytology. *Diagn Cytopathol.* 2012;40(7):639-650.

Yan Z, Grenert JP, Joseph NM, et al. Hepatic angiomyolipoma: mutation analysis and immunohistochemical pitfalls in diagnosis. *Histopathology.* 2018;73(1):101-108.

Epithelioid Hemangioendothelioma

Antonescu CR, Le Loarer F, Mosquera JM, et al. Novel YAP1-TFE3 fusion defines a distinct subset of epithelioid hemangioendothelioma. *Genes Chromosomes Cancer.* 2013;52(8):775-784.

Doyle LA, Fletcher CD, Hornick JL. Nuclear expression of CAMTA1 distinguishes epithelioid hemangioendothelioma from histologic mimics. *Am J Surg Pathol.* 2016;40(1):94-102.

Errani C, Sung YS, Zhang L, Healey JH, Antonescu CR. Monoclonality of multifocal epithelioid hemangioendothelioma of the liver by analysis of WWTR1-CAMTA1 breakpoints. *Cancer Genet.* 2012;205(1-2):12-17.

Flucke U, Vogels RJ, de Saint Aubain Somerhausen N, et al. Epithelioid hemangioendothelioma: clinicopathologic, immunohistochemical, and molecular genetic analysis of 39 cases. *Diagn Pathol.* 2014;9:131.

Ishak KG, Sesterhenn IA, Goodman ZD, Rabin L, Stromeyer FW. Epithelioid hemangioendothelioma of the liver: a clinicopathologic and follow-up study of 32 cases. *Hum Pathol.* 1984;15(9):839-852.

Jurczyk M, Zhu B, Laskin W, Lin X. Pitfalls in the diagnosis of hepatic epithelioid hemangioendothelioma by FNA and needle core biopsy. *Diagn Cytopathol.* 2014;42(6):516-520.

Lee SJ, Yang WI, Chung WS, Kim SK. Epithelioid hemangioendotheliomas with TFE3 gene translocations are compossible with CAMTA1 gene rearrangements. *Oncotarget.* 2016;7(7):7480-7488.

Makhlouf HR, Ishak KG, Goodman ZD. Epithelioid hemangioendothelioma of the liver: a clinicopathologic study of 137 cases. *Cancer.* 1999;85(3):562-582.

Shibuya R, Matsuyama A, Shiba E, Harada H, Yabuki K, Hisaoka M. CAMTA1 is a useful immunohistochemical marker for diagnosing epithelioid haemangioendothelioma. *Histopathology*. 2015;67(6):827-835.

Tanas MR, Sboner A, Oliveira AM, et al. Identification of a disease-defining gene fusion in epithelioid hemangioendothelioma. *Sci Transl Med*. 2011;3(98):98ra82.

Weiss SW, Enzinger FM. Epithelioid hemangioendothelioma: a vascular tumor often mistaken for a carcinoma. *Cancer*. 1982;50(5):970-981.

Chronic Pancreatitis

Klöppel G. Chronic pancreatitis, pseudotumors and other tumor-like lesions. *Mod Pathol*. 2007;20(1):S113-S131. Available at: https://doi.org/10.1038/modpathol.3800690.

Singh VK, Yadav D, Garg PK. Diagnosis and management of chronic pancreatitis: a review. *JAMA*. 2019;322(24):2422-2434. Available at: https://doi.org/10.1001/jama.2019.19411.

Kleeff J, Whitcomb DC, Shimosegawa T, et al. Chronic pancreatitis. *Nat Rev Dis Primers*. 2017;3:17060. Available at: https://doi.org/10.1038/nrdp.2017.60.

Autoimmune Pancreatitis

Schneider A, Michaely H, Rückert F, et al. Diagnosing autoimmune pancreatitis with the Unifying-Autoimmune-Pancreatitis-Criteria. *Pancreatology*. 2017;17(3):381-394. Available at: https://doi.org/10.1016/j.pan.2017.03.005.

Shimosegawa T, Chari ST, Frulloni L, et al. International consensus diagnostic criteria for autoimmune pancreatitis: Guidelines of the International Association of Pancreatology. *Pancreas*. 2011;40(3):352-358. Available at: https://doi.org/10.1097/MPA.0b013e3182142fd2.

Klöppel G, Lüttges J, Sipos B, Capelli P, Zamboni G. Autoimmune pancreatitis: pathological findings. *JOP*. 2005;6(suppl 1):97-101.

Paraduodenal Pancreatitis

Casetti L, Bassi C, Salvia R, et al. "Paraduodenal" pancreatitis: results of surgery on 58 consecutives patients from a single institution. *World J Surg*. 2009;33(12):2664-2669. Available at: https://doi.org/10.1007/s00268-009-0238-5.

Adsay NV, Zamboni G. Paraduodenal pancreatitis: a clinico-pathologically distinct entity unifying "cystic dystrophy of heterotopic pancreas," "para-duodenal wall cyst," and "groove pancreatitis." *Semin Diagn Pathol*. 2004;21(4):247-254. Available at: https://doi.org/10.1053/j.semdp.2005.07.005.

Lymphoepithelial Cyst

Policarpio-Nicolas ML, Shami VM, Kahaleh M, et al. Fine-needle aspiration cytology of pancreatic lymphoepithelial cysts. *Cancer*. 2006;108(6):501-506. Available at: https://doi.org/10.1002/cncr.22289.

Adsay NV, Hasteh F, Cheng JD, et al. Lymphoepithelial cysts of the pancreas: a report of 12 cases and a review of the literature. *Mod Pathol*. 2002;15(5):492-501. Available at: https://doi.org/10.1038/modpathol.3880553.

VandenBussche CJ, Maleki Z. Fine-needle aspiration of squamous-lined cysts of the pancreas. *Diagn Cytopathol*. 2014;42(7):592-599. Available at: https://doi.org/10.1002/dc.23080.

Squamoid Cyst

Othman M, Basturk O, Groisman G, Krasinskas A, Adsay NV. Squamoid cyst of pancreatic ducts: a distinct type of cystic lesion in the pancreas. *Am J Surg Pathol*. 2007;31(2):291-297. Available at: https://doi.org/10.1097/01.pas.0000213349.42143.ec.

Yoo DG, Hwang S, Hwang DW, et al. Case report of a pancreatic squamoid cyst. *Korean J Hepatobiliary Pancreat Surg*. 2013;17(4):181-185. Available at: https://doi.org/10.14701/kjhbps.2013.17.4.181.

Intrapancreatic Accessory Spleen

Li BQ, Xu XQ, Guo JC. Intrapancreatic accessory spleen: a diagnostic dilemma. *HPB*. 2018;20(11):1004-1011. Available at: https://doi.org/10.1016/j.hpb.2018.04.004.

Jang KM, Kim SH, Lee SJ, Park MJ, Lee MI I, Choi D. Differentiation of an intrapancreatic accessory spleen from a small (<3-cm) solid pancreatic tumor: value of diffusion-weighted MR imaging. *Radiology*. 2013;266(1):159-167. Available at: https://doi.org/10.1148/radiol.12112765.

Pancreatic Ductal Adenocarcinoma

Ren B, Liu X, Suriawinata AA. Pancreatic ductal adenocarcinoma and its precursor lesions. *Am J Pathol*. 2019;189(1):9-21. Available at: https://doi.org/10.1016/j.ajpath.2018.10.004.

Stark AP, Sacks GD, Rochefort MM, et al. Long-term survival in patients with pancreatic ductal adenocarcinoma. *Surgery*. 2016;159(6):1520-1527. Available at: https://doi.org/10.1016/j.surg.2015.12.024.

Oshima M, Okano K, Muraki S, et al. Immunohistochemically detected expression of 3 major genes (CDKN2A/P16, TP53, and SMAD4/DPC4) strongly predicts survival in patients with resectable pancreatic cancer. *Ann Surg*. 2013;258(2):336-346. Available at: https://doi.org/10.1097/SLA.0b013e3182827a65.

Gonzalez RS, Bagci P, Basturk O, et al. Intrapancreatic distal common bile duct carcinoma. *Mod Pathol*. 2016;29(11):1358-1369. Available at: https://doi.org/10.1038/modpathol.2016.125.

Acinar Cell Carcinoma

La Rosa S, Sessa F, Capella C. Acinar cell carcinoma of the pancreas: overview of clinicopathologic features and insights into the molecular pathology. *Front Med*. 2015;2:41. Available at: https://doi.org/10.3389/fmed.2015.00041.

Chmielecki J, Hutchinson KE, Frampton GM, et al. Comprehensive genomic profiling of pancreatic acinar cell carcinomas identifies recurrent RAF fusions and frequent inactivation of DNA repair genes. *Cancer Discov*. 2014;4(12):1398-1405. Available at: https://doi.org/10.1158/2159-8290.CD-14-0617.

Schempf U, Sipos B, König C, Malek NP, Bitzer M, Plentz RR. FOLFIRINOX as first-line treatment for unresectable acinar cell carcinoma of the pancreas: a case report. *Z Gastroenterol*. 2014;52(2):200-203. Available at: https://doi.org/10.1055/s-0033-1356439.

Pancreatoblastoma

Abraham SC, Wu TT, Klimstra DS, et al. Distinctive molecular genetic alterations in sporadic and familial adenomatous polyposis-associated pancreatoblastomas: frequent alterations in the APC/beta-catenin pathway and chromosome 11p. *Am J Pathol*. 2001;159(5):1619-1627. Available at: https://doi.org/10.1016/S0002-9440(10)63008-8.

Reid MD, Bhattarai S, Graham RP, et al. Pancreatoblastoma: cytologic and histologic analysis of 12 adult cases reveals helpful criteria in their diagnosis and distinction from common mimics. *Cancer Cytopathol*. 2019;127(11):708-719. Available at: https://doi.org/10.1002/cncy.22187.

Salman B, Brat G, Yoon YS, et al. The diagnosis and surgical treatment of pancreatoblastoma in adults: a case series and review of the literature. *J Gastrointest Surg*. 2013;17(12):2153-2161. Available at: https://doi.org/10.1007/s11605-013-2294-2.

Undifferentiated Carcinoma With Osteoclast-Like Giant Cells

Sakhi R, Hamza A, Khurram MS, Ibrar W, Mazzara P. Undifferentiated carcinoma of the pancreas with osteoclast-like giant cells reported in an asymptomatic patient: a rare case and literature review. *Autops Case Rep*. 2017;7(4):51-57. Available at: https://doi.org/10.4322/acr.2017.042.

Tanaka M, Masashi F, Noriyoshi F. Undifferentiated carcinoma of the pancreas with/without osteoclast-like giant cells. *Pathol Case Rev*. 2010;15(6):210-214. Available at: https://doi.org/10.1097/PCR.0b013e3181ffb8ac.

Muraki T, Reid MD, Basturk O, et al. Undifferentiated carcinoma with osteoclastic giant cells of the pancreas: clinicopathological analysis of 38 cases highlights a more protracted clinical course than currently appreciated. *Am J Surg Pathol*. 2016;40(9):1203-1216. Available at: https://doi.org/10.1097/PAS.0000000000000689.

Well-Differentiated Pancreatic Neuroendocrine Tumor

Shi C, Klimstra DS. Pancreatic neuroendocrine tumors: pathologic and molecular characteristics. *Semin Diagn Pathol*. 2014;31(6):498-511. Available at: https://doi.org/10.1053/j.semdp.2014.08.008.

Basturk O, Yang Z, Tang LH, et al. The high grade (WHO G3) pancreatic neuroendocrine tumor category is morphologically and biologically heterogeneous and includes both well differentiated and poorly differentiated neoplasms. *Am J Surg Pathol.* 2015;39(5):683-690. Available at: https://doi.org/10.1097/PAS.0000000000000408.

Tang LH, Basturk O, Sue JJ, Klimstra DS. A practical approach to the classification of WHO Grade 3 (G3) Well Differentiated Neuroendocrine Tumor (WD-NET) and Poorly Differentiated Neuroendocrine Carcinoma (PD-NEC) of the pancreas. *Am J Surg Pathol.* 2016;40(9):1192-1202. Available at: https://doi.org/10.1097/PAS.0000000000000662.

Poorly Differentiated Neuroendocrine Carcinoma

Basturk O, Tang L, Hruban RH, et al. Poorly differentiated neuroendocrine carcinomas of the pancreas: a clinicopathologic analysis of 44 cases. *Am J Surg Pathol.* 2014;38(4):437-447. Available at: https://doi.org/10.1097/PAS.0000000000000169.

Tang LH, Untch BR, Reidy DL, et al. Well-differentiated neuroendocrine tumors with a morphologically apparent high-grade component: a pathway distinct from poorly differentiated neuroendocrine carcinomas. *Clin Cancer Res.* 2016;22(4):1011-1017. Available at: https://doi.org/10.1158/1078-0432.CCR-15-0548.

Serous Cystic Neoplasm

Charville GW, Kao CS. Serous neoplasms of the pancreas: a comprehensive review. *Arch Pathol Lab Med.* 2018;142(9):1134-1140. Available at: https://doi.org/10.5858/arpa.2017-0195-RS.

Hammel PR, Vilgrain V, Terris B, et al. Pancreatic involvement in von Hippel–Lindau disease. *Gastroenterology.* 2000;119(4):1087-1095. Available at: https://doi.org/10.1053/gast.2000.18143.

Mucinous Cystic Neoplasm

Fukushima N, Fukayama M. Mucinous cystic neoplasms of the pancreas: pathology and molecular genetics. *J Hepatobiliary Pancreat Surg.* 2007;14(3):238-242. Available at: https://doi.org/10.1007/s00534-006-1168-3.

Jang KT, Park SM, Basturk O, et al. Clinicopathologic characteristics of 29 invasive carcinomas arising in 178 pancreatic mucinous cystic neoplasms with ovarian-type stroma: implications for management and prognosis. *Am J Surg Pathol.* 2015;39(2):179-187. Available at: https://doi.org/10.1097/PAS.0000000000000357.

Intraductal Papillary Mucinous Neoplasm

Rezaee N, Barbon C, Zaki A, et al. Intraductal papillary mucinous neoplasm (IPMN) with high-grade dysplasia is a risk factor for the subsequent development of pancreatic ductal adenocarcinoma. *HPB.* 2016;18(3):236-246. Available at: https://doi.org/10.1016/j.hpb.2015.10.010.

Kallen ME, Naini BV. Intraductal oncocytic papillary neoplasms of the pancreas. *Arch Pathol Lab Med.* 2016;140(9):992-996. Available at: https://doi.org/10.5858/arpa.2014-0595-RS.

Motosugi U, Yamaguchi H, Furukawa T, et al. Imaging studies of intraductal tubulopapillary neoplasms of the pancreas: 2-tone duct sign and cork-of-wine-bottle sign as indicators of intraductal tumor growth. *J Comput Assist Tomogr.* 2012;36(6):710-717. Available at: https://doi.org/10.1097/RCT.0b013e31826d1fc8.

Jang KT, Park SM, Basturk O, et al. Clinicopathologic characteristics of 29 invasive carcinomas arising in 178 pancreatic mucinous cystic neoplasms with ovarian-type stroma: implications for management and prognosis. *Am J Surg Pathol.* 2015;39(2):179-187. Available at: https://doi.org/10.1097/PAS.0000000000000357.

5

Genitourinary: Prostate, Bladder, and Kidney Pathology

Jane K. Nguyen • Rajal B. Shah

PROSTATE

1) POST-ATROPHIC HYPERPLASIA

DIFFERENTIAL DIAGNOSIS: ATROPHIC PROSTATIC ADENOCARCINOMA (Table 5.1)

Clinical Features

Post-atrophic hyperplasia (PAH) of the prostate is a benign lesion that may be encountered incidentally or as potential target of directed biopsies after MRI imaging. Typical mean age of presentation is 50, but can be seen at any age. PAH is typically encountered in the peripheral zone (PZ) compared with the transition zone (TZ) of the prostate.

Pathologic Features (Fig. 5.1)

LOW-POWER ARCHITECTURAL FEATURES

This lesion maintains preservation of lobular architecture with a dilated central duct surrounded by proliferation of small round distorted acini. Stroma typically shows sclerosis and chronic inflammation.

HIGH-POWER CYTOLOGIC FEATURES

Nuclei occupy full cell height with lack of appreciable cytoplasm. Prominent nucleoli can be common with mitotic figures, which are usually seen in the presence of an inflammatory milieu.

IMMUNOHISTOCHEMICAL FEATURES

Basal cell markers are positive. AMACR is typically not expressed.

TABLE 5.1

Post-atrophic Hyperplasia Versus Atrophic Prostatic Adenocarcinoma (PAC)

	Post-Atrophic Hyperplasia (Fig. 5.1)	Atrophic PAC (Fig. 5.2)
Location	PZ > TZ	PZ > TZ
Histologic features Low power	Lesion appears basophilic at low power due to nuclei occupying full cell height with scant cytoplasm	Less basophilic at low power due to scant yet appreciable cytoplasm
	Preservation of lobular architecture containing central dilated duct with surrounding proliferation of small round acini	Infiltrative or haphazard process between benign acinar structures
		Sclerotic stromal response typically not present
	Often associated with sclerotic stromal response	
High power	Occasional prominent nucleoli and mitotic figures commonly seen in association with inflammatory milieu	Cytologic atypia with nuclear enlargement and prominent nucleoli is required for the diagnosis
		Frequently associated with conventional acinar PAC
Immunohistochemistry stains	Positive for basal cell markers (p63, HMWCK) Negative for AMACR	Negative for basal cell markers (p63, HMWCK) AMACR is variably positive

PZ, Peripheral zone; *TZ*, transition zone.

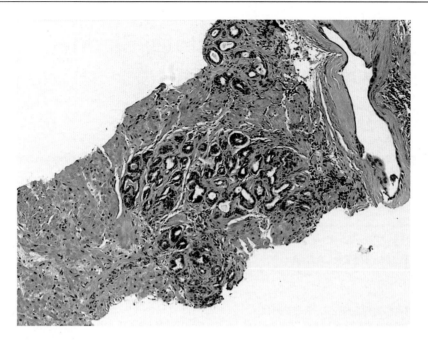

FIG. 5.1

At low power, post-atrophic hyperplasia is characterized by a circumscribed/lobulated collection of small dark atrophic acini with round to distorted contours arranged around a larger dilated duct. The dark appearance of the lesion at low power may arouse a suspicion for cancer but is due to scant cytoplasm rather than abundant amphophilic/granular cytoplasm seen in cancer. The stroma surrounding acini is usually sclerotic.

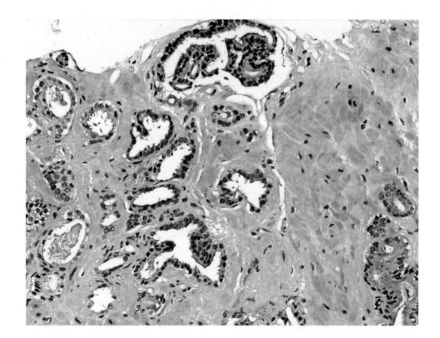

FIG. 5.2

In atrophic cancer, glands demonstrate marked reduction in cytoplasm mimicking completely atrophic glands. However, in contrast to complete atrophy, there is still relatively abundant amphophilic cytoplasm. Significant cytologic atypia argues against the diagnosis of benign atrophy. Glands also impart an infiltrative growth. The presence of conventional acinar adenocarcinoma *(lower right corner)* may be present and provides an additional diagnostic clue.

TABLE 5.2

Partial Atrophy Versus Prostatic Adenocarcinoma (PAC)

	Partial Atrophy (Fig. 5.3, 5.4A–C)	PAC
Location	PZ > TZ	PZ > TZ
Histologic features Low power	Crowded small-/medium-caliber glands with reduced cytoplasm, placed laterally to nuclei giving a distinct pale appearance	Crowded small/medium caliber glands exhibiting cytoplasmic amphophilia
	Haphazard or disorganized growth common but lacks infiltrative architecture	Infiltrative between benign acinar structures
	Luminal borders range from undulated to straight with poorly formed glands appearance	Typically "punched out"/straight luminal borders
High power	Slight nuclear enlargement with frequent small nucleoli but lacks prominent nucleoli, mitoses, apoptosis	Nuclear enlargement, prominent nucleoli and hyperchromasia. Mitosis may be occasionally present
	Occasional blue mucin and crystalloids can be present	Luminal secretions, crystalloids, blue mucin common
Immunohistochemistry stains	Frequent patchy positivity for basal cell markers; may entirely lack basal cell staining AMACR expression is frequently seen. Lacks ERG overexpression	Negative for basal cell markers AMACR is expressed in majority of cases ERG overexpression seen in up to 50% of cases

PZ, Peripheral zone; *TZ,* transition zone.

2) PARTIAL ATROPHY

DIFFERENTIAL DIAGNOSIS: PROSTATIC ADENOCARCINOMA (Table 5.2)

Clinical Features

Partial atrophy of the prostate is a benign entity that is one of the most common and troublesome benign mimickers of prostate cancer. Typical mean age of presentation is 50. Partial atrophy is typically encountered in the PZ.

Pathologic Features (Figs. 5.3 and 5.4A–C)

LOW-POWER ARCHITECTURAL FEATURES

This lesion comprises small-/medium-caliber pale glands that often present with disorganized or haphazard growth. Glands have reduced cytoplasm, placed laterally to nuclei giving a distinct pale appearance at low power. The luminal borders of the acini range from star shaped with undulated borders to poorly formed.

HIGH-POWER CYTOLOGIC FEATURES

Nuclei may be slightly enlarged with frequent small nucleoli but lack prominent nucleoli, mitoses, and

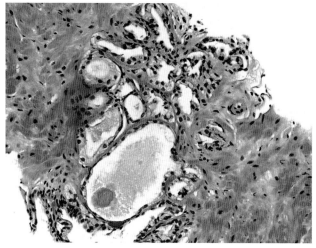

FIG. 5.3

Most partial atrophy lesions are composed of a lobular arrangement of crowded glands with lumina ranging from round to stellate/undulating. Note pale, clear cytoplasm placed laterally to the nuclei, lack of nuclear enlargement and macro-nucleoli, as well as the presence of few completely atrophic glands within the focus.

apoptosis. Occasional intraluminal blue mucin can be present.

IMMUNOHISTOCHEMICAL FEATURES

Basal cell markers frequently demonstrate patchy positivity with some may entirely lacking basal cell staining. AMACR can be also frequently expressed. Small proportion of lesion may demonstrate immunophenotype of prostatic adenocarcinoma (PAC) characterized by lack

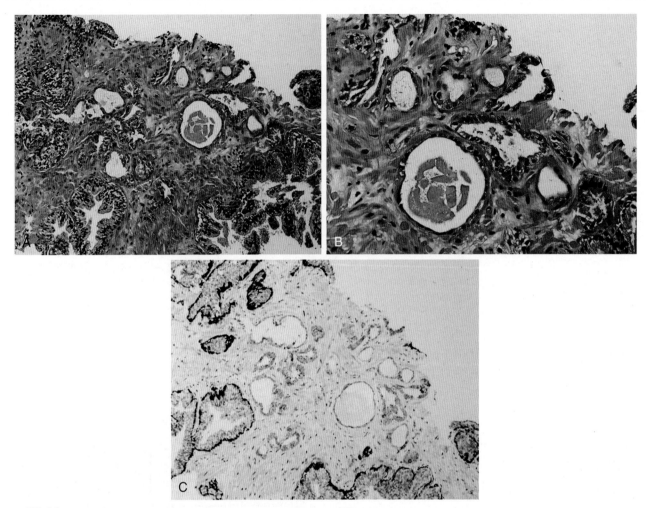

FIG. 5.4
Partial atrophy composed of a crowded proliferation of predominantly small glands with pale cytoplasm similar to the adjacent benign glands. In addition to partially atrophic glands, there are several completely atrophic glands, a very useful diagnostic clue **(A)**. At high power, small micro-nucleoli are visible **(B)**. Immunohistochemistry for PIN cocktail antibodies (brown chromogen = p63; red chromogen = AMACR) demonstrate rare basal cells and weak AMACR expression, important pitfalls. Such immunostaining pattern in the context of appropriate morphology is acceptable for the diagnosis of partial atrophy **(C)**.

of basal cells with AMACR overexpression, an important pitfall to keep in mind (Fig. 5.4A–C). ERG overexpression is not seen.

3) BENIGN PROSTATIC TISSUE WITH RADIATION THERAPY EFFECT

DIFFERENTIAL DIAGNOSIS: PROSTATIC ADENOCARCINOMA WITH RADIATION THERAPY EFFECT (Table 5.3)

Clinical Features

Benign prostatic tissue with radiation therapy effect (RTE) typically presents in patients treated with radiation therapy. RTE can be seen many years after therapy. Patients frequently present with asymptomatic hematuria due to radiation necrosis. The clinical history of prior radiation therapy, either brachytherapy or external beam radiation, for treatment of PAC is pertinent. Marked epithelial atypia tends to persist for a longer time (up to 6 years), particularly in patients treated with brachytherapy. Can occur equally in the PZ and TZ.

Pathologic Features (Fig. 5.5)

LOW-POWER ARCHITECTURAL FEATURES

This lesion usually maintains the overall lobular architecture of glands. Glands are atrophic and reduced, with an increased stromal component due to RTE.

TABLE 5.3

Benign Prostatic Tissue (BPT) With Radiation Therapy (RTE) Effect Versus Prostatic Adenocarcinoma (PAC) With RTE

	BPT With RTE (Fig. 5.5)	PAC With RTE (Fig. 5.6)
Location	PZ = TZ	PZ > TZ
Histologic features Low power	Maintains lobular architecture	Infiltrating pattern of poorly formed glands or single cell pattern
	Atrophic and reduced glands with increased stroma	Abundant cytoplasmic vacuoles with partially atrophic appearance
High power	Epithelium with random cytologic atypia with some nuclei exhibiting bizarre pleomorphism and smudgy chromatin	Nuclei may appear pyknotic. Atypia typically is uniform with frequent prominent nucleoli
		Gleason score is not provided for PAC exhibiting RTE
Immunohistochemistry stains	Positive for basal cell markers. AMACR is negative	Negative for basal cell makers. AMACR is positive

PZ, Peripheral zone; *TZ*, transition zone.

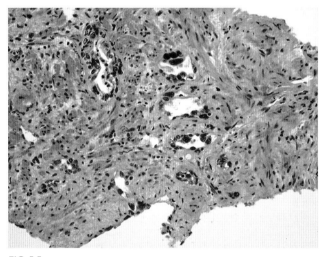

FIG. 5.5

In post-radiation biopsies, there is an overall paucity of glands. Glands are atrophic and exhibit random cytologic atypia including occasional markedly enlarged nuclei, a tell-tale feature for radiation atypia. However, the cytologic atypia is random and degenerative in nature, and is characterized by hypochromatic nuclei with frequent cytoplasmic vacuolization.

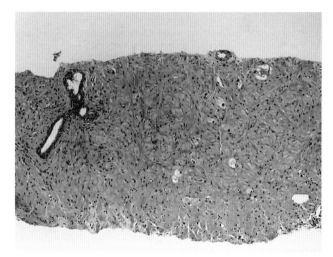

FIG. 5.6

In residual adenocarcinoma demonstrating radiation treatment effect, cancer glands grow in a haphazard manner, show frequent tumor breakdown with poorly formed glands and single cells, relatively abundant cytoplasm, and uniform cytologic atypia. Nuclei are small and frequently shrunken.

HIGH-POWER CYTOLOGIC FEATURES

The epithelium of the acini displays marked random nuclear atypia in which some nuclei have bizarre pleomorphism and smudgy chromatin. PAC that is sufficiently well differentiated rarely would produce this degree of atypia. The acini maintain the basal cell layer, which is helpful in distinguishing from malignancy.

IMMUNOHISTOCHEMICAL FEATURES

Basal cell markers are positive in prostatic tissue with RTE, and AMACR is not expressed.

4) BASAL CELL HYPERPLASIA

DIFFERENTIAL DIAGNOSIS: HIGH-GRADE PROSTATIC INTRAEPITHELIAL NEOPLASIA, BASAL CELL CARCINOMA, P63 POSITIVE ADENOCARCINOMA (PAC) (Table 5.4)

Clinical Features

Basal cell hyperplasia is a benign entity that is typically associated with benign prostatic hyperplasia. Typically

TABLE 5.4

Basal Cell Hyperplasia Versus High-grade Prostatic Intraepithelial Neoplasia (HGPIN) Versus Basal Cell Carcinoma Versus p63-Positive Prostatic Adenocarcinoma (PAC)

	Basal Cell Hyperplasia (Fig. 5.7A and B)	HGPIN (Fig. 5.8)	Basal Cell Carcinoma (Fig. 5.9A and B)	p63-Positive PAC (Fig. 5.10A–C)
Location	TZ > PZ	PZ > TZ	TZ > PZ	PZ > TZ
Histologic features Low power	Maintains lobular architecture or may show proliferation of isolated large glands	Isolated or crowded glands	Infiltrative process	Infiltrative
	Solid and incomplete nests or large glands with undulating lumina; cellular proliferation is away from luminal aspect; hypercellular stromal cells characteristic of BPH often present	Large glands with tufting, micropapillary or flat architecture	Variably sized nests, cribriforming glands and trabeculae in an infiltrative process. Desmoplastic stroma, perineural invasion, extraprostatic extension, and necrosis are common	Atrophic individual glands with cord-like pattern
High power	Multilayering of basal cells with scant cytoplasm and frequent prominent nucleoli. Nuclei are ovoid, "coffee bean–like" with frequent grooves	Luminal proliferation of columnar secretory cells with relatively abundant cytoplasm. Prominent nucleoli visible at 20×, occasional mitotic activity	Basal cells with multilayering with prominent nucleoli	Nuclei may show stratification, lack pleomorphism; may be admixed with usual PAC
Immunohistochemistry stains	Positive for basal cell markers; negative for AMACR, typically lacks diffuse positivity for BCL2	Frequently patchy positive for basal cell markers; positive for AMACR	Positive for basal cell markers; diffusely positive for BCL2, prostate markers including NKX3.1 are negative	Positive p63 and AMACR, negative for HMWCK, prostate markers including NKX3.1 are positive

BPH, Benign prostatic hyperplasia; *PZ,* peripheral zone; *TZ,* transition zone.

occurs in the TZ. Can be associated with androgen deprivation therapy (ADT) effect.

Pathologic Features (Fig. 5.7A and B)

LOW-POWER ARCHITECTURAL FEATURES

This lesion shows a nodular proliferation composed of both completely solid nests admixed with incomplete nests that often exhibit small gland or large gland architecture, including cribriform architecture. Overall, the proliferation consists of multilayered basal cells and lacks an infiltrative pattern.

HIGH-POWER CYTOLOGIC FEATURES

The proliferation of basaloid cells typically undermines the secretory cells and can have prominent nucleoli. Nuclei are oriented like a "pack of cigar" with scant cytoplasm. Nuclei are ovoid, coffee bean-like with frequent grooves.

IMMUNOHISTOCHEMICAL FEATURES

Basal cell markers are positive. AMACR is typically not expressed.

5) HIGH-GRADE PROSTATIC INTRAEPITHELIAL NEOPLASIA

DIFFERENTIAL DIAGNOSIS: CENTRAL ZONE GLANDS (Table 5.5)

Clinical Features

High-grade prostatic intraepithelial neoplasia (HGPIN) is a putative neoplastic precursor lesion that is seen in the 50s to elderly men, although it is not rare in 40s. Detected as an incidental finding and by itself, does not elevate serum prostate-specific antigen (PSA). Clinical significance of HGPIN as a marker of unsampled PAC

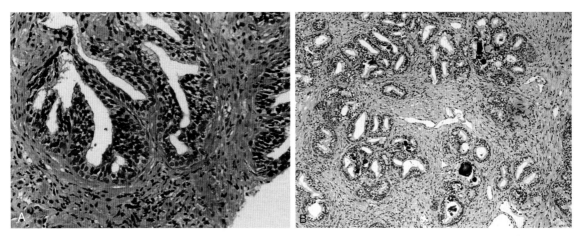

FIG. 5.7

In basal cell hyperplasia, a range of growth patterns is observed. Isolated large glands with nuclear stratification mimic high-grade prostatic intraepithelial neoplasia. Nuclei are arranged like a pack of cigars without visible cytoplasm and are coffee bean–like with frequent grooves and vesicular glassy chromatin. Prominent nucleoli are frequently seen. Nuclear proliferation is seen away from lumen **(A)**. In resection specimens, a nodular architecture suggestive of benign prostate enlargement is typically present. Calcifications are common. Note the presence of background cellular spindle cells, suggestive of a benign proliferative process and is a useful diagnostic clue **(B)**.

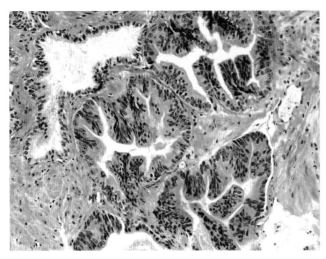

FIG. 5.8

At scanning power, high-grade prostatic intraepithelial neoplasia glands are architecturally similar to but appear darker than the adjacent benign glands. At 20× magnification, the secretory cells have crowded and stratified nuclei that are enlarged and have coarse and clumpy chromatin with relatively more cytoplasm between nuclei. Importantly, large and conspicuous nucleoli are present in the secretory cells.

on repeat biopsy has been substantially reduced in the contemporary extended biopsy. However, multiple cores involvement (involving >1 core) and/or multifocal HGPIN and ERG overexpression is still considered important risk factors for unsampled cancer and in this setting a repeat biopsy is recommended.

Pathologic Features

LOW-POWER ARCHITECTURAL FEATURES

This lesion consists of medium to large glands of the size of normal prostate acini, lined by crowded epithelial

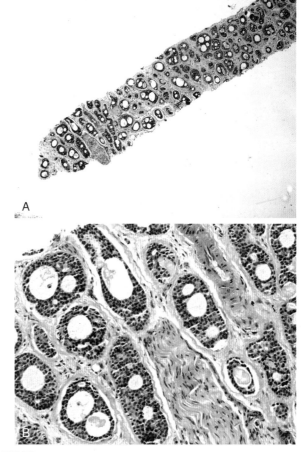

FIG. 5.9

Basal cell carcinoma (BCC) with a solid and cribriform architecture, mimicking basal cell hyperplasia **(A)**. The distinction from basal cell hyperplasia is especially difficult in needle biopsy samples, as cells can be relatively bland and infiltrative features may not be easily appreciated. In contrast to basal cell hyperplasia, tumor cells in BCC are dense, haphazardly arranged with infiltrative features characterized by edematous desmoplastic stroma, destruction of smooth muscle, and perineural invasion **(B)**. Infiltrative growth is the hallmark of BCC and is required to differentiate from florid basal cell hyperplasia.

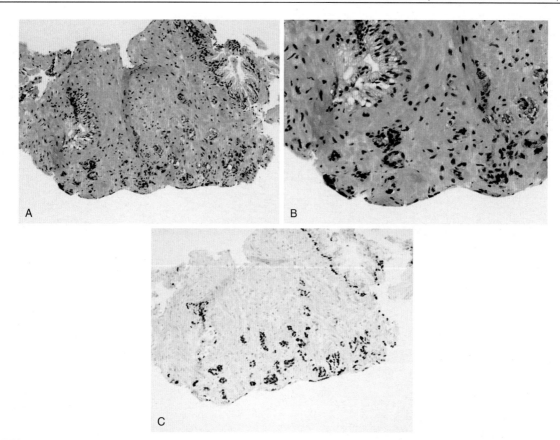

FIG. 5.10

Prostate cancer positive for p63. Atrophic-appearing glands with stratification infiltrate between benign prostate glands **(A)**. They are lined with several layers of cancer cells with poorly formed lumen. The nucleoli are prominent **(B)**. All the cancer glands were negative for HMWCK (34βE12, not shown) but were uniformly positive for p63 **(C)**. Rather than being in basal cell distribution, the staining is found in all the cancer cells. Prostate cancer positive for p63 is exceedingly rare and probably represents a form of prostate cancer with basal cell differentiation.

TABLE 5.5

High-grade Prostatic Intraepithelial Neoplasia (HGPIN) Versus Central Zone (CZ)

	HGPIN	CZ (Fig. 5.11A and B)
Location	PZ > TZ	CZ, base of prostate
Histologic features Low power	Medium to large prostatic glands of size of normal glands lined by crowded epithelial cells with cytologic atypia	Medium to large prostate glands of size of normal prostate glands. May have papillary infolding, cribriform formation, and roman bridges
	Increased cytoplasmic amphophilia gives a distinct darker appearance at low power than adjacent benign glands	Lined by tall pseudostratified epithelium with distinct cytoplasmic eosinophilia (a helpful feature)
	Architectural patterns: tufted, micropapillary, flat, and loose cribriform. The diagnosis of cribriform HGPIN is discouraged. Nuclei in roman bridges are round and lack streaming in relation to bridges	Nuclei in roman bridges stream parallel in relation to bridges (a helpful feature)
High power	Hyperchromasia, nuclear overlap, enlarged nuclei, prominent nucleoli that are easily observed at 20× magnification and infrequent mitosis. Cytologic atypia is of secretory cells involving luminal cells	Atypia seen is typically basal cell in nature. Secretory cells lacks prominent nucleoli
Immunohistochemistry stains	A patchy or continuous basal cell layer seen with basal cell markers; variable AMACR expression common; small subset may exhibit ERG overexpression typically in setting of adjacent ERG-positive PAC	Positive basal cell markers; negative for AMACR and ERG

PZ, Peripheral zone; *TZ,* transition zone.

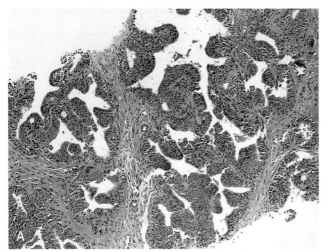

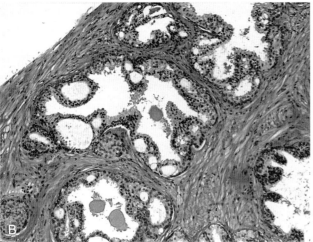

FIG. 5.11

Central zone histology is typically a mimicker of high-grade prostatic intraepithelial neoplasia (HGPIN); however, prominent cribriform architecture in some cases may mimic cancer. This histology is typically seen in biopsies from the base of the prostate. In the central zone, glands are complex with frequent papillation and undulating architecture with pseudostratified lining epithelium. At low magnification, glands demonstrate distinct cytoplasmic eosinophilia **(A)**. Roman bridges and cribriform architecture are common. In contrast to HGPIN, nuclei stream parallel to bridges in comparison with perpendicular orientation in HGPIN **(B)**.

cells that demonstrate cytologic atypia. There are four major architectural patterns: tufted, micropapillary, flat, and rarely loose cribriform. The diagnosis of cribriform HGPIN in biopsy setting is not discouraged and such lesion is often classified as atypical intraductal proliferation (AIP; see Section 10 on page 237 for further discussion). Glands stand out as being darker than normal glands with prominent cytoplasmic amphophilia. May have papillary infolding and roman bridges, but nuclei lack streaming in relation to the bridges to distinguish from normal central zone glands.

HIGH-POWER CYTOLOGIC FEATURES

The abnormal cytologic features include: hyperchromasia, nuclear overlap, enlarged nuclei, prominent nucleoli

that are easily observed at 20× magnification, and rarely mitoses. A basal cell layer is typically preserved but may be indistinct.

IMMUNOHISTOCHEMICAL FEATURES

Basal cell markers highlight intact or a discontinuous basal cell layer around the involved ducts or acini. AMACR is expressed in acinar cells variably. ERG overexpression is seen in about 18% of cases that typically have adjacent ERG-positive PAC. ERG overexpression in isolated HGPIN is typically not seen.

6) PROSTATE ADENOSIS (ADENOMATOUS HYPERPLASIA)

DIFFERENTIAL DIAGNOSIS: PROSTATIC ADENOCARCINOMA (Table 5.6)

Clinical Features

Prostatic adenosis is a benign entity that is more commonly seen in transurethral resection or radical prostatectomy specimens. Typically occurs in the TZ but can be seen in the PZ when diffuse, and referred to as diffuse adenosis of the peripheral zone (DAPZ). DAPZ has an increased risk of PAC on subsequent re-biopsy.

Pathologic Features (Fig. 5.12A–C)

LOW-POWER ARCHITECTURAL FEATURES

This lesion shows a lobular collection of glands. Glands can be crowded and appear back-to-back when diffuse. Smaller glands are admixed with larger benign-appearing glands and are similar in appearance without any cytoplasmic or cytologic differences. Commonly associated with corpora amylacea and rarely, intraluminal blue mucin can be present. DAPZ involves multiple cores. Hypercellular stroma, characteristic of benign prostate enlargement, is often present and provides a useful clue to the diagnosis.

HIGH-POWER CYTOLOGIC FEATURES

The cytoplasm is pale-clear with indistinct or small nucleoli.

IMMUNOHISTOCHEMICAL FEATURES

Basal cell markers are frequently patchy positive with some glands retaining basal cells, while some may entirely lack

TABLE 5.6
Prostate Adenosis Versus Prostatic Adenocarcinoma (PAC)

	Prostate Adenosis (Fig. 5.12A–C)	PAC
Location	TZ > PZ	PZ > TZ
Histologic features Low power	Maintains lobular architecture. DAPZ has diffuse involvement in multiple cores	Infiltrating pattern
	Smaller glands are admixed with larger benign-appearing glands without any cytoplasmic or cytologic differences. Hypercellular stroma, characteristic of benign prostate enlargement is often present and provides a useful clue to the diagnosis.	Small glands infiltrating between benign glands differ in cytoplasmic and cytologic characteristics
	Corpora amylacea and intraluminal crystalloids are common	Corpora amylacea is not seen
	Intraluminal blue mucin may be present	Intraluminal blue mucin common
High power	Pale-clear cytoplasm	Cytoplasm is amphophilic
	Indistinct or small nucleoli	Nuclear enlargement, hyperchromasia, and prominent nucleoli are present
Immunohistochemistry stains	Frequent patchy or fragmented positivity for basal cell markers. Weak to moderate AMACR can be present, ERG is not expressed	Negative for basal cell makers. AMACR is positive, ERG overexpression in up to 50% cases

DAPZ, Diffuse adenosis of the peripheral zone; *PZ*, peripheral zone; *TZ*, transition zone.

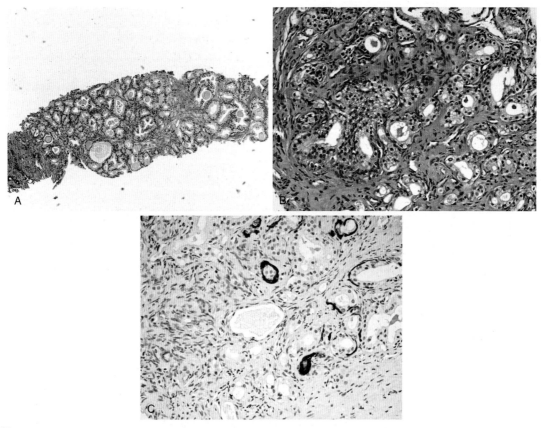

FIG. 5.12

At low power, adenosis is characterized by a circumscribed collection of variably sized glands **(A)**. Within the nodule, small round acini are admixed with larger benign-appearing glands with papillary infolding. There are no obvious cytoplasmic or cytologic differences between them. Essentially, small and large glands merge with each other imperceptibly. At high power, the columnar cells have abundant pale to clear cytoplasm and bland-appearing nuclei with inconspicuous to small nucleoli **(B)**. The stroma between the glands is densely cellular, a feature to suggest a benign reactive nature. Basal cell markers typically demonstrate a discontinuous/patchy-staining pattern, with some glands lacking the staining **(C)**.

basal cells. As long as glands that have positive basal cells and glands that are negative have a similar appearance, this staining pattern is considered compatible with the diagnosis of adenosis (Fig. 5.12C). Weak to moderate AMACR expression is seen in subset of cases. ERG overexpression is not seen.

7) SCLEROSING ADENOSIS

DIFFERENTIAL DIAGNOSIS: HIGH-GRADE PROSTATIC ADENOCARCINOMA (Table 5.7)

Clinical Features

Sclerosing adenosis of the prostate is a benign entity that is more commonly seen in transurethral resection or radical prostatectomy specimens, and rarely on needle core biopsy. Typically occurs in the TZ.

Pathologic Features (Fig. 5.13A and B)

LOW-POWER ARCHITECTURAL FEATURES

This lesion is relatively well circumscribed and is composed of a mixture of well-formed glands, poorly formed or compressed glands, single epithelial cells, and cellular spindled cells. A hyaline sheath of collagen can be seen surrounding glands. A striking feature of this lesion is the dense spindle cell component. The

presence of few well-circumscribed cellular nodules in the TZ mimicking high-grade prostate cancer is a typical finding and should prompt a consideration for the diagnosis of sclerosing adenosis.

HIGH-POWER CYTOLOGIC FEATURES

The glandular component has pale-clear cytoplasm and bland nuclei. The single cell component may have prominent nucleoli.

IMMUNOHISTOCHEMICAL FEATURES

Basal cell markers are positive in the glandular component. Basal cells exhibit myoepithelial differentiation and are positive for smooth muscle actin (SMA) and S100 protein.

8) PSEUDOHYPERPLASTIC PROSTATIC ADENOCARCINOMA

DIFFERENTIAL DIAGNOSIS: CROWDED BENIGN PROSTATIC GLANDS (Table 5.8)

Clinical Features

Pseudohyperplastic PAC is a variant morphology of PAC that may be a mimic of crowded benign prostate glands or benign prostate hyperplasia. It typically occurs in the PZ.

TABLE 5.7
Sclerosis Adenosis Versus High-grade Prostatic Adenocarcinoma (PAC)

	Sclerosing Adenosis (Fig. 5.13A and B)	High-grade PAC
Location	TZ > PZ	PZ > TZ
Histologic features Low power	The presence of few well-circumscribed cellular nodules composed of a mixture of well-formed and poorly formed glands, single epithelial cells, and cellular spindled cells, mimicking high-grade PAC is a typical finding	Infiltrating pattern with single cell or poorly formed/fused gland pattern
	Hyaline sheath of collagen can be seen surrounding glands	Lacks collagen sheath
	Dense spindle cell component	Usually lacks stromal response
High power	Glandular component with pale-clear cytoplasm and bland nuclei; blue mucin can be seen	Glandular component with amphophilic cytoplasm and prominent nucleoli
	Single cell component with occasional prominent nucleoli	Single cell component with prominent nucleoli
Immunohistochemistry stains	Positive for basal cell markers, SMA and S100 highlights myoepithelial cells	Negative for basal cell makers, AMACR is positive, SMA is negative

PZ, Peripheral zone; *TZ*, transition zone.

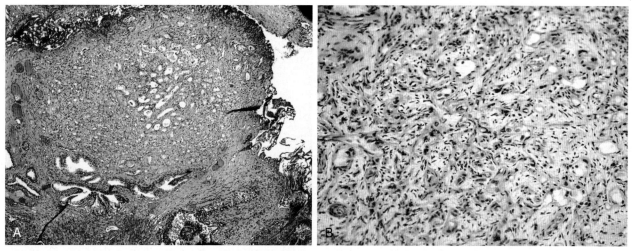

FIG. 5.13

This transurethral resection of the prostate (TURP) specimen demonstrates a proliferation of poorly formed and complex glands mimicking high-grade prostate carcinoma. Low-power recognition is a key. It typically forms a well-circumscribed nodule of tightly packed glands **(A)**. At high magnification, glands demonstrate complex proliferation, poorly formed glands with slit-like lumina, fused glands, and even single cells with signet ring cell–like features, mimicking high-grade cancer. Stroma surrounding the glands is cellular and hyalinized **(B)**. Prominent nucleoli, crystalloids, and blue mucin are common. When one or more well-circumscribed cellular lesions mimicking high-grade prostate cancer are encountered in TURP or biopsies from the transition zone of the prostate, sclerosing adenosis should be ruled out.

TABLE 5.8

Pseudohyperplastic Prostatic Adenocarcinoma (PAC) Versus Crowded Benign Glands

	Pseudohyperplastic PAC (Fig. 5.14A–D)	Crowded Benign Glands
Location	PZ > TZ	TZ > PZ
Histologic features Low power	Crowded larger glands with branching and papillary infolding of the lumen that mimic as benign prostate hyperplasia or crowded benign glands. Conventional PAC often is present and provide a useful clue	Crowded glands of variable size with branching and papillary infolding
	Tall columnar cells with abundant mildly amphophilic cytoplasm and basally located nuclei along the basement membrane	Large benign glands with abundant pale-clear cytoplasm and undulating luminal borders
	Pink secretions with crystalloids	Corpora amylacea common
	Intraluminal blue mucin rare	Intraluminal blue mucin rare
High power	Nuclear atypia including prominent nucleoli	Lacks nuclear atypia and prominent nucleoli
Immunohistochemistry stains	Negative for basal cell makers, AMACR is variably positive	Positive for basal cell makers, AMACR is typically negative

PZ, Peripheral zone; *TZ*, transition zone.

Pathologic Features (Fig. 5.14A–D)

LOW-POWER ARCHITECTURAL FEATURES

This lesion shows several crowded or haphazardly arranged large glands with branching and papillary infolding of the lumen. The large glands have tall columnar cells with abundant mildly amphophilic cytoplasm and basally located nuclei along the basement membrane.

Often times associated with pink secretions within the lumen and crystalloids. Conventional acinar PAC is frequently present.

HIGH-POWER CYTOLOGIC FEATURES

Nuclear atypia in form of nuclear enlargement and prominent nucleoli is typically present and is required to make the diagnosis.

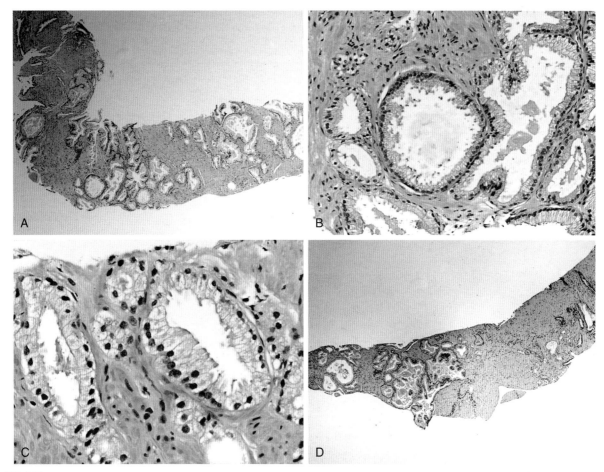

FIG. 5.14

An example of pseudohyperplastic carcinoma in needle biopsy. Note relatively deceptive, bland appearance of large glands at low power. Crowding, admixture with some small glands, and differences in cytoplasmic characteristics bring attention to these glands at low power **(A)**. At higher magnification, single layer of nuclei, with nuclear enlargement and prominent nucleoli, are visible **(B, C)**. The lack of basal cell markers (HMWCK and p63) in numerous glands along with strong internal control supports the diagnosis of pseudohyperplastic prostate carcinoma **(D)**. AMACR expression can be variable.

IMMUNOHISTOCHEMICAL FEATURES

Basal cell markers are negative and AMACR is variably positive. The diagnosis requires the presence of several glands showing the above features. In a small focus, immunohistochemistry is not reliable.

9) FOAMY GLAND PROSTATIC ADENOCARCINOMA

DIFFERENTIAL DIAGNOSIS: XANTHOMA, COWPER GLANDS (Table 5.9)

Clinical Features

Foamy gland PAC is a variant morphology of PAC. Typically occurs in the PZ. Well-formed foamy gland

PAC may mimic Cowper glands, mucinous metaplasia, poorly formed adenocarcinoma, or xanthoma.

Pathologic Features (Fig. 5.15A and B)

LOW-POWER ARCHITECTURAL FEATURES

This lesion shows crowded or infiltrative glands with abundant xanthomatous bubbly cytoplasm that resemble xanthoma cells/histiocytes. Architecturally, can vary from well-formed glands, nests, cords, and single cells. Intraluminal amorphous secretions are common. Conventional acinar PAC is frequently present.

HIGH-POWER CYTOLOGIC FEATURES

A key cytologic feature is the presence of hyperchromatic pyknotic nuclei pushed to one side (typically basal). The overall nuclear-to-cytoplasmic (N:C) ratio is

TABLE 5.9

Foamy Gland Prostatic Adenocarcinoma (PAC) Versus Cowper Glands Versus Xanthoma

	Foamy Gland PAC (Fig. 5.15A and B)	Cowper Glands (Fig. 5.16A and B)	Xanthoma (Fig. 5.17)
Location	PZ > TZ	Striated muscles of urogenital diaphragm lateral to the membranous urethra	PZ > TZ
Histologic features Low power	Abundant xanthomatous bubbly cytoplasm that resembles xanthoma cells. Intraluminal amorphous secretions are common. Conventional acinar PAC may be present	Lobulated collection of glands with abundant mucinous cytoplasm. Dimorphic appearance of central ducts surrounded by acini	Diffuse infiltration of xanthoma cells in small clusters or aggregates. Mixed inflammatory cell infiltrate common and provides a useful diagnostic clue. Cells lack glandular differentiation
	Architecturally, can vary from well-formed glands, nests, cords, and single cells	Smooth muscle cells commonly present	
High power	Hyperchromatic pyknotic nuclei; mucin when present is luminal	Bland nuclei, mucin is intracellular	Bland nuclei
Immunohistochemistry stains	Negative for basal cell makers, AMACR is variably positive	Basal cells are retained, AMACR is negative	Positive for CD68, negative for keratins

PZ, Peripheral zone; *TZ,* transition zone.

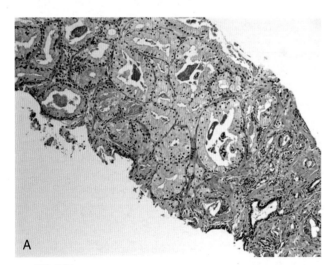
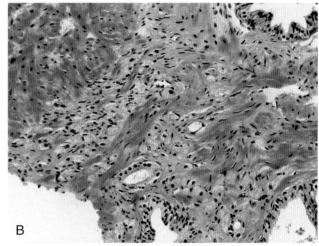

FIG. 5.15

At low power, a foamy gland carcinoma is characterized by abundant xanthomatous cytoplasm with low nuclear-to-cytoplasmic ratio, simulating a benign process. Intraluminal, dense, pink, acellular secretions are common. Conventional acinar differentiation is also common in foamy carcinoma. The nuclei are small and dense; typical malignant nuclear features of prostate cancer are only variably present **(A)**. A poorly differentiated foamy gland carcinoma simulating xanthomatous inflammation in needle biopsy. Presence of cytologic atypia and/or any glandular differentiation support the diagnosis of foamy gland carcinoma. An immunohistochemistry panel consisting of histiocytic markers and pancytokeratin may be needed to arrive at a definitive diagnosis in such cases, particularly in small needle biopsy samples **(B)**.

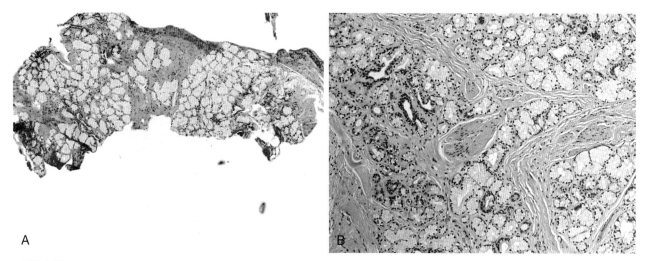

FIG. 5.16

At low power, Cowper glands are composed of tightly circumscribed or lobulated proliferation of small, uniform acini lined by mucin-containing cells with a central duct. This dimorphic population of ducts surrounded by acini is a characteristic feature. Cytologic features are bland, including small nuclei and inconspicuous nucleoli. Mucin is present in the intracellular compartment in contrast to intraluminal mucin in prostate cancer **(A)**. Skeletal muscle is frequently present in the stroma **(B)**.

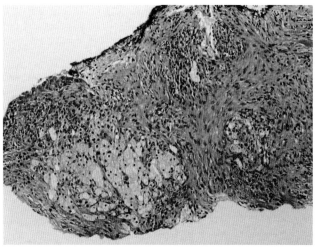

FIG. 5.17

In small needle biopsy samples, xanthomatous inflammation may mimic high-grade foamy carcinoma. Lack of any glandular differentiation, relatively bland nuclear features, and other inflammatory cells suggests the diagnosis of xanthomatous infiltrate. A panel of immunohistochemical markers of histiocytic lineage (CD68) and pancytokeratin may be necessary to rule out carcinoma.

low, giving it a bland cytologic appearance. Intraluminal mucin may be present.

IMMUNOHISTOCHEMICAL FEATURES

Basal cell markers are negative with variable positivity for AMACR. Negative for CD68.

10) INTRADUCTAL CARCINOMA OF THE PROSTATE

DIFFERENTIAL DIAGNOSIS: CLEAR CELL CRIBRIFORM HYPERPLASIA, HIGH-GRADE PROSTATIC INTRAEPITHELIAL NEOPLASIA, INTRADUCTAL SPREAD OF UROTHELIAL CARCINOMA, HIGH-GRADE (CRIBRIFORM) PAC, DUCTAL ADENOCARCINOMA (Table 5.10)

Clinical Features

Intraductal carcinoma of the prostate (IDC-P) is characterized by an expansile intraductal proliferation of malignant cells usually in dense cribriform or solid pattern. It typically represents a retrograde spread of associated high-grade and high-volume advanced PAC. Rarely, IDC-P may be identified in the absence of infiltrating carcinoma. Typically occurs in the PZ.

Pathologic Features (Fig. 5.18A–C)

LOW-POWER ARCHITECTURAL FEATURES

This lesion consists of medium- to large-caliber glands with expansile intraductal growth of carcinoma. Glands often have a branching pattern. Partial involvement of the gland is a common feature. Architectural growth

TABLE 5.10

Intraductal Carcinoma of the Prostate (IDC-P) Versus Clear Cell Cribriform Hyperplasia Versus High-grade Prostatic Intraepithelial Neoplasia (HGPIN) Versus High-grade (Cribriform) Prostatic Adenocarcinoma (PAC) Versus Ductal PAC Versus Intraductal Spread of Urothelial Carcinoma (UCa)

	IDC-P (Fig. 5.18A–C)	Clear Cell Cribriform Hyperplasia (Fig. 5.20)	HGPIN	High-Grade (Cribriform) PAC (Fig. 5.21)	Ductal PAC (Fig. 5.22)	Intraductal Spread of UCa (Fig. 5.23)
Location	PZ > TZ	TZ>PZ	PZ > TZ	PZ > TZ	Urethral mass or PZ when admixed with acinar PAC	TZ > PZ
Histologic features Low power	Medium- to large-caliber glands with expansile growth exhibiting frequent branching pattern	Numerous medium- to large-caliber cribriform glands with usually round contour in a pattern of nodular hyperplasia or rarely infiltrative	Glands of normal size with non-expansile growth	Small-, medium-, large-caliber glands with expansile growth	Large-caliber glands with expansile growth	Normal to expanded glands
	Comedo necrosis is a frequent finding	Necrosis absent	Necrosis absent	Can have necrosis	Can have necrosis	Can have necrosis
Architectural patterns	Dense cribriform, solid, loose cribriform, and rarely micropapillary	Glands lined by clear to mildly eosinophilic cytoplasm; glands exhibit roman bridges with nuclei streaming parallel to bridges	Tufted, flat, and micropapillary; cribriform architecture is typically not allowed in biopsy; such lesions often referred to as atypical intraductal proliferation	Cribriform glands of varying size and contour. Often confluent and infiltrative in nature. Solid nests and single cells if associated with a component of Gleason pattern 5	Cribriform, papillary and solid patterns; cribriform glands have slit-like compressed lumina	Solid nests with colonizing of high-grade cells
High power	Cytologic atypia present; Marked nuclear pleomorphism six times or greater than the size of a normal nucleus seen in subset of cases	Small bland nuclei with inconspicuous or small nucleoli; a strikingly prominent basal cell layer	Nuclei enlarged with prominent nucleoli, but lacks pleomorphism	Nuclear atypia present, but marked nuclear pleomorphism is uncommon	Columnar epithelium with elongated pseudostratified nuclei is a characteristic feature	Marked nuclear pleomorphism common
Immunohistochemistry stains	Positive for basal cell markers; variable AMACR positivity; PTEN loss and ERG overexpression in majority of cases	Positive for basal cell markers; negative for AMACR	Frequent patchy positive basal cells; variable AMACR positivity; intact PTEN; small subset with intermingling adjacent adenocarcinoma (18%) may express ERG	Negative for basal cell markers; positive for AMACR	Patchy retention of basal cells common in areas of intraductal growth; positive for AMACR; frequent ERG overexpression	Positive for p63 and GATA-3; negative for prostate-specific markers: PSA and NKX3.1

PZ, Peripheral zone; *TZ,* transition zone.

patterns include dense cribriform (intraluminal cellular proliferation exceeding >50% of luminal space), solid, loose cribriform (intraluminal cellular proliferation <50% of luminal space), and rarely micropapillary. The presence of comedo necrosis in lesions with solid and/or dense cribriform is a frequent feature. Marked nuclear pleomorphism in some cases may be seen. In the presence of only loose cribriform or micropapillary architecture, the presence of non-focal comedo necrosis or marked nuclear pleomorphism is required to make

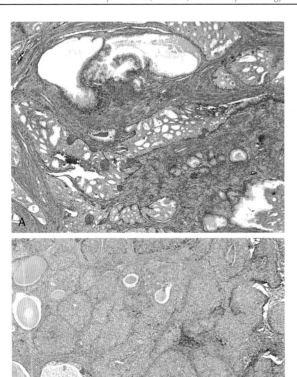

FIG. 5.18

A wide range of morphologic patterns may be seen in intraductal carcinoma, including loose cribriform, dense cribriform (cellular proliferation >50% of luminal spaces) with punched out or irregular lumina **(A)**, solid **(B)**, glands with comedo necrosis, partial involvement of benign gland, pleomorphic nuclei that are ≥6× of the adjacent nuclei and neoplastic cells exhibiting marked variation in nuclear size. For lesion lacking dense or solid architecture, the presence of either non-focal comedo necrosis or marked nuclear atypia is required to make the diagnosis of intraductal carcinoma. Glands are typically large and have branching architecture, a useful clue. Basal cells are usually visible but may require basal cell staining in some cases. Dense cribriform architecture is the most common presentation.

the diagnosis. Borderline cases, specifically exhibiting loose cribriform growth or nuclear atypia that exceeds that of HGPIN but falls short of the diagnosis of IDC-P, should be referred to as AIP (Fig. 5.19).

HIGH-POWER CYTOLOGIC FEATURES

Cytologic features include nuclear enlargement, hyperchromasia, and frequent prominent nucleoli. Marked nuclear pleomorphism that is six times or greater than the size of a normal nucleus is seen in some cases. Infrequently, dimorphic population of central small monomorphic cells and outer pleomorphic cells is present.

IMMUNOHISTOCHEMICAL FEATURES

Basal cells are uniformly retained with variable AMACR positivity. PTEN loss and ERG overexpression are seen in

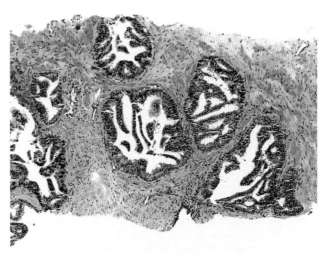

FIG. 5.19

Atypical intraductal proliferation (AIP) is morphologically more atypical than high-grade prostatic intraepithelial neoplasia (HGPIN) but lacks characteristic features of intraductal carcinoma of the prostate (IDC-P). Several glands present with lumen-spanning proliferation exhibiting loose cribriform architecture (luminal spaces account >50% of cellular proliferation) with morphologic features worse than HGPIN but falling short of IDC-P. AIP in biopsy should not be simply regarded as HGPIN, which may be conservatively followed. On the contrary, immediate repeat biopsy is warranted in this setting to rule out unsampled invasive carcinoma.

majority of cases, and can be helpful in borderline cases in the differential of HGPIN.

11) DUCTAL ADENOCARCINOMA OF THE PROSTATE

DIFFERENTIAL DIAGNOSIS: PIN-LIKE ADENOCARCINOMA, HIGH-GRADE PROSTATIC INTRAEPITHELIAL NEOPLASIA, PAPILLARY UROTHELIAL CARCINOMA (Table 5.11)

Clinical Features

Ductal adenocarcinoma of the prostate typically occurs in 50s to elderly age range. It arises in the verumontanum in the prostatic urethra and underlying periurethral prostatic ducts but also commonly arises in the peripheral prostatic ducts and acini. When presenting as a urethral lesion, it typically is associated with gross or microscopic hematuria, dysuria, and frequency. Can be associated with a variable rise in PSA. Pure ductal adenocarcinoma is rare. Majority have a component of mixed ductal and acinar adenocarcinoma. Papillary and cribriform ductal adenocarcinoma is considered a Gleason pattern 4 or 5 if associated with necrosis. PIN-like ductal adenocarcinoma is considered Gleason pattern 3.

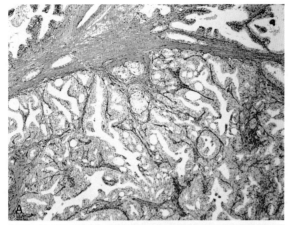

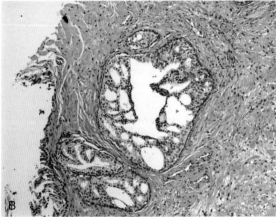

FIG. 5.20

Clear cell cribriform hyperplasia represents a spectrum of benign prostate hyperplasia and therefore is typically encountered in the transition zone of the prostate. In this transurethral resection specimen, there is a nodular proliferation of non-confluent large cribriform glands with clear to eosinophilic cytoplasm **(A)**. The cells forming the central lumina are cuboidal to low columnar secretory-type cells, with uniform round nuclei and clear cytoplasm. The glands are rimmed with a prominent basal cell layer **(B)**.

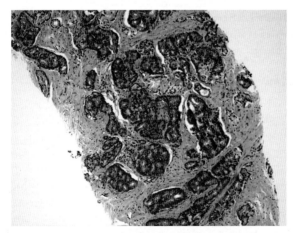

FIG. 5.21

In this prostate biopsy sample, many confluent atypical cribriform glands of varying size and shape are seen in an infiltrative pattern, suggestive of Gleason score 4 + 4 = 8. Basal cells to distinguish intraductal carcinoma of the prostate (IDC-P) from invasive cribriform glands should be utilized only when there is a concern whether the biopsy contains IDC-P only or when the Gleason grade could significantly change with the diagnosis of IDC-P.

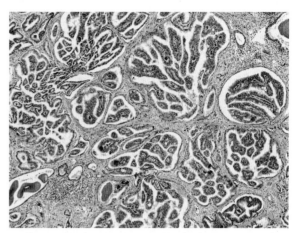

FIG. 5.22

Ductal adenocarcinoma typically grows within preexisting ducts in cribriform and papillary patterns (prominent papillary pattern shown in this example). Glands and papillae are lined by tall pseudostratified columnar cells with elongated nuclei, a definitional feature. Basal cells may be preserved which should not be misinterpreted as high-grade prostatic intraepithelial neoplasia or intraductal carcinoma of the prostate .

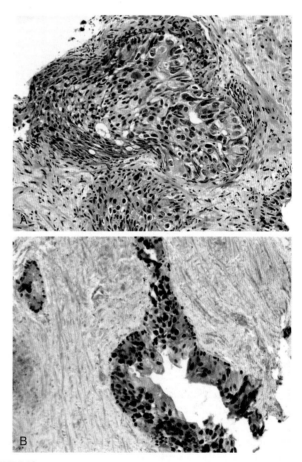

FIG. 5.23

In urothelial carcinoma of the prostate, preexisting acini/ducts are expanded by high-grade pleomorphic cells without evidence of stromal invasion. Cytologic pleomorphism of tumor cells and scattered peripheral basal cells are visible **(A)**. This presentation mimics intraductal spread of high-grade prostate cancer. Strong reactivity for p63 in tumor cells supports the diagnosis of urothelial carcinoma; benign prostate glands demonstrate a peripheral layer of basal cells **(B)**.

TABLE 5.11

Ductal Prostatic Adenocarcinoma (PAC) Versus Prostatic Intraepithelial Neoplasia (PIN)-like PAC Versus High-grade Prostatic Intraepithelial Neoplasia (HGPIN) Versus Papillary Urothelial Carcinoma (UCa)

	Ductal PAC (Fig. 5.24A and B)	PIN-like PAC (Fig. 5.25)	HGPIN	Papillary UCa
Location	Verumontanum and periure-thral ducts Mixed acinar and ductal forms involve peripheral ducts	PZ > TZ	PZ > TZ	TZ > PZ
Histologic features Low power	Cribriform or papillary growth with true fibrovas-cular cores	Crowded proliferation of back-to-back darker than normal glands with frequent cystic dilatation	Scattered darker than normal glands with intra-luminal proliferation	Papillary growth with true fibrovascular cores
Architectural patterns	Cribriform, papillary, and solid slit-like lumina	Tufted, flat, and micropapillary. Crib-riform or papillary architecture is not compatible with the diagnosis. Strips of epithelium at the edge of the biopsy are a frequent finding and a useful clue to the diagnosis	Tufted, flat, and micropap-illary. Rarely cribriform	Papillary fronds with high-grade cells
High power	Pseudostratified columnar nuclei with elongated nu-clei; nuclear enlargement and prominent nuclei	PIN-like ductal adenocarcinoma have glands lined by elongated pseudostratified nuclei with hy-perchromasia but lack prominent nucleoli; PIN-like acinar form has rounder nuclei and lack columnar appearance	Round enlarged nuclei with prominent nucleoli	Marked nuclear pleomor-phism common
Immunohisto-chemistry stains	Can be positive for basal cell markers (in areas show-ing spread in ducts) or negative; variable AMACR positivity	Negative for basal cell markers; vari-able AMACR positivity	Patchy positive for basal cell markers; variable AMACR positivity	Positive for p63 and GATA-3; negative for prostate-specific mark-ers: PSA and NKX3.1

PZ, Peripheral zone; *TZ*, transition zone.

Pathologic Features (Fig. 5.24A and B)

LOW-POWER ARCHITECTURAL FEATURES

This lesion consists of papillary, cribriform, or solid growth patterns. Papillary fronds and glands are lined by pseudostratified columnar epithelium. Glands often have slit-like compressed lumina.

HIGH-POWER CYTOLOGIC FEATURES

The cells lining papillae and cribriform glands have pseu-dostratified columnar epithelium with tall/elongated nu-clei with cytologic atypia, a definitional feature of ductal differentiation. May show preservation of basal cell layer when arising or spreading in large ducts.

IMMUNOHISTOCHEMICAL FEATURES

Can be positive for basal cell markers (in areas showing spread within ducts), an important pitfall that should not be misinterpreted as HGPIN. Variable AMACR positivity.

12) SMALL CELL (NEUROENDOCRINE) CARCINOMA

DIFFERENTIAL DIAGNOSIS: POORLY DIFFERENTIATED UROTHELIAL CARCINOMA, POORLY DIFFERENTIATED PROSTATIC ADENOCARCINOMA (Table 5.12)

Clinical Features

Small cell carcinoma is a high-grade aggressive tumor defined by characteristic nuclear features. Approxi-mately 40% to 50% of small cell carcinomas have a history of conventional PAC. The interval between the diagnosis of small cell carcinoma and prior conven-tional PAC ranges from 1 to 300 months with median of 25 months. Patients with this aggressive disease have frequent systemic disease and less often paraneoplastic

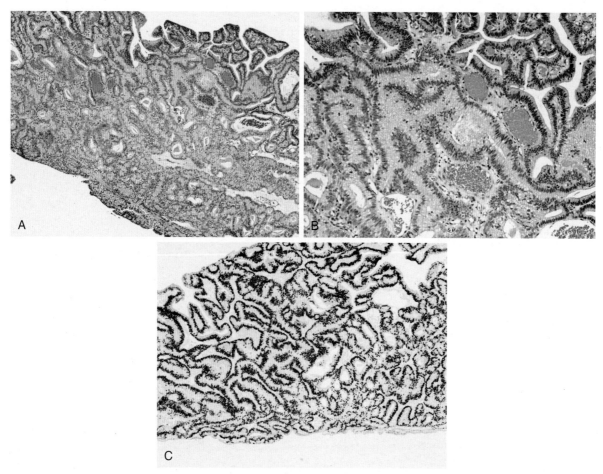

FIG. 5.24

Ductal adenocarcinoma often grows within the urethra as a papillary or polypoid mass. The tumor often has prominent papillary, cribriform or solid architecture that is typically encountered in transurethral resection specimens where the distinction from urothelial carcinoma could be problematic (**A**). Glands and papillae are lined by characteristic ductal epithelium and have prominent slit-like lumina (**B**). An immunohistochemical panel of prostate and urothelial markers should be performed to rule out high-grade urothelial carcinoma. The tumor in this example is seen diffusely positive for NKX3.1 (**C**).

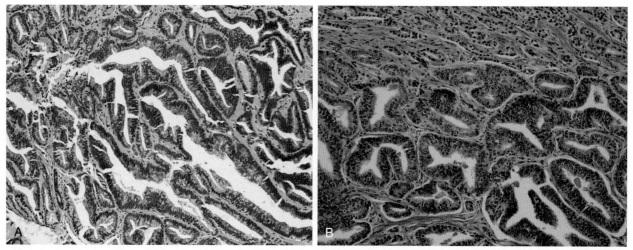

FIG. 5.25

Prostatic intraepithelial neoplasia (PIN)–like adenocarcinoma appears as a focus of crowded large glands. Each individual cancer gland is large and has flat or irregular contours with tufted and micropapillary lumens lined with pseudostratified cells similar to high-grade prostatic intraepithelial neoplasia (HGPIN) glands (**A**). However, cancer glands are more crowded than HGPIN. Nuclei are either round or elongated similar to ductal adenocarcinoma (**B**). Some tumors show less prominent nucleoli than HGPIN. Cribriform or papillary architecture is not compatible with the diagnosis. Cancer glands are devoid of basal cells.

TABLE 5.12

Small Cell Carcinoma Versus Poorly Differentiated Urothelial Carcinoma (UCa) Versus Poorly Differentiated Prostatic Adenocarcinoma (PAC)

	Small Cell Carcinoma (Fig. 5.26)	Poorly Differentiated UCa	Poorly Differentiated PAC (Fig. 5.27A and B)
Location	PZ > TZ	Bladder neck	PZ > TZ
Histologic features Low power	Very blue due to high N:C ratio; geographic necrosis	Darker than normal glands	Eosinophilic appearance due to the low N:C ratio, relatively abundant cytoplasm
Architectural patterns	Sheets of cells without glandular differentiation	Lacks cribriform architecture; typically solid nests	Cribriform glands, large solid nests, and cords and sheets of cells
High power	Salt-and-pepper chromatin with lack of prominent nucleoli, nuclear molding, with very little cytoplasm	Nuclear pleomorphism with hyperchromasia	Nuclei with prominent nucleoli
	Numerous mitoses and apoptotic bodies	Increased mitotic figures with necrosis common	Can have variable mitotic figures and focal necrosis
Immunohistochemistry stains	Positive for at least one NE marker in over 90% of cases; high Ki-67 > 70%; PSA and other prostatic markers negative or only focally positive; p63 and high-molecular-weight cytokeratin positive in subset of cases. TTF1 frequently positive and does not differentiate primary from metastasis	Positive keratin, GATA-3, P63; variable AMACR positivity; negative for prostate markers	PSA and other prostate markers are typically retained and diffusely expressed, neuroendocrine markers can be variably positive, typically lack p63 and high-molecular-weight cytokeratins, Ki-67 < 50%

N:C ratio, Nuclear-to-cytoplasmic ratio; *PZ,* peripheral zone; *TZ,* transition zone.

syndromes. In cases of advanced disease, urinary obstructive symptoms and hematuria, in addition to distant metastases seen on imaging, may occur. Typically occurs in the PZ. Treatment includes multimodality therapy with platinum-based chemotherapy and ADT for associated conventional PAC. Small cell or large cell neuroendocrine (NE) carcinoma is not Gleason graded.

Pathologic Features (Fig. 5.26)

LOW-POWER ARCHITECTURAL FEATURES

This tumor is characterized by diffuse proliferation of sheets and nests of very blue cells with high N:C ratio, separated by geographic areas of necrosis. A starry sky pattern is common due to high cellular proliferation.

HIGH-POWER CYTOLOGIC FEATURES

Characteristic nuclear features include salt-and-pepper–type chromatin with lack of prominent nucleoli, nuclear molding, fragility, and crush artifact. High mitotic rate and apoptotic bodies are common. Morphologic variations include intermediate cell type with slightly more open chromatin and visible small nucleoli, seen in about 30% to 40% of cases.

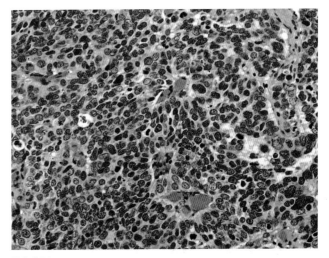

FIG. 5.26
Pure small cell carcinoma involving the prostate shows basophilic tumor cells arranged in haphazard nests and trabeculae. Cytologic features are identical to its pulmonary counterpart with scant cytoplasm, spindling of nuclei with salt-and-pepper chromatin, indistinct nucleoli, increased mitosis, apoptosis, and geographic areas of necrosis.

IMMUNOHISTOCHEMICAL FEATURES

Small cell carcinomas are positive for one or more NE markers (synaptophysin, chromogranin, CD56, INSM-1) in almost 90% of cases. PSA and other prostatic markers

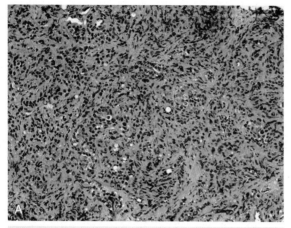

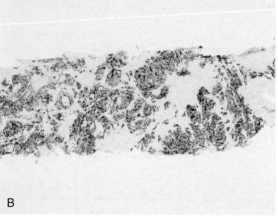

FIG. 5.27

Poorly differentiated prostatic adenocarcinoma, Gleason score 5 + 5 = 10 in prostate biopsy with crush artifact, mimics small cell (neuroendocrine) carcinoma. Despite crush artifact, tumor cells exhibit relatively abundant cytoplasm and focal glandular differentiation **(A)**. Prostate-specific antigen was diffusely positive **(B)**. Focal neuroendocrine markers expression was noted and Ki-67 demonstrated moderate proliferation of about 40% (not shown).

are typically negative or focally positive. In up to 30% of cases, positivity for basal cell markers can be present. TTF-1 is positive in up to 50% of cases. Ki-67 demonstrates high proliferation rate, typically >70%.

13) PROSTATE STROMAL SARCOMA

DIFFERENTIAL DIAGNOSIS: SARCOMATOID CARCINOMA, GASTROINTESTINAL STROMAL TUMOR, MALIGNANT SOLITARY FIBROUS TUMOR, LEIOMYOSARCOMA (Table 5.13)

Clinical Features

Prostatic stromal sarcoma typically presents with lower urinary tract obstruction, abnormal digital rectal exam,

and hematuria. Patients may exhibit symptoms of rectal fullness and/or a palpable rectal mass. Serum PSA levels are often within normal limits. Age of presentation is before the age of 50. Can occur in the PZ or TZ. Treatment includes radical prostatectomy; however, optimal therapy for metastatic disease is unknown.

Pathologic Features (Fig. 5.28A and B)

LOW-POWER ARCHITECTURAL FEATURES

The tumor is characterized by hypercellular stroma. Stromal overgrowth, infiltration, and extraprostatic extension is frequently present. It can resemble stromal tumor of uncertain malignant potential (STUMP) with scattered atypical, but degenerative-appearing stromal cells. However, intervening stroma is too hypercellular for STUMP. Biphasic malignant phyllodes pattern with hypercellular mitotically active stroma with atypia covered by benign-appearing prostatic epithelium can also be present. Myxoid stroma is uncommon. Other patterns include: storiform, epithelioid, fibrosarcomatous, and patternless.

HIGH-POWER CYTOLOGIC FEATURES

Nuclear features of malignancy include marked nuclear pleomorphism, increased mitoses, necrosis, and apoptotic bodies. Epithelial component if present is typically benign in nature.

IMMUNOHISTOCHEMICAL FEATURES

Immunohistochemical stains are generally not helpful with this diagnosis. Tumor cells are positive for CD34 and frequently for progesterone receptor (PR).

BLADDER

1) UROTHELIAL CARCINOMA *IN SITU*

DIFFERENTIAL DIAGNOSIS: REACTIVE UROTHELIAL ATYPIA, RADIATION/CHEMOTHERAPY UROTHELIAL ATYPIA (Table 5.14)

Clinical Features

Primary or de novo urothelial carcinoma *in situ* (CIS) is exceedingly rare. It is typically detected with a high-grade

TABLE 5.13

Prostatic Stromal Sarcoma Versus Sarcomatoid Carcinoma Versus Gastrointestinal Stromal Tumor (GIST) Versus Malignant Solitary Fibrous Tumor (SFT) Versus Leiomyosarcoma

	Prostatic Stromal Sarcoma (Fig. 5.28A and B)	Sarcomatoid Carcinoma (Fig. 5.29)	GIST (Fig. 5.30A and B)	Malignant SFT (Fig. 5.31)	Leiomyosarcoma (Fig. 5.32)
Location	PZ = TZ	TZ > PZ	Posterior of the prostate, arising from rectum or perirectal space. No convincing case of intraprostatic GIST reported	Most arise in prostate but can occur from secondary extension	Prostate or periprostatic mesenchymal elements
Gross features	Solid or partially cystic mass			Well circumscribed, firm with white-tan cut surface	Large, solid mass; may have cystic degeneration
Histologic features Low power	May resemble STUMP, however, intervening stroma is very hypercellular and shows stromal overgrowth with infiltration, hypercellularity, and EPE	Identifiable adenocarcinomatous and mesenchymal component	Fascicle or palisading growth pattern of cellular uniform spindle cells that lack pleomorphism and collagen deposition between tumor cells; biopsy typically lacks prostate glands	Ropey collagen and thick-walled irregular staghorn-shaped blood vessels	Sweeping intersecting fascicles of spindle cells, Lacks an adenocarcinomatous component
	Biphasic growth pattern resembling malignant phyllodes pattern with hypercellular mitotically active stroma with atypia; covered by benign-appearing prostate epithelium can be seen	Adenocarcinomatous component can be acinar, ductal, squamous, or small cell type		Patternless pattern	May have an epithelioid morphology
High power	Nuclear hyperchromasia and pleomorphism, mitotic activity, and necrosis. Epithelial component if present is typically benign in nature	High-grade spindle cells with or without heterologous elements and epithelioid component	Occasional perinuclear vacuoles	Haphazardly arranged spindled cells with oval nuclei and scant cytoplasm	Varying nuclear atypia, mitotic activity, and necrosis; can be low grade or high grade
Immunohistochemistry stains	Positive for CD34 and PR; variable positivity for SMA and desmin	Spindle cell component variably positive for keratins, especially HMWCK; p63 is a sensitive marker for epithelial differentiation in the spindle cell component; variably positive for PSA, PSAP, NKX3.1, SMA and desmin; negative for CD34	Positive for CD34; diffusely and strongly positive for CD117 (CKIT) and DOG1; S100, SMA and desmin are typically negative	Positive for CD34 and STAT6; negative for SMA and desmin; variable positivity for PR	Positive for SMA and desmin; one quarter of cases express cytokeratin (an important pitfall); p63 typically negative

EPE, Extraprostatic extension; *PZ*, peripheral zone; *STUMP*, stromal tumor of uncertain malignant potential; *TZ*, transition zone.

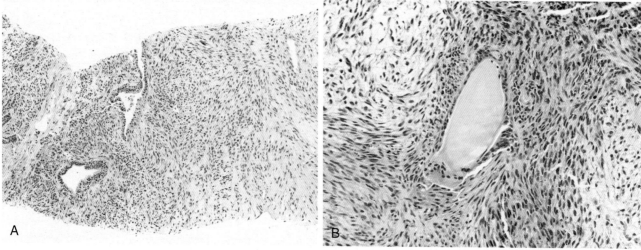

FIG. 5.28

In contrast to stromal tumor of uncertain malignant potential (STUMP), the prostatic stromal sarcoma demonstrates high cellularity **(A)** and obvious cytologic atypia with frequent mitoses **(B)**. Tumor cells may be seen proliferating between preexisting benign glands, similar to STUMP.

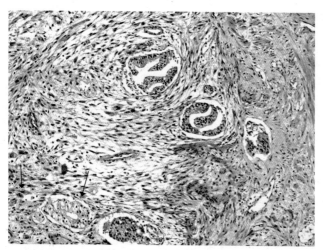

FIG. 5.29

Sarcomatoid carcinoma has high-grade undifferentiated spindle cell sarcoma with a myxoid background. Acinar carcinoma is present *(arrows)* and is intimately admixed with the sarcomaotid component. In contrast to prostate stromal sarcoma, epithelial component in sarcomatoid carcinoma is malignant. Extensive sampling is usually required to document the presence of the epithelial component. History of previous prostate carcinoma is also very useful to diagnose a sarcomatoid carcinoma and rule out primary sarcoma.

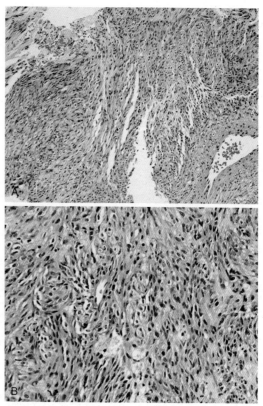

FIG. 5.30

Gastrointestinal stromal tumor (GIST) in a prostate core biopsy often represents rectal-based tumors that compress and displace the prostate gland. These GISTs, similar to other sites of origin, may have a variety of histologic patterns, including spindled and epithelioid morphology **(A, B)**. The spindle cell morphology may have significant overlap with that of prostatic stromal proliferations, which are more common. Immunophenotypically, GISTs characteristically express CD34, CD117, and DOG-1. One must remember to consider this diagnostic possibility in prostate biopsies. GISTs involving the prostate gland should be evaluated using standard prognostic stratification proposed by WHO.

urothelial carcinoma (UCa) component. Most commonly seen in the sixth or seventh decade of life. Patients may present asymptomatically, or with dysuria, nocturia, and microscopic hematuria. Cystoscopic appearance can range from normal, to frequently erythematous velvety lesion, to edematous or erosive. It commonly presents as multifocal disease.

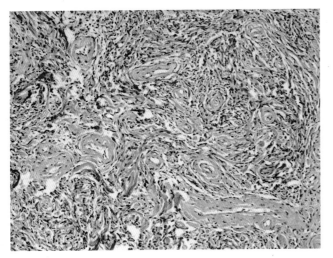

FIG. 5.31

Solitary fibrous tumor (SFT) involving the prostate gland demonstrates proliferation of bland spindle cells with a "patternless" pattern of stroma that is collagenized. Lack of admixed prostate glands and prominent collagen deposition in the stroma distinguishes it from a prostate stromal tumor. Vessels are abundant, hyalinized, and vary from small capillaries to characteristic larger hemangiopericytoma-like staghorn vessels. Strong and diffuse nuclear reactivity of STAT6 monoclonal antibody, suggestive of *NAB2-STAT6* gene fusion, is characteristic and confirms the diagnosis of SFT.

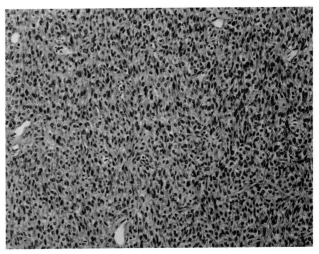

FIG. 5.32

The transurethral resection of the prostate (TURP) specimen from a 58-year-old man demonstrated diffuse proliferation of high-grade spindle and epithelioid cells in a fascicular growth pattern. Some nuclei have a cigar shape and demonstrate frequent atypical mitoses. The differential diagnosis included prostatic stromal sarcoma, sarcomatoid carcinoma, and leiomyosarcoma. Tumor cells were diffusely and strongly positive for several muscle markers including desmin, calponin, and muscle-specific actin (*not shown*). The tumor cells also demonstrated focal aberrant reactivity for pan cytokeratin. The diagnosis of high-grade leiomyosarcoma was made.

TABLE 5.14

Carcinoma *In Situ* (CIS) Versus Reactive Urothelium Versus Radiation/Chemotherapy (RT/CT) Urothelial Atypia

	CIS (Fig. 5.33A–C)	Reactive Urothelium (Fig. 5.34)	RT/CT Urothelial Atypia (Fig. 5.35A and B)
Cystoscopic features	Flat lesion with erythematous, edematous, or erosive appearance	Flat lesion with erythematous, edematous, or erosive appearance	Flat lesion with erythematous, edematous, or erosive appearance
Histologic features Low power	Morphologic patterns include: pleomorphic, pagetoid, "clinging" or denuding, small cell, plasmacytoid type	Degree of reactive changes proportional to extent of inflammation	Flat mucosa and von Brunn nests exhibit marked random and degenerative-type atypia
	Loss of cellular cohesion and polarity to basement membrane common	Intraepithelial inflammation is prominent. Cellular cohesion and polarity maintained	Surrounding stroma shows reactive changes including hemorrhage, fibrin thrombi, and atypical stromal cells. Cellular cohesion and polarity maintained
	Thickness variable	Thickness variable	Thickness variable
High power	Nucleomegaly more than five times normal lymphocyte nucleus	Enlarged nuclei	Nuclei are bizarre with multinucleation and vacuolization
	Coarse, condensed nuclear chromatin	Nuclei uniform in size and shape, nuclei vesicular with central prominent nucleoli.	Nuclei often have degenerative atypia, cytoplasm abundant with spindled appearance
	Mitoses variable, with atypical forms that frequently present in upper layer	Mitotic figures may be numerous, lacks atypical mitoses	Mitoses variable, lacks atypical mitosis
Immunohistochemistry stains	CK20 full thickness positivity; CD44 negative or restricted to basal cells; p53 aberrant expression is specific but lacks sensitivity	CK20 confined to the umbrella cell layer; CD44 positive in basal and upper layers	CK20 confined to the umbrella cell layer; CD44 positive in basal and upper layers

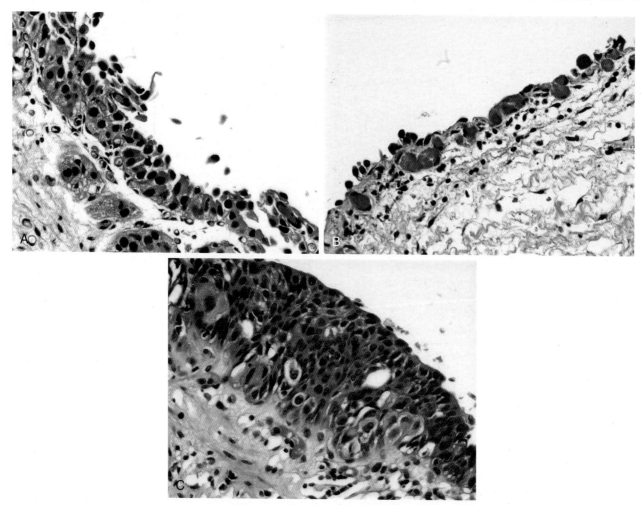

FIG. 5.33

A, In carcinoma *in situ* (CIS), cells are discohesive with markedly enlarged hyperchromatic nuclei relative to stromal lymphocytes. Nuclei are variable in size and shape. Mitosis including atypical forms are seen. **B**, CIS with marked denudation of urothelium. Remaining cells are loosely cohesive with markedly enlarged and hyperchromatic cells, characteristic of "clinging" or "denuding" type. **C**, In pagetoid CIS, few markedly atypical cells with abundant cytoplasm are seen dispersed throughout otherwise a normal-appearing epithelium.

Pathologic Features (Fig. 5.33A–C)

LOW-POWER ARCHITECTURAL FEATURES

Urothelial CIS has various morphologic patterns: pleomorphic, pagetoid, "clinging" (denuding), small cell, and plasmacytoid. Urothelial thickness varies from denuded to normal to hyperplastic. Loss of cellular cohesion and polarity is frequently observed.

HIGH-POWER CYTOLOGIC FEATURES

There is marked nucleomegaly of more than five times the size of a normal lymphocyte nucleus. Nuclear chromatin is coarse, condensed with frequent pleomorphism. Mitoses are variable, with atypical forms, frequently extending to the upper layer of urothelium. A strict diagnostic threshold is maintained for this diagnosis. For a lesion that appears worse than reactive/inflammatory atypia but falls short of diagnostic

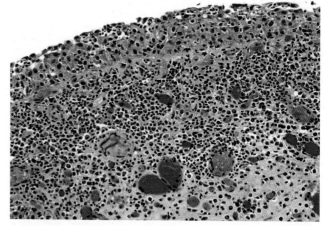

FIG. 5.34

In reactive urothelial atypia, polarity of cells is well maintained. Nuclei are uniformly enlarged with vesicular chromatin and single prominent nucleoli. Numerous intramucosal neutrophils are present with background inflammation.

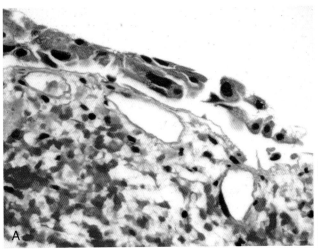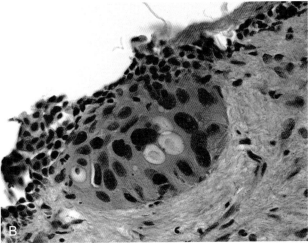

FIG. 5.35

In treatment-induced cytologic atypia, polarity of cells is maintained. Nuclei show random degenerative-type marked cytologic atypia. Stroma shows reactive changes **(A)**. Cells have abundant often vacuolated cytoplasm with frequent multinucleation. Mitotic activity, specifically atypical forms, not seen **(B)**.

criteria of CIS, the diagnosis of dysplasia should be considered in the differential. The term flat urothelial atypia of unknown significance is utilized when cytologic atypia cannot be distinguished between dysplasia from a reactive/inflammatory process.

IMMUNOHISTOCHEMICAL FEATURES

CK20 demonstrates full-thickness positivity. Full-thickness staining does not distinguish dysplasia from CIS. Additionally, loss of CD44 expression or expression confined to the basal cell layer is seen. P53 aberrant expression (diffuse positive or null phenotype) is a specific staining pattern of CIS but lacks sensitivity. Immunohistochemical markers are not helpful in differential of dysplasia from CIS.

2) LOW-GRADE PAPILLARY UROTHELIAL CARCINOMA

DIFFERENTIAL DIAGNOSIS: PAPILLARY UROTHELIAL NEOPLASM OF LOW MALIGNANT POTENTIAL, UROTHELIAL PAPILLOMA (Table 5.15)

Clinical Features

UCa has a male predominance (M:F, 3:1). Mean age of presentation is in the seventh decade of life. Patients present with gross or microscopic hematuria. Stage progression is very rare, but recurrence or new occurrence is common. Cystoscopic examination shows exophytic fronds of tumor that can vary from solitary or multiple with a wide range of size.

Pathologic Features (Fig. 5.36)

LOW-POWER ARCHITECTURAL FEATURES

The papillae of this lesion are long and slender with frequent branching and fusion. It is lined by hyperplastic urothelium that has increased cell layers and/or increased cell density. The level of cytoarchitectural disorder is minimal to mild. Cells have minimal loss of polarity and can have a "streaming" appearance with a general maintenance of the basal cell layer.

HIGH-POWER CYTOLOGIC FEATURES

Cells are relatively uniform in size without significant nuclear pleomorphism or nucleomegaly. Nuclei are often rounded and bland in appearance. Nuclear chromatin is relatively fine to slightly abnormal. Mitotic figures are rare, and usually confined to basal cell layer. Cases with focal high-grade atypia, typically ≥5% of tumor is overall classified as high grade using the 2014 International Society of Urologic Pathology (ISUP)/World Health Organization (WHO) criteria.

IMMUNOHISTOCHEMICAL FEATURES

Immunohistochemical features of papillary tumors are typically not reliable.

TABLE 5.15

Low-grade Papillary Urothelial Carcinoma (UCa) Versus Papillary Urothelial Neoplasm of Low Malignant Potential (PUNLMP) Versus Urothelial Papilloma

	Low-grade Papillary UCa (Fig. 5.36)	PUNLMP (Fig. 5.37)	Urothelial Papilloma (Fig. 5.38)
Cystoscopic features	Exophytic papillary lesion	Small exophytic papillary lesion	Small exophytic/papillary lesion
Histologic features Low power	Urothelium overtly thick	Urothelium overtly thick	Urothelium normal in thickness
	Focal architectural abnormality including papillary fusion common	Discrete papillae lined by hyper-plastic urothelium	Discrete papillae
	May present with inverted growth	May present with inverted growth	Exophytic growth pattern
	Polarity mostly maintained but can have regions of streaming appearance	Polarity strictly maintained	Well-maintained polarity
High power	Mild cytologic atypia	Cytology is normal with minimal atypia	Cytology is normal
	Nucleoli range from indistinct to small	Nuclei uniform in size and shape with indistinct nucleoli	Umbrella cells vary from inconspicuous to prominent with degenerative-type atypia
	Few mitoses are allowed for the diagnosis	Mitoses absent to rare	Mitoses absent
Immunohistochemistry stains	Not reliable in this differential	Not reliable in this differential	Not reliable in this differential

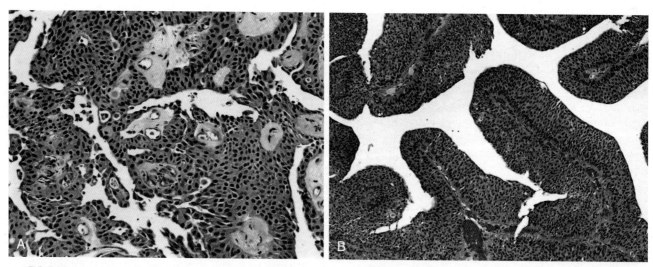

FIG. 5.36

A, In low-grade papillary urothelial carcinoma, mild to moderate architectural atypia characterized by few fused papillae may be present. **B,** The lining urothelium is thickened with mild cytologic atypia characterized by slightly enlarged hyperchromatic nuclei with minimum variation is size and shape. Few mitotic figures are permissible for the diagnosis.

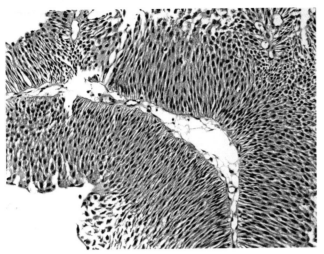

FIG. 5.37
In papillary urothelial neoplasm of low malignant potential, papillae are discrete, typically non-fused. The urothelium is overtly thick, even at low magnification. Cytology is normal or at most slightly enlarged nuclei with virtually absent mitotic activity.

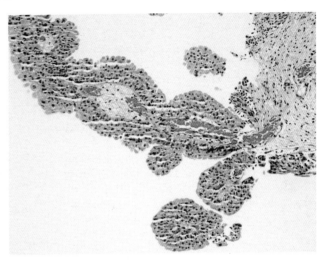

FIG. 5.38
In urothelial papilloma, well-defined papillary fronds with fibrovascular cores are present. No significant architectural complexity is present. Papillae are lined by normal thickness urothelium with benign cytology. Prominent umbrella cells with reactive cytologic atypia may be present.

3) PAPILLARY/POLYPOID CYSTITIS

DIFFERENTIAL DIAGNOSIS: PAPILLARY UROTHELIAL NEOPLASM, PAPILLARY NEPHROGENIC ADENOMA (Table 5.16)

Clinical Features

Papillary/polypoid cystitis often times is related to indwelling catheter, vesicle fistula, or post-radiation therapy. It can occur in any age group. Patient presents with hematuria and irritative bladder symptoms. Cystoscopic appearance is of edematous broad, elongated papillae with friable mucosal irregularity.

Pathologic Features (Fig. 5.39)

LOW-POWER ARCHITECTURAL FEATURES

Polypoid cystitis is usually small in size (<1 cm) but may involve the mucosa more diffusely. It is characterized by exophytic projections of urothelium secondary to underlying edema within the lamina propria. Papillae lack complex branching. Stromal cores are composed of edema and fibrosis with a broad base. Background mucosa shows reactive changes, including acute and chronic inflammation. Occasional small papillary structures can be present. The presence of reactive background stroma is typically seen and is a useful diagnostic clue.

HIGH-POWER CYTOLOGIC FEATURES

Overlying urothelium can be hyperplastic in appearance with urothelial atypia that is reactive/inflammatory in nature.

IMMUNOHISTOCHEMICAL FEATURES

Immunohistochemical studies are not helpful in differential of the urothelial neoplasia spectrum. However, PAX8 can be helpful in distinction from papillary nephrogenic adenoma (NA) as papillary/polypoid cystitis is negative for PAX8.

4) NEPHROGENIC ADENOMA

DIFFERENTIAL DIAGNOSIS: CLEAR CELL ADENOCARCINOMA OF URINARY TRACT, NESTED AND TUBULAR VARIANT OF UROTHELIAL CARCINOMA, PROSTATIC ADENOCARCINOMA (Table 5.17)

Clinical Features

NA is typically seen secondary to longstanding urothelial injury such as calculi, infection, neurogenic bladder, and instrumentation. It can also be seen in association with diverticuli. It is usually an incidental finding. Patients can have irritative symptoms from an underlying

TABLE 5.16

Polypoid/Papillary Cystitis Versus Papillary Urothelial Neoplasm Versus Papillary Nephrogenic Adenoma (NA)

	Polypoid/Papillary Cystitis (Fig. 5.39)	Papillary Urothelial Neoplasm (Fig. 5.40)	Papillary NA (Fig. 5.41)
Cystoscopic features	Edematous broad, elongated papillae with friable mucosal irregularity	Papillary tumor	Variably, papillary or nodular; velvety lesion, can be multifocal
Histological features Low power	Simple folds/pseudopapillae of pale, edematous urothelium	Well-defined finger-like and branching papillae with delicate fibrovascular cores	Smooth with focal exophytic fronds
	Papillae are wide based with edematous stroma that lack discrete fibrovascular core	Base of papillary fronds are typically narrow	Papillary surface lined by attenuated cuboidal epithelium
	Background stroma has reactive changes, which often provides important diagnostic clue		Multilayered lining epithelium is not seen, a useful feature to separate from papillary urothelial neoplasm
	In older lesions, stroma can be densely fibrotic with associated inflammation	Stalks with loose stroma, small well-defined fibrovascular core; without inflammation	May also exhibit tubular component. Tubules are often surrounded by hyaline connective tissue sheath
High power	Urothelium has reactive-type atypia	Urothelial atypia with enlarged nuclei with variable size and hyperchromasia	Cuboidal cells may have prominent nucleoli with hobnailing
	Mitoses can be seen	Mitoses can be seen	Mitoses rare or absent
Immunohistochemistry stains	Not reliable in this differential	Not reliable in this differential	Positive for PAX8

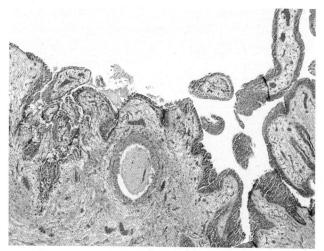

FIG. 5.39

In polypoid cystitis, simple folds of pale, edematous urothelium containing inflammatory cells with wide base are characteristically present. Folds lack well-defined fibrovascular cores. Occasional smaller edematous papillary structures could be misdiagnosed as papillary urothelial neoplasm.

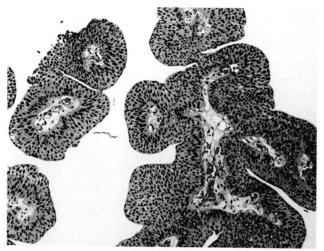

FIG. 5.40

In papillary urothelial neoplasm, stalk may appear edematous, yet is not inflamed, and exhibit numerous prominent capillaries. Urothelium is markedly thickened. Complex branching pattern including multiple "free-floating" fronds are frequently present.

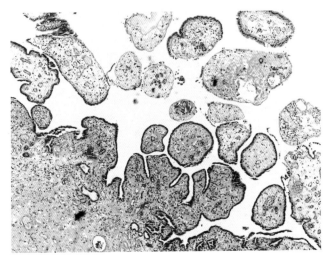

FIG. 5.41

In papillary nephrogenic adenoma, simple folds of urothelium without well-defined fibrovascular cores are present, lined by attenuated bland cuboidal lining epithelium. Multilayered lining epithelium is absent.

inflammatory process. Cystoscopic appearance of a papillary/polypoid lesion or irregular flat velvety lesion.

Pathologic Features (Fig. 5.42A–C)

LOW-POWER ARCHITECTURAL FEATURES

Variety of architectural patterns can be observed and is often admixed: tubular/glandular, papillary, cystic, nested, fibromyxoid, and flat. The most common pattern seen is tubular/glandular with admixed papillary pattern which on low power may appear pseudoinfiltrative. The lesion should be restricted to the superficial lamina propria.

HIGH-POWER CYTOLOGIC FEATURES

Lining cells may have a hobnail and atrophic appearance. It can also show single cells with small lumen with

TABLE 5.17

Nephrogenic Adenoma (NA) Versus Clear Cell Adenocarcinoma Versus Nested and Tubular Variant of Urothelial Carcinoma (UCa) Versus Prostatic Adenocarcinoma (PAC)

	NA (Fig. 5.42A–C)	Clear Cell Adenocarcinoma (Fig. 5.43A and B)	Nested and Tubular Variant of UCa	PAC
Cystoscopic features	Variably, papillary or nodular; velvety lesion, frequently is multifocal	Large unifocal exophytic tumor	Nodular surface lacking an exophytic papillary component	Nodular surface lacking an exophytic papillary component, typically encountered in prostatic urethra
Histological features Low power	Tubular, papillary, nests, fibromyxoid, and signet ring cell–like patterns; lesion may appear pseudoinfiltrative but invasion in muscularis propria is not compatible with the diagnosis	Solid, tubular, and papillary patterns; superficially resembles NA but is typically an infiltrative process with jagged borders and/or muscularis propria invasion	May have a coexisting component of papillary UCa; nests and tubules often are confluent	Typically lacks exophytic component
	Eosinophilic cytoplasm with rare focal clear cytoplasm	Variably eosinophilic and/or clear cytoplasm	Lamina propria filled with small crowded tubules and small nests	Crowded small-/medium-caliber glands exhibiting cytoplasmic amphophilia
	Lined by a single cuboidal epithelium with a collar of hyaline connective tissue sheath	Lacks hyaline connective tissue sheath and secretions	Jagged/irregular base with infiltrative tubules extending deep, often within the muscularis propria	Typically "punched out"/straight luminal borders
High power	Cuboidal cells may have prominent nucleoli with hobnailing	Prominent cytologic atypia with hyperchromatic nuclei, may also exhibit hobnailing	Lacks cytologic atypia in areas, but deeper nests may have random cytologic atypia	Nuclear enlargement with prominent nucleoli
	Mitoses rare or absent	Mitotic figures common	Occasional mitotic figures	Mitotic figures can be seen
	Necrosis absent, inflammation is common	Necrosis common	Lacks desmoplastic stroma and inflammatory response	Luminal secretions, crystalloids, blue mucin common

Continued

TABLE 5.17

Nephrogenic Adenoma (NA) Versus Clear Cell Adenocarcinoma Versus Nested and Tubular Variant of Urothelial Carcinoma (UCa) Versus Prostatic Adenocarcinoma (PAC)—cont'd

	NA (Fig. 5.42A–C)	Clear Cell Adenocarcinoma (Fig. 5.43A and B)	Nested and Tubular Variant of UCa	PAC
Immunohistochemistry stains	Positive for PAX8, cytokeratin, EMA, and AMACR	Positive for CK7, CEA, PAX8, AMACR. High Ki67. Immunohistochemical markers are not reliable to distinguish it from NA	Positive for GATA3 and P63. Negative for NKX3.1. Up to 50% of nested UCa may express PAX8, an important diagnostic pitfall. *TERT* mutations are common in nested UCa and may be helpful in distinction from benign mimics in difficult cases in superficial biopsy	Positive for NKX3.1 and AMACR. Negative for PAX8

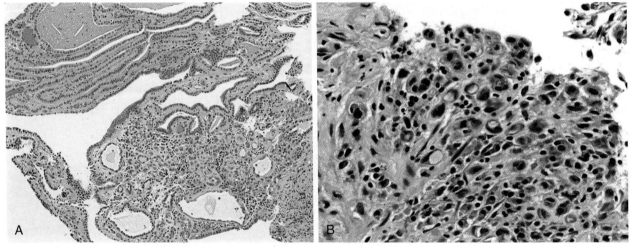

FIG. 5.42

A, Nephrogenic adenoma may exhibit variety of growth patterns including tubules, papillae, vascular-like, fibromyxoid, signet ring cell–like, and nests. Tubulopapillary growth is the most common presentation. Lining epithelium exhibits hobnail changes with frequent reactive epithelial atypia. **B**, Some tubules are surrounded by hyaline connective tissue sheath, a useful diagnostic feature. Necrosis is absent. Pseudoinfiltrative growth pattern can be seen, but muscle invasion is not permissible for the diagnosis.

eccentric nuclei that mimic signet ring cells. May contain basophilic or eosinophilic intraluminal secretions. A thick basement membrane/hyalinized sheath often surrounds epithelium. Lining cells are usually bland with eosinophilic to clear cytoplasm but may demonstrate prominent nucleoli due to the reactive changes and background inflammation. Degenerative-type atypia is common.

IMMUNOHISTOCHEMICAL FEATURES

NA is diffusely positive for PAX8, cytokeratins, and EMA. Majority of lesions also express AMACR (P504S), an important pitfall while working up for a differential diagnosis of PAC.

5) PSEUDOCARCINOMATOUS EPITHELIAL HYPERPLASIA

DIFFERENTIAL DIAGNOSIS: SUPERFICIALLY INVASIVE UCA (Table 5.18)

Clinical Features

Pseudocarcinomatous epithelial hyperplasia or proliferation is a term utilized to describe an epithelial proliferation that usually is seen following radiation or chemotherapy.

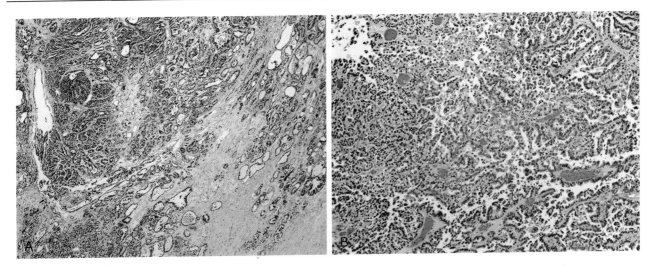

FIG. 5.43

A, In clear cell adenocarcinoma, tubulopapillary proliferation superficially mimics nephrogenic adenoma. **B,** Tubules and papillae exhibit prominent cytologic atypia characterized by hyperchromatic hobnail nuclei with clear to eosinophilic cytoplasm. Mitoses are frequently observed and necrosis is common. Deep invasion into muscularis propria may be present but usually not evident on limited biopsy.

TABLE 5.18

Pseudocarcinomatous Epithelial Hyperplasia Versus Superficially Invasive Urothelial Carcinoma (UCa)

	Pseudocarcinomatous Epithelial Hyperplasia (Fig. 5.44)	Superficially Invasive UCa (Fig. 5.45)
Cystoscopic features	Localized or diffuse erythematous lesion, can appear polypoid	Polypoid or mass lesion
Histological features Low power	Background stroma provides important clues to the diagnosis with numerous vessels having fibrin thrombi, vascular congestion, and hemorrhage	Stroma shows desmoplastic or myxoid/inflammatory response. Stroma lacks fibrin thrombi within vessels, hemorrhage, and edema
	Prominent acute and chronic inflammation within intervening stroma	May have inflammatory response, but often not pronounced
	Ulceration common	Ulceration common
	Nests of urothelial cells within in the lamina propria	Nests of urothelial cells within in the lamina propria with frequent retraction artifact; proliferation is haphazard with irregular or infiltrative interface
High power	Lack of overlying associated CIS or papillary carcinoma component	Overlying urothelium may exhibit associated CIS or papillary carcinoma component
	Urothelium with mild to moderate nuclear pleomorphism	Urothelium with moderate to marked nuclear pleomorphism
	Mitotic figures can be seen	Mitotic figures can be seen
Immunohistochemistry stains	Not helpful in this differential	Not helpful in this differential

CIS, Carcinoma *in situ.*

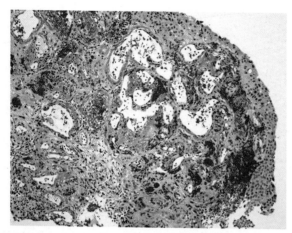

FIG. 5.44

In pseudocarcinomatous epithelial hyperplasia, irregular nests proliferate into the lamina propria. Stroma provides important diagnostic clues. Between nests, numerous dilated blood vessels, fibrin thrombi, and hemorrhage/vascular congestion are typically seen. Admixed acute and chronic inflammation is frequently present.

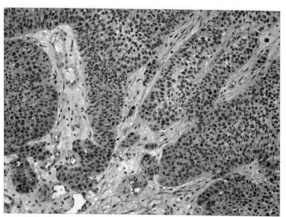

FIG. 5.45

In superficially invasive urothelial carcinoma, overlying carcinoma *in situ* or papillary carcinoma is typically present. Stroma may show desmoplastic or myxoid changes. Retraction spaces surrounding invading nests are frequently seen, while vascular congestion, dilated blood vessels with thrombi are typically not present.

However, morphologic manifestations following radiation and/or chemotherapy could be much broader than seen in pseudocarcinomatous hyperplasia. Can also be seen in low-flow or ischemia-inducing conditions. Patients present with symptoms of radiation cystitis and hematuria. Cystoscopic appearance is of an erythematous polypoid lesion. It can have associated ulceration, edema, and trabeculations.

Pathologic Features (Fig. 5.44)

LOW-POWER ARCHITECTURAL FEATURES

Urothelial proliferation is composed of small nests with rounded or irregular borders. Prominent cytoplasmic

eosinophilia imparting a "squamous" appearance is common. Often times is associated with ulceration. Characteristic stromal changes provide important clues to the diagnosis, which includes vascular congestion/ectasia, stromal hemorrhage, hemosiderin deposition, fibrin thrombi, and hyalinization.

HIGH-POWER CYTOLOGIC FEATURES

Cytologic features in keeping with radiation-induced changes such as cytoplasmic ballooning and multilobulated nuclei may be appreciated. Smudgy nuclear chromatin with associated cytoplasmic vacuoles and karyorrhectic debris is common.

IMMUNOHISTOCHEMICAL FEATURES

Immunohistochemical markers are not helpful in diagnosis or differential diagnosis of this entity.

6) FLORID VON BRUNN NEST PROLIFERATION

DIFFERENTIAL DIAGNOSIS: NESTED VARIANT OF UROTHELIAL CARCINOMA, NEPHROGENIC ADENOMA WITH SOLID NESTS (Table 5.19)

Clinical Features

Florid von Brunn nest proliferation may occur as a result of local inflammation and is considered a variant of normal histology. It increases in frequency with age. Typically occurs in the bladder trigone, renal pelvis, and ureter. Most are cystoscopically not visible but can appear as mucosal blebs when prominent.

Pathologic Features (Fig. 5.46)

LOW-POWER ARCHITECTURAL FEATURES

Florid von Brunn nest proliferations are composed of solid nests of urothelial cells within the superficial lamina propria. Nests have smooth, round contours with occasional confluence and/or branching. Overall has an orderly arrangement with a lobular configuration. Overall, Florid von Brunn nest proliferations have an orderly arrangement with a lobular configuration, and they lack a stromal reaction. Base of lesion has a sharp linear border distinguishing it specifically from nested and/or tubular variant of UCa.

TABLE 5.19

Florid von Brunn Nest Proliferation Versus Nested Variant of Urothelial Carcinoma (UCa) Versus Nephrogenic Adenoma (NA) With Solid Nests

	Florid von Brunn Nest Proliferation (Fig. 5.46)	Nested Variant of UCa (Fig. 5.47A and B)	NA with Solid Nests (Fig. 5.42C)
Cystoscopic features	Tumor-like polypoid mass with smooth surface	Nodular surface, with or without exophytic papillary component	Nodular surface, with or without exophytic papillary component
Histological features Low power	Lamina propria filled with round nests of urothelium	Lamina propria filled with small crowded/confluent nests of urothelium	Lamina propria filled with solid or cord-like pattern; imparts a diffuse pattern when back to back
	Nests are linear or lobular without an infiltrative border	Nests have an irregular base with infiltration into different depths; muscle invasion is common in deeper biopsy	Other admixed patterns often present including papillary and tubular
	Nests evenly spaced without stromal reaction		Prominent basement membrane surrounds nests
High power	Lacks cytologic atypia unless seen with background of inflammation	Lacks cytologic atypia in areas, but deeper nests may have random cytologic atypia with prominent nucleoli	Cuboidal cells may have prominent nucleoli with hobnailing
	Mitotic figures may be seen in the setting of inflammation	Occasional mitotic figures	Mitotic figures absent/rare
Immunohistochemistry stains	Typically, not required in the diagnosis. P63 positive and PAX8 is typically negative. Lacks *TERT* mutations	Not helpful in this differential. Up to 50% of nested UCa may express PAX8, an important diagnostic pitfall. The presence of *TERT* mutation may be helpful in distinction from proliferative von Brunn nests in difficult cases	Positive for PAX8. P63 negative

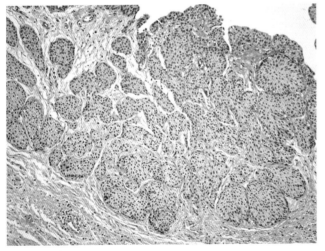

FIG. 5.46

In florid proliferative von Brunn nests, lamina propria is filled with small to large rounded nests of the urothelium with bland cytology. Nests are evenly spaced with linear or rounded borders. One can mentally draw a line at the base of the lesion.

HIGH-POWER CYTOLOGIC FEATURES

Von Brunn nests have small nuclei and bland cytologic features. Cytologic features are similar to the overlying normal urothelium.

IMMUNOHISTOCHEMICAL FEATURES

Immunohistochemical markers are not helpful in diagnosis of this entity. However, in the diagnostic differential with NA with solid nests, florid von Brunn nest proliferation would be negative for PAX8. Von Brunn nest proliferation lacks *TERT* mutations which may be helpful in distinction from nested UCa in difficult cases and/or superficial biopsy specimens.

7) PLASMACYTOID VARIANT OF UROTHELIAL CARCINOMA

DIFFERENTIAL DIAGNOSIS: PLASMACYTOMA, REACTIVE PLASMA CELL PROLIFERATION (Table 5.20)

Clinical Features

Plasmacytoid variant of UCa is a rare variant morphology that is composed of cells that resemble plasma cells and/or signet ring cells. Clinical presentation is similar

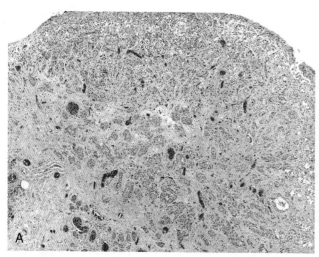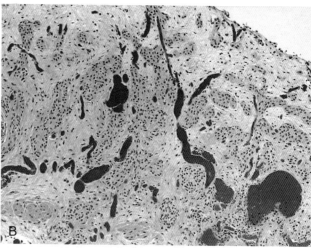

FIG. 5.47

A, In nested urothelial carcinoma, there is proliferation of small to large nests with bland cytology, mimicking proliferative von Brunn nests. **B,** In contrast to von Brunn nests proliferation, nests are often crowded, confluent, and haphazardly placed with infiltrative borders. In deeper biopsy, invasion into muscularis propria is frequently appreciated.

TABLE 5.20

Plasmacytoid Variant of Urothelial Carcinoma (UCa) Versus Plasmacytoma Versus Reactive Cell Proliferation

	Plasmacytoid of Variant UCa (Fig. 5.48A and B)	Plasmacytoma	Reactive Plasma Cell Proliferation
Cystoscopic features	May present with diffuse "linitis plastica–like" disease; typically does not make an exophytic mass	Variable	Does not make an exophytic mass
Histological features Low power	Infiltrative loosely cohesive individual cells that resemble plasma cells or signet ring cells; undermines the surface urothelium	Loosely cohesive individual cells that form a mass lesion	Loosely cohesive individual cells, often admixed with other inflammatory cells
	May co-exist with conventional UCa or other morphologic variants of UCa	Lacks an *in situ* or invasive conventional UCa component	Lacks an *in situ* or invasive conventional UCa component
High power	Individual cells lack pleomorphism and have eosinophilic cytoplasm with eccentrically placed hyperchromatic nuclei	Cells exhibit classic plasmacytoid appearance with basophilic cytoplasm, eccentrically placed nuclei with frequent binucleation and perinuclear halo	Cells exhibit classic plasmacytoid appearance but lacks significant cytologic atypia
	Usually deeply invasive into the muscularis propria	Cytologic atypia is seen but usually lacks pleomorphism	Usually located near the surface urothelium, admixture with other inflammatory infiltrate is common
Immunohistochemistry stains	Positive for GATA3, p63, cytokeratin; may express CD138. Loss of membranous E-cadherin positivity	Positive for CD138; negative for cytokeratin; kappa or lambda restriction may be helpful	Positive for CD138; lacks kappa or lambda restriction

to that of UCa, with hematuria being the main presenting symptom; however, majority present with advanced disease. May present with diffuse "linitis plastica-like" disease; typically does not make an exophytic mass. Extravesical involvement including peritoneal spread is common. It is considered to be one of the most aggressive variants of UCa.

Pathologic Features (Fig. 5.48A and B)

LOW-POWER ARCHITECTURAL FEATURES

Plasmacytoid variant of UCa is characterized by the presence of discohesive malignant cells in a loose myxoid stroma. A component of high-grade UCa is present

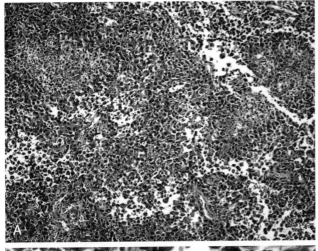

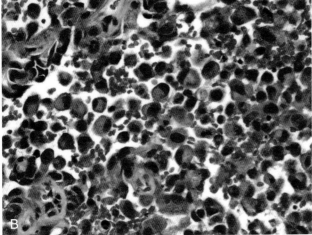

FIG. 5.48

In plasmacytoid urothelial carcinoma, loosely cohesive individual infiltrating cells are present **(A)**. Cells have plasmacytoid or sometimes signet ring cell features with hyperchromatic eccentrically pushed nuclei. Cells typically lack pleomorphism **(B)**. It may coexist with usual urothelial carcinoma. Cells are usually deeply invasive into the muscularis propria with a linitis plastica pattern.

in about 50% of cases. UCa previously diagnosed as signet ring cell adenocarcinoma without extracellular blue mucin is now included within the spectrum of plasmacytoid UCa.

HIGH-POWER CYTOLOGIC FEATURES

The tumor cells have eosinophilic cytoplasm and eccentrically placed enlarged, hyperchromatic nuclei with small nucleoli. Cytologic atypia can be minimal. In addition to the plasmacytoid component, a number of single cells with cytoplasmic vacuoles imparting a signet ring appearance may be seen.

IMMUNOHISTOCHEMICAL FEATURES

Tumor cells are positive for CK7, pancytokeratin, p63, and GATA3. It is characterized by loss of E-cadherin

expression due to truncating mutation of the gene. It frequently expresses plasma cell marker CD138, an important diagnostic pitfall.

8) MICROPAPILLARY VARIANT OF UROTHELIAL CARCINOMA

DIFFERENTIAL DIAGNOSIS: INVASIVE UROTHELIAL CARCINOMA WITH RETRACTION ARTIFACT, UROTHELIAL CARCINOMA WITH LYMPHOVASCULAR INVASION (Table 5.21)

Clinical Features

Micropapillary variant of UCa is a well-recognized variant morphology, constituting 0.6% to 2.2% of all UCa. There is a male predominance with an M:F ratio of 3:1. Peak incidence is in the sixth decade of life. Clinically, it often presents with advanced disease including nodal metastasis. Patients with micropapillary UCa without muscle invasion may be offered an early cystectomy for disease management.

Pathologic Features (Fig. 5.49)

LOW-POWER ARCHITECTURAL FEATURES

Micropapillary UCa displays multiple small filiform nests, without vascular cores, in the same lacunar space. This feature is considered to be a definitional feature. Other features include back-to-back lacunae, ring forms, and cytoplasmic vacuolization. Lymphovascular invasion is present in more than 50% of cases. A component of conventional UCa and/or CIS when present is a helpful feature to suggest the primary process.

HIGH-POWER CYTOLOGIC FEATURES

The nuclei are peripherally oriented with atypia. Cytoplasmic vacuoles with distortion of the nuclear contours are common.

IMMUNOHISTOCHEMICAL FEATURES

Micropapillary UCa shows similar immunophenotype as conventional UCa. HER2/neu overexpression is frequently present and may be helpful in management of advanced cases.

TABLE 5.21

Micropapillary Variant of Urothelial Carcinoma (UCa) Versus Invasive UCa With Retraction Artifact Versus UCa With Lymphovascular Invasion (LVI)

	Micropapillary Variant of UCa (Fig. 5.49)	Invasive UCa With Retraction Artifact (Fig. 5.50)	UCa With LVI (Fig. 5.51)
Cystoscopic features	Nodular or papillary tumor	Nodular or papillary tumor	Nodular or papillary tumor
Histological features Low power	Typically extensive tumor with frequent muscularis propria invasion	Nests are variably sized with each surrounded by its own individual space or lacuna. Shapes of nests conform to the shape of the space	Shape and size of nests within space differ from surrounding infiltrating tumor
	Small filiform nests do not necessarily conform to the shape of the space	Shape and size of nests within space do not differ from surrounding infiltrating tumor	Typically seen as isolated foci, consistent with a distribution of vessels
High power	Numerous uniformly sized nests of carcinoma with peripheral localization of nuclei and central cytoplasm in a large lacuna	Nests within spaces lacking endothelial cells	Nests of carcinoma within spaces lined by endothelial cells
	Back-to-back lacunae and cytoplasmic vacuolization is frequently seen		
Immunohistochemistry stains	Not helpful in this differential	IHC is negative for vascular markers	Typically not helpful in this differential but vessels can be highlighted by CD31 and ERG

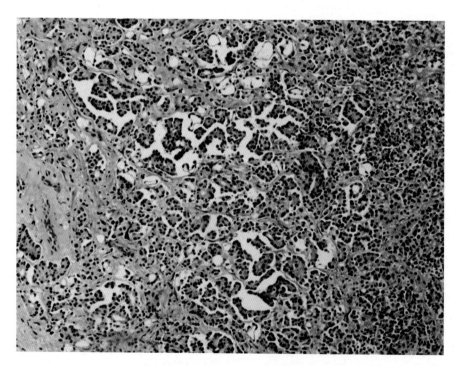

FIG. 5.49

In micropapillary urothelial carcinoma, numerous small uniform filiform nests are seen floating within the same lacunar space, a characteristic feature. Lacunae are back to back. Urothelial nests show peripheral localization of nuclei and cytoplasmic vacuolization.

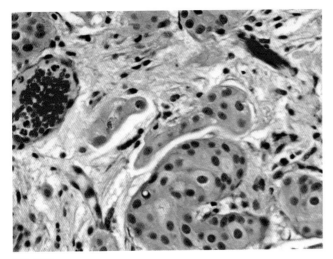

FIG. 5.50
Infiltrating urothelial carcinoma with retraction artifact. The spaces lack an endothelial lining and the have the same shape as the nests of carcinoma.

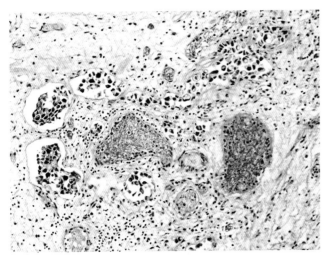

FIG. 5.51
Vascular invasion within a blood vessel. The intravascular nest's shape is different from the shape of the vessel and from the surrounding tumor.

9) INFLAMMATORY MYOFIBROBLASTIC TUMOR OR POSTOPERATIVE SPINDLE-CELL NODULE

DIFFERENTIAL DIAGNOSIS: LEIOMYOSARCOMA, SARCOMATOID UROTHELIAL CARCINOMA (Table 5.22)

Clinical Features

Inflammatory myofibroblastic tumor (IMT) or postoperative spindle-cell nodule has no known inflammatory

or infectious etiology. It presents usually in the second to fourth decade of life but can also be seen in children. Patients may have a history of trauma or prior instrumentation. It may present with clinical symptoms of gross hematuria, abdominal pain, irritative, or obstructive voiding symptoms. Cystoscopic appearance is that of a polypoid or submucosal nodule. IMT has wide ranging clinical behavior. Recurrence and metastasis may occur.

Pathologic Features (Fig. 5.52A and B)

LOW-POWER ARCHITECTURAL FEATURES

Characterized by proliferation of spindle cells in a loose fascicular or "tissue culture"–like architecture. Individual cells with tapered elongated cytoplasmic processes are present. Cellularity is variable with admixture of edematous and/or myxoid stroma. Areas of zonation of superficial hypocellularity and deeper hypercellularity are commonly present. Admixed inflammatory infiltrate is commonly seen. Prior instrumentation may create a keloid-like collagenous response.

HIGH-POWER CYTOLOGIC FEATURES

Spindle cells have fine and evenly distributed nuclear chromatin. Mitotic activity may be brisk, but atypical mitoses are usually not seen. Necrosis may be present.

IMMUNOHISTOCHEMICAL FEATURES

Spindle cells are positive for SMA and desmin. Strong cytokeratin positivity is common, especially low molecular weight, an important diagnostic pitfall. Two third of cases are positive for ALK. FISH has higher sensitivity than IHC stain.

10) PARAGANGLIOMA

DIFFERENTIAL DIAGNOSIS: INVASIVE UROTHELIAL CARCINOMA, GRANULAR CELL TUMOR (Table 5.23)

Clinical Features

Paragangliomas of the urinary bladder are often associated with a germline mutation in *SDH* genes. Therefore, patients present at a younger age and may have association with other neoplasms such as paragangliomas of other sites, SDH-deficient renal cell carcinoma (RCC),

TABLE 5.22

Inflammatory Myofibroblastic Tumor (IMT) Versus Leiomyosarcoma Versus Sarcomatoid Urothelial Carcinoma (UCa)

	IMT (Fig. 5.52A and B)	Leiomyosarcoma	Sarcomatoid UCa (Fig. 5.53)
Cystoscopic features	Pedunculated mass	Large exophytic mass	Large exophytic mass
Histological features Low power	Plump, stellate, or elongated spindle cells that have a "tissue culture"–like appearance	Compact fascicles of spindle cells that lack "tissue culture"–like appearance	Composed of an epithelial and mesenchymal component, but may lack epithelial component altogether
	Myxoid stroma with prominent vascularity with extravasated erythrocytes and interspersed inflammatory cells	Lacks myxoid stroma; without much vascularity or associated inflammation	Myxoid and sclerosing patterns can mimic IMT; deeply invasive but can be superficial in some cases
High power	Nuclei enlarged yet relatively uniform in size and shape with vesicular chromatin and distinct nucleoli	Nuclei enlarged with pleomorphism and scattered hyperchromatic nuclei	Nuclear pleomorphism and hyperchromasia
	Variable mitotic activity, but typically lacks atypical ones	Variable mitotic activity, with atypical ones	Variable mitotic activity, with atypical ones
Immunohistochemistry stains	Positive for SMA and desmin; strong positivity for cytokeratins is common and important diagnostic pitfall; two third of cases are positive for ALK	Diffusely positive for desmin, SMA; aberrant reactivity for cytokeratin seen in 25%–50% of cases; negative for p63 and high-molecular-weight cytokeratin (CK903 or CK5/6), ALK negative	Positive for high-molecular-weight cytokeratin and CK5/6, and p63 in both epithelial and spindled components. Epithelial differentiation in nonspecific malignant spindle cells is diagnostic of sarcomatoid carcinoma. Mesenchymal components demonstrate reactivity specific to sarcoma component

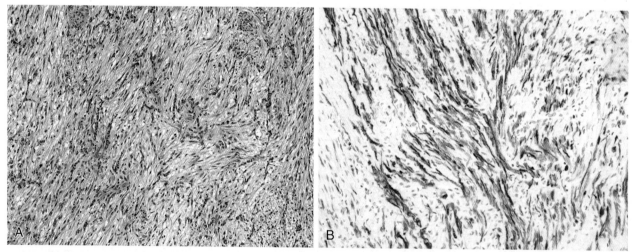

FIG. 5.52

In inflammatory myofibroblastic tumor, "tissue culture"–like fibroblasts in a myxoid background with inflammatory cells are present. Spindle cells proliferate haphazardly in a loose background. Variable mitotic activity is present, but atypical forms are usually not seen **(A)**. Cytokeratins, especially low-molecular-weight, are frequently strongly and diffusely positive, an important diagnostic pitfall **(B)**.

gastrointestinal stromal tumors of stomach, and pituitary adenomas. Less commonly can be associated with von Hippel-Lindau (VHL) disease. Patients present with hematuria and can have associated headache, hypertension, and palpitations. Clinical workup may reveal elevated serum and urine catecholamines. Cystoscopic appearance is usually of a submucosal nodule.

Pathologic Features (Fig. 5.54)

LOW-POWER ARCHITECTURAL FEATURES

Majority of cases show well-delineated/circumscribed submucosal nodules of tumor cells arranged in a zell-ballen/nested pattern with a surrounding prominent

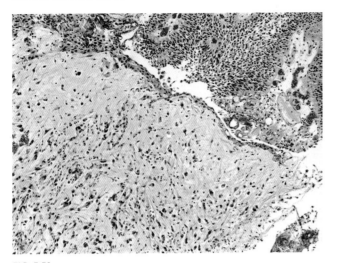

FIG. 5.53
Sarcomatoid carcinoma showing malignant spindle cell proliferation in a myxoid background. A component of conventional urothelial carcinoma is also present, confirming the diagnosis and primary process.

vascular network. Intervening extravasated red blood cells can be seen. Overlying surface urothelium is normal in appearance. Neoplastic cells are round and monomorphic.

HIGH-POWER CYTOLOGIC FEATURES

Nuclear contours are typically round and sharp but can have scattered individual pleomorphic cells characteristic of endocrine-type atypia. Nuclear chromatin is vesicular. Nucleoli are typically not prominent. Cytoplasm

is abundant, eosinophilic to clear, and may be occasionally basophilic. Mitoses may be present.

IMMUNOHISTOCHEMICAL FEATURES

Tumor cells are positive for NE markers: synaptophysin, chromogranin, and CD56. S100 highlights sustentacular cells. Tumor cells are negative for cytokeratins, EMA, and p63. GATA3 is positive, an important diagnostic pitfall.

11) SMALL CELL CARCINOMA

DIFFERENTIAL DIAGNOSIS: POORLY DIFFERENTIATED UROTHELIAL CARCINOMA, LYMPHOMA (Table 5.24)

Clinical Features

Small cell carcinoma of the bladder is rare, accounting for less than 1% of malignant bladder tumors. It affects males more than females, with an M:F ratio of 3:1. Age at presentation is the sixth or seventh decade of life. The most common clinical presenting symptom is hematuria, followed by dysuria and obstructive symptoms. Cystoscopic appearance of the tumor includes large, solid, solitary, polypoid, nodular mass with or without ulceration. It often presents as a systemic disease. Patients

TABLE 5.23			
Paraganglioma Versus Invasive Urothelial Carcinoma (UCa) Versus Granular Cell Tumor			
	Paraganglioma (Fig. 5.54)	Invasive UCa	Granular Cell Tumor
Cystoscopic features	Exophytic mass with intact smooth mucosa	Exophytic mass with irregular mucosa	Exophytic with intact smooth mucosa
Histological features Low power	Well-delineated submucosal nodule of uniformly sized and shaped nests delineated by delicate fibrovascular septae in a "zellballen" pattern	Irregular sized and shaped nests without fibrovascular septae	Lacks fine vascular network
	Can also have small nests with associated surrounding dense collagen	Diffuse to infiltrative type growth pattern common	Sheet-like growth pattern
High power	Nuclei are uniform but endocrine-type random marked nuclear atypia can be seen; atypia is degenerative type	Nuclei with atypia and hyperchromasia	Nuclei are uniform without atypia
	Abundant amphophilic granular cytoplasm	Eosinophilic cytoplasm without granular appearance	Abundant eosinophilic granular cytoplasm
	Mitotic figures are uncommon	Mitotic figures are common	Mitotic figures are rare
Immunohistochemistry stains	Positive for synaptophysin, chromogranin CD56, and GATA3. S100 highlights sustentacular cells. Negative for cytokeratins, EMA and p63	Positive for GATA3 and p63. Negative for NE markers	Diffusely positive for S100

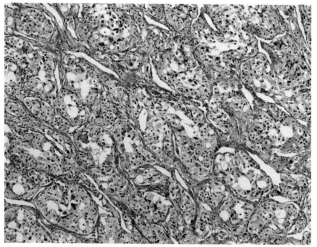

FIG. 5.54

In paraganglioma, large nests are separated by thin vascular network. Tumor cells have densely amphophilic cytoplasm with endocrine-type degenerative nuclear atypia.

often are treated with platinum-based neoadjuvant chemotherapy followed by cystectomy.

Pathologic Features (Fig. 5.55A and B)

LOW-POWER ARCHITECTURAL FEATURES

The tumor is composed of sheets of small cells with high N:C ratio, separated by scant stroma. For designation of a pure small cell carcinoma, the small cell histology must constitute the majority of the tumor. Majority of cases have an associated component of conventional UCa. Necrosis is common.

HIGH-POWER CYTOLOGIC FEATURES

The tumor cells demonstrate salt-and-pepper–like fine chromatin without prominent nucleoli and nuclear molding. The cytoplasm is sparse and mitoses are numerous and readily identifiable.

IMMUNOHISTOCHEMICAL FEATURES

Majority of cases demonstrate positivity for NE markers: synpatophysin, chromogranin, CD56, and/or INSM1. CD56 is the most sensitive marker. TTF1 is positive in over 40% of cases and does not differentiate primary from a secondary process. Ki-67 demonstrates high proliferation activity.

12) INVERTED UROTHELIAL PAPILLOMA

DIFFERENTIAL DIAGNOSIS: NONINVASIVE UROTHELIAL CARCINOMA WITH INVERTED GROWTH PATTERN, FLORID VON BRUNN NEST PROLIFERATION
(Table 5.25)

Clinical Features

Inverted urothelial papilloma is a very uncommon urothelial lesion and accounts for <1% of urothelial lesions. Age at presentation is the fifth or sixth decade of life. Males are more frequently affected, with an M:F ratio of 5.8:1. Patients most commonly present with hematuria. Most tumors are

---

TABLE 5.24

Small Cell Carcinoma Versus Poorly Differentiated Urothelial Carcinoma (UCa) Versus High-grade Lymphoma

	Small Cell Carcinoma (Fig. 5.55A and B)	Poorly Differentiated UCa	High-Grade Lymphoma
Cystoscopic features	Large polypoid mass	Exophytic with irregular mucosa	Large polypoid mass
Histological features Low power	"Dark blue" appearance with sheets of cells	Eosinophilic appearance with sheets of cells	"Dark blue" appearance with sheets of cells
	Associated geographic necrosis	Can have associated necrosis but more focal	Cells are discohesive
High power	High nuclear-to-cytoplasmic ratio, nuclear molding, nuclear hyperchromasia without prominent nucleoli	Enlarged nuclei with prominent nucleoli and abundant cytoplasm	Nuclear pleomorphism with open chromatin and prominent nucleoli
	Brisk mitotic activity with apoptotic bodies	Frequent mitotic figures with infrequent apoptotic bodies	Numerous mitotic figures with apoptotic bodies
Immunohistochemistry stains	Positive for synaptophysin, chromogranin, CD56, INSM1; high Ki67	Positive for GATA, p63, HMWCK	Positive for hematopoietic markers

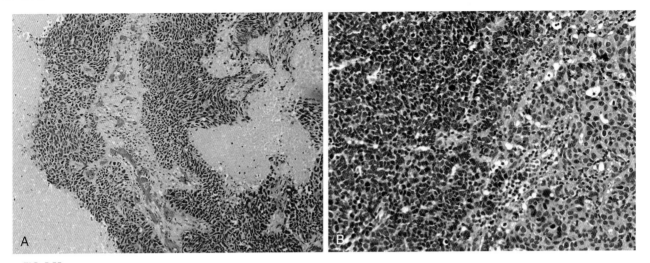

FIG. 5.55

A, In small cell carcinoma, nests/sheets of tumor cells with high nuclear-to-cytoplasmic ratio, salt-and-pepper chromatin, brisk mitotic activity, and geographic areas of tumor necrosis are present. **B,** A component of conventional urothelial carcinoma *(right)* is frequently present and suggests the primary process.

TABLE 5.25

Inverted Urothelial Papilloma Versus Non-invasive Urothelial Carcinoma (UCa) With Inverted Growth Pattern Versus Florid von Brunn Nest Proliferation

	Inverted Urothelial Papilloma (Fig. 5.56A and B)	Non-invasive UCa With Inverted Growth Pattern (Fig. 5.57A and B)	Florid von Brunn Nest Proliferation (Fig. 5.46)
Cystoscopic features	Polypoid tumor with a smooth mucosal surface	Polypoid tumor with a smooth mucosal surface	Tumor-like polypoid mass with smooth surface
Histological features Low power	Smooth pushing borders, tumor, and stromal interface smooth and rounded	Pushing borders, nests are thicker and nodular/bulbous	Lamina propria filled with round uniform nests of urothelium, cystitis cystica changes common
	Lacks exophytic papillary growth	Rounded bulbous nests are of varying size and separated by variable stroma	Nests are linear or lobular without an infiltrative border
	Tight proliferation of thin interconnecting cords/trabeculae with palisading of the basal cells in a "jigsaw puzzle"–like growth pattern	Areas of expansile nests typically present and a component of exophytic papillary fronds may be seen	Lacks trabecular or cord-like pattern; nests separated by variable stroma and lacks tight jigsaw pattern of growth
High power	Central aspect of nests/trabeculae demonstrate spindling. No or minimal cytologic atypia	Cytologic atypia frequently present, lacks peripheral palisading and central spindling	Lacks cytologic atypia unless seen with background of inflammation
	Degenerative type atypia may be seen	Cells have architectural disorder	Mitotic figures may be seen in the setting of inflammation
Immunohistochemistry stains	Not helpful in this differential	Not helpful in this differential.	Typically, not required in the diagnosis. P63 positive; PAX8 is typically negative. Lacks *TERT* mutations

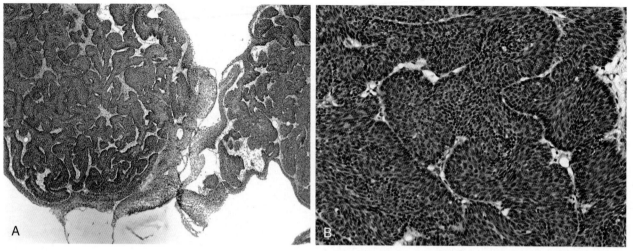

FIG. 5.56

In inverted urothelial papilloma, at low magnification, surface is smooth without exophytic papillary fronds. The lamina propria is filled with anastomosing cords and trabeculae of urothelium in a tight "jig-saw puzzle" pattern **(A)**. Peripheral aspects of columns are lined by cells with a palisading appearance and cells stream parallel to the basement membrane in center of nests. No cytologic atypia is present. Intervening stroma is delicate with lack of inflammation **(B)**.

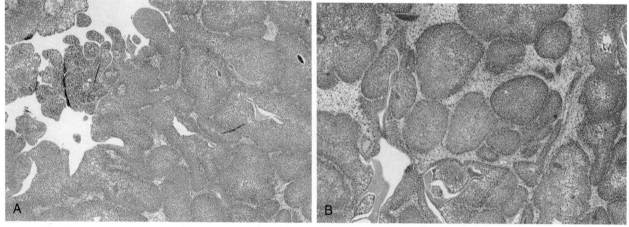

FIG. 5.57

In noninvasive urothelial carcinoma with inverted growth pattern, an exophytic component is often present **(A)**. The lamina propria is filled with variable size and placed, large rounded nests of the urothelium. There is lack of peripheral palisading and streaming of cells in center of nests **(B)**. Cytologic atypia and mitotic figures vary depending on the grade. Intervening stroma may show inflammation.

solitary and commonly occur in the trigone and bladder neck region. Cystoscopic appearance is of a polypoid tumor with a smooth mucosal surface. Inverted papilloma is a benign neoplasm with rare or no recurrence.

Pathologic Features (Fig. 5.56)

LOW-POWER ARCHITECTURAL FEATURES

The tumor has a trabecular growth pattern, which can sometimes be associated with cystic change and vacuolization of the luminal cells. The urothelial proliferation invaginates into the lamina propria and forms tight thin interconnecting cords/trabeculae with palisading of the basal cells in a "jigsaw puzzle" pattern. Cords and trabeculae are typically thin. Central areas of the cords may impart a spindled appearance. Overall, the lesion has a smooth pushing border. Tumor and stroma interface is regular and smooth. The overlying urothelium can be normal, attenuated, or hyperplastic.

HIGH-POWER CYTOLOGIC FEATURES

The tumor cells show no or minimal cytologic atypia, but degenerative type atypia may be seen. Rare mitotic figures may be present within the basal cell layer.

IMMUNOHISTOCHEMICAL FEATURES

Immunohistochemical markers are not helpful in diagnosis of this entity.

13) MUSCULARIS PROPRIA (DETRUSOR MUSCLE) INVASION

DIFFERENTIAL DIAGNOSIS: MUSCULARIS MUCOSAE INVASION (Table 5.26)

Clinical Features

The identification of muscularis propria (detrusor muscle) invasion is clinically significant as this parameter for clinicians defines management between conservative and definitive treatment modalities on biopsy or transurethral resection specimens. The designation of muscularis propria invasion would give a pathologic stage of pT2 indicating the need for definitive management (i.e., cystectomy, neoadjuvant chemotherapy, and/or radiation therapy).

Pathologic Features (Fig. 5.58A and B)

LOW-POWER ARCHITECTURAL FEATURES

The muscularis propria consists of three smooth muscle layers: inner and outer longitudinal layers and a central circular layer. The muscularis propria is typically arranged in bundles in horizontal and vertical orientation, forming layers with a distinct round thick muscle bundle with smooth outlines. Muscle bundles with tumor invasion are typically not associated with rows of dilated veins, which is typically seen in the lamina propria. In cases where each muscle bundle is thin, there are numerous thin muscle fibers invaded by extensive solid sheets of tumor. In trigone and bladder neck areas, there is lack of muscularis mucosae. Muscularis propria in this area is characterized by small regular rows of muscle bundles.

HIGH-POWER CYTOLOGIC FEATURES

No distinguishing features.

IMMUNOHISTOLOGIC FEATURES

Immunohistochemical markers are generally not helpful in identification of this entity. SMA and demsin would demonstrate diffuse and strong positivity in both the muscularis mucosae and muscularis propria and can help in distinction from desmoplastic stroma. Smoothelin can demonstrate differential immunoreactivity, with strong and diffuse positivity in muscularis propria and negative in muscularis mucosae; however, in challenging cases it can be quite variable in immunoreactivity and overall are not helpful.

14) BLADDER ADENOCARCINOMA

DIFFERENTIAL DIAGNOSIS: EXTENSIVE CYSTITIS CYSTICA ET GLANDULARIS WITH INTESTINAL METAPLASIA, MULLERIANOSIS (Table 5.27)

Clinical Features

Adenocarcinoma involving the urinary tract has many faces which includes primary urothelial type, urachal

---

TABLE 5.26

Muscularis Propria Invasion Versus Muscularis Mucosae Invasion

	Muscularis Propria Invasion (Fig. 5.58A and B)	Muscularis Mucosae Invasion (Fig. 5.59)
Cystoscopic features	No distinguishing features seen	No distinguishing features seen
Histological features Low power	Tumor infiltrating round thick muscle bundle with smooth outlines; lack row of dilated veins characteristic of lamina propria	Limited tumor that is infiltrating superficial thin, wispy/pointed, and discontinuous muscle bundles; the presence of thick dilated veins is a helpful clue of lamina propria if present
	Infiltrating between multiple rows of muscle bundles and/or thin muscle bundles with extensive solid sheets of tumor	Infrequently can be hypertrophic. In this situation, bundles of muscularis mucosae have haphazard orientation and irregular outlines
	In trigone and bladder neck, muscularis propria is characterized by multiple small regular rows of muscle bundles	Trigone and bladder neck lack muscularis mucosae; diverticulum demonstrates thick muscularis mucosae and lack muscularis propria
High power	No distinguishing features	No distinguishing features
Immunohistochemistry stains	Not helpful in this differential	Not helpful in this differential

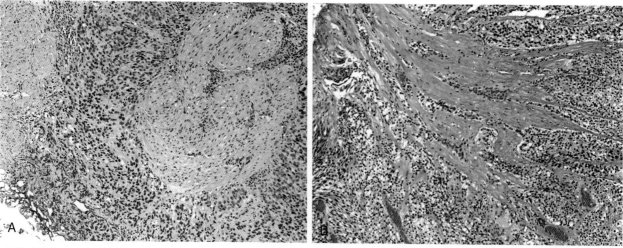

FIG. 5.58

In muscularis propria invasion, tumor cells infiltrate thick round muscle bundles. Invaded muscle is not associated with row of dilated veins **(A)**. In some cases, although each muscle bundle is thin, there are numerous thin muscles invaded by extensive solid sheets of tumor **(B)**.

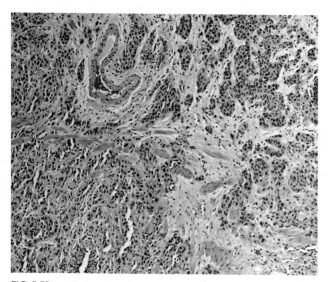

FIG. 5.59

In muscularis mucosae, tumor infiltrates thin, discontinuous, wispy, and pointed superficial muscle bundles. Row of dilated veins corresponding to the midlevel of the lamina propria is frequently present.

based, mullerian type, and metastatic origin. Urachal tumors originate in the dome, whereas non-urachal tumors typically involve the posterior wall and trigone. Non-urachal type may arise from intestinal metaplasia, whereas urachal type from urachal remnants. Primary adenocarcinoma of the bladder is rare accounting for <2% of bladder malignancies. The peak incidence of age is in the sixth decade of life. Males are more frequently affected (M:F, 2.6:1). Predisposing factors include bladder extrophy, non-functional bladder, and chronic inflammation. Clinical presentation includes hematuria, dysuria, and mucosuria. Clinical correlations with radiographic studies

are imperative for the diagnostic consideration of secondary site involvement.

Pathologic Features (Fig. 5.60)

LOW-POWER ARCHITECTURAL FEATURES

Primary invasive adenocarcinoma of the bladder demonstrates nearly pure glandular differentiation with varying morphologic patterns seen in intestinal adenocarcinoma: signet ring, colloid/mucinous and enteric non-mucinous carcinoma. Primary urothelial adenocarcinoma can often be seen in association with intestinal metaplasia. If extracellular mucin is present, it is lined by and often present with floating malignant cells. It may be associated with an *in situ* adenocarcinoma, villous adenoma, or UCa.

HIGH-POWER CYTOLOGIC FEATURES

Tumor cells show high-grade cytologic features similar to adenocarcinomas from other organs.

IMMUNOHISTOCHEMICAL FEATURES

Typically expresses CK20, and may express CDX2 and SATB2. CK7 is variable. PAX8, ER, and PR are negative. Metastatic colonic adenocarcinoma usually shows nuclear staining for beta-catenin, whereas primary bladder adenocarcinomas are negative or show cytoplasmic/membranous staining. Co-expression of CK7 and GATA3 in combination with lack of nuclear beta-catenin immunoreactivity strongly favors urothelial primary adenocarcinoma over colonic origin. Primary adenocarcinoma of the bladder is negative for *TERT* mutations.

TABLE 5.27

Bladder Adenocarcinoma Versus Extensive Cystitis Cystica et Glandularis With Intestinal Metaplasia Versus Mullerianosis

	Bladder Adenocarcinoma (Fig. 5.60)	Extensive Cystitis Cystica et Glandularis With Intestinal Metaplasia (Fig. 5.61A and B)	Mullerianosis (Fig. 5.62)
Cystoscopic features	Nodular mass or papillary tumor	Mucosa may show a mass lesion mimicking malignancy	Hemorrhagic spots and/or mass lesion in female patients usually in 30s to 40s
Histological features Low power	Identical to intestinal adenocarcinoma, including signet ring cells, colloid/mucinous and enteric non-mucinous morphology	Resembles normal colon crypts. Lacks any of the patterns that may be seen in intestinal adenocarcinoma. Cells typically are lined by goblet cells	Glands lined by endometrial cells, cuboidal cells, or endocervical cells; may involve the muscularis propria and perivesical adipose tissue without desmoplastic reaction
	May show dirty luminal necrosis	No *in situ* adenocarcinoma, villous adenoma, carcinoma *in situ*, or conventional urothelial carcinoma	Lacks *in situ* urothelial component
	Surface mucosa with *in situ* adeno-carcinoma, villous adenoma, or urothelial carcinoma may be present. Associated stromal desmoplasia around glands	Mucin extravasation is common but is acellular; lacks desmo-plastic stromal reaction	Lacks extracellular mucin; endometriosis in most cases has cuff of cellular stroma surrounding glands
High power	High-grade cytologic features	Bland nuclear cytology	Bland cytology with rare focal reactive-type changes
	Often identical to gastrointestinal tract lesion		Associated hemorrhage and hemosiderin deposition in surrounding stroma in endometriosis
Immunohistochemistry stains	Positive for CK20; variable expression for CK7. PAX8, ER and PR negative. Can be positive for CDX2 and SATB2. Nuclear beta-catenin negative. Primary bladder adenocarcinomas are negative or cytoplasmic/membra-nous staining for beta-catenin. Negative for *TERT* mutations	Not helpful in this differential process	Glands positive for PAX8, ER and PR; endometrial stroma positive for CD10

KIDNEY

1) METANEPHRIC ADENOMA

DIFFERENTIAL DIAGNOSIS: ADULT WILMS' TUMOR, SOLID PAPILLARY RENAL CELL CARCINOMA (Table 5.28)

Clinical Features

Metanephric adenoma usually occurs in adults but can be seen as early as the first decade of life. The tumor arises in the renal cortex. It usually is a unifocal tumor. Symptoms are non-specific, but can been associated with polycythemia. More common in females (M:F, 1:2).

Pathologic Features (Fig. 5.63A and B)

GROSS FEATURES

The tumor is well circumscribed with tan/white solid cut surfaces. The tumor infrequently may show hemorrhage, calcifications, and cystic changes.

LOW-POWER ARCHITECTURAL FEATURES

Metanephric adenoma is a well-circumscribed tumor, merging with the renal cortex imperceptibly without a distinct capsule. Overall, the tumor has a "blue" appearance on low power due to the crowded small tubules and papillae with minimal cytoplasm, a useful diagnostic clue. The glomeruloid structures are frequently seen in areas showing papillary formations. The tumor is often associated with a myxoid stromal component.

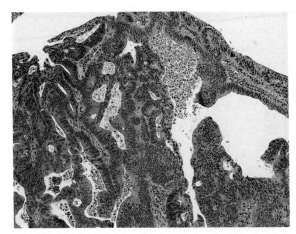

FIG. 5.60

In bladder adenocarcinoma, wide range of growth patterns can be observed. An example of enteric non-mucinous type of primary adenocarcinoma. Glands exhibit columnar lining epithelium with overt cytologic atypia. Intraluminal dirty necrosis is present. Distinction of primary urothelial adenocarcinoma from metastasis relies primarily on careful clinical evaluation. Immunohistochemical markers are usually not reliable.

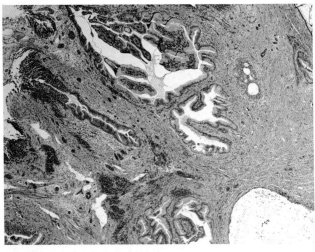

FIG. 5.62

In endocervicosis, glands are lined by mucin-secreting columnar epithelial cells and are deeply placed within muscle, mimicking adenocarcinoma. However, there is lack of stromal reaction and glands are benign cytologically.

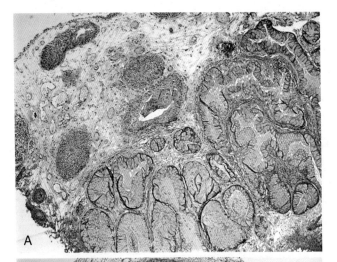

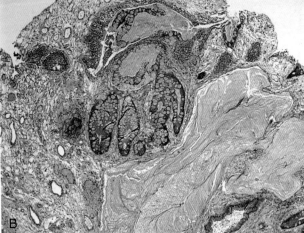

FIG. 5.61

In cystitis glandularis with intestinal metaplasia, glands resemble normal colon crypts with goblet cells. Lining cells are bland and often merge with non-intestinal cystitis cystica et glandularis **(A)**. Extracellular mucin may raise concern for malignancy but is acellular and lacks desmoplastic reaction **(B)**.

HIGH-POWER CYTOLOGIC FEATURES

Tumor nuclei are relatively uniform, round, and bland in appearance. Due to the lack of cytoplasm, has a high N:C ratio. Nucleoli are not present.

IMMUNOHISTOCHEMICAL FEATURES

The tumor demonstrates diffuse nuclear positivity for WT1, granular cytoplasmic positivity for AMACR, and cytoplasmic positivity for CD57 and BRAF V600E. CK7 is negative.

2) CLEAR CELL RENAL CELL CARCINOMA

DIFFERENTIAL DIAGNOSIS: CLEAR CELL PAPILLARY RENAL CELL TUMOR, CHROMOPHOBE RENAL CELL CARCINOMA
(Table 5.29)

Clinical Features

Clear cell renal cell carcinoma (CCRCC) occurs in adults with a peak incidence in the sixth decade. It can present with the classic triad of hematuria, mass lesion, and flank pain. It is usually detected incidentally due to increasing use of imaging techniques. Majority present as a sporadic tumor, but hereditary association with *VHL* syndrome is seen in subset of cases. Presents unifocal but can be multifocal in the setting of familial syndromes.

TABLE 5.28

Metanephric Adenoma Versus Adult Wilms' Tumor Versus Solid Papillary Renal Cell Carcinoma (RCC)

	Metanephric Adenoma (Fig. 5.63A and B)	Adult Wilms' Tumor (Fig. 5.64A and B)	Solid Papillary RCC (Fig. 5.65A and B)
Location	Renal cortex; unilateral, rarely multifocal	Renal cortex or medulla; can be bilateral and multifocal	Renal cortex; unifocal, unless hereditary
Gross features	Well-circumscribed tumor without a capsule; homogeneous and tan-white cut surface	Well delineated or sharply circumscribed, soft, tan mass with bulging cut surface	Solid homogenous cut surface, but degenerative changes are commonly present
Histologic features Low power	"Blue" appearance due to crowded small tubules and papillae with minimal cytoplasm	"Blue" appearance due to minimal cytoplasm	Densely solid areas but relatively abundant cytoplasm gives a "pink" appearance, a useful diagnostic clue
	Glomeruloid appearance is common in areas with papillary formations	Tubules and glomeruloid structures	Tubulopapillary proliferation in solid pattern
	Myxoid stroma; lacks heterologous elements	Triphasic histology—blastemal, stromal, and epithelial elements are commonly present and provide a useful diagnostic clue; heterologous elements are also commonly seen	Foamy histiocytes within fibrovascular cores and hemosiderin-laden macrophages are typically present
High power	Nuclei uniform, round, bland in appearance	Nuclei molded round-oval with coarse chromatin	Nuclei are typically low grade. Rarely may show higher-grade nuclei
	Mitoses rare	Frequent mitoses	Mitoses can be seen
Immunohistochemistry stains	Negative CK7; Positive for WT1, CD57 and BRAF	Positive for WT1; usually positive for PAX8; cytokeratin positive in epithelial components	Positive for CK7; negative for WT1

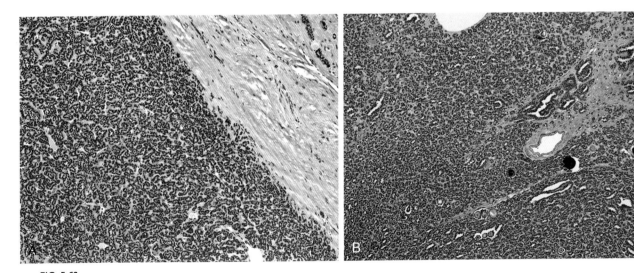

FIG. 5.63

Metanephric adenoma. **A,** A well-circumscribed tumor without a distinct capsule with tightly packed small tubules separated by scant stroma. **B,** In addition to small tubules, glomeruloid formations, elongated tubules with branching morphology, and psammomatous calcifications are also seen.

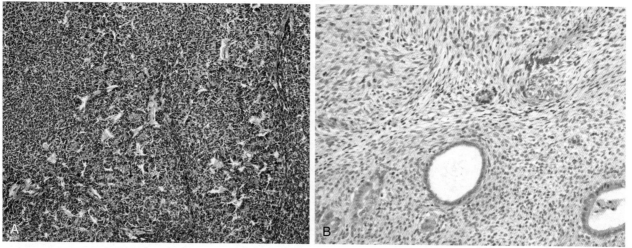

FIG. 5.64

Adult Wilms' tumor. **A,** The morphology showing the typical blastemal and epithelial components are readily identified. Closely packed cells with scant cytoplasm are appreciated. **B,** The stromal component of adult Wilms' tumor consists of nondescript spindle cells with an admixed epithelial component.

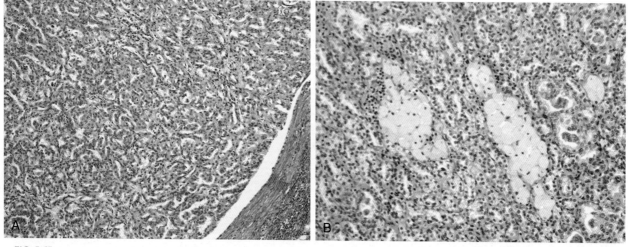

FIG. 5.65

Solid papillary renal cell carcinoma. **A,** There are tightly packed papillae, resulting in a solid appearance. Multiple tubular and glomeruloid architectural patterns are present. **B,** The presence of foamy macrophages are a diagnostic clue and helpful in this entity.

Sporadic VHL gene inactivation is present in approximately two thirds of cases. In VHL syndrome, inherited germline inactivation occurs in vHL 3p25-26.

Pathologic Features (Fig. 5.66)

GROSS FEATURES

This tumor can present as a solid or cystic mass with distinct pushing borders. Cut surface of solid areas are golden yellow. CCRCC is typically associated with hemorrhage and necrosis in larger masses.

LOW-POWER ARCHITECTURAL FEATURES

The tumor is composed of polygonal cells with optically clear to granular eosinophilic cytoplasm, arranged in acini, tubules, nests, or solid sheets. Cells are surrounded by intricate delicate branching fibrovascular pattern. Such pattern is typically seen in low-grade areas and is considered characteristic for the diagnosis of CCRCC. Extensive sampling may be required to demonstrate such areas in an otherwise poorly differentiated tumor. Stromal hyalinization and regression changes are common. Tumor necrosis characterized by dirty granular debris is an important adverse prognostic parameter.

TABLE 5.29

Clear Cell Renal Cell Carcinoma (CCRCC) Versus Clear Cell Papillary Renal Cell Tumor (CCPRCT) Versus Chromophobe Renal Cell Carcinoma (ChRCC)

	CCRCC (Fig. 5.66)	CCPRCT (Fig. 5.67A–C)	ChRCC (Fig. 5.68)
Location	Unifocal; multifocal or bilateral in familial syndrome	Unifocal; multifocal in setting of ESRD	Unifocal; multifocal or bilateral in setting of Birt-Hogg-Dube (BHD) syndrome
Gross features	Solid and cystic; golden-yellow; often with associated hemorrhage and necrosis	Solid with cystic change; white-pale yellow; hemorrhage or necrosis are typically not seen	Solid, well-circumscribed unencapsulated tumor; light brown cut surface
Histologic features Low power	Polygonal cells with optically clear to granular eosinophilic cytoplasm, arranged in acini, tubules, nests or solid sheets	Branching tubules and papillary structures with cuboidal cell lining with clear cytoplasm and luminal (apical) polarization of nuclei. Tubules are short and branching, referred to as "shark smile." Apical snouts are also observed.	Large polygonal cells with pale and lightly reticulated cytoplasm; admixed with eosinophilic cytoplasm
	Surrounded by delicate intricate branching fibrovascular pattern	Cystic spaces with lining of cuboidal to flat cells with clear cytoplasm	Arranged in nests or solid sheets; plant-like prominent/thick cell membranes
High power	Nuclear grading follows ISUP grading system. High nuclear grade seen in areas of granular/eosinophilic cytoplasm.	Low nuclear grade. Histologic grade 1–2, but ISUP grading not applicable	Koilocytotic atypia characterized by raisinoid nuclei with perinuclear halos and frequent binucleation; high nuclear and nucleolar features, but ISUP grading not applicable
Immunohistochemistry stains	CK7 is typically negative but can be variable; diffusely positive membranous staining pattern for CA9	Diffusely positive for CK7; CA9 expression is often observed in "cup-shaped" pattern	Diffusely positive for CK7 and CD117; negative for CA9

ESRD, End-stage renal disease; *ISUP,* International Society of Urologic Pathology.

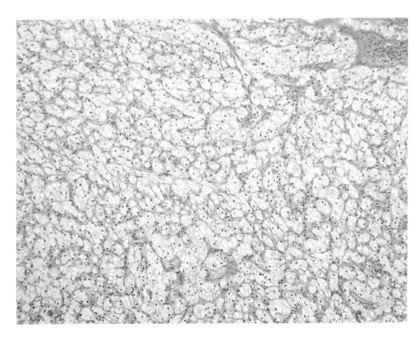

FIG. 5.66

In clear cell renal cell carcinoma, nests of clear cells surrounded by intricate branching fibrovascular septations are an important diagnostic feature of this entity.

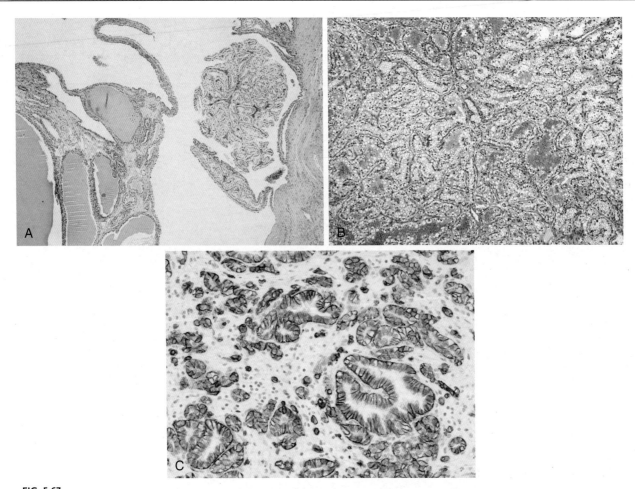

FIG. 5.67

Clear cell papillary renal cell tumor. **A,** Composed of branching tubules and papillary structures with cuboidal cell lining with clear cytoplasm. **B,** Tubules are short and branching creating a "shark smile" effect. The linear arrangement of the nuclei away from the basement membrane is a helpful diagnostic feature. **C,** CA9 expression is often observed in "cup-shaped" pattern.

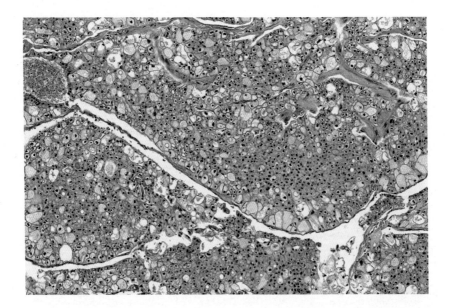

FIG. 5.68

In chromophobe renal cell carcinoma, there is a predominantly solid pattern of growth, separated by thin and incomplete vascular septations. There is a mixture of larger cells with reticular/granular cytoplasm and plant-like cell wall appearance, and smaller eosinophilic cells with perinuclear halos. Nuclei often have a raisinoid appearance with associated binucleation.

HIGH-POWER CYTOLOGIC FEATURES

Nuclear grading follows ISUP grading system. CCRCC typically shows nuclear and cytoplasmic synchronization where clear cell areas show lower nuclear grade while high nuclear grade seen in areas of granular/eosinophilic cytoplasm.

IMMUNOHISTOCHEMICAL FEATURES

Tumor is diffusely positive for PAX8, cytokeratins, and CA9. CA9 expression is seen in a diffuse membranous pattern. CK7 is negative but can be variable.

3) MULTICYSTIC RENAL CELL NEOPLASM OF LOW MALIGNANT POTENTIAL

DIFFERENTIAL DIAGNOSIS: CLEAR CELL RCC WITH PROMINENT CYSTIC CHANGE, ATYPICAL RENAL CYST, CYSTIC CLEAR CELL PAPILLARY RENAL CELL TUMOR
(Table 5.30)

Clinical Features

Multicystic renal cell neoplasm of low malignant potential (MCN-LMP) occurs with a peak incidence in the sixth decade. Usually presents as a unifocal lesion. Typically asymptomatic but can present with pain and hematuria. Local recurrence and metastasis are not observed with this entity.

Pathologic Features (Fig. 5.69)

GROSS FEATURES

This lesion has a gross appearance of a multilocular cystic mass. The cysts have a smooth lining and are filled with a straw-colored fluid.

LOW-POWER ARCHITECTURAL FEATURES

The cyst walls have a smooth lining of flattened to cuboidal cells, frequently with clear cytoplasm. Within the septate are rare small non-expansile aggregates of cells with clear cytoplasm, a characteristic feature. Any expansile nodule of clear cells is considered incompatible with the diagnosis. Evaluation of entire cystic mass is often required to establish the diagnosis.

HIGH-POWER CYTOLOGIC FEATURES

Nuclei are round to oval with low nuclear grade, ISUP grade 1–2. No necrosis is seen.

IMMUNOHISTOCHEMICAL FEATURES

MCN-LMP has immunohistochemical features identical to CCRCC. Cytokeratin stain may help in identification of small clusters of clear cells within septae.

TABLE 5.30

Multicystic Renal Cell Neoplasm of Low Malignant Potential (MCN-LMP) Versus Cystic Clear Cell Renal Cell Carcinoma (CCRCC) Versus Atypical Renal Cyst Versus Cystic Clear Cell Papillary Renal Cell Tumor (CCPRCT)

	MCN-LMP (Fig. 5.69)	Cystic CCRCC (Fig. 5.70)	Atypical Renal Cyst (Fig. 5.71)	Cystic CCPRCT (Fig. 5.72)
Location	Unifocal	Unifocal	Often multifocal	Unifocal; multifocal in setting of ESRD
Gross features	Well circumscribed with fibrous capsule; multicystic cut surface	Predominately cystic with fibrosis and hyalinization, solid areas are usually present	Unilocular or multilocular cystic lesion	Predominantly cystic tumor, small in size, well circumscribed with a well-defined capsule
Histological features Low power	Cysts have a smooth lining of flattened to cuboidal clear cells	Variable sized cysts lined by cuboidal clear cells often within a prominent vasculature, degenerative changes are common	Variable sized unilocular or multilocular cysts lined by heaped up cells with eosinophilic to clear cytoplasm imparting a "tufted" appearance	Common architectural patterns include: short tubules with branching, papillary, tubulocystic, and compact nested
	Cyst walls/septae have small non-expansile aggregates of cells with clear cytoplasm	Septae/cyst walls contain sheets of cells with expansile solid appearance	Lacks solid clusters/aggregates of clear cells in the cyst walls	Cuboidal cell lining with clear cytoplasm and reverse polarity due to luminal/apical polarization of nuclei

Continued

TABLE 5.30

Multicystic Renal Cell Neoplasm of Low Malignant Potential (MCN-LMP) Versus Cystic Clear Cell Renal Cell Carcinoma (CCRCC) Versus Atypical Renal Cyst Versus Cystic Clear Cell Papillary Renal Cell Tumor (CCPRCT)—cont'd

	MCN-LMP (Fig. 5.69)	Cystic CCRCC (Fig. 5.70)	Atypical Renal Cyst (Fig. 5.71)	Cystic CCPRCT (Fig. 5.72)
High power	Nuclei with low nuclear grade, histologic grade 1–2	Nuclei with low nuclear grade, ISUP grade 1–2	Nuclei are cytologically bland	Low nuclear grade. Almost always histologic grade 1–2
Immunohistochemistry stains	Cytokeratin stain may help in documenting small clusters of clear cells within septae, overall identical to CCRCC	Positive for PAX8, CA9, CD10, vimentin; CK7 is typically negative but can be variable	Not helpful	Diffusely positive for CK7; frequent "cup"-shaped membranous CA9 positivity. CD10 is typically negative

ESRD, End-stage renal disease; *ISUP,* International Society of Urologic Pathology.

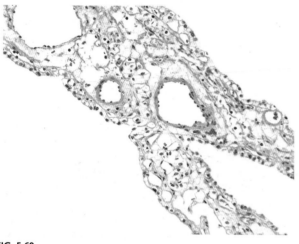

FIG. 5.69

In multicystic renal cell neoplasm of low malignant potential, the cysts are lined by clear cells with small clusters of tumor within septae.

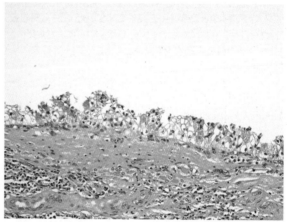

FIG. 5.71

In atypical renal cyst, the cyst wall is lined with stratified clear cells and/or eosinophilic epithelium with low nuclear grade.

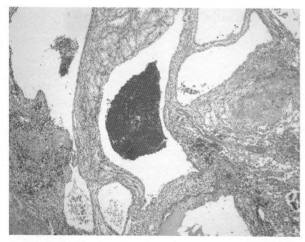

FIG. 5.70

In a predominantly cystic clear cell renal cell carcinoma, the septations have expansile nests of clear cells.

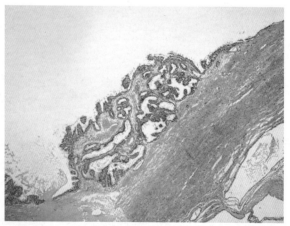

FIG. 5.72

In a predominantly cystic clear cell papillary renal cell tumor, within the cystic component, there is a papillary or tubulopapillary proliferation that demonstrates linear arrangement of nuclei away from the basement membrane.

TABLE 5.31

Tubulopapillary Adenoma Versus Papillary Renal Cell Carcinoma (RCC)

	Tubulopapillary Adenoma (Fig. 5.73)	Papillary RCC
Location	Unifocal or multifocal	Unifocal; multifocal/bilateral in hereditary syndromes
Gross features	Unencapsulated and ≤15 mm diameter	Encapsulated with cystic change
Histological features Low power	Papillae and tubules lined by single layer of polygonal cells with granular/eosinophilic cytoplasm.	Papillae and tubules lined by single layer of polygonal cells with granular/eosinophilic or pale/clear cytoplasm
	No cystic change, necrosis, and hemorrhage	Cystic change, necrosis, and hemorrhage common
	Typically lacks foamy histiocytes and hemosiderin	Foamy histiocytes, cholesterol clefts, and hemosiderin frequently seen
High power	Nuclei with low nuclear grade, ISUP grade 1–2	Nuclei with low or high nuclear grade, ISUP grade 2–4
	No mitoses	Mitoses in higher grade lesions
Immunohistochemistry stains	Not helpful, identical to papillary RCC	Positive for CK7

ISUP, International Society of Urologic Pathology.

4) TUBULOPAPILLARY ADENOMA

DIFFERENTIAL DIAGNOSIS: PAPILLARY RENAL CELL CARCINOMA (Table 5.31)

Clinical Features

Tubulopapillary adenomas occur in adults. They are more commonly seen in association with end-stage renal disease (ESRD) or in association with papillary RCCs. Patients are asymptomatic and tubulopapillary adenoma usually does not present as a mass lesion.

Pathologic Features (Fig. 5.73)

GROSS FEATURES

This lesion is well circumscribed with grayish-white to yellow nodules that are unencapsulated and ≤15 mm in diameter.

Low-power architectural features. Tubulopapillary adenomas are benign epithelial proliferations that have a papillary, tubular, or tubulopapillary configuration and are ≤15 mm in diameter and without a capsule. Papillae and tubules are lined by a single layer of polygonal cells with granular/eosinophilic cytoplasm. Cystic change, necrosis, and hemorrhage are not seen. Calcifications may be seen. Rare foamy histiocytes and

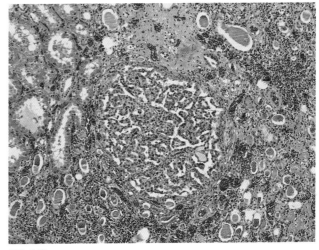

FIG. 5.73

Tubulopapillary adenoma is a well-circumscribed and non-encapsulated lesion with a prominent tubular or tubulopapillary architecture. By definition, must be ≤15 mm and without a capsule.

hemosiderin deposition may be present in tubulopapillary adenomas.

HIGH-POWER CYTOLOGIC FEATURES

Nuclear features are of low nuclear grade with ISUP grade 1–2. No mitoses are seen.

IMMUNOHISTOLOGIC FEATURES

Not helpful in this entity as staining is identical to papillary RCC.

5) ONCOCYTOMA

DIFFERENTIAL DIAGNOSIS: EOSINOPHILIC VARIANT OF CHROMOPHOBE RENAL CELL CARCINOMA, SDHB-DEFICIENT RENAL CELL CARCINOMA, EOSINOPHILIC SOLID AND CYSTIC RENAL CELL CARCINOMA, LOW-GRADE ONCOCYTIC FUMARATE HYDRATASE–DEFICIENT RENAL CELL CARCINOMA (Table 5.32)

Clinical Features

Oncocytoma is a benign tumor that typically presents in the sixth decade of life. Usually presents as a unifocal mass, however, can be multifocal/bilateral. Patients may present with the classic triad of hematuria, flank pain, and renal mass. Tumor showing mixture of renal onco-cytoma with focal clear cells or classic chromophobe tumor-like areas is referred to as a hybrid oncocytic tumor. Such changes with or without renal oncocytosis should raise consideration of familial hereditary Birt-Hogg-Dube syndrome. Patients with this syndrome also present with fibrofolliculomas, lung cysts, and pneumothorax.

Pathologic Features (Fig. 5.74A–C)

GROSS FEATURES

This tumor is well circumscribed and unencapsulated. Gross appearance on cut surface is mahogany brown to tan-yellow in color and can be associated with a central scar.

TABLE 5.32

Oncocytoma Versus Eosinophilic Variant of Chromophobe Renal Cell Carcinoma (ChRCC) Versus SDHB-deficient RCC Versus Eosinophilic Solid and Cystic Renal Cell Carcinoma (ESCRCC) Versus Low-grade Oncocytic Fumarate hydratase (FH)-deficient RCC

	Oncocytoma (Fig. 5.74A–C)	Eosinophilic Variant of ChRCC (Fig. 5.75)	SDHB-Deficient RCC (Fig. 5.76A–C)	ESCRCC (Fig. 5.77A–D)	Low-grade Onco-cytic FH-deficient RCC
Location	Unifocal; can be multi-focal/bilateral	Unifocal; rarely multifocal/bilateral	Unifocal	Unifocal	Unifocal
Gross features	Mahogany brown to tan-yellow; can be associated with a central scar	Light-brown cut surface	Tan-brown to red cut surface	Tan mass, solid and macrocystic	Multinodular solid mass; can have cystic change
Histological features Low power	Cells arranged in nests, acini, tubules in prominent fibromyx-oid stroma	Cells arranged in compact nests or solid sheets	Well-circumscribed tumor with lobulated or pushing borders without capsule	Solid areas with sheets of eosinophilic cells admixed with variably sized macro- and microcysts	Solid, nested, focally tubular architecture
	Large, round, polygo-nal cells with eosino-philic cytoplasm	Large polygonal cells with pale and reticulated cytoplasm, admixed with cells with eosinophilic cytoplasm	Diffuse sheet-like or compact nested growth pattern with scattered cysts con-taining pale eosino-philic material. Cells lined by abundant pale eosinophilic cytoplasm	Cyst septae vary in thickness and lined with neoplastic cells with voluminous eosinophilic cyto-plasm and hobnail arrangement	Sometimes may exhibit a microcytic pattern with pink luminal contents
High power	Nuclei are bland and uniform with fine chromatin and vari-able nucleoli	Raisinoid nuclei with irregular, wrinkled nuclear membranes and perinuclear halos; binucleation is a characteristic nuclear feature	Smooth nuclear contours, evenly dispersed chromatin, and inconspicuous nucleoli	Solid areas of growth with admixed histio-cytes and lympho-cytes	Uniform cytology of polygonal cells with flocculent, vacuolated eosinophilic cyto-plasm with scattered inclusions

TABLE 5.32

Oncocytoma Versus Eosinophilic Variant of Chromophobe Renal Cell Carcinoma (ChRCC) Versus SDHB-deficient RCC Versus Eosinophilic Solid and Cystic Renal Cell Carcinoma (ESCRCC) Versus Low-grade Oncocytic Fumarate hydratase (FH)-deficient RCC—cont'd

	Oncocytoma (Fig. 5.74A–C)	Eosinophilic Variant of ChRCC (Fig. 5.75)	SDHB-Deficient RCC (Fig. 5.76A–C)	ESCRCC (Fig. 5.77A–D)	Low-grade Oncocytic FH-deficient RCC
	Can have degenerative-type atypia with multinucleation; dense hyperchromatic nuclei of oncoblasts	Features of plant-like, thick cell membranes, may not be conspicuous	Cytoplasmic vacuoles or flocculent inclusions that impart a bubbly appearance	Prominent granular cytoplasmic stippling consisting of basophilic to purple cytoplasmic granules, reminiscent of leishmaniasis	Fine chromatin with inconspicuous nucleoli
Immunohistochemistry stains	Positive CD117; patchy positive CK7	Positive CK7 and CD117	Loss of expression for SDHB; typically negative for CD117 and CK7	Positive for CK20; negative for CK7	Retained expression of SDHB; loss of expression of FH

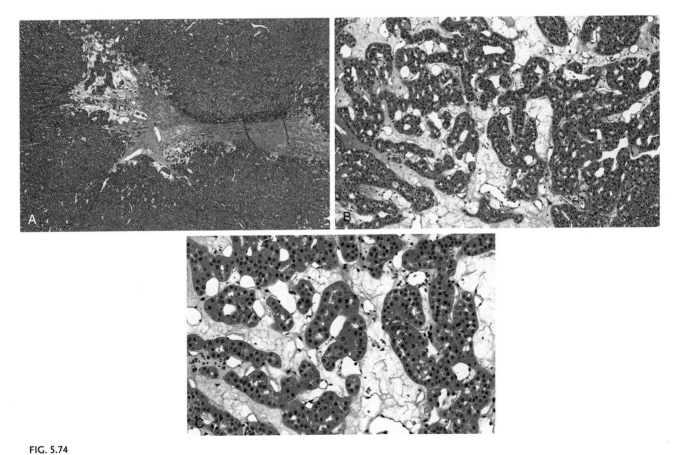

FIG. 5.74

Oncocytoma. **A,** Typical architecture of solid nests with a central scar. **B,** Nests of cells are arranged in discrete archipelagous pattern that is separated by loose stroma. **C,** Tumor cells with eosinophilic, granular cytoplasm, uniform and round nuclei, with a prominent central nucleoli.

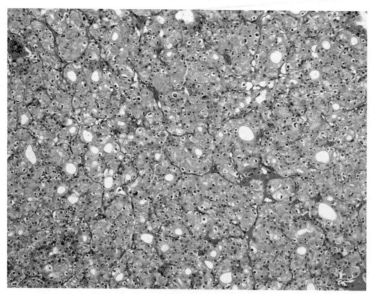

FIG. 5.75
Eosinophilic variant of chromophobe renal cell carcinoma has an acinar architectural pattern of eosinophilic cells with perinuclear halos and raisinoid nuclei.

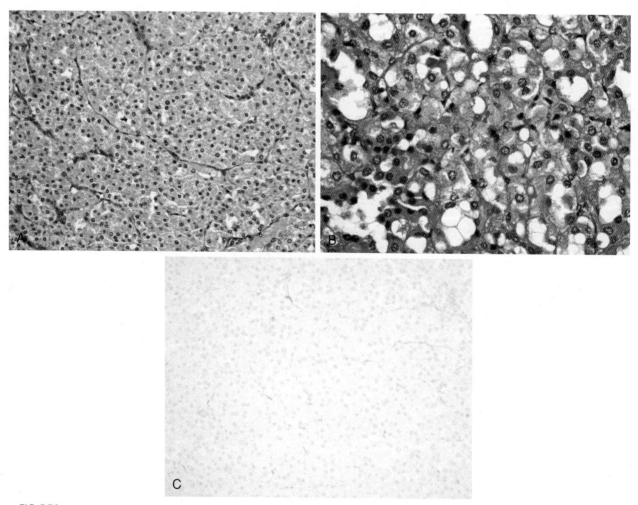

FIG. 5.76
SDHB-deficient renal cell carcinoma. **A,** Diffuse sheet-like and/or nested morphology composed of cells with pale eosinophilic cytoplasm. **B,** Cytoplasmic vacuoles or flocculent eosinophilic inclusions that impart a bubbly appearance. **C,** Immunohistochemical stains for SDH-B demonstrate loss of expression.

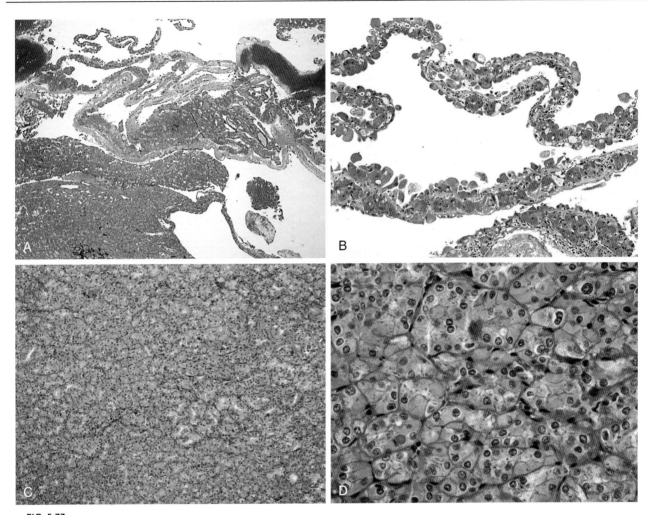

FIG. 5.77

Eosinophilic solid and cystic renal cell carcinoma (ESCRCC). **A,** Solid areas with sheets of eosinophilic cells admixed with variably sized macrocysts and microcysts. **B,** Cyst septae vary in thickness and lined with neoplastic cells with voluminous eosinophilic cytoplasm and hobnail arrangement. **C,** The solid areas of ESCRCC can be a diagnostic challenge in oncocytic renal neoplasia. **D,** Prominent granular cytoplasmic stippling consisting of basophilic to purple cytoplasmic granules, reminiscent of leishmaniasis, is a helpful feature.

LOW-POWER ARCHITECTURAL FEATURES

Architecturally, the tumor is composed of solid nests but may have micro- and macrocysts and tubules. Nests/tubules are lined by cells with abundant eosinophilic granular cytoplasm. Edematous myxoid or hyalinized stroma representing scar-like area is a frequent finding (Fig. 5.74A). Perirenal, renal sinus or small vessels invasion rarely may be present and is a permissible feature for the diagnosis. Renal vein involvement is not permissible for the diagnosis.

HIGH-POWER CYTOLOGIC FEATURES

Cell nuclei are uniform and round with vesicular chromatin and central prominent nucleoli. Occasional groups of cells with hyperchromasia, degenerative-type atypia, and multinucleation may be seen. Oncoblasts,

characterized by smaller cells with higher N:C ratio and dense hyperchromatic nuclei may be present. Atypical mitoses, papillary architecture, and necrosis are not allowed for the diagnosis. Borderline tumors that cannot be distinguished from eosinophilic variant of chromophobe RCC or other low-grade oncocytic tumors are termed as "oncocytic renal neoplasm of low malignant potential, not further classified" or "renal oncocytic neoplasm of low malignant potential." A conservative approach is especially recommended on needle core biopsy specimens.

IMMUNOHISTOCHEMICAL FEATURES

The tumor usually has patchy CK7 staining but can be negative. Oncocytomas are typically positive for CD117, Ksp-cadherin, and S100A1.

6) FUMARATE HYDRATASE–DEFICIENT/ HEREDITARY LEIOMYOMATOSIS AND RENAL CELL CARCINOMA–ASSOCIATED RENAL CELL CARCINOMA

DIFFERENTIAL DIAGNOSIS: RENAL CELL CARCINOMA, PAPILLARY TYPE (EOSINOPHILIC) (Table 5.33)

Clinical Features

Patients with renal tumors confirmed as having a *fumarate hydratase* (*FH*) mutation are referred to as having "FH-deficient RCC," as well as "HLRCC-associated RCC," if the patient's syndromic setting or germline *FH* mutation is known. However, syndromic setting is not always present and such tumors may occur sporadically. Therefore, FH-deficient RCC is a preferred term to describe these tumors. Usually occurs in the renal cortex but can involve the medulla. Patients in the hereditary setting may present with cutaneous lesions, commonly on the arms or thorax due to familiar leiomyomatosis cutis et uteri or Reed syndrome. Affected women may develop early-onset uterine leiomyomas.

Pathologic Features (Fig. 5.78A–D)

GROSS FEATURES

These tumors may be cystic, solid, and homogeneous but also can present as a predominantly cystic mass.

LOW-POWER ARCHITECTURAL FEATURES

Majority of cases present with a papillary appearance with large cells with abundant eosinophilic cytoplasm. FH-deficient RCCs can have a variety of morphologic pattern including tubular, tubulocystic, solid, and mixed.

HIGH-POWER CYTOLOGIC FEATURES

Cells have large nuclei with prominent inclusion-like eosinophilic nucleoli, a characteristic feature. Typically has an associated perinucleolar halo. Tumors previously regarded as type 2 papillary RCC and dedifferentiated tubulocystic RCC (tubulocystic RCC "gone bad"; Fig. 5.78C and D) often are reclassified as FH-deficient RCC. FH-deficient RCC may also rarely present with low-grade oncocytic tumor features, indistinguishable from SDHB-deficient RCC (see Table 5.32).

IMMUNOHISTOCHEMICAL FEATURES

The tumor demonstrates loss of FH expression and positive staining for 2SC. The sensitivity of the FH immunostain for detecting an underlying mutation, whether somatic or germline, is approximately 85%.

7) RENAL CELL CARCINOMA WITH LEIOMYOMATOUS STROMA

DIFFERENTIAL DIAGNOSIS: CLEAR CELL PAPILLARY RENAL CELL TUMOR, CYSTIC CLEAR CELL RENAL CELL CARCINOMA (Table 5.34)

Clinical Features

Renal cell carcinoma with leiomyomatous stroma usually presents as an incidental mass. Morphologically identical appearing tumors occur in the hereditary setting of tuberous sclerosis complex (TSC) and have been described under terms: "renal adenomyomatous tumor" or

---

TABLE 5.33

Fumarate Hydratase (FH)-deficient Renal Cell Carcinoma (RCC) Versus RCC Papillary Type

	FH-deficient RCC (Fig. 5.78A–D)	RCC Papillary Type (Fig. 5.79)
Location	Unifocal	Unifocal
Gross features	Cystic and solid	Solid and cystic cavitary mass with a friable consistency, often associated hemorrhage and central necrosis
Histological features Low power	Papillary with eosinophilic cytoplasm, most common presentation; however, mixture of growth patterns can be observed	Papillae and tubules lined by single layer of polygonal cells with granular/eosinophilic cytoplasm
	Morphologic patterns including tubular, tubulocystic, solid, and mixed	Foamy macrophages, cholesterol clefts, and hemosiderin
High power	Large nuclei with prominent inclusion-like eosinophilic nucleoli with perinucleolar halos	Nuclear grade ranges from low to high, high-grade cases more commonly with this differential
Immunohistochemistry stains	Loss of FH expression; positive for 2SC	Variably positive for CK7. Retained FH expression

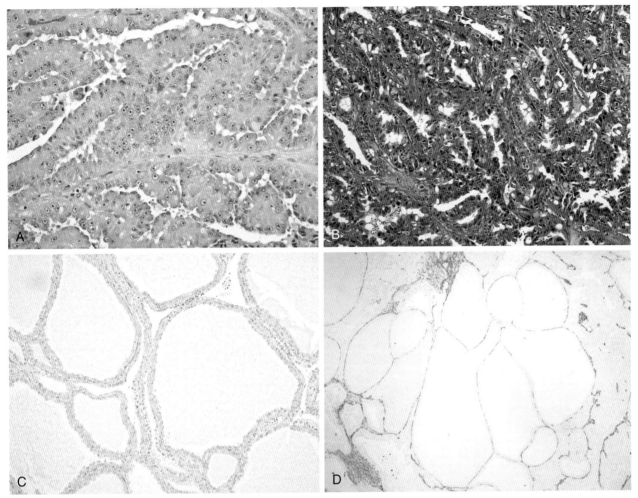

FIG. 5.78

Fumarate hydratase (FH)–deficient renal cell carcinoma. **A,** Papillary tumor with eosinophilic cytoplasm and large nuclei with prominent inclusion-like eosinophilic nucleoli. **B,** Tubular morphologic pattern with eosinophilic cytoplasm. Note the presence of perinucleolar halos. **C,** In an area of tubulocystic pattern, the cells demonstrate eosinophilic cytoplasm with large nuclei with prominent inclusion-like eosinophilic nucleoli, which is a diagnostic feature that is helpful in this entity. **D,** Loss of expression of FH by immunohistochemistry.

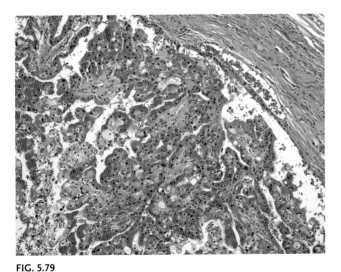

FIG. 5.79

In papillary renal cell carcinoma, a single layer of polygonal cells with eosinophilic cytoplasm lines the papillae and tubules. The presence of foamy macrophages and hemosiderin are a helpful feature.

"papillary-like". Sporadically occurring tumors show recurrent *TSC/MTOR* mutations. A small subset with overlapping morphology, fibrous stroma, and CK7 reactivity exhibit *TCEB1(ELOC)* mutations. It is currently unclear whether *TCEB-1*–mutated RCC represents a distinct tumor type.

Pathologic Features (Fig. 5.80A–C)

GROSS FEATURES

Tumors are typically small, solitary with tan/red solid cut surfaces.

LOW-POWER ARCHITECTURAL FEATURES

This tumor shows two distinct components (epithelial and stromal) which are often times admixed. The epithelial

TABLE 5.34

Renal Cell Carcinoma With Leiomyomatous Stroma (RCCLMS) Versus Cell Papillary Renal Cell Tumor (CCPRCT) Versus Cystic Clear Cell Renal Cell Carcinoma (CCRCC)

	RCCLMS (Fig. 5.80A–C)	CCPRCT	Cystic CCRCC
Location	Unifocal	Unifocal; multifocal in setting of ESRD	Unifocal; multifocal or bilateral in familial syndrome
Gross features	Solitary, tan/red solid tumor with a well-defined capsule	Predominantly cystic tumors, small in size, well-circumscribed with a well-defined capsule	Solid and cystic; golden-yellow; often with associated hemorrhage and necrosis
Histological features Low power	Nodules of elongated frequently branching tubules, lined by abundant clear to mildly eosinophilic cytoplasm separated by variable smooth muscle stroma; variable papillary architecture component also common	Cystic with a prominent tubulo-papillary architecture. Tubules are short and branching giving a "shark smile" appearance	Polygonal cells with optically clear to granular eosinophilic cytoplasm, arranged in acini, tubules, nests, or solid sheets and separated by delicate, intricately branching vasculature
	Amount of smooth muscle can be focal to prominent	Abundant smooth muscle may be present, tightly packed, collapsed acini/tubules may impart a solid appearance	Abundant smooth muscle may be present
High power	Tubules lined by voluminous clear to occasionally mildly eosinophilic cytoplasm	Relatively less amount of clear cytoplasm with frequent apical snouts. Nuclei arranged linearly away from the basal aspect of the cell.	Nuclear grading follows ISUP grading system. High nuclear grade seen in areas of granular/eosinophilic cytoplasm.
Immunohistochemistry stains	Diffusely positive for CK7; CD10 usually positive; "cup"-shaped membranous positivity for CA9 may be present	Diffusely positive for CK7; CA9 (cup-like pattern); negative for CD10 and AMACR	Typically negative for CK7 but can be variable; diffusely positive membranous staining for CA9

ESRD, End-stage renal disease; *ISUP,* International Society of Urologic Pathology.

component classically forms nodules of elongated tubules with variable papillary architecture separated by stromal component that can vary from focal to prominent. Elongated tubules exhibit frequent branching. The epithelial and stromal interface often contains hemosiderin-laden macrophages and lymphoid aggregates.

HIGH POWER CYTOLOGIC FEATURES

The tubules are lined by voluminous clear to mildly eosinophilic cytoplasm. Cells have low N:C ratio due to voluminous clear to mildly eosinophilic cytoplasm. Nuclear grade is usually low but occasionally may show ISUP/WHO grade 3 nuclei.

IMMUNOHISTOCHEMICAL FEATURES

The tumor is diffusely positive for CK7 and is a required feature for the diagnosis. CD10 is usually positive.

8) ACQUIRED CYSTIC DISEASE–ASSOCIATED RENAL CELL CARCINOMA

DIFFERENTIAL DIAGNOSIS: RENAL CELL CARCINOMA, PAPILLARY TYPE; ATYPICAL RENAL CYST (Table 5.35)

Clinical Features

Acquired cystic disease–associated renal cell carcinoma (ACDRCC) is the most common tumor in the kidney of patients with ESRD and acquired cystic disease. Usually, it is encountered in patients undergoing long-term hemodialysis. Background kidney has multiple cysts, in which the tumor is found to arise within. Typically multifocal in nature and can present bilaterally.

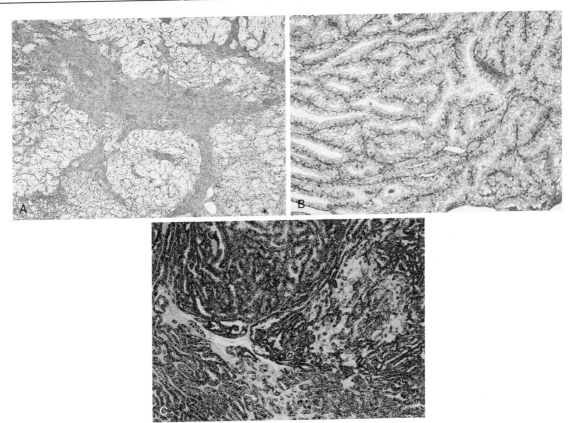

FIG. 5.80

Renal cell carcinoma with leiomyomatous stroma. **A,** Nodules of elongated frequently branching tubules, lined by abundant clear to mildly eosinophilic cytoplasm separated by variable smooth muscle stroma is a characteristic feature. **B,** Tubules lined by voluminous clear to occasionally mildly eosinophilic cytoplasm with a variable papillary architecture. **C,** The tumor is diffusely positive for CK7 and is a required feature for the diagnosis.

TABLE 5.35

Acquired Cystic Disease–associated Renal Cell Carcinoma (ACDRCC) Versus RCC Papillary Type Versus Atypical Renal Cyst

	ACDRCC (Fig. 5.81A–C)	RCC Papillary Type	Atypical Renal Cyst
Location	Multifocal, can be bilateral	Majority unifocal, but can be bilateral and multifocal	Multifocal
Gross features	Multiple complex cysts and associated solid tumors	Cystic cavitary mass with a friable consistency, often associated hemorrhage and central necrosis	Unilocular or multilocular cystic lesion
Histological features Low power	Combination of acinar, solid alveolar, solid sheet-like, microcystic or macrocystic and papillary architectures	Papillae and tubules lined by single layer of polygonal cells with granular/eosinophilic cytoplasm	Variable sized unilocular or multilocular cysts lined by heaped up cells with eosinophilic to clear cytoplasm imparting a "tufted" appearance
	Intra- and intercytoplasmic microscopic lumina imparting a cribriform/sieve-like appearance; intratumoral oxalate crystals	Foamy histiocytes, cholesterol clefts, and hemosiderin frequently seen	Lacks solid clusters/aggregates of cells in the cyst walls
High power	Abundant eosinophilic granular cytoplasm with round, centrally located nucleus; prominent nucleoli	Nuclei with low or high nuclear grade, ISUP grade 2–4	Nuclei are cytologically bland
Immunohistochemistry stains	Positive for AMACR; negative for CK7 and CA9	Positive for CK7	Not helpful

ISUP, International Society of Urologic Pathology.

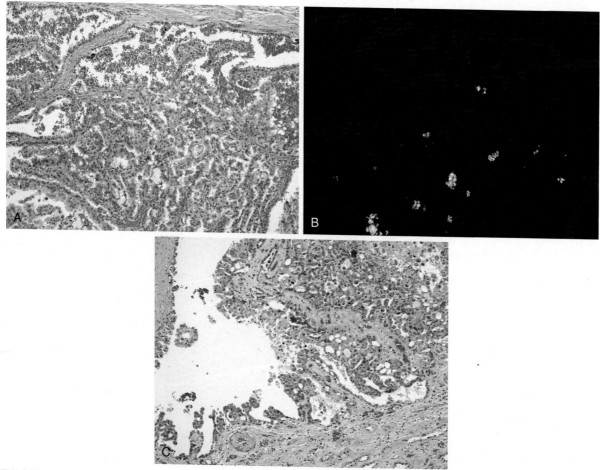

FIG. 5.81

Acquired cystic disease–associated renal cell carcinoma. **A,** Predominant tubulopapillary and papillary architecture with scattered identifiable oxalate crystals are a diagnostic clue to this entity. **B,** Polarization highlights the intratumoral oxalate crystals. **C,** Cytologic features include abundant eosinophilic cytoplasm with prominent nucleoli. Note the prominent intercellular and intracellcular lumina imparting a sieve-like appearance, which is a characteristic feature of this entity.

Pathologic Features (Fig. 5.81A–C)

GROSS FEATURES

This tumor is well-circumscribed multicystic with solid areas, with a tan to yellow cut surface. Hemorrhage and necrosis may be present.

LOW-POWER ARCHITECTURAL FEATURES

This tumor has a variety of growth patterns: acinar, alveolar, tubular, microcystic, papillary, and solid. A distinguishing feature is the presence of intra- or intercytoplasmic lumina imparting a sieve-like/cribriform architecture. Background kidney exhibits end-stage renal changes including multiple cysts.

HIGH-POWER CYTOLOGIC FEATURES

Tumor cells show abundant eosinophilic cytoplasm and prominent nucleoli. Cells of ACDRCC may show cytoplasmic clearing, and background calcium oxalate crystals may be present.

IMMUNOHISTOCHEMICAL FEATURES

The tumor is positive for AMACR and typically negative for CK7.

9) MITF FAMILY TRANSLOCATION–ASSOCIATED RENAL CELL CARCINOMA

DIFFERENTIAL DIAGNOSIS: CLEAR CELL RENAL CELL CARCINOMA; PAPILLARY RENAL CELL CARCINOMA (Table 5.36)

Clinical Features

MiTF family translocation RCC harbors gene fusions involving *TFE3* and *TFEB*. The RCCs associated with Xp11 translocation harbor gene fusions with *TFE3*

TABLE 5.36
MiTF Family Renal Cell Carcinoma (RCC) Versus Clear Cell Renal Cell Carcinoma (CCRCC) Versus Papillary RCC

	MiTF Family RCC (Fig. 5.82A–D)	CCRCC	Papillary RCC
Location	Unifocal	Unifocal	Majority unifocal, but can be bilateral and multifocal
Gross features	Solid mass with a tan-yellow cut surface	Solid and cystic mass with golden to yellow cut surface	Encapsulated mass with a variegated cut surface
Histological features Low power	Clear/pale or eosinophilic cells growing in a nested, alveolar, and papillary architecture	Polygonal cells with optically clear to granular eosinophilic cytoplasm, arranged in acini, tubules, nests, or solid sheets	Broad spectrum of morphologic patterns: papillary, tubular, and solid
	Biphasic appearance of larger epithelioid cells at the periphery of nests with smaller clustered cells with hyaline membranes is present especially in TFEB RCC		Papillary cores composed of loose, fibrovascular tissue, with variable amount of foamy macrophages
	Frequent psammoma bodies	Delicate intricately branching vasculature is typically present at least in low-grade areas	Associated with psammoma bodies and hemosiderin-laden macrophages
High power	Higher nuclear grade, usually ISUP grade 3–4	Conspicuous to prominent nucleoli seen in ISUP grade 3–4	Nuclear grade ranges from ISUP grade 2–4
Immunohistochemistry stains	Negative for CAM5.2, epithelial markers and vimentin. Cathepsin K is usually diffusely positive; TFE3 and TFEB antibodies are not reliable. FISH study for *TFE3/TFEB* rearrangement is necessary for confirmation	Positive for CAM5.2 and vimentin. Negative for cathepsin K	Positive for PAX8 and cytokeratins. CK7 is frequently diffusely positive; negative for cathepsin K

ISUP, International Society of Urologic Pathology.

and the RCCs with t(6:11) harbor a *TFEB* gene fusion. Fusion genes for *TFE3* include: 17q25 (*ASPSCR1* or *ASPL*), 1q21 (*PRCC*), 1p34 (*PSF*), Xq12 (*NONO*), 17q23 (*CLTC*), 17q25 (*RCC17*), 3q23 (unknown); and for *TFEB*: 11q12 (*MALAT1* or *a*). Approximately 40% of pediatric RCCs are Xp11 translocation RCCs. However, these tumors are increasingly recognized in elderly patients with the median patient age of 31 years. In children, TFE3 RCCs, particularly *ASPSCR1* or *ASPL-TFE3* carcinomas, usually present at advanced stage. TFEB-amplified RCC with or without *TFEB* rearrangement often presents with an aggressive clinical course.

Pathologic Features (Fig. 5.82A–D)

GROSS FEATURES

These tumors are well-circumscribed, non-encapsulated solid mass with a tan-yellow cut surface. It can also have irregular infiltrative borders.

LOW-POWER ARCHITECTURAL FEATURES

The most common morphologic pattern of this family of tumors is that of mixture of areas that partly resemble clear cell and partly papillary RCC (Fig. 5.82A and B). Variety of growth patterns including epithelioid cells with voluminous clear cytoplasm in an alveolar pattern (Fig. 5.82C), nested architecture with granular/eosinophilic cytoplasm, and psammoma bodies can be seen. Other distinguishing features include the presence of melanin pigment in tumors with *TFE3* gene fusions. In t(6:11) RCCs, a biphasic appearance of larger epithelioid cells at the periphery of nests with smaller clustered cells with hyaline membranes is typically encountered (Fig. 5.82D). However, this feature is not specific to *TFEB* RCC; can be seen with *TFE3* fusion RCC. TFEB-amplified RCCs often exhibit variable growth patterns. Tumor cells are typically lined by prominent eosinophilic cytoplasm.

HIGH-POWER CYTOLOGIC FEATURES

TFE3 gene fusion–associated RCCs typically are high nuclear grade, typically ISUP grade 3–4.

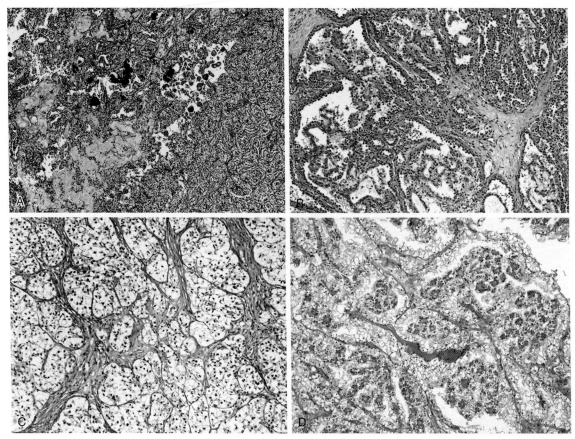

FIG. 5.82

MiTF family renal cell carcinoma (RCC). **A** and **B,** The most common morphologic pattern of this family of tumors is that of mixture of areas that partly resemble clear cell and partly papillary RCC. Additionally, frequent psammoma bodies are seen. **C,** Variety of growth patterns including epithelioid cells with voluminous clear cytoplasm in an alveolar pattern **(D)** A biphasic appearance of larger epithelioid cells at the periphery of nests with smaller clustered cells with hyaline membranes is a unique morphologic pattern that can be seen in this family of tumors.

Immunohistochemical features. The tumor is positive for PAX8 and negative for CAM5.2 and epithelial markers. Small subset is positive for melan A and HMB45 in t(6;11) RCCs. Cathepsin K is usually diffusely positive. TFE3 and TFEB antibodies are not reliable. FISH study for *TFE3/TFEB* rearrangement is usually necessary for confirmation.

10) MEDULLARY RENAL CELL CARCINOMA

DIFFERENTIAL DIAGNOSIS: UROTHELIAL CARCINOMA, COLLECTING DUCT RENAL CELL CARCINOMA, FH-DEFICIENT RENAL CELL CARCINOMA (Table 5.37)

Clinical Features

Medullary RCC has a predilection for young adults and an M:F ratio of 2:1. Most tumors present in the second or third decade of life. Most cases have been reported in African-American decent. Virtually all patients present with flank or abdominal pain and gross hematuria. At the time of presentation, the majority of cases already have metastases. These tumors are centered in the region of the medulla. It is associated with sickle cell trait and related hemoglobinopathies.

Pathologic Features (Fig. 5.83A–C)

GROSS FEATURES

These tumors are centered around the medulla and are poorly circumscribed. Cut surface is grayish-white and sclerotic with softening due to necrosis.

LOW-POWER ARCHITECTURAL FEATURES

Overall, the tumor has an infiltrating appearance with variable morphologic patterns including tubules, glands, and tubulopapillary structures and is often associated with necrosis, desmoplasia, and a background of inflammation.

TABLE 5.37

Medullary Renal Cell Carcinoma (RCC) Versus Urothelial Carcinoma (UCa) Versus Collecting Duct RCC Versus Fumarate Hydratase (FH)-deficient RCC

	Medullary RCC (Fig. 5.83A–C)	UCa	Collecting Duct RCC	FH-Deficient RCC
Location	Unifocal; medulla/sinus mass	Medulla/renal pelvis location	Unifocal; medulla/sinus	Unifocal
Gross features	Infiltrative, centered around medullary region	Large filling tumor within renal pelvis, can be infiltrative	Infiltrative with satellite nodules around medullar	Cystic and solid
Histological features Low power	High-grade infiltrative tumor with tubulopapillary morphology, cords, glands imparting adenoid cystic morphology, and/or solid sheets.	Papillae, irregular nests, cords, glandular, and solid sheets can be seen. High-grade tumors are frequently infiltrative into preexisting structures	High-grade infiltrative tumor with tubulo-papillary structures, cords, glandular, and/or solid sheets	Papillary morphology with abundant eosinophilic cytoplasm; frequently in an infiltrative pattern
	Basophilic or eosinophilic cytoplasm with frequent rhabdoid cell morphology	Basophilic or eosinophilic cytoplasm with occasional squamous differentiation	Basophilic or eosinophilic cytoplasm	Morphologic patterns including tubular, tubulocystic, solid, and mixed
High power	Vesicular pleomorphic nuclei with prominent nucleoli; frequent mitoses	Vesicular pleomorphic nuclei, nuclear hyperchromasia; frequent mitoses	Vesicular pleomorphic nuclei with prominent nucleoli; frequent mitoses	Large nuclei with prominent inclusion-like eosinophilic nucleoli with perinucleolar halos is
	Admixed inflammatory infiltrate of neutrophils	Inflamed desmoplastic stroma	Lacks inflammatory infiltrate but can be seen	Lacks inflammatory infiltrate but can be seen
Immunohistochemistry stains	Positive for PAX8. Loss of INI1 and acquired OCT3/4 expression	Positive for p63, GATA3. Small subset of UCa (specifically nested) can be positive for PAX8. Retained INI1 expression	Positive for PAX8 and cytokeratins. Negative for p63 and GATA3. Retained INI1 expression	Lost expression of FH. Retained INI1 expression

Adenoid cystic, reticular, and microcystic appearances are common. Rhabdoid cell differentiation is also commonly seen.

HIGH-POWER CYTOLOGIC FEATURES

Cells have pronounced cytologic atypia with prominent nucleoli and eosinophilic cytoplasm. Medullary RCC is commonly seen with associated intracytoplasmic mucin.

IMMUNOHISTOCHEMICAL FEATURES

The tumor is positive for PAX8 and usually positive for CAM5.2 and CK7. In addition, will demonstrate loss of INI1 expression and acquired expression of OCT3/4, which are diagnostically helpful.

11) MUCINOUS TUBULAR SPINDLE CELL CARCINOMA

DIFFERENTIAL DIAGNOSIS: SOLID PAPILLARY RENAL CELL CARCINOMA, SARCOMATOID RENAL CELL CARCINOMA
(Table 5.38)

Clinical Features

Mucinous tubular and spindle cell carcinoma has a female predilection with F:M ratio of 3:1. The tumor generally occurs in the cortex but can arise in the

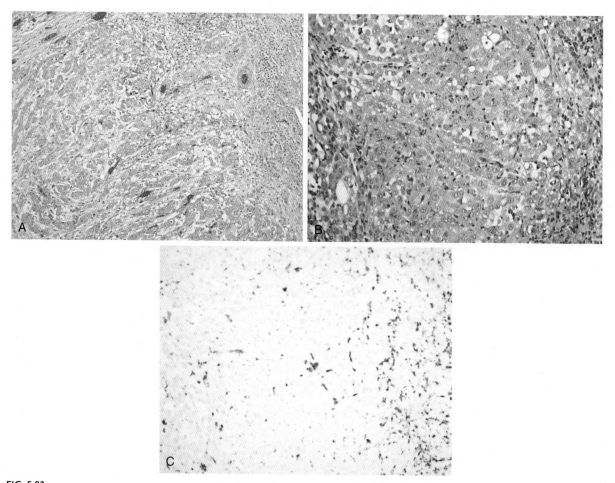

FIG. 5.83

Medullary renal cell carcinoma. **A,** Prominent inflammatory infiltrate within an infiltrative growth pattern with a myxoid stroma is commonly seen in this entity. The presence of sickled RBCs can be a helpful clue to this diagnosis. **B,** On biopsy, a high-grade carcinoma with mixture of neutrophilic rich inflammatory infiltrate points a clue to this entity. **C,** Loss of INI1 expression is diagnostically helpful in this entity.

TABLE 5.38

Mucinous Tubular and Spindle Cell Carcinoma (MTSCC) Versus Solid Papillary Renal Cell Carcinoma (RCC) Versus Sarcomatoid RCC

	MTSCC (Fig. 5.84)	Solid Papillary RCC	Sarcomatoid RCC (Fig. 5.85)
Location	Unifocal	Cortical	Cortical and medulla
Gross features	Solid tan mass	Cystic cavitary mass with a friable consistency, often associated with hemorrhage and central necrosis	Bulging, fleshy gray-white mass. May have associated necrosis
Histological features Low power	Compressed elongated tubular and spindle cells with light eosinophilic cytoplasm	Usually has "pink" appearance due to relatively abundant cytoplasm even in densely solid areas	Arranged in haphazard spindle cells
	Stromal mucin	Glomeruloid/papillary structures with tubular proliferation; can have associated luminal mucin	Can be a component of another subtype of RCC or pure sarcomatoid RCC
High power	Bland epithelial cells with small round nuclei	Majority present with low nuclear grade, ISUP/WHO grade 3 can be present	By definition high nuclear grade, ISUP grade 4
	Low mitoses	Variable mitoses	Frequent mitoses
Immunohistochemistry stains	Positive for CK7, PAX8 and AMACR	Positive for CK7	Usually positive for PAX8; pancytokeratin can also be positive

ISUP, International Society of Urologic Pathology.

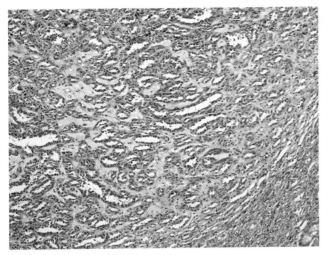

FIG. 5.84

In mucinous tubular and spindle cell carcinoma, there are variably shaped tubules with low-grade spindle areas and stromal mucin that are typical features of this entity.

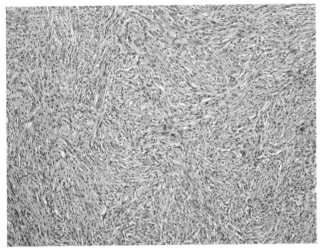

FIG. 5.85

Sarcomatoid renal cell carcinoma should be considered in a field of haphazardly arranged atypical spindle cells.

medulla. These tumors can be associated with nephrolithiasis.

Pathologic Features (Fig. 5.84)

GROSS FEATURES

The tumor is well circumscribed and solid. The cut surface is yellow to tan-brown and pink.

Low-power architectural features. The tumor is composed of bland tubular structures that are elongated and/or anastomosing and transition to a spindled component. The stroma has a basophilic mucinous appearance.

HIGH-POWER CYTOLOGIC FEATURES

The tubular cells are usually cuboidal and may focally show clear cells, oncocytic change, or cytoplasmic vacuolization. The nuclei are typically low grade.

IMMUNOHISTOCHEMICAL FEATURES

The tumor is positive for CK7, PAX8, and AMACR.

12) ANGIOMYOLIPOMA

DIFFERENTIAL DIAGNOSIS: LEIOMYOSARCOMA; RENAL CELL CARCINOMA, UNCLASSIFIED TYPE (Table 5.39)

Clinical Features

Angiomyolipoma (AML) has a female predilection. Peak incidence is in the fifth decade of life. Earlier onset, multifocality, and bilaterality are seen in the setting of TSC. In sporadic cases, AML is most often unifocal. Tumors can occur in the cortex or medulla. AML is a benign tumor unless associated with predominant atypical and/or epithelioid morphology.

Pathologic Features (Fig. 5.86A–C)

GROSS FEATURES

The tumor is well circumscribed but not encapsulated. Cut surface is variable, reflecting the proportion of fat, smooth muscle, or vessels within the tumor.

LOW-POWER ARCHITECTURAL FEATURES

The tumor is composed of variable proportion of adipose tissue, smooth muscle, and vessels. Architecture can vary in composition from tumors with prominent smooth muscle component to prominent lipomatous component. Smooth muscle component can be fascicular, indistinguishable from smooth muscle tumor. Smooth muscle cells often appear to radiate from the vessel walls. Most cases show thickened and hyalinized vessels.

HIGH-POWER CYTOLOGIC FEATURES

AMLs can have spindle cell component that show focal nuclear atypia. Epithelioid AMLs can have bizarre nuclear atypia. Necrosis, increased mitoses, and atypical mitoses can be seen in the epithelioid variant. Cytoplasm often exhibits filamentous appearance.

TABLE 5.39

Angiomyolipoma (AML) Versus Leiomyosarcoma Versus Renal Cell Carcinoma (RCC) Unclassified Type

	AML (Fig. 5.86A–C)	Leiomyosarcoma	RCC Unclassified Type
Location	Unifocal in sporadic; multifocal in setting of TSC	Unifocal	Unifocal
Gross features	Well circumscribed, not encapsulated	Large nodular mass	Variable from organ confined with tan-brown cut surface to large and multinodular with hemorrhage and necrosis
Histological features Low power	Composed of variable mixture of adipose tissue, smooth muscle, and vessels. Tumors can be predominant lipomatous, smooth muscle rich or epithelioid. Smooth muscle rich tumors come in differential of leiomyosarcoma and epithelioid variant may get misdiagnosed as RCC.	Compact well-formed fascicles of spindle cells that lack focal admixture of fat and abnormal vascular structures	Variable morphology, may range from low- to high-grade morphology that is not classifiable into a specific tumor type; may show sheets of anaplastic polygonal cells with eosinophilic cytoplasm lacking acinar or tubular arrangement
	Smooth muscle cells often appear to radiate from the vessel walls and have filamentous appearance	No intratumoral fat or dysmorphic vessels present	Frequently associated with necrosis and hemorrhage
High power	Spindle cell component can show focal nuclear atypia. Epithelioid areas with bizarre nuclei can also be seen. The presence of three of the following four features correlate with recurrence and metastasis in epithelioid variant: The presence of >70% epithelioid areas, ≥2 mitoses per 10 HPF, atypical mitoses or necrosis	Nuclei enlarged with pleomorphism and scattered hyperchromatic nuclei; frequent necrosis	Typically of higher grade morphology with prominent nucleoli, large nuclei with multinucleated tumor cells, ISUP grade 3–4
	May show high mitotic activity and atypical mitotic forms in epithelioid variant	Variable mitotic activity, with atypical mitoses	Mitoses frequent
Immunohisto-chemistry stains	Positive for HMB-45, melan A, cathepsin K. Smooth muscle actin and desmin also frequently positive. Cytokeratins and PAX8 negative	Positive for desmin, SMA; aberrant LMWCK; Negative for melanocytic markers.	Positive for PAX8 and cytokeratins. Negative for cathepsin K. HMB-45, melan A, and tyrosinase negative

HPF, High-power field; *ISUP*, International Society of Urologic Pathology; *TSC*, tuberous sclerosis complex.

IMMUNOHISTOCHEMICAL FEATURES

The tumor is positive for HMB-45, melan A, and cathepsin K. S100 can be positive. Smooth muscle markers are positive. Negative for epithelial markers (cytokeratin, EMA) and PAX8 in spindle cells.

13) ANASTOMOSING HEMANGIOMA

DIFFERENTIAL DIAGNOSIS: ANGIOSARCOMA (Table 5.40)

Clinical Features

Anastomosing hemangioma has no sex predominance and occurs in adults from 40s to elderly. Typically presents as a unifocal tumor. Tumors can occur in the kidney, perinephric adipose tissue, and renal hilum.

Pathologic Features (Fig. 87A and B)

GROSS FEATURES

The tumor is well circumscribed but unencapsulated with a hemorrhagic-mahogany and spongy appearance reflecting the vascularity.

LOW-POWER ARCHITECTURAL FEATURES

The tumor has a loosely lobulated architecture with anastomosing capillary sized blood vessels. These hemangiomas can have a focally infiltrative pattern of growth. Fibrin thrombi, extramedullary hematopoiesis, and hyaline globules are often identified and are useful

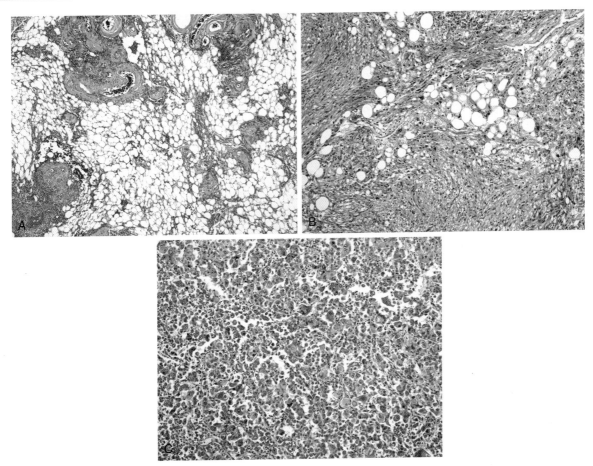

FIG. 5.86

Angiomyolipoma (AML). **A,** Typical triphasic pattern composed of fat, spindled smooth muscle fascicles, and dysmorphic blood vessels. **B,** The presence of adipocytes are a diagnostic clue to this entity, in a background of atypical spindled cells. **C,** In sheet-like growth pattern of epithelioid AML shows a lack of prominent vasculature. Intranuclear inclusions and pleomorphic giant cells are not uncommon.

TABLE 5.40

Anastomosing Hemangioma Versus Angiosarcoma

	Anastomosing Hemangioma (Fig. 5.87A and B)	Angiosarcoma (Fig. 5.88A and B)
Location	Kidney, perinephric adipose tissue, and renal hilum	Kidney, perinephric adipose tissue, and renal hilum
Gross features	Well circumscribed, unencapsulated; hemorrhagic-mahogany and spongy appearance	Large, necrotic mass; hemorrhagic cut surface
Histological features Low power	Loose lobulated architecture with associated anastomosing capillary-sized vessels. Loose stromal edema and/or stromal hyalinization between cellular zones of vascular proliferation	Vasoformative lesion with vascular spaces lined by high-grade cells
	Focal infiltrative pattern can be present	Diffusely infiltrative with parenchymal destruction
	Fibrin thrombi, extramedullary hematopoiesis and hyaline globules are often identified and are considered helpful features	Can have pronounced epithelioid features
High power	Anastomosing sinusoidal capillary-sized vessels with endothelial cells demonstrating "hobnail" morphology	Pleomorphic spindled and epithelioid cells
	Lacks cellular atypia. Mitoses are absent or rare	Numerous mitoses are typically appreciated
Immunohistochemistry stains	Negative for cytokeratin, EMA, and HMB45; Positive for CD31 and ERG highlighting endothelial cells	Negative for cytokeratin, EMA, and HMB45. Positive for CD34 and FLI-1. Epithelioid variant can be keratin positive

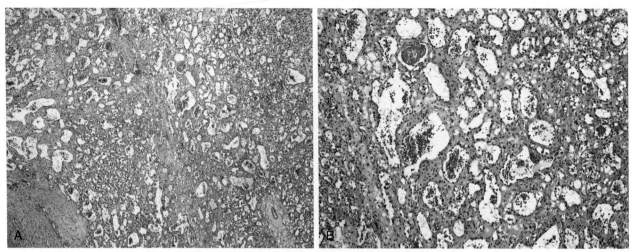

FIG. 5.87

Anastomosing hemangioma. **A,** Composed of anastomosing channels of vessels in a background of hyalinized stroma. **B,** Scattered hobnail endothelial cells lining the vessels, with otherwise bland cytology.

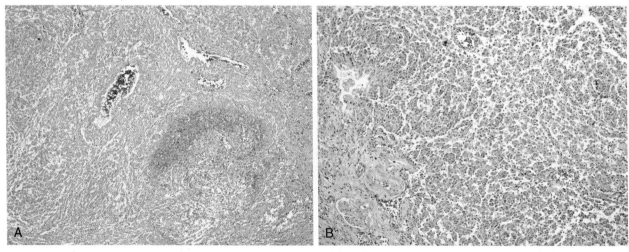

FIG. 5.88

Angiosarcoma. **A,** Infiltrative tumor that is composed of pleomorphic cells with associated necrosis. **B,** Higher magnification demonstrates a vasoformative neoplasm with high-grade tumor cells, providing a clue to this diagnosis.

features. It can be associated with zones of infarction with variable sclerosis.

HIGH-POWER CYTOLOGIC FEATURES

The tumor often shows prominent endothelial cells with "hobnail" morphology imparting a sieve-like appearance. Mitoses are absent or rare.

IMMUNOHISTOCHEMICAL FEATURES

The tumor is negative for keratin AE1/3, EMA, HHV8, and HMB45. CD31 and ERG highlights endothelial cells.

14) ADULT CYSTIC NEPHROMA/MIXED EPITHELIAL AND STROMAL TUMOR FAMILY TUMORS

DIFFERENTIAL DIAGNOSIS: MULTILOCULAR CYSTIC RENAL NEOPLASM OF LOW MALIGNANT POTENTIAL, TUBULOCYSTIC CARCINOMA (Table 5.41)

Clinical Features

Adult cystic nephroma (CN)/mixed epithelial and stromal tumor (MEST) family tumors have a female predilection

TABLE 5.41

Adult Cystic Nephroma/Mixed Epithelial and Stromal Tumor (CN/MEST) Family Tumors Versus Multicystic Renal Cell Neoplasm of Low Malignant Potential (MCN-LMP) Versus Tubulocystic Carcinoma

	Adult CN/MEST Family Tumors (Fig. 5.89A and B)	MCN-LMP	Tubulocystic Carcinoma (Fig. 5.90A and B)
Location	Unifocal	Unifocal	Unifocal
Gross features	Variably solid and cystic, well circumscribed	Well circumscribed with fibrous capsule; multicystic cut surface	Tan/white multicystic mass with sponge-like cut surfaces
Histological features Low power	Varying stromal patterns: ovarian-type, loose fibrous, dense fibrous, or smooth muscle–type. Ovarian-type stroma is a useful diagnostic clue Epithelial component: flat, hobnailed, cuboidal, columnar, urothelial like or clear cell type.	Cysts have a smooth lining of flattened to cuboidal clear cells	Small to intermediate-sized tubules admixed with larger cysts lined by single cuboidal/columnar epithelium with frequent hobnailing
	May be associated with prominent vasculature	Cyst walls/septae have small non-expansile aggregates of cells with clear cytoplasm	Abundant eosinophilic cytoplasm with associated fibrotic stroma
High power	No nuclear atypia or prominent nucleoli within the epithelial cells	Nuclei with low nuclear grade, ISUP grade 1–2	Nuclei are enlarged and irregular with large nucleoli; high nuclear grade
Immunohistochemistry stains	Stromal cells positive for ER and PR.	Lining cells positive for cytokeratins. No stromal reactivity for ER and PR.	Lining cells positive for CK7. No stromal reactivity for ER and PR.

ISUP, International Society of Urologic Pathology.

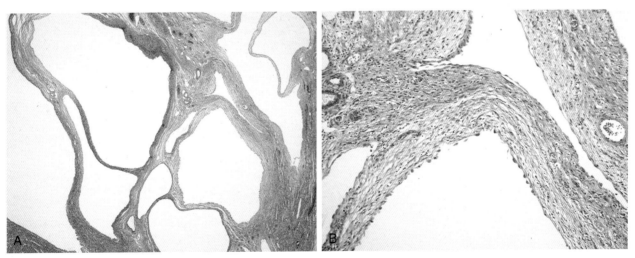

FIG. 5.89

Adult cystic nephroma/mixed epithelial and stromal tumor. **A,** Predominantly cystic areas with septa composed of cellular ovarian-type stroma. **B,** Epithelium shows prominent hobnailing with overall bland cytologic features.

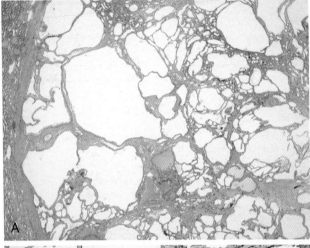

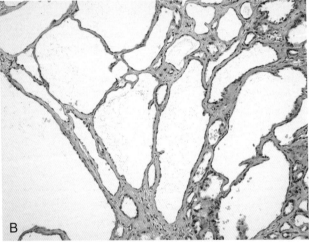

FIG. 5.90

Tubulocystic carcinoma. **A,** Tubulocystic carcinoma by definition is well circumscribed without solid areas. Composed of small to medium-sized tubules admixed with cystically dilated tubules in a background of fibrotic stroma. **B,** Cysts lined by cells with abundant eosinophilic cytoplasm imparting a hobnail appearance.

and are typically solitary tumors that are most often located close to the renal hilum but can involve renal cortex. CN and MEST are considered to represent a morphologic spectrum of one entity.

Pathologic Features (Fig. 5.89A and B)

GROSS FEATURES

The tumor is well circumscribed, confined to the kidney, and is variably solid and cystic. Sometimes, they can have a predominant cystic or solid component. The majority of cysts contain clear serous fluid.

LOW-POWER ARCHITECTURAL FEATURES

The tumor has a varying stroma that can be ovarian-type hypercellular spindled, loose fibrous and edematous,

dense fibrous and sclerotic, or smooth muscle type. The ovarian-type stroma provides a useful diagnostic clue and may show luteinized stromal cells. Often has a prominent vasculature. The tumor cells in the epithelial component can be flat, hobnailed, cuboidal, columnar, urothelial-like, or clear cell.

HIGH-POWER CYTOLOGIC FEATURES

There is no nuclear atypia or nucleolar prominence appreciated. They are often associated with calcifications and foamy histiocytes within the background.

IMMUNOHISTOCHEMICAL FEATURES

The tumor stromal cells are positive for ER, PR, and less commonly inhibin and calretinin.

SUGGESTED READINGS

Prostate

De Marzo AM, Platz EA, Epstein JI, et al. A working group classification of focal prostate atrophy lesions. *Am J Surg Pathol.* 2006;30:1281-1291.

Oppenheimer JR, Wills ML, Epstein JI. Partial atrophy in prostate needle cores: another diagnostic pitfall for the surgical pathologist. *Am J Surg Pathol.* 1998;22:440-445.

Przybycin CG, Kunju LP, Wu AJ, et al. Partial atrophy in prostate needle biopsies: a detailed analysis of its morphology, immunophenotype, and cellular kinetics. *Am J Surg Pathol.* 2008;32:58-64.

Bostwick DG, Egbert BM, Fajardo LF. Radiation injury of the normal and neoplastic prostate. *Am J Surg Pathol.* 1982;6:541-551.

Magi-Galluzzi C, Sanderson H, Epstein JI. Atypia in nonneoplastic prostate glands after radiotherapy for prostate cancer: duration of atypia and relation to type of radiotherapy. *Am J Surg Pathol.* 2003;27:206-212.

Yang XJ, Laven B, Tretiakova M, et al. Detection of alpha-methylacyl-coenzyme A racemase in postradiation prostatic adenocarcinoma. *Urology.* 2003;62:282-286.

Hosler GA, Epstein JI. Basal cell hyperplasia: an unusual diagnostic dilemma on prostate needle biopsies. *Hum Pathol.* 2005;36:480-485.

Epstein JI, Armas OA. Atypical basal cell hyperplasia of the prostate. *Am J Surg Pathol.* 1992;16:1205-1214.

Ali TZ, Epstein JI. Basal cell carcinoma of the prostate: a clinicopathologic study of 29 cases. *Am J Surg Pathol.* 2007;31:697-705.

McKenney JK, Amin MB, Srigley JR, et al. Basal cell proliferations of the prostate other than usual basal cell hyperplasia: a clinicopathologic study of 23 cases, including four carcinomas, with a proposed classification. *Am J Surg Pathol.* 2004;28:1289-1298.

Netto GJ, Epstein JI. Widespread high-grade prostatic intraepithelial neoplasia on prostatic needle biopsy: a significant likelihood of subsequently diagnosed adenocarcinoma. *Am J Surg Pathol.* 2006; 30:1184-1188.

Perner S, Mosquera J-M, Demichelis F, et al. TMPRSS2-ERG Fusion Prostate Cancer: an early molecular event associated with invasion. *Am J Surg Pathol.* 2007;31:882-888.

Shah RB, Li J, Dhanani N, et al. ERG overexpression and multifocality predict prostate cancer in subsequent biopsy for patients with high-grade prostatic intraepithelial neoplasia. *Urol Oncol.* 2016;34: 120.e1-e7.

Gaudin PB, Epstein JI. Adenosis of the prostate. Histologic features in transurethral resection specimens. *Am J Surg Pathol.* 1994;18:863-870.

Gaudin PB, Epstein JI. Adenosis of the prostate. Histologic features in needle biopsy specimens. *Am J Surg Pathol.* 1995;19:737-747.

Lotan TL, Epstein JI. Diffuse adenosis of the peripheral zone in prostate needle biopsy and prostatectomy specimens. *Am J Surg Pathol.* 2008;32:1360-1366.

Grignon DJ, Ro JY, Srigley JR, et al. Sclerosing adenosis of the prostate gland. A lesion showing myoepithelial differentiation. *Am J Surg Pathol.* 1992;16:383-391.

Sakamoto N, Tsuneyoshi M, Enjoji M. Sclerosing adenosis of the prostate. Histopathologic and immunohistochemical analysis. *Am J Surg Pathol.* 1991;15:660-667.

Humphrey PA, Kaleem Z, Swanson PE, et al. Pseudohyperplastic prostatic adenocarcinoma. *Am J Surg Pathol.* 1998;22:1239-1246.

Levi AW, Epstein JI. Pseudohyperplastic prostatic adenocarcinoma on needle biopsy and simple prostatectomy. *Am J Surg Pathol.* 2000;24:1039-1046.

Cina SJ, Silberman MA, Kahane H, et al. Diagnosis of Cowper's glands on prostate needle biopsy. *Am J Surg Pathol.* 1997;21:550-555.

Nelson RS, Epstein JI. Prostatic carcinoma with abundant xanthomatous cytoplasm. Foamy gland carcinoma. *Am J Surg Pathol.* 1996;20:419-426.

Saboorian MH, Huffman H, Ashfaq R, et al. Distinguishing Cowper's glands from neoplastic and pseudoneoplastic lesions of prostate: immunohistochemical and ultrastructural studies. *Am J Surg Pathol.* 1997;21:1069-1074.

Guo CC, Epstein JI. Intraductal carcinoma of the prostate on needle biopsy: histologic features and clinical significance. *Mod Pathol.* 2006;19:1528-1535.

Zhou M. High-grade prostatic intraepithelial neoplasia, PIN-like carcinoma, ductal carcinoma, and intraductal carcinoma of the prostate. *Mod Pathol.* 2018;31:S71-S79.

Robinson BD, Epstein JI. Intraductal carcinoma of the prostate without invasive carcinoma on needle biopsy: emphasis on radical prostatectomy findings. *J Urol.* 2010;184:1328-1333.

Shah RB, Nguyen JK, Przybycin CG, et al. Atypical intraductal proliferation detected in prostate needle biopsy is a marker of unsampled intraductal carcinoma and other adverse pathological features: a prospective clinicopathological study of 62 cases with emphasis on pathological outcomes. *Histopathology.* 2019;75:346-353.

Hameed O, Humphrey PA. Stratified epithelium in prostatic adenocarcinoma: a mimic of high-grade prostatic intraepithelial neoplasia. *Mod Pathol.* 2006;19:899-906.

Tavora F, Epstein JI. High-grade prostatic intraepithelial neoplasialike ductal adenocarcinoma of the prostate: a clinicopathologic study of 28 cases. *Am J Surg Pathol.* 2008;32:1060-1067.

Bostwick DG, Kindrachuk RW, Rouse RV. Prostatic adenocarcinoma with endometrioid features. Clinical, pathologic, and ultrastructural findings. *Am J Surg Pathol.* 1985;9:595-609.

Herawi M, Epstein JI. Immunohistochemical antibody cocktail staining (p63/HMWCK/AMACR) of ductal adenocarcinoma and Gleason pattern 4 cribriform and noncribriform acinar adenocarcinomas of the prostate. *Am J Surg Pathol.* 2007;31:889-894.

Chuang AY, DeMarzo AM, Veltri RW, et al. Immunohistochemical differentiation of high-grade prostate carcinoma from urothelial carcinoma. *Am J Surg Pathol.* 2007;31:1246-1255.

Wang W, Epstein JI. Small cell carcinoma of the prostate. A morphologic and immunohistochemical study of 95 cases. *Am J Surg Pathol.* 2008;32:65-71.

Owens CL, Epstein JI, Netto GJ. Distinguishing prostatic from colorectal adenocarcinoma on biopsy samples: the role of morphology and immunohistochemistry. *Arch Pathol Lab Med.* 2007;131:599-603.

Hansel DE, Epstein JI. Sarcomatoid carcinoma of the prostate: a study of 42 cases. *Am J Surg Pathol.* 2006;30:1316-1321.

Gaudin PB, Rosai J, Epstein JI. Sarcomas and related proliferative lesions of specialized prostatic stroma: a clinicopathologic study of 22 cases. *Am J Surg Pathol.* 1998;22:148-162.

McKenney JK. Mesenchymal tumors of the prostate. *Mod Pathol.* 2018;31:S133-S142.

Herawi M, Epstein JI. Solitary fibrous tumor on needle biopsy and transurethral resection of the prostate: a clinicopathologic study of 13 cases. *Am J Surg Pathol.* 2007;31:870-876.

Bladder

Amin MB, McKenney JK. An approach to the diagnosis of flat intraepithelial lesions of the urinary bladder using the World Health Organization/ International Society of Urological Pathology consensus classification system. *Adv Anat Pathol.* 2002;9:222-232.

McKenney JK, Desai S, Cohen C, et al. Discriminatory immunohistochemical staining of urothelial carcinoma in situ and non-neoplastic urothelium: an analysis of cytokeratin 20, p53, and CD44 antigens. *Am J Surg Pathol.* 2001;25:1074-1078.

Nguyen JK, Przybycin CG, McKenney JK, et al. Immunohistochemical staining patterns of Ki-67 and p53 in florid reactive urothelial atypia and urothelial carcinoma in situ demonstrate significant overlap. *Hum Pathol.* 2020;98:81-88.

McKenney JK, Amin MB, Young RH. Urothelial (transitional cell) papilloma of the urinary bladder: a clinicopathologic study of 26 cases. *Mod Pathol.* 2003;16:623-629.

Magi-Galluzzi C, Epstein JI. Urothelial papilloma of the bladder: a review of 34 de novo cases. *Am J Surg Pathol.* 2004;28:1615-1620.

Pich A, Chiusa L, Formiconi A, et al. Biologic differences between non-invasive papillary urothelial neoplasms of low malignant potential and low-grade (grade 1) papillary carcinomas of the bladder. *Am J Surg Pathol.* 2001;25:1528-1533.

Young RH. Papillary and polypoid cystitis. A report of eight cases. *Am J Surg Pathol.* 1988;12:542-546.

Oliva E, Young RH. Nephrogenic adenoma of the urinary tract: a review of the microscopic appearance of 80 cases with emphasis on unusual features. *Mod Pathol.* 1995;8:722-730.

Lane Z, Epstein JI. Polypoid/papillary cystitis: a series of 41 cases misdiagnosed as papillary urothelial neoplasia. *Am J Surg Pathol.* 2008;32:758-764.

Allan CH, Epstein JI. Nephrogenic adenoma of the prostatic urethra: a mimicker of prostate adenocarcinoma. *Am J Surg Pathol.* 2001;25:802-808.

Young RH, Scully RE. Clear cell adenocarcinoma of the bladder and urethra. A report of three cases and review of the literature. *Am J Surg Pathol.* 1985;9:816-826.

Huang Q, Chu PG, Lau SK, et al. Urothelial carcinoma of the urinary bladder with a component of acinar/tubular type differentiation simulating prostatic adenocarcinoma. *Hum Pathol.* 2004;35:769-773.

Herawi M, Drew PA, Pan CC, et al. Clear cell adenocarcinoma of the bladder and urethra: cases diffusely mimicking nephrogenic adenoma. *Hum Pathol.* 2010;41:594-601.

Wasco MJ, Daignault S, Bradley D, et al. Nested variant of urothelial carcinoma: a clinicopathologic and immunohistochemical study of 30 pure and mixed cases. *Hum Pathol.* 2010;41:163-171.

Taylor AS, McKenney JK, Osunkoya AO, et al. PAX8 expression and TERT promoter mutations in the nested variant of urothelial carcinoma: a clinicopathologic study with immunohistochemical and molecular correlates. *Mod Pathol.* 2020;33:1165-1171.

Baker PM, Young RH. Radiation-induced pseudocarcinomatous proliferations of the urinary bladder: a report of 4 cases. *Hum Pathol.* 2000;31:678-683.

Chan TY, Epstein JI. Radiation or chemotherapy cystitis with "pseudocarcinomatous" features. *Am J Surg Pathol.* 2004;28:909-913.

Lane Z, Epstein JI. Pseudocarcinomatous epithelial hyperplasia in the bladder unassociated with prior irradiation or chemotherapy. *Am J Surg Pathol.* 2008;32:92-97.

Cox R, Epstein JI. Large nested variant of urothelial carcinoma: 23 cases mimicking von Brunn nests and inverted growth pattern of noninvasive papillary urothelial carcinoma. *Am J Surg Pathol.* 2011;35:1337-1342.

Volmar KE, Chan TY, De Marzo AM, et al. Florid von Brunn nests mimicking urothelial carcinoma: a morphologic and immunohistochemical comparison to the nested variant of urothelial carcinoma. *Am J Surg Pathol.* 2003;27:1243-1252.

Fine SW, Epstein JI. Inverted urothelial papillomas with foamy or vacuolated cytoplasm. *Hum Pathol.* 2006;37:1577-1582.

Keck B, Stoehr R, Wach S, et al. The plasmacytoid carcinoma of the bladder—rare variant of aggressive urothelial carcinoma. *Int J Cancer.* 2011;129:346-354.

Nigwekar P, Tamboli P, Amin MB, et al. Plasmacytoid urothelial carcinoma: detailed analysis of morphology with clinicopathologic correlation in 17 cases. *Am J Surg Pathol.* 2009;33:417-424.

Ricardo-Gonzalez RR, Nguyen M, Gokden N, et al. Plasmacytoid carcinoma of the bladder: a urothelial carcinoma variant with a predilection for intraperitoneal spread. *J Urol.* 2012;187:852-855.

Compérat E, Roupret M, Yaxley J, et al. Micropapillary urothelial carcinoma of the urinary bladder: a clinicopathological analysis of 72 cases. *Pathology.* 2010;42:650-654.

Ramani P, Birch BR, Harland SJ, et al. Evaluation of endothelial markers in detecting blood and lymphatic channel invasion in pT1 transitional carcinoma of bladder. *Histopathology.* 1991;19:551-554.

Samaratunga H, Khoo K. Micropapillary variant of urothelial carcinoma of the urinary bladder; a clinicopathological and immunohistochemical study. *Histopathology*. 2004;45:55-64.

Harik LR, Merino C, Coindre JM, et al. Pseudosarcomatous myofibroblastic proliferations of the bladder: a clinicopathologic study of 42 cases. *Am J Surg Pathol*. 2006;30:787-794.

Montgomery EA, Shuster DD, Burkart AL, et al. Inflammatory myofibroblastic tumors of the urinary tract: a clinicopathologic study of 46 cases, including a malignant example inflammatory fibrosarcoma and a subset associated with high-grade urothelial carcinoma. *Am J Surg Pathol*. 2006;30:1502-1512.

Young RH, Wick MR, Mills SE. Sarcomatoid carcinoma of the urinary bladder. A clinicopathologic analysis of 12 cases and review of the literature. *Am J Clin Pathol*. 1988;90:653-661.

Cheng L, Zhang S, Alexander R, et al. Sarcomatoid carcinoma of the urinary bladder: the final common pathway of urothelial carcinoma dedifferentiation. *Am J Surg Pathol*. 2011;35:e34-e46.

Cheng L, Leibovich BC, Cheville JC, et al. Paraganglioma of the urinary bladder: can biologic potential be predicted? *Cancer*. 2000;88:844-852.

Zhou M, Epstein JI, Young RH. Paraganglioma of the urinary bladder: a lesion that may be misdiagnosed as urothelial carcinoma in transurethral resection specimens. *Am J Surg Pathol*. 2004;28:94-100.

Abrahams NA, Moran C, Reyes AO, et al. Small cell carcinoma of the bladder: a contemporary clinicopathological study of 51 cases. *Histopathology*. 2005;46:57-63.

Cheng L, Pan CX, Yang XJ, et al. Small cell carcinoma of the urinary bladder: a clinicopathologic analysis of 64 patients. *Cancer*. 2004;101:957-962.

Amin MB, Gómez JA, Young RH. Urothelial transitional cell carcinoma with endophytic growth patterns: a discussion of patterns of invasion and problems associated with assessment of invasion in 18 cases. *Am J Surg Pathol*. 1997;21:1057-1068.

Hodges KB, Lopez-Beltran A, Maclennan GT, et al. Urothelial lesions with inverted growth patterns: histogenesis, molecular genetic findings, differential diagnosis and clinical management. *BJU Int*. 2011;107:532-537.

Sweeney MK, Rais-Bahrami S, Gordetsky J. Inverted urothelial papilloma: a review of diagnostic pitfalls and clinical management. *Can Urol Assoc J*. 2017;11:66-69.

Paner GP, Ro JY, Wojcik EM, et al. Further characterization of the muscle layers and lamina propria of the urinary bladder by systematic histologic mapping: implications for pathologic staging of invasive urothelial carcinoma. *Am J Surg Pathol*. 2007;31:1420-1429.

Paner GP, Shen SS, Lapetino S, et al. Diagnostic utility of antibody to smoothelin in the distinction of muscularis propria from muscularis mucosae of the urinary bladder: a potential ancillary tool in the pathologic staging of invasive urothelial carcinoma. *Am J Surg Pathol*. 2009;33:91-98.

Miyamoto H, Sharma RB, Illei PB, et al. Pitfalls in the use of smoothelin to identify muscularis propria invasion by urothelial carcinoma. *Am J Surg Pathol*. 2010;34:418-422.

Lopez-Beltran A, Henriques V, Montironi R. Variants and new entities of bladder cancer. *Histopathology*. 2019;74:77-96.

Zhai QJ, Black J, Ayala AG, et al. Histologic variants of infiltrating urothelial carcinoma. *Arch Pathol Lab Med*. 2007;131:1244-1256.

Branca G, Barresi V. Müllerianosis of the urinary bladder: a rare tumor-like lesion. *Arch Pathol Lab Med*. 2014;138:432-436.

Rao Q, Williamson SR, Lopez-Beltran A, et al. Distinguishing primary adenocarcinoma of the urinary bladder from secondary involvement by colorectal adenocarcinoma: extended immunohistochemical profiles emphasizing novel markers. *Mod Pathol*. 2013;26:725-732.

Grignon DJ, Ro JY, Ayala AG, et al. Primary adenocarcinoma of the urinary bladder. A clinicopathologic analysis of 72 cases. *Cancer*. 1991;67:2165-2172.

Kidney

Argani P, Netto GJ, Parwani AV. Papillary renal cell carcinoma with low-grade spindle cell foci: a mimic of mucinous tubular and spindle cell carcinoma. *Am J Surg Pathol*. 2008;32:1353-1359.

Wobker SE, Matoso A, Pratilas CA, et al. Metanephric Adenoma-Epithelial Wilms tumor overlap lesions: an analysis of BRAF status. *Am J Surg Pathol*. 2019;43:1157-1169.

Vujanić GM, Sandstedt B. The pathology of Wilms' tumour (nephroblastoma): the International Society of Paediatric Oncology approach. *J Clin Pathol*. 2010;63:102-109.

Williamson SR, Eble JN, Cheng L, et al. Clear cell papillary renal cell carcinoma: differential diagnosis and extended immunohistochemical profile. *Mod Pathol*. 2013;26:697-708.

Dhakal HP, McKenney JK, Khor LY, et al. Renal neoplasms with overlapping features of clear cell renal cell carcinoma and clear cell papillary renal cell carcinoma: a clinicopathologic study of 37 cases from a single institution. *Am J Surg Pathol*. 2016;40:141-154.

Przybycin CG, Cronin AM, Darvishian F, et al. Chromophobe renal cell carcinoma: a clinicopathologic study of 203 tumors in 200 patients with primary resection at a single institution. *Am J Surg Pathol*. 2011;35:962-970.

Matoso A, Chen YB, Rao V, et al. Atypical renal cysts: a morphologic, immunohistochemical, and molecular study. *Am J Surg Pathol*. 2016;40:202-211.

Suzigan S, López-Beltrán A, Montironi R, et al. Multilocular cystic renal cell carcinoma : a report of 45 cases of a kidney tumor of low malignant potential. *Am J Clin Pathol*. 2006;125:217-222.

Tretiakova M, Mehta V, Kocherginsky M, et al. Predominantly cystic clear cell renal cell carcinoma and multilocular cystic renal neoplasm of low malignant potential form a low-grade spectrum. *Virchows Arch*. 2018;473:85-93.

Wang KL, Weinrach DM, Luan C, et al. Renal papillary adenoma—a putative precursor of papillary renal cell carcinoma. *Hum Pathol*. 2007;38:239-246.

Alomari AK, Nettey OS, Singh D, et al. Clinicopathological and immunohistochemical characteristics of papillary renal cell carcinoma with emphasis on subtyping. *Hum Pathol*. 2015;46:1418-1426.

Tickoo SK, Amin MB. Discriminant nuclear features of renal oncocytoma and chromophobe renal cell carcinoma. Analysis of their potential utility in the differential diagnosis. *Am J Clin Pathol*. 1998; 110:782-787.

Amin MB, Crotty TB, Tickoo SK, et al. Renal oncocytoma: a reappraisal of morphologic features with clinicopathologic findings in 80 cases. *Am J Surg Pathol*. 1997;21:1-12.

Williamson SR, Eble JN, Amin MB, et al. Succinate dehydrogenase-deficient renal cell carcinoma: detailed characterization of 11 tumors defining a unique subtype of renal cell carcinoma. *Mod Pathol*. 2015;28:80-94.

Trpkov K, Hes O, Bonert M, et al. Eosinophilic, solid, and cystic renal cell carcinoma: clinicopathologic study of 16 unique, sporadic neoplasms occurring in women. *Am J Surg Pathol*. 2016;40:60-71.

Kuroda N, Tanaka A, Yamaguchi T, et al. Chromophobe renal cell carcinoma, oncocytic variant: a proposal of a new variant giving a critical diagnostic pitfall in diagnosing renal oncocytic tumors. *Med Mol Morphol*. 2013;46:49-55.

Smith SC, Sirohi D, Ohe C, et al. A distinctive, low-grade oncocytic fumarate hydratase-deficient renal cell carcinoma, morphologically reminiscent of succinate dehydrogenase-deficient renal cell carcinoma. *Histopathology*. 2017;71:42-52.

Trpkov K, Hes O, Agaimy A, et al. Fumarate hydratase-deficient renal cell carcinoma is strongly correlated with fumarate hydratase mutation and hereditary leiomyomatosis and renal cell carcinoma syndrome. *Am J Surg Pathol*. 2016;40:865-875.

Hes O, Brunelli M, Michal M, et al. Oncocytic papillary renal cell carcinoma: a clinicopathologic, immunohistochemical, ultrastructural, and interphase cytogenetic study of 12 cases. *Ann Diagn Pathol*. 2006;10:133-139.

Sarungbam J, Mehra R, Tomlins SA, et al. Tubulocystic renal cell carcinoma: a distinct clinicopathologic entity with a characteristic genomic profile. *Mod Pathol*. 2019;32:701-709.

Smith SC, Trpkov K, Chen YB, et al. Tubulocystic carcinoma of the kidney with poorly differentiated foci: a frequent morphologic pattern of fumarate hydratase-deficient renal cell carcinoma. *Am J Surg Pathol*. 2016;40:1457-1472.

Shah RB, Stohr BA, Tu ZJ, et al. "Renal cell carcinoma with leiomyomatous stroma" harbor somatic mutations of TSC1, TSC2, MTOR, and/or ELOC (TCEB1): clinicopathologic and molecular characterization of 18 sporadic tumors supports a distinct entity. *Am J Surg Pathol*. 2020;44:571-581.

Gobbo S, Eble JN, Grignon DJ, et al. Clear cell papillary renal cell carcinoma: a distinct histopathologic and molecular genetic entity. *Am J Surg Pathol*. 2008;32:1239-1245.

Williamson SR, Gupta NS, Eble JN, et al. Clear cell renal cell carcinoma with borderline features of clear cell papillary renal cell carcinoma: combined morphologic, immunohistochemical, and cytogenetic analysis. *Am J Surg Pathol*. 2015;39:1502-1510.

Przybycin CG, Harper HL, Reynolds JP, et al. Acquired cystic disease-associated renal cell carcinoma (ACD-RCC): a multiinstitutional study of 40 cases with clinical follow-up. Am J Surg Pathol. 2018;42:1156-1165.

Argani P, Hicks J, De Marzo AM, et al. Xp11 translocation renal cell carcinoma (RCC): extended immunohistochemical profile emphasizing novel RCC markers. Am J Surg Pathol. 2010;34:1295-1303.

Argani P, Zhong M, Reuter VE, et al. TFE3-Fusion variant analysis defines specific clinicopathologic associations among Xp11 translocation cancers. Am J Surg Pathol. 2016;40:723-737.

Liu Q, Galli S, Srinivasan R, et al. Renal medullary carcinoma: molecular, immunohistochemistry, and morphologic correlation. Am J Surg Pathol. 2013;37:368-374.

MacLennan GT, Farrow GM, Bostwick DG. Low-grade collecting duct carcinoma of the kidney: report of 13 cases of low-grade mucinous tubulocystic renal carcinoma of possible collecting duct origin. Urology. 1997;50:679-684.

Ohe C, Smith SC, Sirohi D, et al. Reappraisal of morphologic differences between renal medullary carcinoma, collecting duct carcinoma, and fumarate hydratase-deficient renal cell carcinoma. Am J Surg Pathol. 2018;42:279-292.

Fine SW, Argani P, DeMarzo AM, et al. Expanding the histologic spectrum of mucinous tubular and spindle cell carcinoma of the kidney. Am J Surg Pathol. 2006;30:1554-1560.

Brimo F, Robinson B, Guo C, et al. Renal epithelioid angiomyolipoma with atypia: a series of 40 cases with emphasis on clinicopathologic prognostic indicators of malignancy. Am J Surg Pathol. 2010;34:715-722.

Nese N, Martignoni G, Fletcher CD, et al. Pure epithelioid PEComas (so-called epithelioid angiomyolipoma) of the kidney: a clinicopathologic study of 41 cases: detailed assessment of morphology and risk stratification. Am J Surg Pathol. 2011;35:161-176.

Zisman A, Chao DH, Pantuck AJ, et al. Unclassified renal cell carcinoma: clinical features and prognostic impact of a new histological subtype. J Urol. 2002;168:950-955.

Miller JS, Zhou M, Brimo F, et al. Primary leiomyosarcoma of the kidney: a clinicopathologic study of 27 cases. Am J Surg Pathol. 2010;34:238-242.

Montgomery E, Epstein JI. Anastomosing hemangioma of the genitourinary tract: a lesion mimicking angiosarcoma. Am J Surg Pathol. 2009;33:1364-1369.

Brown JG, Folpe AL, Rao P, et al. Primary vascular tumors and tumor-like lesions of the kidney: a clinicopathologic analysis of 25 cases. Am J Surg Pathol. 2010;34:942-949.

Turbiner J, Amin MB, Humphrey PA, et al. Cystic nephroma and mixed epithelial and stromal tumor of kidney: a detailed clinicopathologic analysis of 34 cases and proposal for renal epithelial and stromal tumor (REST) as a unifying term. Am J Surg Pathol. 2007;31:489-500.

Zhou M, Kort E, Hoekstra P, et al. Adult cystic nephroma and mixed epithelial and stromal tumor of the kidney are the same disease entity: molecular and histologic evidence. Am J Surg Pathol. 2009;33:72-80.

COMPLEX SCLEROSING LESION/RADIAL SCAR

DIFFERENTIAL DIAGNOSES: TUBULAR CARCINOMA AND LOW-GRADE ADENOSQUAMOUS CARCINOMA

Clinical Features

Complex sclerosing lesions and radial scars (CSLs/RSs) are benign sclerosing lesions which may be encountered incidentally or as the targets of directed biopsies after imaging. Incidence varies depending upon the mode of detection, with most lesions today being identified by mammography. These sclerosing lesions account for 5% to 9% of cases in large case-control studies of open biopsies and approximately 2% of cases in core needle biopsy studies. CSLs/RSs may be multifocal and bilateral. The most commonly reported age at diagnosis varies from 47 to 54 years; however, a wide age range is noted, with greater incidence of intrinsic epithelial proliferation described in older, postmenopausal women.

Pathologic Features

GROSS FINDINGS

No grossly identifiable lesion may be visualized or palpated with small benign sclerosing lesions. When a gross lesion is noted, a stellate mass with intrinsic tan-yellow streaks may be encountered, and the appearance may grossly mimic a small invasive carcinoma.

MICROSCOPIC FINDINGS

These lesions are characterized by the presence of benign epithelial elements (typically glands and tubules) entrapped within or distorted by fibrous or fibroelastotic tissue. The terminology of radial scar is preferred when the lesion is centered around a sclerotic fibroelastotic nidus with the intrinsic epithelial elements radiating circumferentially outward (Fig. 6.1). The terminology of complex sclerosing lesion is preferred when lesions are larger and when the admixture of fibrous tissue and entrapped benign epithelium is less well organized, lacking a radial distribution. The ducts entrapped within the fibroelastotic stroma of a CSL/RS may become angulated and stretched in appearance but will in general maintain intimate myoepithelial investitures.

Ancillary Studies

Immunohistochemical characterization of investing myoepithelial cells in CSLs/RSs can be valuable in confirming diagnoses. Immunoreactivity for p63, SMMS1, and other myoepithelial markers will be positive in cases of CSL/RS, although it is important to note that such reactivity may be incomplete or reduced and patchy in comparison with non-neoplastic ducts and lobules outside of the lesion proper (Fig. 6.2).

Differential Diagnosis

Perhaps the most important light microscopic differential diagnosis for CSL/RS is tubular carcinoma with other mimics including but not necessarily limited to invasive low-grade adenosquamous carcinoma and bland examples of fibromatosis-like metaplastic carcinoma. Epithelial proliferations such as usual ductal hyperplasia (UDH), atypical ductal hyperplasia (ADH), ductal carcinoma *in situ* (DCIS), atypical lobular hyperplasia (ALH), and lobular carcinoma *in situ* (LCIS) may also arise within CSLs/RSs. Tubular carcinomas are characterized at low power by an infiltrative appearance with haphazard arrangements of cytologically bland tubules set in a desmoplastic stroma (Fig. 6.3). The tubules are often angular and show open lumens, occasionally with small cytoplasmic snouts pushing into the lumens. No myoepithelial cells are visible on routine sections or by ancillary immunohistochemical

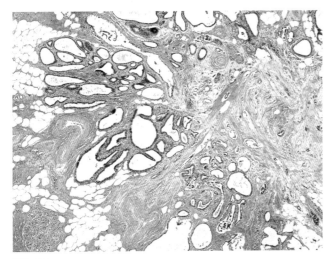

FIG. 6.1
Radial scar at low magnification demonstrating a central fibroelastotic nidus with small entrapped epithelial tubules and a circumferentially outwardly radiating rim of somewhat larger dilated duct spaces.

methods. Tubular carcinomas are sometimes accompanied by ADH and/or low-grade DCIS (Table 6.1). Low-grade adenosquamous carcinomas are composed of infiltrating glandular structures with varying degrees of squamous differentiation and cytologically bland nuclear features (Fig. 6.4). In these malignant tumors, the neoplastic glands vary from elongated to ovoid to compressed and are often noted to percolate around non-neoplastic glands and lobules. The degree of squamoid differentiation varies from case to case, with most cases containing individual squamoid cells and nests and with some cases showing pearl formation and squamous lined microcysts. Clusters of lymphocytes may be present at the periphery of low-grade adenosquamous carcinomas (Table 6.2). Fibromatosis-like metaplastic carcinomas can entrap benign angulated ducts and terminal duct lobular units (TDLUs), also mimicking CSLs/RSs. *In situ* proliferations and even invasive carcinomas may arise in association with otherwise benign sclerosing lesions (Fig. 6.5).

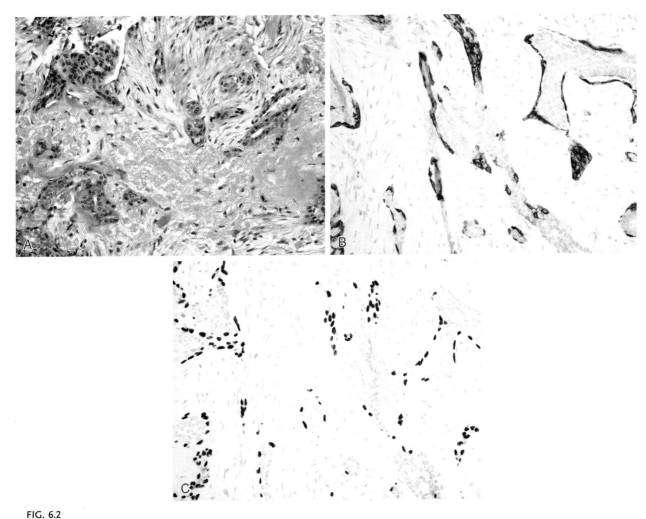

FIG. 6.2
Complex sclerosing lesion at intermediate magnification showing a central fibroelastotic area with small entrapped and angulated glands **(A)** with patchy/discontinuous immunoreactivity for SMMS1 **(B)** and for p63 **(C)** supporting the morphologic impression of a benign sclerosing process and helping to exclude a low-grade (tubular-type) invasive carcinoma.

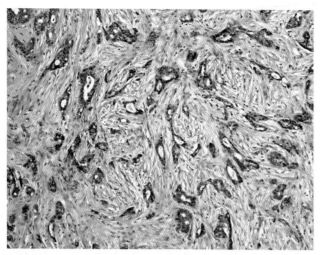

FIG. 6.3

Tubular carcinoma (invasive ductal carcinoma, grade 1 with tubular features) at low magnification showing a desmoplastic-appearing stroma lacking a central nidus of fibroelastosis and showing a haphazard arrangement of small teardrop-like angulated glands lacking myoepithelial investitures.

Prognosis and Therapy

In most centers, management of CSLs/RSs diagnosed by core biopsy has historically been complete surgical excision. Reported upgrade rates for these sclerosing lesions have varied widely, with small lesions lacking associated atypical epithelial proliferation being upgraded to *in situ* or invasive carcinoma in <2% of cases. Recommendations for management should be considered on a case-by-case basis, and surveillance may be appropriate for some patients with small incidental CSLs/RSs without atypia.

COMPLEX SCLEROSING LESIONS/RADIAL SCAR – DISEASE FACT SHEET

Definition

▶▶ Benign sclerotic breast lesions characterized by central nidus of fibroelastotic connective tissue with peripherally arranged intrinsic benign epithelium often shaped as tubules and angulated glands

▶▶ Radial scar terminology favored when small (<10 mm) and well organized with epithelial elements radiating circumferentially

▶▶ Complex sclerosing lesion terminology favored with larger (>10 mm) and less well-organized masses, often with more fibrosis, less elastosis, and lacking an ordered radial appearance

Incidence and Location

▶▶ Varies widely based upon means of detection. Most lesions currently identified by imaging.

▶▶ May be multiple and/or bilateral

Age Distribution

▶▶ Peak age of incidence varies between 47 and 54 years of age

▶▶ Wide age distribution with greater degrees of associated epithelial proliferation reported in older, postmenopausal patients

Clinical Features

▶▶ Most often incidentally discovered.

Radiologic Features

▶▶ Classic radiologic description of lesions large enough for detection by mammography is of spiculated process with central radiolucency analogous to fibroelastotic nidus

Prognosis and Therapy

▶▶ Historical recommendation has been to excise CSLs/RSs identified by core biopsy because of literature suggesting mildly increased risk of associated *in situ* and/or invasive carcinoma

▶▶ Some authors suggest that risk of malignancy is tied to risk of associated proliferative breast disease and not CSLs/RSs themselves

▶▶ Surveillance may be appropriate management for small lesions without associated epithelial atypia diagnosed on core biopsies

---

TABLE 6.1

Histologic Features of Complex Sclerosing Lesion/Radial Scar Compared With Tubular Carcinoma

Complex Sclerosing Lesion/Radial Scar	Tubular Carcinoma
• Fibroelastotic stroma with central nidus	• Desmoplastic stroma throughout lesion
• Stellate appearance with circumferential radial glands and tubules	• Infiltrative appearance with randomly arranged glands and tubules
• Associated cystic changes possible	• Associated cystic changes less likely
• Small tubules generally confined to stroma	• Neoplastic tubules may extend into surrounding adipose tissue
• Entrapped glands distorted by fibrosis and variable in size and shape	• Intrinsic tubules often monotonous and angulated/tear drop with open lumens
• Epithelium not polarized	• Epithelium polarized and may have apical snouts
• Myoepithelial investitures present (although sometimes attenuated)	• Myoepithelial investitures absent
• Associated apocrine changes possible	• Associated apocrine changes less likely
• Associated benign epithelial proliferations more common	• Associated ADH and/or low-grade DCIS more common

ADH, Atypical ductal hyperplasia; *DCIS*, ductal carcinoma *in situ*.

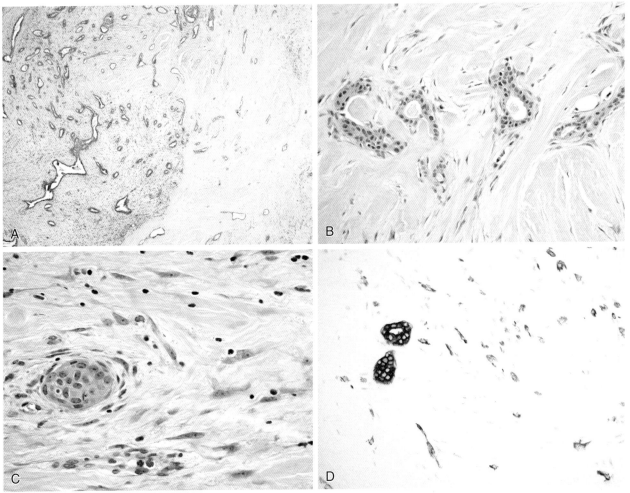

FIG. 6.4

Low-grade adenosquamous carcinoma at low magnification with deceptively bland small angulated gland structures varying from elongated to ovoid in appearance and set in a variably cellular stroma **(A)** with the lesional stroma varying from elastotic to hyalinized **(B)** and with some of the epithelial nests taking on a squamoid appearance **(C)**. Ancillary CAM5.2 immunohistochemical testing **(D)** confirms immunoreactivity in both the lesional epithelial nests as well as in many of the background atypical spindled cells, supporting categorization as a form of metaplastic carcinoma. Low-grade adenosquamous carcinomas can mimic complex sclerosing lesions and radial scars, especially at low-power magnifications.

TABLE 6.2

Histologic and Immunohistochemical Features of Complex Sclerosing Lesion/Radial Scar Compared With Invasive Low-Grade Adenosquamous Carcinoma

Complex Sclerosing Lesion/Radial Scar	Low-grade Adenosquamous Carcinoma
• Fibroelastotic stroma with central nidus	• Spindle cell background with intrinsic atypia
• Stellate appearance with circumferential radial glands and tubules	• Infiltrative appearance with random arrangement of tubules and squamoid nests
• Entrapped glands distorted by fibrosis and variable in size and shape	• Intrinsic neoplastic glands varying from elongated to ovoid to compressed, some blending with normal breast elements and insinuating around non-neoplastic structures
• Squamous differentiation uncommon	• Intrinsic squamous cells, nests, pearls and microcysts classically anticipated
• Peripheral lymphocytes not classically described	• Peripheral lymphoid infiltrates common
• Myoepithelial investitures present (although sometimes attenuated)	• Myoepithelial investitures absent (although in some glands attenuated)
• Immunohistochemistry for myoepithelial markers valuable	• Immunohistochemistry for myoepithelial markers and keratins valuable with some luminal glands p63 positive and with luminal glandular cells more intensely positive with keratins than basally located cells

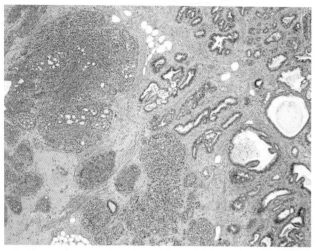

FIG. 6.5

Low-power magnification of lobular carcinoma *in situ* involving a complex sclerosing lesion with intrinsic entrapped terminal duct lobular units filled and distended by a monotonous population of lesional cells of *in situ* lobular neoplasia.

COMPLEX SCLEROSING LESIONS/RADIAL SCAR – PATHOLOGIC FEATURES

Gross Findings

▸▸ Incidental microscopic lesions may not be grossly identifiable

▸▸ If large enough for detection, may appear as a firm mass with a stellate cut surface and radiating tan-yellow streaks

▸▸ May mimic small invasive carcinomas

Microscopic Findings

▸▸ Benign fibroelastotic nidus with entrapped and sometimes angulated tubules and ducts

▸▸ Stellate appearance with circumferentially radiating ducts emanating from area of fibrosis

▸▸ Larger lesions may be less well organized

▸▸ Cystic change possible (particularly at periphery)

▸▸ May contain apocrine metaplasia

▸▸ Intrinsic epithelial structures invested by myoepithelial cells throughout

▸▸ May be associated with epithelial hyperplasias, *in situ* carcinomas, and invasive carcinomas

Pathologic Differential Diagnoses

▸▸ Tubular carcinoma

▸▸ Low-grade adenosquamous metaplastic carcinoma

▸▸ Fibromatosis-like metaplastic carcinoma

CYSTIC NEUTROPHILIC GRANULOMATOUS MASTITIS

DIFFERENTIAL DIAGNOSES: IDIOPATHIC GRANULOMATOUS LOBULAR MASTITIS AND SARCOIDOSIS

Clinical Features

Cystic neutrophilic granulomatous mastitis (CNGM) is a rare subacute to chronic inflammatory condition of the breast. Several small retrospective series detailing patients with CNGM have been published. Most reported patients are parous and range in age from 25 to 50 years, with a mean age of approximately 35 years. No association with tobacco products is known, and some but not all patients report previous history of breast injury. Patients commonly present with pain, palpable areas of tenderness, and abscess formations. Imaging studies may raise differential diagnoses of centrally necrotic malignancies.

Pathologic Features

GROSS FINDINGS

Gross findings in CNGM are non-specific. Imaging studies frequently identify lobulated irregular mass lesions, and central fluid collections are sometimes reported, with masses ranging from less than 1 cm to 10 cm in size. While not common, both cutaneous erythema and associated nipple discharge have been reported. Resected specimens show irregular abscess cavities that often coalesce and may display semisolid central regions with suppuration.

MICROSCOPIC FINDINGS

CNGM is characterized by lobulocentric granulomatous inflammation with small punched-out clear vacuolar spaces lined by neutrophils and containing intravacuolar gram-positive bacilli (Fig. 6.6). At scanning magnification, expanses of mononuclear inflammatory cells (histiocytes predominating) are noted. Superimposed suppuration with collections of neutrophils surrounding vacuolar microcysts (200–800 microns) are noted (Fig. 6.7). While granulomata can be well formed and discrete, vague collections of spindled and epithelioid macrophages are more common.

Ancillary Studies

Tissue Gram staining sometimes allows for identification of gram-positive bacilli within otherwise cleared vacuolar spaces. Routine cultures and molecular sequencing methods also sometimes confirm concurrent microbiological evidence of *Corynebacterium* species. Some authors suggest that thick section Gram staining (6 micron) improves both detection and ease of identification of gram-positive bacilli in CNGM.

Differential Diagnosis

Granulomatous processes of the breast are encountered in clinical practice with some frequency. Certain

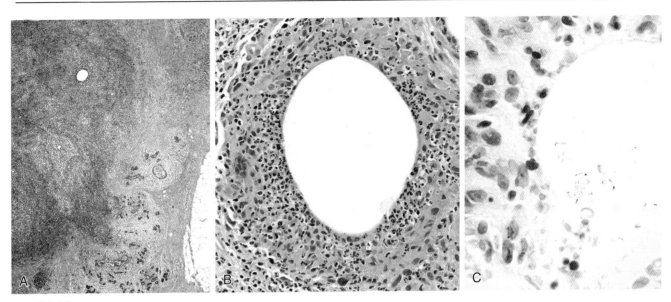

FIG. 6.6

A, Cystic neutrophilic granulomatous mastitis at low histologic power demonstrating diffuse inflammation with involvement of a lobular unit. This inflammatory process includes coalescent spindled and epithelioid macrophages and a mixture of lymphoid and neutrophilic cells. Focal punched-out clear vacuolar spaces can be identified at low power. **B,** On higher power, these clear spaces are rimmed by neutrophils. **C,** Gram staining of histologic sections confirms multiple gram-positive bacilli within the cleared vacuolar spaces.

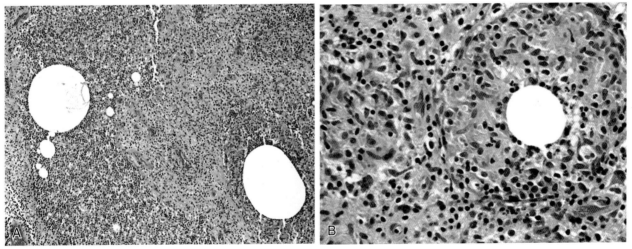

FIG. 6.7

Cleared vacuolar spaces within a subacute to chronic inflammatory background **(A)** are characteristic of cystic neutrophilic granulomatous mastitis. Spindled and epithelioid macrophages creating vague granulomatous island sometimes surround the cleared spaces **(B)** with neutrophils being classically reported at the rims of these spaces.

granulomatous conditions may be anticipated based upon relevant patient history. These include but are not necessarily limited to suture granulomata, silicone granulomata, and fat necrosis following trauma. While patients with conventional mastitis (often associated with lactation and breast feeding) may experience duct rupture and associated host response to extravasated secretions, mastitis associated with breast feeding is most commonly not granulomatous. Lactational mastitis is most commonly associated with staphylococcal or streptococcal infections (gram-positive cocci). Two of the main histologic differential diagnoses for CNGM

are idiopathic granulomatous lobular mastitis (IGLM) and breast involvement by system granulomatous conditions such as sarcoidosis (Fig. 6.8). IGLM does not appear to have a strong tie to lactation or breast feeding and often presents with a firm palpable mass. Histologically, IGLM is classically lobulocentric but like CNGM may obliterate microanatomy and histoarchitecture as it progresses to involve larger areas of parenchyma (Table 6.3). Involvement of the breast by systemic granulomatous diseases (such as sarcoidosis and Sjögren syndrome) may in some instances be suspected based upon patient history. Sarcoid-related

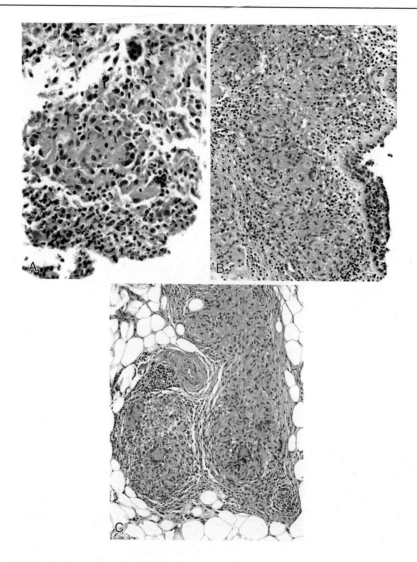

FIG. 6.8

Granulomata composed of cohesive aggregates of spindled and epithelioid macrophages and occasional multinucleated giant cells are present in cystic neutrophilic granulomatous mastitis (CNGM) **(A)**, idiopathic granulomatous lobular mastitis (IGLM) **(B)** and sarcoidosis of the breast **(C)**. The granulomata in CNGM and IGLM are morphologically similar with cases of IGLM lacking associated cleared spaces containing gram-positive bacilli. Granulomata in sarcoidosis are typically small in size but may coalesce and are more well-formed and discrete than in IGLM or CNGM. Sarcoid-related granulomata typically lack necrotizing changes and acute inflammation. Langhans-type giant cells are often present within sarcoidal granulomata **(C)**.

TABLE 6.3

Histologic Features of Cystic Neutrophilic Granulomatous Mastitis Compared With Idiopathic Granulomatous Lobular Mastitis

Cystic Neutrophilic Granulomatous Mastitis	Idiopathic Granulomatous Lobular Mastitis
• Lobulocentric mastitis	• Lobulocentric mastitis
• With enlargement may create diffuse fields of inflammation including macrophages, lymphocytes, and neutrophils	• With enlargement may create diffuse fields of inflammation including macrophages, lymphocytes, and neutrophils
• Few scattered Langhans-type giant cells	• Perhaps more scattered giant cells
• Loose collections of spindled and epithelioid macrophages result in scattered less well-formed granulomata	• Somewhat better formed and more prevalent granulomata, sometimes surrounding epithelial-lined ducts and lobular structures
• Characteristic punched-out vacuolar spaces with spindled and epithelioid macrophages yielding vague granulomatous encasements rimmed by neutrophils	• Absence of punched-out vacuolar spaces
• Gram-positive bacilli identified within cleared vacuolar spaces	• No microorganisms identified by special stains, cultures or molecular sequencing

TABLE 6.4

Histologic Features of Cystic Neutrophilic Granulomatous Mastitis Compared With Sarcoidosis

Cystic Neutrophilic Granulomatous Mastitis	Sarcoidosis of Breast
• Lobulocentric mastitis	• Epithelioid granulomata involving ducts, lobules, and interlobular stroma
• With enlargement may create diffuse fields of inflammation including macrophages, lymphocytes, and neutrophils	• Neutrophilic infiltrates not expected
• Few scattered Langhans-type giant cells	• Numerous Langhans-type giant cells
• Loose collections of spindled and epithelioid macrophages result in scattered less well-formed granulomata	• Well-formed and coalescent non-necrotizing microgranulomata with attendant lymphoplasmacytic reaction
• Characteristic punched-out vacuolar spaces with spindled and epithelioid macrophages yielding vague granulomatous encasements rimmed by neutrophils	• Absence of punched-out vacuolar spaces
• Gram-positive bacilli identified within cleared vacuolar spaces	• No microorganisms identified by special stains, cultures or molecular sequencing

granulomata are often small, well formed, associated with intrinsic Langhans-type giant cells, and non-necrotizing (Table 6.4). Because physical examination and imaging studies are unable to distinguish breast involvement from sarcoidosis, and because patients with sarcoidosis are felt to develop breast cancer at the same frequency as the general population, biopsy of breast lesions in patients with sarcoidosis is recommended. Combining histomorphologic data, results of special studies, imaging findings, and results of other laboratory tests increases the likelihood of accurately classifying mammary granulomatous conditions (Fig. 6.9).

Prognosis and Therapy

Treatment for patients with CNGM can be prolonged due to a combination of both delays in establishment of a specific diagnosis and intrinsic difficulty in management. Multimodal therapeutics including surgical debridement, antimicrobial therapies, and corticosteroids are commonly employed in the management of CNGM. Once accurate classification of CNGM occurs, therapies targeting the specific offending organism can be instituted. After treatments are optimized, most patients experience resolution of symptoms and disease abatement. The time from initial presentation to resolution of symptoms can span several months to a year. Breast disfigurement can occur in severe cases, and multiple surgical procedures may be necessary. When CNGM is originally labeled as IGLM, empiric therapies may result in management dilemmas and uncertain outcomes.

CYSTIC NEUTROPHILIC GRANULOMATOUS MASTITIS – DISEASE FACT SHEET

Definition
- ▶▶ Lobulocentric mastitis with granulomatous features and microabscess formations
- ▶▶ Distinct histologic pattern characterized by suppurative lipogranulomata with punched-out clear spaces rimmed by neutrophils and an outer cuff of spindled and epithelioid macrophages
- ▶▶ Surrounding mixed inflammatory infiltrates contain a few Langhans-type giant cells, lymphocytes, neutrophils, macrophages, and possibly a few plasmacytoid cells and eosinophils
- ▶▶ Some cleared vacuolar spaces may contain gram-positive bacilli
- ▶▶ Culture and molecular sequencing studies sometimes help in identifying *Corynebacterium* species

Incidence and Location
- ▶▶ Can involve any region of the breast and can be multifocal

Age Distribution
- ▶▶ Age of incidence varies between 25 and 50 years of age
- ▶▶ Mean age of incidence approximately 35 years

Clinical Features
- ▶▶ Most patients present with painful breast mass, some but not all patients report prior history of trauma

Radiologic Features
- ▶▶ Irregular mass lesions most commonly reported, some with fluid-filled central regions

Prognosis and Therapy
- ▶▶ Optimal treatment often delayed secondary to lack of specific diagnosis
- ▶▶ Multimodal therapies often employed including debridement, antimicrobials, and corticosteroids
- ▶▶ May lead to breast disfigurement, especially if entity not accurately identified

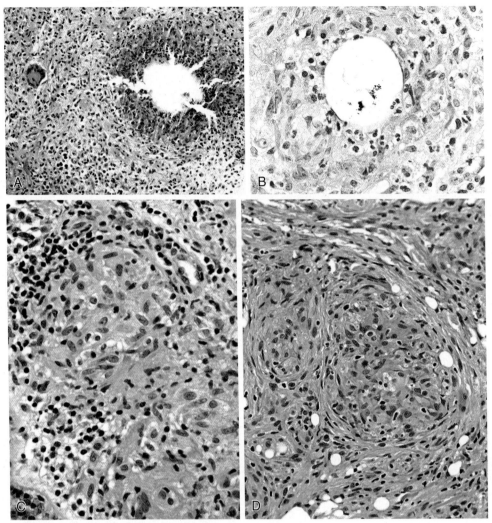

FIG. 6.9

Special stains for microorganisms may be helpful in supporting a morphologic impression of cystic neutrophilic granulomatous mastitis **(A)**. Tissue Gram staining highlights blue-colored gram-positive bacilli within a punched-out vacuolar space rimmed by neutrophils and spindled macrophages **(B)**. In cases of idiopathic granulomatous lobular mastitis **(C)** and mammary sarcoidosis **(D)**, special stains for organisms will be negative in the granulomata as well as in associated fields of mononuclear inflammatory cells.

CYSTIC NEUTROPHILIC GRANULOMATOUS MASTITIS – PATHOLOGIC FEATURES

Gross Findings

▶▶ Mass lesions with irregular indurated borders
▶▶ Highly variable in size ranging from <1 cm to 10 cm with larger lesions likely representing coalescence of smaller foci
▶▶ Central suppuration and semisolid nature may mimic invasive carcinoma with central necrosis

Microscopic Findings

▶▶ Lobulocentric granulomatous mastitis with small characteristic punched-out clear vacuolar spaces containing spindled and epithelioid macrophages and rimmed by neutrophils
▶▶ Intervening expanses of mixed inflammatory cells including macrophages, lymphocytes, neutrophils, a few Langhans-type giant cells, and possibly a few plasmacytoid cells and eosinophils
▶▶ Gram staining may confirm gram-positive bacilli within vacuolar spaces rimmed by neutrophils

---

Pathologic Differential Diagnoses

▶▶ Idiopathic granulomatous lobular mastitis (IGLM), lacks vacuolar spaces rimmed by neutrophils and microorganisms not identified
▶▶ Sarcoidosis involving the breast, lacks vacuolar spaces rimmed by neutrophils, masses composed of coalescing well-formed and non-necrotizing microgranulomata

CELLULAR FIBROADENOMA

DIFFERENTIAL DIAGNOSIS: PHYLLODES TUMOR

Clinical Features

Fibroadenomas (FAs) are the most common benign tumors of the breast, identified in up to one-half of all targeted breast biopsies. These fibroepithelial lesions typically present as slowly enlarging, mobile, painless nodules, often <3 cm in size. They may occur anywhere in the breast and may be solitary, multiple, and/or bilateral. They are identified on imaging studies as round to oval, well-delineated nodular masses with relatively uniform hypoechogenicity or hypodensity. Those with increased cellularity may show hypervascularity. Classic and cellular FAs (CFAs) are most commonly identified in female adolescents and adults <35 years of age, while complex FAs, which account for up to 23% of all FAs, tend to occur in women in their 50s. Juvenile FAs typically occur in young African-Americans, although they may present at any age and may rapidly grow to relatively larger sizes (>5 cm). While juvenile FAs have cellular stroma, they also show intrinsic epithelial proliferation with prominent UDH that is sometimes described as "gynecomastoid-type."

FAs are hormone-sensitive, with the potential to enlarge rapidly during pregnancy or with estrogen therapy, and may regress during menopause. They may also occur in men with gynecomastia. Cyclosporin has been associated with the development of large, multifocal FAs that stop growing or regress following cessation of the drug. The vast majority of FAs are sporadic, with a small proportion of myxoid FAs occurring in association with the Carney complex.

Pathologic Features

GROSS FINDINGS

FAs appear macroscopically as solid, well-circumscribed masses that are typically <3 cm in size. The cut surface is usually white-tan and solid with slit-like spaces and tends to appear whorled and bosselated. Calcified, fibrotic, or myxoid areas may be present.

MICROSCOPIC FINDINGS

FAs are benign biphasic fibroepithelial lesions that arise from the glandular epithelium and intralobular stroma of the breast TDLU. They typically exhibit a balanced distribution of cytologically bland, mitotically inactive epithelial and stromal components. They may display pericanalicular architecture with stromal proliferation around open ducts, and/or intracanalicular architecture with stromal proliferation around compressed ducts. They may show myxoid changes, hyalinization, dystrophic calcifications, bizarre multinucleated giant cells, apocrine metaplasia, squamous metaplasia, apical snouting, and fibrocystic changes including UDH, sclerosing adenosis, and myoepithelial proliferation, as well as involvement by ADH. Rarely, metaplastic changes including smooth muscle, lipomatous, osseous, and chondroid metaplasia may be seen. Invasive carcinoma may also be identified, which typically involves FAs secondarily.

CFAs often display an intracanalicular architectural pattern, mild to moderate increase in stromal cellularity, and a low stromal mitotic rate (≤2 mitoses per 10 high-power fields [HPFs]) (Fig. 6.10). They lack cytologic atypia, periductal stromal condensation, exuberant intracanalicular architecture, stromal overgrowth (absence of epithelium in at least one low-power [4×] field), and intratumoral heterogeneity. Increased stromal cellularity and mitoses may be observed in FAs of young females (<20 years). Occasionally, pleomorphic-appearing multinucleated stromal giant cells may be seen, which should not be overinterpreted as a feature of malignancy, particularly in the absence of other worrisome histologic features.

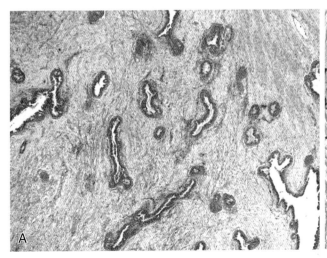
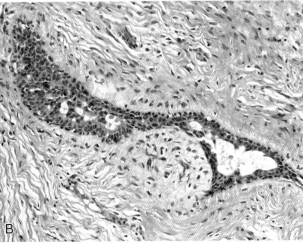

FIG. 6.10
Cellular fibroadenoma at intermediate magnification depicting a biphasic proliferation of uniformly distributed epithelial and stromal elements with increased stromal cellularity and no stromal overgrowth **(A)** and at high magnification demonstrating cytologically bland epithelial and stromal components without associated mitotic activity **(B)**.

Juvenile FAs display increased stromal cellularity, pericanalicular growth, and micropapillary/"gynecomastoid"-type UDH. Complex FAs display one or more of the following: epithelial calcifications, sclerosing adenosis, cysts >3 mm, and/or papillary apocrine metaplasia (Fig. 6.11).

Ancillary Studies

Ancillary immunohistochemical and molecular studies are generally not utilized in the diagnosis of FA. FAs are typically composed of non-clonal epithelium and stroma. However, monoclonality has been demonstrated in areas with cellular stromal expansion or "phyllodal" features, including aberrations in chromosomes 16, 18, and 21. Mutations in exon 2 of *MED12* have been demonstrated within the stromal component in up to 65% of FAs (exclusive of the myxoid variant), particularly in cases with intracanalicular growth, and

have also been identified in up to 74% of phyllodes tumors (PTs) of all grades.

Differential Diagnosis

The most important light microscopic differential diagnosis for CFA is benign PT. These two cellular fibroepithelial lesions are challenging to distinguish due to their overlapping and often subjective histologic features, particularly in the context of intralesional heterogeneity and limited sampling in core biopsies. Prior studies have demonstrated poor interobserver variability in distinguishing CFAs from PTs, even amongst subspecialty breast pathologists.

While both CFAs and benign PTs display mild to moderate stromal cellularity, key histologic features distinguishing the two include differences in stromal architecture, mitotic activity, and atypia (Table 6.5). CFA shows absent or very focal leaf-like stromal expansion

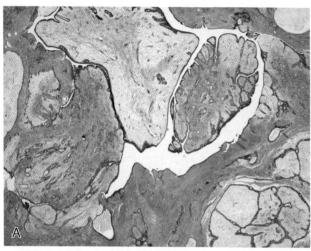 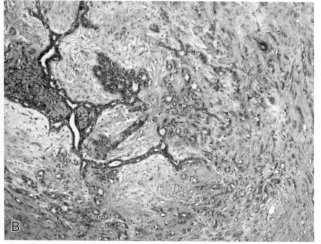

FIG. 6.11
Complex fibroadenoma at low magnification demonstrating focal phyllodal architecture, as seen with focal leaf-like stromal frondular projections **(A)** and at higher magnification showing intracanalicular architecture with increased stromal cellularity and adenosis **(B)**.

TABLE 6.5

Histologic Features of Cellular Fibroadenoma Compared With Benign Phyllodes Tumor

Cellular Fibroadenoma	Benign Phyllodes Tumor
• Absent or focal stromal leaf-like architecture	• Well-developed stromal leaf-like architecture
• ≤2 stromal mitoses/10 HPF (may be more increased in children and young adults)	• 0–4 stromal mitoses/10 HPF
• Lacks stromal atypia (may show pleomorphic-appearing multinucleated giant cells)	• May show mild stromal atypia
• Lacks periductal stromal condensation	• May show periductal stromal condensation
• Typically lacks stromal heterogeneity, pseudoangiomatous stromal hyperplasia, and squamous metaplasia	• May show stromal heterogeneity, pseudoangiomatous stromal hyperplasia, and squamous metaplasia

with lack of periductal stromal condensation, ≤2 stromal mitoses per 10 HPF, and no significant stromal atypia. In contrast, benign PT displays well-formed leaf-like stromal fronds that protrude into dilated cyst-like spaces and may show periductal stromal condensation, up to 4 mitoses per 10 HPF, and mild stromal atypia (Fig. 6.12). Benign PT may also exhibit stromal heterogeneity, pseudoangiomatous stromal hyperplasia (PASH), and squamous metaplasia, whereas CFA typically lacks these features. Similar to CFAs, benign PTs have circumscribed borders and lack stromal overgrowth.

Borderline PTs usually show moderate stromal cellularity, mild to moderate stromal atypia, 5 to 9 mitoses per 10 HPFs, well-defined to focally infiltrative borders, and absent or focal stromal overgrowth. Malignant PTs display marked, typically diffuse stromal cellularity and atypia, ≥10 mitoses per 10 HPFs, infiltrative borders, and frequently show stromal overgrowth. The presence of any malignant heterologous component also denotes malignancy, regardless of the absence of other malignant features. The vast majority of PTs are benign (60%–75%) and are less commonly borderline (15%–26%) or malignant (8%–20%).

It is important to note that pediatric FAs, in addition to increased stromal cellularity, may also display ill-defined borders and focal, small leaf-like stromal fronds. FAs in adolescents <20 years of age may also show increased mitotic activity (up to 6 mitoses per 10 HPF). In the absence of other worrisome histologic features, these findings are subdiagnostic of PT and should not be misdiagnosed as such.

Clinically, PTs differ from FAs in that they have a tendency to present as an enlarging mass with accelerated growth, often exceeding 3 cm in size. They may occasionally arise from a previously stable lesion. The average age at presentation of PTs is 40 to 50 years, which is one to two decades later than that of most FAs.

Particularly on core biopsies with limited tumor sampling, the distinction between CFA and PT is often not possible. Further confounding the issue, up to 36% of PTs have been reported to show FA-like areas; similarly, FAs may display phyllodal-like areas. Features that may favor PT on core biopsies are findings of ≥3 mitoses per 10 HPF, stromal overgrowth, stromal atypia, stromal heterogeneity, subepithelial stromal condensation, and infiltration into adipose tissue. If a distinction is unable to be made, a diagnosis of "benign fibroepithelial

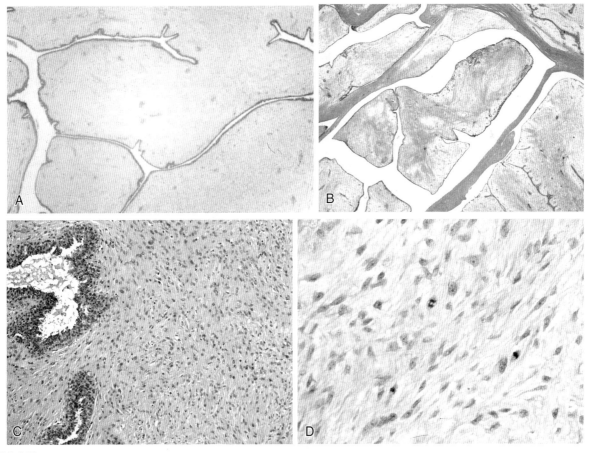

FIG. 6.12

Benign phyllodes tumor at low magnification displaying leaf-like stromal expansion **(A)** with well-developed stromal fronds projecting into dilated cleft-like spaces **(B)**, stromal hypercellularity **(C)**, and stromal atypia with increased mitotic activity **(D)**.

lesion/neoplasm" may be rendered, and final characterization may be deferred to an excisional specimen.

Prognosis and Therapy

FAs are considered benign, and most do not recur following complete surgical excision. However, new lesions may develop in proximity to a prior FA excision site. Most pediatric FAs show increased stromal cellularity and focal leaf-like fronds, which does not correlate with recurrence. ADH confined within FAs reportedly has no association with relative cancer risk.

When a cellular fibroepithelial lesion is encountered on core biopsy, the most common differential diagnoses are CFA and PT. Due to the difficulty in distinction between these two entities on small biopsies, complete surgical excision is typically recommended. However, more recent studies have demonstrated that CFAs and benign PTs confer similarly low rates of recurrence, even with enucleated close or positive margins, suggesting that definitive distinction may not be critical and that 10 mm margins (as recommended for borderline and malignant PTs) may not be required for benign PT.

FIBROADENOMA – DISEASE FACT SHEET

Definition
- Benign biphasic fibroepithelial tumor with circumscribed borders that lacks stromal overgrowth, well-developed stromal fronds, stromal atypia, and significant stromal mitoses (≤2/10 HPF)

Incidence and Location
- Identified in up to 50% of all targeted breast biopsies, and comprises up to 70%–95% of all biopsied breast masses in adolescents
- May occur in any region within the breast
- May be unifocal, multifocal, and/or bilateral

Age Distribution
- Peak incidence in adolescents and young women between 15 and 35 years of age
- Wide age distribution, including children, young adults, and postmenopausal women

Clinical Features
- Typically firm, solitary, slowly enlarging, mobile, painless masses, usually <3 cm
- Giant FAs (>5 cm) and juvenile FAs may enlarge rapidly and cause breast distortion
- Usually present in women, but may also develop in men with gynecomastia
- Hormone-sensitive; may enlarge rapidly during pregnancy or with estrogen therapy

---

- Cyclosporin may induce large, multifocal FAs that stop enlarging or regress with cessation of therapy
- Typically sporadic; myxoid FAs may be associated with the Carney complex

Radiologic Features
- Nodular, round to oval densities or calcified nodules with relatively uniform hypoechogenicity or hypodensity on mammography, ultrasound, or MRI
- Cellular FAs may display hypervascularity

Prognosis and Therapy
- Complete excision is recommend for cellular fibroepithelial lesions identified on core biopsy, as it is often difficult to definitively distinguish cellular FA and benign PT on small biopsies with limited tumor sampling
- Most FAs do not recur; cellular FAs and benign PTs confer similarly low rates of recurrence

---

CELLULAR FIBROADENOMA – PATHOLOGIC FEATURES

Gross Findings
- Solid, well-circumscribed masses
- Typically <3 cm
- Whitish, bosselated, and whorled solid cut surface with slit-like spaces
- Calcified, fibrotic, and myxoid areas may be present

Microscopic Findings
- Biphasic fibroepithelial tumor with a relatively uniform distribution of glandular epithelial and interlobular stromal elements
- Mild to occasionally moderate stromal hypercellularity
- Pericanalicular and/or intracanalicular architecture
- Circumscribed tumor borders
- Absent to minimal stromal mitoses (≤2/HPF; may be increased in children and young adults)
- Lacks stromal overgrowth (4× field), well-developed stromal fronds, and stromal atypia

Pathologic Differential Diagnoses
- Phyllodes tumor (most often benign; occasionally borderline)

MYOFIBROBLASTOMA

DIFFERENTIAL DIAGNOSIS: PSEUDOANGIOMATOUS STROMAL HYPERPLASIA

Clinical Features

Myofibroblastoma is a benign stromal tumor of the breast that typically presents as a solitary, painless, slowly enlarging parenchymal mass. While this entity was initially described in the breast in 1987, subsequent studies report a greater frequency of this tumor at extramammary sites ("mammary-type myofibroblastoma"), the most common being the inguinal region. The incidence of these tumors in the breast is relatively low. Imaging modalities depict non-specific findings of a solid, non-calcified, homogeneous mass with lobulations and circumscribed borders. Although historically considered to have a male predominance, current data demonstrate an equal sex predilection, with most cases presenting in elderly men and postmenopausal women (range, 1–87 years). As myofibroblastoma typically expresses estrogen (ER), progesterone (PR), and/or androgen receptors (AR) and has been observed in association with gynecomastia and PASH, hormonal factors have been etiologically implicated in these tumors. They are considered to represent an entity within the spectrum of the 13q/*Rb* family of tumors with similar histomorphology, immunophenotype, and 13q/*Rb* deletion, which includes spindle cell/pleomorphic lipoma and cellular angiofibroma.

Pathologic Features

GROSS FINDINGS

Most lesions present as ovoid, variably lobulated masses with circumscribed, unencapsulated borders. Sectioning reveals yellow, white, pink, or gray cut surfaces with variably rubbery to mucilaginous consistency, which may mimic the gross appearance of FA or mass-forming PASH.

MICROSCOPIC FINDINGS

Myofibroblastoma arises from precursor mammary stromal cells and histologically appears as a proliferation of cytologically bland, ovoid to spindled myofibroblasts and fibroblasts arranged in short, interlacing fascicles or a haphazard pattern. Characteristically, the lesional cells are admixed with relatively thick, variably hyalinized collagen bands (Fig. 6.13). Focal areas of

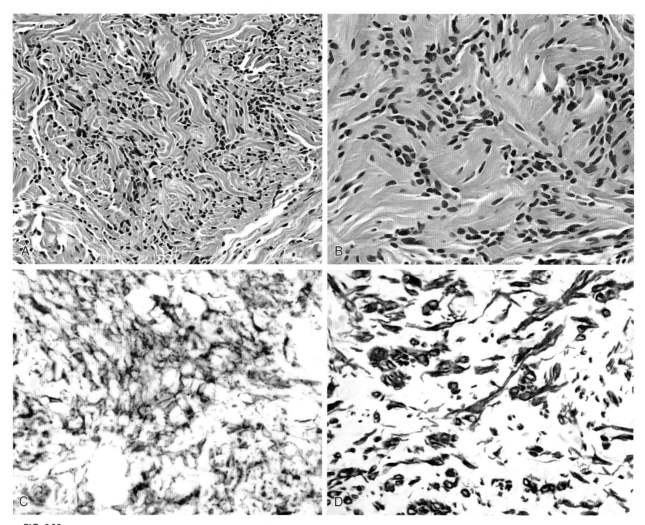

FIG. 6.13

Classic appearance of myofibroblastoma at intermediate magnification, demonstrating a haphazard to fascicular pattern of spindled cells separated by thick, hyalinized collagen bundles **(A)**. High magnification depicts cytologically bland, ovoid to fusiform cells with intervening dense collagen **(B)**. The lesional cells show strong, diffuse expression of CD34 **(C)**, desmin **(D)**,

Continued

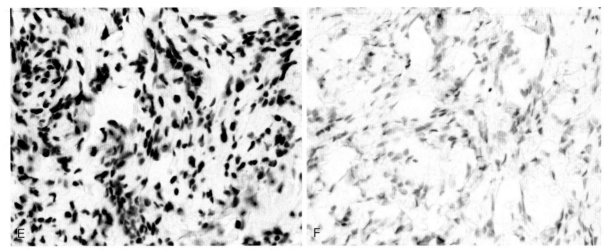

FIG. 6.13, cont'd

ER **(E)**, and loss of expression of RB1 **(F)**.

intralesional mature adipose tissue or neural-like or storiform architecture may be appreciated (Fig. 6.14). Epithelial and myoepithelial elements are absent. Although the mammary ducts and lobules are typically spared, some infiltrating variants may exhibit entrapment of TDLUs (see Fig. 6.14). The bland neoplastic cells may variably display nuclear grooves, pseudoinclusions, and small nucleoli. Occasional cases may depict focal nuclear pleomorphism and floret-like giant cells. Mitotic activity is rarely present. Although uncommon, some tumors may display focally permeative borders, intracytoplasmic and extracellular hyaline globules, myxoid stroma, dense cellularity, and focal myoid, chondroid, or osseous metaplasia. Necrosis, extensively permeating borders, and increased or atypical mitoses are consistently absent. Morphologic patterns of myofibroblastoma include fibrous/collagenized, myxoid, lipomatous, epithelioid/deciduoid, and palisading/Schwannian-like with Verocay-like bodies. Epithelioid-type myofibroblastomas may show few or attenuated collagen bundles, and the lesional cells may be arranged in linear arrays that mimic lobular carcinoma (see Fig. 6.14).

Ancillary Studies

Myofibroblastoma classically coexpresses CD34, desmin, and steroidal hormone receptors including ER, PR,

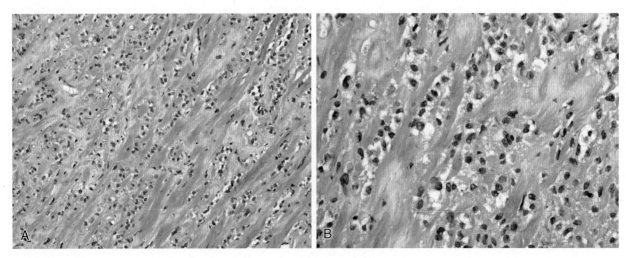

FIG. 6.14

Epithelioid-type myofibroblastoma at low magnification imparting a linear architectural array of epithelioid cells, reminiscent of lobular carcinoma of the breast **(A)** with high magnification demonstrating relatively polygonal lesional cells with more abundant eosinophilic cytoplasm that are admixed with intervening dense collagen **(B)**.

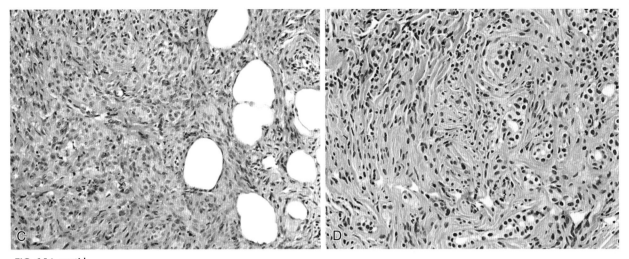

FIG. 6.14, cont'd

Some cases of myofibroblastoma may display hypercellularity with attenuated collagen fibers or intralesional mature adipose tissue **(C)** or, more uncommonly, distortion of terminal duct lobular units **(D)**.

and AR (see Fig. 6.13). Rarely, they may be CD34 and/or desmin negative. The tumors also less consistently express alpha-SMA, calponin, BCL2, CD10, and CD99. They are negative for cytokeratins, EMA, S100, STAT6, ALK1, and beta-catenin.

Approximately 90% of cases show loss of RB1 by immunohistochemistry (Fig. 6.13) as a result of monoallelic or biallelic deletions of 13q14, which may be identified using fluorescence *in situ* hybridization (FISH).

Differential Diagnosis

A major histologic differential diagnosis for myofibroblastoma of the breast is psueodangiomatous stromal hyperplasia (PASH). Like myofibroblastoma, PASH arises from the mammary stroma. PASH is composed of cytologically bland, spindled myofibroblasts distributed in anastomosing networks of compressed, slit-like channels in a background of thick, collagenous stroma. The slit-like spaces are devoid of cellular contents and are lined by flattened myofibroblasts (Fig. 6.15). The spindled cells of PASH possess somewhat more compressed nuclei than the relatively plumper fusiform cells often observed in myofibroblastoma. Both PASH and myofibroblastoma lack significant cytologic atypia and mitotic activity.

A particular less common architectural variant of PASH, "fascicular PASH," may especially mimic myofibroblastoma. In this variant, PASH exhibits a fascicular pattern in which the myofibroblasts are arranged in short fascicles separated by intervening bands of dense, eosinophilic collagen fibers, closely mimicking myofibroblastoma (Fig. 6.19). In such instances, fascicular PASH may be distinguished from myofibroblastoma

by the presence of conventional PASH merging with epithelial mammary structures bordering the lesion, as PASH is often intermixed with TDLUs.

While the spindled cells of PASH, like myofibroblastoma, coexpress CD34, desmin, and hormone receptors, PR is more frequently expressed in PASH than is ER. SMA is also more often positive in PASH than in myofibroblastoma. Furthermore, no molecular underpinnings have been identified in PASH, such as 13q deletion with loss of RB1 in myofibroblastoma, which can further aid in distinguishing the two entities (Table 6.6).

Although PASH is usually identified as an incidental finding on biopsy, it may occasionally present as a firm, circumscribed, non-calcified mass-like lesion, particularly in males with gynecomastia, further mimicking myofibroblastoma. Like myofibroblastoma, PASH is also etiologically purported to be related to hormonal factors that induce an aberrant myofibroblastic proliferation. In contrast to the equal sex distribution of myofibroblastoma, PASH is more often encountered in women and typically presents at a younger mean age of 30 to 40 years, although it may also occur in children, men, and postmenopausal women. When PASH is identified on core biopsy with radiologic concordance, excision is not required.

Prognosis and Therapy

Myofibroblastoma of the breast has an excellent prognosis. Excisional surgery is curative, with subsequent recurrences being uncommon even in the presence of positive resection margins.

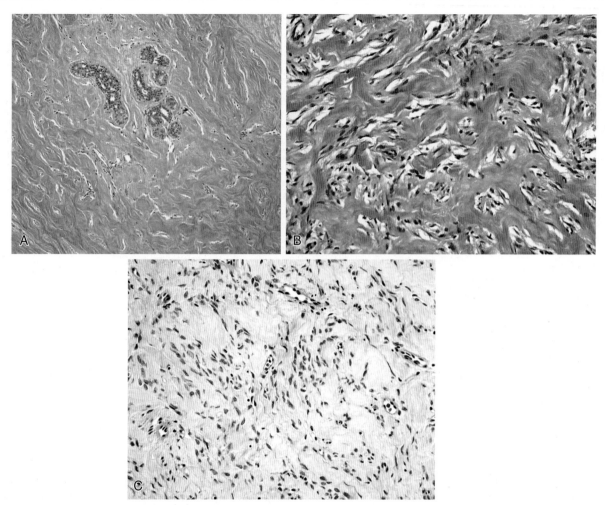

FIG. 6.15

A, Pseudoangiomatous stromal hyperplasia (PASH) at low magnification, surrounding a terminal duct lobular unit. **B,** Increasing magnification demonstrating compressed, slit-like, empty spaces lined by bland, spindled myofibroblasts and surrounded by dense collagenous stroma. **C,** Fascicular pattern of PASH displaying spindled cells arranged in short fascicles separated by collagenous stroma, mimicking myofibroblastoma.

TABLE 6.6

Histologic and Immunohistochemical Features of Myofibroblastoma Compared With Pseudoangiomatous Stromal Hyperplasia (PASH)

Myofibroblastoma	PASH
• Spindled cells arranged in short, interlacing fascicles or a haphazard pattern	• Spindled cells arranged in anastomosing networks of compressed, slit-like spaces
• Associated PASH may be present, but typically does not intermix with the tumor	• Although the more uncommon pattern of "fascicular PASH" comprises short fascicles that mimic myofibroblastoma, it often merges with areas of conventional PASH
• Usually located apart from mammary ducts and lobules	• Surrounding epithelial mammary structures are usually present
• Comparatively plumper fusiform nuclei	• Comparatively compressed fusiform nuclei
• Coexpress CD34, desmin, and hormone receptors; less consistently express SMA	• Coexpress CD34, desmin, and hormone receptors (more often PR than ER); consistently express SMA
• Approximately 90% show loss of RB1 by immunohistochemistry due to 13q14 deletion	• No known molecular aberrations

COLUMNAR CELL LESION

DIFFERENTIAL DIAGNOSES: FLAT EPITHELIAL ATYPIA

Clinical Features

Columnar cell lesions (CCLs) are within the spectrum of benign fibrocystic changes. They are characterized by enlargement of the terminal ductal lobular units (TDLUs) with variably distended acini lined by columnar cells. CCLs are seen with increasing frequency in biopsies performed for mammographic calcifications. CCLs are further classified into columnar cell change (CCC) and columnar cell hyperplasia (CCH).

Pathologic Features

GROSS FINDINGS

CCLs do not have a specific gross finding. They are only identified on microscopy.

MICROSCOPIC FINDINGS

CCLs are identified by their classic appearance of enlarged TDLUs with cystically dilated acinar spaces lined by columnar cells (Figs. 6.16 and 6.17). The cells are uniform with ovoid to elongated nuclei, with fine and even chromatin pattern and inconspicuous nucleoli. The nuclei are perpendicular to the basement membrane, and the arrangement is somewhat reminiscent of a "picket fence" (see Figs. 6.16 and 6.17). The luminal surface of the acini in CCLs often shows apical cytoplasmic blebs or snouts. The lumens frequently contain calcifications and may contain secretions and mucin. CCC is lined by one to two layers of columnar cells (see Fig. 6.16), and CCH is lined by more than two layers of cells, showing varying degrees of stratification (see Fig. 6.17). Mitoses are not frequent in either CCC or CCH. CCH may show micropapillary architecture, but unlike ADH, the tips of the micropapillae have pinched tops and broad bases (see Fig. 6.17).

Ancillary studies

The diagnosis of CCLs is usually made on hematoxylin and eosin (H&E)–stained sections. Ancillary studies are not necessarily used for rendering the diagnosis. CCLs are generally strongly positive for ER (Fig. 6.18) and low-molecular-weight cytokeratin (such as CK7 and CK8/18), whereas negative for high-molecular-weight

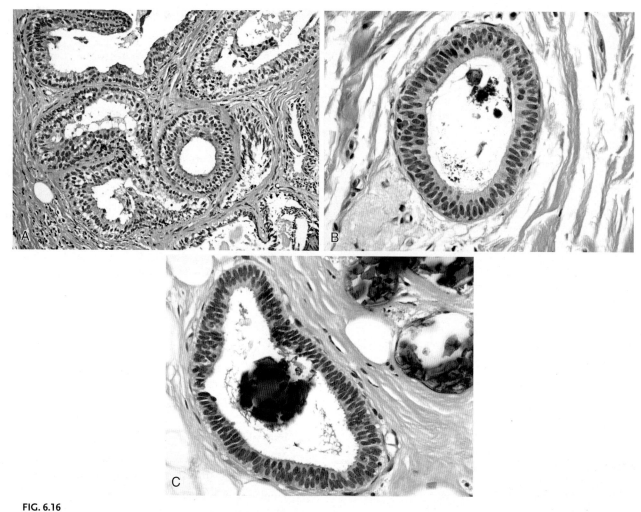

FIG. 6.16
Columnar cell change at intermediate **(A)** and high magnifications **(B, C)** demonstrating terminal duct lobular units with cystically dilated acinar spaces lined by one to two layers of columnar cells with apical cytoplasmic blebs, luminal secretions, and calcifications.

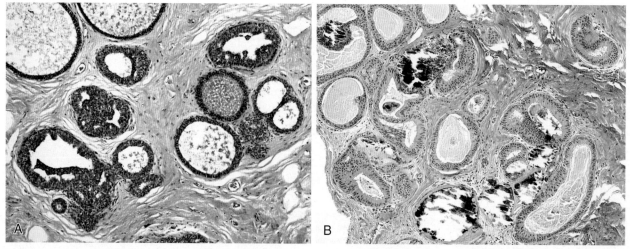

FIG. 6.17
Columnar cell hyperplasia at low **(A, B)** and high magnifications

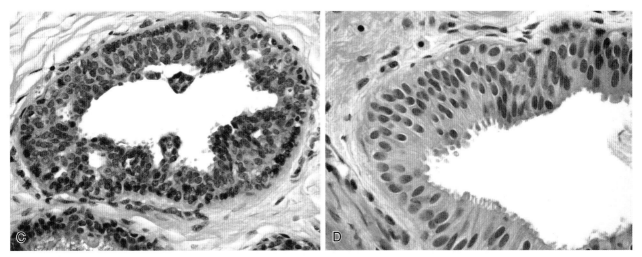

FIG. 6.17, cont'd

(C, D) demonstrating terminal duct lobular units with cystically dilated acinar spaces lined by two or more layers of columnar cells with apical cytoplasmic blebs, luminal secretions, and calcifications.

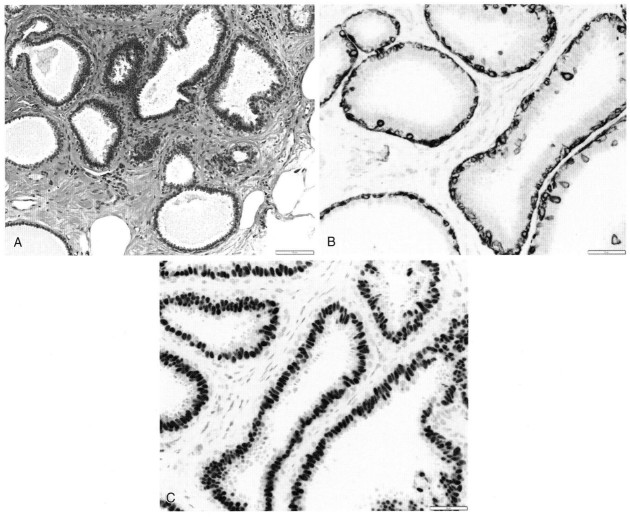

FIG. 6.18

Columnar cell change at intermediate magnification **(A)** and high magnifications **(B, C)** showing absent luminal epithelial staining for CK5 **(B)** and strong diffuse staining with ER **(C)**.

TABLE 6.7

Histologic and Immunohistochemical Features of Columnar Cell Lesion (CCL) Compared With Flat Epithelial Atypia (FEA)

Columnar Cell Lesion	Flat Epithelial Atypia
• Dilated acini lined by columnar cells	• Dilated acini lined by rounded cells (flat type)
• No cytologic atypia	• Low-grade cytologic atypia similar to atypical ductal hyperplasia (ADH) or low-grade ductal carcinoma *in situ*
• Nuclei perpendicular (polarized) to the basement membrane	• Loss of nuclear polarity
• Oval to elongated nuclei with fine chromatin and inconspicuous nucleoli	• Rounded enlarged nuclei with hyperchromasia, increased nuclear-to-cytoplasmic ratio and variably prominent nucleoli
• Micropapillary projections with pinched tips and broad bases	• Flat epithelium with atypia; if micropapillae present then no longer characterized as FEA (characterized as ADH)

Both CCL and FEA can have the following features
• Apical cytoplasmic blebs/snouts
• Nuclear stratification
• Luminal calcifications, secretions, mucin
• ER: strong diffuse staining
• CK5/6 (HMW keratin): absent staining
• CK7 or CK8/18: positive staining

cytokeratin (such as CK5/6) (see Fig. 6.18). This immunoprofile is similar to that of ADH/low-grade DCIS.

Differential Diagnosis

The most common entity in the differential diagnosis of CCLs is flat epithelial atypia (FEA) (Table 6.7). FEA is seen in 1% to 2% of biopsies performed for mammographic calcifications. FEA is a clonal proliferation that is characterized by monomorphic-appearing epithelial cells with low-grade cytologic atypia (Figs. 6.19 and 6.20). The cells

have rounded enlarged nuclei with hyperchromasia, increased nuclear-to-cytoplasmic ratio and variably prominent nucleoli (Fig. 6.20). There is loss of polarity, unlike the perpendicular arrangement of cells as seen in CCLs (Fig. 6.19). The cytologic features in FEA are morphologically similar to that of ADH or low-grade DCIS. However, FEA does not show any architectural complexity, so-called "flat atypia" (Fig. 6.21). The luminal surface may show apical cytoplasmic snouts/blebs similar to CCLs. The lumen often contains calcifications and secretions. Similar to CCLs, nuclei in FEA can show stratification, but the presence of nuclear atypia favors the diagnosis of FEA. The immunophenotype and genetic changes seen in FEA

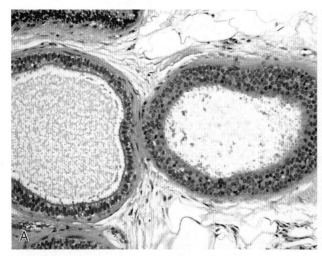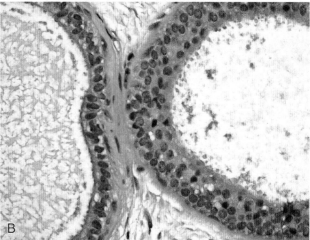

FIG. 6.19

Flat epithelial atypia and columnar cell change at low **(A)** and intermediate magnifications **(B)**. The duct on the left shows columnar cell change with long columnar cells without any atypia. The duct on the right shows monotonous epithelial cells with low-grade atypia characterized by rounding of nuclei and loss of polarity.

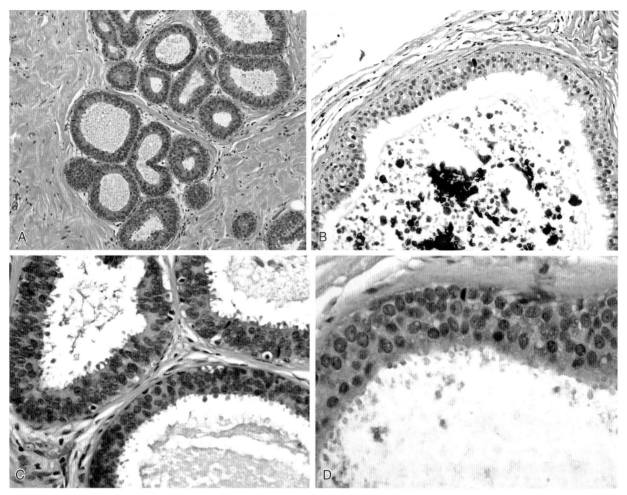

FIG. 6.20

Flat epithelial atypia (FEA) at low **(A)** and intermediate **(B, C)**, and high magnifications **(D)**. FEA shows cystically dilated ductal spaces lined by monotonous-appearing epithelial cells with low-grade cytologic atypia characterized by rounding of nuclei, hyperchromasia, and loss of nuclear polarity.

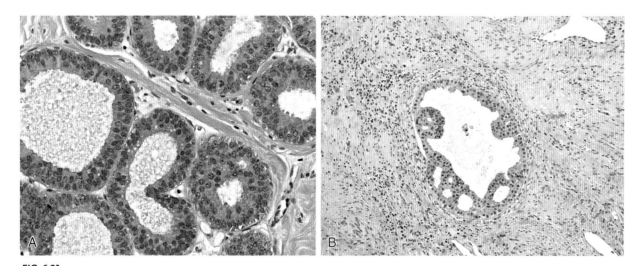

FIG. 6.21

Flat epithelial atypia **(A)** is a flat lesion without any architectural atypia, in contrast to atypical ductal hyperplasia **(B)** that may show bulbous-tipped micropapillae, arches, bridges, and cribriforming. Note that the cytologic atypia in both lesions is low grade.

are similar to that of CCLs, and ADH/low-grade DCIS. Available evidence suggests that CCL and FEA are likely non-obligate precursors to ADH/low-grade DCIS.

Prognosis and Therapy

When found in isolation, studies show that CCLs and FEA may be associated with a 1.5 to 2.5 times increase in the subsequent risk of developing invasive carcinoma. This risk is similar to that of other benign proliferative lesions but lower than that of ADH or ALH. CCLs and FEA May be associated with more aggressive lesions at the time of diagnosis; therefore, the finding of CCL or FEA should prompt a careful examination of the biopsy material, which may include additional levels to evaluate for lesions such as ADH, low-grade DCIS, or invasive carcinoma. Radiologic correlation is of utmost importance in evaluation of lesions diagnosed as FEA. Evidence suggests that up to 30% of patients with FEA on biopsy will be upgraded to a worse lesion on excision. It is still up to debate if surgical excision is necessary for an isolated finding of FEA on biopsy. Studies suggest that FEA in isolation may be left alone after good radiologic and pathologic correlation.

COLUMNAR CELL LESIONS (COLUMNAR CELL CHANGE AND COLUMNAR CELL HYPERPLASIA) – DISEASE FACT SHEET

Definition
▸▸ A benign epithelial lesion with enlargement of terminal ductal lobular units (TDLUs) with variably distended acini lined by one or more layers of columnar cells
▸▸ Studies suggest that CCLs may be a non-obligate precursor of low-grade breast neoplasia pathway

Incidence
▸▸ Most lesions are currently identified on mammography

Age Distribution
▸▸ The peak age of incidence is between 40 and 50 years of age

Clinical Features
▸▸ Identified incidentally on mammography

Radiologic Features
▸▸ Usually identified in biopsies performed for mammographic calcification
▸▸ Often associated with grouped amorphous calcifications

Prognosis and Therapy
▸▸ CCLs are associated with increased risk of breast cancer by 1.5-fold
▸▸ Risk is similar to other benign proliferative lesions such as UDH
▸▸ Can often be associated with FEA, ADH, low-grade DCIS
▸▸ Careful examination of material is required to rule out a worse lesion
▸▸ CLLs when found in isolation and with good radiologic and pathologic correlation, excision is not necessary

COLUMNAR CELL LESIONS (COLUMNAR CELL CHANGE AND COLUMNAR CELL HYPERPLASIA) – PATHOLOGIC FEATURES

Gross Findings
▸▸ Not grossly identifiable

Microscopic Findings
▸▸ Enlarged terminal ductal lobular units (TDLUs) with cystically dilated acini lined by columnar cells
▸▸ Columnar cell change: one or two layers of cells
▸▸ Columnar cell hyperplasia: more than two layers of cells with varying degrees of stratification
▸▸ Uniform appearance with nuclear polarization toward basement membrane (nuclei are perpendicular to basement membrane)
▸▸ Oval to elongated nuclei show even chromatin pattern and inconspicuous nucleoli
▸▸ Mitoses are infrequent
▸▸ Apical cytoplasmic blebs/snouts toward luminal surface
▸▸ Luminal calcifications and secretions are common
▸▸ Mucin production may be present
▸▸ CCH: Micropapillary architecture may be seen: Micropapillae have pinched tops and broad bases.
▸▸ No cytologic atypia

Pathologic Differential Diagnoses
▸▸ Flat epithelial atypia

ATYPICAL DUCTAL HYPERPLASIA

DIFFERENTIAL DIAGNOSES: USUAL DUCTAL HYPERPLASIA, DUCTAL CARCINOMA *IN SITU*

Clinical Features

ADH is a proliferative epithelial lesion often associated with calcifications that may arise in a background of fibrocystic changes. ADH can occur in both men and women and is associated with a fourfold increased risk of subsequent breast cancer development. ADH is most commonly diagnosed in women between 40 and 50 years of age. ADH is identified in 10% of biopsies performed for calcifications seen on screening mammography.

Pathologic Features

GROSS FINDINGS

May not be grossly identifiable unless associated with/involving a papilloma or sclerosing lesion.

MICROSCOPIC FINDINGS

ADH is characterized by intraductal proliferation of monomorphic-appearing epithelial cells that demonstrate

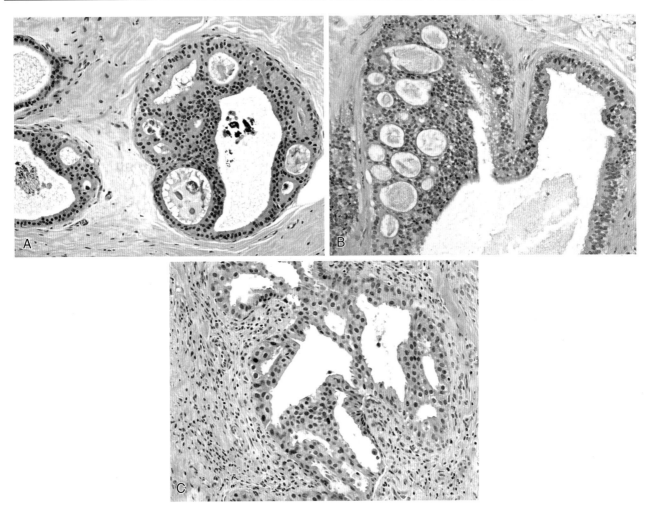

FIG. 6.22

Atypical ductal hyperplasia at intermediate magnification showing monomorphic epithelial cells with low-grade cytologic atypia with luminal calcifications **(A)**, cribriform growth pattern **(B)**, and bridging and arch formation **(C)**. The cells are spaced evenly with round nuclei, inconspicuous nucleoli, and variable amounts of cytoplasm.

low-grade cytologic atypia (Fig. 6.22). The cells are evenly spaced and have round nuclei, inconspicuous nucleoli, and variable amounts of cytoplasm. Often the ducts contain luminal calcifications. The ducts involved by ADH may show partial or complete involvement by the atypical cells. Architectural complexity ranging from bulbous-tipped micropapillary projections, bridge formations, arches, and cribriform spaces can be identified (see Fig. 6.22). The lumens appear rigid with the orientation of the nuclei perpendicular to the lumens. Studies have suggested that the diagnosis of ADH should not be rendered if lesion of interest is more than 2 mm in dimension or shows continuous involvement of more than two contiguous ducts.

Ancillary Studies

Immunohistochemical staining can be extremely helpful in borderline cases. ADH is a clonal lesion and usually shows strong diffuse staining with ER and demonstrates loss of mosaic staining pattern with high-molecular-weight cytokeratins such as CK5/6 (Fig. 6.23). The presence of myoepithelial cells in the periphery of ADH can be highlighted by p63, calponin, and other myoepithelial markers. Interestingly, CK5 will highlight myoepithelial cells in the periphery of ADH while absent staining in the epithelial cells (see Fig. 6.23).

Differential Diagnosis

Two of the most common differentials that are encountered in the diagnosis of ADH are UDH and DCIS (Tables 6.8 and 6.9). While UDH is the benign end of the spectrum of hyperplastic lesions and DCIS is the malignant end, distinguishing ADH from these entities is often challenging. UDH is a lesion composed of epithelial cells that have a heterogeneous appearance in contrast to the monoclonal-appearing cells in ADH (Fig. 6.24). The epithelial cells are round to oval

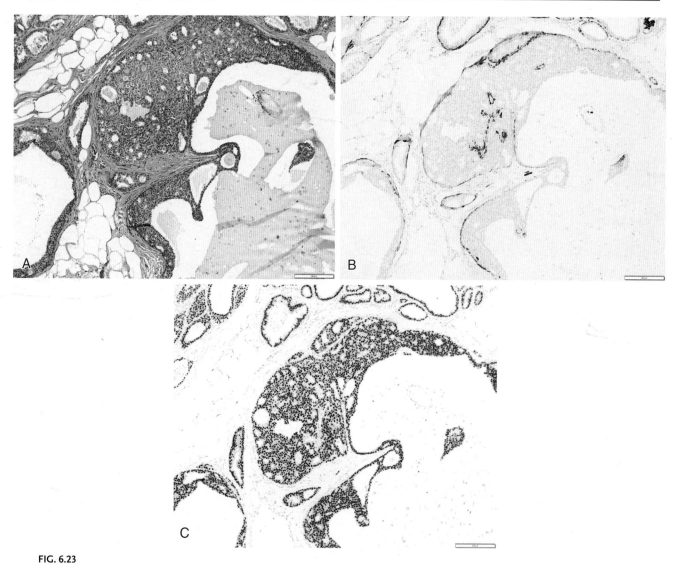

FIG. 6.23

Atypical ductal hyperplasia involving a papilloma at low magnification **(A)** showing loss of mosaic staining pattern with high-molecular-weight keratin (CK5) **(B)**, and strong diffuse staining with ER **(C)**.

TABLE 6.8

Histologic and Immunohistochemical Features of Atypical Ductal Hyperplasia Compared With Usual Ductal Hyperplasia

Atypical Ductal Hyperplasia	Usual Ductal Hyperplasia
• Clonal/monotonous appearance	• Heterogeneous appearance of cells
• Usually evenly spaced cells with prominent cell membranes	• Haphazard arrangement with overlapping nuclei and streaming appearance
• Micropapillary projections with bulbous tips	• Micropapillary projections with pinched tips
• Rigid bridge formation, arches, cribriform spaces	• Slit-like spaces usually in the periphery of the duct
• Epithelium polarized with nuclei perpendicular to the lumens	• Epithelium not polarized: nuclei parallel to lumens
• ER: strong diffuse nuclear staining	• ER: heterogeneous staining pattern
• CK5/6 (HMW keratin): absent staining	• CK5/6: heterogeneous or mosaic staining

TABLE 6.9

Histologic and Immunohistochemical Features of Atypical Ductal Hyperplasia Compared With Ductal Carcinoma *In Situ*

Atypical Ductal Hyperplasia	Ductal Carcinoma *In Situ*
• Complete involvement of ducts (<2 mm in size or involving <2 ductal spaces) or lesion of any size with partial involvement of ducts with clonal/monotonous appearing cells with low-grade atypia	• Complete involvement of ducts with clonal/monotonous appearing cells with low-grade atypia measuring >2 mm or involving >2 ductal spaces
• Cannot have intermediate-grade or high-grade atypia (irrespective of size)	• Can be intermediate-grade or high-grade (irrespective of size)
• ER: strong diffuse nuclear staining	• ER: strong to negative staining depending on the nuclear grade

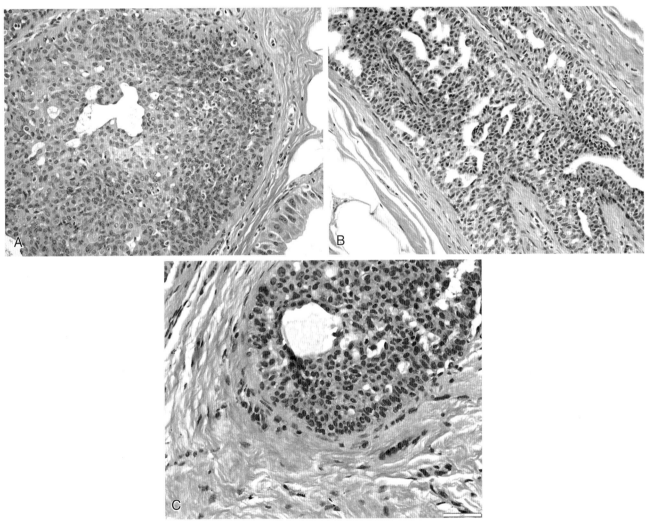

FIG. 6.24

Usual ductal hyperplasia showing intraductal proliferation of heterogeneous-appearing epithelial cells with overlapping, slit-like spaces, nuclear streaming at intermediate magnification **(A, B)** and at high magnification **(C)**.

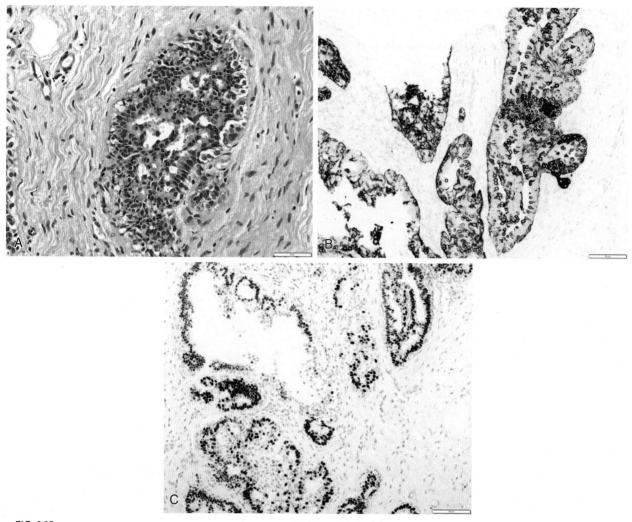

FIG. 6.25

Usual ductal hyperplasia **(A)** at intermediate magnification. Note the mosaic-like staining pattern **(B)** and heterogeneous staining with ER **(C)**.

and have overlapping nuclei with streaming appearance, and rigid bridge formation is not usually present. When lumens are identified, they are more often slit-like with nuclei parallel to the luminal surface (see Fig. 6.24). Often, intranuclear inclusions are present within UDH. In challenging cases, immunohistochemistry with CK5/6 and ER can be very helpful in distinguishing between the two. In UDH, ER demonstrates a heterogeneous staining pattern, and CK5/6 shows a mosaic-like staining pattern (Fig. 6.25).

On the other hand, the differentiation between ADH and low-grade DCIS is based on size and cytologic atypia. Any lesion with cytologic features of ADH, if more than 2 mm or involving more than two contiguous ducts, qualifies for a diagnosis of DCIS (Fig. 6.26). On the contrary, the size criteria do not apply to lesions showing more than low-grade nuclear atypia. Intermediate and high- nuclear-grade lesions are automatically considered carcinoma *in situ* irrespective of their sizes (Fig. 6.27). Low-grade DCIS shows strong diffuse ER staining similar to ADH. However, intermediate- and

high-grade DCIS can have differential staining pattern with ER. Intermediate and high nuclear grade DCIS can form a mass and can also be associated with calcifications and necrosis. Importantly, when associated with a papilloma, the size threshold of 3 mm is used. Any proliferation of atypical epithelial cells within a papilloma is diagnosed as ADH if less than 3 mm. It is, however, essential to note that there is still debate on whether these criteria should be used as a result of significant variations in observer reproducibility.

Prognosis and Therapy

Lesions diagnosed as ADH on biopsies may eventually get upgraded to DCIS on excision specimens. Multiple studies have shown upgrade rates between 12% and 36%. As a result, the diagnosis of ADH on a biopsy is an indication for surgical excision. If a worse lesion is not present on excision, adjuvant antiestrogen therapy, and more

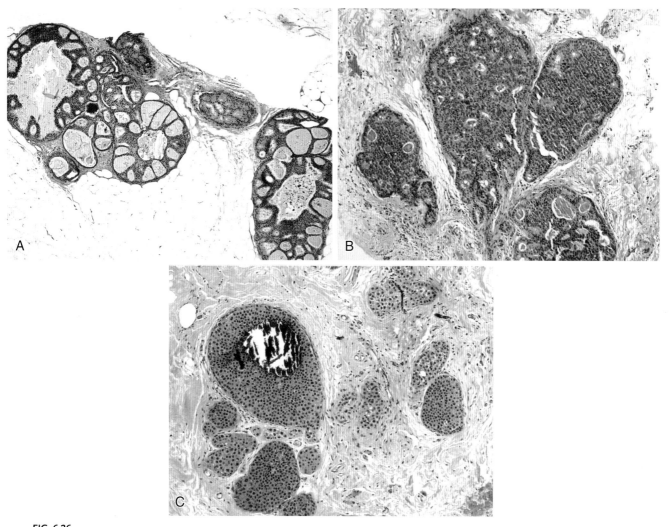

FIG. 6.26

A–C, Low-grade ductal carcinoma *in situ* shows monotonous epithelial cellular proliferation similar to atypical ductal hyperplasia but involving >2 mm and/or involving ≥2 contiguous ductal spaces.

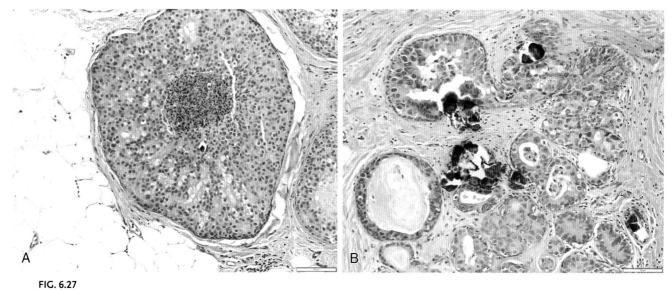

FIG. 6.27

Intermediate-grade **(A)** and high-grade **(B)** ductal carcinoma *in situ* does not need any size criteria for diagnosis.

intensive screening and follow-up is the recommendation for breast cancer prevention. The NSABP trial P-1 studied over 13,000 women with a diagnosis of ADH and demonstrated an 86% reduction in risk of subsequent invasive carcinoma in patients receiving tamoxifen.

ATYPICAL DUCTAL HYPERPLASIA – DISEASE FACT SHEET

Definition
▸▸ Proliferative clonal ductal epithelial lesions with low-grade atypia involving terminal ductal lobular units (TDLUs)
▸▸ Defined as having some but not all microscopic features of DCIS

Incidence
▸▸ Most lesions are currently identified by imaging

Age Distribution
▸▸ The peak age of incidence is between 40 and 50 years of age

Clinical Features
▸▸ Maybe palpable when associated with a papilloma

Radiologic Features
▸▸ Usually identified in 10%–20% biopsies performed for mammographic calcification
▸▸ Often associated with clustered calcifications

Prognosis and Therapy
▸▸ ADH on biopsy is an indication for surgical excision
▸▸ Upgrade rate to DCIS is 15%–20% in excisional specimens
▸▸ Adjuvant anti-estrogen therapy with tamoxifen is associated with a significant reduction in risk of malignancy
▸▸ ADH on excision usually does not need any further surgical management

---

ATYPICAL DUCTAL HYPERPLASIA – PATHOLOGIC FEATURES

Gross Findings
▸▸ May not be grossly identifiable
▸▸ If associated with a larger papilloma, may present as a palpable nodule

Microscopic Findings
▸▸ Clonal intraductal proliferation of monomorphic-appearing epithelial cells
▸▸ Evenly spaced cells with prominent membranes, round nuclei, and variable cytoplasm
▸▸ No more than low-grade cytologic atypia
▸▸ Partial or complete involvement of ducts
▸▸ Micropapillary projections with bulbous tips, arches, bridge formation, and even solid or cribriform architecture
▸▸ Complete involvement of ducts should be less than 2 mm and less than two contiguous ducts
▸▸ When involving a papilloma should measure less than 3 mm
▸▸ May arise in a background of columnar cell alteration and flat epithelial atypia

Pathologic Differential Diagnoses
▸▸ Usual ductal hyperplasia
▸▸ Ductal carcinoma *in situ*

PLEOMORPHIC LOBULAR CARCINOMA *IN SITU*

DIFFERENTIAL DIAGNOSES: SOLID DUCTAL CARCINOMA *IN SITU*

Clinical Features

LCIS of the breast is a non-invasive proliferation of neoplastic cells that both fills and distends pre-existing TDLUs. LCIS can be categorized into subtypes based upon morphology and biology/phenotype. These subtypes include classical LCIS (CLCIS), pleomorphic LCIS (PLCIS), apocrine pleomorphic LCIS (APLCIS), and florid LCIS (FLCIS). CLCIS is often an incidental and multicentric finding. PLCIS and FLCIS are more often radiologically diagnosed at the time of screening mammography with targeted biopsies and may be seen in association with microcalcifications. While CLCIS is most commonly diagnosed in premenopausal patients, PLCIS and FLCIS are encountered more frequently in the postmenopausal age group (mean age of 60 years). LCIS, like DCIS, is a clonal non-obligate precursor and risk factor for invasive breast carcinoma.

Pathologic Features

GROSS FINDINGS

LCIS is in general not associated with grossly identifiable abnormalities.

MICROSCOPIC FINDINGS

CLCIS can be morphologically subdivided into type A (nuclear grade 1 with small bland nuclei 1.5× the size of lymphocytes) and type B (nuclear grade 2 with slightly larger nuclei 2× the size of lymphocytes). To qualify as LCIS, at least 50% of the acini within a TDLU should be both filled and distended by a monotonously uniform population of dyscohesive lesional epithelial cells (Fig. 6.28). These cells may also percolate into or undermine the non-neoplastic epithelium of adjacent ducts (pagetoid spread) and/or directly involve adenosis or other lesions. Cells in all forms of LCIS may contain discrete targetoid intracytoplasmic mucin vacuoles. Such vacuoles are not specific for LCIS. PLCIS has a similar histoarchitectural appearance to CLCIS but comprises cells with a nuclear grade 3 appearance (nuclei 3–4× the size of lymphocytes; Fig. 6.29). In PLCIS, the cytoplasm of the lesional cells is somewhat more abundant, and necrosis and associated calcifications are more common. APLCIS has similar features but with more abundant finely granular eosinophilic

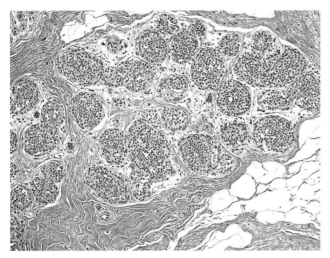

FIG. 6.28

Classical lobular carcinoma *in situ* with essentially all acini of a terminal duct lobular unit filled and distended by monotonous, dyscohesive, low nuclear grade epithelial cells.

cytoplasm. FLCIS is a proliferation comprising bland (CLCIS-like) cells with marked distension of acini/TDLUs/ducts that results in a mass-like histoarchitecture. FLCIS should show little or no intervening stroma between distended acini and expanses of greater than 40 cells across (marked distension).

Ancillary Studies

E-cadherin loss (absence of circumferential membrane expression) by immunohistochemistry is the hallmark of all forms of LCIS (Fig. 6.30). *CDH1* inactivation (a common early event in lobular neoplasia) is identified in more than 80% of LCIS lesions, and mutations in this gene encoding the cell adhesion protein E-cadherin have been found to be associated with age-related profiles in invasive lobular carcinomas. P120 catenin (alone or in combination with E-cadherin) is used in some centers to

assist in diagnosing LCIS. P120 catenin shows diffuse strong cytoplasmic immunoreactivity in LCIS lesions. Immunohistochemical characterization of investing peripheral myoepithelial cells can be useful in confirming the *in situ* nature of LCIS with markers such as p63, smooth muscle myosin, calponin, and others sometimes proving useful. CLCIS and FLCIS subtypes are generally strongly and diffusely positive with both ER and PR. PLCIS cases are often less intensely ER and PR positive, or even ER and PR negative. PLCIS may also show HER2 overexpression.

Differential Diagnosis

Perhaps the most important light microscopic differential diagnosis for PLCIS is intermediate-grade solid-type DCIS (Table 6.10). The category of DCIS encompasses a diverse group of lesions with heterogeneous morphologies and mixed biological potentials. Intermediate-grade solid-type DCIS is an *in situ* disease process most often seen in the terminal ducts and possibly involving TDLUs (cancerization of lobules). In solid DCIS, the cells are more cohesive than in PLCIS and may show abortive microacini/subluminal formations with some polarization at the periphery of involved spaces. Necrosis is less common in low- to intermediate-grade DCIS but microcalcifications may be present, as in many cases of PLCIS. Ancillary studies for E-cadherin (membranous positivity in DCIS with absence of membranous staining in LCIS) (Fig. 6.31) and P120 catenin (membranous positivity in DCIS with cytoplasmic positivity in LCIS) (Fig. 6.32) may be of value in separating PLCIS from DCIS. PLCIS and DCIS can coexist in up to 15% of patients.

Prognosis and Therapy

In most centers, the current management practice for a diagnosis of LCIS is conservative with active surveillance

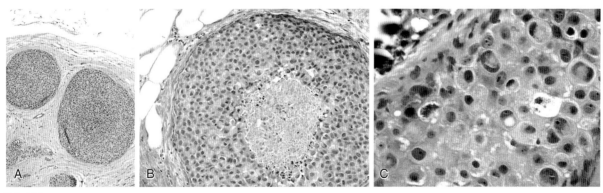

FIG. 6.29

Classical lobular carcinoma *in situ* with small repetitive nuclei **(A)** compared with pleomorphic lobular carcinoma *in situ* (PLCIS) with larger cells having larger nuclei and associated central necrosis **(B)**. The lesional cells in PLCIS show greater anisonucleosis, nucleomegaly, readily discernable nucleoli, mitotic figures, and occasional binucleation or multinucleation **(C)**.

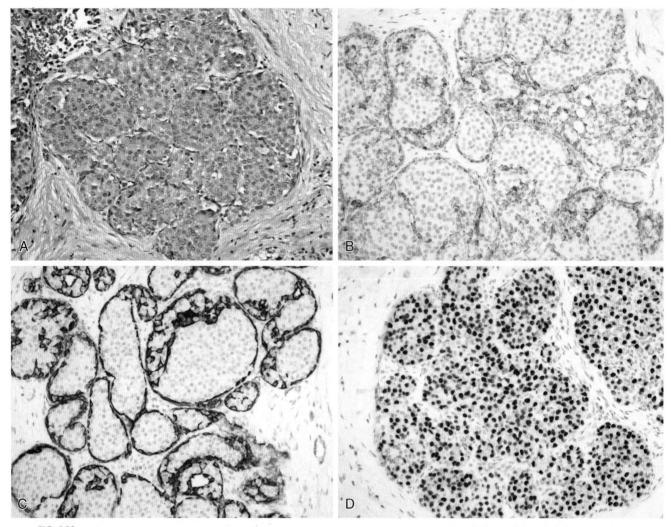

FIG. 6.30

Classical type B lobular carcinoma *in situ* with distension of acini by monotonous epithelial cells **(A)** with absence of E-cadherin expression (no membranous reactivity) by immunohistochemistry **(B)**. Ancillary smooth muscle myosin testing **(C)** confirms peripheral intact myoepithelial investitures supporting the morphologic impression of an *in situ* process, and nearly all nuclei show positivity for estrogen receptors **(D)**.

TABLE 6.10

Histologic and Immunohistochemical Features of Pleomorphic Lobular Carcinoma *In Situ* Compared With Solid Ductal Carcinoma *In Situ*

Pleomorphic Lobular Carcinoma *In Situ*	Solid Ductal Carcinoma *In Situ*
• Classically centered in the acini of terminal duct lobular units	• Classically centered in terminal ducts
• Dyscohesive appearance of cells	• More cohesive appearance of cells
• Greater cellular monotony	• More variability in nuclei
• Necrosis and calcifications possible	• Necrosis and calcifications possible
• Less tendency toward microacinar formations	• More tendency for microacinar structures
• Absence of membranous E-cadherin reactivity	• E-cadherin membranous staining present
• Cytoplasmic P120 catenin reactivity	• P120 membranous staining present

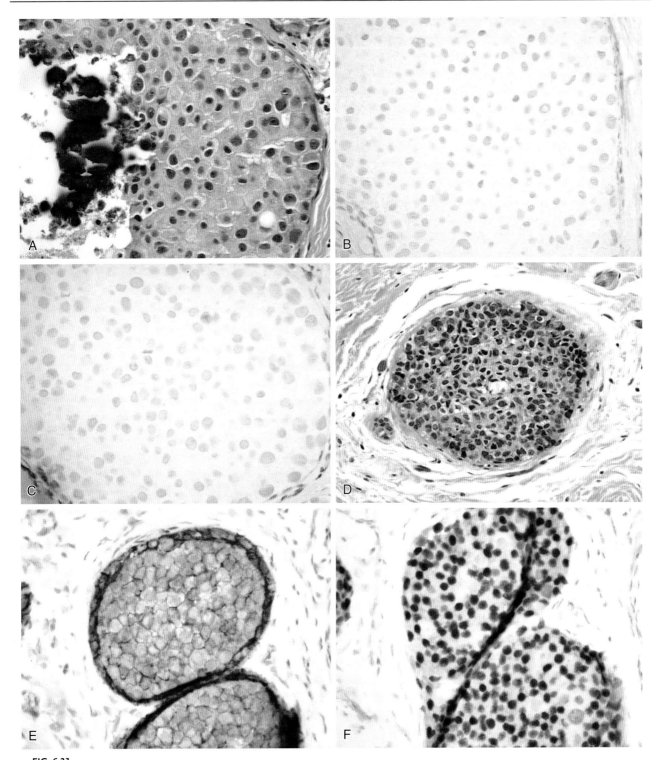

FIG. 6.31

Pleomorphic lobular carcinoma *in situ* with apocrine features (APLCIS) showing large cells with somewhat apocrine appearing cytoplasm and associated calcifications **(A)**. The APLCIS cells are negative for both E-cadherin **(B)** and estrogen receptor **(C)**. In contrast, an example of inter-mediate-grade solid-type ductal carcinoma *in situ* **(D)** with positive E-cadherin **(E)** and positive estrogen receptor **(F)** immunohistochemical studies.

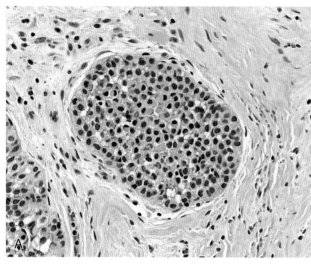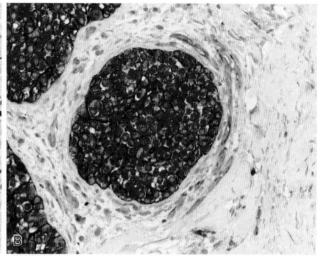

FIG. 6.32

A, Classical lobular carcinoma *in situ* exhibiting circumscription without invasion, cellular/nuclear monotony, and dyscohesion. **B,** Accompanying E-cadherin and P120 catenin cocktail immunohistochemistry study showing diffuse cytoplasmic P120 immunoreactivity in lobular carcinoma *in situ* (red chromogen).

and risk reduction strategies, possibly including anti-estrogen therapies. Surgical excision is generally not pursued for patients with incidental CLCIS who have concordant imaging and histology findings, and CLCIS margins are typically not reported in resections. Excision specimen upgrade rates to invasive carcinoma have been reported at over 50% in some studies when patients have been diagnosed with PLCIS by preoperative core biopsies. Pathologists in many centers standardly report PLCIS and FLCIS margins in resection reports.

▸▸ When associated with necrosis and calcifications can mimic DCIS and even appear as mass-forming lesions

Prognosis and Therapy

▸▸ When PLCIS most serious lesion in excision, extremely low likelihood of metastatic disease
▸▸ PLCIS excision margins standardly reported in many centers
▸▸ Surgical and medical (anti-estrogen) therapies tailored to the individual patient

---

PLEOMORPHIC LOBULAR CARCINOMA *IN SITU* (PLCIS) – DISEASE FACT SHEET

Definition

▸▸ Neoplastic proliferation of monotonous, dyscohesive, intralobular epithelial cells that both fills and distends at least 50% of a TDLU
▸▸ Nuclei 3–4× the size of lymphocytes with greater anisonucleosis than CLCIS

Incidence and Location

▸▸ PLCIS is uncommon, incidence has increased in association with greater population screening
▸▸ LCIS is commonly multifocal (70%) and often bilateral (30%)

Age Distribution

▸▸ Most common in postmenopausal women, mean age of 60 years (10–15 years older than CLCIS)

Clinical Features

▸▸ Excision upgrades to invasive carcinoma following core biopsy of PLCIS of ≥50%

Radiologic Features

▸▸ Can be incidentally discovered in biopsy (as for most cases of CLCIS)

PLEOMORPHIC LOBULAR CARCINOMA *IN SITU* (PLCIS) – PATHOLOGIC FEATURES

Gross Findings

▸▸ Incidental microscopic lesions often not grossly identifiable
▸▸ Examples with central necrosis and calcifications may grossly mimic comedo DCIS

Microscopic Findings

▸▸ At least 50% of a TDLU both filled and expanded by a monotonous, dyscohesive population of rounded cells with eccentric nuclei
▸▸ Peripheral myoepithelial investitures preserved
▸▸ Cells do not form secondary lumina
▸▸ Possible but not requisite discrete targetoid intracytoplasmic mucin droplets
▸▸ Cells with high nuclear grade (nuclei 3–4× the size of lymphocytes)
▸▸ Nuclei often eccentric within cells
▸▸ Greater variation in nuclear size than CLCIS
▸▸ Apoptosis, central necrosis and associated calcifications possible
▸▸ Mitoses identified
▸▸ Possible binucleation/multinucleation of lesional epithelial cells
▸▸ May have apocrine cytoplasmic features (APLCIS)

Pathologic Differential Diagnoses

▸▸ Classical lobular carcinoma *in situ* (CLCIS) composed of type B cells
▸▸ Solid ductal carcinoma *in situ* (DCIS)

INTRADUCTAL PAPILLOMA

DIFFERENTIAL DIAGNOSES: ENCAPSULATED PAPILLARY CARCINOMA AND PAPILLARY DUCTAL CARCINOMA *IN SITU*

Clinical Features

Intraductal papilloma (IDP) is a benign proliferative lesion that may occur in the central or peripheral ducts of the breast. Papillomas most commonly come to clinical attention between 30 and 50 years of age, although they may present over a wide age range. Central ("large duct") IDPs, which are most common, are often solitary and most often present with unilateral clear to serosanguinous nipple discharge. Those large enough to be identified on imaging appear on mammography as a retroareolar circumscribed mass or ductal dilatation, on ultrasound as a hypoechoic, solid to cystic mass with vascular pedicles on Doppler, on MRI as a potentially enhancing mass, and on galactography as ductal dilatation or a luminal filling defect. Peripheral ("microscopic") IDPs are often multiple, arise from the TDLUs, and are most often clinically and radiologically occult. Peripheral IDPs may rarely also present as nipple discharge or as mass lesions with imaging demonstrating nodular ductal prominence or multiple circumscribed masses. Both central and peripheral IDPs may show calcifications on imaging. In a study including a cohort of more than 9000 women, IDPs, either with or without atypia, were identified in approximately 5% of benign breast biopsies.

Pathologic Features

GROSS FINDINGS

Central IDPs may appear as a round, circumscribed mass attached by vascular pedicles to the wall of a dilated duct. Larger lesions may demonstrate areas of hemorrhage or necrosis. They may range in size from subcentimeter nodules to masses >5 cm. Unless associated with other lesions, peripheral IDPs are often macroscopically occult.

MICROSCOPIC FINDINGS

Both central and peripheral IDPs demonstrate papillary architecture comprising broad, fibrotic fibrovascular cores lined by a dual layer of myoepithelial and epithelial cells, with the periphery of the involved ducts also exhibiting myoepithelial investitures (Fig. 6.33). The myoepithelial cells may be subtle and attenuated, in which case immunohistochemical stains may be helpful, or they may be conspicuous or hyperplastic. The overlying epithelial cells form a monolayer of heterogeneous cuboidal to columnar cells and may show apocrine metaplasia or UDH. Infarcted papillomas may display squamous metaplasia. Less commonly, sebaceous, mucinous, and clear cell metaplasia may be seen. Mitotic figures are typically absent or rarely encountered. When encountered on core biopsy, the size of a papillary lesion should be documented to correlate with radiologic findings and to guide further management.

Following needle biopsy or torsion of a fibrovascular core, an IDP may undergo infarction, developing sclerosis or fibrosis that may obscure its papillary architecture. Such sclerosing papillomas and biopsy

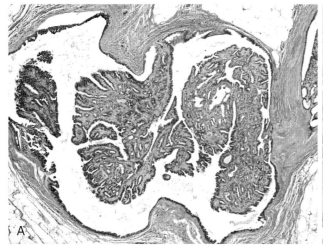
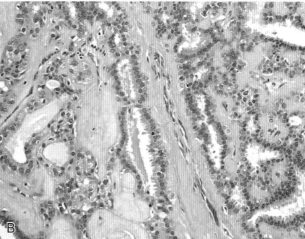

FIG. 6.33

Intraductal papilloma at low magnification demonstrating an intraductal proliferation of well-developed, broad fibrovascular cores **(A)**, rimmed by a dual lining of cytologically bland myoepithelial cells and overlying epithelial cells **(B)**.

Continued

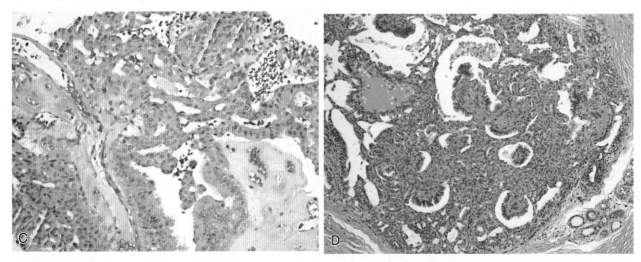

FIG. 6.33, cont'd
On occasion, papillomas may contain intrinsic apocrine metaplasia **(C)** or usual ductal hyperplasia **(D)**.

needle tracts may exhibit entrapped or displaced epithelial nests within areas of sclerosis, mimicking invasive carcinoma. Myoepithelial markers are useful in confirming benignity in these areas. Of note, IDPs may display involvement by atypical lesions including ADH, DCIS, ALH, or LCIS (Fig. 6.34). Much less commonly, IDPs may be involved by invasive carcinoma. Atypical foci are more commonly observed in peripheral IDPs. Foci of ADH and low to intermediate nuclear grade DCIS may demonstrate attenuated or absent myoepithelial cells and often show diffuse expression of ER and absence of high-molecular-weight keratins. The distinction between ADH and DCIS involving an IDP is dependent upon the size of the atypical focus, with <3 mm of involvement considered ADH and ≥3 mm of involvement considered DCIS. Most atypical lesions involving IDPs are of low nuclear grade; should intermediate or high nuclear grade be encountered, a diagnosis of DCIS involving an IDP should be rendered regardless of extent.

Ancillary Studies

Immunohistochemistry is helpful in confirming the presence of myoepithelial cells in cases equivocal for carcinoma. IDPs should demonstrate the presence of myoepithelial cells both surrounding the papillae and rimming the periphery of the duct. These areas express myoepithelial markers such as p63, calponin, CK5/6, and SMMS1, although immunoreactivity may be patchy and/or attenuated in some cases.

IDPs are clonal proliferations that frequently demonstrate activating point mutations in the PIK3CA/AKT1 pathway. Losses of heterozygosity on 16q23 have been demonstrated in malignant papillary lesions, but such losses are absent in benign papillary lesions.

Differential Diagnosis

The differential diagnosis for IDP includes any of several papillary lesions that may occur in the breast, particularly papillary DCIS and encapsulated papillary carcinoma.

Papillary DCIS occurs predominantly in postmenopausal women and is a relatively uncommon subtype of DCIS, accounting for approximately 3% of all DCIS. Papillary DCIS, unlike IDP, exhibits delicate, slender fibrovascular cores devoid of myoepithelial investitures, but similarly to IDP, maintains a myoepithelial lining at the periphery of the involved duct (Fig. 6.35; Table 6.11). Papillary DCIS is most commonly encountered in association with other architectural patterns of DCIS. Particularly in retroareolar locations, papillary DCIS may coexist with encapsulated papillary carcinoma. In previous literature, encapsulated papillary carcinoma and adjacent DCIS, including papillary DCIS, were termed "intracystic papillary DCIS." Both papillary DCIS and encapsulated papillary carcinoma are typically negative for high-molecular-weight cytokeratins and are strongly and diffusely positive for ER, while IDPs without atypia typically display heterogeneous expression of both high-molecular-weight cytokeratins and ER.

Encapsulated papillary carcinoma, like papillary DCIS, occurs most commonly in postmenopausal women, typically in the seventh decade. This tumor characteristically demonstrates a cystically dilated space surrounded by a prominent fibrous capsule and contains finely arborizing papillae lined by low to intermediate-nuclear-grade neoplastic epithelial cells. Unlike IDP, however, both the papillae and the periphery of the cystic spaces lack myoepithelial investitures; however, peripheral myoepithelial cells may appear only attenuated or incomplete in occasional cases

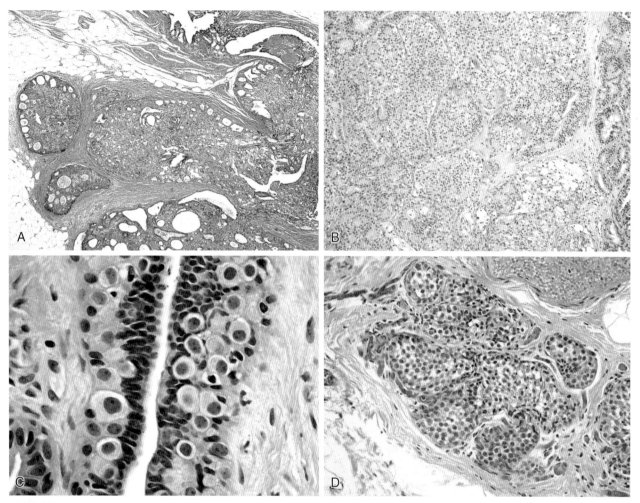

FIG. 6.34

Intraductal papilloma demonstrating involvement by atypical proliferations, including atypical ductal hyperplasia, characterized by a <3 mm extent of ductal atypia **(A, B)** and atypical lobular hyperplasia/lobular carcinoma *in situ* (**C** [pagetoid growth] and **D**).

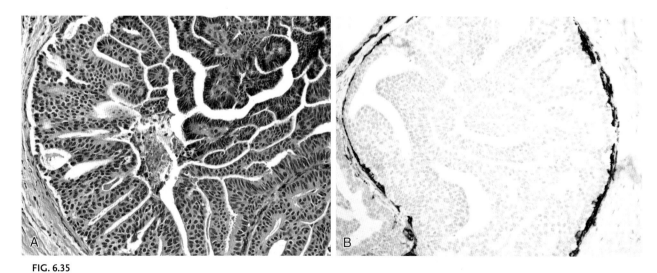

FIG. 6.35

Papillary ductal carcinoma *in situ* at intermediate magnification **(A)**, with an SMMS1 immunostain demonstrating loss of myoepithelial cells surrounding the papillae, but maintaining myoepithelial investitures rimming the periphery of the duct **(B)**.

Continued

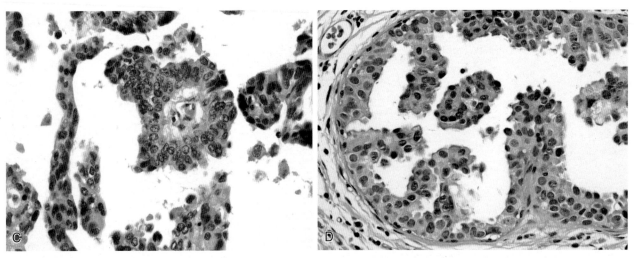

FIG. 6.35, cont'd
High magnification exhibiting fibrovascular cores lined by a monotonous proliferation of epithelial cells **(C)**. Micropapillary ductal carcinoma *in situ* displaying slender pseudopapillae with bulbous tips that lack true fibrovascular cores **(D)**.

TABLE 6.11

Histologic and Immunohistochemical Features of Intraductal Papilloma (IDP) Compared With Papillary Ductal Carcinoma *In Situ* (DCIS)

Intraductal Papilloma	Papillary DCIS
• Lesions may be solitary (central) or multiple (peripheral)	• Typically multiple lesions
• Broad, fibrotic papillae within a duct	• Delicate, slender, variably branching and arborizing papillae within a duct
• Haphazardly arranged, heterogeneous population of luminal cells with normochromatic nuclei	• Uniformly arranged cells with hyperchromatic nuclei, low to intermediate nuclear grade; rarely high nuclear grade
• May display apocrine metaplasia or usual ductal hyperplasia	• Rarely displays apocrine metaplasia or benign proliferative changes
• Both intraductal papillae and duct periphery maintain myoepithelial investitures	• Intraductal papillae show lack or attenuation of myoepithelial cells, while duct periphery maintains myoepithelial investitures
• Adjacent ducts more often demonstrate usual ductal hyperplasia; the IDP itself may occasionally display involvement by ADH, DCIS, ALH, LCIS, or rarely invasive carcinoma	• Adjacent ducts often demonstrate other architectural patterns of DCIS
• Heterogeneous expression of high-molecular-weight cytokeratins (in cases without atypia)	• Negative for high-molecular-weight cytokeratins
• Heterogeneous expression of ER (in cases without atypia)	• Strong, diffuse expression of ER

ADH, Atypical ductal hyperplasia; *ALH*, atypical lobular hyperplasia; *IDP*, intraductal papilloma; *LCIS*, lobular carcinoma *in situ*.

(Fig. 6.36; Table 6.12). Unless frank invasion beyond the fibrous capsule is identified, these lesions are staged as pTis due to their indolent behavior with rare axillary nodal involvement. Solid papillary carcinoma is also occasionally considered in the differential diagnosis of IDP, characterized by nodules expanded by solid sheets of rounded to spindled, low to intermediate nuclear grade cells that frequently express neuroendocrine markers and often demonstrate peripheral palisading around inconspicuous fibrovascular cores.

Prognosis and Therapy

Central IDPs without atypia confer a twofold increased relative risk for invasive breast carcinoma, whereas peripheral IDPs without atypia confer a threefold increased relative risk. IDPs with atypia are reported to have a 5- to 7.5-fold increased relative risk for invasive carcinoma, although the frequent presence of concurrent ADH or DCIS in these cases somewhat confounds these data.

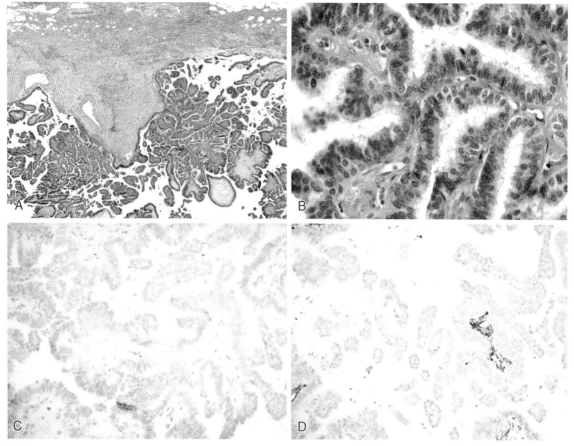

FIG. 6.36

Encapsulated papillary carcinoma at low magnification exhibiting a thick fibrous capsule overlying an intracystic proliferation of complex, finely arborizing papillae **(A)**. High magnification depicting fibrovascular cores lined by cytologically bland epithelial cells **(B)**. The papillae lack myo-epithelial investitures, as evidenced by absent p63 **(C)** and SMA **(D)** immunohistochemical staining, as do the periphery of the cystic spaces.

TABLE 6.12

Histologic and Immunohistochemical Features of Intraductal Papilloma (IDP) Compared With Encapsulated Papillary Carcinoma

Intraductal Papilloma	Encapsulated Papillary Carcinoma
• Lesions may be solitary (central) or multiple (peripheral)	• Typically solitary lesion
• Broad, fibrotic papillae within a duct	• Delicate, slender, variably branching and arborizing papillae within a cystic space surrounded by a prominent fibrous capsule; may also display micropapillary, cribriform, and solid patterns
• Haphazardly arranged, heterogeneous population of luminal cells with normochromatic nuclei	• Uniformly arranged cells with hyperchromatic nuclei, low to intermediate nuclear grade; rarely high nuclear grade
• May display apocrine metaplasia or usual ductal hyperplasia	• Rarely displays apocrine metaplasia or benign proliferative changes
• Both intraductal papillae and periphery of the duct maintain myoepithelial investitures	• Both intralesional papillae and periphery of cystic spaces show lack or attenuation of myoepithelial investitures; may rarely maintain myoepithelial investitures at periphery
• Adjacent ducts more often demonstrate usual ductal hyperplasia; the IDP itself may occasionally display involvement by ADH, DCIS, ALH, LCIS, or rarely invasive carcinoma	• Adjacent ducts more often demonstrate DCIS
• Heterogeneous expression of high-molecular-weight cytokeratins (in cases without atypia)	• Negative for high-molecular-weight cytokeratins
• Heterogeneous expression of ER (in cases without atypia)	• Strong, diffuse expression of ER

ADH, Atypical ductal hyperplasia; *ALH,* atypical lobular hyperplasia; *DCIS,* ductal carcinoma *in situ*; *LCIS,* lobular carcinoma *in situ*.

Although lesional heterogeneity is of concern on core biopsy and upgrade rates of IDPs on excision have ranged between 0% and 29% across series in large cohorts, most studies demonstrate low upgrade rates on excision (≤4%) for IDPs without atypia. This suggests that in cases of IDP without atypia that are radiologically concordant, non-surgical management may be appropriate. Risk factors for malignancy on excision have been reported to include the presence of calcifications, postmenopausal age, peripheral location, and size >5 mm. Should atypical features be identified on core biopsy, such as cytological or architectural atypia or lack of myoepithelial investitures, the lesion should undergo complete excision.

INTRADUCTAL PAPILLOMA – DISEASE FACT SHEET

Definition
▸▸ Benign intraductal lesion of the breast composed of broad, fibrotic papillae with fibrovascular cores lined by a dual population of epithelial and myoepithelial cells

Incidence and Location
▸▸ Present in approximately 5% of benign breast biopsies
▸▸ Central ("large duct") IDPs often present as solitary lesions, and are most common
▸▸ Peripheral ("microscopic") IDPs often present as multiple lesions

Age Distribution
▸▸ Peak age of incidence varies between 30 and 50 years of age
▸▸ May occur over a wide age distribution

Clinical Features
▸▸ Central IDPs are typically solitary and most often present with unilateral clear to serosanguinous nipple discharge
▸▸ Peripheral IDPs are typically multiple and are most often clinically occult, rarely presenting with nipple discharge

Radiologic Features
▸▸ Central IDPs large enough to be identified on imaging appear on mammography as a circumscribed retroareolar mass or ductal dilatation, on ultrasound as a hypoechoic, solid to cystic mass with vascular pedicles demonstrating Doppler expression, on MRI as a potentially enhancing mass, and on galactography as ductal dilatation or a luminal filling defect; calcifications may be present
▸▸ Peripheral IDPs are most often radiologically occult, although they may rarely appear on imaging as nodular ductal prominences, multiple circumscribed masses, or calcifications

Prognosis and Therapy
▸▸ Central IDPs without atypia confer a twofold increased relative risk for invasive carcinoma
▸▸ Peripheral IDPs without atypia confer a threefold increased relative risk for invasive carcinoma
▸▸ IDPs with atypia confer a 5- to 7.5-fold increased relative risk for invasive carcinoma, although these cases frequently demonstrated concurrent ADH or DCIS, somewhat confounding these data

---

▸▸ Most recent studies of IDPs without atypia demonstrate low upgrade rates on excision (≤4%), lending support for surveillance in these cases
▸▸ IDPs with cytological atypia, architectural atypia, or lack of myoepithelial investitures should undergo excision

---

INTRADUCTAL PAPILLOMA – PATHOLOGIC FEATURES

Gross Findings
▸▸ Central IDPs may appear as circumscribed tumors attached to the wall of the dilated duct by vascular pedicles, ranging from subcentimeter nodules to masses >5 cm
▸▸ Peripheral IDPs are most often macroscopically occult, unless associated with other lesions

Microscopic Findings
▸▸ Intraductal papillary proliferation comprising broad, fibrotic fibrovascular cores lined by a dual layer of heterogeneous-appearing epithelial and myoepithelial cells
▸▸ Myoepithelial investitures are present both surrounding the papillae and the duct periphery
▸▸ Myoepithelial cells may be subtle and attenuated or conspicuous and hyperplastic
▸▸ Epithelial cells form a monolayer of cuboidal to columnar cells and may show apocrine metaplasia or usual ductal hyperplasia
▸▸ Squamous metaplasia may be observed in cases with infarction
▸▸ Sebaceous, mucinous, and clear cell metaplasia are less frequently observed
▸▸ Mitotic figures are typically absent or rare
▸▸ Sclerosing papillomas may develop secondary to infarction following needle biopsy or torsion of fibrovascular cores, occasionally obscuring the papillary architecture
▸▸ Sclerosing papillomas and biopsy needle tracts may exhibit entrapped or displaced epithelial nests within areas of sclerosis, mimicking invasive carcinoma
▸▸ Involvement by ADH, DCIS, ALH, and LCIS may be seen and are most commonly observed in peripheral IDPs, most often with low nuclear grade atypia
▸▸ ADH constitutes a focus of involvement <3 mm, whereas DCIS constitutes a focus of involvement ≥3 mm
▸▸ When intermediate or high nuclear grade is encountered, a diagnosis of DCIS involving papilloma should be rendered regardless of extent
▸▸ Foci of ADH and low- to intermediate-grade DCIS show attenuated or absent myoepithelial cells, diffuse expression of ER, and absence of high-molecular-weight keratins

Pathologic Differential Diagnoses
▸▸ Papillary DCIS
▸▸ Encapsulated papillary carcinoma
▸▸ Solid papillary carcinoma

NIPPLE ADENOMA

DIFFERENTIAL DIAGNOSIS: INVASIVE CARCINOMA

Clinical Features

Nipple adenomas are benign epithelial proliferations most often arising immediately beneath the epidermis in the nipple/areola. Patients often present with complaints of serosanguinous nipple discharge and a palpable nodular mass just beneath the nipple. Over time other symptoms such as bleeding, erythema, ulceration, crust formations, and pain may occur. Some lesions may raise differential considerations of Paget disease and even invasive carcinoma as sclerosis and retraction of the nipple may occur. In some instances, large pedunculated exophytic masses develop.

Pathologic Features

GROSS FINDINGS

Most excised nipple adenomas are firm, somewhat irregularly marginated and small (<1 cm). Large pedunculated masses measuring more than 4 cm are known.

MICROSCOPIC FINDINGS

Nipple adenomas appear histologically as relatively well-circumscribed epithelial proliferations, sometimes with associated stromal sclerosis and entrapped-appearing glands at their periphery. While florid papillomatosis is a classically described morphologic feature, architectural complexity and variability are also common (Fig. 6.37). Proliferative histoarchitectural patterns may include tubular formations, papillae, micropapillae, tufts, fronds, arcades, adenosis, and abortive cribriform growth (Fig. 6.38). Some adenomas show cystic areas with associated squamous metaplasia, and internal apocrine metaplasia is also known to happen. Intrinsic UDH is common. Extension of the proliferative glandular epithelium through superficial duct orifices may

result in direct involvement of the epidermis of the overlying skin and lead to frank ulceration. When necessary, ancillary immunohistochemical studies may be helpful in confirming myoepithelial investitures throughout (Fig. 6.39).

Ancillary Studies

Immunohistochemical testing for confirmation of investing myoepithelial cells in nipple adenoma can be valuable in confirming the diagnoses and in excluding the differential diagnosis of an invasive carcinoma. Markers such as p63, calponin, SMMS1, and others are commonly used (Fig. 6.39). Confirmation of cellular heterogeneity (supporting benignity) may in some instances be assessed by performance and interpretation of additional immunohistochemical tests such as CK5/6 and ER.

Differential Diagnosis

Paget disease of the nipple may be an important clinical differential diagnosis for nipple adenoma, as patients with Paget disease often present with erythematous erosion of the nipple as well as scaling and crust formations. The histologic differential diagnosis of Paget disease with nipple adenoma is perhaps less significant than the clinical one, with Paget cells (large intraepidermal malignant cells with abundant pale cytoplasm, pleomorphic nuclei, prominent nucleoli, and mitoses) noted singly and in small nests at the dermal-epidermal

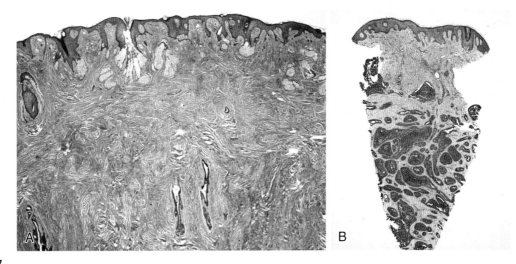

FIG. 6.37

Histologic comparison of resected non-neoplastic nipple tissue from an adult female **(A)** to a core biopsy of a nipple adenoma **(B)**. Both sections show overlying full-thickness stratified squamous epithelium and subjacent dermis. In the non-neoplastic nipple, a few pilosebaceous structures are noted in the dermis and at the dermo-epidermal junction with perpendicularly oriented lactiferous ducts deeper in the tissue. The nipple adenoma core biopsy histology shows intraductal papillomatosis filling and expanding duct spaces and involving both the subcutis and reticular dermis.

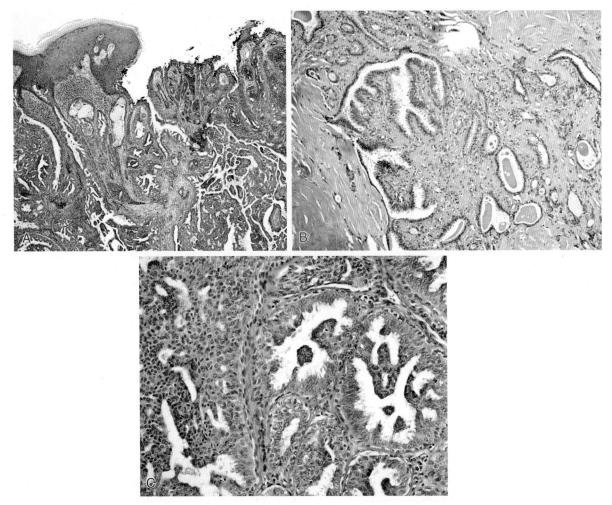

FIG. 6.38

Sections from a nipple adenoma showing erosion of the epidermis with an abrupt demarcation between stratified squamous epithelium and an architecturally complex glandular proliferation **(A)**. The morphology within the lesion is variable, with true papillae having fibrovascular cores and abortive fingertip-like micropapillae also noted. Microcystic spaces distended by eosinophilic secretions **(B)** are common, and foci of usual ductal hyperplasia with slit-like subluminal spaces **(C)** are also frequently seen.

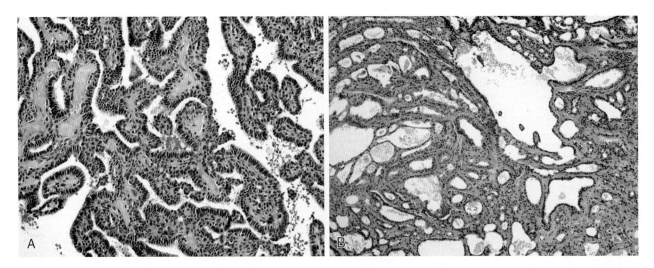

FIG. 6.39

Nipple adenomas are composed of a mixture of fibrous stroma and proliferative epithelium with a predominantly ductal appearance that can be arranged in papillary, bridging, cribriform arcade-like, tufted, solid, adenotic, acinar, frond-like, and other architectural patterns. True papillary architecture with bland cytology **(A)** is reassuring. Areas of cribriform architecture **(B)** may raise concern for an atypical hyperplasia or malignancy, and immunohistochemical

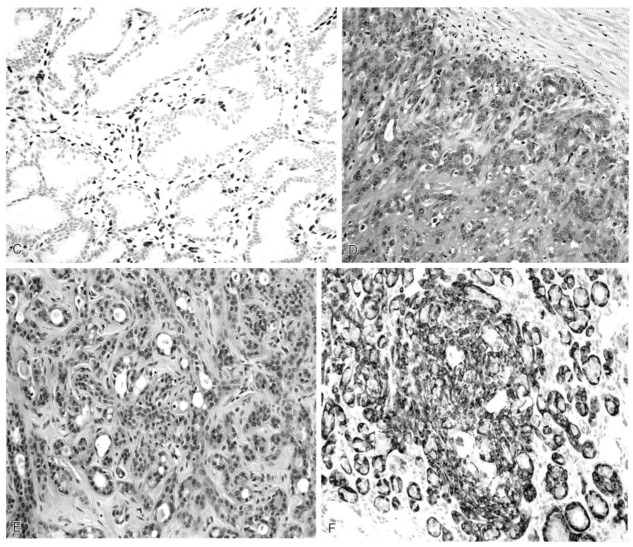

FIG. 6.39, cont'd

(**C**, p63) studies for myoepithelial cells help to confirm a benign process. Adenosis (**D**) and back-to-back acinar architecture (**E**) may raise concerns for an invasive carcinoma. Immunohistochemistry (**F**, calponin) confirming diffuse myoepithelial investitures supports the morphologic impression of small repetitive benign glands within adenosis in a nipple adenoma.

junction with percolation upward between keratinocytes. This appearance is different from that of a usual nipple adenoma. The main and most important differential diagnosis for nipple adenoma is carcinoma. In small biopsies, the complex architectural patterns of nipple adenomas can be mistaken for both *in situ* and invasive ductal carcinoma. Areas of sclerosis with entrapped glands and adenosis at the periphery of adenomas can be especially challenging (Table 6.13). Immunohistochemical studies for calponin, p63, SMMS1, and other myoepithelial markers are especially helpful in confirming a biphenotypic epithelium with intrinsic myoepithelial investitures (Fig. 6.40). Correlations with imaging studies and clinical settings are of paramount importance. Other tumors of the nipple such as central

IDP (which generally does not involve the skin) and syringomatous adenoma (which also does not have an epidermal component) may be differential diagnostic considerations for nipple adenoma.

Prognosis and Therapy

Nipple adenomas are benign. Complete excision is the standard of care in most centers. Recurrences of nipple adenoma have been described following incomplete excisions. Case reports of both associated *in situ* and invasive carcinoma exist. Some literature exists for treatment by Moh's micrographic surgery and cryosurgery.

TABLE 6.13

Histologic Features of Nipple Adenoma Compared With Invasive Ductal Carcinoma

Nipple Adenoma	Invasive Ductal Carcinoma
• Solid mass with irregular margination	• Solid mass with irregular margination
• By definition centered in ducts and stroma immediately subjacent to skin of nipple/areola	• Can be centered in ducts and stroma immediately subjacent to skin of nipple/areola
• Not associated with Paget disease	• May be associated with Paget disease and with ductal carcinoma *in situ*
• Highly variable epithelial proliferation with many patterns of architectural complexity	• More often a single pattern of invasive disease morphology and not associated with diffuse variable background hyperplasia
• Glands entrapped in reactive fibrous stroma	• Glands entrapped in desmoplastic stroma
• Complex glands and areas of cribriform adenosis with associated intrinsic accompanying myoepithelial cells, IHC for myoepithelial markers useful	• Absence of myoepithelial cells in areas of invasion, IHC for myoepithelial markers useful

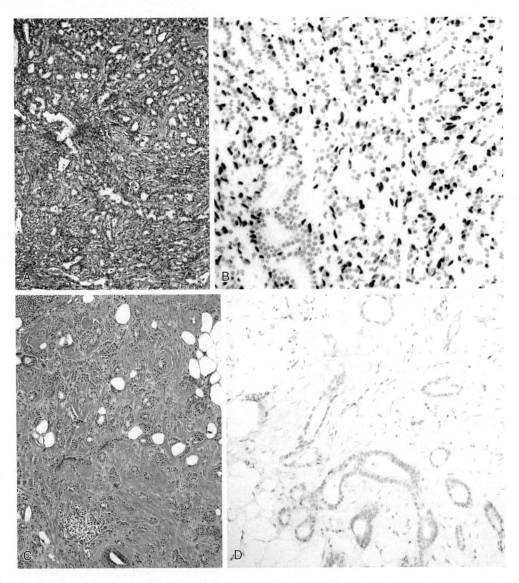

FIG. 6.40

Composite photomicrographic image showing an example of adenosis with abortive cribriform acini within a nipple adenoma **(A)** and p63 immunohistochemistry **(B,** *inset)* confirming uniformly dispersed and diffuse myoepithelial accompaniment. A comparison low-grade invasive ductal carcinoma with prominent tubule formation **(C)** has somewhat more background stroma and completely lacks investing myoepithelial cells by p63 immunohistochemistry **(D,** *inset)*, confirming the diagnosis of an invasive carcinoma.

NIPPLE ADENOMA – DISEASE FACT SHEET

Definition

▸▸ Nipple adenomas, sometimes referred to as florid papillomatosis of the nipple, are benign epithelial proliferations that involve the ducts, superficial duct orifices, stroma, and even contiguous overlying epidermis of the skin of the nipple and areola
▸▸ While some investigators use a langue of epithelial proliferative lesions, others classify as frankly neoplastic

Incidence and Location

▸▸ Rare disease process of the nipple that is typically unilateral
▸▸ More often encountered in females but does arise in males

Age Distribution

▸▸ Can occur at any age. Most commonly reported in the fifth and sixth decades

Clinical Features

▸▸ Early in course identified as small dermal nodule just below the epidermis with associated nipple discharge
▸▸ Over time patients experience tenderness, swelling, ulceration, bleeding, itching, and ulcerative crust formations
▸▸ Can clinically mimic both Paget disease and invasive carcinoma

Radiologic Features

▸▸ Nipple ultrasound may identify circumscribed mass for larger adenomas
▸▸ Some lesions described with an intrinsic cystic component by ultrasound

Prognosis and Therapy

▸▸ Nipple adenoma is a benign entity but can cause symptoms concerning to patients
▸▸ Complete excision is the standard of care
▸▸ Moh's micrographic surgery and cryosurgery have been reported as effective for management
▸▸ Recurrences of nipple adenomas have been reported after incomplete excisions
▸▸ Rare cases known of in situ and invasive carcinoma arising in association with nipple adenomas

---

NIPPLE ADENOMA – PATHOLOGIC FEATURES

Gross Findings

▸▸ Irregularly marginated firm mass, typically <1 cm in greatest dimension
▸▸ May involve epidermis and appear grossly ulcerative

Microscopic Findings

▸▸ Relatively well-circumscribed glandular proliferation involving ducts and stroma of nipple
▸▸ Ductal structures expanded by intrinsic papillomatous hyperplasia
▸▸ Benign and often exuberant proliferative epithelial changes with variable architecture including tubules, papillae, micropapillae, tufts, fronds, arcades, adenosis, and abortive cribriform growth
▸▸ Areas of cystic change with squamous and apocrine metaplasia possible
▸▸ Intrinsic usual ductal hyperplasia common
▸▸ Intrinsic myoepithelial investitures throughout
▸▸ Skin ulceration and involvement of epidermis possible

Pathologic Differential Diagnoses

▸▸ Both glands entrapped in stroma and intrinsic adenosis with areas of sclerosis may mimic invasive carcinoma, especially in small biopsies
▸▸ Glandular epithelium extending into and replacing the overlying squamous epithelium may clinically simulate Paget disease
▸▸ Other morphologic differentials include ductal carcinoma in situ, central intraductal papilloma and syringomatous adenoma

---

ADENOID CYSTIC CARCINOMA

DIFFERENTIAL DIAGNOSIS: COLLAGENOUS SPHERULOSIS

Clinical Features

Adenoid cystic carcinoma (AdCC) of the breast is a biphasic triple-negative breast cancer of low malignant potential in classic cases. They comprise 0.1% to 3.5% of all breast tumors and most frequently occur as a unifocal lesion localized to the retroareolar region. They present most commonly in postmenopausal women (average, 50–65 years) as a palpable mass or in younger women as a smaller nodule detected by mammographic screening. The tumors vary in size based on timing of detection, from subcentimeter nodules to masses greater than 10 cm. Rare cases have been reported in men.

Pathologic Features

GROSS FINDINGS

Most cases present as firm, circumscribed masses with pushing borders. The cut surface may show cystic features. Most tumors measure 1 to 3 cm in greatest dimension, ranging from <1 cm to 12 cm.

MICROSCOPIC FINDINGS

The histologic features of AdCC of the breast are similar to those of its salivary gland counterpart, consisting of a biphasic proliferation of neoplastic epithelial and myoepithelial components associated with basement membrane matrix. The three major histologic subtypes include classic, solid-basaloid, and AdCC with high-grade transformation.

The vast majority of AdCC are of the classic subtype, which typically displays cribriform architecture in the central aspect of the lesion and transitions into tubular formations toward the periphery. The tumors may also exhibit trabecular and solid patterns. The glandular component is lined by ductal epithelial cells that secrete

PAS-positive epithelial mucins into the glandular lumina. The epithelial component is admixed with a myoepithelial component that creates stromal invaginations that form pseudoglandular structures with pseudolumina containing "hyaline cylinders" consisting of duplicated basal lamina and stromal matrix admixed with capillaries and fibroblasts (Fig. 6.41). The pseudoluminal spaces tend to be larger than the true glandular lumina. The neoplastic cells throughout the lesion are relatively uniform and possess scant cytoplasm. The classic subtype lacks significant nuclear atypia, necrosis, and mitotic activity. Perineural invasion may occasionally be seen. Squamous or sebaceous elements may be observed in rare cases. The peripheral tumor borders may be markedly infiltrative, although the tumors are generally grossly well-circumscribed.

The solid-basaloid variant shows solid nests of basaloid cells with high nuclear-to-cytoplasmic ratio consisting of myoepithelial cells with marked nuclear pleomorphism and increased mitotic activity, necrosis, and perineural invasion. Adjacent areas of classic AdCC are

almost invariably present, helping to recognize the entity. Cases of AdCC with high-grade transformation are rare, with literature reports including AdCC associated with invasive ductal carcinoma, small cell carcinoma, and malignant myoepithelioma. Molecular studies have revealed similar molecular aberrations in both the AdCC and transformed components, including the *MYB-NFIB* fusion, which likely results from clonal selection and acquisition of additional mutations.

Ancillary Studies

Immunohistochemistry is helpful in establishing the biphasic cell types of AdCC. The epithelial cells express EMA and low-molecular-weight cytokeratins such as CK7 and CK8 and less often express high-molecular-weight cytokeratins such as CK5/6. The luminal cells also typically demonstrate c-MYB protein overexpression and strong immunoreactivity for c-KIT (CD117),

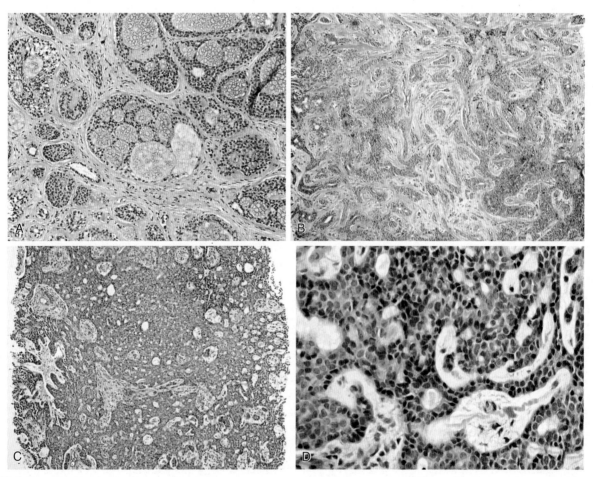

FIG. 6.41

Adenoid cystic carcinoma at low magnification, demonstrating an infiltrative lesion that can display a multitude of growth patterns, including cribriform (A), trabecular (B), and variably solid (C) architecture. High magnification demonstrates an admixture of true glands lined by cytologically bland epithelial cells secreting eosinophilic mucin, intermixed with a cytologically bland myoepithelial proliferation forming pseudolumina containing basement membrane-like material, mucopolysaccharides, capillaries, and fibroblasts (D).

although many other breast tumors, including adeno-myoepithelioma, may exhibit focal c-KIT expression. The myoepithelial cells express CK5/6, CK14, p63, S100, CD10, calponin, and myosin heavy chain (Fig. 6.42). Pseudolumina may be highlighted with basement membrane markers such as laminin and collagen IV. The vast majority of cases are ER, PR, and HER2 negative, with occasional cases demonstrating focal ER and PR expression.

Approximately 90% of cases possess the *MYB-NFIB* fusion gene due to the recurrent chromosomal translocation t(6;9)(q22-23;p23-24), as seen in salivary gland AdCC, and may be detected by FISH or PCR studies. Cases without this fusion may harbor *MYB* amplification or *MYBL1* rearrangements, and less commonly other genetic alterations.

Differential Diagnosis

The major differential diagnosis of AdCC is the benign entity of collagenous spherulosis (CS). While both entities are composed of mucin-producing epithelial cells and matrix-producing myoepithelial cells, in contrast to AdCC, CS is typically encountered as an incidental finding that very infrequently forms a mass-like lesion. Although CS also forms conspicuous cribriform structures, it does not display the other morphologic patterns seen in AdCC (Fig. 6.43). CS may often be seen in association with benign proliferative changes, such as UDH, papillomas, and sclerosing adenosis, and may occasionally be involved by LCIS. Perineural invasion is absent in CS. CS often expresses hormone receptors in its luminal component, in contrast to the infrequent expression of hormone receptors in AdCC. Immunohistochemistry for c-KIT and MYB may be helpful in distinguishing the two lesions, as these stains are negative or only focal and weak in CS (Table 6.14).

Furthermore, the tubular formations in AdCC may mimic those of microglandular adenosis (MGA) or tubular carcinoma. While MGA is also triple negative, tubular carcinoma strongly expresses ER and PR, and both MGA and tubular carcinoma lack the other morphologic features of AdCC and are composed of only epithelial cells. Moreover, the cribriform composition

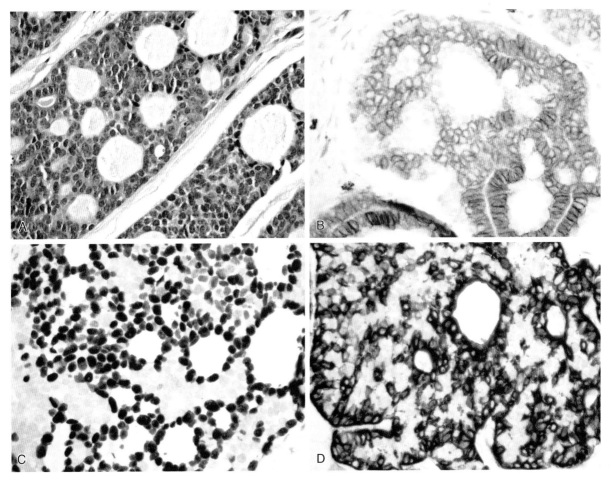

FIG. 6.42

High-magnification view of adenoid cystic carcinoma displaying classic cribriform architecture **(A)**. Immunohistochemistry delineates a biphasic proliferation of luminal cells expressing c-KIT (CD117) **(B)** and myoepithelial cells expressing p63 **(C)** and SMMS1 **(D)**.

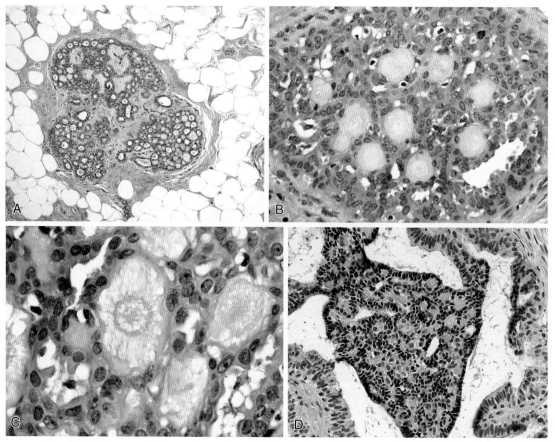

FIG. 6.43

Collagenous spherulosis at low magnification exhibiting a cribriform proliferation with lobulated contours **(A)**. Increasing magnification demonstrates cribriform spherules composed of collagenous- to fibrillary-appearing basement membrane material **(B)** or more mucinous to fibrillary-appearing basement membrane material rimmed by densely pink cuticles **(C)**. The spherules are surrounded by cytologically bland, uniform myoepithelial cells intermixed with true glandular spaces with either empty lumina or occasional apical blebs secreting epithelial mucin **(B, C)**. Collagenous spherulosis may also be observed involving proliferative changes such as papillomas **(D)**.

TABLE 6.14

Histologic and Immunohistochemical Features of Adenoid Cystic Carcinoma (AdCC) Compared With Collagenous Spherulosis

Adenoid Cystic Carcinoma	Collagenous Spherulosis
• Most often palpable, grossly visible mass	• Vast majority are incidentally identified
• Infiltrative microscopic borders	• Circumscribed microscopic borders
• May show a multitude of architectural patterns, including cribriform, tubular, trabecular, and solid	• Typically cribriform architecture, lacking the morphologic variety seen in AdCC
• May have perineural invasion	• Lacks perineural invasion
• May show sebaceous or squamous differentiation	• Lacks sebaceous or squamous differentiation
• May have variably enlarged nuclei with denser chromatin	• Nuclei resemble those of normal ductal epithelial cells
• Relatively uniform deposits of basement membrane material	• Variably collagenous, mucinous, or fibrillary basement membrane material
• Not as often associated with benign proliferative changes or lobular neoplasia	• May often be seen in association with benign proliferative changes, including usual ductal hyperplasia, papilloma, and sclerosing adenosis, as well as lobular carcinoma *in situ*
• Luminal cells strongly and diffusely express c-KIT and MYB	• Luminal cells are usually negative for c-KIT and MYB, although weak and focal expression may be observed
• Majority are negative for ER and PR, although focal expression may infrequently be observed	• Majority express ER and PR in the luminal cells

of AdCC may mimic invasive cribriform carcinoma; however, the latter strongly expresses ER and PR and is composed of only epithelial cells.

Prognosis and Therapy

The prognosis of AdCC of the breast is associated with the histologic subtype. The classic variant typically follows an indolent clinical course, with higher long-term survival rates compared with invasive breast carcinoma of no special type. They tend to present at earlier stages with low rates of axillary metastasis and rarely metastasize to local or distant sites. Radical surgical excision with negative margins is usually curative, with 90% to 100% survival at 10 years. Most studies have shown that grading based on the quantity of the solid component does not correlate well with outcome. The solid-basaloid variant, by contrast, often shows perineural involvement and axillary nodal involvement and may recur several years after excision and follow a prolonged disease course. Distant metastatic disease is more common in the solid-basaloid variant, including to pulmonary, osseous, and cutaneous sites. However, studies have shown that recurrent tumors treated with resection and adjuvant chemotherapy were able to achieve complete remission, and long-term survival has been documented in cases with pulmonary metastasis. Cases with high-grade transformation are rare, with limited cases reported in the literature and most causing death.

Interestingly, studies in microRNA expression have identified similar profiles between normal breast tissue and neoplastic AdCC breast tissue, whereas the profiles of normal salivary and lacrimal gland tissue and neoplastic AdCC salivary and lacrimal gland tissue are distinct from one another. Furthermore, the expression profiles of breast AdCC were different from those of salivary and lacrimal gland AdCC. These findings may offer insight into the divergent biological courses of these tumors based on anatomic site.

ADENOID CYSTIC CARCINOMA – DISEASE FACT SHEET

Definition
▶▶ Invasive biphasic neoplasm composed of epithelial and myoepithelial components, with glandular lumina containing epithelial mucins and pseudolumina containing basement membrane and stromal material

Incidence and Location
▶▶ Comprises 0.1% to 3.5% of all breast tumors
▶▶ Most often localized to the retroareolar region, although any quadrant may be affected
▶▶ The vast majority are unifocal

Age Distribution
▶▶ Peak incidence in postmenopausal women, with an average age of 50–65 years
▶▶ Rare cases occur in adolescents and men

Clinical Features
▶▶ Most often present as a palpable mass in postmenopausal women
▶▶ May present as a smaller nodule on mammographic screening in younger women

Radiologic Features
▶▶ Typically appears as an irregular mass-like lesion or an asymmetrical density that may be heterogeneous or hypoechoic, often with minimal vascularity on Doppler imaging

Prognosis and Therapy
▶▶ Prognosis and management are associated with histologic subtype
▶▶ The classic subtype, which is the most common, is often clinically indolent, with 90%–100% survival at 10 years following radical surgical excision. Most cases present at an early stage, and metastatic involvement is rare.
▶▶ The solid-basaloid variant often shows perineural invasion and axillary nodal metastasis. They more often locally recur and metastasize to distant sites. However, excision and adjuvant chemotherapy have been shown to induce remission, and cases with pulmonary metastasis have been shown to have long-term survival.
▶▶ Only limited cases with high-grade transformation have been reported, with most causing death

---

ADENOID CYSTIC CARCINOMA – PATHOLOGIC FEATURES

Gross Findings
▶▶ Most cases appear as firm, well-circumscribed masses with pushing borders
▶▶ Variably cystic features may be appreciated on cut surfaces
▶▶ Most tumors are between 1 and 3 cm, although they may vary from subcentimeter nodules to masses >12 cm

Microscopic Findings
▶▶ Classic subtype:
  ▶▶ Central cribriform architecture, peripheral tubular architecture
  ▶▶ Trabecular and solid architecture may be seen
  ▶▶ Admixture of epithelial glands that secrete mucins and myoepithelial pseudoglands that contain duplicated basal lamina and stromal matrix
  ▶▶ Cytologically bland neoplastic cells with scant cytoplasm
  ▶▶ Lack significant mitoses
  ▶▶ Occasional perineural invasion
  ▶▶ Squamous or sebaceous elements may be present
▶▶ Solid-basaloid subtype:
  ▶▶ Solid nests of basaloid myoepithelial cells
  ▶▶ Marked nuclear atypia
  ▶▶ Increased mitoses
  ▶▶ May have necrosis
  ▶▶ Perineural invasion more common
  ▶▶ Adjacent morphologically classic AdCC is present

Continued

▶▶ AdCC with high-grade transformation:
  ▶▶ Rare, with literature reports including associated invasive
     ductal carcinoma, small cell carcinoma, and malignant
     myoepithelioma

Pathologic Differential Diagnosis
▶▶ Collagenous spherulosis
▶▶ Less commonly microglandular adenosis, tubular carcinoma, or
   cribriform carcinoma

MICROGLANDULAR ADENOSIS

DIFFERENTIAL DIAGNOSIS: TUBULAR CARCINOMA AND SCLEROSIS ADENOSIS

Clinical Features

MGA of the breast is an exceedingly rare finding that occurs most commonly in the sixth decade of life; however, the entity may be diagnosed over a wide age range. This process is diagnosed in <0.1% of breast biopsies and has been reported only in the female breast. MGA is a bland epithelial proliferation that generally follows an indolent clinical course, most commonly behaving in a benign fashion despite a histomorphologic appearance that may mimic an invasive growth pattern, although MGA has also been considered by some authorities to be a non-obligate precursor of basal-like breast carcinoma. No specific radiologic features are associated with MGA. In many instances, MGA is an incidental microscopic finding. Mammographic microcalcifications and increased tissue density are sometimes described in patients with MGA. A palpable mass may be the presentation for some patients with MGA with a median size of 3 to 4 cm, especially if associated with carcinoma. No specific etiology has been reported to be associated with MGA. Awareness of this entity is important to avoid erroneous overdiagnoses of invasive carcinoma.

Pathologic Features

GROSS FINDINGS

No grossly identifiable lesion may be visualized or palpated in some cases of MGA. When grossly identified, MGA is most often described as an ill-defined area of induration or firmness, typically 3 to 4 cm in size. A mass lesion is usually seen in cases associated with invasive carcinoma.

MICROSCOPIC FINDINGS

MGA appears as an infiltrative, haphazard proliferation of small, rounded glands with open luminal spaces that contain densely eosinophilic, colloid-like, PAS-positive, diastase-resistant secretions. The glands are relatively uniform, comparable in size to a normal breast acinus, and are cytologically bland with uniform nuclei, inconspicuous nucleoli, and amphophilic cytoplasm. The glands are lined by a single layer of flat to cuboidal epithelium, without accompanying myoepithelial cells (Fig. 6.44). However, immunohistochemistry and electron microscopy demonstrate intact basement membranes. Atypical MGA may display cytologic atypia, including vesicular or hyperchromatic nuclei, prominent nucleoli, and nucleomegaly, as well as architectural complexity in the form of glandular crowding, multilayered glandular epithelium, fused or cribriforming glands, lack of intraluminal secretions, and hypercellularity that may obliterate the luminal spaces (Fig. 6.45).

Ancillary Studies

The epithelial cells of MGA usually express cytokeratins, S100, cathepsin D, and EGFR, while they are negative for EMA, ER, PR, and HER2. Myoepithelial cells will be absent by immunohistochemical stains such as p63, calponin, and SMMS1 (Fig. 6.46). Basement membrane markers such as collagen IV and laminin will highlight an intact basement membrane surrounding each individual gland.

Differential Diagnosis

The most important differential diagnosis for MGA is a low-grade invasive ductal carcinoma, particularly tubular carcinoma, given that both entities display non-lobulocentric and infiltrative architecture and lack myoepithelial cells. Although tubular carcinoma is also cytologically bland, the glands in tubular carcinoma display angulated borders and elicit a desmoplastic stromal reaction in comparison with the rounded glands of MGA set in non-desmoplastic stroma (see Fig. 6.8). Furthermore, tubular carcinoma expresses hormone receptors, whereas the vast majority of MGA does not. While basement membranes are absent in tubular carcinoma, they are intact in MGA (Table 6.15). The other major differential diagnosis for MGA is sclerosing adenosis, which is a benign proliferation of small, round to angular tubules compressed by surrounding stromal collagen (Table 6.16). Unlike MGA, the glands in sclerosing adenosis have a lobulocentric distribution, are compressed by sclerosis, and usually possess an easily identifiable myoepithelial cell layer (Fig. 6.47).

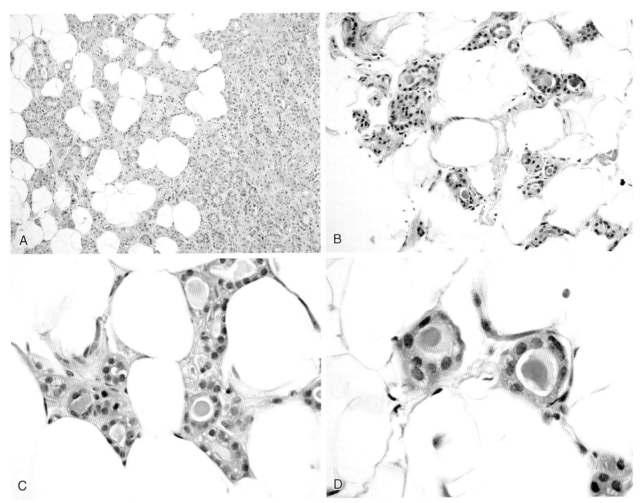

FIG. 6.44

Microglandular adenosis at low magnification with small, round glands dispersed in fibrous tissue that percolate into adjacent adipose tissue **(A)**. These glands are arranged in a non-lobulocentric, haphazard pattern and do not appear compressed by adjacent connective tissue **(B)** with luminal eosinophilic secretory material present in many glands at increasing magnification **(C)**. At high magnification **(D)**, a single layer of epithelial cells is noted without discernable myoepithelial investitures and with bland, flat to cuboidal cells with amphophilic cytoplasm ringing central lumens containing colloid-like eosinophilic material.

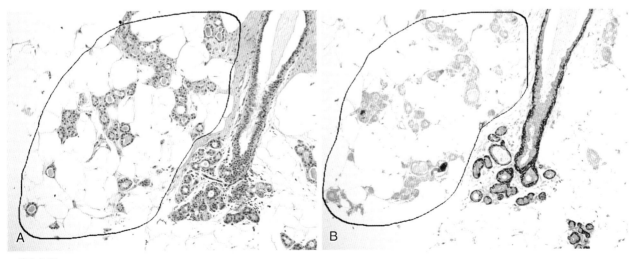

FIG. 6.45

Microglandular adenosis (MGA) at low magnification with small, round glands infiltrating into adipose tissue **(A)** and lacking a myoepithelial cell layer by SMMS1 staining compared with an adjacent benign terminal duct lobular unit **(B)**.

Continued

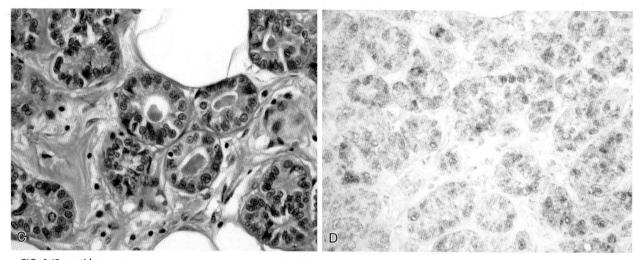

FIG. 6.45, cont'd

Atypical MGA displaying mild nuclear atypia, mild nuclear enlargement, and focal epithelial stratification **(C)**. The epithelial cells of MGA are immunoreactive for S100 **(D)**.

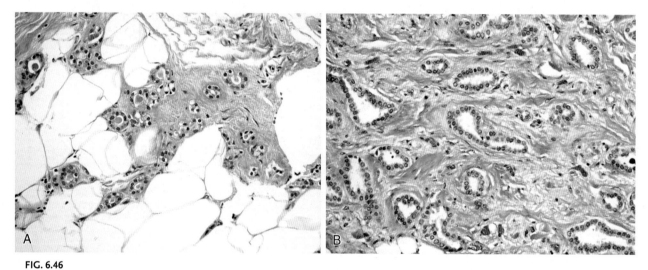

FIG. 6.46

A, Microglandular adenosis at low magnification demonstrating a haphazard proliferation of small, round glands lined by a single layer of cytologically bland epithelial cells percolating through adipose tissue. **B,** Tubular carcinoma (invasive ductal carcinoma, grade 1 with tubular features), by contrast, demonstrating a proliferation of more angulated, teardrop-shaped glands set within a desmoplastic stroma.

TABLE 6.15

Histologic Features of Microglandular Adenosis Compared With Tubular Carcinoma

Microglandular Adenosis	Tubular Carcinoma
• Rounded glands	• Angulated glands
• Dense, eosinophilic luminal secretions	• Less prominent luminal secretions
• No stromal reaction	• Desmoplastic stroma throughout lesion
• Basement membrane intact	• Basement membrane absent
• ER/PR negative; S100 positive	• ER/PR positive; S100 negative
• May be associated with invasive carcinoma	• Associated ADH and/or low-grade DCIS more common

ADH, Atypical ductal hyperplasia; *DCIS,* ductal carcinoma *in situ.*

TABLE 6.16

Histologic Features of Microglandular Adenosis Compared With Sclerosing Adenosis

Microglandular Adenosis	Sclerosing Adenosis
• Non-lobulocentric, haphazard proliferation that may infiltrate into adipose tissue	• Lobulocentric proliferation, but may still extend into adipose tissue
• Rounded glands	• Rounded to angulated glands
• Dense, eosinophilic luminal secretions	• Less prominent luminal secretions
• No glandular compression by stromal collagen	• Compression of glands by intervening stromal collagen
• Myoepithelial investitures absent	• Myoepithelial investitures present
• ER/PR negative; S100 positive	• ER/PR positive; S100 negative
• May be associated with invasive carcinoma	• Associated benign epithelial proliferations more common

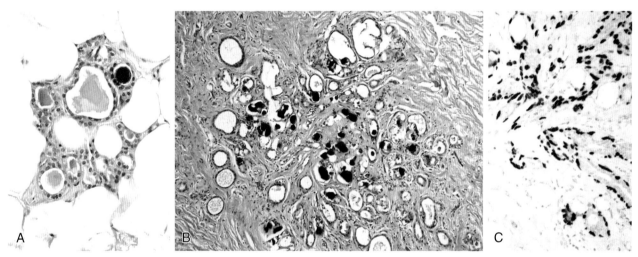

FIG. 6.47

Microglandular adenosis at intermediate magnification with small, round glands containing colloid-like eosinophilic secretions and associated microcalcifications **(A)**. Sclerosing adenosis at low magnification displaying a lobulated arrangement of small, round to angulated epithelial tubules with numerous associated microcalcifications, circumferentially radiating around a central fibroelastotic nidus **(B)** with preserved myoepithelial investitures demonstrated by SMMS1 immunoreactivity **(C)**.

Prognosis and Therapy

Although MGA is considered a benign proliferation, some authorities consider it to be a non-obligate precursor of basal-type breast carcinoma, and rarely of luminal-type breast carcinoma. Studies have reported MGA to be associated with invasive carcinoma in up to 30% of cases, the most common subtypes including basal-like carcinoma, acinic cell carcinoma, AdCC, metaplastic carcinoma, and matrix-producing carcinoma. Array-comparative genomic hybridization-based analyses have demonstrated molecular similarities as well as progressive molecular alterations in MGA/atypical MGA and associated invasive carcinoma.

The prognosis of uncomplicated MGA is favorable. Due to its potential for recurrence and its association with invasive carcinoma, complete excision is recommended.

MICROGLANDULAR ADENOSIS – DISEASE FACT SHEET

Definition

▸▸ Infiltrative, haphazard proliferation of small, rounded glands composed of cytologically bland epithelial cells that lack myoepithelial investitures but retain basement membranes

Incidence and Location

▸▸ Diagnosed in <0.1% of breast biopsies
▸▸ No characteristic location; may be multifocal and/or bilateral

Age Distribution

▸▸ Peak age of incidence in the sixth decade of life
▸▸ Wide age distribution

Clinical Features

▸▸ Most often incidentally diagnosed on breast biopsies performed for other reasons

Continued

MUCOCELE-LIKE LESION

DIFFERENTIAL DIAGNOSES: MUCINOUS CARCINOMA

Clinical Features

Mucocele-like lesion (MLL) is an epithelial lesion characterized by mucin-containing cysts. It is an uncommon lesion with a mammographic finding of pleomorphic or amorphous calcifications or a mass (often produced by clustering of the cysts). Ultrasonography may show a round mass or cystic lesion. In rare instances, they may be palpable. When found in isolation, MLLs are considered benign. In nearly half of the cases, they are associated with atypia or carcinoma. MLLs have a wide age distribution ranging from late 20s to late 70s. A major diagnostic challenge is its distinction from mucinous carcinoma.

Pathologic Features

GROSS FINDINGS

MLLs may not be grossly obvious unless associated with large cysts, gritty calcifications, or grossly distinct lesions.

MICROSCOPIC FINDINGS

MLLs are cystic lesions with small to large cysts most commonly lined by flat to low cuboidal epithelium and containing luminal mucin (Fig. 6.48). MLLs can show a variety of proliferative changes. The epithelial lining is bland in the majority of cases, but in approximately 50% of the cases, association with atypia or carcinoma is reported (Fig. 6.49). Mucin extravasation into the adjacent stroma is not uncommon due to duct rupture and may show detached strips or clusters of epithelial cells floating in the stromal mucin. This feature is particularly challenging on small core biopsy specimens. Multiple levels, and importantly, the cytologic appearance of the epithelial cells, are often helpful in the interpretation of the detached epithelial clusters. Extravasated mucin also contains histiocytes and other inflammatory cells. When not associated with a worse lesion such as ADH or DCIS/invasive carcinoma, the epithelial cells will show bland cytologic features, including uniform oval nuclei and an underlying myoepithelial layer.

Ancillary Studies

Immunohistochemical staining can be helpful in many cases, particularly for demonstrating myoepithelial cells. MLLs have intact myoepithelial layer in the periphery of dilated ducts containing mucin. When epithelial clusters are detached, the myoepithelial cells may not be visualized on H&E-stained sections. Myoepithelial markers, such as p63, calponin, and SMMHC, can be used to demonstrate an intact layer in the periphery. When the epithelium is stripped and floating, myoepithelial cells may be present in association with the floating clusters. Positive staining with myoepithelial markers within the cells floating in mucin may suggest the possibility of MLL. Mucin is usually visible on H&E-stained sections, and immunostaining is not necessary to visualize it. Studies have shown that mucin in MLLs is MUC2 and MUC6 positive. Additionally, MLLs without atypia show heterogeneous staining pattern with ER, similar to benign breast tissue.

Differential Diagnosis

The most common differential and diagnostic dilemma in dealing with MLLs is mucinous carcinoma (Table 6.17).

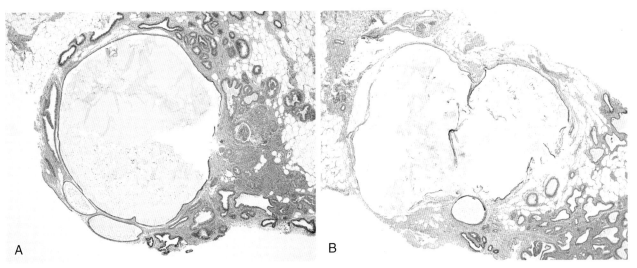

FIG. 6.48

A and B, Mucocele-like lesion at low magnification characterized by small to large cysts lined by flat to low cuboidal epithelium and containing luminal mucin. Areas of acellular stromal mucin extravasation are common. Background breast parenchyma in the right side of both images shows fibrocystic changes, including columnar alteration and usual ductal hyperplasia.

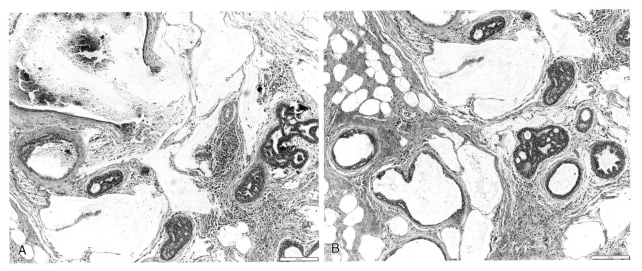

FIG. 6.49

A and B, Mucocele-like lesion with luminal calcifications, extravasated stromal mucin, and associated adjacent atypical ductal hyperplasia.

Mucinous carcinoma is characterized by clusters of neoplastic epithelial cells floating in pools of mucin dissecting through the stroma (Fig. 6.50). While the diagnosis may be more evident on resection specimens, the biggest challenge is making this distinction on biopsy cores, especially in the background of extravasated mucin. The neoplastic cells in mucinous carcinoma usually have low- to intermediate-grade cytologic atypia (Fig. 6.51), which will be very helpful in differentiating from MLLs associated with detached epithelium. Mucinous carcinoma can be associated with low cellularity and making the distinction from MLL even more difficult. The diagnosis becomes particularly more challenging with the detachment of atypical epithelium when MLLs are associated with ADH/DCIS. Using

atypia as criteria may not be ideal in that situation. Often, a background of dilated mucin-containing cysts can help suggest the diagnosis. Ancillary studies can be employed to establish the diagnosis, but in some cases, the differentiation is not possible without the evaluation of an excisional surgical specimen. Myoepithelial markers, such as p63 and calponin, highlight myoepithelial cells around the dilated cysts and within floating epithelial clusters. This finding is of immense help when MLLs are associated with ADH/DCIS. However, it may not always be the case if myoepithelial cells are not present in association with the floating epithelial cells. The ER stain is another marker helpful in the diagnosis. Mucinous carcinoma is strongly and diffusely positive with ER in more than 90% of cases

TABLE 6.17

Clinical, Histologic, and Immunohistochemical Features of Mucocele-like Lesion Compared With Mucinous Carcinoma

Mucocele-like Lesion	Mucinous Carcinoma
• Wide age range at presentation	• Older age at presentation
• A palpable mass is less common	• May present as a palpable mass
• Usually identified on mammography	• Lobulated, round or oval density on imaging
• Cystically dilated ducts containing mucin with stromal extravasation +/– strips of denuded/detached benign epithelial cells	• Floating neoplastic epithelial cell clusters in dissecting pools of mucin
• Uniform cells with ovoid nuclei	• Epithelial cells with low to intermediate grade atypia
• Intact myoepithelial cells around cysts	• Absent myoepithelial cells throughout the lesion
• Myoepithelial cells may be present in floating/detached cell clusters	
• Can be associated with usual ductal hyperplasia, ADH or DCIS	• Frequently associated with ADH or DCIS
• Myoepithelial markers: positive in the periphery of cysts and may be seen in detached clusters	• Myoepithelial markers: Negative
• ER: Heterogeneous staining pattern in pure mucocele-like lesion	• ER: usually strong diffuse staining pattern

ADH, Atypical ductal hyperplasia; *DCIS*, ductal carcinoma *in situ*.

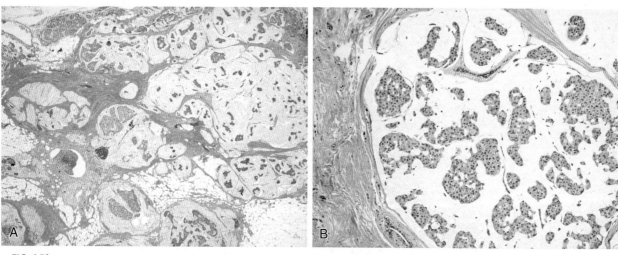

FIG. 6.50

Mucinous carcinoma at low **(A)** and intermediate **(B)** magnification characterized by neoplastic epithelial cells floating in pools of mucin dissecting through the stroma.

(Fig. 6.51), while MLLs without associated ADH/DCIS stain in a heterogeneous pattern similar to benign breast tissue. Correlation with radiologic findings is necessary in challenging cases, especially if the lesion is larger and associated with a mass. When extravasation is extensive, the suspicion of mucinous carcinoma is high, and excision is the most appropriate course or management to rule out that possibility. MLLs associated with ADH or DCIS (see Fig. 6.49) should undergo a complete excision. When a definite diagnosis cannot be rendered, excision is usually recommended. Another entity that may come under the differential diagnosis of the MLL is cystic hypersecretory breast lesions. These lesions are characterized by the presence of cystically dilated ducts containing luminal densely eosinophilic secretions resembling thyroid colloid. The differentiation can be usually made on H&E-stained sections given that the mucin in MLLs is generally pale to bluish.

Prognosis and Therapy

MLLs are associated with ADH/DCIS in nearly half of the cases, and the presence of ADH or DCIS drives the risk of breast cancer development. Lesions definitively diagnosed as MLLs can be left alone as studies suggest, when not associated with atypia and when radiologic

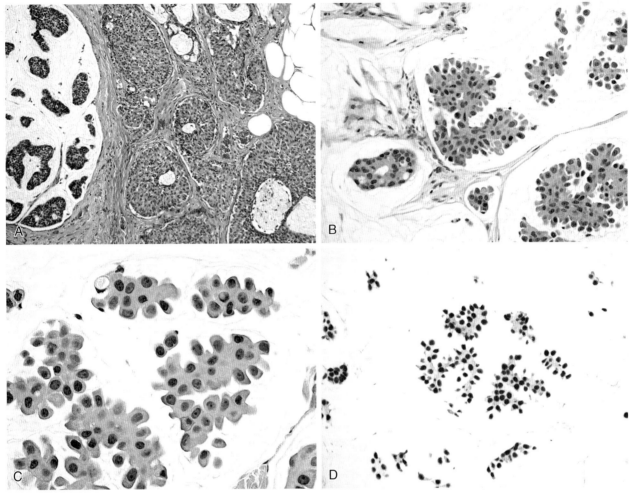

FIG. 6.51
Mucinous carcinoma at low magnification **(A)** demonstrates neoplastic cells freely floating in bluish-appearing mucin *(left)* and carcinoma *in situ* with luminal mucin *(right)*. Intermediate **(B)** and high **(C)** magnification views of floating clusters of neoplastic cells of mucinous carcinoma showing low- to intermediate-grade cytologic atypia with variably prominent nucleoli. Note the fibrous septae between mucin pools **(B)**. Mucinous carcinoma is usually strongly and diffusely estrogen receptor positive **(D)**, unlike the heterogeneous staining pattern in benign mucocele-like lesions.

and clinical findings are not worrisome. Discordant clinicoradiologic results or the presence of atypia warrant an excision to exclude the possibility of invasive carcinoma.

MUCOCELE-LIKE LESION – DISEASE FACT SHEET

Definition
▸▸ Mucin-containing cystic lesion with extravasated stromal mucin

Incidence
▸▸ Most lesions are currently identified by imaging

Age Distribution
▸▸ Wide age range: 20s–70s

Clinical Features
▸▸ Maybe palpable when associated with DCIS or other larger lesion
▸▸ Associated with atypia in 50% cases

Radiologic Features
▸▸ Mammographic findings of cystic lesion
▸▸ Often associated with pleomorphic or clustered calcifications

Prognosis and Therapy
▸▸ Pure MLLs on biopsy do not need excision
▸▸ Risk of cancer is very low when atypia is absent
▸▸ Excision is the treatment of choice when associated with atypia or carcinoma
▸▸ The risk of breast cancer depends on the associated atypical lesion

---

MUCOCELE-LIKE LESION – PATHOLOGIC FEATURES

Gross Findings
▸▸ May not be grossly identifiable
▸▸ If associated with a worse lesion such as DCIS or invasive carcinoma, it may present as a palpable nodule

Continued

ANGIOSARCOMA

DIFFERENTIAL DIAGNOSES: ATYPICAL VASCULAR LESION AND HEMANGIOMA

Clinical Features

Angiosarcoma (AS) is the most common primary and secondary sarcoma to occur in the breast, although it is rare and comprises <1% of all breast malignancies. With increasing implementation of breast-conserving surgery and adjuvant radiation for management of breast cancers, the incidence of postradiation AS is also escalating. Core needle biopsy is recommended for diagnosis, as fine-needle aspiration has a false-negative rate of up to 40%.

Primary AS of the breast is a malignant vascular neoplasm that arises deep within the breast parenchyma and, by definition, is not associated with radiation exposure or chronic lymphedema. Although these tumors may extend into the skin, skin changes are often clinically absent. Most patients present with a rapidly enlarging mass or breast asymmetry, with a median size of 5 cm. Approximately one fifth present with regional disease. These tumors appear on mammography as asymmetrical, non-calcified mass-like lesions, on ultrasound as architectural irregularities with hyperechogenicity or mixed echogenicity, and on contrast-enhanced MRI as heterogeneous enhancements. The median age at presentation is 40 years. Although environmental factors have been implicated, no conclusive etiologies have been established.

Secondary AS of the breast is most commonly attributed to irradiation. Postradiation AS represents an iatrogenic vascular malignancy that develops at a mean latency of 5 to 6 years (ranging from months to decades) following irradiation to the breast and/or chest wall,

most commonly in the setting of breast-conserving surgery and adjuvant radiation therapy for breast carcinoma. Clinically, postradiation AS appears as either single or multiple erythematous skin lesions, ranging from patches and plaques to papules and nodules, or rarely as skin thickening. They tend to present at an older age than primary AS, with a median age of 70 years. More uncommonly, secondary AS of the breast may also arise in the setting of postsurgical chronic lymphedema, known as Stewart-Treves syndrome.

Pathologic Features

GROSS FINDINGS

The gross appearance is variable, ranging from spongy, reddish-brown hemangioma-like lesions in well-differentiated tumors to more solid, fleshy masses with foci of hemorrhage and necrosis with peripherally spongy areas in poorly differentiated tumors. The extent of involvement is unreliable by macroscopic examination.

MICROSCOPIC FINDINGS

Angiosarcomas of the breast display infiltrative tumor borders and may demonstrate a range of histomorphologies. Well-differentiated tumors are composed of well-developed anastomosing, variably compressed to ectatic vascular channels lined by flat to ovoid, mildly atypical endothelial cells (Fig. 6.52). As tumors become higher grade, they exhibit varying combinations of increased cytologic atypia, endothelial hobnailing, multilayering, tufting, intraluminal papillary projections, solid growth, increased mitotic activity, necrosis, and hemorrhagic lakes (see Fig. 6.52). Areas of compressed, slit-like spaces suggestive of vascular differentiation may be noted. Solid architecture is particularly often evident in epithelioid AS, in which the neoplastic endothelial cells exhibit relatively abundant cytoplasm and plump nuclei with nucleomegaly, vesicular chromatin, and macronucleoli.

Primary tumors are usually situated deep within the breast parenchyma with infiltration through fibroadipose tissue and breast lobules. Secondary cutaneous involvement may be noted. Contrastingly, postradiation lesions are centered in the dermis, with variable infiltration into the subcutis and rare infiltration into the mammary parenchyma. Although postradiation lesions typically display some degree of vasoformation, they are often less well-differentiated than primary tumors. As essentially all AS of the breast universally portend an aggressive course, especially those that occur in the postradiation setting, grading of these lesions based on histology is not recommended and they are generally all considered "high grade."

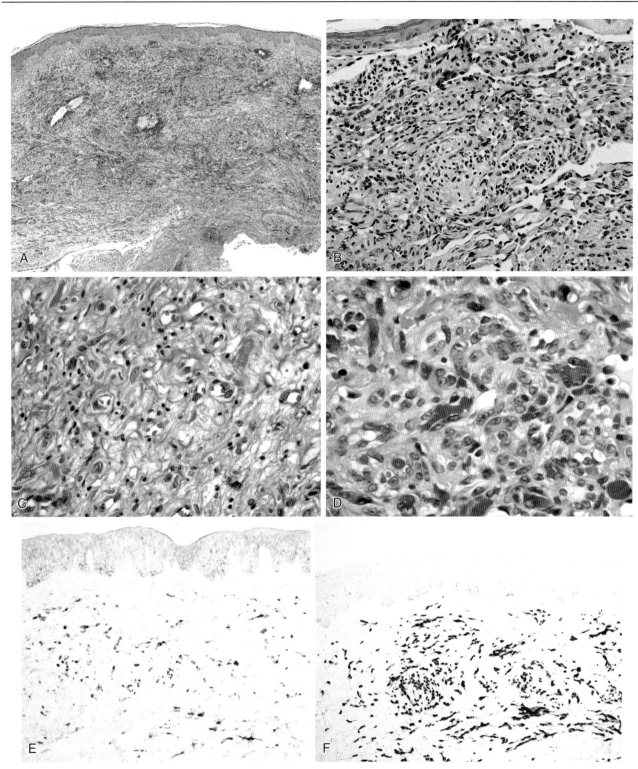

FIG. 6.52

Postradiation angiosarcoma of the breast developing 6 years following irradiation for breast cancer. Low magnification demonstrates an infiltrative, vasoformative neoplastic proliferation dissecting through dermal collagen **(A)**. Increasing magnification displays a haphazard proliferation of variably sized vascular channels **(B)** and more architecturally solid areas composed of cytologically atypical endothelial cells with vesicular to hyperchromatic nuclei, prominent nucleoli, nuclear pleomorphism, and cellular multilayering **(C and D)**. Immunohistochemistry for MYC protein **(E)** and ERG **(F)** demonstrates diffuse expression throughout the tumor.

Ancillary Studies

AS demonstrates strong, diffuse expression of vascular markers including CD31 and ERG, as well as variable expression of CD34, FLI1, and D2-40 (see Fig. 6.52). Focal cytokeratin and rare EMA expression may be observed, particularly in epithelioid subtypes, which poses a major diagnostic pitfall in the differential with carcinoma. Aberrant expression of neuroendocrine markers, CD30, and KIT may also be noted.

Over 90% of postradiation AS demonstrate high-level *MYC* gene amplifications at the 8q24 locus, which may be identified by FISH or by MYC protein overexpression by immunohistochemistry (Table 6.18). A subset of postradiation tumors may also show loss of immunohistochemical expression of H3K27me3. These

studies are useful in distinguishing postradiation AS from postradiation atypical vascular lesions (AVLs), which are consistently MYC negative and H3K27me3 intact. In contrast to postradiation AS, primary AS of the breast rarely harbor *MYC* gene amplification.

Differential Diagnosis

A major diagnostic differential for well-differentiated postradiation AS of the breast is AVLs (Fig. 6.53; Table 6.18). Similar to postradiation AS, AVLs are localized to previously irradiated skin. They present as multiple small (typically up to 0.5 cm), erythematous, papulovesicular cutaneous lesions. Contrary to the cytologically atypical and architecturally infiltrative

---

TABLE 6.18

Histologic and Immunohistochemical Features of Postradiation Angiosarcoma Compared With Atypical Vascular Lesion

Postradiation Angiosarcoma	Atypical Vascular Lesion
• Centered in the dermis, with variable infiltration into the subcutis and rare infiltration into the mammary parenchyma	• Centered in the dermis, predominantly restricted to the superficial to mid dermis with rare involvement of the deep dermis or subcutis
• Infiltrative borders	• Circumscribed borders
• May range from well-differentiated, vasoformative lesions to more poorly differentiated tumors with solid growth	• Consistently form well-formed vascular channels
• May range from well-differentiated tumors with channels lined by a monolayer of atypical endothelial cells to more poorly differentiated tumors displaying increased cytologic atypia, multilayering, tufting, papillary projections, mitoses, necrosis, and hemorrhagic lakes	• Composed of channels lined by a monolayer of variably hyperchromatic, hobnail endothelial cells that lack significant cytologic atypia, multilayering, conspicuous nucleoli, significant mitoses, necrosis, and hemorrhagic lakes
• Over 90% display MYC expression by immunohistochemistry due to high-level gene amplification	• Consistently lack MYC expression by immunohistochemistry
• A subset display loss of H3K27me3	• Retain expression of H3K27me3

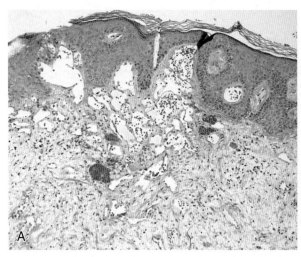 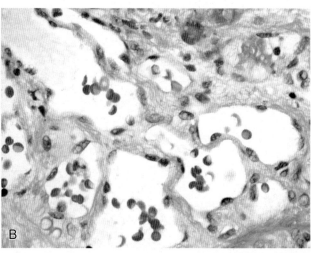

FIG. 6.53

Atypical vascular lesion developing 8 years following irradiation for breast cancer. Low magnification demonstrates a circumscribed proliferation of well-developed, variably ectatic to compressed vascular channels **(A)** lined by a monolayer of variably plump endothelial cells with occasional hobnail morphology and lack of significant cytologic atypia or cellular multilayering **(B)**.

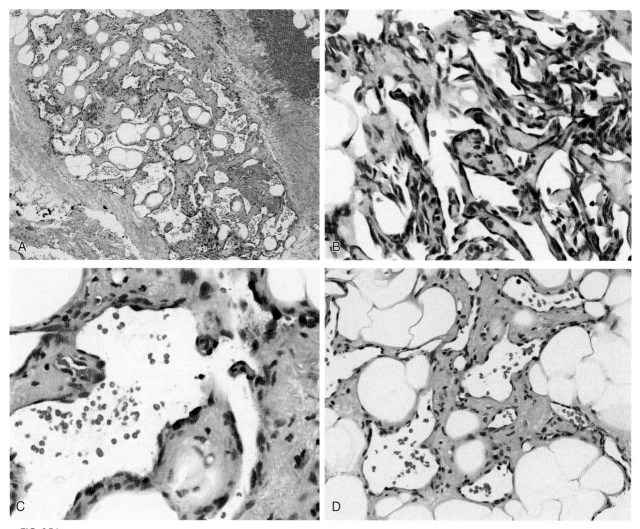

FIG. 6.54

Well-differentiated angiosarcoma of the breast mimicking hemangioma. The lesion is composed of well-formed vascular channels lined by a single layer of relatively inconspicuous endothelial cells at low magnification **(A)**. Increasing magnification shows irregular, anastomosing vascular formations **(B)** composed of a mildly to moderately atypical hyperchromatic endothelial cell proliferation **(C)** that infiltrates through fibroadipose tissue **(D)**.

histologic appearance of postradiation AS, AVL appears as a circumscribed, wedge-shaped, relatively symmetrical proliferation of well-formed vascular channels lined by a single layer of hyperchromatic, hobnail endothelial cells that lack significant cytologic atypia, conspicuous nucleoli, endothelial cell multilayering, necrosis, and mitotic activity (Fig. 6.54). These lesions are typically limited to the superficial and mid dermis, with rare involvement of the deep dermis and subcutis. They consistently lack *MYC* amplification by FISH and MYC overexpression by immunohistochemistry, which are useful ancillary tests to distinguish AVLs from postradiation AS. AVLs are generally considered benign lesions unrelated to AS that may develop secondarily to lymphatic obstruction following radiotherapy. However, some groups suggest that they may represent a precursor of AS, and cases of AS have been reported

to develop in association with AVL. Although the median latency for developing AVL is somewhat shorter (3–6 years) than that of postradiation AS, the causative radiation doses are similar. On core biopsy with limited sampling, the term "atypical vascular proliferation" is preferred, with final classification deferred to an excisional specimen.

Also in the differential diagnosis of well-differentiated AS are other benign entities such as hemangioma and angiomatosis (Table 6.19). Although angiomatosis often displays infiltrative borders, unlike AS, hemangioma and angiomatosis exhibit a relatively uniform distribution of vessels lined by cytologically bland endothelial cells that lack hyperchromasia, significant mitotic activity, lobular disruption, papillae, endothelial tufting, and necrosis (Fig. 6.55). The Ki-67 proliferative index is also generally significantly higher in low-grade AS than in hemangiomas.

TABLE 6.19

Histologic Features of Well-Differentiated Angiosarcoma Compared With Hemangioma

Well-differentiated Angiosarcoma	Hemangioma
• Infiltrative borders	• Circumscribed borders
• Relatively haphazard proliferation of ectatic to compressed vascular channels that dissect through fibroadipose tissue and mammary lobules	• Relatively uniform distribution of well-formed vascular channels that do not disrupt mammary lobules
• Vascular channels lined by a monolayer of mildly to moderately atypical endothelial cells that may display hobnail cytology	• Vascular channels lined by a monolayer of bland endothelial cells that lack hyperchromasia or other cytologic atypia
• More intermediate- to higher-grade lesions display varying degrees and combinations of increased cytologic atypia, multilayering, tufting, papillary projections, mitoses, and necrosis	• Lack cytologic atypia, multilayering, tufting, papillary projections, significant mitoses, and necrosis

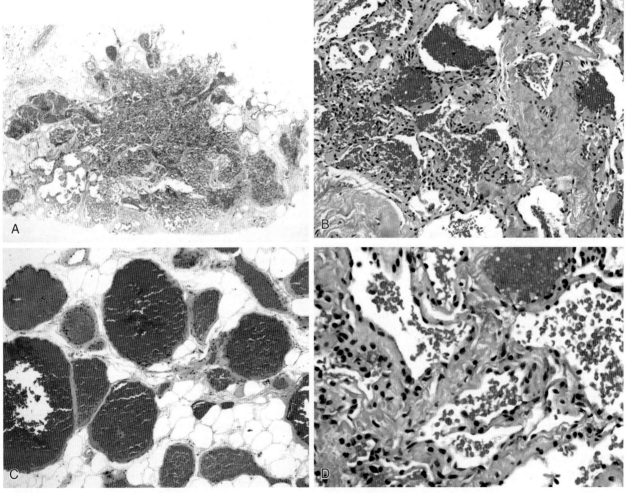

FIG. 6.55

Hemangioma of the breast. Low magnification portraying a lobulated, circumscribed vascular lesion **(A)** that at higher magnification demonstrates a proliferation of well-developed, relatively uniform vascular channels **(B)** with areas of ectatic vessels filled with erythrocytes **(C)** and lining with a monolayer of endothelial cells that lack cytologic atypia and complexity **(D)**.

Importantly, epithelioid AS may be misinterpreted as carcinoma due to its solid growth pattern with limited vasoformation and neoplastic cells that demonstrate polygonal cells with relatively abundant cytoplasm. Moreover, epithelioid AS may also focally express epithelial markers such as cytokeratins and EMA. In contrast to carcinoma, however, epithelioid AS maintains strong and diffuse expression of the vascular markers CD31 and ERG.

Prognosis and Therapy

Primary AS of the breast was historically graded using a three-tier system; however, studies have demonstrated that grade does not correlate with metastatic potential and prognosis. Most cases follow an aggressive course. The most common sites of distant metastasis include the lungs, liver, bones, and central nervous system. Studies have identified genomic alterations involving *KDR (VEGFR2)*, *PIK3CA/PIK3R1*, and *PTPRB*, each occurring at higher frequencies than in AS of other sites, and may guide development of novel targeted therapies.

Postradiation AS is considered universally high grade and portends an aggressive clinical course. Up to half of cases demonstrate local and frequently multiple recurrences, with a median recurrence-free survival of <3 years and a median overall survival of <5 years. Typical sites of metastasis include the lungs, liver, bone, and contralateral breast and skin. In contrast to primary tumors, more than 90% of postradiation AS harbor high-level *MYC* gene amplifications. Reports in the literature vary in regard to potential prognostic differences between primary and secondary AS, with some suggesting that secondary lesions portend a worse prognosis, whereas others report no difference.

AS of the breast is most commonly managed with total mastectomy, although breast-conserving surgery with negative margins may be considered for smaller tumors. However, even with total mastectomy, locoregional recurrences occur in approximately half of cases. As lymph node metastasis is uncommon, with only up to 3.5% of patients having clinical or biopsy-proven nodal metastasis at presentation, prophylactic axillary lymph node dissection without biopsy confirmation is not standardly performed. Various combinations of adjuvant and neoadjuvant radiation and chemotherapy regimens have been utilized in both primary and postradiation AS of the breast. Chemotherapy regimens include anthracycline and taxane-based therapies, which render a 25% (range, 17%–34%) complete or partial response rate in patients with locally advanced or metastatic disease. More novel treatment modalities currently under investigation include targeted therapy with VEGF inhibitors.

ANGIOSARCOMA OF THE BREAST – PATHOLOGIC FEATURES

Gross Findings

▸▸ Variable cut surface, with well-differentiated lesions often imparting a spongy, reddish-brown hemangioma-like appearance and more poorly differentiated lesions displaying a more solid, fleshy appearance with foci of hemorrhage and necrosis and peripherally spongy areas

Microscopic Findings

▸▸ Well-differentiated lesions are composed of variably ectatic and compressed anastomosing vascular channels lined by atypical ovoid endothelial cells that display hyperchromatic to vesicular nuclei, often with prominent small nucleoli

▸▸ Higher-grade lesions demonstrate more solid and cellular growth, increased cytologic atypia, hobnailing, multilayering, tufting, papillary projections, increased mitotic activity, necrosis, and hemorrhagic lakes

▸▸ Epithelioid AS often exhibits a solid proliferation of polygonal endothelial cells with relatively abundant cytoplasm and nuclei displaying nucleomegaly, vesicular chromatin, and macronucleoli

▸▸ Primary AS is more often well-differentiated than secondary AS and infiltrate through fibroadipose tissue and mammary lobules deep within the breast parenchyma

▸▸ Postradiation AS is predominantly centered in the dermis, variably infiltrating into the subcutis and rarely involving the mammary parenchyma

▸▸ The histologic grade of AS of the breast does not seem to correlate with prognosis; most cases follow an aggressive clinical course

Pathologic Differential Diagnoses

▸▸ Atypical vascular lesion
▸▸ Hemangioma/angiomatosis

SUGGESTED READINGS

Complex Sclerosing Lesion/Radial Scar: Tubular Carcinoma and Low-grade Adenosquamous Carcinoma

Aroner SA, Collins LC, Connolly JL, et al. Radial scars and subsequent breast cancer risk: results from the Nurse's Health studies. *Breast Cancer Res Treat*. 2013;139:277-285.

Berg JC, Visscher DW, Vierkant RA, et al. Breast cancer risk in women with radial scars in benign breast biopsies. *Breast Cancer Res Treat*. 2008;108:167-174.

Calhoun BC. Core needle biopsy of the breast an evaluation of contemporary data. *Surg Pathol Clin*. 2018;11:1-16.

Calhoun BC, Collins LC. Recommendations for excision following core needle biopsy of the breast: a contemporary evaluation of the literature. *Histopathology*. 2016;68:138-151.

Conlon N, D'Arcy C, Kaplan JB, et al. Radial scar at image-guided needle biopsy: is excision necessary? *Am J Surg Pathol*. 2015;39:779-785.

Donaldson AR, Sieck L, Booth CN, et al. Radial scars diagnosed on breast core biopsy: frequency of atypia and carcinoma on excision and implications for management. *Breast*. 2016;30:201-207.

Ferreira AI, Borges S, Sous A, et al. Radial scar of the breast: is it possible to avoid surgery? *Eur J Surg Oncol*. 2017;43:1265-1272.

Kawaguchi K, Shin SJ. Immunohistochemical staining characteristics of low-grade adenosquamous carcinoma of the breast. *Am J Surg Pathol*. 2012;36:1009-1020.

Miller CL, West JA, Bettini AC, et al. Surgical excision of radial scars diagnosed by core biopsy may help predict future risk of breast cancer. *Breast Cancer Res Treat*. 2014;145:331-338.

Nassar A, Conners AL, Celik B, et al. Radial scar/complex sclerosing lesions: a clinicopathologic correlation study from a single institution. *Ann Diagn Pathol*. 2015;19:24-28.

Oh EY, Collins LC. Keratin expression patterns in stromal cells of benign sclerosing lesions of the breast. *Arch Pathol Lab Med*. 2015;139: 1143-1148.

Rakha EA, Ahmed MA, Aleskandarany MA, et al. Diagnostic concordance of breast pathologists: lessons from the National Health Service breast screening programme pathology external quality assurance scheme. *Histopathology*. 2017;70:632-642.

Ring NY, DiFlorio-Alexander RM, Bond JS, et al. Papillary and sclerosing lesions of the breast detected and biopsied by MRI: clinical management, upgrade rate and association with apocrine metaplasia. *Breast J*. 2019;25:393-400.

Sanders ME, Page DL, Simpson JF, et al. Interdependence of radial scar and proliferative disease with respect to invasive breast carcinoma risk in patients with benign breast biopsies. *Cancer*. 2006;106:1435-1461.

Cystic Neutrophilic Granulomatous Mastitis: Idiopathic Granulomatous Lobular Mastitis and Sarcoidosis

Benson JR, Dumitru D. Idiopathic granulomatous mastitis: presentation, investigation and management. *Future Oncol*. 2016;11:1381-1394.

D'Alfonso TM, Moo TA, Arleo EK, et al. Cystic neutrophilic granulomatous mastitis: further characterization of a distinctive histopathologic entity not always demonstrable attributable to Corynebacterium infection. *Am J Surg Pathol*. 2015;39:1440-1447.

Endlich JL, Alves Souza J, Ap Bueno de Toledo Osorio C, et al. Breast sarcoidosis as the first manifestation of disease. *Breast J*. 2020;26:543-544.

Gautham I, Radford DM, Kovacs CS, et al. Cystic neutrophilic granulomatous mastitis: the Cleveland Clinic experience with diagnosis and management. *Breast J*. 2019;25:80-85.

Illman JE, Terra SB, Clapp AJ, et al. Granulomatous disease of the breast and axilla: radiological findings with pathological correlation. *Insights Imaging*. 2018;9:59-71.

Johnstone KJ, Robson J, Cherian SG, et al. Cystic neutrophilic granulomatous mastitis associated with Corynebacterium including Corynebacterium kroppenstedtii. *Pathology*. 2017;49:405-412.

Lower EE, Hawkins HH, Baughman RP. Breast disease in sarcoidosis. *Sarcoidosis Vasc Diffuse Lung Dis*. 2001;18:301-306.

Naik MA, Korlimarla A, Shetty ST, et al. Cystic neutrophilic granulomatous mastitis: a clinicopathological study with 16s rRNA sequencing for the detection of Corynebacteria in formalin fixed paraffin embedded tissue. *Int J Surg Pathol*. 2020;28:371-381.

Renshaw AA, Derhagopian RP, Gould EW. Cystic neutrophilic granulomatous mastitis: an underappreciated pattern strongly associated with gram-positive bacilli. *Am J Clin Pathol*. 2011;136:424-427.

Sangoi AR. "Thick section" gram stain yields improve detection of organisms in tissue sections of cystic neutrophilic granulomatous mastitis. *Am J Clin Pathol*. 2020;153:593-597.

Shoyele O, Vidhun R, Dodge J, et al. Cystic neutrophilic granulomatous mastitis: a Clinicopathologic study of a distinct entity with supporting evidence of a role of Corynebacterium targeted therapy. *Ann Diagn Pathol*. 2018;37:51-56.

Troxell ML, Gordon NT, Doggett JS, et al. Cystic neutrophilic granulomatous mastitis: association with gram positive bacilli and Corynebacterium. *Am J Clin Pathol*. 2016;145:635-645.

Wu JM, Turashvili G. Cystic neutrophilic granulomatous mastitis: an update. *J Clin Pathol*. 2020;73:445-453.

Myofibroblastoma: Pseudoangiomatous Stromal Hyperplasia

Boudaouara O, Chaari C, Hassini A, Boudaouara TS. Mammary myofibroblastoma with unusual morphological and immunohistochemical features. *Indian J Med Paediatr Oncol*. 2017;38(2):223-225.

Chen BJ, Mariño-Enríquez A, Fletcher CD, Hornick JL. Loss of retinoblastoma protein expression in spindle cell/pleomorphic lipomas and cytogenetically related tumors: an immunohistochemical study with diagnostic implications. *Am J Surg Pathol*. 2012;36(8):1119-1128.

D'Alfonso TM, Subramaniyam S, Ginter PS, et al. Characterization of CD34-deficient myofibroblastomas of the breast. *Breast J*. 2018; 24(1):55-61.

Howitt BE, Fletcher CD. Mammary-type Myofibroblastoma: clinicopathologic characterization in a series of 143 cases. *Am J Surg Pathol*. 2016;40(3):361-367.

Jung HK, Son JH, Kim WG. Myofibroblastoma of the breast in postmenopausal women: two case reports with imaging findings and review of the literature. *J Clin Ultrasound*. 2020;48(5):279-282.

Krings G, McIntire P, Shin SJ. Myofibroblastic, fibroblastic and myoid lesions of the breast. *Semin Diagn Pathol.* 2017;34(5):427-437.

Magro G, Salvatorelli L, Puzzo L, et al. Practical approach to diagnosis of bland-looking spindle cell lesions of the breast. *Pathologica.* 2019;111(4):344-360.

Magro G. Mammary myofibroblastoma: an update with emphasis on the most diagnostically challenging variants. *Histol Histopathol.* 2016;31(1):1-23.

Magro G. Mammary myofibroblastoma: a tumor with a wide morphologic spectrum. *Arch Pathol Lab Med.* 2008;132(11):1813-1820.

Wargotz ES, Weiss SW, Norris HJ. Myofibroblastoma of the breast. Sixteen cases of a distinctive benign mesenchymal tumor. *Am J Surg Pathol.* 1987;11(7):493-502.

Viswanathan K, Cheng E, Linver MN, Feddersen R, Hoda S. Bilateral multiple mammary myofibroblastomas in an adult male. *Int J Surg Pathol.* 2018;26(3):242-244.

Cellular Fibroadenoma: Benign Phyllodes Tumor

Dessauvagie BF, Lee AHS, Meehan K, et al. Interobserver variation in the diagnosis of fibroepithelial lesions of the breast: a multicentre audit by digital pathology. *J Clin Pathol.* 2018;71(8):672-679.

Durhan G, Önder Ö, Azizova A, et al. Can radiologist and pathologist reach the truth together in the diagnosis of benign fibroepithelial lesions? *Eur J Breast Health.* 2019;15(3):176-182.

Edwards T, Jaffer S, Szabo JR, Sonnenblick EB, Margolies LR. Cellular fibroadenoma on core needle biopsy: management recommendations for the radiologist. *Clin Imaging.* 2016;40(4):587-590.

Jung J, Kang E, Chae SM, et al. Development of a management algorithm for the diagnosis of cellular fibroepithelial lesions from core needle biopsies. *Int J Surg Pathol.* 2018;26(8):684-692.

Krings G, Bean GR, Chen YY. Fibroepithelial lesions; the WHO spectrum. *Semin Diagn Pathol.* 2017;34(5):438-452.

Lawton TJ, Acs G, Argani P, et al. Interobserver variability by pathologists in the distinction between cellular fibroadenomas and phyllodes tumors. *Int J Surg Pathol.* 2014;22(8):695-698.

Loke BN, Md Nasir ND, Thike AA, et al. Genetics and genomics of breast fibroadenomas. *J Clin Pathol.* 2018;71(5):381-387.

Mishima C, Kagara N, Tanei T, et al. Mutational analysis of MED12 in fibroadenomas and phyllodes tumors of the breast by means of targeted next-generation sequencing. *Breast Cancer Res Treat.* 2015; 152(2):305-312.

Tan BY, Acs G, Apple SK, et al. Phyllodes tumours of the breast: a consensus review. *Histopathology.* 2016;68(1):5-21.

Tay TK, Chang KT, Thike AA, Tan PH. Paediatric fibroepithelial lesions revisited: pathological insights. *J Clin Pathol.* 2015;68(8):633-641.

Yasir S, Nassar A, Jimenez RE, et al. Cellular fibroepithelial lesions of the breast: a long term follow up study. *Ann Diagn Pathol.* 2018; 35:85-91.

Yasir S, Gamez R, Jenkins S, Visscher DW, Nassar A. Significant histologic features differentiating cellular fibroadenoma from phyllodes tumor on core needle biopsy specimens. *Am J Clin Pathol.* 2014;142(3):362-369.

Columnar Cell Lesion: Flat Epithelial Atypia

Schnitt SJ, Vincent-Salomon A. Columnar cell lesions of the breast. *Adv Anat Pathol.* 2003;10(3):113-124. doi:10.1097/00125480-200305000-00001.

Datrice N, Narula N, Maggard M, et al. Do breast columnar cell lesions with atypia need to be excised? *Am Surg.* 2007;73(10):984-986.

Lerwill MF. Flat epithelial atypia of the breast. *Arch Pathol Lab Med.* 2008;132(4):615-621. doi:10.1043/1543-2165(2008)132[615:FEAOTB]2.0.CO;2.

Said SM, Visscher DW, Nassar A, et al. Flat epithelial atypia and risk of breast cancer: a Mayo cohort study. *Cancer.* 2015;121(10):1548-1555. doi:10.1002/cncr.29243.

Grabenstetter A, Brennan S, Salagean ED, Morrow M, Brogi E. Flat epithelial atypia in breast core needle biopsies with radiologic-pathologic concordance: is excision necessary? *Am J Surg Pathol.* 2020;44(2):182-190. doi:10.1097/PAS.0000000000001385.

Abdel-Fatah TM, Powe DG, Hodi Z, Reis-Filho JS, Lee AH, Ellis IO. Morphologic and molecular evolutionary pathways of low nuclear grade invasive breast cancers and their putative precursor lesions: further evidence to support the concept of low nuclear grade breast

neoplasia family. *Am J Surg Pathol.* 2008;32(4):513-523. doi:10.1097/PAS.0b013e318161d1a5.

Sudarshan M, Meguerditchian AN, Mesurolle B, Meterissian S. Flat epithelial atypia of the breast: characteristics and behaviors. *Am J Surg.* 2011;201(2):245-250. doi:10.1016/j.amjsurg.2010.02.009.

O'Malley FP, Mohsin SK, Badve S, et al. Interobserver reproducibility in the diagnosis of flat epithelial atypia of the breast. *Mod Pathol.* 2006;19(2):172-179. doi:10.1038/modpathol.3800514.

Calhoun BC, Sobel A, White RL, et al. Management of flat epithelial atypia on breast core biopsy may be individualized based on correlation with imaging studies. *Mod Pathol.* 2015;28(5):670-676. doi:10.1038/modpathol.2014.159.

Jara-Lazaro AR, Tse GM, Tan PH. Columnar cell lesions of the breast: an update and significance on core biopsy. *Pathology.* 2009;41(1):18-27. doi:10.1080/00313020802563486.

Atypical Ductal Hyperplasia: Usual Ductal Hyperplasia and Ductal Carcinoma *In Situ*

Hartmann LC, Degnim AC, Santen RJ, Dupont WD, Ghosh K. Atypical hyperplasia of the breast--risk assessment and management options. *N Engl J Med.* 2015;372(1):78-89. doi:10.1056/NEJMsr1407164.

Vandenbussche CJ, Khouri N, Sbaity E, et al. Borderline atypical ductal hyperplasia/low-grade ductal carcinoma in situ on breast needle core biopsy should be managed conservatively. *Am J Surg Pathol.* 2013;37(6):913-923. doi:10.1097/PAS.0b013e31828ba25c.

Hartmann LC, Radisky DC, Frost MH, et al. Understanding the premalignant potential of atypical hyperplasia through its natural history: a longitudinal cohort study. *Cancer Prev Res (Phila).* 2014;7(2):211-217. doi:10.1158/1940-6207.CAPR-13-0222.

Martinez AP, Cohen C, Hanley KZ, Li XB. Estrogen receptor and cytokeratin 5 are reliable markers to separate usual ductal hyperplasia from atypical ductal hyperplasia and low-grade ductal carcinoma in situ. *Arch Pathol Lab Med.* 2016;140(7):686-689. doi:10.5858/arpa.2015-0238-OA.

Neal L, Sandhu NP, Hieken TJ, et al. Diagnosis and management of benign, atypical, and indeterminate breast lesions detected on core needle biopsy. *Mayo Clin Proc.* 2014;89(4):536-547. doi:10.1016/j.mayocp.2014.02.004.

Wagoner MJ, Laronga C, Acs G. Extent and histologic pattern of atypical ductal hyperplasia present on core needle biopsy specimens of the breast can predict ductal carcinoma in situ in subsequent excision. *Am J Clin Pathol.* 2009;131(1):112-121. doi:10.1309/AJCPGHEJ2R8UYFGP.

Barr FE, Degnim AC, Hartmann LC, et al. Estrogen receptor expression in atypical hyperplasia: lack of association with breast cancer. *Cancer Prev Res (Phila).* 2011;4(3):435-444. doi:10.1158/1940-6207.CAPR-10-0242.

Page DL, Rogers LW. Combined histologic and cytologic criteria for the diagnosis of mammary atypical ductal hyperplasia. *Hum Pathol.* 1992;23(10):1095-1097. doi:10.1016/0046-8177(92)90026-y.

Otterbach F, Bànkfalvi A, Bergner S, Decker T, Krech R, Boecker W. Cytokeratin 5/6 immunohistochemistry assists the differential diagnosis of atypical proliferations of the breast. *Histopathology.* 2000;37(3):232-240. doi:10.1046/j.1365-2559.2000.00882.x.

Page DL, Dupont WD, Rogers LW, Rados MS. Atypical hyperplastic lesions of the female breast. A long-term follow-up study. *Cancer.* 1985;55(11):2698-2708. doi:10.1002/1097-0142(19850601)55: 11<2698::aid-cncr2820551127>3.0.co;2-a.

Fisher B, Costantino JP, Wickerham DL, et al. Tamoxifen for prevention of breast cancer: report of the National Surgical Adjuvant Breast and Bowel Project P-1 Study. *J Natl Cancer Inst.* 1998;90(18):1371-1388. doi:10.1093/jnci/90.18.1371.

Pleomorphic Lobular Carcinoma *In Situ*: Solid Ductal Carcinoma *In Situ*

Blanco LZ, Thurow TA, Mahajan A, et al. Multinucleation is an objective feature useful in the diagnosis of pleomorphic lobular carcinoma in situ. *Am J Clin Pathol.* 2015;144:722-726.

De Brot M, Koslow Mautner S, Muhsen S, et al. Pleomorphic lobular carcinoma in situ of the breast: a single institution experience with clinical follow-up and centralized pathology review. *Breast Cancer Res Treat.* 2017;165:411-420.

Ginter PS, D'Alfonso TM. Current concepts in diagnosis, molecular features and management of lobular carcinoma in situ of the breast with a discussion of morphologic variants. *Arch Pathol Lab Med.* 2017;141:1668-1678.

Harrison BT, Nakhlis F, Dillon, DA, et al. Genomic profiling of pleomorphic and florid lobular carcinoma in situ reveals highly recurrent ERBB2 and ERBB3 alterations. *Mod Pathol.* 2020;33:1287-1297.

King TA, Reis-Filho JS. Lobular neoplasia. *Surg Oncol Clin N Am.* 2014;23:487-503.

Masannat YA, Husain E, Roylance R, et al. Pleomorphic LCIS what do we know? A UK multicenter audit of pleomorphic lobular carcinoma in situ. *Breast.* 2018;38:120-125.

Shamir ER, Chen YY, Chu T, et al. Pleomorphic and florid lobular carcinoma in situ variants of the breast: a Clinicopathologic study of 85 cases with and without invasive carcinoma from a single academic center. *Am J Surg Pathol.* 2019;43:399-408.

Shamir ER, Chen YY, Krings G. Genetic analysis of pleomorphic and florid lobular carcinoma in situ variants; frequent ERBB2/ERBB3 alterations and clonal relationship to classic lobular carcinoma in situ and invasive lobular carcinoma. *Mod Pathol.* 2020;33:1078-1091.

Wazir U, Wazir A, Wells C, et al. Pleomorphic lobular carcinoma in situ: current evidence and a systemic review. *Oncol Lett.* 2016;12: 4863-4868.

Wen HY, Brogi E. Lobular carcinoma in situ. *Surg Pathol Clin.* 2018;11:123-145.

Zhong E, Solomon JP, Cheng E. et al. Apocrine variant of pleomorphic lobular carcinoma in situ. *Am J Surg Pathol.* 2020;44:1092-1103.

Intraductal Papilloma: Encapsulated Papillary Carcinoma and Papillary Ductal Carcinoma *In Situ*

Agoumi M, Giambattista J, Hayes MM. Practical considerations in breast papillary lesions: a review of the literature. *Arch Pathol Lab Med.* 2016;140(8):770-790.

Chen P, Zhou D, Wang C, Ye G, Pan R, Zhu L. Treatment and outcome of 341 papillary breast lesions. *World J Surg.* 2019;43(10):2477-2482.

Genco IS, Tugertimur B, Manolas PA, Hasanovic A, Hajiyeva S. Upgrade rate of intraductal papilloma without atypia on breast core needle biopsy: a clinical, radiological and pathological correlation study. *Am J Surg.* 2020;220(3):677-681.

Hong YR, Song BJ, Jung SS, Kang BJ, Kim SH, Chae BJ. Predictive factors for upgrading patients with benign breast papillary lesions using a core needle biopsy. *J Breast Cancer.* 2016;19(4):410-416.

Jakate K, De Brot M, Goldberg F, Muradali D, O'Malley FP, Mulligan AM. Papillary lesions of the breast: impact of breast pathology subspecialization on core biopsy and excision diagnoses. *Am J Surg Pathol.* 2012;36(4):544-551.

MacColl C, Salehi A, Parpia S, Hodgson N, Ramonas M, Williams P. Benign breast papillary lesions diagnosed on core biopsy: upgrade rate and risk factors associated with malignancy on surgical excision. *Virchows Arch.* 2019;475(6):701-707.

Nasehi L, Sturgis CD, Sharma N, Turk P, Calhoun BC. Breast cancer risk associated with benign intraductal papillomas initially diagnosed on core needle biopsy. *Clin Breast Cancer.* 2018;18(6):468-473.

Oyama T, Koerner FC. Noninvasive papillary proliferations. *Semin Diagn Pathol.* 2004;21(1):32-41.

Pareja F, Corben AD, Brennan SB, et al. Breast intraductal papillomas without atypia in radiologic-pathologic concordant core-needle biopsies: rate of upgrade to carcinoma at excision. *Cancer.* 2016;122(18):2819-2827.

Ueng SH, Mezzetti T, Tavassoli FA. Papillary neoplasms of the breast: a review. *Arch Pathol Lab Med.* 2009;133(6):893-907.

Wei S. Papillary lesions of the breast: an update. *Arch Pathol Lab Med.* 2016;140(7):628-643.

Nipple Adenoma: Invasive Carcinoma

Aftab K, Idrees R. Nipple adenoma of breast: a masquerader of malignancy. *J Coll Physicians Surg Pak.* 2010;20:472-474.

Alhayo ST, Edirimanne S. Clinically challenging case of nipple adenoma. *Breast J.* 2018;24:1084-1085.

Cai S, Wang H, Zhu Q, et al. Clinical and sonographic features of nipple lesions. *Medicine.* 2020;99:1-15.

Di Bonito M, Cantile M, Collina F, et al. Adenoma of the nipple: a clinicopathological report of 13 cases. *Oncol Lett.* 2014;7:1839-1842.

Fernandez-Flores A, Suarez-Penaranda JM. Immunophenotype of nipple adenoma in a male patient. *Appl Immunohistochem Mol Morphol.* 2011;19:190-194.

Owen JL. Successful treatment of nipple adenoma using Mohs micrographic surgery to preserve the nipple-areolar complex. *Dermatol Surg.* 2020;46:132-135.

Pasquali P, Freites-Martinez A, Fortuno A. Nipple adenoma: new images and cryosurgery treatment. *Breast J.* 2016;22:584-585.

Rao P, Shousha S. Male nipple adenoma with DCIS followed 9 years later by invasive carcinoma. *Breast J.* 2010;16:317-318.

Stone K, Wheeler A. A review of anatomy, physiology and benign pathology of the nipple. *Ann Surg Oncol.* 2015;22:3236-3240.

Yang GZ, Li J, Ding HY. Nipple adenoma: a report of 18 cases with review of literature. *Zhonghua Bing Li Xue Za Zhi.* 2009:38;614-616.

Adenoid Cystic Carcinoma: Collagenous Spherulosis

Andreasen S, Tan Q, Agander TK, et al. Adenoid cystic carcinomas of the salivary gland, lacrimal gland, and breast are morphologically and genetically similar but have distinct microRNA expression profiles. *Mod Pathol.* 2018;31(8):1211-1225.

Azoulay S, Laé M, Fréneaux P, et al. KIT is highly expressed in adenoid cystic carcinoma of the breast, a basal-like carcinoma associated with a favorable outcome. *Mod Pathol.* 2005;18(12):1623-1631.

Chae YK, Chung SY, Davis AA, et al. Adenoid cystic carcinoma: current therapy and potential therapeutic advances based on genomic profiling. *Oncotarget.* 2015;6(35):37117-37134.

D'Alfonso TM, Mosquera JM, MacDonald TY, et al. MYB-NFIB gene fusion in adenoid cystic carcinoma of the breast with special focus paid to the solid variant with basaloid features. *Hum Pathol.* 2014;45(11):2270-2280.

Foschini MP, Morandi L, Asioli S, Giove G, Corradini AG, Eusebi V. The morphological spectrum of salivary gland type tumours of the breast. *Pathology.* 2017;49(2):215-227.

Fusco N, Geyer FC, De Filippo MR, et al. Genetic events in the progression of adenoid cystic carcinoma of the breast to high-grade triple-negative breast cancer. *Mod Pathol.* 2016;29(11):1292-1305.

Kim J, Geyer FC, Martelotto LG, et al. MYBL1 rearrangements and MYB amplification in breast adenoid cystic carcinomas lacking the MYB-NFIB fusion gene. *J Pathol.* 2018;244(2):143-150.

Marotti JD, Schnitt SJ. Genotype-phenotype correlations in breast cancer. *Surg Pathol Clin.* 2018;11(1):199-211.

Martelotto LG, De Filippo MR, Ng CK, et al. Genomic landscape of adenoid cystic carcinoma of the breast. *J Pathol.* 2015;237(2): 179-189.

Massé J, Truntzer C, Boidot R, et al. Solid-type adenoid cystic carcinoma of the breast, a distinct molecular entity enriched in NOTCH and CREBBP mutations. *Mod Pathol.* 2020;33(6):1041-1055. doi:10.1038/s41379-019-0425-3.

Pia-Foschini M, Reis-Filho JS, Eusebi V, Lakhani SR. Salivary gland-like tumours of the breast: surgical and molecular pathology [published correction appears in J Clin Pathol. 2003;56(10):804]. *J Clin Pathol.* 2003;56(7):497-506.

Poling JS, Yonescu R, Subhawong AP, et al. MYB Labeling by immunohistochemistry is more sensitive and specific for breast adenoid cystic carcinoma than MYB labeling by FISH. *Am J Surg Pathol.* 2017;41(7):973-979.

Rabban JT, Swain RS, Zaloudek CJ, Chase DR, Chen YY. Immunophenotypic overlap between adenoid cystic carcinoma and collagenous spherulosis of the breast: potential diagnostic pitfalls using myoepithelial markers. *Mod Pathol.* 2006;19(10):1351-1357.

Slodkowska E, Xu B, Kos Z, et al. Predictors of outcome in mammary adenoid cystic carcinoma: a multi-institutional study. *Am J Surg Pathol.* 2020;44(2):214-223.

Treitl D, Radkani P, Rizer M, El Hussein S, Paramo JC, Mesko TW. Adenoid cystic carcinoma of the breast, 20 years of experience in a single center with review of literature. *Breast Cancer.* 2018;25(1):28-33.

Microglandular Adenosis: Tubular Carcinoma and Sclerosing Adenosis

Damron AT, Korhonen K, Zuckerman S, et al. Microglandular adenosis: a possible non-obligate precursor to breast carcinoma with potential to either luminal-type or basal-type differentiation. *Int J Surg Pathol.* 2019;27:781-787.

Foschini MP, Eusebi V. Microglandular adenosis of the breast: a deceptive and still mysterious benign lesion. *Human Pathol.* 2018;82:1-9.

Geyer FC, Berman SH, Marchio C, et al. Genetic analysis of microglandular adenosis and acinic cell carcinoma of the breast provides evidence for the existence of a low-grade triple negative breast neoplasia family. *Mod Pathol.* 2017;30:69-84.

Khalifeh IM, Albarracin C, Diaz LK, et al. Clinical, histopathologic and immunohistochemical features of microglandular adenosis and transition into in situ and invasive carcinoma. *Am J Surg Pathol.* 2008;32:544-552.

Kim GE, Kim NI, Lee JS, et al. Metaplastic carcinoma with chondroid differentiation arising in microglandular adenosis. *J Pathol Transl Med.* 2017;51:418-421.

Kravtsov O, Jorns JM. Microglandular adenosis and associated invasive carcinoma. *Arch Pathol Lab Med.* 2019;144:42-46.

Lea V, Gluch L, Kennedy CW, et al. Tubular carcinoma of the breast: axillary involvement and prognostic factors. *ANZ J Surg.* 2015;85:448-451.

Muller KE, Jorns JM. Metaplastic carcinoma with extensive chondromyxoid differentiation arising in association with microglandular adenosis. *Int J Surg Pathol.* 2017;25:513-514.

Rosen PP. So-called acinic cell carcinoma of the breast arises from microglandular adenosis and is not a distinct entity. *Mod Pathol.* 2017;30:1504.

Salarieh A, Sneige N. Breast carcinoma arising in microglandular adenosis: a review of the literature. *Arch Pathol Lab Med.* 2007; 131:1397-1399.

Schwartz CJ, Dolgalev I, Yoon E, et al. Microglandular adenosis is an advanced precursor breast lesion with evidence of molecular progression to matrix-producing metaplastic carcinoma. *Hum Pathol.* 2019;85:65-71.

Spruill L. Benign mimickers of malignant breast lesions. *Semin Diagn Pathol.* 2016;33:2-12.

Shui R, Yang W. Invasive breast carcinoma arising in microglandular adenosis: a case report and review of the literature. *Breast J.* 2009; 15:653-656.

Tavassoli FA, Bratthauer GL. Immunohistochemical profile and differential diagnosis of microglandular adenosis. *Mod Pathol.* 1993;6:318-322.

Mucocele-like Lesion: Mucinous Carcinoma

Carder PJ, Murphy CE, Liston JC. Surgical excision is warranted following a core biopsy diagnosis of mucocele-like lesion of the breast. *Histopathology.* 2004;45(2):148-154. doi:10.1111/j.1365-2559.2004.01920.x.

Ha D, Dialani V, Mehta TS, Keefe W, Iuanow E, Slanetz PJ. Mucocele-like lesions in the breast diagnosed with percutaneous biopsy: is surgical excision necessary? *AJR Am J Roentgenol.* 2015;204(1):204-210. doi:10.2214/AJR.13.11988.

Weaver MG, Abdul-Karim FW, al-Kaisi N. Mucinous lesions of the breast. A pathological continuum. *Pathol Res Pract.* 1993;189(8):873-876. doi:10.1016/S0344-0338(11)81097-6.

Glazebrook K, Reynolds C. Original report. Mucocele-like tumors of the breast: mammographic and sonographic appearances. *AJR Am J Roentgenol.* 2003;180(4):949-954. doi:10.2214/ajr.180.4.1800949.

Kim SM, Kim HH, Kang DK, et al. Mucocele-like tumors of the breast as cystic lesions: sonographic-pathologic correlation. *AJR Am J Roentgenol.* 2011;196(6):1424-1430. doi:10.2214/AJR.10.5028.

Tan PH, Tse GM, Bay BH. Mucinous breast lesions: diagnostic challenges. *J Clin Pathol.* 2008;61(1):11-19. doi:10.1136/jcp.2006.046227.

Molavi D, Argani P. Distinguishing benign dissecting mucin (stromal mucin pools) from invasive mucinous carcinoma. *Adv Anat Pathol.* 2008;15(1):1-17. doi:10.1097/PAP.0b013e31815e52aa.

Harrison BT, Dillon DA. An update of mucinous lesions of the breast. *Surg Pathol Clin.* 2018;11(1):61-90. doi:10.1016/j.path.2017.09.002.

Ginter PS, Tang X, Shin SJ. A review of mucinous lesions of the breast. *Breast J.* 2020;26(6):1168-1178. doi:10.1111/tbj.13878.

Rakha EA, Shaaban AM, Haider SA, et al. Outcome of pure mucocele-like lesions diagnosed on breast core biopsy. *Histopathology.* 2013;62(6):894-898. doi:10.1111/his.12081.

Angiosarcoma: Atypical Vascular Lesion and Hemangioma

Abdou Y, Elkhanany A, Attwood K, Ji W, Takabe K, Opyrchal M. Primary and secondary breast angiosarcoma: single center report and a meta-analysis. *Breast Cancer Res Treat.* 2019;178(3):523-533.

Alves I, Marques JC. Radiation-induced angiosarcoma of the breast: a retrospective analysis of 15 years' experience at an oncology center. *Radiol Bras.* 2018;51(5):281-286.

Baker GM, Schnitt SJ. Vascular lesions of the breast. *Semin Diagn Pathol.* 2017;34(5):410-419.

Beca F, Krings G, Chen YY, et al. Primary mammary angiosarcomas harbor frequent mutations in KDR and PIK3CA and show evidence of distinct pathogenesis. *Mod Pathol.* 2020;10:1038.

Brenn T, Fletcher CD. Radiation-associated cutaneous atypical vascular lesions and angiosarcoma: clinicopathologic analysis of 42 cases. *Am J Surg Pathol.* 2005;29(8):983-996.

Cornejo KM, Deng A, Wu H, et al. The utility of MYC and FLT4 in the diagnosis and treatment of postradiation atypical vascular lesion and angiosarcoma of the breast. *Hum Pathol.* 2015;46(6):868-875.

Corradini AG, Asioli S, Morandi L, et al. Post-radiotherapy vascular lesions of the breast: immunohistochemical and molecular features of 74 cases with long term follow up and literature review. *Histopathology.* 2020;77(2):293-302. doi:10.1111/his.14090.

Ginter PS, Mosquera JM, MacDonald TY, D'Alfonso TM, Rubin MA, Shin SJ. Diagnostic utility of MYC amplification and anti-MYC immunohistochemistry in atypical vascular lesions, primary or radiation-induced mammary angiosarcoma, and primary angiosarcoma of other sites. *Hum Pathol.* 2014;45(4):709-716.

Nascimento AF, Raut CP, Fletcher CD. Primary angiosarcoma of the breast: clinicopathologic analysis of 49 cases, suggesting that grade is not prognostic. *Am J Surg Pathol.* 2008;32(12):1896-1904.

Ragavan S, Lim HJ, Tan JW, et al. Axillary lymph node dissection in angiosarcoma of the breast: an Asian institutional perspective. *Sarcoma.* 2020;2020:4890803.

Ronen S, Ivan D, Torres-Cabala CA, et al. Post-radiation vascular lesions of the breast. *J Cutan Pathol.* 2019;46(1):52-58.

Salminen SH, Wiklund T, Sampo MM, et al. Treatment and prognosis of radiation-associated breast angiosarcoma in a nationwide population. *Ann Surg Oncol.* 2020;27(4):1002-1010.

Zdravkovic D, Granic M, Crnokrak B. Proper treatment of breast angiosarcoma—mastectomy or breast conserving surgery? *Breast Cancer Res Treat.* 2020;179(3):765.

Bone and Joint

John D. Reith • Scott E. Kilpatrick

DISEASES OF JOINTS

PRIMARY DEGENERATIVE JOINT DISEASE DIFFERENTIAL DIAGNOSIS: SECONDARY DEGENERATIVE JOINT DISEASE OF ANY CAUSE

Clinical Features

Primary degenerative joint disease (DJD) is the most common form of arthritis and causes progressively worsening pain, swelling, and lack of mobility in the affected joint, most often starting in the sixth and seventh decades when the reparative mechanisms can no longer keep pace with the degeneration of the articular cartilage. The large weight-bearing joints—the hips, knees, and spine—are most commonly affected, but DJD can also occur in the hands, wrists, and shoulders.

Secondary DJD, as the name implies, results from an underlying condition that causes destruction of the articular cartilage. Conditions that predispose patients to secondary DJD include osteonecrosis (avascular necrosis [AVN]), hip dysplasia, trauma, crystal deposition disorders, and Paget disease, among others.

Radiographic Features

The loss of articular cartilage manifests radiographically as narrowing of the joint space. The loss of joint space is usually accompanied by osteosclerosis of the subchondral bone on both sides of the joint, subchondral cysts, and reparative osteophytes at the periphery of the joint (Fig. 7.1).

Pathologic Features

GROSS FINDINGS

The gross changes in DJD are similar regardless of which joint is involved (Fig. 7.2). The degree of cartilage damage can vary tremendously from case to case, and early in the course of the disease, the cartilage may appear "velvety" when the superficial aspect of the cartilage is affected. Later, the full thickness of the cartilage is destroyed, and as the subchondral bone on either side of the joint articulates, it becomes thickened and "polished," a gross feature referred to as "eburnation." Subchondral cysts and exaggerated reactive osteocartilaginous excrescences known as osteophytes may also form. The synovium may appear normal or become markedly hyperplastic.

MICROSCOPIC FINDINGS

The microscopic features (Fig. 7.3) very closely mimic the gross and radiographic appearance of the joint. Early, the cartilage develops fibrillations or cracks, which may remain superficial or extend full thickness to the tide mark. The tide mark is often duplicated or even triplicated. At this stage, the chondrocytes become clustered ("cloned") and the proteoglycan ground substance surrounding the chondrocytes may appear more prominent than usual. Reactive fibrocartilaginous nodules frequently extend from the subchondral bone to the articular surface. Eventually the full thickness of the cartilage is destroyed, and the subchondral bone becomes sclerotic, resembling cortical lamellar bone. The content of the subchondral cysts can vary from mucoid material to loose, edematous fibrous tissue. Osteophytes are reparative osteocartilaginous excrescences extending from the peripheral margins of the joint surface. The synovium may appear normal or show papillary hyperplasia, mild chronic synovitis, detritic synovitis (fragments of bone or cartilage buried in the synovium), or hemosiderotic synovitis.

Differential Diagnosis

The distinction between primary and secondary DJD rests on the identification of an underlying process. In primary DJD, there is no evidence of an underlying etiology, whereas in secondary DJD an underlying cause is identified. Some underlying etiologies are more easily detected

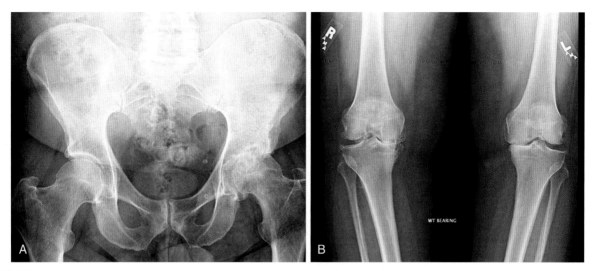

FIG. 7.1

A, Plain radiograph of the pelvis shows loss of the normal joint space in the left hip, as well as patchy sclerosis and subchondral cystic changes in the femoral head and acetabulum, indicative of degenerative joint disease. **B,** Plain radiograph of the knees shows loss of the normal joint space in the medial compartment of both joints, indicating bilateral degenerative joint disease.

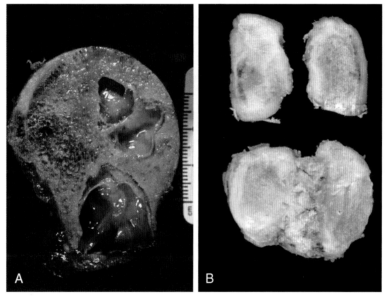

FIG. 7.2

A, A coronally sectioned femoral head shows progressive loss of articular cartilage, marked osteosclerosis in the subchondral region, and large subchondral cysts, characteristic of degenerative joint disease. **B,** Gross photo of a knee arthroplasty specimen shows severe erosion of the articular surface of the femoral condyles and tibial plateau with eburnation of the medial femoral condyle and medial aspect of the tibial plateau.

radiographically (e.g., hip dysplasia), whereas others may be discovered either radiographically or by pathologic examination (e.g., AVN or Paget-associated arthritis).

One of the more common underlying conditions that results in secondary DJD is AVN (Fig. 7.4). AVN can result from both intrinsic and extrinsic compromise of the vascular supply to the end of a bone—most commonly the proximal femur—and there are numerous etiologies for this disorder, including those cases that are idiopathic in nature. When the vascular supply to the end of a bone is compromised, a wedge-shaped infarct develops. In the femoral head, the area of osteonecrosis appears radiodense on radiographs, and a "crescent

sign" may be present representing separation of the subchondral plate and overlying articular cartilage from the remainder of the bone. Nevertheless, osteonecrosis of the femoral head is also easily mistaken for severe osteoarthritis, and the underlying cause not recognized until the femoral head is examined pathologically.

Grossly, the necrotic bone of AVN has a yellow, friable appearance that is easily distinguished from the adjacent unaffected cancellous bone. Characteristically, the articular cartilage and subchondral plate are separated from the underlying necrotic bone, accounting for the radiographic crescent sign. With collapse and the onset of secondary arthritis, the infarct may be difficult

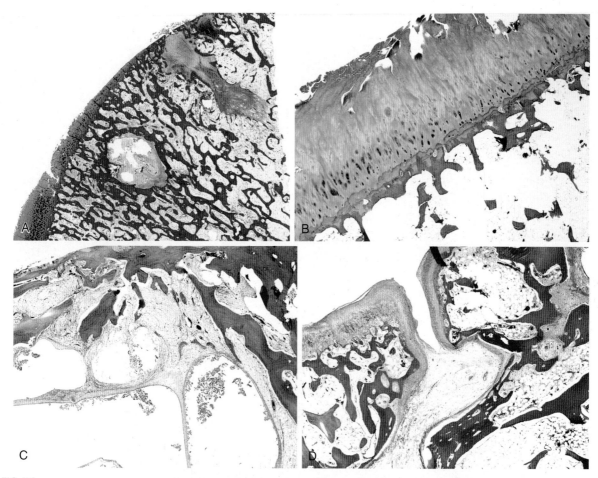

FIG. 7.3
The histologic changes of degenerative joint disease include progressive loss of articular cartilage with subchondral osteosclerosis and cysts **(A)**, fibrillation of the articular cartilage with duplication of the tidemark **(B)**, large subchondral cysts **(C)**, and osteophytes **(D)**.

to identify. Histologically, necrotic bone lacks osteocytes, and calcification develops in the fibrous tissue that invariably replaces marrow fat. The process is surrounded by fibrovascular tissue and reactive bone. The interface between the infarct and viable bone is rich in osteoclastic activity, and necrotic bone is eventually replaced by a process referred to as "creeping substitution," in which woven bone is directly deposited onto necrotic bone trabeculae.

Other underlying etiologies for secondary osteoarthritis include Paget disease (Fig. 7.5), hip dysplasia, and slipped capital femoral epiphysis (SCFE), to include just a few.

Prognosis and Therapy

The initial management of DJD is conservative and consists of a combination of physical therapy, anti-inflammatory medications, and sometimes either steroid or viscosupplement injections. However, many patients ultimately require a joint replacement for full symptom relief. With modern joint prostheses and surgical techniques, long-term outcomes are excellent.

PRIMARY DEGENERATIVE JOINT DISEASE – DISEASE FACT SHEET

Definition
▸▸ Most common form of arthritis in which there is progressive loss of articular cartilage not associated with a predisposing condition

Incidence and Location
▸▸ Extremely common, develops in at least 10% or more of the elderly population
▸▸ Common in large joints, particularly the knees and hips
▸▸ Also common in the hands and spine

Age Distribution
▸▸ Older patients typically develop primary degenerative joint disease

Clinical Features
▸▸ Patients present with pain, swelling, and limitation of motion

Radiologic Features
▸▸ Joint space narrowing
▸▸ Subchondral osteosclerosis
▸▸ Subchondral cysts
▸▸ Peripheral osteophytes

Continued

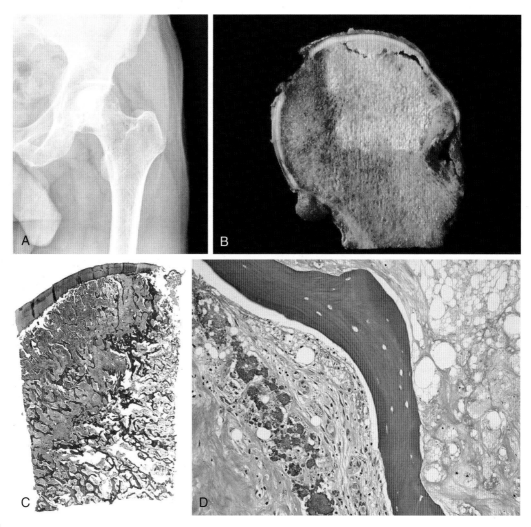

FIG. 7.4

A, Avascular necrosis, a common cause of secondary degenerative joint disease, is characterized by a large, discrete area of radiodensity of the femoral head. **B,** Grossly, avascular necrosis is characterized by a well-defined, wedge-shaped area of yellowish infarction surrounded by a rim of sclerotic bone. Separation of the articular cartilage and subchondral plate, reflected radiographically as a "crescent sign," is also characteristic. **C,** Histologically, the discrete area of osteonecrosis is evident at low power, as is the separation of the articular cartilage and subchondral plate. **D,** Osteonecrosis is characterized by dropout of osteocyte nuclei from the bone trabeculae, necrosis and fibrosis of the fatty marrow, and calcific deposits in the fibrous tissue.

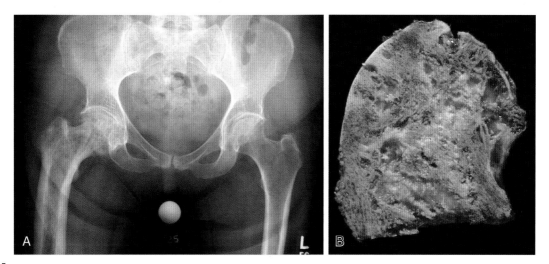

FIG. 7.5

Secondary degenerative joint disease is a common complication of Paget disease, as seen in this radiograph **(A)** and gross photo **(B)** of the right femoral head.

Prognosis and Therapy

▸▸ Therapy can range from conservative management with analgesics or injections to surgical management with arthroplasty
▸▸ Most patients ultimately gain pain relief and full function
▸▸ Prostheses may have to be revised for aseptic reasons or in the event of an infection

---

PRIMARY DEGENERATIVE JOINT DISEASE – PATHOLOGIC FEATURES

Gross Findings

▸▸ Variably severe damage to articular cartilage, ranging from superficial fibrillation to complete destruction with resulting eburnation
▸▸ Sclerosis of subchondral bone
▸▸ Subchondral cysts
▸▸ Peripheral osteophytes

Microscopic Findings

▸▸ Generally closely mirror the gross findings
▸▸ Early, the articular cartilage shows superficial clefts and cloning of chondrocytes with duplication of the tide mark
▸▸ Later, the articular cartilage is eroded full thickness, accompanied by marked subchondral bone sclerosis
▸▸ Subchondral cysts
▸▸ Marginal osteophytes

Pathologic Differential Diagnoses

▸▸ Secondary DJD, which can result from many underlying disorders
▸▸ Avascular necrosis with secondary DJD can be particularly difficult to separate from primary DJD clinically and radiographically

---

TENOSYNOVIAL GIANT CELL TUMOR, DIFFUSE TYPE

DIFFERENTIAL DIAGNOSIS: HEMOSIDEROTIC SYNOVITIS

Clinical Features

Diffuse intra-articular tenosynovial giant cell tumors (GCTs), formerly referred to as "pigmented villonodular synovitis," usually arise in large joints, particularly the hips and knees. Patients are typically young, often less than 40 years of age, and there is a slight female predominance. Their localized counterpart, formerly referred to as "giant cell tumor of tendon sheath," most often occurs in the distal upper extremity and is far more common than the diffuse subtype.

Patients with these neoplasms present with pain, swelling, and loss of motion of the affected joint, and aspiration of the joint yields hemorrhagic fluid.

Radiographic Features

Conventional radiographs typically only reveal a soft tissue density in the region of the affected joint. Erosions can involve both articular and non-articular regions of the joint, resulting in lucencies in the subchondral bone. Both CT and MRI will show the extent of the neoplasm, but MRI is extremely useful in establishing a diagnosis of diffuse type tenosynovial GCT because of the signal characteristics of the lesion (Fig. 7.6). The prominent hemosiderin deposits within the lesion (see Microscopic Findings) are low signal intensity on both T1- and T2-weighted images, whereas fluid and foamy histiocytes lead to high signal intensity on T2-weighted images (Fig. 7.7). Contrast enhancement is noted within the tissue, while fluid in the joint is non-enhancing.

Pathologic Features

GROSS FINDINGS

Diffuse type tenosynovial GCTs have a prominent villous appearance and frequently occupy the entire synovial lining of a joint, resulting in exceptionally large lesions. The cut surface is variegated and may show light-tan, yellow, or brown foci depending on the histologic composition of the lesion.

MICROSCOPIC FINDINGS

Histologically, diffuse type tenosynovial GCTs fill and expand the synovium and can infiltrate adjacent structures (Fig. 7.8). The expansion of individual synovial

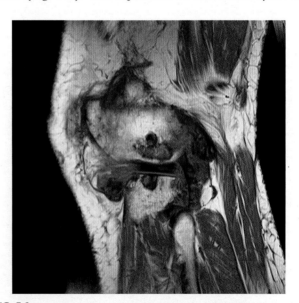

FIG. 7.6

Sagittal MRI of the knee shows a diffuse tenosynovial giant cell tumor filling the knee joint with erosion of the distal femoral and proximal tibial articular cartilage, resulting in subchondral bone lesions.

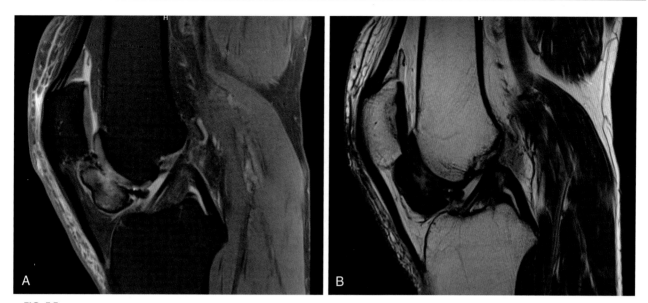

FIG. 7.7

MRI of diffuse tenosynovial giant cell tumor involving the anterior portion of the knee joint. The lesion is variable in signal intensity on proton density **(A)** and T2-weighted **(B)** sequences.

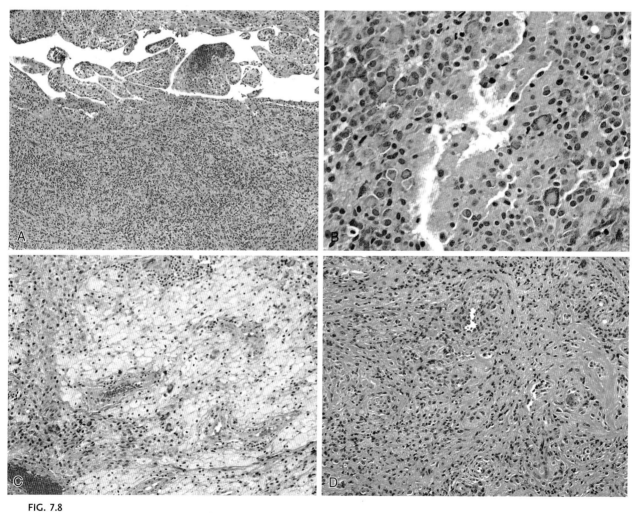

FIG. 7.8

The histologic features of diffuse tenosynovial giant cell tumor include a villous architecture evident on the surface of the lesion **(A)**, giant cells and histiocyte-like mononuclear cells containing rings of iron in their cytoplasm **(B)**, foamy histiocytes, which may be prominent **(C)**, and hyalinization, which may also be prominent **(D)**.

fronds leads to a prominent villous appearance and may result in cleft-like spaces lined by synovium. Pseudoalveolar spaces may also be identified. The cellular composition of a given lesion may be very heterogeneous. The principal tumor cells are mononuclear cells that vary from small to large. These cells are admixed with multinucleated giant cells, foamy histiocytes, chronic inflammatory cells, and hemosiderin. The hemosiderin is occasionally deposited in a ring-like fashion in mononuclear cells. The background stroma may become hyalinized, and individual villi may become necrotic through torsion. Similar to localized tenosynovial GCTs, mitotic activity may be brisk, but cytologic atypia is lacking.

Ancillary Studies

The pathogenesis of tenosynovial GCTs involves an underlying translocation involving the *CSF1* and *COL6A3* genes. The resulting fusion results in the overproduction of CSF1, which in turn binds with the CSF1 receptor found on the neoplastic mononuclear cells, creating an autocrine loop. In select cases or small biopsies, the identification of a *CSF1* rearrangement may be diagnostically useful.

Differential Diagnosis

Diffuse type tenosynovial GCT needs to be differentiated from hemosiderotic synovitis, which represents a reaction to an intra-articular bleed. Hemosiderotic synovitis is characterized by synovial hyperplasia and the deposition of hemosiderin in histiocytes beneath the synovial lining cells, often accompanied by a small amount of chronic inflammation (Fig. 7.9). Multinucleated giant cells, foamy histiocytes, and the neoplastic mononuclear cells of tenosynovial GCTs are absent in hemosiderotic synovitis. However, foci resembling hemosiderotic synovitis can occasionally be found in the synovium adjacent to diffuse type tenosynovial GCT, causing confusion in small biopsy specimens.

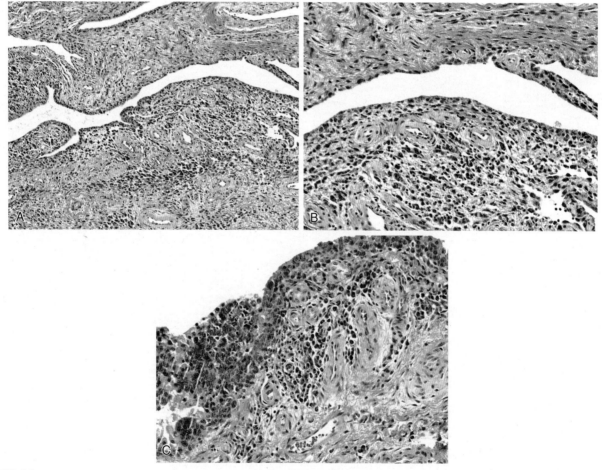

FIG. 7.9

Hemosiderotic synovitis typically shows hyperplastic synovium with hemosiderin deposited in histiocytes beneath the synoviocytes **(A, B)** and small foci of chronic inflammation **(C)**. The prominent mononuclear and multinucleated giant cell population that characterizes diffuse tenosynovial giant cell tumor is absent.

Prognosis and Therapy

Diffuse type tenosynovial GCT is treated by complete surgical excision. The local recurrence rate is extremely high, occurring in greater than 50% of cases, often necessitating complete synovectomy. Tyrosine kinase inhibitors have also been used to disrupt the CSF1-CSF1R pathway. Depending on the underlying cause, hemosiderotic synovitis does not typically require complete synovectomy for treatment, and thus this distinction is important.

TENOSYNOVIAL GIANT CELL TUMOR, DIFFUSE TYPE – DISEASE FACT SHEET

Definition
▸▸ Benign fibrohistiocytic neoplasm arising from synovium, tenosynovium, or bursa lining

Incidence and Location
▸▸ Diffuse tenosynovial giant cell tumor is far less common than the localized type
▸▸ Most cases occur in the large joints, including the hips and knees
▸▸ Less common sites include the temporomandibular joint and facet joint of the spine

Age Distribution
▸▸ Most cases occur in adults in the fourth or fifth decades

Clinical Features
▸▸ Patients present with pain, swelling, or limitations in motion of the affected joint

Radiologic Features
▸▸ Conventional radiographs show only a soft tissue density
▸▸ MRI is the best imaging modality, and will show the local extent of the lesion
▸▸ T1 and T2 both show areas of low signal intensity due to the presence of hemosiderin; bright foci on T2 are related to fluid and collections of foamy histiocytes

Prognosis and Therapy
▸▸ Complete synovectomy is often necessary
▸▸ Local recurrences are common

TENOSYNOVIAL GIANT CELL TUMOR, DIFFUSE TYPE – PATHOLOGIC FEATURES

Gross Findings
▸▸ Diffuse expansion of synovium
▸▸ Cut surface is variegated tan-brown and yellow, but varies with the histologic composition of the lesion

Microscopic Findings
▸▸ Cleft-like spaces are created by opposing synovium-lined fronds
▸▸ Principal tumor cells are small or large histiocytoid mononuclear cells
▸▸ Giant cells, foamy histiocytes, and stromal hyalinization are common
▸▸ Hemosiderin deposition often occurs in characteristic ring-like fashion in histiocytes

Pathologic Differential Diagnoses
▸▸ Hemosiderotic synovitis
▸▸ Malignant tenosynovial giant cell tumor is extremely rare

Ancillary Studies
▸▸ Detection of *CSF1* gene rearrangement may be useful in select cases

---

SYNOVIAL CHONDROMATOSIS

DIFFERENTIAL DIAGNOSIS: OSTEOCARTILAGINOUS LOOSE BODIES, SYNOVIAL CHONDROSARCOMA

Clinical Features

Synovial chondromatosis is an uncommon cartilaginous neoplasm that arises in the connective tissue of the synovium and tenosynovium. The majority of cases involve the large joints of adult patients, particularly the knee and hip. However, smaller joints such as the spinal facet joints, temporomandibular joint, and joints and tenosynovium of the hands and feet can also be affected. The most common presenting symptoms include pain, swelling, and mechanical symptoms.

Radiographic Features

Depending on the degree of calcification or ossification of the cartilage nodules in a given lesion, plain radiographs may show a soft tissue shadow or small radiodense nodules within the joint. CT is often useful in identifying the calcified nodules, and MRI may show low or high signal intensity nodules depending on the degree of mineralized and unmineralized cartilage (Fig. 7.10). The cartilage nodules initially form beneath the synovial surface in subsynovial connective tissue but can be extruded into the joint in later stages.

Pathologic Features

GROSS FINDINGS

In most cases, the nodules of cartilage in synovial chondromatosis have a glistening, smooth, bosselated surface (Fig. 7.11). The cut surface has a white or gray appearance and lacks the concentric rings characteristic of osteocartilaginous loose bodies.

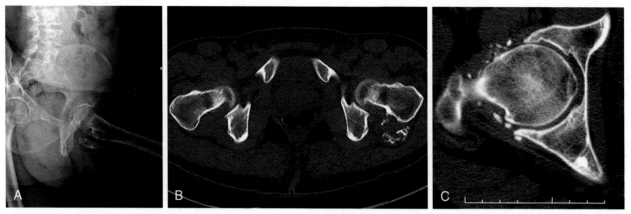

FIG. 7.10

Oblique radiograph **(A)** and CT **(B)** from a case of synovial chondromatosis involving the hip showing a localized area of calcification in the posterior region of the hip joint. CT from another case of synovial chondromatosis involving the hip shows more diffuse involvement of the hip joint, characterized by numerous small, calcified nodules throughout the joint **(C)**.

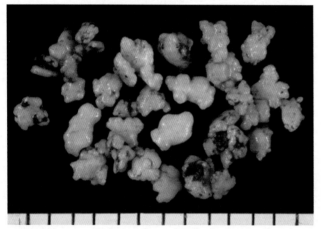

FIG. 7.11

Grossly, the nodules of synovial chondromatosis have a bosselated, glistening surface and grayish color.

MICROSCOPIC FINDINGS

Synovial chondromatosis is composed of nodules of hyaline cartilage, often covered by a thin layer of fibrous tissue or synovium (Fig. 7.12A). The most characteristic finding is the nested or clustered arrangement of the chondrocytes, which may show some degree of cytologic atypia (Fig. 7.12B and C). The hyaline cartilage matrix may be calcified or even ossified if an individual lobule is vascularized. Synovial chondromatosis may cause pressure erosions on adjacent bone, but true permeative invasion, the histologic hallmark of malignant cartilage neoplasms, is not identified.

Ancillary Studies

Both synovial chondromatosis and synovial chondrosarcoma (discussed later) have been shown to harbor *FN1-ACVR2A* and *ACVR2A-FN1* fusions.

Differential Diagnosis

Primary synovial chondromatosis must be distinguished from multiple osteocartilaginous loose bodies, which are most commonly found in severe DJD. Osteocartilaginous loose bodies are more variable in size than the nodules of synovial chondromatosis (Fig. 7.13), and histologically they are composed of concentric rings of cartilage that are often arranged around a central core of necrotic bone (Fig. 7.14). The chondrocytes of osteocartilaginous loose bodies lack the clustered arrangement that is seen in synovial chondromatosis. This distinction is important because synovial chondromatosis is treated with complete synovectomy, whereas synovial loose bodies are treated by removing the nodules and correcting the underlying disease process.

The distinction between synovial chondromatosis with cytologic atypia and synovial chondrosarcoma is extremely difficult. Loss of the clustered arrangement of chondrocytes, marked cytologic atypia, atypical mitotic figures, and permeative invasion of adjacent bone are features that favor a diagnosis of synovial chondrosarcoma (Fig. 7.15).

Synovial chondromatosis involving the tenosynovium in the hands and feet must be distinguished from both soft tissue chondroma and periosteal chondroma. The easiest way to separate these entities from synovial chondromatosis is based on the location of the lesion. Soft tissue chondromas do not involve synovium or tenosynovium, and periosteal chondromas arise between the cortex and periosteum of the involved bone. Separating these entities based solely on histologic features alone is usually difficult. Interestingly, periosteal chondromas have *IDH1/2* mutations, while soft tissue chondromas contain *FN1* rearrangements.

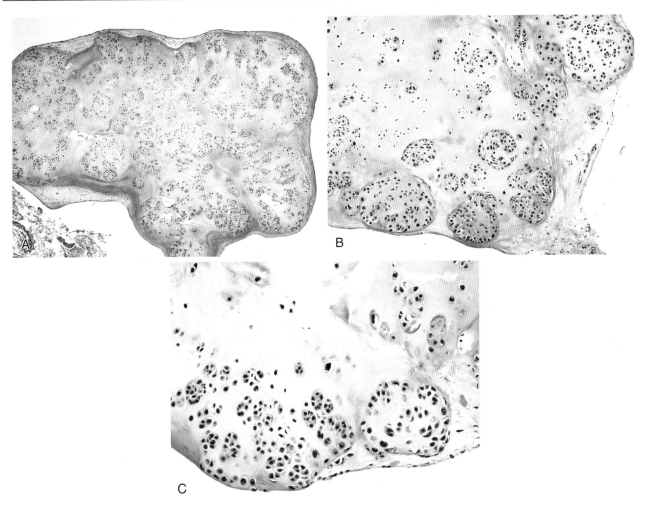

FIG. 7.12

A, At low magnification, the cartilaginous nodules of synovial chondromatosis initially arise beneath an intact synovial layer. **B,** The characteristic clustered arrangement of the chondrocytes is easily appreciated. **C,** In some cases, mild chondrocyte atypia may be found, and binucleate chondrocytes are frequently encountered.

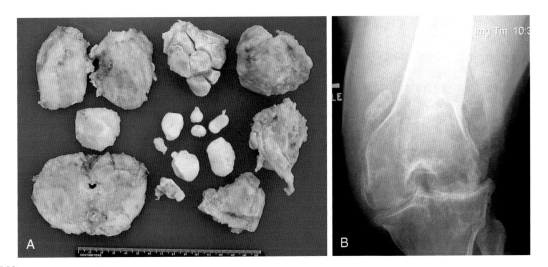

FIG. 7.13

Osteocartilaginous loose bodies are common in the setting of severe degenerative joint disease (DJD). Grossly, the variably sized yellowish nodules in the center of the gross photograph represent loose bodies, and the severity of the DJD in the femoral condyles and tibial plateau can be seen at left **(A)**. Radiographically, loose bodies appear as variably sized, oval to round densities involving the joint **(B)**.

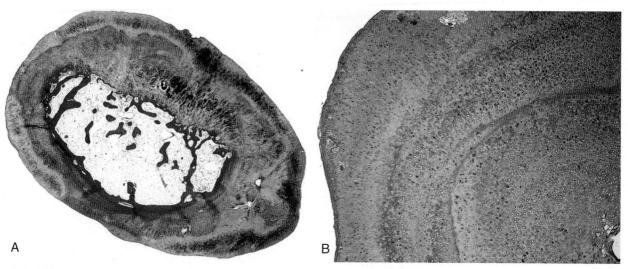

FIG. 7.14

A, Osteocartilaginous loose bodies are characterized by concentric growth of cartilage, typically surrounding a central core of bone. **B,** The concentric pattern of cartilage proliferation is easily seen at slightly higher magnification.

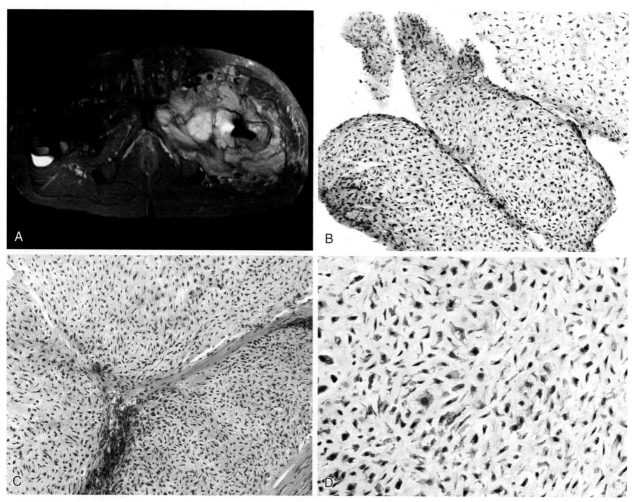

FIG. 7.15

Synovial chondrosarcoma of the hip joint. T2 MRI shows a large mass arising within the hip joint adjacent to a prosthesis **(A).** The mass involves extensive areas of skeletal muscle and invades the adjacent ischium. Histologically, the mass fills fronds of synovium **(B),** forms hypercellular nodules separated by fibrous bands **(C),** and shows severe cytologic atypia at high magnification **(D).**

Prognosis and Therapy

Synovial chondromatosis is a locally aggressive neoplasm with a local recurrence rate of approximately 20%. The standard treatment for this entity is complete synovectomy.

SYNOVIAL CHONDROMATOSIS – DISEASE FACT SHEET

Definition
- ▶▶ Locally aggressive intra-articular or tenosynovial cartilage neoplasm

Incidence and Location
- ▶▶ Relatively rare
- ▶▶ Most commonly affects large joints, including the knee, hip, or shoulder
- ▶▶ Can also arise in the temporomandibular joint or facet joint
- ▶▶ May involve tenosynovium in the hands and feet

Age Distribution
- ▶▶ Most patients are adults between 20 and 40 years of age

Clinical Features
- ▶▶ Typically causes mechanical symptoms in the affected joint, pain, and swelling

Radiologic Features
- ▶▶ Lightly or heavily mineralized nodules within the joint
- ▶▶ May be better visualized with CT or MRI

Prognosis and Therapy
- ▶▶ Locally aggressive, approximately 20% recur following surgery
- ▶▶ Complete synovectomy is the surgical treatment of choice

---

SYNOVIAL CHONDROMATOSIS – PATHOLOGIC FEATURES

Gross Findings
- ▶▶ Multiple smooth, bosselated gray-white nodules

Microscopic Findings
- ▶▶ Mature hyaline cartilage nodules arising in subsynovial connective tissue
- ▶▶ Characteristic clustered or nested arrangement of mildly cytologically atypical chondrocytes embedded in hyaline cartilage stroma

Pathologic Differential Diagnoses
- ▶▶ Osteocartilaginous loose bodies
- ▶▶ Synovial chondrosarcoma (very uncommon)
- ▶▶ Periosteal chondroma or soft tissue chondroma (for tenosynovial chondromatosis in hands or feet)

PERIPROSTHETIC JOINT INFECTION

DIFFERENTIAL DIAGNOSIS: ASEPTIC LOOSENING/ARTHROPLASTY EFFECT

Clinical Features

Periprosthetic joint infection (PJI) is a complex clinical problem that is made even more problematic by the

---

TABLE 7.1

Musculoskeletal Infection Society Criteria for Periprosthetic Joint Infection

Major Criteria (One Necessary)	Minor Criteria (Four Necessary)
1. Sinus tract communicating with the prosthesis	1. Elevated ESR/CRP
2. Pathogen isolated from at least two separate fluid or tissue samples from the affected joint	2. Elevated synovial leukocyte count (>3000 leukocytes/μL in chronic infection, >10,000 in acute infection)
	3. Elevated synovial neutrophil % (80% chronic, 90% acute)
	4. Pathogen isolated one fluid or tissue sample
	5. >5 neutrophils per high-power field in 5 high-power fields
	6. Purulence in affected joint

CRP, C-reactive protein; *ESR*, erythrocyte sedimentation rate.

---

lack of a gold-standard diagnostic test and limited sensitivity and specificity of the various laboratory tests used in the evaluation of these patients. Approximately 1% to 2% of primary arthroplasties are complicated by a PJI. Elbows have the highest incidence of PJI, followed by the knee; the hip and shoulder have the lowest incidence. Infection rates appear to be higher following revision surgery than following the primary arthroplasty. PJI can develop early (<3 months postoperatively), delayed (3 months to 2 years postoperatively), or late (>2 years postoperatively). The organisms most often associated with PJI include *Staphylococcus aureus*, coagulase-negative staphylococci, and *Cutibacterium acnes* (particularly in the shoulder). However, many microorganisms, including fungi, are known to cause PJI.

The symptoms/signs of PJI vary from localized manifestations, such as erythema, pain, loosening of the prosthesis, or the formation of a sinus tract, to systemic findings including fevers and chills and elevated white cell counts. The criteria necessary for a diagnosis of PJI are listed in Table 7.1. A modified version of these criteria incorporates preoperative and intraoperative parameters, including alpha-defensin results.

Pathologic Features

MICROSCOPIC FINDINGS

In addition to histologic findings, numerous laboratory tests are used in the evaluation for PJI (see Table 7.1). The most common screening tests include serum C-reactive protein (CRP) and erythrocyte sedimentation rate (ESR). Tests often obtained preoperatively on synovial fluid include white blood cell count with leukocyte percentage, CRP, culture, and alpha-defensin. Alpha-defensin is a particularly sensitive and specific test that is invaluable in the setting of inflammatory arthropathies and ongoing antibiotic therapy. Several of these tests are also available for use intraoperatively, including alpha-defensin.

Microscopic examination of the tissue surrounding an implant is also important in the evaluation for possible PJI, and intraoperative frozen sections are often requested by the orthopedic surgeon. The most important inflammatory cells to identify are neutrophils, and the threshold for significant acute inflammation is *at least five neutrophils per high-power field in more than five separate high-power fields*, excluding the fibrin layer that develops between the implant and the interface membrane (Fig. 7.16). Other types of inflammatory cells, including lymphocytes, plasma cells, and eosinophils, are not indicative of infection. Care should be taken not to over-interpret neutrophils in the surface fibrin, marginating neutrophils (see Fig. 7.16), neutrophils that are a component of hematopoietic marrow, neutrophils that may be present due to periprosthetic dislocation or fracture, or neutrophils that might be the present as the result of an inflammatory arthropathy. The presence of significant acute inflammation in the periprosthetic tissue or bone is not a sufficient finding in and of itself for a diagnosis of PJI but rather represents one minor criterion according to the Musculoskeletal Infection Society (MSIS).

Differential Diagnosis

PJI must be differentiated from non-infectious causes of prosthesis failure or related symptoms. When loosening is aseptic and the result of an adverse tissue reaction to components of the prosthesis, evidence of this is manifested in the surrounding bone and soft tissue. Microscopically, the tissue may show fibrosis, histiocytes, or foreign body giant cell reaction to foreign materials including metal,

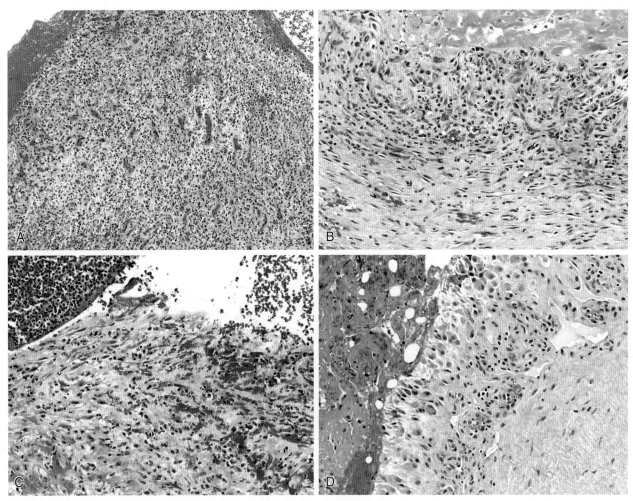

FIG. 7.16

At low magnification, the tissue from a periprosthetic joint infection (PJI) commonly shows inflamed granulation tissue **(A)** with aggregates of neutrophils within the stromal tissue beneath the pseudosynovial layer adjacent to the implant **(B)**. Stromal neutrophils in excess of 5 per high-power field in more than five separate high-power fields and abscesses *(upper left)* are often found histologically in cases of PJI **(C)**. Marginating neutrophils should not be counted during the assessment for PJI **(D)**.

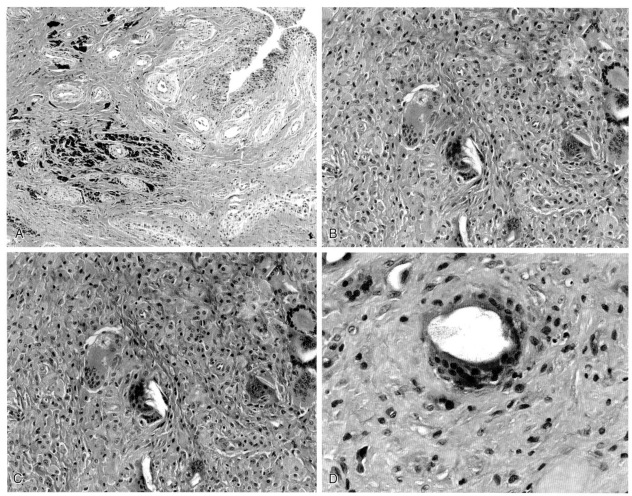

FIG. 7.17
Diverse types of biomaterials are often seen in biopsies from cases of aseptic prosthetic loosening, including metal wear debris **(A)**, polyethylene wear debris that polarizes **(B, C)**, and methylmethacrylate or bone cement; the cement dissolves during routine processing, leaving only the refractile barium that is peripherally distributed around clear spaces surrounded by giant cells **(D)**.

polyethylene, or barium/polymethylmethacrylate, among others (Fig. 7.17). If the reaction is immunologic in nature (so-called aseptic lymphocyte-dominated vasculitis-associated lesion, or ALVAL), large perivascular lymphoid aggregates will be identified deep in the periprosthetic tissue, and a sizable pseudotumor may be present. None of the aseptic causes of prosthetic loosening result in the accumulation of neutrophils in periprosthetic tissue, although it should be remembered that neutrophils may be present in the setting of periprosthetic fracture or dislocation.

Prognosis and Therapy

PJI are treated with a combination of surgery and long-term antibiotics. Surgical options generally include staged revisions with placement of a temporary antibiotic-impregnated spacing device or component exchange with thorough debridement of infected tissue.

PERIPROSTHETIC JOINT INFECTION – DISEASE FACT SHEET

Definition
▶▶ Infection of the bone or soft tissue surrounding a joint prosthesis, often leading to failure of the implant

Incidence and Location
▶▶ Complication that occurs in approximately 1%–2% of all joint arthroplasties, more common in elbow and knee prosthesis than in hip and shoulder prostheses

Age Distribution
▶▶ Any aged patient with a joint prosthesis

Clinical Features
▶▶ Local symptoms including implant loosening, erythema, pain, swelling, or formation of a sinus tract
▶▶ Systemic symptoms also possible

Prognosis and Therapy
▶▶ Treated with a combination of surgery and long-term antibiotic therapy

ENCHONDROMA

DIFFERENTIAL DIAGNOSIS: ATYPICAL CARTILAGINOUS TUMOR/GRADE 1 CHONDROSARCOMA

Clinical Features

Enchondromas are relatively common neoplasms that occur over a wide age range. The most common site of origin is the small tubular bones of the hands and feet, followed by long tubular bones such as the femur, tibia, and humerus. Enchondromas are extremely uncommon in the pelvis and other flat bones. Enchondromas are non-growing lesions that are usually asymptomatic and often discovered incidentally during the workup of other conditions such as arthritis, internal derangement of the knee, rotator cuff tear, or on imaging studies to assess for metastatic carcinoma. Large enchondromas or tumors involving the digits may be complicated by pathologic fracture, resulting in pain.

Enchondromas are usually solitary, and multiple enchondromas are characteristic of Ollier disease and Maffucci syndrome.

Radiographic Features

Conventional radiographs and CT are the best imaging modalities available to evaluate cartilage tumors. Enchondromas are usually radiolucent with areas of mineralization that vary from punctate to ring-like (Figs. 7.18–7.21). Endosteal scalloping may be seen with both enchondromas and atypical cartilaginous tumor (ACT)/grade 1 chondrosarcomas; however, endosteal scalloping associated with other features such as cortical thickening, periosteal reaction, or soft tissue extension is an ominous feature suggesting ACT/grade 1 chondrosarcoma. The most important radiographic features of

enchondromas are those that are *not* present, including extensive bone destruction, cortical destruction, periosteal reaction, and the formation of a soft tissue mass; the presence of these findings strongly suggests the possibility of ACT/grade 1 chondrosarcoma. The radiographic features that help distinguish enchondromas from ACT/low-grade chondrosarcomas in the long bones are not applicable to lesions in three specific instances: (1) lesions involving the small bones of the hands and feet; (2) lesions arising in the setting of enchondromatosis; and (3) lesions occurring in skeletally immature patients.

Pathologic Features

GROSS FINDINGS

Enchondromas are seldom encountered intact in resection specimens. In curettage specimens, enchondromas have a lobular appearance with a white or gray, glistening cut surface. Calcifications are frequently seen and appear as yellowish foci. Intact enchondromas have a sharply circumscribed, lobular border and do not cause significant destruction of cancellous or cortical bone (Fig. 7.22).

MICROSCOPIC FINDINGS

Enchondromas are composed of lobules of hyaline cartilage, often separated by normal cancellous bone or marrow. Many of the lobules are partially or completely surrounded by bone (so-called "encasement pattern"), and endochondral ossification may be present at the periphery of individual lobules. Enchondromas lack invasive properties and do not entrap cancellous bone or invade the cortex or soft tissue, differentiating them from ACT/grade 1 chondrosarcomas. Cytologically, there is significant overlap between enchondromas and ACT/grade 1 chondrosarcomas, and high-magnification evaluation cannot reliably separate these entities. Nonetheless, most enchondromas are paucicellular and contain small, pyknotic chondrocyte nuclei (Fig. 7.23). Lesions arising in the small bones of the hands and feet, those occurring in the setting of enchondromatosis, and those in children may appear somewhat more cellular.

Ancillary Studies

The pathogenesis of enchondromas is related to *IDH1* and *IDH2* mutations. However, identical mutations are also found in chondrosarcomas, so the identification of the gene mutation cannot be used to distinguish these lesions. Enchondromas are immunoreactive for S-100 and ERG, and a small percentage will be positive for the

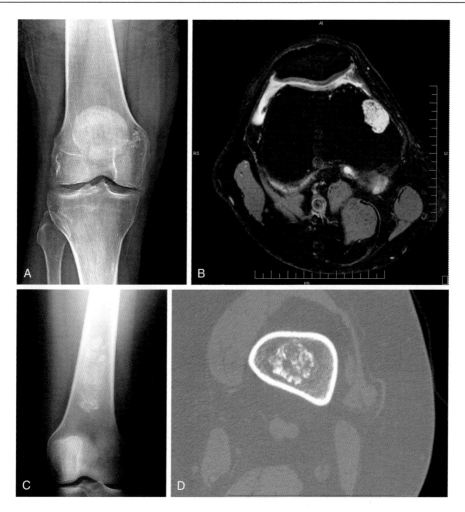

FIG. 7.18

Incidentally discovered enchondroma of the medial femoral metaphysis. **A,** A conventional radiograph shows a small, circumscribed lesion in the medial femoral condyle with punctate calcifications, typical of an enchondroma. **B,** The circumscribed enchondroma shows high signal intensity on axial T2-weighted MRI. **C,** The absence of cortical destruction, soft tissue extension, and periosteal reaction is also typical of an enchondroma. The typical circumscription and calcification pattern are seen in this larger enchondroma arising in the distal femur. **D,** The typical stippled and ring-like pattern of calcification in an enchondroma is often better appreciated on CT.

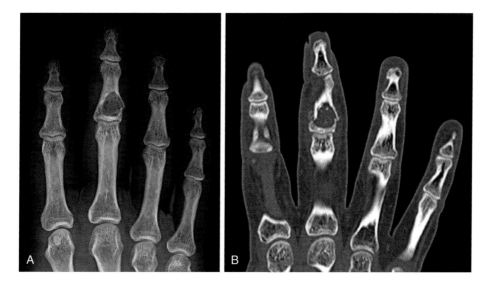

FIG. 7.19

Enchondroma of the middle phalanx of the third finger complicated by a pathologic fracture. **A,** Conventional radiograph shows a well-circumscribed radiolucent lesion with a thin rim of surrounding reactive bone and punctate matrix calcifications. A fracture involves the ulnar side of the cortex adjacent to the lesion. **B,** CT scan also highlights the punctate matrix mineralization within the lesion and the associated pathologic fracture, which involves both the ulnar and radial aspects of the cortex adjacent to the lesion.

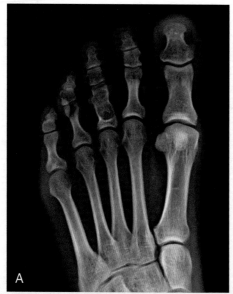

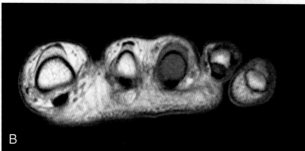

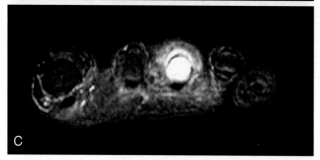

FIG. 7.20

Enchondroma arising in the proximal phalanx of the third toe. A conventional radiograph shows a radiolucent lesion with associated expansile remodeling and a surrounding thin rim of reactive bone **(A)**. The lesion is low signal intensity on T1 MRI **(B)** and high signal intensity on T2 MRI **(C)**.

p.Arg132His IDH1 antibody, but immunohistochemistry is usually not necessary for diagnosis.

Differential Diagnosis

The most important differential diagnosis for enchondroma is ACT/grade 1 chondrosarcoma. According to the WHO, the term ACT should be used synonymously for grade 1 chondrosarcomas arising in the extremities, while the diagnosis of grade 1 chondrosarcoma is retained for lesions arising in the ribs, pelvis, and other

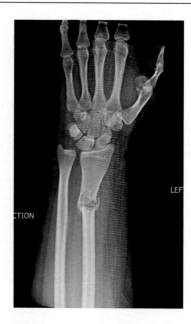

FIG. 7.21

A conventional radiograph of an enchondroma of the distal radial diaphysis with pathologic fracture. It is important not to mistake nodules of cartilage spilled into soft tissue through the fracture site and osteocartilaginous fracture callus as evidence of atypical cartilaginous tumor/grade 1 chondrosarcoma

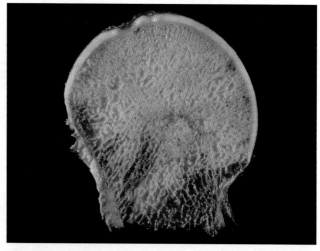

FIG. 7.22

Gross photograph of a small enchondroma identified incidentally in a hip arthroplasty specimen removed for a subcapital fracture. The small, well-circumscribed enchondroma was not identified on preoperative radiographs and was only found by routine examination of the femoral head.

axial sites. The distinction between enchondroma and ACT/grade 1 chondrosarcoma is made using a combination of clinical, radiographic, and histologic information. Clinically, ACT/grade 1 chondrosarcomas are almost always symptomatic and, as opposed to enchondromas, cause pain and sometimes a mass. Radiographically, these tumors show features that are not seen with enchondromas, including ill-defined margins; fusiform, expansile remodeling of the affected bone with endosteal scalloping and associated cortical thickening; cortical destruction with the formation of a soft tissue mass;

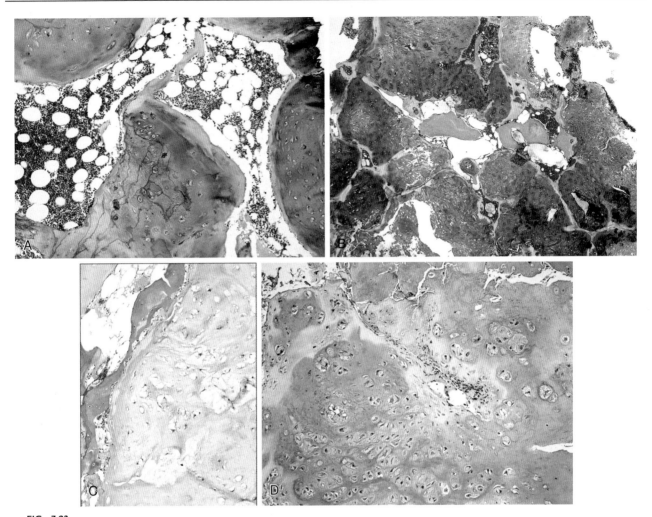

FIG. 7.23

The lobules of mature hyaline cartilage in an enchondroma are often separated by cancellous bone and fatty or hematopoietic marrow **(A, B)**. One of the characteristic histologic findings in enchondroma is encasement of the lobules of cartilage by a thin rim of bone. The paucicellular nature of the lesion and the small, pyknotic chondrocytes are also evident **(C)**. Some enchondromas, particularly those involving the small bones of the hands and feet, can show hypercellularity and mild cytologic atypia, neither of which should be mistaken for evidence of malignancy in these specific locations **(D)**.

and periosteal reaction (Fig. 7.24). Although enchondroma and ACT/grade 1 chondrosarcoma are cytologically similar, the latter is characterized by permeative or invasive growth. This feature is best identified at low power, where lobules of cartilage entrap cancellous bone, extend into cortical vascular canals, or extend into soft tissue (Fig. 7.25). Care should be taken not to overinterpret lobules of enchondroma involving soft tissue in the setting of a pathologic fracture as evidence of soft tissue invasion.

Occasionally, fibrous dysplasia can contain lobules of hyaline cartilage, and rarely the cartilaginous foci can represent the dominant component of the lesion (Fig. 7.26). In such cases, distinction from enchondroma or ACT/grade 1 chondrosarcoma can prove difficult. Careful attention to patient demographics, the location of the lesion and its radiographic appearance, and meticulous examination of biopsy material for a fibro-osseous component will allow for accurate classification as fibrous dysplasia.

Prognosis and Therapy

Enchondromas of long bones are safely managed by observation alone, whereas those in the hands or feet may require curettage when symptomatic or associated with a pathologic fracture. Biopsy of well-differentiated cartilage tumors is of limited utility, and sampling issues often preclude reliably distinguishing enchondromas and ACT/grade 1 chondrosarcomas. It should be emphasized that radiographic and clinical features are extremely valuable in separating enchondroma from ACT/grade 1 chondrosarcomas.

Enchondromas have a minimal risk of progression to ACT/grade 1 chondrosarcoma and are not likely to recur following curettage. ACT/grade 1 chondrosarcoma may recur locally following curettage or resection, and metastases are very uncommon. However, ACT/grade 1 chondrosarcoma can progress in grade following local recurrence and may transform into dedifferentiated chondrosarcoma.

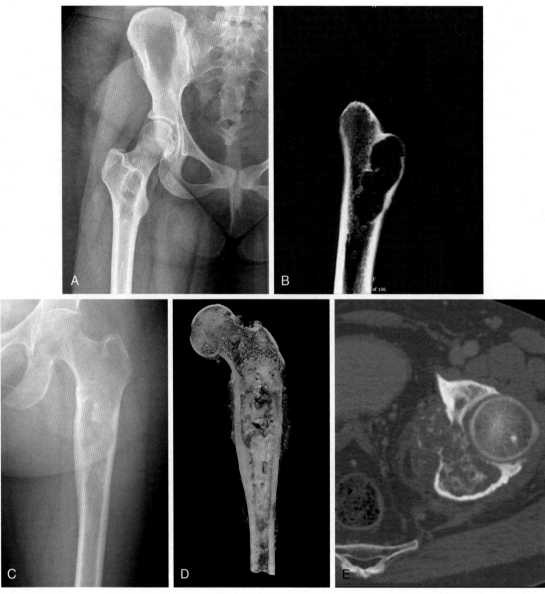

FIG. 7.24

A, A plain radiograph of an atypical cartilaginous tumor (ACT) shows a somewhat ill-defined lesion arising in the intertrochanteric region of the proximal femur. **B,** A CT of the same lesion highlights the calcification pattern typical of a low-grade cartilage neoplasm and shows the ill-defined distal border of the lesion as well as periostitis proximally. The latter two changes suggest the lesion is not likely to be an enchondroma. **C,** Conventional radiograph showing an ACT of the proximal femur. This lesion is ill-defined, focally mineralized, and shows deep endosteal scalloping and cortical remodeling. **D,** The gross features of this ACT perfectly mirror the imaging findings. **E,** This tumor arising in the periacetabular region of the pelvis shows the typical mineralization pattern of a low-grade cartilage neoplasm. The lesion extends through the medial wall of the acetabulum into adjacent soft tissue. Tumors with grade 1 cytomorphology retain the name "chondrosarcoma" (as opposed to ACT) when they arise in the pelvis or other central flat bones.

ENCHONDROMA – DISEASE FACT SHEET

Definition

▶▶ Benign hyaline cartilage neoplasm that arises within the medullary cavity

Incidence and Location

▶▶ Relatively common primary bone neoplasm
▶▶ Most commonly arise within the small bones of the hands and feet (approximately 50%)
▶▶ Can also arise in long bones (proximal humerus, femur, tibia)
▶▶ Rare in flat bones and the craniofacial skeleton

Age Distribution

▶▶ Wide age distribution, can occur in children
▶▶ Usually identified in a younger age group than ACT/grade 1 chondrosarcoma

Clinical Features

▶▶ Asymptomatic, usually discovered incidentally in long bones, during a work-up for unrelated disorders (internal derangement of the knee, arthritis, rotator cuff tear, etc.)
▶▶ Enchondromas in the small bones of the hands and feet may cause pain or undergo pathologic fracture

Continued

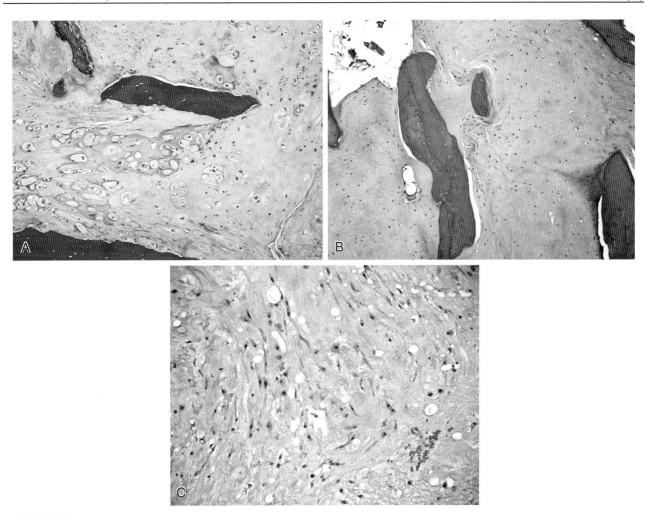

FIG. 7.25

Atypical cartilaginous tumor (ACT)/grade 1 chondrosarcoma is characterized by infiltrative, permeative growth in which lobules of neoplastic cartilage surround cancellous bone trabeculae on at least three sides; the bone entrapped in the cartilage is often necrotic **(A, B)**. Cytologically, ACT/grade 1 chondrosarcomas may show focal myxoid change, but lack cytologic atypia and mitotic activity, and are generally difficult to distinguish from enchondromas histologically **(C)**.

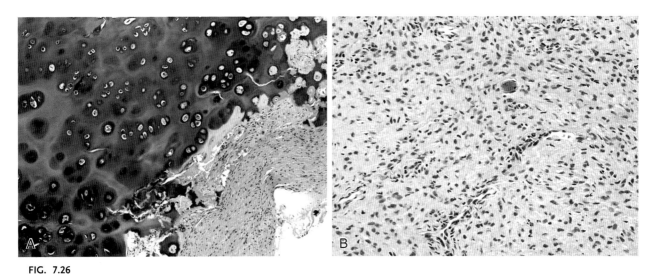

FIG. 7.26

A, Chondroid differentiation can be prominent in some cases of fibrous dysplasia and can occasionally be the dominant histologic feature (so-called "fibrous dysplasia with massive chondroid differentiation" or "fibrocartilaginous dysplasia"). **B,** The diagnosis rests on the careful correlation between the histologic, clinical, and radiographic findings and the recognition of small fibro-osseous foci.

Radiologic Features

▸▸ Well-circumscribed lesion involving the metaphysis or diaphysis

▸▸ Often show dot-like matrix calcification or rings/arcs pattern of mineralization

▸▸ Do not cause bone destruction, and periosteal reaction and soft tissue extension are absent

▸▸ Endosteal scalloping may be present, but the adjacent cortex usually remains thin

▸▸ Lesions in small bones may cause expansile remodeling

▸▸ Low signal intensity on T1 MRI, high signal intensity on fluid-sensitive MRI sequences

Prognosis and Therapy

▸▸ Most enchondromas of long bones do not need to be removed surgically

▸▸ Symptomatic lesions in small bones are curetted

▸▸ Curettage is usually curative, and local recurrence is very uncommon

ENCHONDROMA – PATHOLOGIC FEATURES

Gross Findings

▸▸ Curetted tissue fragments have the typical bluish-gray, firm appearance that articular cartilage has

Microscopic Findings

▸▸ Lobules of mature hyaline cartilage, some myxoid change may be present

▸▸ Lobules are well-circumscribed, often partially or completely surrounded by a shell of bone

▸▸ No permeative growth (invasion of marrow, cancellous bone, haversian canals, soft tissue)

▸▸ Individual neoplastic chondrocyte nuclei are typically small and pyknotic

▸▸ Enchondromas involving small bones or those arising in the setting of enchondromatosis may be more cellular

Pathologic Differential Diagnoses

▸▸ Atypical cartilaginous tumor/grade 1 chondrosarcoma

▸▸ Fibrous dysplasia with chondroid differentiation

OSTEOCHONDROMA

DIFFERENTIAL DIAGNOSIS: PERIOSTEAL CHONDROMA, SECONDARY CHONDRO-SARCOMA/ATYPICAL CARTILAGINOUS TUMOR/GRADE 1 CHONDROSARCOMA ARISING IN OSTEOCHONDROMA, PAROSTEAL OSTEOSARCOMA

Clinical Features

Osteochondroma is one of the most common benign bone tumors encountered in surgical pathology. Most patients present in adolescence or young adulthood, and most osteochondromas are recognized in patients between 10 and 20 years of age. The majority of osteochondromas do not cause symptoms but present as slowly growing painless masses. They may become symptomatic if the stalk fractures, an overlying bursa develops, or if the mass impinges on adjacent neurovascular structures. The most common locations are the metaphyses of the distal femur, proximal tibia, proximal humerus, and within the pelvis. The vast majority of osteochondromas are solitary, but patients with the autosomal dominant condition multiple hereditary exostoses (MHE) have multiple lesions and modeling deformities in affected bones, particularly around the knee.

Radiographic Features

Radiographically, osteochondromas have a very characteristic appearance (Fig. 7.27). These exophytic osteo-cartilaginous neoplasms can be pedunculated (with a thin stalk) or sessile (with a broad base). One key feature of osteochondromas is corticomedullary continuity with the bone of origin. The cortical and medullary portions of the osteochondroma stalk merge with the same structures in the underlying bone. This feature is easily demonstrated on CT and MRI. The cartilage cap of the osteochondroma, best assessed with MRI, seldom exceeds 1 cm, is typically thinner than that in skeletally mature patients, and diminishes as the patient's skeleton matures.

Pathologic Features

GROSS FINDINGS

The gross features of an osteochondroma closely mirror the radiographic findings. The surface of an osteochondroma is covered by a thin layer of fibrous tissue that represents a continuation of the periosteum. The measurable hyaline cartilage cap ranges from a few millimeters to a centimeter in thickness and is often thicker in skeletally immature patients. The surface may appear bosselated in larger sessile osteochondromas. The junction of the cartilage cap and underlying stalk contains calcified cartilage, and the stalk itself is composed of cortical and cancellous bone (Fig. 7.28).

MICROSCOPIC FINDINGS

The cartilage cap appears smooth and is composed of hyaline cartilage; endochondral ossification is evident at the junction of the cap and underlying stalk. The stalk of an osteochondroma is composed of cortical and cancellous bone (Fig. 7.29). The cartilage cap of the osteochondroma actively proliferates until the patient reaches skeletal maturity at which point its growth ceases, similar to the physis. In older patients, an osteochondroma

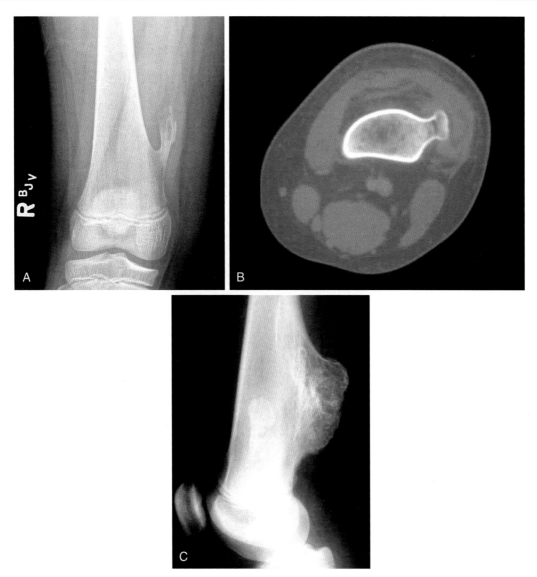

FIG. 7.27

Radiographically, osteochondromas can be pedunculated (on a narrow stalk) **(A, B)** or sessile (broad-based) **(C)**. The corticomedullary continuity between the osteochondroma and underlying bone is easily appreciated on CT **(B)**.

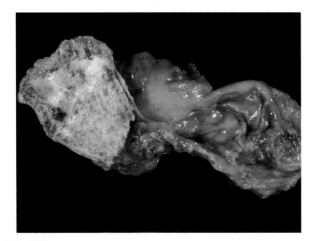

FIG. 7.28

Gross photo of an osteochondroma from an adult showing only a thin cartilage cap, but there is evidence of ossified cartilage in the superficial aspect of the stalk. This osteochondroma was complicated by the development of an overlying bursa, which has been opened *(right)*.

may lack a cartilage cap altogether. A bursa may develop around the head of a long-standing osteochondroma; in turn, this bursa may develop complications such as osteocartilaginous loose bodies or synovial (bursal) chondromatosis (Fig. 7.30).

Ancillary Studies

Ancillary studies are not necessary to diagnose osteochondromas. However, the pathogenesis of osteochondromas is well-known. These neoplasms are caused by mutations in the exostosin (*EXT*) 1 or 2 genes. Mutations in these tumor suppressor genes result in disorganization of the structure in the growth plate, resulting in an exophytic osteocartilaginous mass originating near the zone of Ranvier.

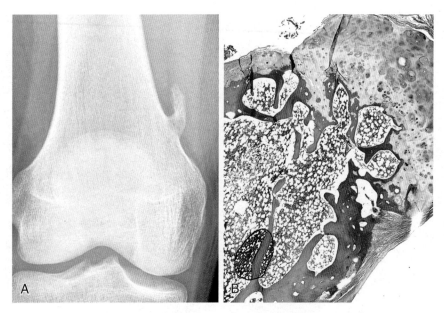

FIG. 7.29

The histologic features of an osteochondroma closely mirror the radiographic findings. This pedunculated osteochondroma of the distal femur **(A)** has a thin, continuous cartilage cap overlying a bony stalk composed of both cortical and cancellous bone and hematopoietic marrow **(B)**.

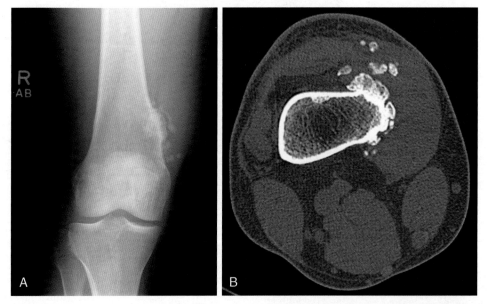

FIG. 7.30

Another complication of osteochondromas is secondary bursal osteochondromatosis. **A,** On plain radiograph, the sessile osteochondroma in the distal femur is somewhat obscured by osteocartilaginous loose bodies. **B,** The loose bodies are more easily appreciated on CT.

Differential Diagnosis

Periosteal chondroma is a benign surface-based cartilage neoplasm that arises between an intact cortex and its periosteum and most commonly involves the proximal humerus, femur, and small bones of the hands and feet. The main radiographic difference between osteochondroma and periosteal chondroma is the lack of corticomedullary continuity in the latter. The cortex is intact beneath periosteal chondromas, which can cause cortical erosions and peripheral buttressing where reactive bone extends over the edges of the lesion. Histologically, periosteal chondromas are composed of lobules of hyaline cartilage but lack a stalk and the prominent endochondral ossification of an osteochondroma (Figs. 7.31 and 7.32).

Malignant transformation in the cap of osteochondromas is seen far less commonly in solitary lesions compared with those occurring in patients with MHE. Most often, the malignant transformation resembles grade 1 chondrosarcoma; according to the WHO, such tumors are referred to as "peripheral ACT" in the appendicular skeleton and "grade 1 peripheral chondrosarcoma" when

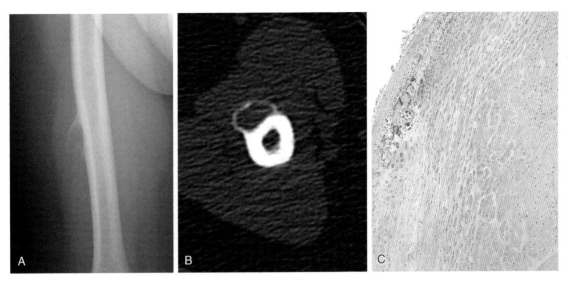

FIG. 7.31

Plain radiograph showing a periosteal chondroma arising in the humeral diaphysis. **A,** The small surface lesion causes broad-based erosion of the underlying cortex and has the typical buttress of reactive bone along its proximal aspect. **B,** These features are more easily appreciated on axial CT, and on this cross-section a reactive rim of bone derived from the periosteum completely encompasses the tumor. **C,** Histologically, this periosteal chondroma is composed of mature hyaline cartilage and is covered by the fibrous periosteum and a thin rim of reactive bone.

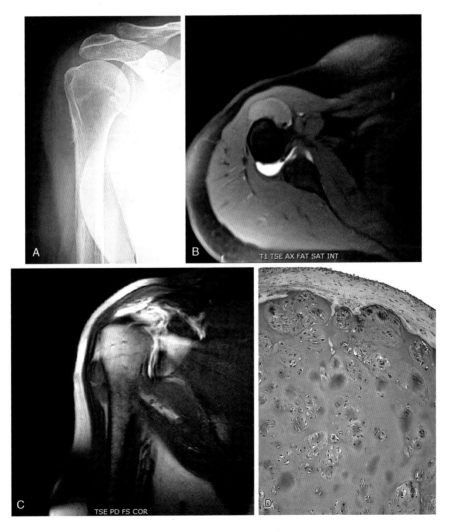

FIG. 7.32

This periosteal chondroma of the proximal humerus is barely perceptible on conventional radiograph, with the exception of a small buttress of reactive bone along the distal aspect of the lesion **(A).** The well-circumscribed periosteal chondroma is intermediate in signal intensity on axial T1 MRI **(B),** and slightly lower in signal intensity on a coronal proton density MRI **(C).** The lesion is composed of mature hyaline cartilage covered by an intact layer of periosteum **(D).**

located in axial skeleton. Transformation into higher-grade chondrosarcomas is uncommon. Rapid growth and new-onset pain after skeletal maturity are clinical indicators of malignant transformation. Radiographically, growth after skeletal maturity, the development of a soft tissue mass, and a thick, irregular cartilage cap also suggest the possibility of malignant transformation (Fig. 7.33). Histologically, loss of the smooth contour in the cap of an osteochondroma, the development of satellite nodules in fibrous tissue adjacent to the cartilage cap, or destruction/invasion of the bone in the stalk of the osteochondroma are features associated with malignant transformation (Fig. 7.34).

The distinction of osteochondroma from parosteal osteosarcoma is discussed later.

Prognosis and Therapy

Small, asymptomatic osteochondromas are safely monitored and do not require excision. Larger, symptomatic

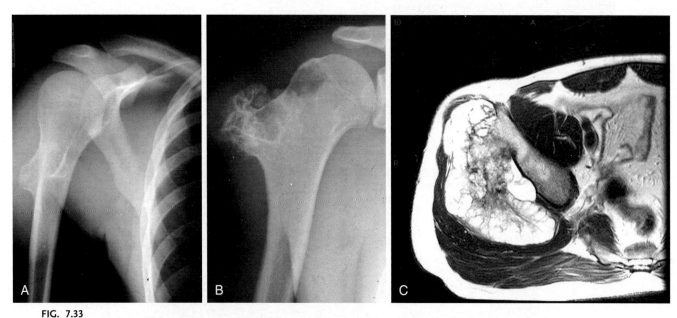

FIG. 7.33
Radiographically, secondary atypical cartilaginous tumor arising in the cap of an osteochondroma is characterized by growth after skeletal maturity, as seen in this sequence of radiographs obtained 6 years apart **(A, B)**. A secondary chondrosarcoma arising in the cap of a solitary pelvic osteochondroma demonstrates the characteristic markedly thickened, irregular cartilage cap indicative of malignant transformation **(C)**.

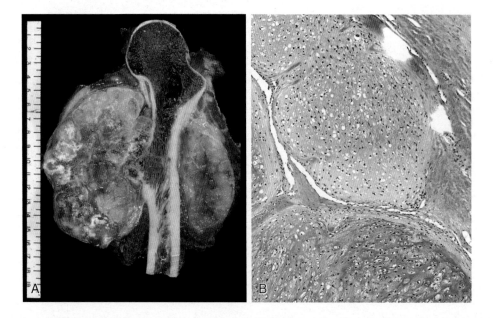

FIG. 7.34
A, In this gross photo, the cap of the secondary atypical cartilaginous tumor (ACT) arising from an osteochondroma is at least 8 cm in thickness and encircles the proximal femur. **B,** The smooth, continuous cartilage cap is lost when secondary ACT/grade 1 chondrosarcomas arise in the cap of an osteochondroma. In this instance, the cartilage grows as small satellite nodules embedded in fibrous tissue.

osteochondromas are almost always cured by surgical resection; however, local recurrences are possible if the cartilage cap is not removed in its entirety.

OSTEOCHONDROMA – DISEASE FACT SHEET

Definition
- ▸▸ A benign cartilage neoplasm composed of a mature bony stalk with a cartilage cap that is in continuity with the bone of origin

Incidence and Location
- ▸▸ One of the most common bone tumors seen in surgical pathology
- ▸▸ Solitary osteochondromas arise from the metaphysis of long bones, particularly around the knee and proximal humerus; the pelvis can also be involved

Age Distribution
- ▸▸ Usually first identified in adolescents or young adults

Clinical Features
- ▸▸ Usually present as asymptomatic, slowly growing masses
- ▸▸ Pain possible with fracture of the stalk, compression of neurovascular structures, or the development of an overlying bursa

Radiologic Features
- ▸▸ Exophytic mass that arises from the metaphysis
- ▸▸ Smooth, variably thick cartilage cap overlying a bone stalk that is either sessile or pedunculated
- ▸▸ There is corticomedullary continuity between the stalk and underlying bone
- ▸▸ Patients with multiple hereditary exostoses have multiple osteochondromas and modeling deformities of the skeleton

Prognosis and Therapy
- ▸▸ Symptomatic lesions should be surgically removed
- ▸▸ Local recurrences are uncommon but possible if the cartilage cap is not removed in its entirety

---

OSTEOCHONDROMA – PATHOLOGIC FEATURES

Gross Findings
- ▸▸ Osteocartilaginous mass with a well-defined cartilage cap of variable thickness
- ▸▸ Pedunculated lesions have a finger-like stalk
- ▸▸ Sessile lesions are cauliflower-like
- ▸▸ The stalk consists of cortical and cancellous bone

Microscopic Findings
- ▸▸ The variably thick cartilage cap (usually less than 2 cm) shows proliferative activity until skeletal maturity
- ▸▸ The cartilage cap is usually smooth and continuous, although it may be nearly absent in adults
- ▸▸ Endochondral ossification occurs at the junction of the cartilage cap and underlying stalk
- ▸▸ The stalk is composed of cortical and cancellous bone, and hematopoietic marrow may also be seen

Pathologic Differential Diagnoses
- ▸▸ Periosteal chondroma
- ▸▸ Secondary ACT/grade 1 chondrosarcoma arising in an osteochondroma
- ▸▸ Parosteal osteosarcoma

CHONDROMYXOID FIBROMA

DIFFERENTIAL DIAGNOSIS: MYXOID CHONDROSARCOMA

Clinical Features

Chondromyxoid fibroma (CMF) of bone is a rare benign tumor of cartilaginous nature. It usually occurs in the long bones of children and young adults but has also been reported in the small bones of the hands and feet, pelvis, ribs, vertebrae, and skull base. CMF in the skull base or flat bones often occur in an older patient population and are sometimes mistaken for myxoid chondrosarcoma or chordoma. Most patients present with pain and swelling.

Radiographic Features

On conventional radiographs, CMF are eccentric, well-circumscribed radiolucent lesions that arise in the metaphysis (Fig. 7.35). They may contain internal septations and often have a coarse rim of surrounding reactive bone. Some CMF may completely erode the cortex, resulting in a characteristic "cookie bite" appearance, but are contained beneath an intact periosteal layer. Far less commonly, CMF may arise on the surface of the bone. Matrix calcifications are uncommon and are more easily detected with CT scan. On MRI, CMF are high signal intensity on T2-weighted images, and intermediate in signal intensity on T1-weighted images.

Pathologic Features

GROSS FINDINGS

It is relatively uncommon to examine intact CMF specimens, and curettage specimens typically show tan, firm, somewhat gelatinous glistening tissue. Intact specimens show a circumscribed border with a prominent rim of reactive bone adjacent to the lesion (Fig. 7.36).

MICROSCOPIC FINDINGS

CMF is a characteristically lobulated neoplasm that is sharply circumscribed from the adjacent bone. The matrix of CMF is more myxoid than chondroid, and hyaline cartilage is an uncommon finding. Centrally, the lobules of CMF are paucicellular, and the cellularity increases at the periphery of individual lobules. The cytoplasm of the tumor cells often extends outward into the

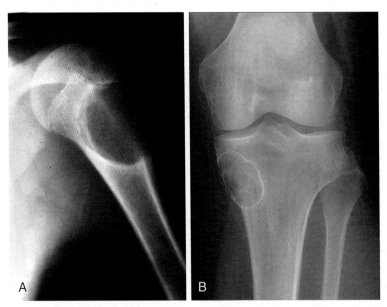

FIG. 7.35

Plain radiographs of chondromyxoid fibroma (CMF) typically show eccentric, metaphyseal lesions which are sharply circumscribed and surrounded by a rim of reactive bone, as seen in these lesions in the proximal humerus in a child **(A)** and proximal tibia of an adult **(B)**. The proximal humeral lesion shows the characteristic "cookie bite" or "shark bite" appearance of a CMF.

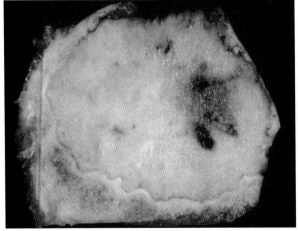

FIG. 7.36

Gross appearance of a chondromyxoid fibroma resected from the pelvis of an elderly patient. The lesion is well-circumscribed, has a thick layer of surrounding reactive bone, and has a somewhat gelatinous cut surface. The hemorrhagic foci are the result of core biopsy.

myxoid matrix, resulting in stellate-appearing tumor cells. Individual lobules are separated by intersecting bands of highly cellular tissue composed of fibroblast-like spindle cells, and osteoclasts are found in and immediately adjacent to these areas when present (Fig. 7.37). Matrix calcification may occur, particularly in juxtacortical CMF. The occasional presence of large pleomorphic cells may result in an erroneous diagnosis of chondrosarcoma, particularly in recurrent lesions. However, mitotic figures are exceptional and, when present, should suggest an alternative diagnosis. Some tumors show a combination of the histologic features of chondroblastoma and CMF, and in such cases radiographic information should be incorporated for diagnosis.

Ancillary Studies

The use of ancillary studies is usually not necessary to render a diagnosis of CMF. However, these neoplasms have been shown to have an immunophenotype which is both chondroid and myofibroblastic in nature. SOX9 and S-100 protein are both immunoreactive in chondrogenic areas, whereas smooth muscle actin or muscle-specific actin expression is present in the myoid spindled cells.

Cytogenetically, clonal rearrangements of chromosome 6 have been identified, and fusions involving the *GRM1* gene with several possible partners are considered the driver mutations for CMF.

Differential Diagnosis

The main differential diagnosis for CMF is myxoid chondrosarcoma. In the usual clinical and radiographic setting, this distinction is not problematic as CMF occurs in a much younger age group and the imaging findings are not aggressive when compared with those of myxoid chondrosarcoma. However, distinguishing CMF from myxoid chondrosarcoma in an older patient with a pelvic lesion can be extremely difficult. Radiographically, myxoid chondrosarcomas are radiolucent but are also extremely destructive, often have a large soft tissue mass, and lack peripheral reactive bone (Fig. 7.38). While myxoid chondrosarcomas are lobular and can have overlapping cytologic features with CMF, they are invasive, permeative neoplasms that lack variable

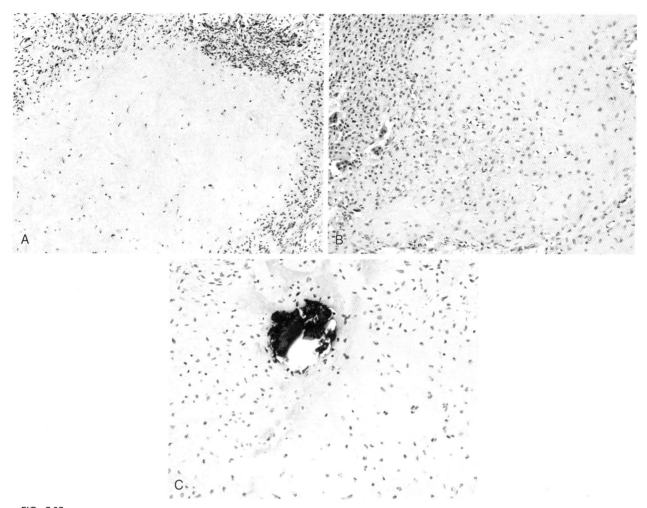

FIG. 7.37

Histologically, chondromyxoid fibroma shows lobular architecture with peripheral hypercellularity **(A)**, stellate spindled cells deposited in a myxochondroid matrix and giant cells within cellular zones **(B)**, and focal coarse calcifications **(C)**.

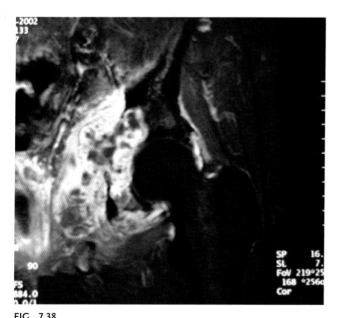

FIG. 7.38

MRI of a myxoid chondrosarcoma of the pelvis shows a highly destructive tumor with a large soft tissue mass.

cellularity and contain at least a low level of mitotic activity (Fig. 7.39).

Prognosis and Therapy

CMF is a benign neoplasm that is usually treated surgically with curettage. They have a modest risk for local recurrence in up to 15% of cases.

CHONDROMYXOID FIBROMA – DISEASE FACT SHEET

Definition

▸▸ A benign cartilaginous neoplasm containing chondromyxoid and myofibroblastic areas

---

Incidence and Location

▸▸ Rare cartilaginous neoplasm
▸▸ Most common in long bones, including the proximal tibia, distal femur, and humerus

Continued

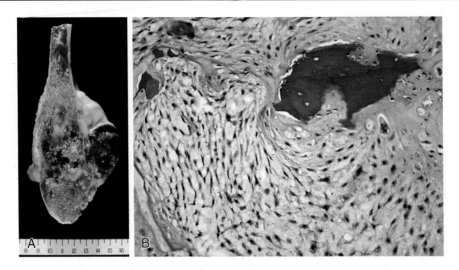

FIG. 7.39

A, Grossly, this myxoid chondrosarcoma of the distal femur is destructive, has a large soft tissue mass, and has a cut surface that appears gelatinous. **B,** Histologically, myxoid chondrosarcomas are permeative neoplasms composed of stellate cells suspended in myxoid matrix. As opposed to chondrosarcomas with hyaline cartilage matrix, the tumor cells in myxoid chondrosarcomas do not occupy lacunae.

▸▸ May occur in small bones of the hands/feet or flat bones, particularly in the pelvis

Age Distribution

▸▸ Occur most commonly in children and young adults, but can also affect older patients

Clinical Features

▸▸ Patients present with slow-onset pain and swelling

Radiologic Features

▸▸ Radiographs show an eccentric metaphyseal radiolucent lesion with a prominent rim of reactive bone
▸▸ Complete cortical erosion results in the typical "cookie bite" appearance
▸▸ Low-to-intermediate signal on T1 MRI, high signal intensity on T2 MRI

Prognosis and Therapy

▸▸ Benign tumor treated with curettage
▸▸ Local recurrence in up to 15% of cases

CHONDROMYXOID FIBROMA – PATHOLOGIC FEATURES

Gross Findings

▸▸ Curettings usually appear solid, tan, and somewhat gelatinous
▸▸ Intact specimens have a layer of reactive bone separating the neoplasm from adjacent bone

Microscopic Findings

▸▸ Distinctly lobular with chondromyxoid stroma
▸▸ Variable cellularity of lobules, paucicellular centrally but hypercellular peripherally
▸▸ Cellular septa containing spindled myofibroblastic cells and occasional giant cells separate lobules

Pathologic Differential Diagnoses

▸▸ Myxoid chondrosarcoma

GIANT CELL TUMOR

DIFFERENTIAL DIAGNOSIS: CHONDROBLASTOMA, CLEAR CELL CHONDROSARCOMA

Clinical Features

Giant cell tumor (GCT) is typically seen in skeletally mature patients over the age of 20 years. It is more common in women than in men and seems to occur more frequently in China than in Western countries. The sites most commonly affected include the distal femur, proximal tibia, and distal radius. GCT may also arise in the humerus, fibula, and skull, particularly the sphenoid bone. Occasionally, GCT is diagnosed in a child and/or in a metaphyseal or diaphyseal location. Involvement of the bones of the hands and feet, jaw, and vertebrae (other than the sacrum) is uncommon. Multicentricity has been reported, particularly in young patients and in the small bones of hands and feet, and pulmonary metastases may develop after surgical manipulation of a GCT. The most common symptoms include pain, swelling, and occasionally pathologic fracture. GCT arising in the spinal column may cause neurologic symptoms.

Radiographic Features

The typical appearance of a GCT is that of a well-circumscribed radiolucent lesion involving the epiphysis and metaphysis that lacks surrounding reactive bone

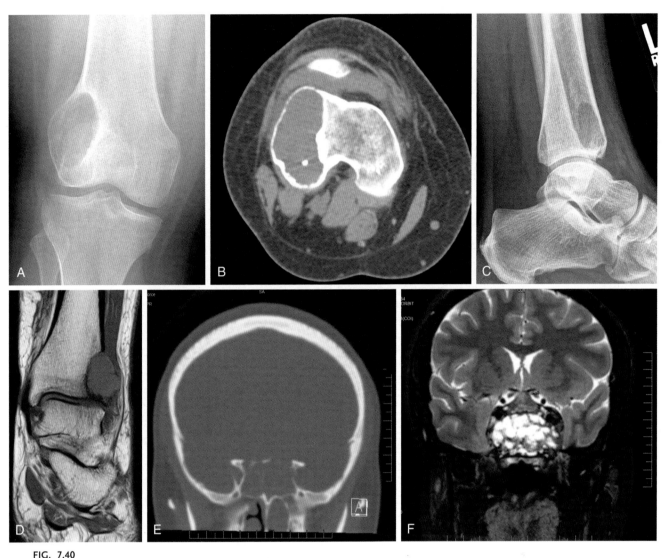

FIG. 7.40

Conventional radiograph **(A)** and CT **(B)** show a sharply circumscribed giant cell tumor (GCT) involving the distal femoral epiphysis/metaphysis partially surrounded by a rim of reactive bone. Lateral radiograph **(C)** and MRI **(D)** showing a GCT of the distal femur. The lesion extends from the subchondral plate proximally into the metaphysis, and soft tissue extension is easily appreciated on the MRI. CT **(E)** and T2-weighted MRI **(F)** showing a GCT involving the base of the skull.

formation (Fig. 7.40). Fine trabeculations often develop with GCT and are evident on conventional radiographs. GCT may be confined to the bone or destroy the cortex; when the cortex is breached, the tumor is typically contained by an intact periosteum, and true soft tissue extension beyond the periosteum is unusual. Cystic changes are best evaluated with either CT or MRI. GCTs treated with denosumab become heavily mineralized.

Pathologic Features

GROSS FINDINGS

The cut surface of a GCT is soft and friable and has a variegated red-brown and yellow appearance. Hemorrhage and necrosis are sometimes prominent. When the cortex is thinned or destroyed, a thin rim of reactive

bone usually surrounds the tumor (Fig. 7.41). Prominent cystic change resembling aneurysmal bone cyst (ABC) may be identified. On rare occasions, GCTs may extend into the joint or even across a joint and into an adjacent bone along an anatomic structure such as the anterior cruciate ligament in the knee or the ligamentum teres in the hip.

MICROSCOPIC FINDINGS

The two main components of GCT are the neoplastic mononuclear stromal cells and multinucleated giant cells. The giant cells are generally large, have over 20 or 30 nuclei, and are evenly dispersed among the stromal cells. The neoplastic mononuclear cells vary from round to ovoid with vesicular nuclei to spindled and embedded in a collagenous stroma. Mitoses can be prominent in the mononuclear stromal cells (Fig. 7.42). Secondary

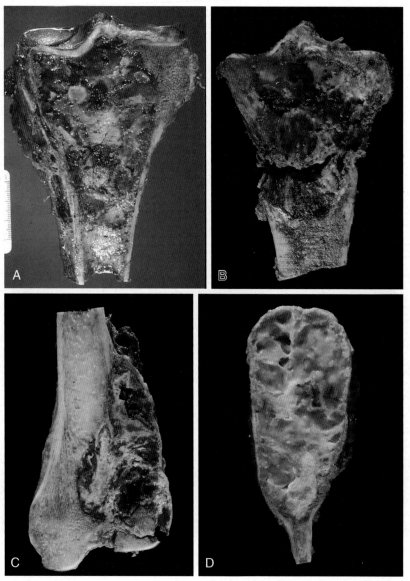

FIG. 7.41
Gross images of giant cell tumor (GCT) in the proximal tibia **(A, B)** showing the heterogeneity of the cut surface, which ranges from red-brown to yellow. The GCT in B was complicated by a pathologic fracture. GCT involving the distal femur **(C)** showing extension beyond the cortex. The periosteum is intact but elevated proximally where the tumor extends through the cortex. GCT of the proximal fibula **(D)** with cystic change and prominent fibrohistiocytic component, represented by the extensive yellow foci.

changes, including hemorrhage, necrosis, fibrohistiocytic change, or hemorrhagic cystic change, may obscure the classic histologic features of GCT (Fig. 7.43). In such cases, careful correlation of the histologic and radiographic features or the use of H3F3 antibodies are important for accurate diagnosis. Additionally, symplastic or pseudoanaplastic changes are present in occasional GCT, and these features may be mistaken for evidence of sarcomatous degeneration. Foci of vascular invasion may be identified in GCTs that extend into extraosseous soft tissue.

Malignant GCTs are uncommon and can show marked cytologic atypia and mitotic activity in a tumor otherwise resembling a GCT or sarcomatous transformation to a sarcoma of differing histologic subtypes (so-called "dedifferentiated GCT").

When GCTs are treated with denosumab (a RANK-ligand inhibitor), the giant cells disappear, the stromal cells become spindled, and abundant woven bone or calcified matrix forms, resulting in a post-therapy appearance reminiscent of a bone-forming neoplasm (see Fig. 7.43) (see later).

Ancillary Studies

Most GCTs harbor mutations in the *H3F3A* gene, the most common of which is p.Gly34Trp, or G34W. Less commonly, G34L, G34R, or G34V mutations are detected. Immunostains that detect the abnormal proteins

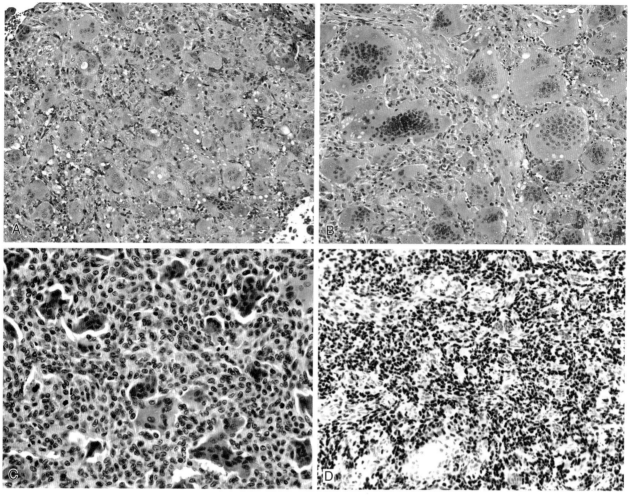

FIG. 7.42

Typical giant cell tumor (GCT) shows diffuse, even distribution of giant cells **(A)**. The giant cells of GCT often contain 25 or more nuclei, and the mononuclear stromal cells are somewhat epithelioid in appearance in this example **(B)**. The neoplastic mononuclear cells can show significant mitotic activity **(C)**. An immunostain for H3G34W is positive in more than 90% of GCT **(D)**.

are an excellent surrogate for the detection of the mutation and can be used to confirm the diagnosis of GCT on small samples, for lesions arising in unusual sites, or when radiology suggests the possibility of GCT but the classic histologic features are obscured by secondary changes.

Differential Diagnosis

Many benign lesions feature abundant multinucleated giant cells and can easily be confused with GCT. However, chondroblastoma and clear cell chondrosarcoma are two primary bone tumors that commonly involve the epiphyses of long bones and also contain large numbers of giant cells.

Chondroblastoma is a benign chondroid neoplasm that preferentially involves the epiphyses of skeletally immature patients and can contain prominent multinucleated giant cells. Chondroblastomas usually arise

in skeletally immature patients in a similar anatomic distribution to GCT. Radiographically, chondroblastomas sometimes contain foci of matrix calcification and typically show intense perilesional edema, two characteristics not seen with GCT (Fig. 7.44). Histologically, chondroblastomas have three main components: mononuclear stromal cells (chondroblasts), immature cartilaginous matrix, and multinucleated giant cells. Chondroblasts have distinct cytologic characteristics including well-defined cytoplasmic borders resulting in a discohesive, "cobblestone-like" appearance (Fig. 7.45). Additionally, the stromal cell nuclei have longitudinal grooves. The characteristic "chicken wire calcification" is seen in a minority of chondroblastomas. Finally, chondroblastomas can harbor mutations in either the *H3F3B* (more common) or *H3F3A* genes, detectable with the H3K36M antibody, further distinguishing chondroblastoma from GCT.

Clear cell chondrosarcoma is an unusual subtype of chondrosarcoma that preferentially involves the epiphyseal/metaphyseal region of long bones, particularly the

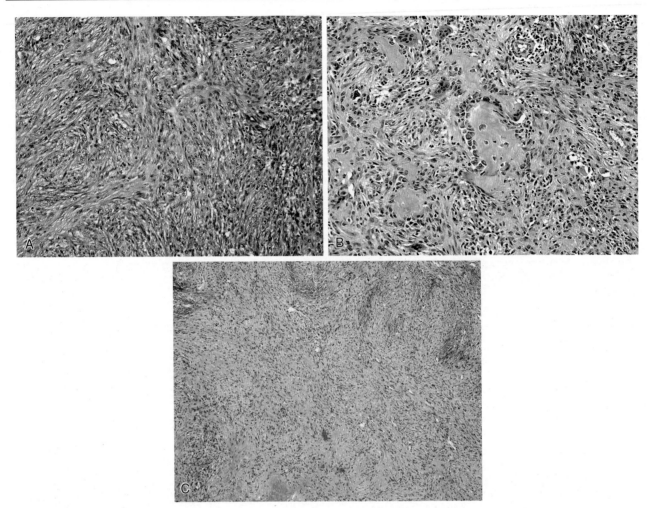

FIG. 7.43

Fibrohistiocytic change (A) and reactive bone (B) are sometimes prominent in giant cell tumor. With denosumab effect, the neoplastic mono-nuclear cells often show spindling, and the stroma becomes ossified or calcified (C).

proximal femur, proximal tibia, and proximal humerus. There is significant overlap in the radiographic features of GCT and clear cell chondrosarcoma. However, clear cell chondrosarcomas have unique histologic features that include cartilage and bone matrix formation, abundant multinucleated giant cells, and distinctive large mononuclear cells with abundant clear or lightly eosinophilic cytoplasm, large central nuclei, and prominent nucleoli (Fig. 7.46).

Prognosis and Therapy

The treatment of GCT is usually surgical for tumors in most sites and involves extended curettage with adjuvants and cementation with or without bone grafting. En bloc excision is utilized less frequently. The use of radiation therapy should be reserved only for cases in which surgical removal is impossible, in view of the relatively high number of reported cases of malignant transformation following this therapeutic modality.

There is growing experience with the treatment of GCT with denosumab, a monoclonal antibody antagonist of RANKL. This drug offers an alternative to radiotherapy for lesions arising in locations not amenable to surgery or for local recurrences and is a highly effective adjuvant for local control. Histologically, denosumab-treated GCTs show a marked diminution in the number of giant cells and an abundance of bone formation or calcification, resulting in an appearance resembling osteosarcoma.

The natural history of GCT is that of a low-grade neoplasm. Local recurrence following curettage is common (approximately 25%–30%). A small number of GCTs (1%–2%) metastasize, almost always following surgical manipulation. No relationship has been found between metastases and the presence of GCT invasion of blood vessels. Metastases are more likely in younger patients, from tumors located in the axial skeleton, following local recurrences, and in lesions that present with extraosseous extension. GCT metastases have a benign histologic appearance and do not ultimately cause death. Nevertheless, all patients with GCT are staged with imaging of the chest.

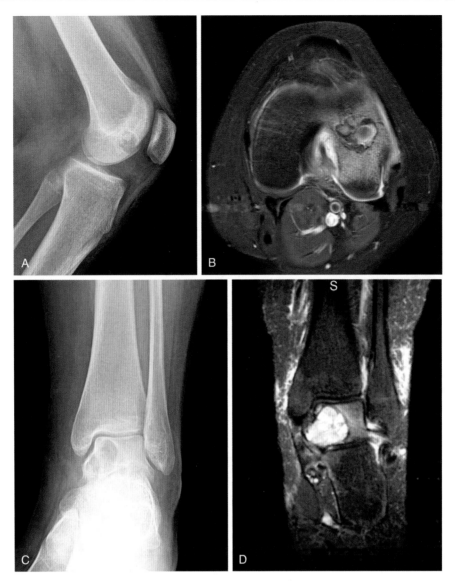

FIG. 7.44

Chondroblastomas also involve the epiphyseal region of the bone, and larger examples can extend into the metaphysis; patients are usually skeletally immature, as in this example in the distal femur **(A, B)**; however, skeletally mature patients can develop chondroblastomas in unusual locations such as the talus **(C, D)**. MRI typically shows extensive perilesional edema, which is not a prominent radiographic feature in giant cell tumor.

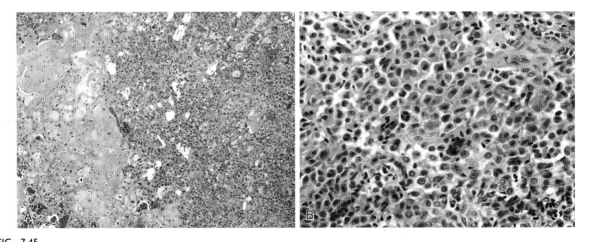

FIG. 7.45

A, Histologically, chondroblastomas contain a mix of eosinophilic chondroid matrix, chondroblasts, and multinucleated giant cells. **B,** The chondroblasts have nuclear cleft and well-defined cytoplasmic borders, resulting in a "cobblestone-like" appearance.

Continued

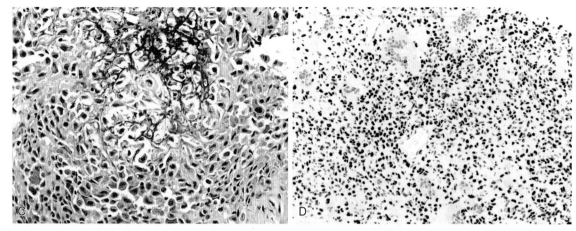

FIG. 7.45, cont'd

C, One of the histologic hallmarks of chondroblastoma is "chicken wire" calcification. **D,** The H3K36M immunostain is almost always positive in chondroblastomas.

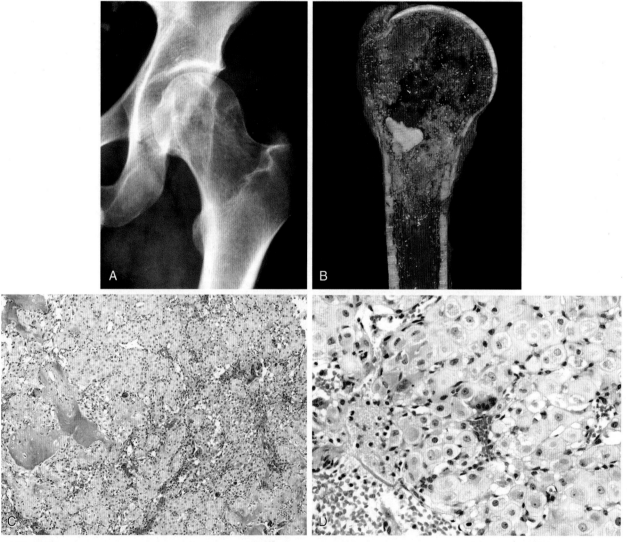

FIG. 7.46

Clear cell chondrosarcomas have imaging findings similar to giant cell tumor and involve the epiphysis and metaphysis as seen in this example in the proximal femur **(A)**. Gross example of a clear cell chondrosarcoma arising in the proximal humerus **(B)**. Histologically, clear cell chondrosarcomas can contain either cartilage or woven bone and have numerous multinucleated giant cells **(C)** but are defined by large, epithelioid cells with clear or eosinophilic cytoplasm, large nuclei, and prominent nucleoli **(D)**.

ANEURYSMAL BONE CYST

DIFFERENTIAL DIAGNOSIS: TELANGIECTATIC OSTEOSARCOMA, SIMPLE BONE CYST (SBC)

Clinical Features

Primary ABC is a benign bone neoplasm not associated with un underlying lesion, whereas secondary ABC (now thought of as ABC-like or hemorrhagic cystic change rather than true ABC) arises in association with a wide variety of benign and malignant neoplasms, including GCT, chondroblastoma, fibrous dysplasia, or osteosarcoma, among others. Primary ABC occurs most commonly in patients between 10 and 20 years of age and is slightly more common in females than in males. Primary ABCs have been reported in nearly all bones but arise mainly in the posterior elements of vertebrae and in the metaphyses of long bones. Vertebral lesions may involve more than one spinal level. The main symptom is pain, and spine lesions can cause symptoms related to compression of the spinal cord.

Radiographic Features

Radiographically, primary ABCs can arise within the medullary cavity or beneath the periosteum (Fig. 7.47). Centrally located lesions are radiolucent and cause expansile remodeling of the affected bone with thinning of the cortex. A thin shell of reactive bone often encompasses ABC, best appreciated on radiograph or CT. Central lesions that erode through the cortex and extend into the soft tissue also have a shell of reactive bone surrounding the soft tissue component. ABCs have a multiloculated appearance on MRI, and the characteristic fluid-fluid levels are best appreciated on this radiographic modality (Fig. 7.48). Secondary ABCs can involve the epiphysis, metaphysis, or diaphysis, depending on the preferred location of the underlying, primary lesion.

Pathologic Features

GROSS FINDINGS

Grossly, ABCs are spongy, hemorrhagic masses surrounded by a thin shell of reactive bone; those cysts that extend into the adjacent soft tissue are also contained by a thin shell of reactive bone derived from the periosteum (Fig. 7.49). Some ABCs, particularly those arising

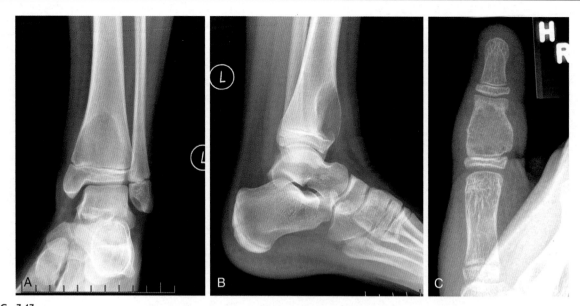

FIG. 7.47

AP **(A)** and lateral **(B)** plain radiographs show a primary aneurysmal bone cyst (ABC) arising in the distal tibia. The lesion arises in the metaphysis, is well-circumscribed, and although the cortex is thinned anteriorly, the lesion is covered by a thin rim of reactive bone. In the small bones of the hands and feet, ABCs are often solid. This example in the proximal phalanx of the tumor causes significant expansile remodeling **(C)**.

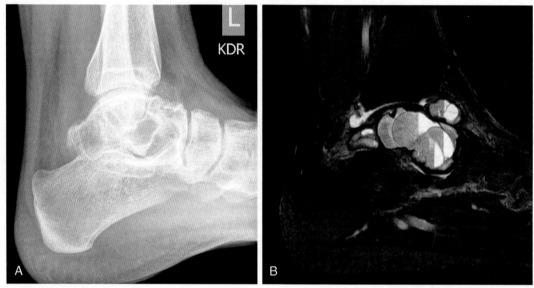

FIG. 7.48

Lateral plain radiograph **(A)** and MRI **(B)** showing an aneurysmal bone cyst arising in the talus. Fluid-fluid levels are easily recognized on MRI.

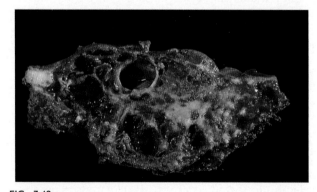

FIG. 7.49

Grossly, aneurysmal bone cysts have large cystic spaces filled with blood with small foci of intervening solid tissue.

in the small bones of the hands and feet, may not appear cystic but contain solid foci of hemorrhagic tissue. These "solid" ABCs have also been referred to as "giant cell reparative granulomas" and "giant cell lesions of the small bones."

MICROSCOPIC FINDINGS

ABC is a blood-filled cystic neoplasm with cellular septa containing fibroblasts, inflammatory cells, giant cells, and woven bone. The woven bone often follows the contour of the individual septum. The fibroblastic foci resemble nodular fasciitis in appearance. Characteristic blue bone ("blue reticulated chondroid-like material")

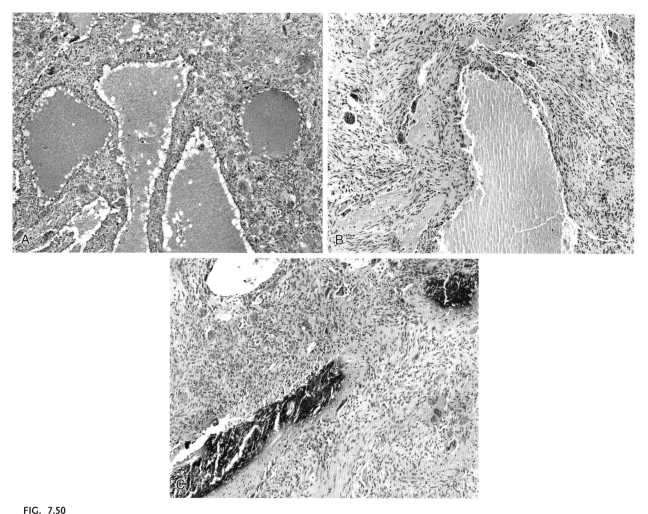

FIG. 7.50

A, Microscopically, aneurysmal bone cysts (ABCs) have prominent pseudocystic spaces containing blood. **B,** The intact tissue surrounding the cystic spaces often appears fasciitis-like and contains numerous giant cells. **C,** Calcified matrix is found in approximately half of ABC.

is present in a minority of ABCs (Fig. 7.50). Mitotic figures are often present and may be numerous; however, atypical mitoses and cytologic atypia should not be identified. Solid foci can be seen in ABCs, especially in lesions arising in the small bones of the hands and feet (so-called "giant cell lesion of the small bones"), which lack cystic spaces and are composed of fibroblasts, clustered multinucleated giant cells, and abundant reactive woven bone.

Ancillary Studies

Approximately 70% of primary ABCs harbor a rearrangement of the *USP6* gene, most commonly involving a t(16;17)(q22;p13), resulting in a *CDH11-USP6* fusion. A variety of other partner genes have been identified, but they are far less common. In difficult cases, particularly those involving small biopsies or primarily solid lesions, evaluation for a *USP6* rearrangement

by fluorescence *in situ* hybridization (FISH) or the identification of a USP6 fusion with next-generation sequencing–based fusion panels can be helpful in establishing the diagnosis.

Differential Diagnosis

Telangiectatic osteosarcomas can have remarkably similar radiographic and gross characteristics to ABCs but are typically far more destructive. Telangiectatic osteosarcomas have a similar low-magnification appearance as ABCs. However, telangiectatic osteosarcomas have significant cytologic atypia, a feature not seen in ABC (Figs. 7.51 and 7.52).

SBCs also appear as radiolucent lesions that initially abut the growth plate but "migrate" away from the physis as the skeleton grows. SBCs can cause expansile remodeling and thinning of the cortex, but not to the degree seen in ABCs. SBC has a single large

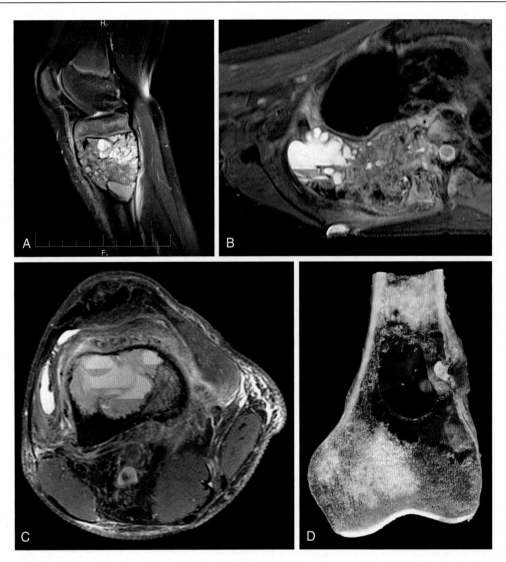

FIG. 7.51

Telangiectatic osteosarcomas can have an MRI appearance similar to aneurysmal bone cyst, as seen in these examples in the proximal tibia **(A)**, chest wall **(B)**, and distal femur **(C)**. Telangiectatic osteosarcomas also have a bloody, cystic appearance grossly **(D)**.

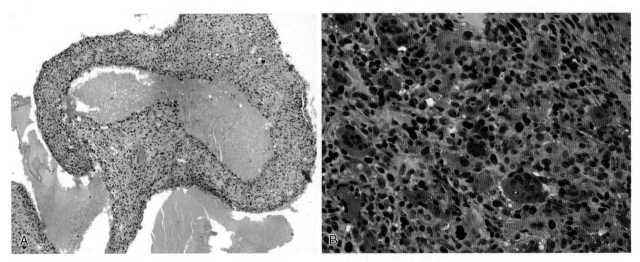

FIG. 7.52

Histologically, telangiectatic osteosarcomas have a low-magnification appearance that is similar to aneurysmal bone cyst **(A)** but show marked cytologic atypia and increased mitotic activity **(B)**.

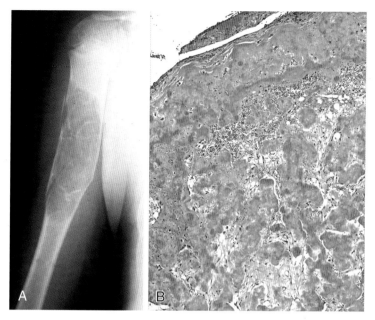

FIG. 7.53

Simple bone cysts (SBCs) also arise in the metaphyseal region of long bones, as in this example in the proximal humerus. Pathologic fracture leads to fragments of cortex falling into the cyst, as seen here, referred to as the "fallen fragment" or "fallen leaf" sign **(A)**. Histologically, SBCs have a fibrous lining, and the wall of the cyst often contains fibrin-like material **(B)**.

chamber and lacks fluid-fluid levels radiographically. After pathologic fracture, fragments of cortex may float freely in the cyst, a pathognomonic finding referred to as the "fallen fragment" sign. Histologically, SBCs have a simple fibrous lining and fibrin-like material can be deposited within the wall of the cyst (Fig. 7.53). As the fibrin-like material calcifies, it can resemble cementum and eventually may ossify. Other histologic features include cholesterol clefts, foamy histiocytes, and chronic inflammation. When SBCs undergo pathologic fracture, ABC-like features may develop, and careful radiographic correlation is necessary for diagnosis. As opposed to *USP6* rearrangements, approximately 30% to 40% of SBC will show *EWSR1-* or *FUS-NFATC2* fusions. SBCs must also be distinguished from cystic fibrous dysplasia, a problematic differential diagnosis more commonly encountered in adults than in children.

Finally, extensive sampling and careful radiographic correlation is necessary in all cases of ABCs to exclude the possibility of an underlying lesion.

Prognosis and Therapy

Although ABC is a locally aggressive neoplasm, most are treated with curettage. Reported local recurrence rates are highly variable, ranging from 25% to 75%. ABCs have also been treated with steroid and doxycycline injections, as well as radiotherapy.

ANEURYSMAL BONE CYST – DISEASE FACT SHEET

Definition

▶▶ A benign neoplasm containing blood-filled cystic spaces and multinucleated giant cells

Incidence and Location

▶▶ Affects the metaphyses of long bone and the posterior elements of vertebrae

▶▶ ABCs in the small bones of the hands and feet are often solid

Age Distribution

▶▶ Can occur in a wide age range, but most commonly affects patients in the first and second decades

Clinical Features

▶▶ ABCs cause pain and swelling, and can cause pathologic fracture

▶▶ Lesions in the spine can lead to neurologic symptoms

Radiologic Features

▶▶ Arise in the metaphyseal region of long bones, posterior elements of vertebrae

▶▶ Radiolucent lesions that can cause significant remodeling of the cortex, but are surrounded by a thin layer of reactive bone when the cortex is thinned or absent

▶▶ Characteristic fluid-fluid levels are best seen on MRI

Prognosis and Therapy

▶▶ Usually treated with curettage, but larger lesions may require resection

▶▶ Intralesional steroid or doxycycline injections are sometimes effective

▶▶ Radiotherapy may be necessary in some sites

FIBROUS DYSPLASIA

DIFFERENTIAL DIAGNOSIS: OSTEOFIBROUS DYSPLASIA, ADAMANTINOMA, LOW-GRADE CENTRAL OSTEOSARCOMA

Clinical Features

Fibrous dysplasia can be monostotic or polyostotic. The monostotic form is usually seen in older children and young adults and most commonly affects the ribs, femur, tibia, and craniofacial bones. The less common polyostotic type may be unilateral or have widespread skeletal involvement. Patients with widespread skeletal involvement may also have associated endocrine dysfunction, precocious puberty in female individuals, and areas of cutaneous hyperpigmentation (McCune-Albright syndrome). Monostotic fibrous dysplasia, polyostotic fibrous dysplasia, and McCune-Albright syndrome all occur sporadically and are caused by postzygotic somatic activating mutations in the *GNAS1* gene, which is located on 20q13 and encodes the α-stimulatory subunit of the heterotrimeric G proteins. The differences in clinical manifestation presumably relate to the timing of the mutation, with mutations occurring during embryonic life being more likely to result in McCune-Albright syndrome, and mutations occurring in postnatal life more likely to cause monostotic disease. The bone lesions of fibrous dysplasia have been found to be

clonal, indicating that fibrous dysplasia is a neoplastic process.

Monostotic fibrous dysplasia may be asymptomatic and discovered incidentally or cause pain. Occasionally, patients will experience a pathologic fracture. Lesions involving craniofacial bone can cause significant deformities. Patients with polyostotic fibrous dysplasia often have significant deformities and suffer repeated fractures.

Radiographic Features

Fibrous dysplasia arises within the medullary cavity and may cause expansile remodeling of the bone. The lesions are usually well-circumscribed and frequently have prominent surrounding reactive bone (Fig. 7.54). The appearance of the lesion on conventional radiographs and CT depends on the relative proportion of bone matrix and fibrous stroma within the lesion but is often described as having "ground-glass opacity" (Fig. 7.55). Punctate areas of calcification may be seen when chondroid differentiation is present. Lesions involving craniofacial bones may appear radiodense. Repeated fractures and repair of the femoral neck cause the typical "shepherd's crook" deformity, a finding often found in polyostotic fibrous dysplasia. Occasionally fibrous dysplasia protrudes far beyond the normal bone contour; such cases are referred to as "fibrous dysplasia protuberans."

Pathologic Features

GROSS FINDINGS

Fibrous dysplasia arises within the medullary cavity and may cause expansile remodeling of the involved bone. The periphery of fibrous dysplasia is well-circumscribed from the surrounding bone and often separated by a rim of reactive bone. The cut surface is grayish-white and cuts with a gritty consistency (Fig. 7.56). Nodules of gray hyaline cartilage are present in cases containing chondroid differentiation. Older lesions may become cystic, and in such cases the possibility of a primary bone cyst may be considered.

MICROSCOPIC FINDINGS

Microscopically, fibrous dysplasia is composed of irregularly shaped trabeculae of woven bone deposited in a fibrous stroma of variable cellularity (Fig. 7.57). The bone trabeculae may have a "C" or "S" shape or can appear round. These bone trabeculae are woven when viewed with polarized light but lack the accompanying osteoblastic rimming that would be expected given the immaturity of the bone. Osteoclasts are sometimes

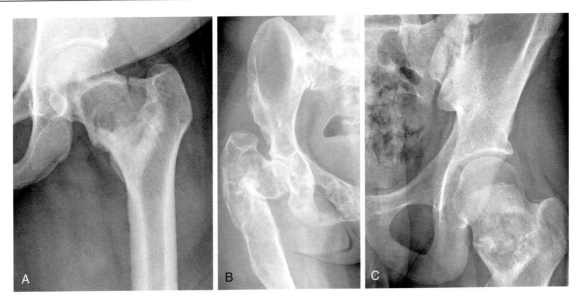

FIG. 7.54

A, Radiographically, this example of monostotic fibrous dysplasia arising in the femoral neck is well-circumscribed, has a surrounding layer of reactive bone, and is complicated by a pathologic fracture. **B,** Plain radiograph showing the severe deformity associated with polyostotic fibrous dysplasia, including a classic "shepherd crook deformity" of the proximal femur. **C,** Fibrous dysplasia with extensive chondroid metaplasia arising in the proximal left femur.

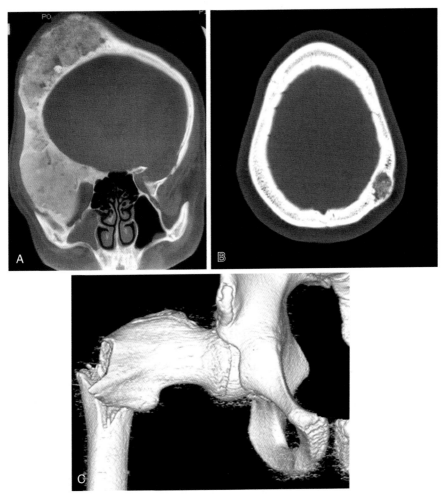

FIG. 7.55

A, CT shows extensive craniofacial involvement by fibrous dysplasia, which has the typical ground-glass appearance in this example. **B,** A solitary focus of fibrous dysplasia in the cranium is well-circumscribed but causes expansile remodeling. **C,** This three-dimensional reconstruction shows a pathologic fracture through fibrous dysplasia in the femoral neck.

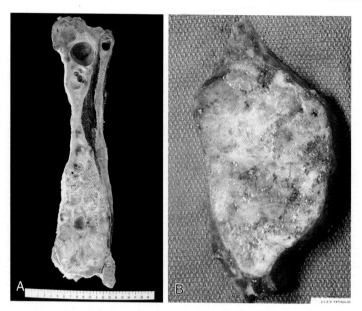

FIG. 7.56

A, Gross example of polyostotic fibrous dysplasia in the tibia and fibula with prominent cystic change. **B,** A gross example of fibrous dysplasia with chondroid differentiation involving the proximal fibula. The gray chondroid nodules are easily appreciated.

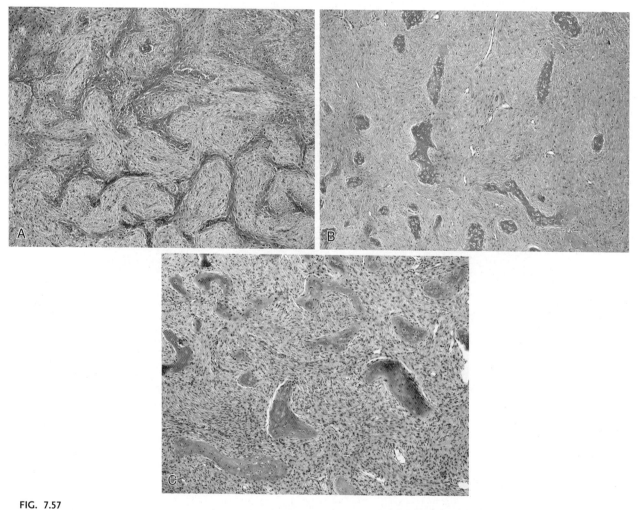

FIG. 7.57

A, At low magnification, fibrous dysplasia is composed of immature woven bone deposited in a fibrous stroma. **B,** The irregularly shaped woven bone trabeculae lack osteoblastic rimming, and the stroma often contains prominent capillaries. **C,** In this example, the fibrous stroma is cellular, but the woven bone trabeculae lack osteoblastic rimming.

numerous. The stromal component of fibrous dysplasia is variably cellular and composed of bland spindled cells deposited in a collagenous or variably myxoid stroma rich in capillaries. Older lesions may become cystic or develop a histiocytic infiltrate. Stromal hemorrhage may elicit a giant cell reaction, and ABC-like changes often accompany fibrous dysplasia.

Occasionally, lesions of fibrous dysplasia show calcified spherules similar to those seen in cemento-osseous jaw lesions. Other cases show highly cellular areas that may be diagnosed incorrectly as sarcoma. Focal areas of hyaline cartilage and cystic areas may also be present (Fig. 7.58). The former is more common in the polyostotic variety and can dominate the microscopic picture to such a degree that a mistaken diagnosis of a cartilaginous tumor can be made.

Ancillary Studies

Fibrous dysplasia does not have a diagnostic immunophenotype, and the vast majority of cases can be confidently diagnosed without the use of ancillary diagnostic tests. Detection of the *GNAS* mutation helps separate fibrous dysplasia from low-grade central osteosarcoma, which is characterized by *MDM2* amplification.

Differential Diagnosis

One of the most important tumors in the differential diagnosis is low-grade central osteosarcoma (Fig. 7.59).

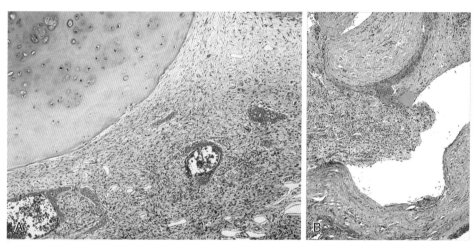

FIG. 7.58
Examples of fibrous dysplasia with chondroid differentiation **(A)** and cystic change **(B)**.

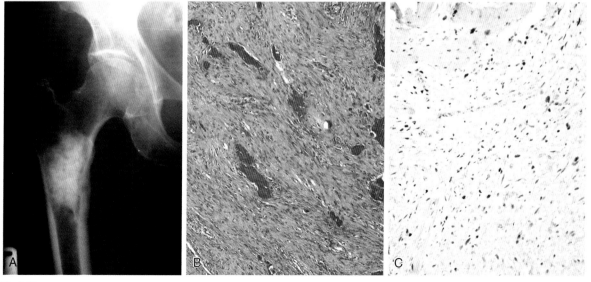

FIG. 7.59
A, Radiographically, this example of low-grade central osteosarcoma is radiodense, has ill-defined borders, and disrupts the cortex medially. **B,** Histologically, low-grade central osteosarcomas resemble parosteal osteosarcomas and are composed of spicules of woven bone deposited in a fibrous stroma with mild cytologic atypia. **(C)** MDM2 immunohistochemistry is usually positive in the fibroblastic stromal cells of low-grade central osteosarcoma and is a useful ancillary study when molecular diagnostic testing is not possible due to the use of decalcifiers.

This variant of osteosarcoma usually arises in long bones. Radiographically, low-grade central osteosarcomas are less circumscribed than fibrous dysplasia and lack surrounding reactive bone. Histologically, these tumors are infiltrative and have a greater degree of cytologic atypia than fibrous dysplasia. A high percentage of low-grade central osteosarcomas show *MDM2* amplification by FISH and are positive for MDM2 immunohistochemistry.

Fibrous dysplasia must also be distinguished from osteofibrous dysplasia (Fig. 7.60) and osteofibrous dysplasia-like adamantinoma (Fig. 7.61). Importantly, both of these tumors arise within the cortex, most commonly the anterior cortex of the tibia or fibula, as opposed to the central medullary cavity epicenter of fibrous dysplasia. Osteoblastic rimming of the bony trabeculae, a prominent feature in osteofibrous dysplasia, is less commonly seen in fibrous dysplasia, and the keratin-immunoreactive stromal cells of osteofibrous dysplasia are never observed in fibrous dysplasia. Nodules of benign hyaline cartilage may be present in a subset of fibrous dysplasia cases but are not encountered in osteofibrous dysplasia. Finally, fibrous dysplasia is characterized at the molecular level by activating missense mutations in *GNAS*, which have not been identified in osteofibrous dysplasia. In addition to being intracortical, osteofibrous dysplasia-like adamantinoma is characterized by isolated nests of keratin-immunoreactive epithelial cells, a feature not found in fibrous dysplasia.

Prognosis and Therapy

Asymptomatic lesions can be safely observed, but larger symptomatic lesions or those with impending pathologic fracture require surgical management, usually curettage. Local recurrence rates are extremely low following curettage. Fibrous dysplasia has a small risk of malignant transformation.

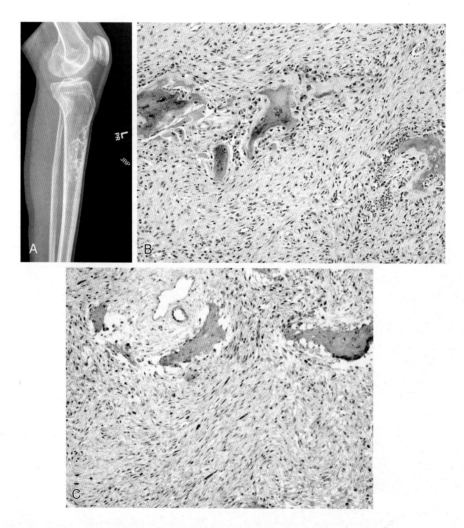

FIG. 7.60

A, Radiographic example of osteofibrous dysplasia showing radiolucencies in the anterior tibial cortex. **B,** Osteofibrous dysplasia is a benign fibro-osseous neoplasm with cellular fibrous stroma and woven bone trabeculae with prominent osteoblastic rimming. **C,** An immunostain for cytokeratin can be used to highlight individual spindle cells in the stroma, but nests of epithelial cells should not be identified.

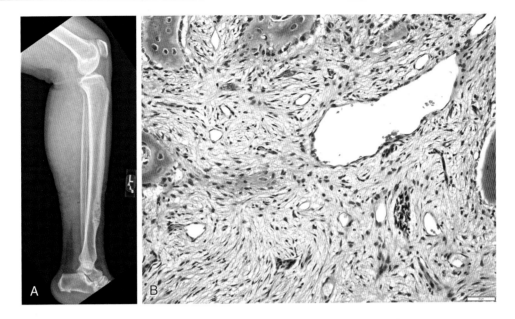

FIG. 7.61

A, Osteofibrous dysplasia-like adamantinoma has radiographic features essentially identical to osteofibrous dysplasia. **B,** In addition to having a predominately fibro-osseous appearance, osteofibrous dysplasia-like adamantinoma also contains isolated nests of epithelial cells.

FIBROUS DYSPLASIA – DISEASE FACT SHEET

Definition
- ▸▸ Benign fibro-osseous neoplasm that can be monostotic or polyostotic

Incidence and Location
- ▸▸ Any bone can be affected by fibrous dysplasia
- ▸▸ Monostotic fibrous dysplasia occurs most commonly in the craniofacial bones and proximal femur
- ▸▸ Polyostotic fibrous dysplasia can range from localized to a single limb to diffuse skeletal involvement

Age Distribution
- ▸▸ Can occur in either children or adults

Clinical Features
- ▸▸ Often asymptomatic
- ▸▸ Symptomatic lesions cause pain and possibly pathologic fracture
- ▸▸ Patients with McCune-Albright syndrome have endocrine abnormalities, pigmented lesions, and polyostotic fibrous dysplasia
- ▸▸ Patients with Mazabraud syndrome have fibrous dysplasia and intramuscular myxomas

Radiologic Features
- ▸▸ Well-circumscribed lesions with ground-glass density
- ▸▸ Surrounding reactive bone is usually prominent
- ▸▸ Shepherd's crook deformity of the proximal femur is essentially pathognomonic

Prognosis and Therapy
- ▸▸ Asymptomatic lesions can be observed
- ▸▸ Symptomatic lesions are typically managed with curettage
- ▸▸ Local recurrence is uncommon following surgery

FIBROUS DYSPLASIA – PATHOLOGIC FEATURES

Gross Findings
- ▸▸ Tissue is tan and gritty, and cysts may be present

Microscopic Findings
- ▸▸ Benign fibro-osseous neoplasm
- ▸▸ Woven bone trabeculae devoid of osteoblastic rimming deposited in a variably cellular fibrous stroma
- ▸▸ Cyst change occurs in longstanding lesions
- ▸▸ Chondroid nodules possible

Pathologic Differential Diagnoses
- ▸▸ Low-grade central osteosarcoma
- ▸▸ Osteofibrous dysplasia
- ▸▸ Osteofibrous dysplasia-like adamantinoma

PAROSTEAL OSTEOSARCOMA

DIFFERENTIAL DIAGNOSIS: PERIOSTEAL OSTEOSARCOMA, HIGH-GRADE SURFACE OSTEOSARCOMA, OSTEOCHONDROMA, JUXTACORTICAL MYOSITIS OSSIFICANS

Clinical Features

Parosteal osteosarcoma is a low-grade, surface-based osteosarcoma variant that is fibro-osseous in histologic appearance. Parosteal osteosarcoma is the most common surface variant of osteosarcoma, represents approximately

5% of osteosarcomas, and arises in patients aged 20 to 40 years. Parosteal osteosarcomas occur most frequently in the distal femur, proximal tibia, and proximal humerus. Most patients present with a long history of a slowly growing mass that sometimes affects range of motion. A small number of parosteal osteosarcomas dedifferentiate into a high-grade sarcoma, often reflected clinically in sudden rapid growth.

Radiographic Features

Conventional radiographs usually have a characteristic appearance. Parosteal osteosarcomas most commonly arise from the posterior cortex in the metaphyseal region of the bone. They are densely ossified, lobular,

spherical masses separated from the underlying cortex by a thin cleft, and sharply circumscribed from adjacent soft tissue (Fig. 7.62). CT and MRI are useful in assessing invasion of the underlying bone (Fig. 7.63). A cartilage cap or cartilaginous nodules within the tumor can also be identified with MRI, appearing as high signal intensity foci within an otherwise low signal intensity mass. Foci of dedifferentiation are identified radiographically as radiolucencies within an otherwise densely ossified mass.

Pathologic Features

GROSS FINDINGS

Parosteal osteosarcomas are dense, lobulated neoplasms attached to the outer surface of the underlying cortex.

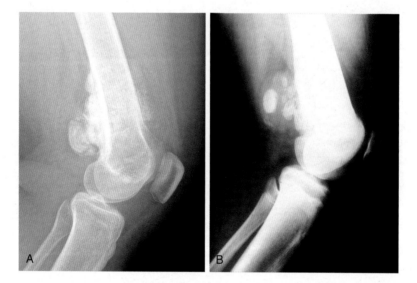

FIG. 7.62

Parosteal osteosarcomas have a characteristic radiographic appearance consisting of one or more heavily ossified nodules adherent to the posterior cortex of the involved bone, most often the distal femur. Parosteal osteosarcomas may encircle the bone **(A)** or have multiple satellite nodules **(B)**.

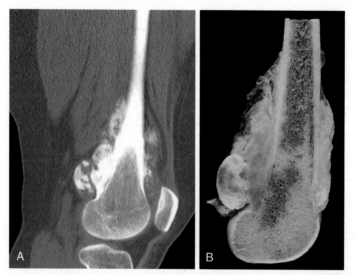

FIG. 7.63

A, CT highlights the ossified nature of a parosteal osteosarcoma of the distal femur. **B,** Grossly, parosteal osteosarcomas appear as densely ossified mass adherent to the surface of the underlying bone. In this example the lesion encircles the distal femur.

Some larger examples will encircle the bone (see Fig. 7.63). The cut surface is firm and tan, and chondroid nodules may be present within the mass or as a cartilage cap. Invasion of the underlying bone may occur with parosteal osteosarcomas, particularly when dedifferentiated foci develop.

MICROSCOPIC FINDINGS

Microscopically, parosteal osteosarcomas are histologically identical to low-grade central osteosarcomas and are composed of a bland fibrous stroma containing disorganized, immature bone that sometimes has a Pagetic appearance (Fig. 7.64). The cytologic features of malignancy in the fibrous stroma are often subtle, thus accounting for the great frequency of misdiagnoses made in this tumor. Some tumors contain large areas of fibroblastic stroma devoid of bone that resemble desmoplastic

fibroma. Cartilage may be present on the periphery of the tumor or embedded deep within it. Foci of high-grade dedifferentiation can resemble undifferentiated pleomorphic sarcoma or osteosarcoma, most commonly.

Ancillary Studies

Parosteal osteosarcomas are characterized cytogenetically by supernumerary giant or ring chromosomes that contain amplified material from 12q13-15, corresponding to the *CDK4* and *MDM2* genes, among others. The evaluation of these gene amplifications by FISH or the detection of their protein products by immunohistochemistry is useful in distinguishing parosteal osteosarcoma from the other lesions in the differential diagnosis that lack these genetic alterations.

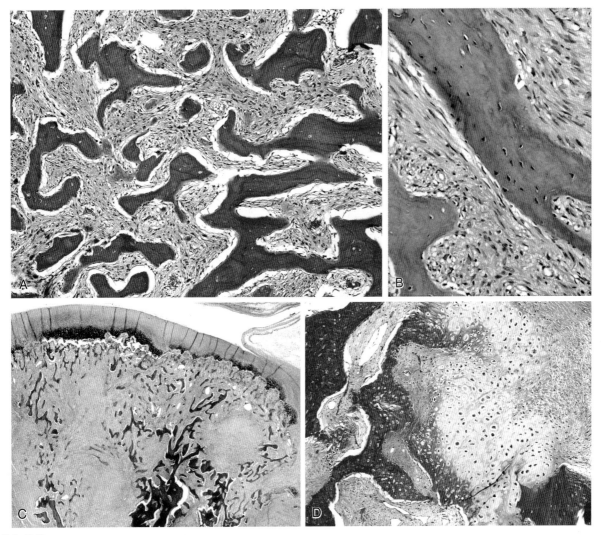

FIG. 7.64

At low magnification, parosteal osteosarcomas resemble fibro-osseous neoplasms are composed of both bone and fibrous stroma. In some cases, the bone is Pagetic in appearance as seen here **(A)**. The bland cytologic features of parosteal osteosarcoma are better appreciated at high magnification **(B)**. A cartilage cap may be present on the surface of a parosteal osteosarcoma **(C)**, or chondroid nodules may occur more centrally within the tumor **(D)**.

Differential Diagnosis

The two other surface variants of osteosarcoma are far less common than parosteal osteosarcomas. High-grade surface osteosarcoma histologically resembles a conventional high-grade osteosarcoma but arises from the surface of the bone, and its distinction from parosteal osteosarcoma is straightforward.

Periosteal osteosarcoma is an intermediate-grade surface osteosarcoma with largely chondroblastic features (Fig. 7.65). Its radiographic features differ significantly from those of parosteal osteosarcoma. Most arise in the diaphysis of long bones and have a lenticular or fusiform shape. There is frequently an associated periosteal reaction, a feature that parosteal osteosarcomas lack, and rather than a dense, lobular appearance, these tumors have hair-on-end mineralization. Because they are

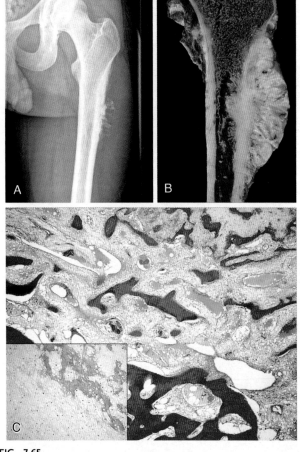

FIG. 7.65

A, Radiographically, periosteal osteosarcomas are usually more diaphyseal in location and often show a sunburst appearance of mineralization. **B,** Grossly, periosteal osteosarcomas have a lens-shaped appearance, are heavily chondroblastic, and arising between the cortex and periosteum. **C,** Histologically, large areas of periosteal osteosarcoma may consist of reactive bone, but the chondroblastic nature of this osteosarcoma variant is evident in the inset photo.

predominately chondroblastic, the signal intensity of periosteal osteosarcomas is bright on water-sensitive sequences, whereas parosteal osteosarcomas are low-to-intermediate in signal intensity on similar sequences. Their chondroblastic appearance also differs significantly from the low-grade fibroblastic appearance of parosteal osteosarcomas.

Because of its bland cytologic features and the occasional presence of a cartilage cap, parosteal osteosarcomas can be confused with osteochondromas. These lesions are easily distinguished with careful radiographic and histologic correlation. Osteochondromas are exophytic osteocartilaginous neoplasms that are in direct continuity with the underlying bone; the cortex of an osteochondroma is continuous with the cortex of the bone of origin, allowing the medullary cavity of the stalk of an osteochondroma to flow directly into the medullary cavity of the bone. In contrast, the cortex underlying a parosteal osteosarcoma is intact. Osteochondromas have an orderly, smooth cartilaginous cap, whereas the cartilaginous foci in a parosteal osteosarcoma are slightly hypercellular, disorganized, and display mild cytologic atypia. The features of osteochondroma are discussed earlier in this chapter.

Myositis ossificans (Fig. 7.66) differs from parosteal osteosarcoma in several ways. Both radiographically and histologically, myositis ossificans shows a distinctive zonal architecture, with bone formation peripherally and a mitotically active spindle cell proliferation centrally. However, the zonal architecture can be subtle on small biopsies, and therefore careful radiographic correlation and testing for *MDM2* and *USP6* gene abnormalities is important. Many cases of myositis ossificans will harbor a *USP6* gene rearrangement but not *MDM2* gene amplification.

Prognosis and Therapy

Parosteal osteosarcomas are low-grade sarcomas that rarely metastasize and have an excellent prognosis. Local recurrence may occur following incomplete excision, and wide surgical margins should be obtained surgically. A small percentage of parosteal osteosarcomas will transform into high-grade sarcomas (so-called dedifferentiated parosteal osteosarcoma).

PAROSTEAL OSTEOSARCOMA – DISEASE FACT SHEET

Definition
▸▸ A low-grade surface variant of osteosarcoma

Incidence and Location
▸▸ The most common surface variant of osteosarcoma
▸▸ Most arise from the posterior metaphyseal surface of the distal femur, proximal tibia, or proximal humerus

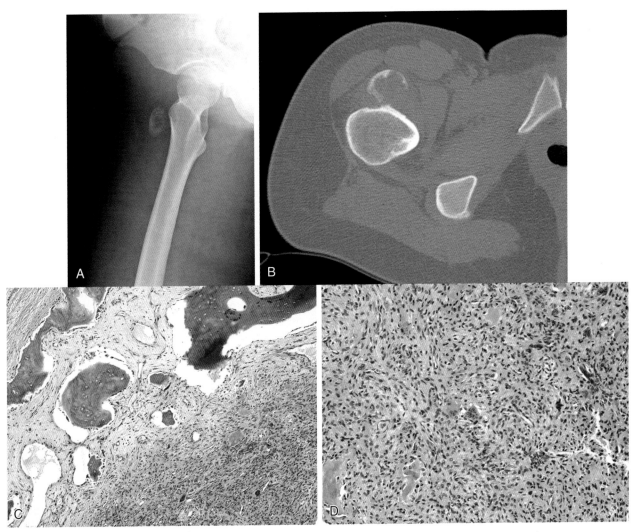

FIG. 7.66

Myositis ossificans has a zonal architecture on both plain radiograph **(A)** and CT **(B)**, with peripheral ossification and central lucency. **(C)** Histologically, the periphery of myositis ossificans shows reactive woven bone that is sharply circumscribed from the adjacent muscle. **(D)** The central radiolucent zone is composed of a mitotically active spindle cell proliferation that lacks cytologic atypia.

Age Distribution

▸▸ Occur most commonly in the third and fourth decades of life

Clinical Features

▸▸ Present as slowly enlarging painless masses

Radiologic Features

▸▸ Plain radiographs and CT show a lobulated, radiodense mass attached to the surface of the bone
▸▸ Often partially separated from the cortex by a thin radiolucent cleft
▸▸ Cartilaginous foci and areas of dedifferentiation may appear radiolucent

Prognosis and Therapy

▸▸ Treated with wide surgical excision
▸▸ Excellent prognosis
▸▸ Dedifferentiated parosteal osteosarcomas behave like high-grade osteosarcomas

PAROSTEAL OSTEOSARCOMA – PATHOLOGIC FEATURES

Gross Findings

▸▸ Densely ossified mass stuck to the surface of the bone
▸▸ Chondroid foci have a grayish appearance
▸▸ May extend through the cortex and into the medullary cavity

Microscopic Findings

▸▸ Low-grade fibroblastic osteosarcoma resembling a fibro-osseous lesion
▸▸ The bone can appear relatively mature and have Pagetic features; osteoblastic rimming is possible
▸▸ The fibroblastic stroma is bland, and mitoses are uncommon
▸▸ Chondroid foci can be present at the periphery of the mass or within the central portion

Ancillary studies

▸▸ Similar to low-grade central osteosarcoma, *MDM2* amplification may be demonstrated by FISH
▸▸ MDM2 immunohistochemistry is usually positive

Continued

DESMOPLASTIC FIBROMA

DIFFERENTIAL DIAGNOSIS: FIBROUS DYSPLASIA, LOW-GRADE CENTRAL OSTEOSARCOMA

Clinical Features

Desmoplastic fibroma is a rare, locally aggressive primary bone neoplasm that most commonly arises in adolescents and young adults. The most common locations for desmoplastic fibroma are the gnathic bones, particularly the mandible, followed by long bones. Patients typically present with a mass, swelling, or long history of pain associated with the lesion.

Radiographic Features

On conventional radiographs, desmoplastic fibromas are radiolucent lesions that may appear well-circumscribed or destroy the cortex and extend into adjacent soft tissue. They cause significant expansile remodeling, lack surrounding reactive bone, and often contain internal trabeculations. CT and MRI are useful for identifying soft tissue extension (Fig. 7.67). Like many fibrous lesions, desmoplastic fibromas tend to be low in signal intensity on T1-weighted MRI and low or intermediate signal intensity on T2-weighted MRI.

Pathologic Features

GROSS FINDINGS

Desmoplastic fibromas have a firm, whitish, trabeculated cut surface. They often appear deceptively well-circumscribed and can appear to have well-defined borders despite having microscopic extension into adjacent soft tissue.

MICROSCOPIC FINDINGS

The microscopic appearance of desmoplastic fibroma is often compared with soft tissue fibromatosis, composed of long, intersecting fascicles of bland fibroblastic or myofibroblastic spindled cells embedded in a dense collagenous stroma (Fig. 7.68). However, some lesions lack the fascicular growth pattern. The lesional spindled cells lack cytologic atypia, and no mitoses or necrosis are present.

Ancillary Studies

Only rare cases of desmoplastic fibroma have been shown to contain *CTNNB1* gene mutations, despite the fact that beta-catenin immunoreactivity is significantly more common. These tumors do not show *MDM2* amplification or *GNAS* mutations, and immunohistochemistry for MDM2 is negative (see below).

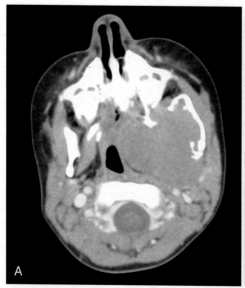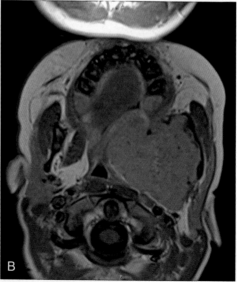

FIG. 7.67

CT **(A)** and MRI **(B)** show a destructive desmoplastic fibroma arising in the mandible of a young child.

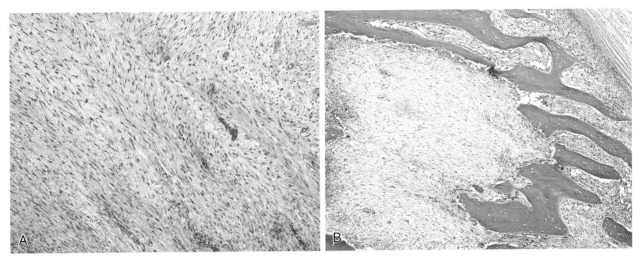

FIG. 7.68

A, At low magnification, desmoplastic fibroma resembles soft tissue fibromatosis and is composed of fascicles of fibroblasts set in abundant collagen. **B,** Desmoplastic fibromas may destroy a portion of the cortex.

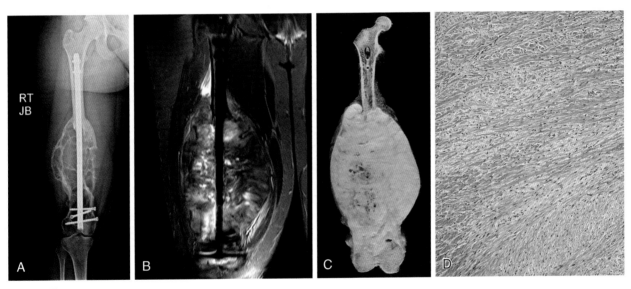

FIG. 7.69

Conventional radiograph **(A)** and MRI **(B)** of an unusual low-grade central osteosarcoma that had undergone prior intramedullary fixation for a presumed diagnosis of aneurysmal bone cyst. **(C)** Grossly, this large, fleshy lesion infiltrated cancellous bone and extended into adjacent soft tissue. **(D)** Histologically, this lesion closely resembled a desmoplastic fibroma; however, the tumor was positive for MDM2 immunohistochemically, and molecular analysis showed *MDM2* amplification.

Differential Diagnosis

Fibrous dysplasia is a benign fibro-osseous neoplasm that can be difficult to distinguish from desmoplastic fibroma, particularly when sampling is limited. Most cases of fibrous dysplasia contain a prominent component of woven bone that is not present in desmoplastic fibroma; however, "bone poor" cases of fibrous dysplasia may contain predominately fibrous stroma. Radiology can be useful in separating these entities. Fibrous dysplasia is a circumscribed lesion often having a prominent shell of surrounding reactive bone, whereas desmoplastic fibromas show considerably more aggressive

radiologic features. Polyostotic bone involvement is also a feature of fibrous dysplasia and not desmoplastic fibroma. In cases where the diagnosis is uncertain, molecular testing for a *GNAS* mutation, which is characteristic of fibrous dysplasia, can be useful.

Low-grade central osteosarcomas can also contain desmoplastic fibroma-like areas (Fig. 7.69), and the overlapping histologic features can result in difficulty separating the two entities. Many low-grade central osteosarcomas have a prominent bony component which is not found in desmoplastic fibromas. However, in ambiguous cases, particularly those arising in long bones, molecular testing may be necessary for definitive diagnosis. Low-grade central osteosarcomas are characterized by *MDM2* gene amplification and may be positive for MDM2 immunohistochemically; desmoplastic fibromas lack both of these features.

Prognosis and Therapy

Desmoplastic fibromas are treated surgically. Curettage is frequently associated with local recurrence, after which formal resection may be necessary. This lesion is considered a locally aggressive neoplasm that does not metastasize.

DESMOPLASTIC FIBROMA – DISEASE FACT SHEET

Definition
▸▸ Locally aggressive fibroblastic neoplasm of bone resembling soft tissue fibromatosis

Incidence and Location
▸▸ Rare
▸▸ Most cases arise in the mandible or long bones

Age Distribution
▸▸ Most cases are found in adolescents and young adults, although the age range is broad

Clinical Features
▸▸ Patients present with pain, swelling, or pathologic fracture

Radiologic Features
▸▸ Can appear as circumscribed or destructive radiolucent lesions on conventional radiographs
▸▸ CT or MRI highlight extraosseous extension
▸▸ Frequently have internal trabeculations

Prognosis and Therapy
▸▸ Treated with surgery alone
▸▸ Recurrences are common following incomplete excision
▸▸ Resection may be necessary

DESMOPLASTIC FIBROMA – PATHOLOGIC FEATURES

Gross Findings
▸▸ White, firm cut surface with trabeculations
▸▸ May extend into soft tissue
▸▸ Little if any surrounding reactive bone

Microscopic Findings
▸▸ Resemble soft tissue fibromatosis
▸▸ Bland spindled cells embedded in a dense collagenous stroma
▸▸ May have a fascicular growth pattern or a haphazard growth pattern
▸▸ No cytologic atypia or significant mitotic activity

Ancillary Studies
▸▸ Rare cases have *CTNNB1* mutations
▸▸ Immunoreactivity for beta-catenin possible

Pathologic Differential Diagnoses
▸▸ Fibrous dysplasia
▸▸ Low-grade central osteosarcoma

OSTEOID OSTEOMA

DIFFERENTIAL DIAGNOSIS: OSTEOBLASTOMA, OSTEOSARCOMA

Clinical Features

Osteoid osteoma and osteoblastoma are now known to be related benign osteoblastic neoplasms. Most patients with osteoid osteomas present between the ages of 10 and 30 years, and they are more common in men than in women by a 2:1 ratio. Most patients have a classic clinical history that includes intense often sharply localized pain that is more severe at night and relieved by non-steroidal anti-inflammatory medications, unaccompanied by clinical or laboratory evidence of infection. Vertebral lesions may be associated with scoliosis, and lesions arising in the hands and feet may mimic osteomyelitis. Intra-articular lesions can cause symptoms resulting in confusion with an inflammatory arthropathy.

Osteoid osteoma has been reported in practically every bone but occurs most frequently in the femur, tibia, humerus, small bones of the hands and feet, vertebrae, and fibula. Lesions of long bones are usually metaphyseal, but they may be epiphyseal and even juxta-/intra-articular (arising within the portion of the bone contained within the joint capsule). Most are centered in the cortex, but they may also occur in the medullary cavity or subperiosteal region. Vertebral lesions typically affect the posterior elements.

Radiographic Features

Osteoid osteomas contain a radiolucent central nidus smaller than 2.0 cm that may or may not contain a radiodense center. This nidus is typically surrounded by a densely sclerotic layer of reactive bone that may extend for several centimeters along both sides of the cortex (Fig. 7.70); however, osteoid osteomas arising within the medullary cavity may lack this reaction. The radiographic differential diagnosis includes Brodie's abscess, sclerosing osteomyelitis, and stress fracture. Juxta-articular lesions may be mistaken for an inflammatory arthropathy due to the induction of a marked chronic synovitis, and lesions in this location may be better visualized with MRI scans.

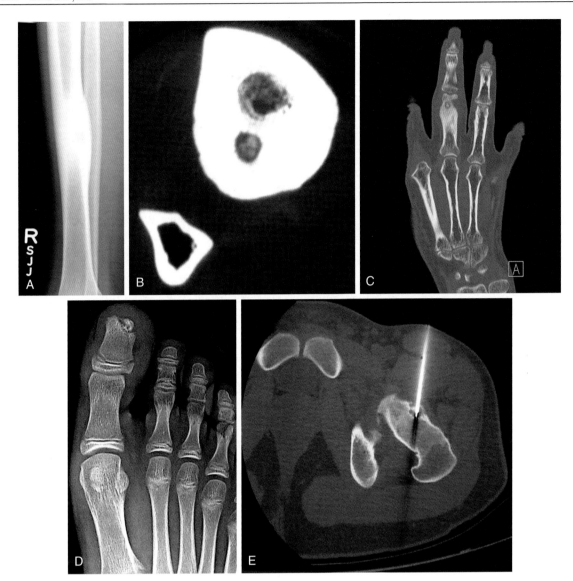

FIG. 7.70

Most osteoid osteomas in the long bones arise within the cortex, where they form a radiolucent nidus surrounded by dense reactive bone that can be seen on conventional radiograph **(A)** but is better visualized on CT **(B)**. CT shows an osteoid osteoma of the third phalanx that has a radiodense nidus surrounded by reactive bone. This lesion was initially mistaken for osteomyelitis with a sequestrum **(C)**. Plain radiograph of an osteoid osteoma involving the distal phalanx of the big toe that caused marked enlargement of the distal portion of the digit **(D)**. Radiofrequency ablation is a non-surgical alternative for the treatment of osteoid osteomas **(E)**.

Pathologic Features

GROSS FINDINGS

Osteoid osteomas are well-circumscribed lesions measuring less than 2.0 cm, and the nidus has a red appearance with central areas of bone formation (Fig. 7.71). The surrounding reactive bone is densely sclerotic, particularly when the lesion arises within the cortex.

MICROSCOPIC FINDINGS

Microscopically, the sharply circumscribed central nidus of an osteoid osteoma is composed of more or less calcified osteoid and woven bone prominently lined by plump osteoblasts, and while osteoclast-like giant cells can vary

significantly in number, they are usually present. The intervening stroma fibrous stroma is highly vascularized (Fig. 7.72). Occasionally, sheet-like osteoid deposits are found. There is a variably thick layer of dense cortical-type bone with widened Haversian canals surrounding the nidus, usually more prominent in cortically based tumors.

Ancillary Studies

Ancillary studies are usually not necessary to establish a diagnosis of osteoid osteoma but can be useful when evaluating osteoblastomas. Both osteoid osteoma and osteoblastoma share common genetic abnormalities, including *FOS* and less commonly *FOSB* gene rearrangements.

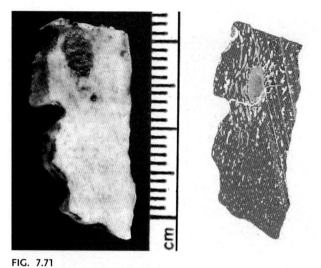

FIG. 7.71

Grossly, the nidus of an osteoid osteoma is circumscribed, has a red gritty appearance, and is surrounded by dense bone *(left)*. The nidus is easily seen at low magnification *(right)*.

Anti-FOS and -FOSB antibodies are also useful for highlighting the neoplastic osteoblasts in both lesions and are not immunoreactive in other lesions in the differential diagnosis.

Differential Diagnosis

It is now accepted that osteoid osteoma and osteoblastoma are closely related benign bone-forming neoplasms linked by common genetic mutations in the *FOS* and *FOSB* genes. While these two neoplasms share remarkably similar histologic features, osteoblastomas are more common in the spine, show variable intralesional maturation and prominent ectatic stromal blood vessels, may contain prominent epithelioid change in the osteoblasts, and exceed 2.0 cm in greatest dimension (Figs. 7.73–7.75). In contrast, osteoid osteomas are

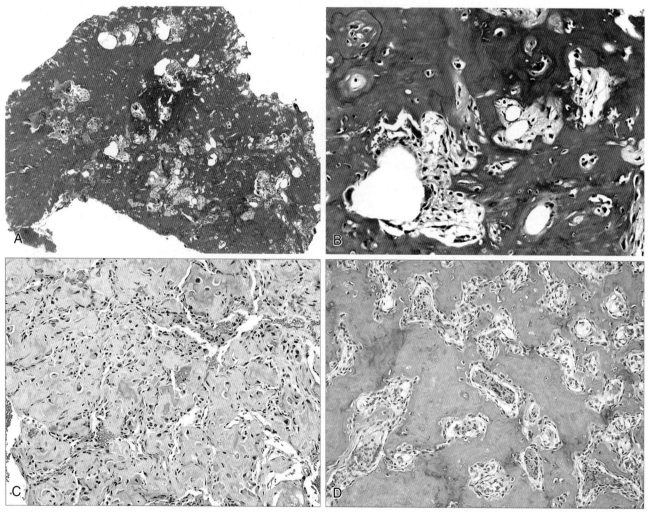

FIG. 7.72

A, At low magnification, the nidus of this osteoid osteoma is composed of dense woven bone with small foci of fibrovascular stroma. **B,** At higher magnification, the nidus shows focal osteoblastic rimming, osteoclastic activity, and bland cytologic features. **C,** This osteoid osteoma contains primitive bone formation and large osteoblasts. **D,** This osteoid osteoma features prominent osteoblastic rimming on nearly every woven bone surface and the stroma contains numerous blood vessels.

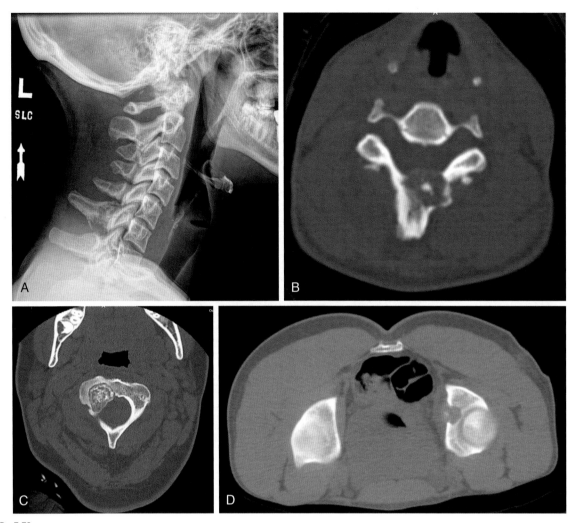

FIG. 7.73

Conventional radiograph **(A)** and CT **(B)** showing an osteoblastoma arising in the posterior elements of C6. The lesion arises at the base of the spinous process, is well-circumscribed, and has a small focus of central ossification best appreciated on the CT. CT of an osteoblastoma in C2 shows a well-circumscribed mass with heavy ossification arising in the right anterior aspect of the axis with slight encroachment on the spinal canal **(C)**. CT of an osteoblastoma arising in the medial wall of the acetabulum **(D)**. Although the lesion extends through the medial cortex, the medullary border is well-circumscribed. The lesion contains faint areas of ossification throughout.

smaller than 2.0 cm, frequently measuring smaller than 1.5 cm in greatest dimension.

When the bone formation in osteoid osteomas and osteoblastomas is primitive, either lesion could be mistaken for an osteosarcoma, particularly if the appropriate radiographic correlation is not obtained. Nevertheless, the degree of cytologic atypia and mitotic activity in osteosarcomas is usually sufficiently severe to allow for straightforward diagnosis. One exception, however, is the osteoblastoma-like variant of osteosarcoma (Fig. 7.76). High-grade osteoblastoma-like osteosarcoma does not cause diagnostic issues provided the lesion is sampled sufficiently because the high-grade component is similar to conventional osteosarcoma. However, low-grade osteoblastoma-like osteosarcoma can be extremely difficult to distinguish from osteoblastoma, and radiographic correlation may or may not help with this differential. The most important feature of low-grade osteoblastoma-like osteosarcoma is poor circumscription and infiltration

around pre-existing cancellous bone, a feature not found in osteoblastoma. Osteoblastoma-like osteosarcomas may also contain sheets of osteoblasts not associated with bone production and lack of peripheral maturation, but these features can be difficult to identify on small samples.

Prognosis and Therapy

CT-guided radiofrequency ablation has largely replaced surgical excision for osteoid osteomas and has proven to be an extremely effective treatment modality for both spinal and extra-spinal tumors. This technique provides excellent pain relief, reduces operative morbidity, and is associated with a low local recurrence rate. Osteoblastomas are usually treated with curettage, but en bloc resection may be necessary in some cases. The local recurrence rate following curettage is approximately 25%.

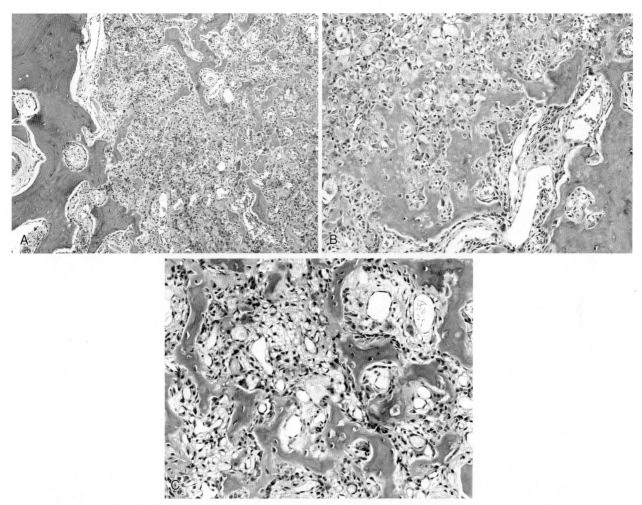

FIG. 7.74

A, Histologically, an important feature in osteoblastomas is the sharp circumscription of the border between the lesion and the host bone. **B,** Osteoblastomas show prominent osteoblastic rimming and frequently contain dilated blood vessels in the stroma. **C,** Osteoblastoma with interconnecting trabeculae of woven bone with prominent osteoblastic rimming and dilated stromal vessels.

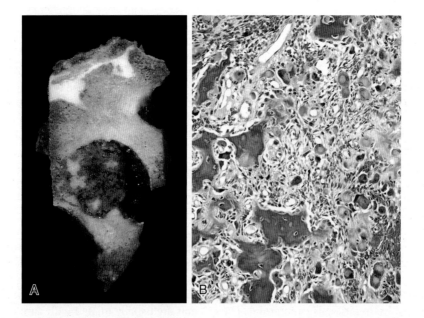

FIG. 7.75

This example of an epithelioid osteoblastoma arose in a sacral nerve root foramen **(A)** and shows the prominent epithelioid morphology of the osteoblasts that is characteristic of this entity **(B)**.

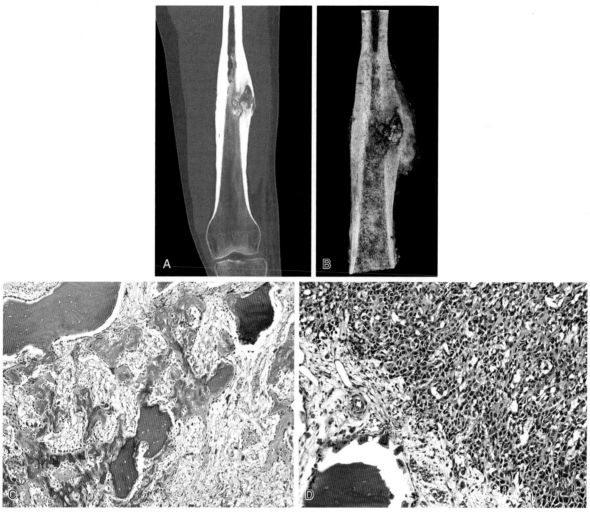

FIG. 7.76

A, CT of an osteoblastoma-like osteosarcoma shows deceptively unaggressive features, including involvement of both the medullary cavity and cortex and a long layer of dense reactive bone proximal and distal to the lesion. **B,** The tumor has a tan-gray, gritty cut surface, involves the cortex and medullary cavity, and is associated with extensive reactive bone. **C,** Areas of the tumor strongly resembling osteoblastoma show a permeative growth pattern and entrap necrotic cancellous bone in the medullary cavity. **D,** In other areas, the tumor has the appearance of a conventional high-grade osteosarcoma.

Low-grade osteoblastoma-like osteosarcoma is sometimes only recognized following multiple local recurrences but is most appropriately treated with en bloc resection. Following biopsy, high-grade osteoblastoma-like osteosarcomas, like conventional osteosarcomas, are appropriately treated with neoadjuvant chemotherapy and resection followed by adjuvant chemotherapy.

OSTEOID OSTEOMA – DISEASE FACT SHEET

Definition
▸▸ A benign bone-forming neoplasm measuring less than 2.0 cm in largest dimension

Incidence and Location
▸▸ Relatively common, accounting for approximately 10% of primary bone tumors
▸▸ Most commonly arise in long bones (50%), usually the femur or tibia
▸▸ Also occur in the posterior elements of the spine

Age Distribution
▸▸ Most common in children and adolescents

Clinical Features
▸▸ Characteristic clinical history that includes pain which is worse at night and relieved by non-steroidal anti-inflammatory medications
▸▸ Lesions arising in the digits can clinically mimic osteomyelitis
▸▸ Lesions arising in the spine can cause painful scoliosis

Radiologic Features
▸▸ In long bones, osteoid osteomas usually arise in the cortex and have a small central nidus surrounded by dense reactive bone that can obscure the nidus
▸▸ The central nidus is more easily seen on CT
▸▸ MRI is useful for the identification of intramedullary osteoid osteomas

Prognosis and Therapy
▸▸ Most spinal and extraspinal osteoid osteomas are treated with radiofrequency ablation and the risk for local recurrence is extremely low (less than 5%)

OSTEOID OSTEOMA – PATHOLOGIC FEATURES

Gross Findings

▶▶ The nidus of an osteoid osteoma measures less than 2.0 cm, is well-circumscribed, and often surrounded by dense reactive bone

▶▶ The cut surface of the nidus is red and gritty

Microscopic Findings

▶▶ The bone matrix deposition in osteoid osteoma can range from dense, sheet-like osteoid to interconnected trabeculae of woven bone

▶▶ Osteoblasts are prominent on the trabecular surface

▶▶ Fibrovascular stroma is between bone trabeculae

▶▶ Dense cortical-type bone surrounds the nidus

Ancillary Studies

▶▶ *FOS* and less commonly *FOSB* rearrangements are common in osteoid osteoma

▶▶ The FOS immunostain highlights the neoplastic cells of osteoid osteoma

Pathologic Differential Diagnoses

▶▶ Osteoblastoma

▶▶ Osteoblastoma-like osteosarcoma

▶▶ Brodie's abscess and stress fracture (radiographic differential diagnosis)

CONVENTIONAL CHORDOMA

DIFFERENTIAL DIAGNOSIS: MYXOID CHONDROSARCOMA, BENIGN NOTOCHORDAL CELL TUMOR

Clinical Features

Conventional chordoma is most frequent in the fifth and sixth decades but can occur in all age groups and in both sexes. Chordomas grow slowly, and the duration of the symptoms before diagnosis is often ≥5 years. Approximately 50% arise in the sacrococcygeal region, 35% in the spheno-occipital area, and the remainder in the mobile spine. The sacrococcygeal tumors are more common in the fifth and sixth decades of life; chordomas arising in children and adolescents are more likely to involve the spheno-occipital region. Extra-axial chordomas are also well-described. Pain is the most common presenting symptom, and neurologic symptoms relative to the specific site of origin in the spine are also frequently reported.

Radiographic Features

Chordomas are destructive, midline lesions that may be extremely difficult to identify on plain radiographs. However, they are readily evident on CT or MRI (Fig. 7.77). In the sacrum and coccyx, chordomas form lobular masses that cause extensive bone destruction and extend into soft tissue anteriorly toward the rectum and bladder. Lesions arising in the skull base involve the midline, destroy surrounding bone, and may encroach on the brainstem or optic nerves. Chordomas arising in the mobile spine may grow eccentrically into adjacent soft tissue (Fig. 7.78).

Pathologic Features

GROSS FINDINGS

Grossly, conventional chordomas are lobulated, gelatinous neoplasms (Fig. 7.79). The cut surface is soft and variegated, with a tan-gray and hemorrhagic appearance.

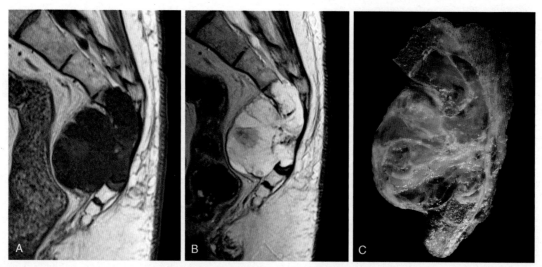

FIG. 7.77

T1 **(A)** and T2 **(B)** MRI show a destructive lesion arising in the distal sacral segments and extending into soft tissue anteriorly. The lesion is low signal intensity on T1 and bright on T2. The gross specimen **(C)** shows a destructive, lobulated, gelatinous neoplasm typical of chordoma.

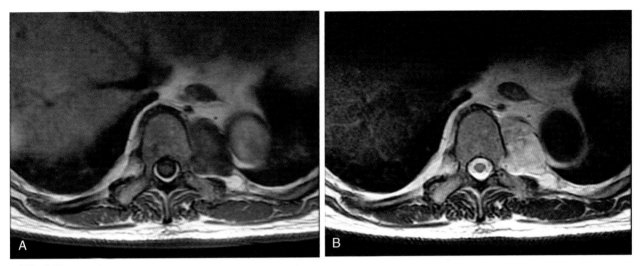

FIG. 7.78

This example of a chordoma arising in T9 shows eccentric soft tissue extension rather than the usual anterior extension. The lesion is low signal intensity on T1 **(A)** and higher in signal intensity on T2 **(B)**.

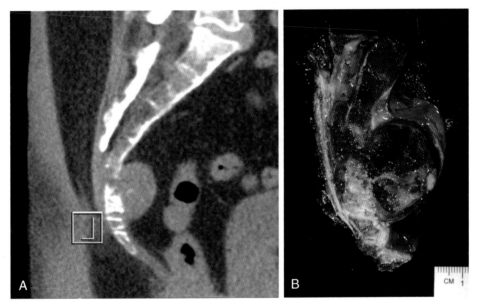

FIG. 7.79

CT **(A)** showing a smaller chordoma arising in the distal aspect of the sacrum and extending anteriorly. Grossly, the tumor is composed of gelatinous lobules with foci of hemorrhage **(B)**.

Intact lesions are typically only encountered with resection specimens from the mobile spine or sacrococcygeal region. Such tumors are often large and extend into extra-osseous soft tissue, particularly anterior to the spine.

MICROSCOPIC FINDINGS

Microscopically, conventional chordomas contain cohesive chords and nests of epithelioid cells deposited in an abundant myxoid stroma, organized into distinct lobules by fibrous septa often containing chronic inflammation. Individual tumor cells have eosinophilic cytoplasm, and those with prominent vacuoles are referred to as "physaliphorous" cells (Fig. 7.80). Tumor cells are variable in size and may have prominent nucleoli;

cytologic atypia may be pronounced. Mitotic figures are generally scant or absent. A variant of conventional chordoma referred to as "chondroid chordoma" may contain foci of hyaline cartilage in place of the usual myxoid stroma.

Ancillary Studies

Chordomas show diffuse immunoreactivity for cytokeratins and patchy immunoreactivity for EMA and S-100. The introduction of the brachyury antibody, which is almost always positive in chordomas, has greatly simplified the workup of chordomas. This transcription factor, which is the product of the *TBXT* gene,

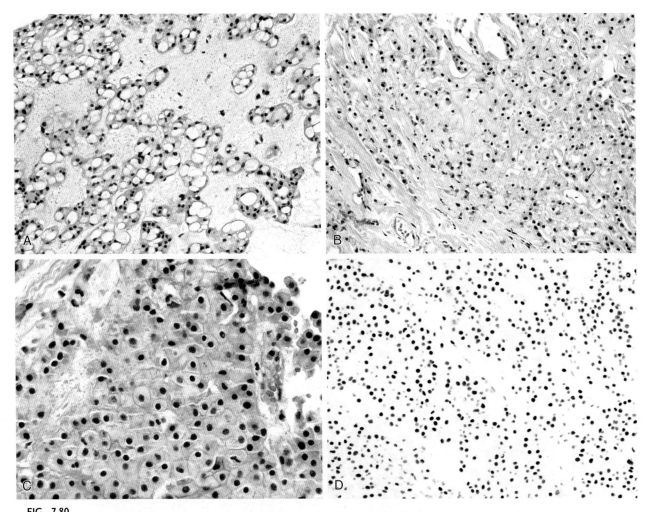

FIG. 7.80

A, Conventional chordomas are composed of chords and nests of cohesive, vacuolated epithelioid cells deposited in a myxoid matrix. **B,** The chord-like arrangement of the cells is evident in the photomicrograph. **C,** Cytologically, the cells in chordoma can have clear or eosinophilic cytoplasm that show variable cytologic atypia and mitotic activity. **D,** An immunostain for brachyury is strongly, diffusely positive in chordoma.

is necessary for notochord formation and is an extremely sensitive and specific marker for chordoma. However, false negatives are known to occur within sections that have been decalcified.

Differential Diagnosis

While neoplasms with epithelioid cytologic features and myxoid or mucinous stroma, such as myoepithelial tumors and metastatic mucinous carcinoma, can mimic conventional chordoma, one of the more difficult differential diagnoses in the spinal axis is chondrosarcoma. Chondrosarcomas have a radiographic appearance that is remarkably similar to chordomas, although they can be eccentric rather than midline in location. The chondroid component of a chondroid chordoma has a histologic appearance essentially identical to a grade 1 chondrosarcoma. Myxoid chondrosarcomas are lobular neoplasms with prominent myxoid stroma. The

cells in a myxoid chondrosarcoma are generally discohesive and generally smaller in size compared with the cohesive groups of large epithelioid cells characteristic of chordoma (Fig. 7.81). Immunostains are extremely helpful in separating these entities. Chordomas are strongly positive for brachyury and show patchy positivity for S-100, whereas chondrosarcomas are generally diffusely positive for S-100 but negative for brachyury.

Another important differential diagnosis is benign notochordal cell tumor (BNCT). BNCTs are generally asymptomatic and found incidentally on imaging studies. They are often difficult to visualize on conventional radiographs and appear as relatively circumscribed sclerotic lesions on CT that lack surrounding bone destruction and importantly lack soft tissue extension (Fig. 7.82). BNCTs have heterogeneous signal intensity on MRI (Fig. 7.83) and lack activity on radioisotope scans. Histologically, BNCTs are deceptive neoplasms that are difficult to recognize because they do not alter the architecture of the cancellous bone, and a population of the neoplastic cells resemble adipocytes with slightly

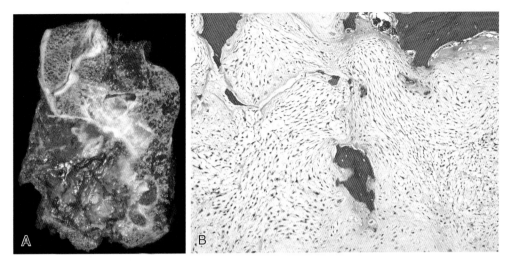

FIG. 7.81

A, Grossly, this myxoid chondrosarcoma of the sacrum is composed of gelatinous lobules, similar to chordoma. **B,** Histologically, the cells of a myxoid chondrosarcoma are discohesive and have a stellate appearance, different from those in a chordoma.

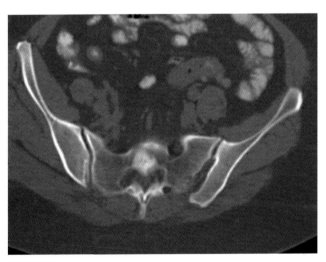

FIG. 7.82

CT scan showing a circumscribed, sclerotic benign notochordal cell tumor in the sacrum. The lesion is small, circumscribed, and does not extend into extraosseous soft tissue.

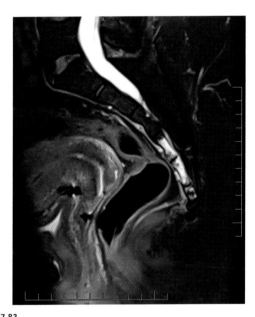

FIG. 7.83

T2 MRI shows a hyperintense benign notochordal cell tumor involving the distal sacral segments.

eosinophilic cytoplasm cytologically. Islands of hematopoietic marrow are frequently trapped within BNCTs (Fig. 7.84). These lesions lack the lobular architecture, cytologic atypia, myxoid matrix, and the bone destruction of a chordoma, although the two lesions have identical immunohistochemical features.

Prognosis and Therapy

Conventional chordomas have a significant risk of local recurrence following surgical excision, particularly when located in the skull base, and adjuvant proton beam radiotherapy may be beneficial for skull base chordomas.

Non-skull base chordomas metastasize to the lung or bone in approximately 40% of cases.

CONVENTIONAL CHORDOMA – DISEASE FACT SHEET

Definition
▸▸ A malignant neoplasm with notochordal differentiation that arises in the spinal column

Incidence and Location
▸▸ Rare
▸▸ Most arise in the sacrococcygeal area or skull base, and less frequently in the mobile spine
▸▸ Rare extra-axial locations have been reported

Continued

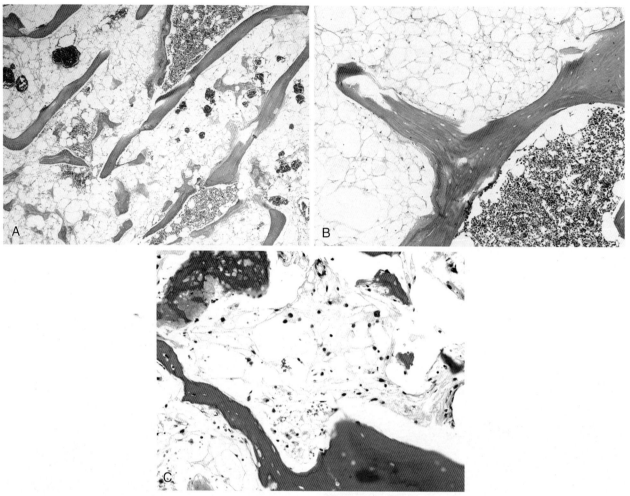

FIG. 7.84

A, At low magnification, the vacuolated cells of a benign notochordal cell tumor (BNCT) extend between trabeculae of bone with little reaction. Entrapped islands of hematopoietic marrow are also seen. **B,** The vacuolated cells of a BNCT adjacent to trabecular bone, which shows slight appositional thickening. **C,** The vacuolated cells of BNCT are easily overlooked and can be mistaken for marrow adipocytes.

Age Distribution

▸▸ Conventional chordomas most commonly arise in the fifth to seventh decades
▸▸ Uncommon in children

Clinical Features

▸▸ Pain and neurologic deficits are the common symptoms

Radiologic Features

▸▸ Destructive midline lesion arising anywhere along the spinal axis
▸▸ May be difficult to visualize on conventional radiographs
▸▸ CT or MRI is necessary to visualize soft tissue extension
▸▸ Sacro-coccygeal chordomas often extend anteriorly and abut the bladder or rectum

Prognosis and Therapy

▸▸ Local recurrences are common following surgical excision
▸▸ Adjuvant radiotherapy is effective in helping control local disease
▸▸ Metastases develop in approximately 40% of cases, particularly from non-skull base tumors

CONVENTIONAL CHORDOMA – PATHOLOGIC FEATURES

Gross Findings

▸▸ Multilobulated, gelatinous tumors that extend into extra-osseous soft tissue

Microscopic Findings

▸▸ Lobulated tumors with abundant extracellular myxoid matrix
▸▸ Fibrous septa often contain chronic inflammation
▸▸ Cohesive nests or chords of tumor cells
▸▸ Individual tumor cells are epithelioid and may have cytoplasmic vacuoles ("physaliphorous cells")
▸▸ Cytologic atypia may be pronounced, but mitotic activity is limited

Pathologic Differential Diagnosis

▸▸ Benign notochordal cell tumor (BNCT)
▸▸ Myxoid chondrosarcoma
▸▸ Metastatic mucinous adenocarcinoma

Ancillary Studies

▸▸ Keratins and brachyury are typically diffusely positive, S-100 is patchy positive

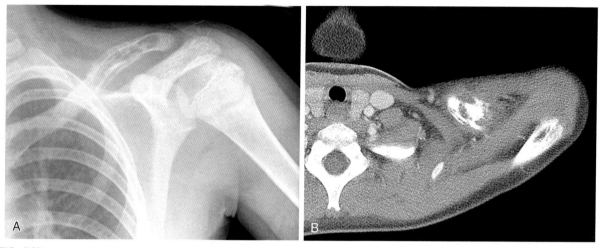

FIG. 7.85

Conventional radiograph **(A)** and CT **(B)** showing Langerhans cell histiocytosis in the distal clavicle. The lesion causes permeative destruction of bone and is accompanied by a prominent periosteal reaction, mimicking an aggressive neoplasm such as Ewing sarcoma.

LANGERHANS CELL HISTIOCYTOSIS

DIFFERENTIAL DIAGNOSIS: OSTEOMYELITIS

Clinical Features

Langerhans cell histiocytosis (LCH) arising in bone occurs most commonly as a solitary lesion but can also be multifocal and simultaneously involve other organs such as skin, lung, liver, spleen, and others.

LCH with solitary bone involvement, which represents the most common variety, has traditionally been referred to as eosinophilic granuloma. Children and young adults are most commonly affected. Any bone can be involved, although solitary lesions arising in the hands and feet are rare. The most common osseous sites are the skull, jaw, humerus, ribs, and femur.

Multiple bone lesions can be accompanied by proptosis, diabetes insipidus, chronic otitis media, or a combination of these conditions, historically referred to as Hand-Schüller-Christian disease. This form is characterized by a prolonged clinical course, often marked by alternating episodes of regressions and recurrences, although the eventual outcome is favorable in most cases. By contrast, Letterer-Siwe disease, characterized by the development of LCH in multiple organ systems, follows a more aggressive clinical course and can be fatal.

Radiographic Features

LCH is often referred to as "the great imitator." Most lesions appear as well-circumscribed, punched-out radiolucent lesions. In flat bones, LCH can have an

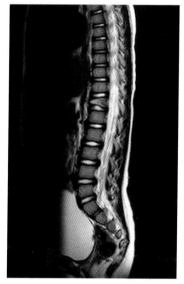

FIG. 7.86

An example of vertebra plana involving the T12 vertebral body, caused by Langerhans cell histiocytosis.

aggressive pattern of bone destruction reminiscent of Ewing sarcoma, lymphoma, or osteomyelitis that can be accompanied by periosteal reaction (Fig. 7.85). In the spine, LCH causes marked flattening of the vertebral body, a finding referred to as vertebra plana (Fig. 7.86). In the jaw, bone destruction spares the teeth, a finding referred to as "floating teeth." Many lesions spontaneously regress, particularly following biopsy.

Pathologic Features

MICROSCOPIC FINDINGS

LCH is a dendritic cell neoplasm characterized by the accumulation of Langerhans cells and other inflammatory cells, including eosinophils, multinucleated giant cells, neutrophils, and foamy histiocytes and often accompanied by areas of fibrosis. Eosinophils are sometimes sufficiently prominent to form eosinophilic microabscesses. The diagnostic Langerhans cells have a characteristic cytologic appearance, with nuclei that are lobulated or indented, sometimes with a longitudinal groove; their cytoplasm is, for the most part, distinctly eosinophilic (Fig. 7.87). In some cases, cytologic atypia and mitotic activity may be prominent, and necrosis may be present. The healing phase of LCH is characterized by fibrosis, histiocytic inflammation, and these changes can obscure the diagnostic features of LCH.

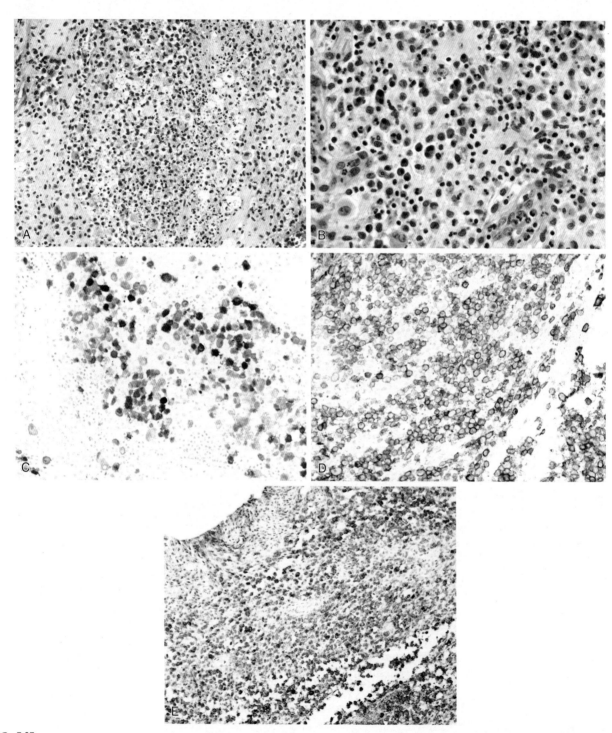

FIG. 7.87

At low magnification, Langerhans cell histiocytosis is composed of a polymorphous infiltrate consisting of Langerhans cells, neutrophils, eosinophils, and other inflammatory cells, mimicking inflammatory conditions such as osteomyelitis and neoplasms such as lymphoma **(A)**. Higher magnification shows a mixture of eosinophils and Langerhans cells, which have characteristic grooves and clefts **(B)**. Langerhans cells are immunoreactive for S-100 **(C)** and CD1a **(D)**. Many cases of Langerhans cell histiocytosis are immunoreactive for BRAF **(E)**, which is an excellent surrogate for the *BRAF* V600E mutation.

Ancillary Studies

The diagnostic Langerhans cells can be highlighted with immunostains for S-100 protein, CD1a, or langerin (CD207). A specific intracytoplasmic organelle, known as a Langerhans or Birbeck granule, is regularly present on electron microscopic examination. It has been shown that a relatively high percentage of cases of LCH (50%) harbor *BRAF* V600E mutations, resulting in activation of the MAPK pathway. A smaller percentage of lesions have mutations in the *MAP2K1* gene; these mutations are mutually exclusive.

Differential Diagnosis

Because a prominent inflammatory cell component is seen in LCH, one of the main entities to consider in the differential diagnosis is osteomyelitis. Hematogenous osteomyelitis most commonly affects children, the same age group that develops LCH. Much like LCH, osteomyelitis can cause ill-defined, aggressive-appearing radiographic findings with associated periosteal reaction (Fig. 7.88). Acute osteomyelitis is characterized by a dense inflammatory infiltrate rich in neutrophils accompanied by necrotic bone (Fig. 7.89). The eosinophils that are

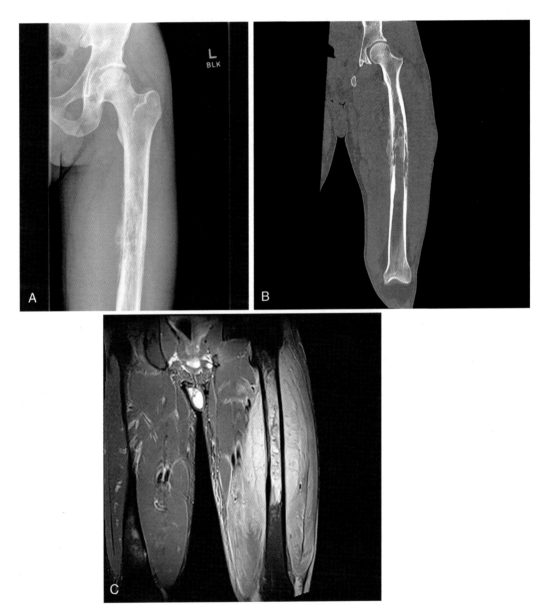

FIG. 7.88

A, Acute osteomyelitis has an aggressive appearance radiographically and shows permeative destruction of bone accompanied by periosteal reaction, mimicking neoplasms such as Langerhans cell histiocytosis, Ewing sarcoma, and lymphoma. **B,** Coronal CT highlights the bone destruction and periosteal reaction of osteomyelitis. **C,** On T1 MRI, there is extensive edema in the medullary cavity and adjacent skeletal muscle.

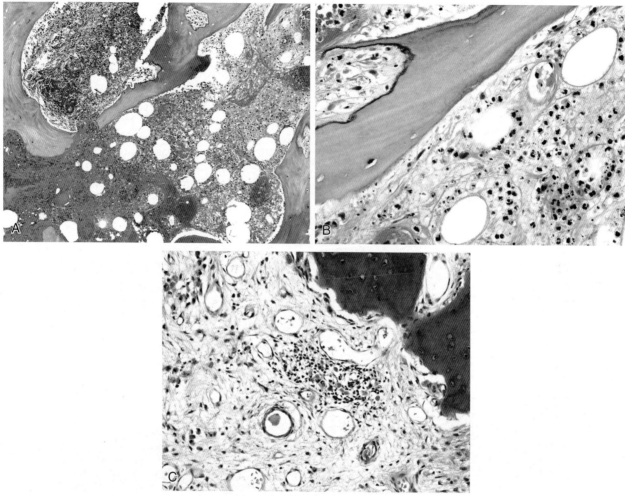

FIG. 7.89

In acute osteomyelitis, there is bone destruction, and the marrow space is filled by an inflammatory infiltrate rich in neutrophils **(A)**. Acute osteomyelitis can be difficult to distinguish from Langerhans cell histiocytosis, particularly on frozen section. Higher magnification showing the neutrophilic infiltrate characteristic of acute osteomyelitis **(B)**. Chronic osteomyelitis is characterized by fibrosis of the marrow space accompanied by an infiltrate of lymphocytes and plasma cells, which can be difficult to distinguish from Langerhans cell histiocytosis in the healing phase **(C)**.

characteristic of the infiltrate are seen with LCH not typically a component of the inflammatory infiltrate in osteomyelitis; however, their presence or absence can be difficult to appreciate, particularly on frozen sections. Therefore, touch preparations—which preserve the granules of eosinophils—can be valuable in this differential diagnosis at the time of frozen section. Equivocal cases can usually be solved with immunostains for CD1a or langerin. Chronic osteomyelitis, which mimics the healing phase of LCH, may also necessitate an immunohistochemical workup to exclude the possibility of LCH. Correlating microbiology culture results is often helpful when osteomyelitis is a diagnostic possibility.

Prognosis and Therapy

The treatment for LCH can include observation, surgery, radiotherapy, or chemotherapy, depending on the extent of the disease. Many solitary lesions regress following biopsy. The long-term prognosis, particularly for solitary lesions, is excellent. It is exceptional for these patients to develop other bone lesions or involvement of other organs. Lesions with *BRAF* mutations are successfully treated with BRAF inhibitors.

LANGERHANS CELL HISTIOCYTOSIS – DISEASE FACT SHEET

Definition

▶▶ Neoplasm of Langerhans cells that can involve bone, skin, and other organs

▶▶ Caused by mutations in *BRAF* or *MAP2K1* genes

Incidence and Location

▶▶ Can involve any bone, particularly the craniofacial bones, spine, and long bones

Age Distribution

▸▸ Usually diagnosed in the first three decades, but more severe forms arise in children

Clinical Features

▸▸ Solitary bone lesions present as pain
▸▸ Disseminated forms present with a wide variety of symptoms and vary in severity

Radiologic Features

▸▸ "The great imitator"
▸▸ Discrete punched out radiolucent lesions are common
▸▸ Can cause permeative bone destruction accompanied by periosteal reaction, mimicking a malignant neoplasm

Prognosis and Therapy

▸▸ Solitary lesions often regress following biopsy
▸▸ Disseminated disease can cause death
▸▸ Therapy varies depending on severity and distribution of lesions, but chemotherapy and radiotherapy are effective, as are BRAF inhibitors

---

LANGERHANS CELL HISTIOCYTOSIS – PATHOLOGIC FEATURES

Microscopic Findings

▸▸ Langerhans cells admixed with a variety of other inflammatory cell types
▸▸ Langerhans cells have eosinophilic cytoplasm and nuclei with grooves
▸▸ Eosinophils are usually prominent
▸▸ Healing lesions have fibrosis and histiocytes which may obscure the diagnostic features

Pathologic Differential Diagnoses

▸▸ Osteomyelitis (acute and chronic)

EPITHELIOID HEMANGIOMA

DIFFERENTIAL DIAGNOSS: EPITHELIOID HEMANGIOENDOTHELIOMA, PSEUDO-MYOGENIC HEMANGIOENDOTHELIOMA, ANGIOSARCOMA

Clinical Features

Epithelioid hemangioma is a distinctive variant of hemangioma that may present as a solitary lesion or in a regionally multifocal distribution. This variant is locally aggressive compared with the typical hemangioma of bone, which is completely benign. Epithelioid hemangioma can occur over a very wide age range, from childhood to late adulthood. Lesions can arise in a variety of skeletal sites, but the long bones are most commonly affected, followed by the flat bones and vertebrae. Most patients are symptomatic and present with pain.

Radiographic Features

On conventional radiographs, epithelioid hemangiomas are sharply circumscribed lesions that arise in the metaphysis or diaphysis. Locally aggressive lesions may erode the cortex and extend into soft tissue. Multifocal lesions may involve one bone or multiple bones regionally.

Pathologic Features

GROSS FINDINGS

Epithelioid hemangiomas can range from small to multiple centimeters in greatest dimension. They are well-circumscribed, soft, red, and hemorrhagic (Fig. 7.90). A subset of these lesions is locally aggressive, eroding through the cortex and into adjacent soft tissue.

MICROSCOPIC FINDINGS

Epithelioid hemangiomas can be either circumscribed or have infiltrative borders. They are lobular neoplasms composed of well-formed vascular channels lined by epithelioid endothelial cells often described as "hobnail" or "tombstone-like" in appearance. The endothelial cells often contain intracytoplasmic vacuoles or blisters. They lack stromal matrix deposition but frequently have a prominent inflammatory background that is rich in eosinophils (Fig. 7.91). A subset of epithelioid hemangiomas has atypical features, such as increased cellularity, mild cytologic atypia, and necrosis.

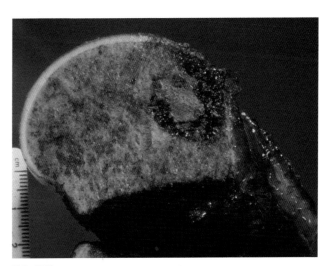

FIG. 7.90

Gross photo of an epithelioid hemangioma of the femoral condyle. The lesion is circumscribed and has a red cut surface. The central gray material indicates the site of prior biopsy.

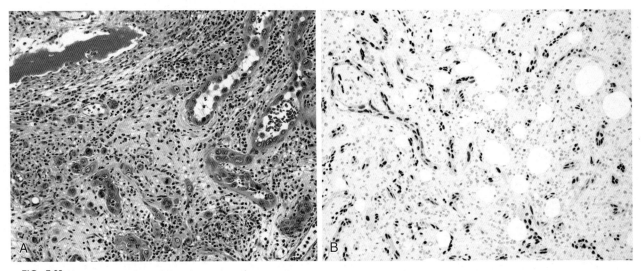

FIG. 7.91
Epithelioid hemangiomas are composed of vessels lined by prominent epithelioid endothelial cells that protrude into the vessel lumen. **(A)** The stroma is rich in eosinophils. **(B)** Epithelioid hemangiomas are positive for a variety of endothelial markers, including ERG.

Ancillary Studies

Epithelioid hemangiomas are immunoreactive for all endothelial markers, including CD31, CD34, ERG, and FLI1. Immunostains for keratin are also frequently positive. Surrounding pericytes can be identified with smooth muscle actin.

A majority of epithelioid hemangiomas harbor fusions of the *FOS* gene, and several partner genes have been identified. Less frequently, *FOSB* fusions are encountered. Immunostains for FOS or FOSB are useful in a subset of epithelioid hemangiomas.

Differential Diagnosis

Epithelioid hemangioma must be differentiated from several benign and malignant vascular neoplasms that feature epithelioid endothelial cells. Epithelioid hemangioendothelioma (EHE) is a rare malignant epithelioid vascular neoplasm that can arise in both viscera and bone, and the bone involvement can be multifocal. Skeletal EHE has clinical and radiographic features that overlap with epithelioid hemangioma. Histologically, however, they have a distinct appearance that is quite different than epithelioid hemangioma. The tumor cells of EHE are arranged in cords and nests, which are deposited in a myxoid, hyaline, or chondroid matrix. Well-formed vessels are not a feature of EHE, which more closely resembles metastatic carcinoma than a vascular neoplasm. Characteristic intracytoplasmic vacuoles sometimes contain erythrocytes (Fig. 7.92). Cytologic atypia and mitotic activity are not prominent in EHE. Most EHEs have a *WWTR1-CAMTA1* fusion, and less commonly a *YAP1-TFE3* fusion. As a result, immunostains for CAMTA1 or TFE3 can be used to confirm the diagnosis. EHE is also immunoreactive for CD34, CD31, ERG, and keratins.

Pseudomyogenic hemangioendothelioma is also a rare malignant epithelioid vascular neoplasm that is sometimes confused with epithelioid hemangioma. Pseudomyogenic hemangioendothelioma shares some clinical and radiographic similarities with epithelioid hemangioma and EHE in that it can be multifocal within bone; however, while it may involve soft tissue, it does not involve the viscera like EHE does. Histologically, pseudomyogenic hemangioendothelioma is not obviously vasoformative, and is composed of fascicles of spindled and epithelioid cells, a subset of which contain brightly eosinophilic cytoplasm reminiscent of rhabdomyoblasts. Neutrophils are often scattered throughout the stroma, as opposed to the prominent stromal eosinophils of epithelioid hemangioma (Fig. 7.93). Pseudomyogenic hemangioendotheliomas harbor *FOSB* rearrangements, usually *SERPINE1-FOSB* or *ACTB-FOSB* fusions, although other partner genes have also been reported. The resulting upregulation of *FOSB* can be identified immunohistochemically, and FOSB is a sensitive immunostain for pseudomyogenic hemangioendothelioma.

Angiosarcoma arising in bone can also be multifocal; however, angiosarcomas show a variable degree of vasoformation and typically demonstrate significant cytologic atypia and mitotic activity, allowing for accurate diagnosis (Fig. 7.94).

Prognosis and Therapy

Epithelioid hemangioma is a locally aggressive neoplasm most often treated with curettage. Radiotherapy has been used successfully for lesions arising in inaccessible sites. The local recurrence rate following curettage is low.

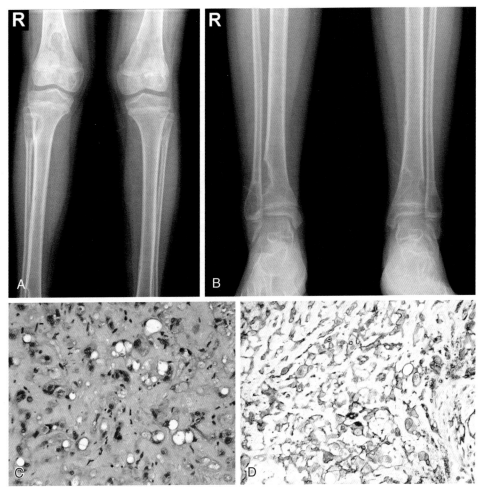

FIG. 7.92

A case of multifocal epithelioid hemangioendothelioma (EHE) in which individual lesions appear as punched-out radiolucencies in nearly every bone of the lower extremity **(A, B)**. EHEs are composed of cords and nests of epithelioid endothelial cells deposited in a myxochondroid background stroma. Individual tumor cells have intracytoplasmic vacuoles, some of which contain erythrocytes **(C)**. EHEs are also positive for a variety of endothelial markers, including CD31 **(D)**.

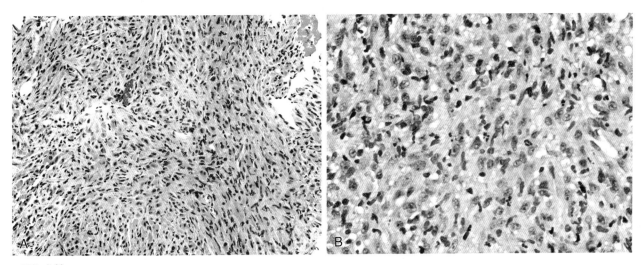

FIG. 7.93

Pseudomyogenic hemangioendothelioma is composed of fascicles of spindled cells, many of which have brightly eosinophilic cytoplasm reminiscent of rhabdomyoblasts. Scattered neutrophils are present in the stroma **(A, B)**.

Continued

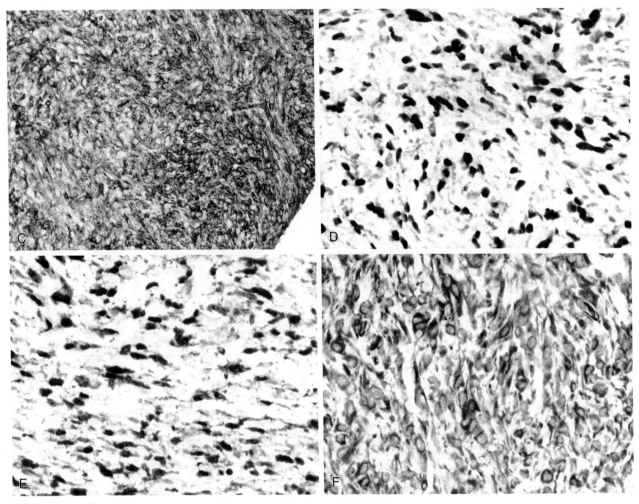

FIG. 7.93, cont'd
Pseudomyogenic hemangioendotheliomas are positive for CD31 **(C)**, ERG **(D)**, FOSB **(E)**, and keratin **(F)**.

EPITHELIOID HEMANGIOMA – DISEASE FACT SHEET

Definition
▶▶ Benign epithelioid vascular neoplasm that can arise in bone, soft tissue, skin, and parenchymal organs
▶▶ Can be multifocal in bone and locally aggressive

Incidence and Location
▶▶ Uncommon neoplasm that more commonly involve the long and short tubular bones of the extremities than flat bones

Age Distribution
▶▶ Very wide age range

Clinical Features
▶▶ Bone lesions present as pain

Radiologic Features
▶▶ Usually cause one or more circumsribed radiolucent lesions in the metaphysis or diaphysis
▶▶ Occasionally destroy the cortex and extend into soft tissue

Prognosis and Therapy
▶▶ Treated surgically with curettage or resection
▶▶ Radiotherapy is effective
▶▶ Local recurrence rate is low, lymph node metastases are uncommon

EPITHELIOID HEMANGIOMA – PATHOLOGIC FEATURES

Microscopic Findings
▶▶ Lobular vasoformative neoplasm with prominent epithelioid endothelial cells
▶▶ Solid, less obviously vasoformative foci are possible
▶▶ Epithelioid endothelial cells have abundant eosinophilic cytoplasm and cytoplasmic vacuoles or blisters
▶▶ Stroma is often rich in eosinophils

Ancillary Studies
▶▶ Endothelial nature can be demonstrated with immunostains for CD31, CD34, and ERG; keratins may be immunoreactive
▶▶ FOS or FOSB immunostains may be positive; *FOS* or *FOSB* rearrangements are commonly detected

Pathologic Differential Diagnoses
▶▶ Angiosarcoma and epithelioid hemangioendothelioma

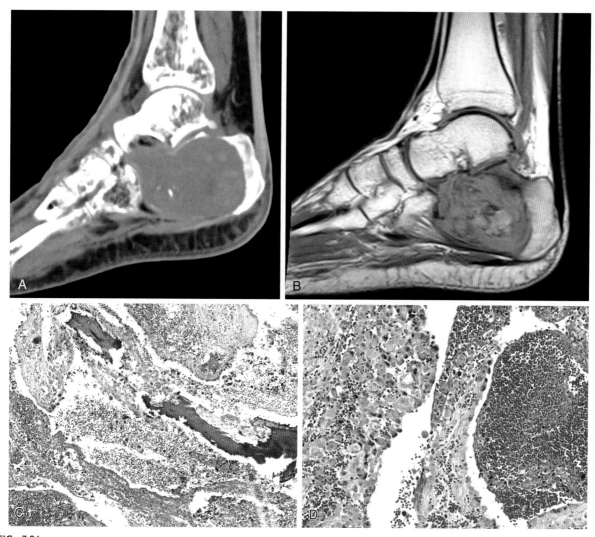

FIG. 7.94

Sagittal CT **(A)** and T1-weighted MRI **(B)** showing a destructive angiosarcoma arising in the talus. Histologically, angiosarcomas of bone are destructive, bloody, and hemorrhagic **(C)**. Highly atypical, mitotically active endothelial cells form solid nodules and line spaces containing blood **(D)**.

EWING SARCOMA

DIFFERENTIAL DIAGNOSIS: OTHER FUSION-DRIVEN ROUND CELL SARCOMAS, LYMPHOBLASTIC LYMPHOMA, SMALL CELL OSTEOSARCOMA, METASTATIC NEUROBLASTOMA

The group of round cell sarcomas has grown increasingly complex since 2010, owing largely to the rapid expansion of genetic information, the increasing use of molecular diagnostic techniques, and the identification of new immunohistochemical markers. In fact, confidently diagnosing this complex group of neoplasms almost always requires the judicious use of ancillary diagnostic tools. The prototype round cell sarcoma is Ewing sarcoma, a neoplasm historically characterized by the t(11;22)(q24;q12), and more

recently fusions of either *EWSR1* or *FUS* with ETS genes, most commonly *FLI1*.

Clinical Features

Ewing sarcoma is the most common round cell sarcoma of bone and represents the second most common primary bone sarcoma in the children after osteosarcoma. It is usually seen in patients between the ages of 5 and 20 years, with only a minority of the cases presenting in early infancy or adulthood. Clinically, Ewing sarcoma can simulate osteomyelitis because patients frequently experience pain, fever, and leukocytosis. It can arise in virtually any bone in the body but occurs most often in long bones (femur, tibia, humerus, and fibula) and in bones of the pelvis, ribs, vertebrae, and clavicle.

Radiographic Features

Radiographically, Ewing sarcoma causes permeative destruction of bone, usually accompanied by an aggressive periosteal reaction often described as "onion skin" in appearance. There is intense uptake of isotope on scintigraphy, and CT and MRI typically show extensive soft tissue involvement that is often underappreciated on plain radiographs (Figs. 7.95–7.97). The differential diagnosis for these changes includes a variety of benign and malignant processes, including osteomyelitis, lymphoma, LCH, and even osteosarcoma.

Pathologic Features

GROSS FINDINGS

Ewing sarcoma is seldom examined intact prior to radiotherapy and/or chemotherapy. The cut surface has a tan, fleshy appearance, and hemorrhage and necrosis can be prominent.

MICROSCOPIC FINDINGS

Ewing sarcoma is composed of a monotonous population of primitive small round cells that grow in either

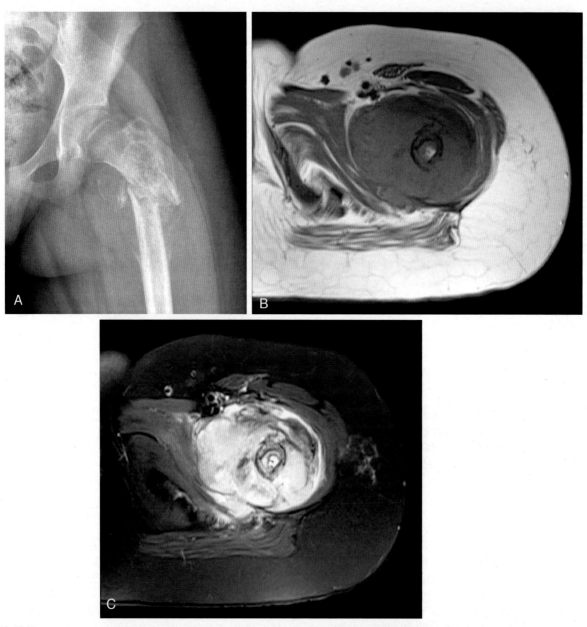

FIG. 7.95

Ewing sarcoma arising in the proximal femur. Conventional radiograph **(A)** shows a destructive lesion with an associated pathologic fracture. T1 **(B)** and T2 **(C)** MRI shows a large, concentric soft tissue mass surrounding the proximal femur that is not evidence of plain film images.

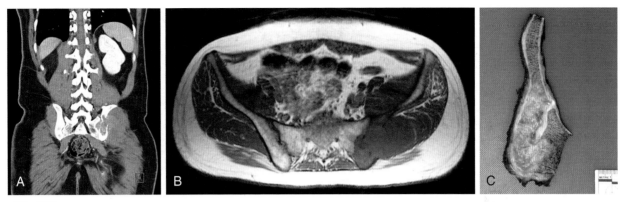

FIG. 7.96

Ewing sarcoma arising in the ilium. Coronal CT **(A)** shows a destructive lesion arising in the ilium that extends into soft tissue and erodes into the sacrum. MRI **(B)** highlights the extent of the tumor and involvement of the sacrum. Following chemotherapy, the soft tissue mass is considerably smaller, but residual Ewing sarcoma has a tan, fleshy cut surface and extends through the sacro-iliac joint into the sacrum **(C)**.

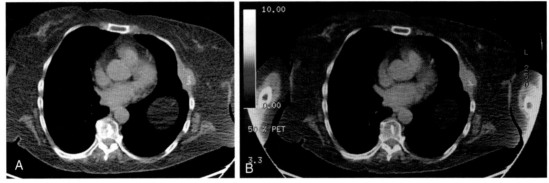

FIG. 7.97

Ewing sarcoma arising in a rib. CT **(A)** shows a destructive lesion in the rib extending into soft tissue. The lesion is highly PET-avid **(B)**.

sheets or nests that are separated by fibrous septa. Large areas of necrosis may be evident at low magnification (Fig. 7.98). Evidence of neural differentiation includes rosette formation in lesions formerly referred to as "primitive neuroectodermal tumor." Cytologically, individual tumor cells are uniform, have minimal eosinophilic to clear cytoplasm, and nuclei have stippled chromatin and occasional nucleoli. Mitotic activity is highly variable from tumor to tumor. Some examples of Ewing sarcoma are composed of larger cells (so-called "atypical Ewing sarcoma").

Ancillary Studies

Ancillary testing is required for a diagnosis of Ewing sarcoma. Immunohistochemically (Table 7.2), Ewing sarcoma usually shows diffuse membranous immunoreactivity for CD99, although this antibody is not specific. NKX2.2 is also usually positive in Ewing sarcoma and has better specificity than CD99 (Fig. 7.99). Depending

on the specific gene fusion, FLI1 or ERG might be positive, as well as neuroendocrine markers and keratins.

Molecular pathology is usually required to confirm the diagnosis of Ewing sarcoma, which is characterized by FET-ETS gene fusions (*EWSR1* or *FUS* fused with *FLI1*, *ERG*, and others) (see Table 7.2).

Differential Diagnosis

The differential diagnosis for Ewing sarcoma is broad and includes a variety of mesenchymal and non-mesenchymal neoplasms. Three fusion-driven sarcomas that commonly arise in bone include BCOR sarcomas, *EWSR1/FUS-NFATC2* fusion tumors, and mesenchymal chondrosarcoma. BCOR (BCL6 Corepressor) sarcomas are rare neoplasms that can arise in both bone and soft tissue. They occur in a broad age group but are most common in children and adolescents (Fig. 7.100), and patients present with symptoms similar to those seen with Ewing sarcoma. Histologically, BCOR sarcomas

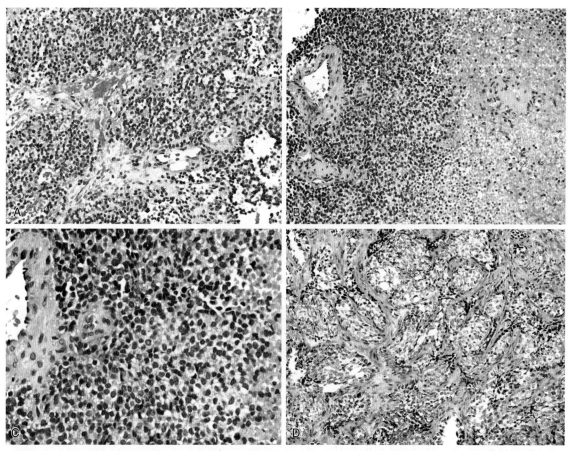

FIG. 7.98

A, Histologically, Ewing sarcoma is composed of sheets of primitive round cells at low magnification. **B,** Necrosis may be a prominent feature. **C,** Ewing sarcoma cells are primitive and have a small amount of eosinophilic or clear cytoplasm; mitotic activity can vary significantly between tumors. **D,** The adamantinoma-like variant of Ewing sarcoma shows distinct nests of tumor with peripheral palisading.

TABLE 7.2

Molecular and Immunohistochemical Features of Selected Round Cell Sarcomas Involving Bone

	Ewing Sarcoma	BCOR Sarcoma	EWSR1/FUS-NFATC2 Sarcoma	Mesenchymal Chondrosarcoma
Molecular alteration	EWSR1 or FUS fused with ETS family gene (most commonly FLI1 or ERG)	BCOR-CTNNB3 fusion or BCOR ITD	EWSR1 or FUS fused with NFATC2	HEY1-NCOA2 fusion
CD99	+	+/−	+	+
NKX2.2	+	−	+/−	−
NXK3.1	−	−	+	+
PAX7	+	−	+/−	−
Keratin	+/−	−	Rare	−
S-100	Rare	−	Rare	+
FLI1	+/−	−	−	−
ERG	+/−	−	−	−
SATB2	−	+	−	−
BCOR	−	+	−	−
Cyclin D1	−	+	−	−
Aggrecan	−	−	+	+/−

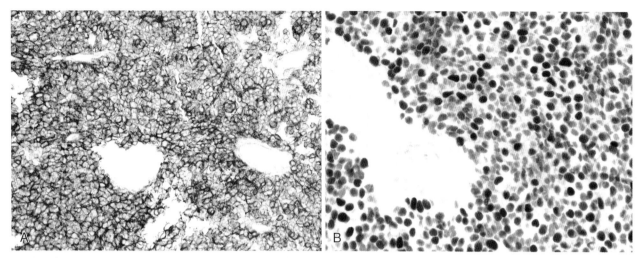

FIG. 7.99

Ewing sarcoma shows diffuse membranous immunoreactivity for CD99 **(A)** and strong nuclear immunoreactivity for NKX2.2 **(B)**.

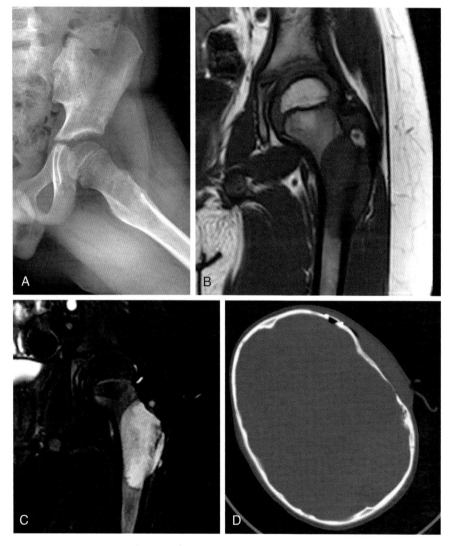

FIG. 7.100

BCOR sarcoma arising in the proximal femur of a child. Conventional radiographs show a destructive radiolucent lesion with associated periosteal reaction **(A)**. The lesion is low signal intensity on T1 MRI **(B)** and bright on T2 MRI **(C)**. The patient later developed a metastasis to the cranium **(D)**.

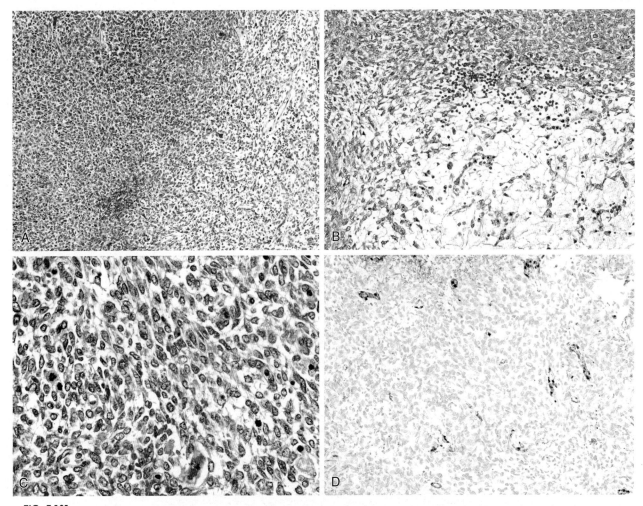

FIG. 7.101

A, *BCOR-CCNB3* fusion sarcoma showing both cellular and loosely myxoid areas at low magnification. **B,** A cellular area surrounding a myxoid focus. **C,** This tumor is characterized by short fascicles of uniform, mitotically active ovoid cells. **D,** An immunostain for CD99 was negative in this example.

show highly variable features, as opposed to the monotonous small round cell appearance of Ewing sarcoma. Most examples contain sheets or fascicles of round to spindled cells that are uniform in appearance, and the stroma is often myxoid (Fig. 7.101). Immunohistochemically, they are usually positive for BCOR, cyclin D1, and SATB2. CD99 is positive in only 50% of BCOR sarcomas. The most common *BCOR* rearrangement is a *BCOR-CCNB3* fusion, although a variety of other partners have been reported. *BCOR* internal tandem duplication (ITD) has also been described but is more commonly identified in soft tissue tumors. Limited data suggest that the prognosis for BCOR sarcomas is similar to Ewing sarcoma.

Another fusion-driven Ewing-like sarcoma is the *EWSR1/FUS-NFATC2* tumor. These tumors also have demographics and presenting symptoms similar to Ewing sarcoma and can occur more commonly in bone than soft tissue (Fig. 7.102). Tumors with this fusion can have a wide spectrum of histologic findings, but the most characteristic feature is groups of small cells arranged in cords or nests deposited in a fibrous, myxoid, or chondroid stroma, reminiscent of a myoepithelial tumor (Fig. 7.103). Focal or extensive areas of the tumor can be composed of round to spindled cells lacking matrix. *EWSR1/FUS-NFATC2* tumors also lack a specific immunohistochemical profile but are typically immunoreactive for CD99 and aggrecan, and keratins can also be positive. *EWSR1-NFATC2* fusions are more common than *FUS-NFATC2* fusions, and the latter fusion has also been identified in SBCs. Recognition of this tumor is important because these tumors do not respond to chemotherapy and their prognosis is extremely poor.

The non-chondroid component of mesenchymal chondrosarcomas can also closely resemble Ewing sarcoma. These tumors arise in a slightly older age group than Ewing sarcoma, and those that arise in bone have a predilection for the craniofacial bones, spine, ribs, and pelvis. Mesenchymal chondrosarcomas are biphasic neoplasms that contain chondroid foci admixed with Ewing-like primitive round cell component or a

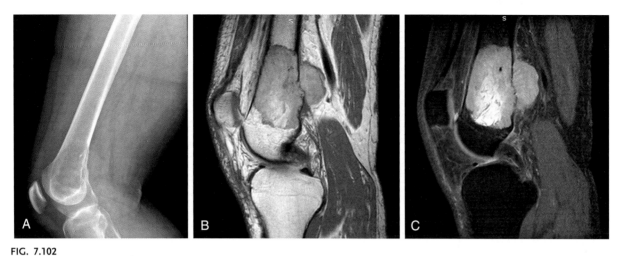

FIG. 7.102

An example of a *FUS-NFATC2* sarcoma. Lateral radiograph shows a destructive tumor arising in the distal femur **(A)**. On T1 **(B)** and T2 **(C)** MRI, the lesion has well-defined medullary borders but aggressively extends through the posterior cortex into soft tissue.

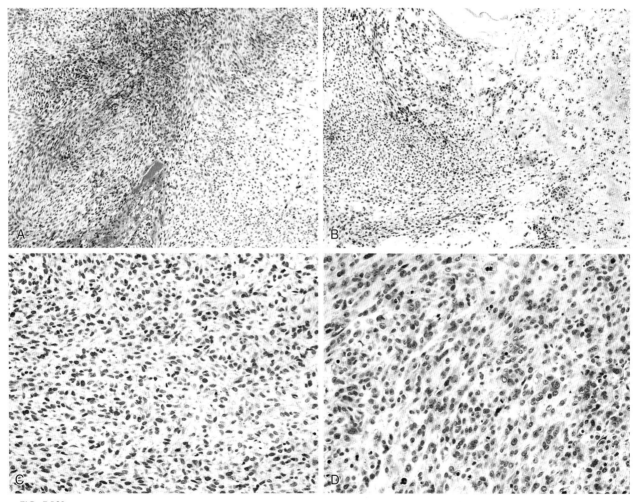

FIG. 7.103

NFATC2 sarcomas are variable in composition. This example contained areas composed of fascicles of monotonous spindled cells adjacent to foci with vaguely chondroid stroma **(A)**. In some areas, the tumor contained foci reminiscent of chordoma or a myoepithelial neoplasm **(B)**. Other areas were composed of ovoid to spindle cells with slightly more pleomorphism and mitotic activity **(C, D)**.

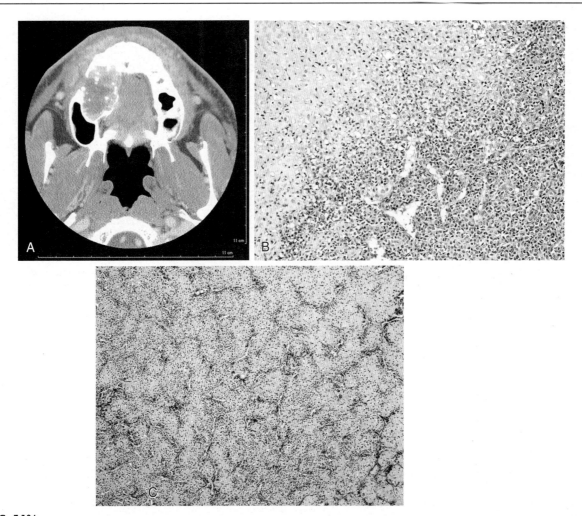

FIG. 7.104

CT of a mesenchymal chondrosarcoma of the mandible, a common location for this lesion **(A)**. Histologically, mesenchymal chondrosarcomas show areas of cartilage formation adjacent to foci composed of round cells resembling Ewing sarcoma **(B)**, often containing a prominent hemangiopericytoma-like vascular pattern **(C)**.

primitive spindle cell component containing a hemangiopericytoma-like vascular proliferation (Fig. 7.104). When appropriately sampled, the diagnosis is typically straightforward. However, when the chondroid component is not present, mesenchymal chondrosarcoma can be mistaken for other round cell neoplasms. Immunohistochemically, the primitive component is often positive for CD99 and SOX9, whereas the chondroid component is positive for S-100. Most mesenchymal chondrosarcomas harbor a *HEY1-NCOA2*, and the identification of this fusion can be helpful in diagnostically challenging cases.

Neuroblastoma frequently presents with solitary or multiple, typically lytic, bone lesions. This tumor has a unique predilection to metastasize to the orbit, jaws, and metaphyseal parts of long tubular bones. Neuroblastoma is one example of a pediatric malignancy that can present as a solitary bone metastasis with a clinically occult primary lesion. Discrete diffuse involvement of bone marrow in bone marrow biopsy samples is frequently seen and can be documented in nearly 50% of neuroblastomas. On the other hand, radiographically demonstrable destructive bone lesions are seen less frequently in approximately 25% of children with neuroblastoma. In typical cases, the presence of neuropil and ganglionic differentiation are microscopic features diagnostic of neuroblastoma. PHOX2B is a dependable immunostain for the diagnosis of neuroblastoma.

Lymphoblastic lymphoma of precursor B-cell type can present as a solitary bone tumor and very closely simulates Ewing sarcoma histologically and immunohistochemically (Fig. 7.105). Immunohistochemically, the tumor cells are diffusely positive for CD99, but are also positive for terminal deoxynucleotidyl transferase (TdT), PAX5, CD43, CD34, CD79a, and variably positive for CD20. This diagnosis should always be entertained in the differential diagnosis of Ewing sarcoma, and ancillary immunohistochemistry, molecular diagnostic testing, and flow cytometry must be used to separate these entities.

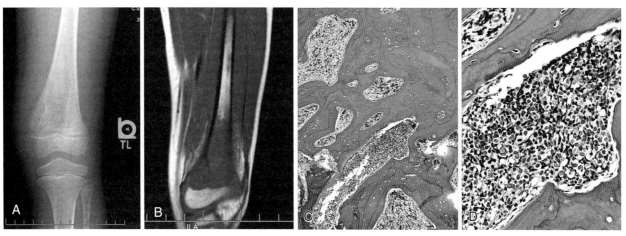

FIG. 7.105

Example of acute lymphoblastic lymphoma initially appearing as a solitary bone lesion. Plain radiograph **(A)** and MRI **(B)** show a destructive lesion arising in the distal femoral metaphysis **(A, B)**. Histologically, the lesion strongly resembles Ewing sarcoma and is composed of primitive round cells surrounded by sclerotic bone **(C, D)**. This lesion was strongly immunoreactive for CD99, TdT, CD79A, and CD43, confirming the diagnosis.

Prognosis and Therapy

Like osteosarcoma, the prognosis for Ewing sarcoma has improved dramatically with current chemotherapy and radiotherapy regimens. Patients with Ewing sarcoma are treated with a specific chemotherapy regimen, and local control is achieved with surgery, radiotherapy, or a combination of the two, depending on the expendability of the bone. Patients with localized Ewing sarcoma have a 70% cure rate, but patients presenting with metastatic disease have a 5-year survival of less than 50%.

>> MRI frequently shows a soft tissue mass far larger than is evident on conventional radiographs

Prognosis and Therapy

>> With current multimodal chemotherapy, radiotherapy, and surgery, approximately 70% of patients with localized disease are cured
>> Patients with metastatic disease have a poor prognosis

EWING SARCOMA – DISEASE FACT SHEET

Definition

>> A small round cell sarcoma containing an FET-ETS family fusion, most commonly *EWSR1-FLI1*

Incidence and Location

>> Second most common primary bone sarcoma in children
>> Can arise in any portion of any bone
>> Long bone lesions are often diaphyseal
>> Bones of pelvis and rib are also common locations

Age Distribution

>> Usually occurs during the first two decades
>> Uncommon after the age of 30

Clinical Features

>> Causes symptoms similar to osteomyelitis, including pain, fever, and leukocytosis
>> Pathologic fracture possible

Radiologic Features

>> Cause aggressive, permeative bone destruction associated with periosteal reaction resembling "onion skin"

EWING SARCOMA – PATHOLOGIC FEATURES

Gross Findings

>> Tan-gray fleshy cut surface, often with necrosis

Microscopic Findings

>> Primitive, uniform small round cell tumor, individual tumor cells may have clear cytoplasm
>> Necrosis is common
>> Mitotic activity variable
>> Cases with neuroectodermal differentiation have rosettes and/or immunohistochemical evidence of neuroectodermal differentiation
>> Atypical Ewing sarcoma is characterized by larger cells

Ancillary Studies

>> CD99 is diffusely positive in a membranous pattern
>> NKX2.2 often strongly positive
>> Molecular diagnostic testing evidence of an FET-ETS fusion, most commonly *EWSR1-FLI1* (85%) or *EWSR1-ERG* (10%).
>> *FUS* gene fusions also possible

Pathologic Differential Diagnoses

>> *BCOR-CCNB3* sarcomas
>> *EWSR1/FUS-NFATC2* sarcoma
>> Mesenchymal chondrosarcoma
>> Lymphoblastic lymphoma
>> Metastatic neuroblastoma

SUGGESTED READINGS

Degenerative Joint Disease

Dermawan J, Reith J, Kilpatrick S. Accurate and reliable diagnosis of avascular necrosis of the femoral head from total hip arthroplasty specimens requires pathologic examination. *Am J Clin Pathol.* 2021;155:565-574.

DiCarlo EF, Klein MJ. Arthritis pathology. *Surg Pathol.* 2012;5:15-65.

DiCarlo EF, Klein MJ. Comparison of clinical and histologic diagnoses in 16,587 total joint arthroplasties. *Am J Clin Pathol.* 2014;141:111-118.

Hamerman D. The biology of osteoarthritis. *N Engl J Med.* 1989;320:1322-1330.

Malfait AM. Osteoarthritis year in review 2015: biology. *Osteoarthritis Cartilage.* 2016:24:21-26.

Manenti G, Altobelli S, Pugliese L, Tarantino V. The role of imaging in diagnosis and management of femoral head osteonecrosis. *Clin Cases Miner Bone Metab.* 2015;12(suppl 1):31-38.

Mankin HJ. Nontraumatic necrosis of bone (osteonecrosis). *N Engl J Med.* 1992;326:1473-1479.

Yamamoto T, Yamaguchi T, Lee KB, Bullough PG. A clinicopathologic study of osteonecrosis in the osteoarthritic hip. *Osteoarthritis Cartilage.* 2000;8:303-308.

Yamamoto T, DiCarlo EF, Bullough PG. The prevalence and clinicopathological appearance of extension of osteonecrosis in the femoral head. *J Bone Joint Surg Br.* 1999;81:328-332.

Tenosynovial Giant Cell Tumor, Diffuse Type (PVNS)

Al-Ibraheemi A, Ahrens WA, Fritchie K, et al. Malignant tenosynovial giant cell tumor: the true "synovial sarcoma?" A clinicopathologic, immunohistochemical, and molecular cytogenetic study of 10 cases, supporting origin from synoviocytes. *Mod Pathol.* 2019;32: 242-251.

Bertoni F, Unni KK, Beabout JW, Sim FH. Malignant giant cell tumor of the tendon sheaths and joints (malignant pigmented villonodular synovitis). *Am J Surg Pathol.* 1997;21:153-163.

Cupp JS, Miller MA, Montgomery KD, et al. Translocation and expression of CSF1 in pigmented villonodular synovitis, tenosynovial giant cell tumor, rheumatoid arthritis and other reactive synovitides. *Am J Surg Pathol.* 2007;31:970-976.

Folpe AL, Weiss SW, Fletcher D, Gown AM. Tenosynovial giant cell tumors: evidence for a desmin-positive dendritic cell subpopulation. *Mod Pathol.* 1998;11:939-944.

Layfield LJ, Meloni-Ehrig A, Liu K, Shepard R, Harrelson JM. Malignant giant cell tumor of synovium (malignant pigmented villonodular synovitis). *Arch Pathol Lab Med.* 2000;124:1636-1641.

Li CF, Wang JW, Huang WW, et al. Malignant diffuse-type tenosynovial giant cell tumors: a series of 7 cases comparing with 24 benign lesions with review of the literature. *Am J Surg Pathol.* 2008;32:587-599.

Mendenhall WM, Mendenhall CM, Reith JD, et al. Pigmented villonodular synovitis. *Am J Clin Oncol.* 2006;29:548-550.

Murphey MD, Rhee JH, Lewis RB, et al. Pigmented villonodular synovitis: radiologic-pathologic correlation. *Radiographics.* 2008;28:1493-1518.

O'Connell JX, Fanburg JC, Rosenberg AE. Giant cell tumor of tendon sheath and pigmented villonodular synovitis: immunophenotype suggests a synovial cell origin. *Hum Pathol.* 1995;26:771-775.

Oda Y, Izumi T, Harimaya K, et al. Pigmented villonodular synovitis with chondroid metaplasia, resembling chondroblastoma of the bone: a report of three cases. *Mod Pathol.* 2007;20:545-551.

Ottaviani S, Ayral X, Dougados M. et al. Pigmented villonodular synovitis: a retrospective single center study of 122 cases and review of the literature. *Semin Arthritis Rheum.* 2011;40:539-546.

West RB, Rubin BP, Miller MA, et al. A landscape effect in tenosynovial giant-cell tumor from activation of CSF1 expression by a translocation in a minority of tumor cells. *Proc Natl Acad Sci USA.* 2006;103:690-695.

Primary Synovial Chondromatosis

Agaram NP, Zhang L, Dickson BC, et al. A molecular study of synovial chondromatosis. *Genes Chromosomes Cancer.* 2020;59:144-151.

Amary F, Perez-Casanova L, Ye H, et al. Synovial chondromatosis and soft tissue chondroma: extra-osseous cartilaginous tumors defined by FN1 gene rearrangement. *Mod Pathol.* 2019;32:1762-1771.

Bertoni F, Unni KK, Beabout JW, Sim FH. Chondrosarcomas of the synovium. *Cancer.* 1991;67:155-162.

Evans S, Boffano M, Chaudhry S, et al. Synovial chondrosarcoma arising in synovial chondromatosis. *Sarcoma.* 2014;2014:647939.

Fetsch JF, Vinh TN, Remotti F, Walker EA, Murphey MD, Sweet DE. Tenosynovial (extraarticular) chondromatosis: an analysis of 37 cases of an underrecognized clinicopathologic entity with a strong predilection for the hands and feet and a high local recurrence rate. *Am J Surg Pathol.* 2003;27:1260-1268.

Murphey MD, Vidal JA, Fanburg-Smith JC, et al. Imaging of synovial chondromatosis with radiologic-pathologic correlation. *Radiographics.* 2007;27:1465-1488.

Sah AP, Geller DS, Mankin HJ, et al. Malignant transformation of synovial chondromatosis of the shoulder to chondrosarcoma. A case report. *J Bone Joint Surg.* 2007;89:1321-1328.

Sciot R, Dal Cin P, Bellemans J, Samson I, Van den Berghe H, Van Damme B. Synovial chondromatosis: clonal chromosome changes provide further evidence for a neoplastic disorder. *Virchows Archn.* 1998;433:189-191.

Villacin AB, Brigham LN, Bullough PG. Primary and secondary synovial chondrometaplasia: histopathologic and clinicoradiologic differences. *Hum Pathol.* 1979;10:439-451.

Prosthesis Pathology

Abdul-Karim FW, McGinnis MG, Kraay M, Emancipator SN, Goldberg V. Frozen section biopsy assessment for the presence of polymorphonuclear leukocytes in patients undergoing revision of arthroplasties. *Mod Pathol.* 1998;11:427-431.

Bauer TW, Hayashi R. The role of the pathologist in diagnosing periprosthetic infection. *Surg Pathol Clin.* 2012;5:67-77.

Bauer TW, Schils J. The pathology of total joint arthroplasty. II. Mechanisms of implant failure. *Skel Radiol.* 1999;28:483-497.

Bauer TW, Bedair H, Creech JD, et al. Hip and knee section, diagnosis, laboratory tests: Proceedings of International Consensus on orthopedic infections. *J Arthroplasty.* 2019;34(suppl 2):S351-S359.

Bingham J, Clarke H, Spangehl M, Schwartz A, Beauchamp C, Goldberg B. The alpha defensin-1 biomarker assay can be used to evaluate the potentially infected total joint arthroplasty. *Clin Orthop Rel Res.* 2014;472:4006-4009.

Corvec S, Portillo ME, Pasticci BM, Borens O, Trampuz A. Epidemiology and new developments in the diagnosis of prosthetic joint infection. *Int J Artif Organs.* 2012;35:923-934.

Krenn V, Morawietz L, Perino G, et al. Revised histopathological consensus classification of joint implant related pathology. *Pathol Res Pract.* 2014;210:779-786.

Mirra JM, Marder RA, Amstutz HC. The pathology of failed total joint arthroplasty. *Clin Orthop Rel Res.* 1982;170:175-183.

Parvizi J, Tan TL, Goswami K, et al. The 2018 definition of periprosthetic hip and knee infection: an evidence-based and validated criteria. *J Arthroplasty.* 2018;33:1309-1314.

Parvizi J, Zmistowski BS, Berbari EF, et al. New definition for periprosthetic joint infection. From the workgroup of the Musculoskeletal Infection Society. *Clin Orthop Rel Res.* 2011;469:2992-2994.

Renz N, Yermak K, Perka C, Trampuz A. Alpha defensin lateral flow test for diagnosis of periprosthetic joint infection. Not a screening but a confirmatory test. *J Bone Joint Surg Am.* 2018;100:742-750.

Shohat N, Tan, TL, Della Valle CJ, et al. Development and validation of an evidence-based algorithm for diagnosing periprosthetic joint infection. *J Arthroplasty.* 2019;34:2730-2736.

Enchondroma

Afonso PD, Isaac A, Villagran JM. Chondroid tumor as incidental findings and differential diagnosis between enchondromas and low-grade chondrosarcomas. *Semin Musculoskel Radiol.* 2019;23:3-18.

Amary MF, Bacsi K, Maggiani F, et al. IDH1 and IDH2 mutations are frequent events in central chondrosarcoma and central and periosteal chondromas but not in other mesenchymal tumors. *J Pathol.* 2011;224:334-343.

Brien EW, Mirra JM, Kerr R. Benign and malignant cartilage tumors of bone and joint: their anatomic and theoretical basis with an emphasis on radiology, pathology, and clinical biology. I. The intramedullary tumors. *Skeletal Radiol.* 1997;26:325-353.

Duckworth LV, Reith JD. Well-differentiated central cartilage tumors of bone: an overview. *Surg Pathol.* 2012;5:147-161.

Fanburg JC, Meis-Kindblom JM, Rosenberg AE. Multiple enchondromas associated with spindle-cell hemangioendotheliomas. An overlooked variant of Maffucci's syndrome. *Am J Surg Pathol.* 1995;19: 1029-1038.

Greenspan A. Tumors of cartilage origin. *Orthop Clin North Am.* 1989;20:347-366.

Ishida T, Dorfman HD. Massive chondroid differentiation in fibrous dysplasia of bone (fibrocartilaginous dysplasia). *Am J Surg Pathol.* 1993;17:924-930.

Marco RAW, Gitelis S, Brabach GT, Healey JH. Cartilage tumors: Evaluation and treatment. *J Am Acad Orthop Surg.* 2000;8:292-304.

McCarthy EF, Tyler WK. Distinguishing enchondroma from low-grade central chondrosarcoma. *Pathol Case Rev.* 2001;6:8-13.

Mirra JM, Gold R, Downs J, Eckardt JJ. A new histologic approach to the differentiation of enchondroma and chondrosarcoma of the bones. A clinicopathologic analysis of 51 cases. *Clin Orthop.* 1985;201:214-237.

Mohler DG, Chiu R, McCall DA, Avedian RS. Curettage and cryosurgery for low-grade cartilage tumors is associated with low recurrence and high function. *Clin Orthop Rel Res.* 2010;468:2765-2773.

Murphey MD, Flemming DJ, Boyea SR, et al. Enchondroma versus chondrosarcoma in the appendicular skeleton: Differentiating features. *Radiographics.* 1998;18:1213-1237.

Ogose A, Unni KK, Swee RG, et al. Chondrosarcoma of small bones of the hands and feet. *Cancer.* 1997;80:50-59.

Pansuriya TC, Kroon HM, Bovee JVMG. Enchondromatosis: insights on the different subtypes. *Int J Clin Exp Pathol.* 2010;3:557-569.

Scarborough MT, Moreau G. Benign cartilage tumors. *Orthop Clin North Am.* 1996;27:583-589.

Schiller AL. Diagnosis of borderline cartilage lesions of bone. *Semin Diagn Pathol.* 1985;2:42-62.

Shon W, Folpe AL, Fritchie KJ. ERG expression in chondrogenic bone and soft tissue tumors. *J Clin Pathol.* 2015;68:125-129.

Silve C, Juppner H. Ollier disease. *Orphanet J Rare Dis.* 2006;1:37.

Suster D, Hung YP, Nielsen GP. Differential diagnosis of cartilaginous lesions of bone. *Arch Pathol Lab Med.* 2020;144:71-82.

Osteochondroma

Bauer TW, Dorfman HD, Latham JT. Periosteal chondroma: a clinicopathologic study of 23 cases. *Am J Surg Pathol.* 1982;6:631-637.

Bernard SA, Murphey MD, Flemming DJ, et al. Improved differentiation of benign osteochondromas from secondary chondrosarcomas with standardized measurement of cartilage cap at CT and MRI imaging. *Radiology.* 2010;255:857-865.

Boriani S, Bacchini P, Bertoni F, Campanacci M. Periosteal chondroma. A review of twenty cases. *J Bone Joint Surg Am.* 1983;65:205-212.

Bovee JV, Cleton-Jansen AM, Wuyts W, et al. EXT-mutation analysis and loss of heterozygosity in sporadic and hereditary osteochondromas and secondary chondrosarcomas. *Am J Hum Genet.* 1999;65: 689-698.

De Andrea CE, Reijnders CM, Kroon HM, et al. Secondary peripheral chondrosarcoma evolving from osteochondroma as a result of outgrowth of cells with functional EXT. *Oncogene.* 2012;31:1095-1104.

De Santos LA, Spjut HG. Periosteal chondroma: a radiologic spectrum. *Skeletal Radiol.* 1981;6:15-20.

Lewis MM, Kenan S, Yabut SM, et al. Periosteal chondroma. A report of ten cases and review of the literature. *Clin Orthop Rel Res.* 1990;256:185-192.

Chondromyxoid Fibroma

Bahk WJ, Mirra JM, Sohn KR, Shin DS. Pseudoanaplastic chondromyxoid fibroma. *Ann Diagn Pathol.* 1998;2:241-246.

Baker AC, Rezeanu L, O'Laughlin S, Unni K, Klein MJ, Siegal GP. Juxtacortical chondromyxoid fibroma of bone: a unique variant: a case study of 20 patients. *Am J Surg Pathol.* 2007;31:1662-1668.

Baumhoer D, Amary F, Flanagan AM. An update of molecular pathology of bone tumors. Lessons learned from investigating samples by next generation sequencing. *Genes Chromosomes Cancer.* 2019;58:88-99.

Bleiweiss IJ, Klein MJ. Chondromyxoid fibroma: report of six cases with immunohistochemical studies. *Mod Pathol.* 1990;3:664-666.

Keel SB, Bhan AK, Liebsch NJ, Rosenberg AE. Chondromyxoid fibroma of the skull base: a tumor which may be confused with chordoma and chondrosarcoma. A report of three cases and review of the literature. *Am J Surg Pathol.* 1997;21:577-582.

Nielsen GP, Keel SB, Dickersin GR, Selig MK, Bhan AK, Rosenberg AE. Chondromyxoid fibroma: a tumor showing myofibroblastic, myochondroblastic, and chondrocytic differentiation. *Mod Pathol.* 1999;12:514-517.

Wu CT, Inwards CY, O'Laughlin S, Rock MG, Beabout JW, Unni KK. Chondromyxoid fibroma of bone: a clinicopathologic review of 278 cases. *Hum Pathol.* 1998;29:438-446.

Yasuda T, Nishio J, Sumegi J, et al. Aberrations of 6q13 mapped to the COL12A1 locus in chondromyxoid fibroma. *Mod Pathol.* 2009;11: 1499-1506.

Zillmer DA, Dorfman HD. Chondromyxoid fibroma of bone: thirty-six cases with clinicopathologic correlation. *Hum Pathol.* 1989;20: 952-964.

Giant Cell Tumor

Amary MF, Berish F, Mozela R, et al. The H3F3 K36M mutant antibody is a sensitive and specific marker for the diagnosis of chondroblastoma. *Histopathology.* 2016;69:121-127.

Behjati S, Tarpey PS, Presneau N, et al. Distinct H3F3A and H3F3B driver mutations define chondroblastoma and giant cell tumor of bone. *Nat Genet.* 2013;45:1479-1482.

Bertoni F, Bacchini P, Staals EL. Malignancy in giant cell tumor of bone. *Cancer.* 2003;97:2520-2529.

Bjornsson J, Unni KK, Dahlin DC, Beabout JW, Sim FH. Clear cell chondrosarcoma of bone. Observations in 47 cases. *Am J Surg Pathol.* 1984;8:223-230.

Branstetter DG, Nelson SD, Manivel JC, et al. Denosumab induces tumor reduction and bone formation in patients with giant cell tumor of bone. *Clin Cancer Res.* 2012;18:4415-4424.

Chan CM, Adler Z, Reith JD, Gibbs CP. Risk factors for pulmonary metastases from giant cell tumor of bone. *J Bone Joint Surg Am.* 2015;97:420-428.

de Silva MV, Reid R. Chondroblastoma: varied histologic appearance, potential diagnostic pitfalls, and clinicopathologic features associated with local recurrence. *Ann Diagnost Pathol.* 2003;7: 205-213.

Hoch BL, Inwards C, Sundaram M, Rosenberg AE. Multicentric giant cell tumor of bone: a clinicopathologic analysis of thirty cases. *J Bone Joint Surg Am.* 2006;88:1998-2008.

Hudson TM, Scheibler M, Springfield DS, et al. Radiology of giant cell tumors of bone: computed tomography, arthro-tomography, and scintigraphy. *Skeletal Radiol.* 1984;11:85-95.

James SL, Panicek DM, Davies AM. Bone marrow oedema associated with benign and malignant bone tumours. *Eur J Radiol.* 2008;67:11-21.

Laitinen MK, Stevenson JD, Evans S, et al. Chondroblastoma in pelvis and extremities – a single center study of 177 cases. *J Bone Oncol.* 2019;17:100248.

Lucas DR. Giant cell tumor of bone. *Surg Pathol.* 2012;5:183-200.

Nishio J, Reith JD, Ogose A, et al. Cytogenetic findings in clear cell chondrosarcoma. *Cancer Genet Cytogenet.* 2005;162:74-77.

Presneau N, Baumhoer D, Behjati S, et al. Diagnostic value of H3H3A mutations in giant cell tumour of bone compared to osteoclast-rich mimics. *J Pathol Clin Res.* 2015;1:113-123.

Sarungbam J, Agaram N, Hwang S, et al. Symplastic/pseudoanaplastic giant cell tumor of the bone. *Skeletal Radiol.* 2016;45:929-935.

Schaefer IM, Fletcher JA, Neilsen, et al. Immunohistochemistry for histone H3G34W and H3K36M is highly specific for giant cell tumor of bone and chondroblastoma, respectively, in FNA and core needle biopsy. *Cancer Cytopathol.* 2018;126:552-566.

Shi W, Indelicato DJ, Reith JD, et al. Radiotherapy in the management of giant cell tumor of bone. *Am J Clin Oncol.* 2013;36:505-508.

Thomas D, Henshaw R, Skubitz K, et al. Denosumab in patients with giant cell tumor of bone: an open-label, phase 2 study. *Lancet Oncol.* 2010;11:275-280.

Wojcik J, Rosenberg AE, Brandella, MA, et al. Denosumab-treated giant cell tumor of bone exhibits morphologic overlap with malignant giant cell tumor of bone. *Am J Surg Pathol.* 2016;40:72-80.

Aneurysmal Bone Cyst

Althof PA, Ohmori K, Zhou M, et al. Cytogenetic and molecular cytogenetic findings in 43 aneurysmal bone cysts: aberrations of 17p mapped to 17p13.2 by fluorescence in situ hybridization. *Mod Pathol.* 2004;17:518-525.

Bahk WJ, Mirra JM. Differential diagnostic value of "blue reticulated chondroid-like material" in aneurysmal bone cysts: a classic histopathologic analysis of 215 cases. *Am J Clin Pathol*. 2015;143:823-829.

Baumhoer D, Smida J, Nathrath M, et al. The nature of the characteristic cementum-like matrix deposits in the walls of simple bone cysts. *Histopathology*. 2011;59:390-396.

Campanacci M, Capanna R, Picci P. Unicameral and aneurysmal bone cysts. *Clin Orthop Rel Res*. 1986;(204):25-36.

Li L, Bui MM, Zhang M, et al. Validation of Fluorescence in situ hybridization testing of USP6 gene rearrangement for diagnosis of primary aneurysmal bone cyst. *Ann Clin Lab Sci*. 2019;49:590-597.

Mascard E, Gomez-Brouchet A, Lambot K. Bone cysts: unicameral and aneurysmal bone cyst. *Orthop Traumatol Surg Res*. 2015;101(suppl 1):S119-S127.

Oliveira AM, Perez-Atayde AR, Inwards CY, et al. USP6 and CDH11 oncogenes identify the neoplastic cell in primary aneurysmal bone cysts and are absent in so-called secondary aneurysmal bone cysts. *Am J Surg Pathol*. 2004;165:1773-1780.

Struhl S, Edelson C, Pritzker H, et al. Solitary (unicameral) bone cyst: The fallen fragment sign revisited. *Skeletal Radiol*. 1989;18:261-265.

Vergel De Dios AM, Bond JR, Shives TC, McLeod RA, Unni KK. Aneurysmal bone cyst. A clinicopathologic study of 238 cases. *Cancer*. 1992;69:2921-2931.

Wold LE, Dobyns JH, Swee RG, Dahlin DC. Giant cell reaction (giant cell reparative granuloma) of the small bones of the hands and feet. *Am J Surg Pathol*. 1986;10:491-496.

Yamaguchi T, Dorfman HD. Giant cell reparative granuloma: a comparative clinicopathologic study of lesions in gnathic and extragnathic sites. *Int J Surg Pathol*. 2001;9:189-200.

Zishan US, Pressney I, Khoo M, Saifuddin A. The differentiation between aneurysmal bone cyst and telangiectatic osteosarcoma: a clinical, radiographic and MRI study. *Skeletal Radiol*. 2020;49:1375-1386.

Fibrous Dysplasia

Aoki T, Kouho H, Hisaoka M, Hashimoto H, Nakata H, Sakai A. Intramuscular myxoma with fibrous dysplasia: a report of two cases with a review of the literature. *Pathol Int*. 1995;45:165-171.

de Sanctis L, Delmastro L, Russo MC, Matarazzo P, Lala R, de Sanctis C. Genetics of McCune-Albright syndrome. *J Ped Endocrinol Metab*. 2006;19(suppl 2):577-582.

Dorfman HD, Ishida T, Tsuneyoshi M. Exophytic variant of fibrous dysplasia (fibrous dysplasia protuberans). *Hum Pathol*. 1994;25:1234-1237.

Duhamel LA, Ye H, Halai D, et al. Frequency of Mouse Double Minute 2 (MDM2) and Mouse Double Minute 4 (MDM4) amplification in parosteal and conventional osteosarcoma subtypes. *Histopathology*. 2012;60:357-359.

Dujardin F, Binh MB, Bourier C, et al. MDM2 and CDK4 immunohistochemistry is a valuable tool in the differential diagnosis of low-grade osteosarcomas and other primary fibro-osseous lesion of the bone. *Mod Pathol*. 2011;24:624-637.

Ishida T, Dorfman HD. Massive chondroid differentiation in fibrous dysplasia of bone (fibrocartilaginous dysplasia). *Am J Surg Pathol*. 1993;17:924-930.

Matsuba A, Ogose A, Tokunaga K, et al. Activating Gs alpha mutation at the Arg201 codon in, liposclerosing myxofibrous tumor. *Hum Pathol*. 2003;34:1204-1209.

Nascimento A, Kilpatrick SE, Reith JD. Osteofibrous dysplasia and adamantinoma. *Surg Pathol Clin*. 2021;14:723-735.

Ruggieri P, Sim FH, Bond JR, Unni KK. Malignancies in fibrous dysplasia. *Cancer*. 1994;73:1411-1424.

Yoshida A, Ushiku T, Motoi T, et al. Immunohistochemical analysis of MDM2 and CDK4 distinguishes low-grade osteosarcoma from benign mimics. *Mod Pathol*. 2010;23:1279-1288.

Parosteal Osteosarcoma

Bertoni F, Present D, Hudson T, et al. The meaning of radiolucencies in parosteal osteosarcoma. *J Bone Joint Surg Am*. 1985;67-A:901-910.

Campanacci M, Picci P, Gherlinzoni F, Guerra A, Bertoni F, Neff JR. Parosteal osteosarcoma. *J Bone Joint Surg Br*. 1984;66:313-321.

deSantos LA, Murray JA, Finklestein JB, Spjut HJ, Ayala AG. The radiographic spectrum of periosteal osteosarcoma. *Radiology*. 1978;127:123-129.

Dujardin F, Binh MB, Bourier C, et al. MDM2 and CDK4 immunohistochemistry is a valuable tool in the differential diagnosis of low-grade osteosarcomas and other primary fibro-osseous lesion of the bone. *Mod Pathol*. 2011;24:624-637.

Duhamel LA, Ye H, Halai D, et al. Frequency of Mouse Double Minute 2 (MDM2) and Mouse Double Minute 4 (MDM4) amplification in parosteal and conventional osteosarcoma subtypes. *Histopathology*. 2012;60:357-359.

Hall RB, Robinson LH, Malawar MM, Dunham WK. Periosteal osteosarcoma. *Cancer*. 1985;55:165-171.

Okada K, Unni KK, Swee RG, Sim FH. High grade surface osteosarcoma: a clinicopathologic study of 46 cases. *Cancer*. 1999;85:1044-1054.

Salinas-Souza C, De Andrea C, Bihl M, et al. GNAS mutations are not detected in parosteal and low-grade central osteosarcoma. *Mod Pathol*. 2015;28:1336-1342.

Sheth DS, Yasko AW, Raymond AK, et al. Conventional and dedifferentiated parosteal osteosarcoma. Diagnosis, treatment, and outcome. *Cancer*. 1996;78:2136-2145.

Unni KK, Dahlin DC, Beabout JW. Periosteal osteogenic sarcoma. *Cancer*. 1976;37:2476-2485.

Unni KK, Dahlin DC, Beabout JW, Ivins JC. Parosteal osteogenic sarcoma. *Cancer*. 1976;37:2466-2475.

Wold LE, Unni KK, Beabout JW, Pritchard DJ. High-grade surface osteosarcomas. *Am J Surg Pathol*. 1984;8:181-186.

Wold LE, Unni KK, Beabout JW, Sim FH, Dahlin DC. Dedifferentiated parosteal osteosarcoma. *J Bone Joint Surg Am*. 1984;66:53-59.

Yoshida A, Ushiku T, Motoi T, et al. Immunohistochemical analysis of MDM2 and CDK4 distinguishes low-grade osteosarcoma from benign mimics. *Mod Pathol*. 2010;23:1279-1288.

Desmoplastic Fibroma

Bertoni F, Calderoni P, Bacchini P, Campanacci M. Desmoplastic fibroma of bone. A report of six cases. *J Bone Joint Surg Br*. 1984;66:265-268.

Bohm P, Krober S, Greschniok A, Laniado M, Kaiserling E. Desmoplastic fibroma of the bone. A report of two patients, review of the literature, and therapeutic implications. *Cancer*. 1996;78:1011-1023.

Cho S, Bean G, Charville S, et al. Molecular genetics of desmoplastic fibroma of bone. *Mod Pathol*. 2020;33:174-239.

Gebhardt MC, Campbell CJ, Schiller AL, Mankin HJ. Desmoplastic fibroma of bone. A report of eight cases and review of the literature. *J Bone Joint Surg Am*. 1985;67:732-747.

Hauben EI, Jundt G, Cleton-Jansen AM, et al. Desmoplastic fibroma of bone: an immunohistochemical study including beta-catenin expression and mutational analysis for beta-catenin. *Hum Pathol*. 2005;36:1025-1030.

Inwards CY, Unni KK, Beabout JW, Sim FH. Desmoplastic fibroma of bone. *Cancer*. 1991;68:1978-1983.

Song W, van den Berg E, Keww TC, et al. Low-grade central fibroblastic osteosarcoma may be differentiated from its mimicker desmoplastic fibroma by genetic analysis. *Clin Sarcoma Res*. 2018;8:16. doi:10.1186/s13569-018-0104-z.

Osteoid Osteoma

Amary F, Markert E, Berisha F, et al. FOS expression in osteoid osteoma and osteoblastoma: a valuable ancillary diagnostic tool. *Am J Surg Pathol*. 2019;43:1661-1667.

Barei DP, Moreau G, Scarborough MT, Neel MD. Percutaneous radiofrequency ablation of osteoid osteoma. *Clin Orthop Relat Res*. 2000;373:115-124.

Bauer TW, Zehr RJ, Belhobek GH, Marks KE. Juxta-articular osteoid osteoma. *Am J Surg Pathol*. 1991;15:381-387.

Bertoni F, Bacchini P, Donati D, Martini A, Picci P, Campanacci M. Osteoblastoma-like osteosarcoma. The Rizzoli Institute experience. *Mod Pathol*. 1993;6:707-716.

Bertoni F, Unni KK, McLeod RA, Dahlin DC. Osteosarcoma resembling osteoblastoma. *Cancer*. 1985;55:416-426.

Dorfman HD, Weiss SW. Borderline osteoblastic tumors: problems in the differential diagnosis of aggressive osteoblastoma and low-grade osteosarcoma. *Sem Diagnostic Pathol*. 1984;1:215-234.

Fittall MW, Mifsud, W, Pillay N, et al. Recurrent rearrangements of FOS and FOSB define osteoblastoma. *Nat Commun*. 2018;9:2150.

Gambarotti M, Dei Tos AP, Vanel D, et al. Osteoblastoma-like osteosarcoma: high-grade or low-grade osteosarcoma? *Histopathology*. 2019; 74:494-503.

Garcia RA, Inwards CY, Unni KK. Benign bone tumors – recent developments. *Semin Diagn Pathol*. 2011;28:73-85.

Loizaga JM, Calvo M, Lopez Barea F, Martinez Tello FJ, Perez Villanueva J. Osteoblastoma and osteoid osteoma. Clinical and morphological features of 162 cases. *Pathol Res Pract*. 1993;189:33-41.

Lucas DR. Osteoblastoma. *Arch Pathol Lab Med*. 2010;134:1460-1466.

Lucas DR, Unni KK, McLeod RA, O'Connor MI, Sim FH. Osteoblastoma: clinicopathologic study of 306 cases. *Hum Pathol*. 1994;25:117-134.

Weber MA, Springel SD, Omlor GW, et al. Clinical long-term outcome, technical success, and cost analysis of radiofrequency ablation for the treatment of osteoblastomas and spinal osteoid osteomas in comparison to open surgical resection. *Skeletal Radiol*. 2015;44:981-993.

Yalcinkaya U, Doganavsargil B, Sezak M, et al. Clinical and morphologic characteristics of osteoid osteoma and osteoblastoma: a retrospective single-center analysis of 204 patients. *Ann Diagn Pathol*. 2014;18:319-325.

Chordoma

Angelini A, Pala E, Calabro E, et al. Prognostic factors in surgical resection of sacral chordoma. *J Surg Oncol*. 2015;112:344-351.

Bjornsson J, Wold LE, Ebersold MJ, Laws ER. Chordoma of the mobile spine. A clinicopathologic analysis of 40 patients. *Cancer*. 1993;71: 735-740.

Deshpande V, Nielsen GP, Rosenthal DI, Rosenberg AE. Intraosseous benign notochord cell tumors (BNCT): further evidence supporting a relationship to chordoma. *Am J Surg Pathol*. 2007;31:1573-1577.

Hoch BL, Nielsen GP, Liebsch NJ, Rosenberg AE. Base of skull chordomas in children and adolescents: a clinicopathologic study of 73 cases. *Am J Surg Pathol*. 2006;30:811-818.

Indelicato DJ, Rotondo RL, Begosh-Mayne D, et al. A prospective outcomes study of proton therapy for chordomas and chondrosarcomas of the spine. *Int J Radiat Oncol Biol Phys*. 2016;95:297-303.

Jambhekar NA, Rekhi B, Thorat K, et al. Revisiting chordoma with brachyury, a "new age" marker: analysis of a validation study on 51 cases. *Arch Pathol Lab Med*. 2010;134:1181-1187.

Lalam R, Cassar-Pullicino VN, McClure J, Singh J. Entrapped intralesional marrow: a hitherto undescribed imaging features of benign notochordal cell tumor. *Skeletal Radiol*. 2012;41:725-731.

Miettinen M, Wang Z, Lasota J, et al. Nuclear brachyury expression is consistent in chordoma, common in germ cell tumors and small cell carcinomas, and rare in other carcinomas and sarcomas. *Am J Surg Pathol*. 2015;39:1305-1312.

O'Connell JX, Renard LG, Liebsch NJ, Efird JT, Munzenrider JE, Rosenberg AE. Base of skull chordoma. A correlative study of histologic and clinical features of 62 cases. *Cancer*. 1994;74: 2261-2267.

Rosenberg AE, Brown GA, Bhan AK, Lee JM. Chondroid chordoma—a variant of chordoma. A morphologic and immunohistochemical study. *Am J Clin Pathol*. 1994;101:36-41.

Rosenthal DI, Scott JA, Mankin HJ, et al. Sacrococcygeal chordoma: Magnetic resonance imaging and computed tomography. *Am J Roentgenol*. 1985;148:143-147.

Sangoi AR, Karamchandani J, Lane B, et al. Specificity of brachyury in the distinction of chordoma from clear cell renal cell carcinoma and germ cell tumors: a study of 305 cases. *Mod Pathol*. 2011;24:425-429.

Tauziede-Esperiat D, Bresson D, Polivka M, et al. Prognostic and therapeutic markers in chordomas: a study of 287 tumors. *J Neuropathol Exp Neurol*. 2016;75:111-120.

Tirabosco R, Mangham DC, Rosenberg AE, et al. Brachyury expression in extra-axial skeletal and soft tissue chordomas: a marker that distinguishes chordoma from mixed tumor/myoepithelioma/parachordoma in soft tissue. *Am J Surg Pathol*. 2008;32:572-580.

Vujovic S, Henderson S, Presneau N, et al. Brachyury, a crucial regulator of notochordal development, is a novel biomarker for chordoma. *J Pathol*. 2006;209:157-165.

Yamaguchi T, Iwata J, Sugihara S, et al. Distinguishing benign notochordal cell tumors from vertebral chordoma. *Skeletal Radiol*. 2008;37:291-299.

Yamaguchi T, Suzuki S, Ishiiwa H, Shimizu K, Ueda Y. Benign notochordal cell tumors: a comparative histological study of benign notochordal cell tumors, classic chordomas, and notochordal vestiges of fetal intervertebral discs. *Am J Surg Pathol*. 2004;28:756-761.

Yamaguchi T, Suzuki S, Ishiiwa H, Ueda Y. Intraosseous benign notochordal cell tumours: overlooked precursors of classic chordomas? *Histopathology*. 2004;44:597-602.

Langerhans Cell Histiocytosis

Beck-Broichsitter BE, Smeets R, Heiland M. Current concepts in pathogenesis of acute and chronic osteomyelitis. *Curr Opin Infect Dis*. 2015;28:240-245.

El Demellawy D, Young JL, de Nanassy J, et al. Langerhans cell histiocytosis: a comprehensive review. *Pathology*. 2015;47:294-301.

Gibson SE, Prayson RA. Primary skull lesions in the pediatric population: a 25-year experience. *Arch Pathol Lab Med*. 2007;131:761-766.

Harmon CM, Brown N. Langerhans cell histiocytosis. A clinicopathologic review and molecular pathogenetic update. *Arch Pathol Lab Med*. 2015;139:1211-1214.

Howarth DM, Gilchrist GS, Mullan BP, Wiseman GA, Edmonson JH, Schomberg PJ. Langerhans cell histiocytosis: diagnosis, natural history, management, and outcome. *Cancer*. 1999;85:2278-2290.

Lau SK, Chu PG, Weiss LM. Immunohistochemical expression of Langerin in Langerhans cell histiocytosis and non-Langerhans cell histiocytic disorders. *Am J Surg Pathol*. 2008;32:615-619.

Epithelioid Hemangioma

Antonescu CR, Chen HW, Zhang L, et al. ZFP36-FOSB fusion defines a subset of epithelioid hemangioma with atypical features. *Genes Chromosomes Cancer*. 2014;53:951-959.

Antonescu CR, Le Loarer F, Mosquera JM, et al. Novel YAP1-TFE3 fusion defines a distinct subset of epithelioid hemangioendothelioma. *Genes Chromosomes Cancer*. 2013;52:775-784.

Deshpande V, Rosenberg AE, O'Connell JX, Nielsen GP. Epithelioid angiosarcoma of the bone: a series of 10 cases. *Am J Surg Pathol*. 2003;27:709-716.

Deyrup AT, Montag AG. Epithelioid and epithelial neoplasms of bone. *Arch Pathol Lab Med*. 2007;131:205-216.

Doyle LA, Fletcher CD, Hornick JL. Nuclear expression of CAMTA1 distinguishes epithelioid hemangioendothelioma from histologic mimics. *Am J Surg Pathol*. 2016;40:94-102.

Errani C, Zhang L, Sung YS, et al. A novel WWTR1-CAMTA1 gene fusion is a consistent abnormality in epithelioid hemangioendothelioma of different anatomical sites. *Genes Chromosomes Cancer*. 2011;50: 644-653.

Gill R, O'Donnell RJ, Horvai A. Utility of immunohistochemistry for endothelial markers in distinguishing epithelioid hemangioendothelioma from carcinoma metastatic to bone. *Arch Pathol Lab Med*. 2009;133:967-972.

Hasegawa T, Fujii Y, Seki K, et al. Epithelioid angiosarcoma of bone. *Hum Pathol*. 1997;28:985-989.

Huang SC, Zhang L, Sung YS, et al. Frequent FOS gene rearrangements in epithelioid hemangioma: a molecular study of 58 cases with morphologic reappraisal. *Am J Surg Pathol*. 2015;39:1313-1321.

Hung YP, Fletcher CD, Hornick JL. FOSB is a useful diagnostic marker for pseudomyogenic hemangioendothelioma. *Am J Surg Pathol*. 2017;41:596-606.

Inyang A, Mertens F, Puls F, et al. Primary pseudomyogenic hemangioendothelioma of bone. *Am J Surg Pathol*. 2016;40:587-598.

Kleer CG, Unni KK, McLeod RA. Epithelioid hemangioendothelioma of bone. *Am J Surg Pathol*. 1996;20:1301-1311.

Lau K, Massad M, Pollak C, et al. Clinical patterns of outcome in epithelioid hemangioendothelioma with or without pulmonary involvement: insights from an internet registry in the study of a rare cancer. *Chest*. 2011;140:1312-1318.

Mitsuhashi T, Shimizu Y, Ban S, et al. Multicentric contiguous variant of epithelioid angiosarcoma of the bone. A rare variant showing angiotropic spread. *Ann Diagn Pathol*. 2005;9:33-37.

Nielsen GP, Srivastava A, Kattapuram S, et al. Epithelioid hemangioma of bone revisited. A study of 50 cases. *Am J Surg Pathol*. 2009;33:270-277.

O'Connell JX, Nielsen GP, Rosenberg AE. Epithelioid vascular tumors of bone: a review and proposal of a classification scheme. *Adv Anat Pathol*. 2001;8:74-82.

Righi A, Sbaraglia M, Gambarotti M, et al. Primary vascular tumors of bone: a monoinstitutional morphologic and molecular analysis of

427 cases with emphasis on epithelioid variants. *Am J Surg Pathol.* 2020;44:1192-1203.

Scott MT, Indelicato DJ, Morris CG, et al. Radiation therapy for hemangioendothelioma: the University of Florida experience. *Am J Clin Oncol.* 2014;37:360-363.

Tusda Y, Suurmeijer AJH, Sung YS, et al. Epithelioid hemangioma of bone harboring FOS and FOSB gene rearrangements: a clinicopathologic and molecular study. *Genes Chromosomes Cancer.* 2021;60:17-25.

van Ijzendoorn DGP, de Jong D, Romagosa C, et al. Fusion events lead to truncation of FOS in epithelioid hemangioma of bone. *Genes Chromosomes Cancer.* 2015;54:565-574.

Zhang HZ, Dong L, Wang SY, et al. TFE3 rearranged epithelioid hemangioendothelioma of bone: a clinicopathological, immunohistochemical and molecular study of two cases. *Ann Diagn Pathol.* 2020;46:151487.

Round Cell Tumors

Bishop JA, Alaggio R, Zhang L, et al. Adamantinoma-like Ewing family tumors of the head and neck: a pitfall in the differential diagnosis of basaloid and myoepithelial carcinomas. *Am J Surg Pathol.* 2015;39:1267-1274.

Bridge JA, Fidler ME, Neff JR, et al. Adamantinoma-like Ewing's sarcoma: genomic confirmation, phenotypic drift. *Am J Surg Pathol.* 1999;23:159-165.

Chen S, Deniz K, Sung Y, et al. Ewing sarcoma with ERG gene rearrangements: a molecular study focusing on the prevalence of FUS-ERG and common pitfalls in detecting EWSR1-ERG by FISH. *Am J Surg Pathol.* 2016;55:340-349.

Diaz-Perez JA, Nielsen GP, Antonescu C, et al. *EWSR1/FUS-NFATc2* rearranged round cell sarcoma: clinicopathological series of 4 cases and literature review. *Hum Pathol.* 2019;90:45-53.

Ewing J. Diffuse endothelioma of bone. *Proc NY Path Soc.* 1921;12:17-24.

Folpe AL, Goldblum JR, Rubin BP, et al. Morphologic and immunophenotypic diversity in Ewing family tumors: a study of 66 genetically confirmed cases. *Am J Surg Pathol.* 2005;29:1025-1033.

Fujii H, Honoki K, Enomoto Y, et al. Adamantinoma-like Ewing's sarcoma with EWS-FLI1 fusion gene: a case report. *Virchows Arch.* 2006;449:579-584.

Kallen ME, Hornick JL. From the ashes of "Ewing-like" sarcoma: a contemporary update of the classification, immunohistochemistry, and molecular genetics of round cell sarcomas. *Sem Diagn Pathol.* 2022;39:29-37.

Le Loarer F, Baud J, Azmani R, et al. Advances in the classification of round cell sarcomas. *Histopathology.* 2022;80:33-53.

Llombart-Bosch A, Machado I, Navarro S, et al. Histological heterogeneity of Ewing's sarcoma/PNET: an immunohistochemical analysis of 415 genetically confirmed cases with clinical support. *Virchows Arch.* 2009;455:397-411.

Ma Y, Feng J, Zhao J, et al. PHOX2B as a reliable marker for neuroblastoma in tissue and cytology specimens. *J Neuropathol Exp Neurol.* 2021;80:1108-1116.

Perret R, Escuriol J, Velasco V, et al. NFATC2-rearranged sarcomas: clinicopathologic, molecular, and cytogenetic study of 7 cases with evidence of AGGRECAN as a novel diagnostic marker. *Mod Pathol.* 2020;33:1930-1944.

Picci P, Bohling T, Bacci G, et al. Chemotherapy-induced tumor necrosis as a prognostic factor in localized Ewing's sarcoma of the extremities. *J Clin Oncol.* 1997;15:1553-1559.

Puls F, Niblett A, Marland G, et al. BCOR-CCNB3 (Ewing-like) sarcoma: a clinicopathologic analysis of 10 cases in comparison with conventional Ewing sarcoma. *Am J Surg Pathol.* 2014;38:1307-1318.

Sbaraglia M, Righi A, Gambarotti M, Dei Tos AP. Ewing sarcoma and Ewing-like tumors. *Virchows Arch.* 2020;476:109-119.

Wang WL, Patel NR, Caragea M, et al. Expression of ERG, an ETS family transcription factor, identifies ERG-rearranged Ewing sarcoma. *Mod Pathol.* 2012;25:1378-1383.

Wang GY, Thomas DG, Davis JL, et al. EWSR1-NFATC2 translocation-associated sarcoma. Clinicopathologic findings in a rare aggressive primary bone or soft tissue sarcoma. *Am J Surg Pathol.* 2019;43:1112-1122.

Wei S, Siegal GP. Round cell tumors of bone: an update on recent molecular genetic advances. *Adv Anat Pathol.* 2014;21:359-372.

Yoshida K, Machado I, Motoi T, et al. NKX3-1 is a useful immunohistochemical marker of *EWSR1-NFATC2* sarcoma and mesenchymal chondrosarcoma. *Am J Surg Pathol.* 2020;44:719-728.

8 Soft Tissue Neoplasms

Sandra Gjorgova Gjeorgjievski • John D. Reith • Scott E. Kilpatrick

ADIPOCYTIC TUMORS

LIPOMA

DIFFERENTIAL DIAGNOSIS: ATYPICAL LIPOMATOUS TUMOR/WELL-DIFFERENTIATED LIPOSARCOMA

Clinical Features

Lipoma represents the most common mesenchymal soft tissue tumor of adults. Most commonly, lipomas are localized to the subcutaneous adipose tissue, presenting as a painless mass/swelling, although examples may arise in intramuscular locations and intrathoracic/intra-abdominal/retroperitoneal regions. If associated with peripheral nerves, there may be tenderness. Unlike ordinary lipomas, angiolipomas present as small and often painful subcutaneous masses, frequently in adolescence and young adults. Myolipomas (extrauterine lipoleiomyomas) are typically an incidental finding, originating in the abdominal cavity (usually retroperitoneum), but may also be found in the soft tissues of the trunk and extremities. Chondroid lipomas are generally deep-seated, painless lesions, most commonly occurring in the proximal extremities and limb girdles.

Pathologic Features

GROSS FINDINGS

Lipomas are well-circumscribed fatty lesions with white-yellow discoloration, commonly encapsulated by a thin glistening fibrous membrane. Within skeletal muscle, intramuscular lipomas are infiltrative, entrapping skeletal muscle fibers within the tumor proper. Depending on their location and potential to remain undetected, lipomas may become quite large, exceeding 20 cm. Angiolipomas produce small, subcutaneous tan-yellow to red nodules. Chondroid lipomas are very well defined, with yellow-tan to mucinous cut surfaces. Gross inspection can help identify the "myo" component of myolipomas, especially when prominent, as tan whorled nodules admixed with yellow-tan adipose tissue. These tumors may become quite large (>10 cm), particularly when deep.

MICROSCOPIC FINDINGS

Lipomas are benign tumors composed of mature adipocytes, with little to no variation in size and shape (Fig. 8.1). Some have thin fibrous septa dissecting the tumor proper. There is no to minimal cytologic atypia, and mitotic activity is virtually non-existent. Because of their infiltrative nature, intramuscular lipomas commonly entrap skeletal muscle fibers (Fig. 8.2). Variable amounts of fat necrosis may occur.

Angiolipomas (Fig. 8.3) are well circumscribed and characterized by variable numbers and aggregates of small caliber, thin-walled capillary vessels, often containing microthrombi (Fig. 8.3B). These vessels are lined by bland endothelial cells and surrounded by a pericytic layer. Thick, muscular-walled blood vessels are not a feature of angiolipoma.

Myolipomas are mature adipocytic neoplasms that contain variable amounts of well-differentiated smooth muscle. There is no cytologic atypia or increased mitotic activity.

Chondroid lipomas (Fig. 8.4) are lobulated, well-encapsulated masses with a characteristic histologic presentation of mature adipose tissue admixed with cords and nests of vacuolated cells (lipoblasts), embedded in a chondromyxoid to hyalinized matrix.

Ancillary Studies

The adipocytes are positive for S100. The smooth muscle component in a myolipoma is diffusely positive for SMA, desmin, and caldesmon. In addition to S100 protein, keratins are rarely expressed in chondroid lipoma, but EMA is negative.

FISH analysis for *MDM2* gene amplification is negative among all lipomas and variants. Angiolipomas usually have a normal karyotype.

Chondroid lipomas have a recurrent t(11;16) (q13;p130), associated with the *C11orf95-MKL2* gene rearrangement.

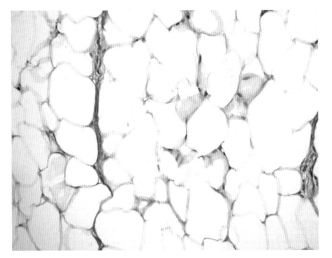

FIG. 8.1

Lipoma is composed of mature adipocytes, with little to no variation in size and shape and often thin fibrous septa.

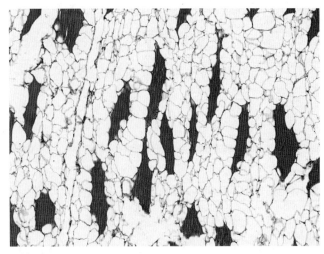

FIG. 8.2

Intramuscular lipoma, with mature adipose tissue entrapping skeletal muscle fibers.

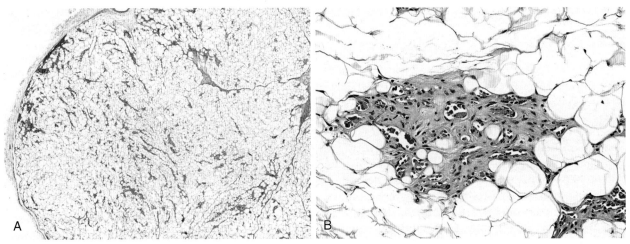

FIG. 8.3

Angiolipoma with sharp circumscription and variable numbers of characteristic small caliber blood vessels **(A)** with occasional microthrombi **(B)**.

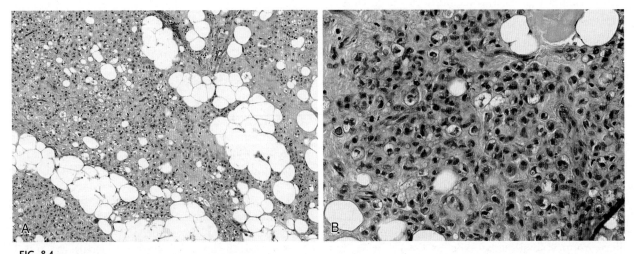

FIG. 8.4

(A, B) Chondroid lipoma showing mature adipose tissue admixed mononuclear chondroblastoma-like cells and lipoblasts within a chondroid to myxohyaline stroma.

Differential Diagnosis

The most important differential diagnosis, especially among deeply-seated benign adipocytic neoplasms, is atypical lipomatous tumor/well-differentiated liposarcoma (ALT/WDL). The presence of large and atypical, often multinucleated hyperchromatic cells is diagnostic of the latter, most frequently seen in the non-lipogenic fibrous tissue. FISH analysis for *MDM2* gene amplification may be necessary in difficult cases, deep-seated tumors, especially in the abdominal and retroperitoneal regions, and among small needle biopsy specimens, primarily composed of normal-appearing adipose tissue.

In angiolipomas with a dominating "angio" component, the differential may include hemangioma. The presence of circumscription and interspersed adipose tissue will help establish the diagnosis of angiolipoma.

The extrauterine location of a myolipoma supports the diagnosis of myolipoma over leiomyoma with increased intralesional adipose tissue.

The differential diagnosis of chondroid lipoma includes myxoid liposarcoma (ML). Circumscription and encapsulation and absence of ML vascular pattern, accompanied by the characteristic epithelioid cells, lipoblasts, and mature fat, helps establish the diagnosis of chondroid lipoma.

Prognosis and Therapy

Overall, local recurrences are rare in lipomas (<5%) and mainly seen in incompletely excised deeply seated lesion. In the absence of more obvious diagnostic features, locally recurrent "lipomas" probably should be evaluated for *MDM2* gene amplification, to fully exclude an under-sampled ALT/WDL. Like ordinary lipomas, chondroid lipomas rarely locally recur. Surgical excision is curative for angiolipomas and myolipomas.

LIPOMAS AND VARIANTS – DISEASE FACT SHEET

Definition
- ▶▶ Lipoma is a benign tumor composed almost exclusively of mature adipocytes
- ▶▶ Angiolipoma is a subcutaneous tumor composed of mature adipocytes intermingled with small, thin-walled capillaries, some of which contain fibrin microthrombi
- ▶▶ Myolipoma is a benign extrauterine tumor composed of mature adipose tissue and variably amounts of well-differentiated smooth muscle
- ▶▶ Chondroid lipoma is a benign adipose tissue tumor composed of variable numbers of lipoblasts, mature adipocytes, and epithelioid cells, embedded in a myxohyaline to chondroid matrix

Incidence and Location
- ▶▶ Lipoma is the most common mesenchymal neoplasm in adults, seen in the upper back, proximal extremities, and abdomen, ranging from cutaneous to deep

- ▶▶ Angiolipomas are relatively common, mostly seen in the subcutis of the forearm, followed by the trunk
- ▶▶ Myolipoma, rare tumor, typically retroperitoneum, abdominal cavity, and pelvis, less commonly trunk or extremities
- ▶▶ Chondroid lipoma, rare tumor, usually deep-seated involving skeletal muscle of proximal extremities and limb girdles

Age Distribution
- ▶▶ Lipoma, fifth to seventh decade of life
- ▶▶ Angiolipoma, second to fourth decades of life
- ▶▶ Myolipoma, adulthood
- ▶▶ Chondroid lipoma, adulthood

Clinical Features
- ▶▶ Lipoma, commonly painless mass, symptomatic if associated with nerves or vital structures, occurs virtually anywhere
- ▶▶ Angiolipoma, painful, often multiple, extremity subcutaneous masses
- ▶▶ Myolipoma, retroperitoneal and extrauterine, incidental
- ▶▶ Chondroid lipoma, painless, well-defined, deep-seated, extremity

Prognosis and Therapy
- ▶▶ Surgical excision is curative. Rare local recurrences if incomplete excision.

LIPOMAS AND VARIANTS – PATHOLOGIC FEATURES

Gross Findings
- ▶▶ Lipomas are well-circumscribed, white-yellow encapsulated fatty lesions. Intramuscular lipomas are not well circumscribed and entrap skeletal muscle within the tumor proper
- ▶▶ Angiolipoma, tan-yellow to red circumscribed nodules
- ▶▶ Myolipoma, white-yellow adipose tissue with tan whorled nodules
- ▶▶ Chondroid lipoma typically very well defined, fatty to glistening myxoid

Microscopic Findings
- ▶▶ Lipomas are exclusively mature adipocytes without cytologic atypia
- ▶▶ Angiolipoma, mature adipocytes admixed with small thin-walled capillary vessels with occasional fibrin microthrombi
- ▶▶ Myolipoma, extrauterine, mature adipocytes admixed with variable amounts of smooth muscle
- ▶▶ Chondroid lipoma, lipoblasts, mature adipocytes, and occasional epithelioid cells, embedded in a chondromyxoid matrix

Pathologic Differential Diagnoses
- ▶▶ Atypical lipomatous tumor/well-differentiated liposarcoma, hemangioma (angiolipoma), uterine or parasitic leiomyoma (myolipoma), and myxoid liposarcoma (chondroid lipoma)

LIPOBLASTOMA/LIPOBLASTOMATOSIS

DIFFERENTIAL DIAGNOSIS: MYXOID LIPOSARCOMA

Clinical Features

Lipoblastoma/lipoblastomatosis is a benign neoplasm of embryonal white fat that may present as a lobulated and localized, well-circumscribed mass (lipoblastoma) or, alternatively, a diffuse and infiltrative lesion (lipoblastomatosis). Most examples present in infancy and early childhood, before 5 years of age. There appears to be a slightly male predilection. The extremities and the trunk are the most common anatomic sites.

Pathologic Features

GROSS FINDINGS

Usually lipoblastomas are <5 cm, although lesions larger than 10 cm have been described. They are typically well circumscribed and lobulated, and the cut surface is white-yellow often with prominent fibrous trabeculae separating myxoid areas, cystic spaces, or fat nodules.

MICROSCOPIC FINDINGS

Lipoblastomas are characterized by nodules of adipocytes of variable maturation embedded in a lightly myxoid stroma and separated by variably thick fibrous septa (Fig. 8.5). The adipocytic maturation may represent a somewhat zonal maturation, ranging from primitive mesenchymal cells, to univacuolated (signet-ring like) lipoblasts, multivacuolated lipoblasts to mature adipocytes. The background myxoid stroma often exhibits thin-walled plexiform vessels, mimicking ML (Fig. 8.5B). Occasionally, heterologous elements can be seen, such as chondroid metaplasia, extramedullary hematopoiesis, and chronic inflammation. There is no significant cytologic atypia or mitotic activity.

Ancillary Studies

As with ordinary adult lipomas, the adipocytes in lipoblastoma also are positive for S100. CD34 reactivity is seen in the more spindled cells in myxoid and fibrous regions, and desmin positivity is sometimes observed. Lipoblastomas typically contain structural alterations or gene fusions involving 8q12 (*PLAG1*). One or more extra copies of chromosome 8 may occur with or without the associated gene fusion.

Differential Diagnosis

The most important differential diagnosis is ML. However, the presence of lobulation and more mature nonmyxoid areas, especially when associated with a child, helps establish the diagnosis of lipoblastoma.

Prognosis and Therapy

Surgical resection of the localized form (lipoblastoma) generally results in complete cure. Local recurrences are more likely to be associated with the diffuse form (lipoblastomatosis), ranging up to 50% of cases, when incompletely excised. Dedifferentiation does not occur, and there is no risk of distant metastases.

LIPOBLASTOMA – DISEASE FACT SHEET

Definition
▸▸ Benign tumor of embryonal white fat which may be localized or diffuse (lipoblastomatosis)

Incidence and Location
▸▸ Rare neoplasm most commonly arising in the trunk and extremities

Age Distribution
▸▸ Children, <3 years, rarely adolescents and adults

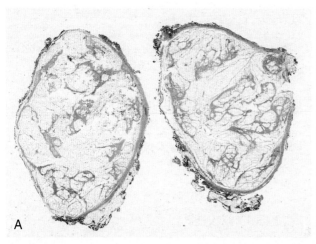
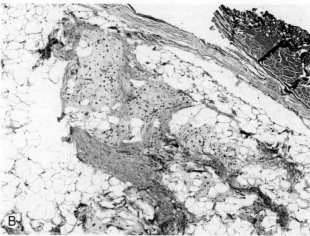

FIG. 8.5

Lipoblastoma is a well-circumscribed, lobulated adipocytic neoplasm with thick fibrous septa **(A)** composed of variably mature adipocytes intermixed with less mature cells and variably myxoid stroma **(B)**. The latter appearance can mimic myxoid liposarcoma.

HIBERNOMA

Clinical Features

Hibernomas are benign, slowly growing, painless neoplasms, most often arising in young to middle-aged adults, with a slight male predominance. The most common anatomic location is the thigh, followed by the trunk and upper extremity. Radiographically, many will display a signal intensity within the tumor proper described as intermediate between mature adipose tissue and skeletal muscle.

Pathologic Features

GROSS FINDINGS

Most are well circumscribed and lobular adipocytic lesions, yellow to brown.

MICROSCOPIC FINDINGS

Hibernomas display varying proportions of brown fat admixed with mature, white adipose tissue. At low power, a distinct lobulation is evident. Cytologically, the brown fat cells exhibit a centrally placed nucleus and a prominent nucleolus, surrounded by a cytoplasm ranging from granular and eosinophilic to uniformly multi-vacuolated (Fig. 8.6). Rarely, myxoid change and spindled cell areas occur. Mitotic figures are absent, and significant nuclear atypia is not a feature.

Ancillary Studies

S100 protein is strongly and diffusely positive within both brown and white fat cells. CD10 has recently been noted to be expressed and may be helpful in distinguishing hibernoma from potential fatty lesion mimics. Desmin and SMA are negative.

Cytogenetic analysis reveals structural rearrangements, including translocations and deletions, involving chromosome 11q13. *MDM2* gene amplification is not present.

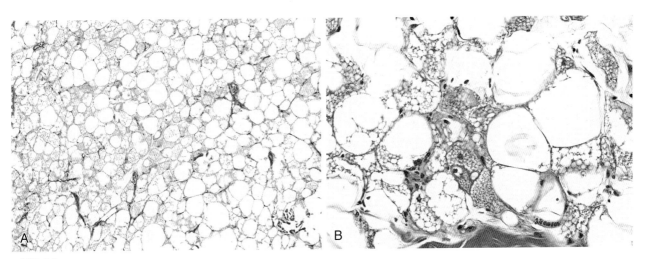

FIG. 8.6
A variable mixture of mature adipocytes and multivacuolated brown fat is characteristic for a hibernoma (**A**). Many of multivacuolated cells appear eosinophilic, with centrally placed, round nuclei with fine chromatin material and prominent nucleoli (**B**).

Differential Diagnosis

The most important differential diagnosis is ALT/WDL. The enlarged atypical and often multi-nucleated cells and lipoblasts associated with it are not seen in hibernoma. When hibernomas are composed of a predominance of brown fat with eosinophilic cells, rhabdomyoma may also be considered within the differential diagnosis. Desmin positivity excludes hibernoma.

Prognosis and Therapy

Surgical resection is curative.

HIBERNOMA – DISEASE FACT SHEET

Definition
▸▸ Benign lobular adipocytic neoplasm with multivacuolated brown fat differentiation

Incidence and Location
▸▸ Rare, thigh, trunk, chest, and upper extremity

Age Distribution
▸▸ Young to middle-aged adults

Clinical Features
▸▸ Slow-growing, painless, mobile and usually subcutaneous, less commonly intramuscular

Radiologic Features
▸▸ MRI: Hibernomas are T1 iso- to hypointense and T2 iso- to hyperintense compared with the normal fat; often described as intermediate between normal subcutaneous fat and skeletal muscle

Prognosis and Therapy
▸▸ Benign neoplasm, complete excision is curative

HIBERNOMA – PATHOLOGIC FEATURES

Gross Findings
▸▸ Well-circumscribed, lobulated, brown-yellow fatty mass

Microscopic Findings
▸▸ Circumscribed and lobulated, fibrous septa, mixture of varying proportions of mature white and brown adipocytes, with extensive cytoplasmic multi-vacuolation to eosinophilic granular change, centrally placed nuclei, prominent nucleoli

Pathologic Differential Diagnoses
▸▸ Atypical lipomatous tumor/well-differentiated liposarcoma and adult rhabdomyoma, especially if predominantly eosinophilic brown fat cells

---

SPINDLE CELL/PLEOMORPHIC LIPOMA

DIFFERENTIAL DIAGNOSIS: ATYPICAL SPINDLE CELL/PLEOMORPHIC LIPOMATOUS TUMOR

Clinical Features

Most common presentation for spindle cell/pleomorphic lipoma is the posterior neck, back, and shoulders of elderly males. In women, these lipomas are frequently found outside the shawl region, often at younger ages and with a wider anatomic distribution, such as the extremities and the face.

Pathologic Features

GROSS FINDINGS

Well-circumscribed, ovoid mass with yellow-to-white and myxoid cut surface. Based on the proportion of the adipose and fibrous tissue, it may be firmer than a lipoma.

MICROSCOPIC FINDINGS

Spindle cell lipomas and pleomorphic lipomas represent spectrums of a similar neoplasm, both being well circumscribed and often encapsulated, usually subcutaneous, less commonly dermal or intramuscular. "Spindle" cell lesions are composed of mature adipocytes and various amounts of intermingled fibrous to myxoid tissue (Fig. 8.7), within which are bland spindle cells, admixed with scattered variably thick, eosinophilic collagen fibers ("ropy collagen") and mast cells. At the opposite end, "pleomorphic" forms are further characterized by the additional presence of randomly distributed multinucleated, "floret-like" giant cells (Fig. 8.8).

Occasionally, there may be little to no adipocytes, so-called "fat-poor" spindle cell/pleomorphic lipoma. Rare examples display branching and dilated vascular-like spaces that separate the tumor to form pseudopapillary projections, designated as the pseudoangiomatous subtype.

Ancillary Studies

The spindled and pleomorphic cells are diffusely and strongly positive for CD34 (Fig. 8.7C) and usually have loss of nuclear RB1 protein expression. As expected, the adipocytes express S100 protein.

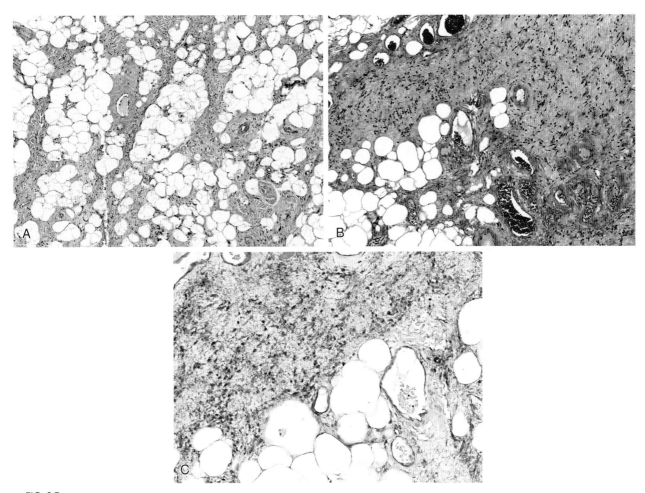

FIG. 8.7

Spindle cell lipomas are characterized by variable proportions of mature adipocytes and uniform, bland spindled cells **(A)** embedded in myxoid stroma with scattered thick collagen fibers and occasional mast cell **(B)**. The spindled cells are diffusely positive for CD34 **(C)**.

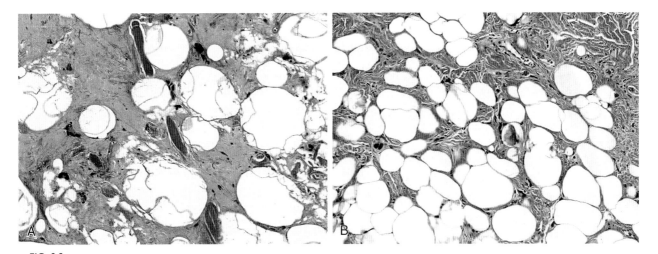

FIG. 8.8

A and **B,** Pleomorphic lipomas represent a spectrum of spindle cell lipomas being additionally defined by the presence of multinucleated giant "floret-like" cells within a variably fibromyxoid stroma.

Differential Diagnosis

The recently described atypical spindle cell/pleomorphic lipomatous tumor represents a benign adipocytic neoplasm, characterized by ill-defined tumor margins, mild to moderate nuclear atypia, enlarged and bizarre lipoblasts, and occasional presence of pleomorphic, multinucleated cells. Admittedly, some examples may be indistinguishable from spindle cell/pleomorphic lipoma. There is no *MDM2* gene amplification, low tendency to locally recur (10%–15%) if incompletely excised, but no risk for dedifferentiation. CD34 positivity and RB1 loss can be shared by both atypical spindle cell/pleomorphic lipomatous tumor and spindle cell/pleomorphic lipoma.

ALT/WDL is only rarely seen in the superficial soft tissues of the head and neck and shoulder regions; more often arises in deeply seated extremities, abdominal cavity, or retroperitoneum; and is characterized by *MDM2* gene amplification. The atypical and enlarged, multinucleated cells in the latter exhibit some morphologic overlap with the floret cells seen in spindle cell/pleomorphic lipoma.

Prognosis and Therapy

Local recurrences are rare, even with incomplete resection.

SPINDLE CELL/PLEOMORPHIC LIPOMA – DISEASE FACT SHEET

Definition
▶▶ Benign adipocytic neoplasm composed of varying proportions of adipocytes and spindled cells embedded in fibromyxoid stroma with scattered ropy collagen and mast cells
▶▶ Pleomorphic, multinucleated "floret-like" giant cells in addition to the abode histology, may be present

Incidence and Location
▶▶ Elderly men, back, shoulders, and neck. <10% of cases occur in females, often in unusual locations (such as extremities and face)

Age Distribution
▶▶ Males, 50–75 years

Clinical Features
▶▶ Subcutaneous, rarely intramuscular, well-circumscribed lesion

Prognosis and Therapy
▶▶ Benign lesion, surgical excision is curative

SPINDLE CELL/PLEOMORPHIC LIPOMA – PATHOLOGIC FEATURES

Gross Findings
▶▶ Well-circumscribed nodule, yellow to white, can present as myxoid and firmer than conventional lipoma

Microscopic Findings
▶▶ Various proportions of adipocytes and spindled cells embedded in myxoid to fibromyxoid stroma with scattered ropy collagen and mast cells

Pathologic Differential Diagnoses
▶▶ Atypical spindle cell/pleomorphic lipomatous tumor and atypical lipomatous tumor/well-differentiated liposarcoma

ATYPICAL LIPOMATOUS TUMOR/ WELL-DIFFERENTIATED LIPOSARCOMA

DIFFERENTIAL DIAGNOSIS: LIPOMA AND VARIANTS

Clinical Features

ALT/WDL is a potentially locally aggressive mature adipocytic neoplasm characterized by variably thick fibrous septa and enlarged, atypical and often multinucleated cells, predominantly within fibrous tissue and occasionally mature adipocytes. Intersecting adipocytic proliferation. It most commonly is deeply seated, arising bellow the fascia of the extremities. The retroperitoneum and the paratesticular soft tissues are common areas where ALT/WDL arises. Less common anatomic sites include the mediastinum, distal extremities, and rarely the head and neck region.

Pathologic Features

GROSS FINDINGS

Well-circumscribed and lobulated yellow fatty mass. Some areas of myxoid changes and, rarely, typically within retroperitoneum, areas of infarct-like necrosis may be focally observed.

MICROSCOPIC FINDINGS

The adipocytes show heterogeneity in size and shape, usually separated in lobules by variably thick fibrous septa (Fig. 8.9). The scattered atypical and often multinucleated stromal cells are significantly pleomorphic (even bizarre), characterized by nuclei with irregular nuclear membranes and dense hyperchromatic chromatin pattern, giving the impression of "smudged" cells (Fig. 8.9B). Most are seen within the fibrous tissue, less commonly mature adipocytes and muscular walls of blood vessels. Lipoblasts are less commonly observed (Fig. 8.9C). Fat necrosis rarely dominates.

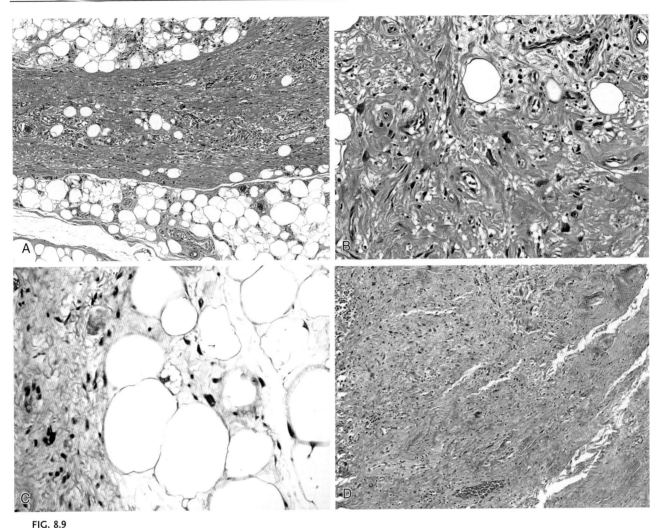

FIG. 8.9

At low power, atypical lipomatous tumor/well-differentiated liposarcoma (ALT/WDL) is characterized by variably amounts of fibrous and adipose tissue, often displaying heterogeneity within individual adipocytes **(A)**. Atypical, enlarged, and often multinucleated cells are within fibrous tissue and adjacent to adipocytes **(B)**. Less commonly, multivacuolated lipoblasts are seen **(C)**. The sclerosing variant of ALT/WDL is composed predominantly of dense, hypocellular fibrous tissue but retains the characteristic atypical and enlarged multinucleated cells **(D)**.

When fibrous tissue predominates, some designate these as "sclerosing" WDL (Fig. 8.9D). Even more rare, abundant lymphocytes and plasma cells within the fibrous tissue may obscure the background atypical cells/lipoblasts; this form has been referred to as "inflammatory" WDL.

Mature heterologous features, usually in the form of osseous, cartilaginous, or myogenic differentiation, are rare but should not be confused with dedifferentiation.

Mitotic figures tend to be rare, but, in more cellular examples, should never exceed 4 mitoses/10 high-power fields (HPF).

Ancillary Studies

Immunohistochemistry usually shows MDM2 nuclear expression, particularly with the larger atypical cells.

More sensitive, especially in lipoma-like WDL, and more specific is confirmation of *MDM2* (12q15) gene amplification via FISH analysis. On cytogenetic analysis, karyotyping of ALT/WDL is characterized by supernumerary ring chromosomes and/or giant marker chromosomes, involving chromosome 12.

Differential Diagnosis

The differential diagnosis includes most commonly lipoma, hibernoma, and spindle cell/pleomorphic lipoma. The deeper location, especially when seen in the retroperitoneum, presence of enlarged, atypical and hyperchromatic cells, less commonly lipoblasts, and, when necessary, *MDM2* gene amplification help establish the diagnosis.

Prognosis and Therapy

Lesions that arise in the retroperitoneum, paratesticular soft tissue, mediastinum, and similar places where complete excision is challenging, the term WDL is better used given the higher potential for local recurrence and progression compared with lesions arising within the extremities for which the term atypical lipomatous neoplasm is better applied. ALT/WDL has no metastatic potential, unless it has undergone dedifferentiation.

The risk for dedifferentiation varies depending on location, exceeding 20% for retroperitoneal forms but less than 2% when arising in the extremities. Consequently, the risk of mortality and metastases is greater for retroperitoneal and paratesticular lesions than for those localized to the extremities.

ATYPICAL LIPOMATOUS TUMOR/WELL-DIFFERENTIATED LIPOSARCOMA – DISEASE FACT SHEET

Definition
▶▶ Locally aggressive adipocytic neoplasm, usually predominantly fatty and characterized by variably thick fibrous septa with atypical, enlarged to multinucleated cells and, less commonly, lipoblasts

Incidence and Location
▶▶ Rare, deep soft tissues of the extremities, retroperitoneum, and paratesticular regions

Age Distribution
▶▶ Middle-aged to older adults

Clinical Features
▶▶ Deep-seated, painless, slowly enlarging mass
▶▶ Often asymptomatic, large, when arising in retroperitoneum and abdominal cavity

Prognosis and Therapy
▶▶ Complete resection, when possible, potentially lowers the risk for local recurrence and potential for dedifferentiation, representing transformation to a higher-grade neoplasm
▶▶ Metastases only occur with dedifferentiation

ATYPICAL LIPOMATOUS TUMOR/WELL-DIFFERENTIATED LIPOSARCOMA – PATHOLOGIC FEATURES

Gross Findings
▶▶ Well-circumscribed, lobulated fatty lesion, yellow to firm white and gelatinous
▶▶ Areas of myxoid changes, fat necrosis, and sclerosis may be seen

Microscopic Findings
▶▶ Adipocytes of varying size and shapes (heterogeneity) separated by variably thickened fibrous septa
▶▶ Randomly distributed, atypical, enlarged and often multinucleated cells and, less common, multivacuolated lipoblasts

Pathologic Differential Diagnoses
▶▶ Lipomas and variants

DEDIFFERENTIATED LIPOSARCOMA

DIFFERENTIAL DIAGNOSIS: UNDIFFERENTIATED PLEOMORPHIC SARCOMA

Clinical Features

Dedifferentiated liposarcoma (DL) is defined as a high-grade sarcoma arising concomitantly from an ALT/WDL (most common) or occurring in the same anatomic site as a previously resected ALT/WDL. In cases where the precursor ALT/WDL is not present, the diagnosis can be confirmed molecularly, namely amplification of *MDM2* via FISH analysis. The vast majority are found in older adults, especially in the deep soft tissues of the proximal extremities, intra-abdominal, and retroperitoneal locations.

Pathologic Features

GROSS FINDINGS

DL usually presents as a large fleshy mass, juxtaposed to a smaller yellow-tan lipoma or lipoma-like lesion. Calcifications and even ossification are rarely present. Necrosis and hemorrhage are commonly seen.

MICROSCOPIC FINDINGS

Most commonly, the transition of the ALT/WDL and DL components is sharply demarcated (Fig. 8.10A), but a gradual transition from the well-differentiated component to the high-grade, non-lipogenic areas is rarely present. Usually, the hypercellular dedifferentiated component is composed of atypical and pleomorphic spindled cells, arranged in fascicles and whorls (Fig. 8.10B), resembling undifferentiated pleomorphic sarcoma (UPS), without further defining features. However, in about 5% to 10% of cases, the dedifferentiated component exhibits varying degrees of heterologous differentiation including osteosarcoma/chondrosarcoma, leiomyosarcoma, myxofibrosarcoma, and rhabdomyosarcoma. So-called "homologous" lipoblastic differentiation, mimicking pleomorphic liposarcoma (PLS), is characterized by the presence of isolated and/or groups of lipoblasts. By definition, the dedifferentiated component should have at least ≥5 mitoses/10 HPF to qualify as "dedifferentiated," separating it morphologically and prognostically from cellular forms of ALT/WDL.

Ancillary Studies

MDM2 immunohistochemistry may be helpful (Fig. 8.10D), especially in small biopsy specimen and in

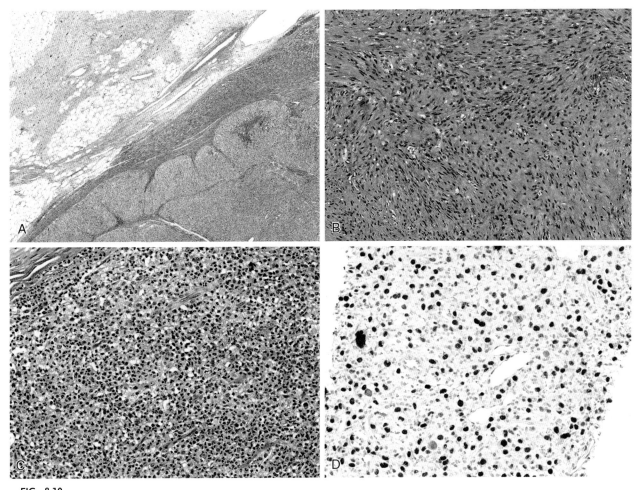

FIG. 8.10

Dedifferentiated liposarcoma is defined by the presence of high-grade sarcoma juxtaposed to atypical lipomatous tumor/well-differentiated liposarcoma **(A)**. The histologic features of the high-grade component can be diverse, but most resemble an undifferentiated pleomorphic sarcoma or fibrosarcoma **(B)**. Abundant background inflammation may confound the diagnosis **(C)**. An MDM2 immunohistochemical stain can be helpful in highlighting the neoplastic cells in dedifferentiated liposarcoma **(D)**.

instances where the low-grade component is not obviously present. Confirmation of *MDM2* gene amplification by FISH analysis represents the gold standard.

Differential Diagnosis

UPS is a diagnosis of exclusion, does not have *MDM2* gene amplification, or is evidence of a concomitant or pre-existing ALT/WDL.

Primary PLS, leiomyosarcoma, rhabdomyosarcoma, and extraskeletal osteosarcoma can be excluded if the low-grade ALT/WDL component is confirmed or in the presence of MDM2 immunoexpression and/or *MDM2* gene amplification via FISH.

Prognosis and Therapy

Prognosis is significantly related to anatomic site, with retroperitoneal/intra-abdominal and paratesticular origins

correlated with a worse survival than those localized to the deep soft tissues of the extremities. Local recurrence rates range up to 40%, while distant metastasis occurs in approximately 15% to 20% of cases. Overall mortality is estimated at 28% to 30% at 5 years.

There appears to be no association between the extent of the dedifferentiated component and survival, although data is limited. However, the presence of myogenic differentiation is associated with a worse clinical outcome.

DEDIFFERENTIATED LIPOSARCOMA – DISEASE FACT SHEET

Definition

▶▶ High-grade spindled to epithelioid sarcoma, with at least 5 mitoses/10 HPF, arising concomitantly or in the setting of a previously resected ALT/WDL, or, in the absence of a known low-grade component, confirmed by molecular evidence of *MDM2* gene amplification, with or without evidence of heterologous differentiation

Continued

MYXOID LIPOSARCOMA

DIFFERENTIAL DIAGNOSIS: MYXOMA AND MYXOFIBROSARCOMA

Clinical Features

ML presents as a large soft tissue mass, usually involving the deep soft tissues of the extremities. The most common anatomic location is the posterior thigh. Retroperitoneal ML most often represents either metastasis or evidence of a DL.

Pathologic Features

GROSS FINDINGS

MLs are large (>10 cm), typically well-demarcated, myxoid, and multinodular neoplasms.

MICROSCOPIC FINDINGS

ML presents as a lobulated neoplasm, variably cellular, with often noticeable increased cellularity at the periphery of the nodules. The background stroma is abundant and myxoid accompanied by a delicate network of plexiform and arborizing vessels (Fig. 8.11). Sometimes foci of extracellular mucinous matrix appear extremely paucicellular, giving a pulmonary edema appearance. The uniform neoplastic cells have small, bland round to oval nuclei with minimal amounts of eosinophilic cytoplasm. Signet ring cell univacuolated lipoblasts are often present, at least focally (Fig. 8.11B).

High-grade ML (also known as round cell liposarcoma) is defined as ML with more than 5% of round cell component (Fig. 8.11C). The histologic features of the round cell component are characterized by marked hypercellularity, diminished background myxoid stroma, and a population of larger, round cells with prominent nucleoli and increased mitotic activity. Pure high-grade ML (round cell liposarcoma), especially in small biopsy specimens, may lack an obvious myxoid stroma, making the diagnosis difficult to establish by routine microscopy alone (Fig. 8.11D).

Ancillary Studies

Immunohistochemistry is not generally helpful. In difficult cases, demonstration of a *DDIT3* gene rearrangement, most often combined with *FUS*, associated with the t(12;16)(q13;p11) translocation, and, less often with *EWSR1*, t(12;22)(q13;q12), is helpful in establishing the diagnosis. Generally, the diagnosis of ML, especially when low grade, does not require further ancillary studies.

Differential Diagnosis

Intramuscular myxoma may be confused with ML, but is typically less cellular, lacks the characteristic vascular network, and does not display signet ring cell lipoblasts.

Myxofibrosarcoma is a relatively common sarcoma, most commonly arising in the superficial soft tissues of the extremities in elderly patients. The tumors are highly infiltrative and show significant nuclear pleomorphism and cytologic atypia, background curvilinear blood vessels, and an absence of *DDIT3* gene fusions.

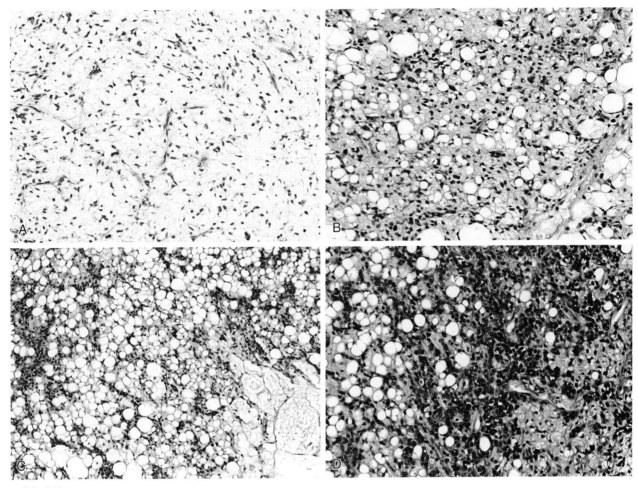

FIG. 8.11
Myxoid liposarcoma is composed of bland spindled to stellate cells embedded in a myxoid stroma with prominent delicate ("chicken wire"-like) vasculature (**A**) and variable amounts of monovacuolated (signet ring cell–like) lipoblasts (**B**). High-grade myxoid liposarcomas, also known as round cell liposarcoma, display a population of larger cells with round nuclei and occasional prominent nucleoli, often clustering and covering the underlying myxoid stroma (**C**, low power; **D**, high power).

Lipoblastoma, commonly seen in infants and children, may focally mimic ML but is usually easily distinguished if attention is paid to the age of the patient and the presence of extensive mature fat.

ML-like lesions arising in the retroperitoneum should be considered ALT/WDL or, if higher grade, DL until proven otherwise.

Prognosis and Therapy

Local recurrence is commonly seen (up to 25% per some studies) as well as distal metastasis (up to 60%). Distant metastasis can be seen many years after the initial diagnosis. The most common location for the distant metastases is bone, followed by the lung. The presence of a round cell component (hypercellularity) >5% and/or tumor necrosis correlates with increased risk of metastases and poor survival. Mainstay of treatment is surgical excision, but the tumor is very radiosensitive, responding well to radiation therapy.

MYXOID LIPOSARCOMA – DISEASE FACT SHEET

Definition
▸▸ Myxoid liposarcoma is malignant neoplasm arising in the deep soft tissues of the extremities, composed of nodules of uniform, small oval to round, bland cells embedded in abundant myxoid matrix with variable amounts of univacuolated/bivacuolated lipoblasts admixed with a prominent and delicate branching vascular network.

Incidence and Location
▸▸ Rare, deep soft tissues of the extremities, most commonly in the posterior thigh, rarely in subcutaneous locations and retroperitoneum

Age Distribution
▸▸ Peak age fourth to fifth decades

Clinical Features
▸▸ Large soft tissue mass involving the deep soft tissues of the proximal extremities

Continued

Prognosis and Therapy

▸▸ Local recurrences and distant metastases are commonly seen, especially if a round cell component is present

▸▸ Surgical excision is the optimal treatment, but tumors also respond to radiation therapy

Gross Findings

▸▸ Large, well-circumscribed and multinodular mass with gelatinous/myxoid cut surface

Microscopic Findings

▸▸ Lobulated neoplasm with tendency toward increased cellularity at the periphery of the lobules, composed of remarkably uniform, round to ovoid cells

▸▸ The background stroma is myxoid and associated with a network of delicate and arborizing blood vessels, accompanied by scattered uni- to multivacuolated lipoblasts

▸▸ High-grade ML (round cell liposarcoma) is characterized by larger, round cells with irregular nuclear membranes, significant hypercellularity, prominent nucleoli, resulting in a diminished background myxoid matrix

Pathologic Differential Diagnoses

▸▸ Intramuscular myxoma, myxofibrosarcoma, and lipoblastoma

▸▸ If retroperitoneal or intra-abdominal, atypical lipomatous tumor/well-differentiated liposarcoma and dedifferentiated liposarcoma

PLEOMORPHIC LIPOSARCOMA

DIFFERENTIAL DIAGNOSIS: DEDIFFERENTIATED LIPOSARCOMA, UNDIFFERENTIATED PLEOMORPHIC SARCOMA

Clinical Features

PLS presents as a rapidly growing, often painless mass, most commonly involving the deep soft tissues of the extremities, followed by the trunk, retroperitoneum, and spermatic cord. Up to 25% of cases arise in the subcutaneous tissues. By definition, there are no areas of concomitant ALT/WDL.

Pathologic Features

GROSS FINDINGS

PLS are typically large neoplasms, non-encapsulated, often with ill-defined and infiltrative borders. Myxoid change and necrosis are commonly seen.

MICROSCOPIC FINDINGS

Histologically, PLS is a high-grade sarcoma, predominantly pleomorphic undifferentiated-appearing spindle to epithelioid cells with variable numbers of diagnostic multivacuolated lipoblasts (Fig. 8.12). There is usually significantly increased mitotic activity with many atypical mitotic forms. Necrosis and myxoid stromal change, sometimes mimicking myxofibrosarcoma, are commonly seen. The lipoblasts are frequently quite large with multiple, variably sized intracytoplasmic vacuoles, usually indenting the large, central to para-centrally placed nucleus. Dominating epithelioid features, resembling a carcinoma, are seen in a minority of cases. The presence of at least focal lipoblasts is absolutely necessary for establishing the diagnosis.

Ancillary Studies

There are no immunohistochemical or molecular features pathognomonic for PLS. In the absence of an obvious ALT/WDL liposarcomatous component, evaluation for *MDM2* gene amplification may be useful to fully exclude DL with a homologous PLS component, especially among intra-abdominal and retroperitoneal tumors.

Differential Diagnosis

DL should have a concomitant, often juxtaposed low-grade component, ALT/WDL, and *MDM2* gene amplification. PLS with epithelioid features may express keratins, potentially confounding the diagnosis with "carcinoma." The presence of lipoblasts helps establish the diagnosis of PLS.

UPS is a diagnosis of exclusion, by definition lacking lipoblastic differentiation.

Prognosis and Therapy

PLS are aggressive sarcomas, commonly exhibiting local recurrence and metastatic events; overall 5-year survival rates approach 60%. Distant metastases are mostly seen in the lungs and pleura.

Definition

▸▸ High grade pleomorphic, usually spindled to epithelioid sarcoma, with at least focal lipoblastic differentiation and an absence of an associated ALT/WDL

Incidence and Location

▸▸ Rare sarcoma, deep soft tissues of the extremities, followed by the trunk/chest wall, retroperitoneum, and spermatic cord

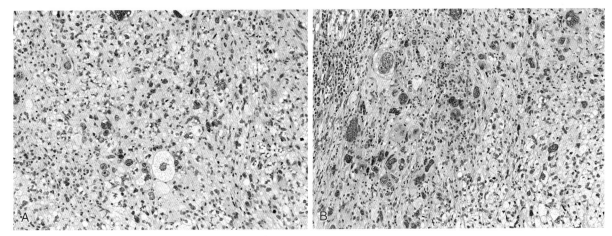

FIG. 8.12

A and **B**, Pleomorphic liposarcoma is a high-grade, pleomorphic spindled to epithelioid sarcoma defined by the presence of diagnostic multi-vacuolated lipoblasts.

Age Distribution
▸▸ Adults, peak incidence in seventh decade

Clinical Features
▸▸ Rapidly growing, commonly painless mass with symptoms related to anatomic location

Prognosis and Therapy
▸▸ Aggressive sarcoma with common local recurrences and distant metastases to lung and pleura
▸▸ Surgical resection with negative margins is the therapy of choice

PLEOMORPHIC LIPOSARCOMA – PATHOLOGIC FEATURES

Gross Findings
▸▸ Large, well-demarcated to infiltrative, fleshy to white-yellow neoplasm, with necrosis

Microscopic Findings
▸▸ High-grade sarcoma, resembling undifferentiated pleomorphic sarcoma, composed at least focally of multi-vacuolated lipoblasts, and often necrosis

Pathologic Differential Diagnoses
▸▸ Dedifferentiated liposarcoma, undifferentiated pleomorphic sarcoma, rarely poorly differentiated carcinoma

FIBROBLASTIC/MYOFIBROBLASTIC TUMORS

NODULAR FASCIITIS

DIFFERENTIAL DIAGNOSIS: LOW-GRADE FIBROMYXOID SARCOMA

Clinical Features

Nodular fasciitis is a benign, rapidly growing, and often self-limiting, typically subcutaneous lesion in the upper extremities, trunk, and head and neck, almost never exceeding 5 cm. Most patients are between 20 and 40 years of age. Occasionally, it localizes to intramuscular areas, but intradermal lesions tend to be rare. Head and neck localization is often seen in children.

Pathologic Features

GROSS FINDINGS

Well-circumscribed, usually subcutaneous white to slightly myxoid lesion, typically 1 to 2 cm.

MICROSCOPIC FINDINGS

Nodular fasciitis is a circumscribed, but non-encapsulated, neoplasm, composed of plump, uniform, and proliferating spindled cells, arranged loosely in short fascicles (Fig. 8.13) and storiform patterns, creating a "tissue culture" appearance. The stroma is variably collagenous to myxoid with microcysts and frequent extravasated red blood cells and lymphocytes. The borders of nodular fasciitis can be infiltrative (Fig. 8.13C). Mitotic activity may be prominent; however, atypical mitotic figures are never seen.

Ancillary Studies

Immunohistochemistry is generally not required for the diagnosis. The spindled cells display a myofibroblastic phenotype, virtually always diffuse smooth muscle actin positivity, variable to negative desmin expression, but negativity for S100, cytokeratin, EMA, and CD34. At the molecular level, most examples harbor a *USP6* (17p13.2) gene rearrangement, most commonly

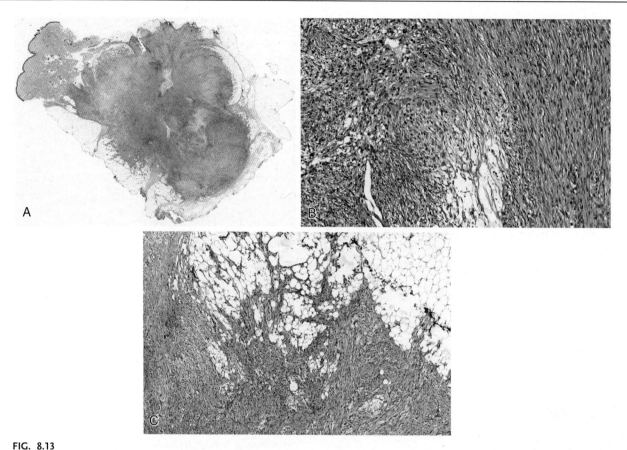

FIG. 8.13

Nodular fasciitis is a circumscribed, non-encapsulated neoplasm **(A)**, composed of plump, uniform and proliferating spindled cells, arranged loosely in short loose fascicles within a variably collagenous to myxoid stroma, often associated with microcysts and extravasated RBCs **(B)**. Despite appearing circumscribed grossly, it tends to show minor degrees of infiltration **(C)**.

t(17;22)(p13.2;q12.3) with the *USP6-MYH9* gene fusion, supporting the concept of a neoplasm.

Differential Diagnosis

Various spindle cell sarcomas, typically dermatofibrosarcoma protuberans (DFSP) and low-grade fibromyxoid sarcoma (LGFS), represent the most important differential diagnoses for nodular fasciitis. Nevertheless, the characteristic superficial location and circumscription, loose tissue culture-like growth pattern, uniformity of the tumor cells without significant atypia, and the presence of SMA but absence of CD34 expression is diagnostic of nodular fasciitis. MUC-4 positivity, characteristic of LGFS, is not seen in nodular fasciitis, and diffuse CD34 expression is characteristic of DFSP.

Intravascular fasciitis has virtually identical histologic features to nodular fasciitis but, as the name implies, involves blood vessels, typically intravascular and muscular walled veins.

Cranial fasciitis refers to a rapidly growing, nodular fasciitis-like lesion, involving the skull outer table of infants within the first year of life. It is commonly associated with myxoid stroma and foci of osseous metaplasia.

Prognosis and Therapy

Self-limiting and spontaneous resolution, even following incomplete excision, is typical, leading to the designation of "transient neoplasia." Local recurrence (or persistence) is very rare, less than 1%.

NODULAR FASCIITIS – DISEASE FACT SHEET

Definition
▶▶ Well-circumscribed, subcutaneous, <2 cm, cellular myofibroblastic lesion with a tissue culture-like growth pattern, microcysts, and often myxoid stroma, arising in the extremities of young adults

Incidence and Location
▶▶ Subcutaneous, occasionally intramuscular, upper extremities, trunk, and, especially in children, head and neck

Age Distribution
▶▶ Young adults, but may occur at any age

Clinical Features
▶▶ Rapidly growing, superficial, commonly painless soft tissue swelling, <2 cm

Prognosis and Therapy
▶▶ Benign, often spontaneous resolution, local recurrences rare

---

NODULAR FASCIITIS – PATHOLOGIC FEATURES

Gross Findings

▸▸ Circumscribed to slightly infiltrative, fibrous to myxoid, <2 cm, subcutaneous

---

Microscopic Findings

▸▸ Unencapsulated but sharply demarcated, cellular myofibroblastic proliferation, uniform spindled cells, arranged in sheets and fascicles with a tissue culture-like growth pattern, microcysts, extravasated lymphocytes and red blood cells, and collagenous to myxoid stroma

---

Pathologic Differential Diagnoses

▸▸ Cranial fasciitis (newborns), intravascular fasciitis, low-grade fibromyxoid sarcoma, and dermatofibrosarcoma protuberans

---

ISCHEMIC FASCIITIS (ATYPICAL DECUBITAL FIBROPLASIA)

DIFFERENTIAL DIAGNOSIS: PROLIFERATIVE FASCIITIS AND MYOSITIS

Clinical Features

Ischemic fasciitis, also known as atypical decubital fibroplasia, is a reactive pseudosarcomatous fibroblastic/myofibroblastic proliferation commonly arising in areas of constant pressure and/or injury, frequently associated with immobilization (sacral region, limb girdles, greater trochanter). Most cases are elderly patients, over 60 years of age, and it tends to be more common in males.

Pathologic Features

GROSS FINDINGS

White fibrous to yellow ill-defined lesion with central necrosis and often cystic changes. May be associated with an overlying ulcer.

MICROSCOPIC FINDINGS

It is poorly circumscribed but there is a distinct zonal appearance. Central hypocellular areas are characterized by fibrinoid degeneration/necrosis and pseudocyst formation (Fig. 8.14), transitioning to a granulation tissue-like vascular proliferation with large ganglion-like reactive fibroblasts (Fig. 8.14B), similar to that seen in proliferative fasciitis and myositis.

Ancillary Studies

Sometimes SMA and less often desmin are observed in the lesional cells. S100 is negative.

Differential Diagnosis

Proliferative fasciitis and myositis, although associated with similar ganglion-like fibroblasts, lack the distinct zoning appearance and are found exclusively in subcutaneous fat and skeletal muscle, respectively. Proliferative fasciitis, typically seen in the upper extremities of middle-aged to older adults, forms poorly circumscribed lesions in subcutaneous tissue, resembling nodular fasciitis but associated with ganglion-like fibroblasts. Proliferative myositis shows virtually identical morphologic features in the same age group but more frequently involves the

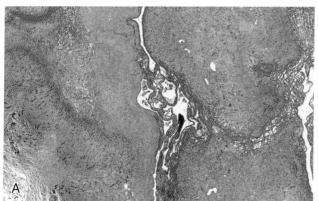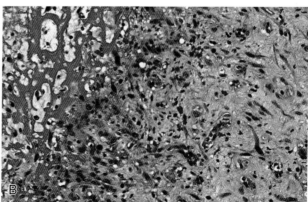

FIG. 8.14

Ischemic fasciitis has distinct zonal appearance **(A)** with areas of fibrinoid degeneration/necrosis and pseudocyst formation transitioning to a granulation tissue–like vascular proliferation with large ganglion-like reactive fibroblasts **(B)**.

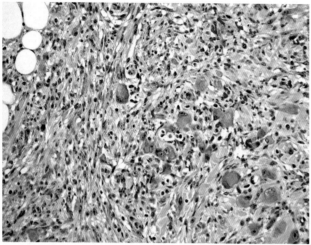

FIG. 8.15
Proliferative fasciitis is composed of similar ganglion-like fibroblasts within the subcutis but lacks the distinct zoning appearance of ischemic fasciitis.

trunk and shoulder girdles and is typically larger, and the ganglion-like fibroblasts are more prominent (Fig. 8.15). Neither are associated with overlying ulceration of the skin. *FOS/FOSB* gene rearrangements have been documented in proliferative fasciitis and myositis.

Prognosis and Therapy

Local excision is usually curative but may persist if underlying cause is not addressed.

ISCHEMIC FASCIITIS – DISEASE FACT SHEET

Definition
▸▸ Reactive pseudosarcomatous fibroblastic/myofibroblastic proliferation, characterized by zonal fibrinoid necrosis/cystic changes, ganglion-like fibroblasts, and commonly found in areas of pressure, associated with immobilization

Incidence and Location
▸▸ Tends to occur in the deep subcutis in areas subjected to trauma or constant pressure (sacral region, limb girdles, and greater trochanter)

Age Distribution
▸▸ Elderly, between seventh and ninth decades

Clinical Features
▸▸ Often bed-ridden, frequently but not always associated with debilitation, ulcerated, painless mass

Prognosis and Therapy
▸▸ Local excision is usually curative
▸▸ May persist in disabled patients if underlying cause is not addressed

---

ISCHEMIC FASCIITIS – PATHOLOGIC FEATURES

Gross Findings
▸▸ Ill-defined, deep-seated lesion, sometimes underlying an ulcer

Microscopic Findings
▸▸ Distinct zonal appearance with more central hypocellular areas characterized by fibrinoid degeneration, necrosis, and/or pseudocyst formation, transitioning to a granulation tissue-like proliferation with large ganglion-like reactive fibroblasts

Pathologic Differential Diagnoses
▸▸ Proliferative fasciitis and myositis

MYOSITIS OSSIFICANS AND FIBRO-OSSEOUS PSEUDOTUMOR OF DIGITS

DIFFERENTIAL DIAGNOSIS: CALCIFYING APONEUROTIC FIBROMA AND EXTRASKELETAL OSTEOSARCOMA

Clinical Features

Myositis ossificans (MO) is a benign, rapidly growing but self-limited neoplasm, usually occurring in areas susceptible to trauma. It may develop anytime from early childhood and until late adulthood, but most arise in active young adults. On radiology, the early phases are characterized by well-demarcated, soft tissue fullness and edema. Focal (flocculent) mineralization in the periphery of the neoplasm begins after 2–6 weeks, evolving into an eggshell-like mineralized layer of bone with a radiolucent center. In the latest stages, MO becomes circumscribed, entirely mineralized, and hard.

Fibro-osseous pseudotumor of digits (FOPD), also known in the literature as florid reactive periostitis, is related to MO but represents a benign neoplasm specifically of the subcutaneous tissues of the phalanges and metatarsals/metacarpals of the fingers and, less frequently, the toes. Formation of a peripheral eggshell-like bone does not generally occur. Radiologically, a characteristic fusiform swelling is associated with juxtacortical calcifications and a periosteal reaction. The mineralization tends to be randomly distributed.

Pathologic Features

GROSS FINDINGS

MO and FOPD are usually well-circumscribed, round to ovoid, hard masses with variable amounts of bone,

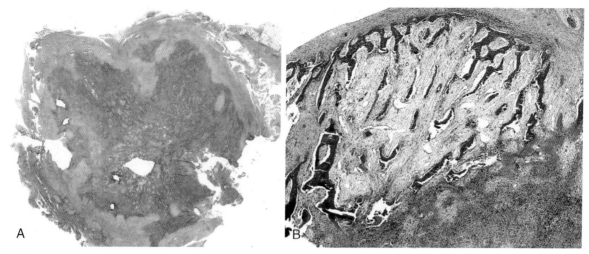

FIG. 8.16

Myositis ossificans is well circumscribed with a classical zonal appearance, most often composed of a more mature peripheral rim of osteoid to woven bone trabeculae merging to a central, more densely cellular, non-ossified spindled nodular to proliferative fasciitis-like proliferation (**A,** low power; **B,** high power).

depending on the age of the neoplasm. The center of MO is usually soft, consistent with a zonal growth pattern.

MICROSCOPIC FINDINGS

A typical zonal appearance is characteristic of in MO (Fig. 8.16). The periphery is composed of at least a partial rim of osteoid to woven bone trabeculae, rimmed by osteoblasts, merging centrally with a densely cellular but uniform spindled to ganglion-like cell proliferation, often devoid of osteoid/bone, closely resembling nodular/proliferative fasciitis. These latter cells often are haphazardly arranged, have eosinophilic cytoplasm, plump to ovoid nuclei with open chromatin, and may be quite mitotically active. The background stroma is variably fibrous to edematous with increased vascularity. Extravasated erythrocytes, lymphocytes, and osteoclast-type giant cells are frequent. Rarely, MO undergoes central cystic degeneration, resembling an aneurysmal bone cyst. In FOPD, the bone does not usually form a peripheral outer layer, but instead, the bone and fibrous tissue are admixed and randomly distributed (Fig. 8.17).

Ancillary Studies

Immunohistochemically, the spindled cells often express SMA but are generally negative for desmin and CD34. As in nodular fasciitis, *USP6* gene (17p13) arrangements are characteristic, but most commonly associated with the *COL1A1* (17q21) gene.

Differential Diagnosis

Calcifying aponeurotic fibroma (CAF) may be mistaken for FOPD. CAF is a rare benign neoplasm, most commonly

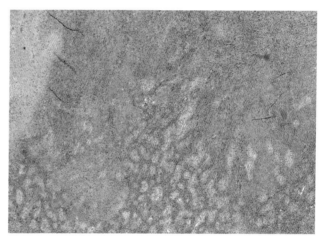

FIG. 8.17

Fibro-osseous pseudotumor of digits lacks the typical zonal morphology of usual myositis ossificans, with admixtures of bone trabecula and bland fibrous tissue, arising as a fusiform swelling of a digit.

seen in children, between 5 and 15 years of age, arising in association with fibro-tendinous tissues on the distal extremities, palmar, and plantar surfaces. There is no involvement of underlying bone or periosteal reaction. It has high risk of local recurrence (50%) if incompletely excised. The tumors are variably cellular with infiltrative fibromatosis-like spindle cell areas admixed with less cellular zones, characterized by plump epithelioid fibroblasts admixed with zones of calcification, sometimes appearing hyalinized to chondroid (Fig. 8.18). CAF is not associated with *USP6* gene rearrangements.

Extraskeletal osteosarcomas form deeply seated masses, arising in older adults, lacking the characteristic zonal pattern of MO. Microscopically, they appear obviously malignant, with significant cytologic atypia and pleomorphism along with other signs of malignancy (increased mitotic activity, necrosis, infiltration) (Fig. 8.19).

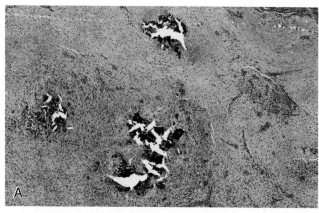
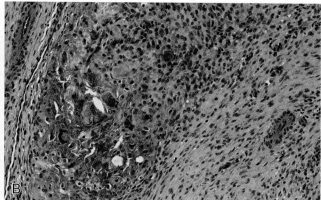

FIG. 8.18

Calcifying aponeurotic fibroma has infiltrative fibromatosis–like spindled cell areas admixed with less cellular areas of plump epithelioid fibroblasts with zones of calcification (**A,** low power; **B,** high power).

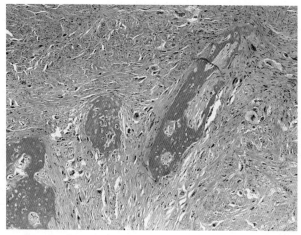

FIG. 8.19

Extraskeletal osteosarcoma has obvious malignant features, with significant cytologic atypia and nuclear pleomorphism, increased mitotic activity, and bone production by the malignant cells.

There is no characteristic gene fusion associated with extraskeletal osteosarcoma.

Prognosis and Therapy

Although clinical follow-up without further therapy is a reasonable decision, the preferred treatment for MO and FOPD is simple excision, and both entities have an excellent prognosis. Local recurrence rarely occurs in FOPD.

MYOSITIS OSSIFICANS/FIBRO-OSSEOUS PSEUDOTUMOR – DISEASE FACT SHEET

Definition
▸▸ MO is a rapidly growing and self-limited neoplasm, sometimes associated with trauma, characterized by a zonation, with a more mature, ossified periphery and a less mature, often non-ossified center

▸▸ FOPD is a benign neoplasm in the subcutaneous tissues/periosteum, arising as a fusiform lesion of the small tubular bones of the digits, characterized as a non-zonal fibro-osseous process

Incidence and Location
▸▸ Extremities, typically proximal (MO) and acral (FOPD)

Age Distribution
▸▸ Wide age distribution, but most commonly adolescents and young adults

Clinical Features
▸▸ Well circumscribed, rapidly growing
▸▸ Zonation may be radiographically evident with MO, while a periosteal reaction and fusiform mass swelling are classical for FOPD

Prognosis and Therapy
▸▸ Excellent prognosis, simple excision generally curative

MYOSITIS OSSIFICANS/FIBRO-OSSEOUS PSEUDOTUMOR – PATHOLOGIC FEATURES

Gross Findings
▸▸ Well circumscribed, firm masses

Microscopic Findings
▸▸ MO, well circumscribed peripheral osteoid/bone shell, transitioning to less mature, hypercellular nodular/proliferative fasciitis-like centrally
▸▸ FOPD, well-demarcated fusiform swelling/periosteal reaction from small tubular bones of the digits, associated with a benign-appearing fibro-osseous proliferation, without zonation

Pathologic Differential Diagnoses
▸▸ CAF, especially for FOPD, and extraskeletal osteosarcoma

ELASTOFIBROMA

DIFFERENTIAL DIAGNOSIS: DESMOID-TYPE FIBROMATOSIS

Clinical Features

Elastofibroma presents as an ill-defined, slowly growing, and painless solid tissue proliferation, which on MRI has a signal intensity similar to skeletal muscle with interspersed adipose tissue, commonly seen in the deep connective tissues between the lower scapula and the thoracic wall. Females older than 50 years of age are more commonly afflicted than males. Extrascapular localization has been described but is considered exceedingly rare.

Pathologic Features

GROSS FINDINGS

Poorly defined rubbery fibrous tissue with interspersed fat is classically observed.

MICROSCOPIC FINDINGS

Elastofibromas form bland, ill-defined masses composed of mixtures of adipose and fibromyxoid tissue, with the latter containing haphazardly arranged abnormal and dystrophic elastic fibers (Fig. 8.20). The background fibroblasts lack cytologic atypia, and mitotic activity is essentially non-existent.

Ancillary Studies

Elastin stains highlight the abnormal elastic fibers, described as coarse, deeply eosinophilic, and fragmented

into linear beads of serrated discs. There is no characteristic gene fusion diagnostic of elastofibroma.

Differential Diagnosis

The most important differential diagnosis is desmoid-type fibromatosis, which is significantly more cellular and composed of sweeping fascicles of uniform spindled cells infiltrating fat and skeletal muscle.

Prognosis and Therapy

Elastofibroma is an entirely benign lesion. Local recurrence is exceptionally rare after simple excision.

ELASTOFIBROMA – DISEASE FACT SHEET

Definition
▶▶ Benign, slowly growing fibroadipose tissue lesion, associated with abundant but abnormal elastic fibers, involving the connective tissues between the inferior scapula and thoracic wall of older females

Incidence and Location
▶▶ Deep connective tissues between the scapula and thoracic wall

Age Distribution
▶▶ Elderly (almost all older than 50 years)

Clinical Features
▶▶ Benign, poorly defined and painless soft tissue mass, localized between the lower scapular and chest wall

Prognosis and Therapy
▶▶ Benign, local excision is curative

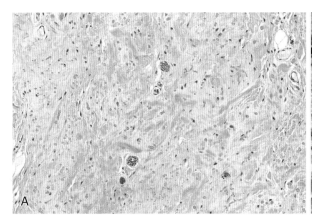 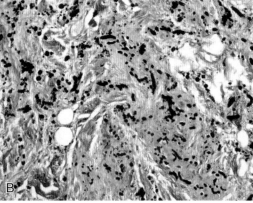

FIG. 8.20

Elastofibroma is an ill-defined mass, with variable amount of adipose and fibromyxoid tissue accompanied by increased abnormal and dystrophic elastic fibers **(A)**, highlighted by Elastin stain **(B)**.

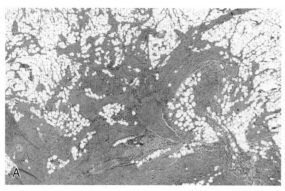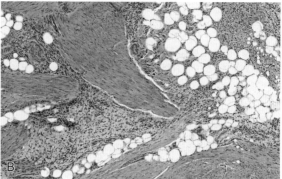

FIG. 8.21

Fibrous hamartoma of infancy has triphasic morphology with variable proportions of three distinct components: bland fibroblastic/myofibroblastic fascicles, primitive myxoid mesenchymal cells, and mature adipose tissue **(A)**. The primitive mesenchymal component consists of primitive, rounded to stellate cells within the myxoid stroma **(B)**.

ELASTOFIBROMA – PATHOLOGIC FEATURES

Gross Findings

▸▸ Ill-defined rubbery fibroadipose tissue

Microscopic Findings

▸▸ Poorly demarcated fibroadipose tissue lesion, variably myxoid, and associated with abundant and abnormal elastic fibers

Pathologic Differential Diagnoses

▸▸ Desmoid-type fibromatosis

FIBROUS HAMARTOMA OF INFANCY

DIFFERENTIAL DIAGNOSIS: LIPOFIBROMATOSIS

Clinical Features

Fibrous hamartoma of infancy (FHI) typically presents as a small, superficial and mobile, painless mass, arising in the anterior and posterior axillary folds of infants and young children (<2 years old). Other common locations include the upper arm, trunk, inguinal region, and external genitalia.

Pathologic Features

GROSS FINDINGS

Most are ill-defined with variably amounts of fibrous and adipose tissue.

MICROSCOPIC FINDINGS

FHI is characterized by a typical triphasic morphology with variable proportions of three distinct components: bland fibroblastic/myofibroblastic fascicles, primitive

myxoid mesenchymal cells, and mature adipose tissue (Fig. 8.21). The bland fibroblastic/myofibroblastic cell proliferation is composed of monomorphic spindled cells with dense eosinophilic collagenous background stroma. Hyalinization also may occur. The primitive mesenchymal component consists of primitive, rounded to stellate cells within myxoid stroma (Fig. 8.21B). Mitotic figures are rare.

Ancillary Studies

SMA is variably positive in the fibroblastic areas and occasionally in the primitive mesenchymal zones, which also are positive for CD34. S100 is absent.

Differential Diagnosis

Lipofibromatosis also is composed of mixtures of fat and cellular fascicles of fibromatosis-like tissue, arising in subcutaneous tissues of children (Fig. 8.22).

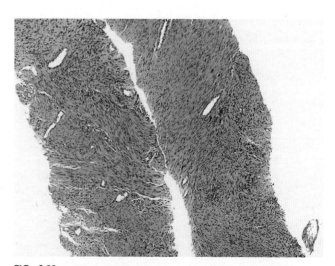

FIG. 8.22

Lipofibromatosis is characterized by cellular fascicles of fibromatosis-like tissue and fat infiltrating surrounding soft tissues. Small biopsy samples may not contain all components.

However, it has a predilection for the hands and feet and lacks the classic triphasic organoid appearance of FHI.

Prognosis and Therapy

Simple excision with potential for local recurrence if incompletely excised is usual for FHI.

FIBROUS HAMARTOMA OF INFANCY – DISEASE FACT SHEET

Definition
▸▸ Triphasic, hamartoma-like neoplasm composed of variably amounts of admixed bland fibroblastic/myofibroblastic fascicles, immature mesenchymal zones, and mature adipose tissue, arising in the superficial soft tissues of the trunk and extremities of infants and young children

Incidence and Location
▸▸ Rare tumor, most commonly seen in the anterior/posterior axillary folds, trunk, extremities, and external genitalia

Age Distribution
▸▸ Infants and young children (<2 years of age)

Clinical Features
▸▸ Painless, mobile superficial nodule

Prognosis and Therapy
▸▸ Local recurrence may be seen in up to 15% of patients, but simple excision remains treatment of choice

---

FIBROUS HAMARTOMA OF INFANCY – PATHOLOGIC FEATURES

Gross Findings
▸▸ Ill-defined rubbery fibrous tissue

Microscopic Findings
▸▸ Triphasic morphology of varying admixed amounts of bland fibroblastic/myofibroblastic fascicles, mature adipose tissue, and immature mesenchymal nests with lightly myxoid stroma

Pathologic Differential Diagnoses
▸▸ Lipofibromatosis

DESMOID FIBROMATOSIS

DIFFERENTIAL DIAGNOSIS: PALMAR AND PLANTAR FIBROMATOSIS

Clinical Features

Desmoid fibromatosis presents as a deeply seated, painless but non-mobile mass typically arising in the extremities, trunk, retroperitoneum or abdominal cavity and, less commonly, in the head and neck, paraspinal and flank regions, of young to middle aged adults, especially females. It may be associated with prior trauma and/or surgery. A minority of patients with familial adenomatous polyposis (Gardner syndrome) develop intra-abdominal fibromatosis, usually multifocal, involving children and young adults.

Superficial fibromatoses represent a spectrum of similar nodular fibroblastic/myofibroblastic proliferations involving the hands (palmar fibromatosis, Dupuytren contracture.) and feet (plantar fibromatosis, Ledderhose disease). Palmar disease forms painless nodules and cords, causing contractures in the palms and fingers of older adults, usually males. The plantar form is more often seen in young to middle-aged adults, typically females. It is associated with painless swelling and no contractures.

Pathologic Features

GROSS FINDINGS

Desmoid fibromatosis forms solid, usually large and infiltrative masses, with ill-defined margins and a fibrous, white to whorled cut surface. Superficial fibromatoses are small, rubbery fibrous nodules, intimately associated with fibro-tendinous tissues on the hands and feet.

MICROSCOPIC FINDINGS

Both desmoid and superficial fibromatosis have overlapping morphologic features, characterized by long sweeping fascicles of elongated and uniform spindled cells. Cytologically, the cells have eosinophilic cytoplasm and elongated nuclei with open chromatin, without significant pleomorphism. The cellular proliferation in superficial fibromatoses, particularly the palmar form, often are confined to the fibro-tendinous and fascial tissues. Desmoid fibromatosis exhibits widespread infiltration, entrapping fat and skeletal muscle (Fig. 8.23A). At the periphery of the lesion, lymphoid aggregates often are seen (Fig. 8.23B). The background is commonly uniformly collagenous but rarely may exhibit keloid-like areas and myxoid changes, more common in intra-abdominal and mesenteric forms. The scattered background blood vessels have thin walls with characteristic perivascular edema (Fig. 8.23C). Mitotic figures tend to be uncommon, and tumor necrosis is not present.

Ancillary Studies

Immunohistochemical stains are not necessary for diagnosis. SMA is usually expressed by the lesional

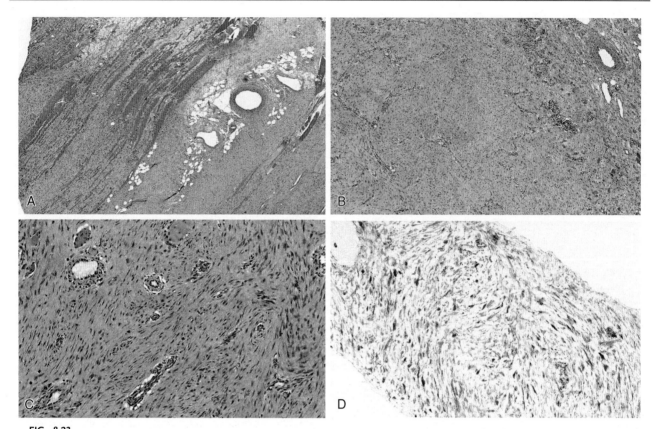

FIG. 8.23

Desmoid fibromatosis with long sweeping fascicles infiltrating the surrounding soft tissues and skeletal muscle **(A)**, often accompanied by lymphoid aggregates, peripherally **(B)**. The background stroma is usually uniformly collagenous with thin-walled blood vessels and characteristic perivascular edema **(C)**. Nuclear beta-catenin positivity may be helpful but is often inconsistently expressed **(D)**.

cells, but desmin positivity is variable. CD117 expression represents a potential diagnostic pitfall in intra-abdominal lesions, but cytokeratin, CD34, DOG1, and S100 are negative. Nuclear β-catenin positivity (Fig. 8.23D) is considered characteristic, but, in our experience, interpretation can be challenging. Somatic *CTNNB1* mutations (β-catenin gene) and, in patients with Gardner syndrome, germline *APC* gene mutation are seen.

Differential Diagnosis

Superficial fibromatoses, despite morphologic overlap, have characteristic and distinct locations and presentations. Both plantar and palmar forms are commonly negative for β-catenin (Fig. 8.24).

When involving viscera, sarcomatoid carcinoma should be considered; however, it is keratin positive and typically exhibits more significant cytologic atypia and pleomorphism.

DL may have fibromatosis-like areas, but the presence of a low-grade lipomatous component and, when necessary, confirmation of *MDM2* gene amplification, helps to confirm this diagnosis.

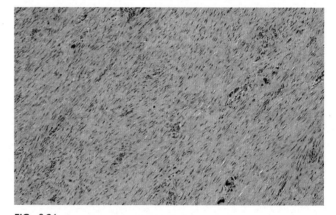

FIG. 8.24

Superficial (palmar/plantar) fibromatosis has overlapping morphologic features with desmoid fibromatosis, characterized by long sweeping fascicles of elongated and uniform spindled cells, enclosed within fibrotendinous and fascial tissues.

Prognosis and Therapy

The prognosis is variable, depending on the location, size, involvement of viscera, and resectability. Desmoid fibromatosis is an aggressive tumor, so wide surgical resection with negative margins is required. However, up to one third of the patients develop local recurrences, but distant metastases do not occur. The most important prognostic factor is adequacy of surgical excision. The goal of achieving negative margins should be balanced with a desire to preserve function.

DESMOID FIBROMATOSIS – DISEASE FACT SHEET

Definition
▸▸ Locally aggressive, recurring, and non-metastasizing deep-seated neoplasm, composed of long sweeping infiltrative fascicles of monotonous spindled cells within dense fibrous stroma, thin-walled blood vessels with perivascular edema, and peripheral lymphoid aggregates

Incidence and Location
▸▸ Rare, deep soft tissues of the extremities, abdomen, retroperitoneum, and trunk

Age Distribution
▸▸ Young to middle-aged adults, usually female

Clinical Features
▸▸ Deep-seated and large mass, densely adherent/fixed to the surrounding tissues
▸▸ Prior history of trauma and/or surgery is common

Prognosis and Therapy
▸▸ Aggressive and commonly locally recurs
▸▸ Wide surgical excision with negative margins is the preferred approach

---

DESMOID FIBROMATOSIS – PATHOLOGIC FEATURES

Gross Findings
▸▸ Solid, infiltrative mass, with white fibrous to whorled cut surface

Microscopic Findings
▸▸ Long sweeping fascicles composed of monomorphic spindled cells, with eosinophilic cytoplasm and elongated nuclei, infiltrating the surrounding adipose tissue and skeletal muscle
▸▸ Peripheral lymphoid aggregates and perivascular edema
▸▸ Collagenous to slightly myxoid stroma

Pathologic Differential Diagnoses
▸▸ Superficial (palmar or plantar) fibromatosis, sarcomatoid carcinoma, and dedifferentiated liposarcoma

FIBROMA OF TENDON SHEATH

DIFFERENTIAL DIAGNOSIS: NODULAR FASCIITIS

Clinical Features

Fibroma of tendon sheath presents as a slowly growing nodule, usually <3 cm and associated with tendon sheaths of fingers, involving patients, between the ages of 20 and 50 years.

Pathologic Features

GROSS FINDINGS

Rounded, firm to lobular nodule, associated with tendons.

MICROSCOPIC FINDINGS

Well circumscribed and nodular, bland spindle cell proliferation (Fig. 8.25), arranged in short fascicles within dense collagenous stroma, accompanied by thin-walled blood vessels with slit-like appearance (Fig. 8.25B). Cytologically the cells do not exhibit significant cytologic atypia and pleomorphism.

Ancillary Studies

Immunohistochemically, most express SMA but are negative for S100 and desmin. A subset of more cellular

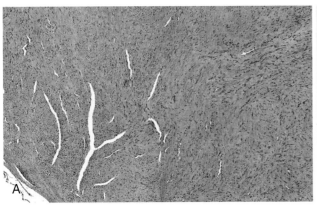
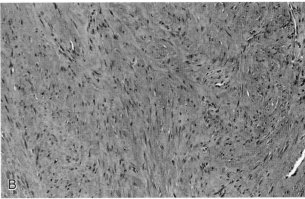

FIG. 8.25
Fibroma of tendon sheath is a well-circumscribed and nodular spindle cell proliferation **(A)** composed of bland spindled cells arranged as short fascicles within densely collagenous to hyalinized stroma with slit-like thin-walled blood vessels **(B)**.

examples, possibly representing a spectrum with nodular fasciitis, display *USP6* gene rearrangements.

Differential Diagnosis

Nodular fasciitis is typically significantly more cellular, displaying a loose tissue culture appearance, variably collagenous stroma, extravasated red blood cells and lymphocytes, and predominantly occurs in the subcutis. More cellular forms of fibroma of tendon sheath, especially those with *USP6* gene rearrangements, likely represent rare examples of tenosynovial nodular fasciitis.

Tenosynovial giant cell tumor (TGCT; localized type) may exhibit a virtually identical clinical presentation. However, TGCTs are not spindled cell lesions, being instead composed of mostly uniform epithelioid to histiocytoid mononuclear cells, scattered multinucleated osteoclast-type giant cells, and hemosiderin pigment.

Prognosis and Therapy

Fibroma of tendon sheath is a benign tumor but may locally recur in up to 25% of cases. Surgical resection should be undertaken with the aim to preserve function.

FIBROMA OF TENDON SHEATH – DISEASE FACT SHEET

Definition
- ▸▸ Benign well circumscribed and lobular, usually hypocellular spindle cell proliferation associated with dense collagen and arising in tendons, especially fingers

Incidence and Location
- ▸▸ Rare, associated with tendons of hands and, less commonly, feet

Age Distribution
- ▸▸ Young to middle-aged adults

Clinical Features
- ▸▸ Painless soft tissue mass, associated with finger tendons

Prognosis and Therapy
- ▸▸ Benign lesion, potential for local recurrences, with surgical excision

---

FIBROMA OF TENDON SHEATH – PATHOLOGIC FEATURES

Gross Findings
- ▸▸ Lobulated firm and circumscribed nodule

Microscopic Findings
- ▸▸ Well-demarcated, lobulated lesion with spindled cells arranged in short fascicles within a densely collagenous background, containing slit-like blood vessels

Pathologic Differential Diagnoses
- ▸▸ Nodular fasciitis and tenosynovial giant cell tumor (localized type)

MYOFIBROBLASTOMA

DIFFERENTIAL DIAGNOSIS: CELLULAR ANGIOFIBROMA

Clinical Features

Myofibroblastoma is a benign neoplasm, originally described as arising in the mammary regions, within the superficial soft tissues of mostly males. However, mammary-type myofibroblastomas appear more common in extramammary sites, primarily the inguinal and groin areas, including the vulva/vaginal region and scrotum. Less common anatomic sites are extremities, viscera, and retroperitoneum. Most present as painless masses of older patients, although the age range is wide.

Pathologic Features

GROSS FINDINGS

Myofibroblastoma forms well-circumscribed masses, white whorled to yellowish, with variable amounts of fat component.

MICROSCOPIC FINDINGS

Myofibroblastoma is a well-circumscribed but unencapsulated spindled cell neoplasm composed of short and stubby spindled cells with indistinct cell borders and eosinophilic cytoplasm. The cells are usually arranged in short fascicles and sheets (Fig. 8.26). Their nuclei are oval with even chromatin and occasional pinpoint nucleoli. The background stroma is myxoid with scattered ropy to thick collagenous bundles and randomly distributed mast cells.

Ancillary Studies

Immunohistochemically, the spindled cells are diffusely and strongly positive for ER (Fig. 8.26C), CD34 (Fig. 8.26D), and desmin, but usually negative for SMA. Loss of RB1 also is present. At the molecular level, myofibroblastomas have loss of 13q14 (*RB1* gene), a shared genetic abnormality with spindle cell/pleomorphic lipoma and cellular angiofibroma.

Differential Diagnosis

Spindle cell lipomas typically arise in the neck, shoulder, and upper back subcutis of elderly adults. Desmin always is negative.

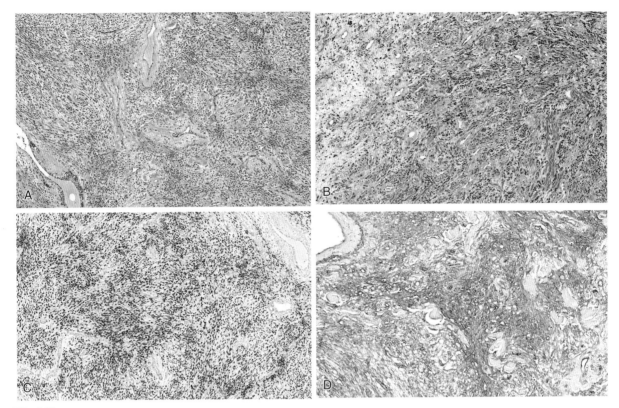

FIG. 8.26

Myofibroblastoma is a well-circumscribed, unencapsulated spindle cell neoplasm composed of short and stubby, uniform spindled cells with indistinct cell borders and eosinophilic cytoplasm arranged in short fascicles and sheets embedded in a variably myxoid stroma with scattered thick collagen fibers (**A,** low power; **B,** high power). The cells are usually positive for desmin, ER **(C),** and CD34 **(D).**

Cellular angiofibroma is a benign, hypercellular, and vascular neoplasm, located commonly in the superficial soft tissues of the scrotal and vulvar region, characterized by circumscription and uniform, short, spindled cells within an edematous stroma with admixed collagen bundles and medium-sized blood vessels with irregular branching lumina (Fig. 8.27). Variable expression of SMA, desmin, as well as ER and PR, are described. CD34 may be positive in up to 30% of cases, but nuclear RB1 is lost.

Angiofibroma of soft tissue also is a benign, slowly growing, and painless neoplasm, most commonly arising in the extremities (legs) of middle-aged males. Histologically, they form well-demarcated lesions composed of uniform spindled cells, abundant myxoid to fibromyxoid stroma, and a prominent network of innumerable branching, thin-walled blood vessels (Fig. 8.28). These tumors have near-diploid karyotypes with a recurrent t(5;8) (p15;q13) and *AHRR-NCOA2* gene fusion.

Prognosis and Therapy

Myofibroblastomas are benign neoplasms with exceptionally rare recurrence potential, even after marginal excision.

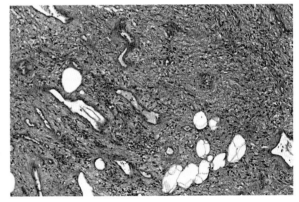

FIG. 8.27

Cellular angiofibroma is a circumscribed, hypercellular, and vascular neoplasm with an edematous to lightly myxoid stroma, accompanied by collagen bundles and prominent branching blood vessels.

MYOFIBROBLASTOMA – DISEASE FACT SHEET

Definition

▶▶ Benign soft tissue neoplasm occurring in superficial tissues, less often deep, characterized by short stubby spindled cells, arranged in haphazard fascicles within myxoid stroma with admixed thick collagenous fibers and mast cells

▶▶ Lesional cells show diffuse and strong expression of CD34, desmin, and ER, with loss of nuclear RB1

Continued

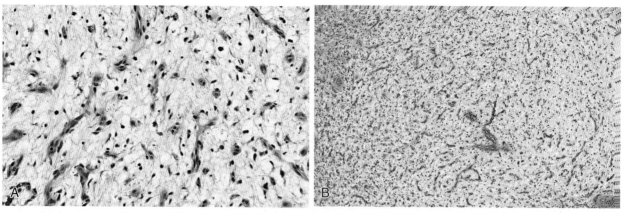

FIG. 8.28

Angiofibroma of soft tissue also is composed of uniform spindled cells (**A,** high power), modestly cellular, in an abundant myxoid stroma with a more prominent network of innumerable branching, thin-walled blood vessels (**B,** low power).

MYOFIBROBLASTOMA – DISEASE FACT SHEET—cont'd

Incidence and Location
▸▸ Rare, inguinal and groin

Age Distribution
▸▸ Wide age range, peak in middle-aged to older adults

Clinical Features
▸▸ Painless soft tissue nodule

Prognosis and Therapy
▸▸ Benign neoplasm, exceptionally rare potential for local recurrences, even after marginal excision

---

MYOFIBROBLASTOMA – PATHOLOGIC FEATURES

Gross Findings
▸▸ Well-delineated, nodular firm lesion with variable yellowish fat component

Microscopic Findings
▸▸ Well-circumscribed, non-encapsulated spindled cell neoplasm composed of short and stubby spindled cells, arranged in fascicles, within a lightly myxoid stroma with admixed scattered thick collagenous fibers and mast cells

Pathologic Differential Diagnoses
▸▸ Spindle cell lipoma, cellular angiofibroma, and angiofibroma of soft tissue

---

ANGIOMYOFIBROBLASTOMA

DIFFERENTIAL DIAGNOSIS: DEEP ANGIOMYXOMA

Clinical Features

Angiomyofibroblastomas present as well-circumscribed and painless masses, arising in the subcutis of pelvic region, most commonly seen in the vulva and vagina of middle-aged females, typically premenopausal. A subset occurs in males, in the paratesticular region and scrotum.

Pathologic Features

GROSS FINDINGS

Well-delineated, non-encapsulated soft tissue mass, red-tan and soft, are usual gross features.

MICROSCOPIC FINDINGS

Histologically, angiomyofibroblastomas are well-circumscribed lesions, composed of spindled to epithelioid cells, often concentrated around blood vessels, within an edematous to lightly myxoid stroma with prominent vascularity (Fig. 8.29). A minority display an adipocytic component. The epithelioid cells are frequently multi-nucleated and plasmacytoid. The background can be loose and edematous with scattered small vessels that can have hyalinized walls.

Ancillary Studies

Immunohistochemically, strong and diffuse desmin and ER co-expression is typical, often accompanied by CD34 positivity. SMA may be focally positive.

Differential Diagnosis

Deep angiomyxoma is the most important differential diagnosis. Although benign, deep angiomyxomas are "aggressive" infiltrative neoplasms, arising within the

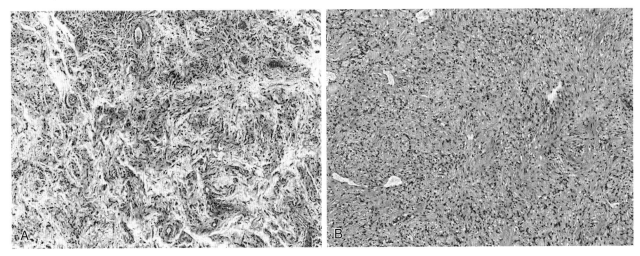

FIG. 8.29

A and **B,** Angiomyofibroblastoma is a well-circumscribed lesion, composed of spindled to epithelioid cells, often concentrated around blood vessels, within an edematous to lightly myxoid stroma with prominent vascularity.

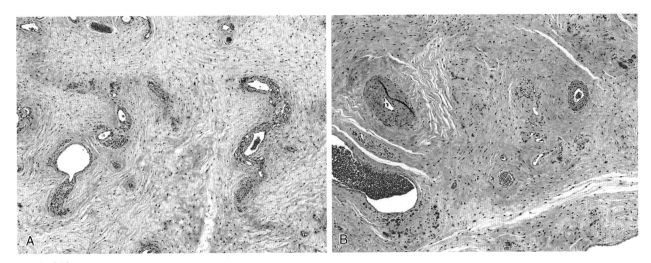

FIG. 8.30

A and **B,** Deep angiomyxoma is a relatively hypocellular but infiltrative spindled cell neoplasm, with abundant edematous to lightly myxoid stroma, admixed with medium to large muscular-walled blood vessels.

deep soft tissues of the pelvis/perineum of young to middle-aged females. Histologically they are relatively hypocellular spindled cell neoplasms with abundant edematous to myxoid stroma, accompanied by medium to large muscular-walled blood vessels (Fig. 8.30). The cells are most often randomly distributed, uniform, and may be associated with entrapment of fat. Diffuse co-expression of desmin and ER is typical, with positivity for CD34 and SMA less consistent. *HMGA2* (12q14) gene rearrangements have been confirmed by FISH analysis.

Prognosis and Therapy

Marginal excision is rarely associated with local recurrence.

ANGIOMYOFIBROBLASTOMA – DISEASE FACT SHEET

Definition

▸▸ Uncommon, benign and circumscribed neoplasm arising from the subcutis of the pelvic/perineal region, composed of spindled to epithelioid cells, often aggregating around blood vessels, within an edematous to lightly myxoid stroma

Incidence and Location

▸▸ Pelvic/inguinal region, most commonly vulvar/vaginal

Age Distribution

▸▸ Females of reproductive age, rarely postmenopausal females and males

Clinical Features

▸▸ Pelvic/perineal subcutaneous nodule, circumscribed and painless

Prognosis and Therapy

▸▸ Benign neoplasm, rare local recurrences following excision

NUCHAL-TYPE FIBROMA

DIFFERENTIAL DIAGNOSIS: GARDNER FIBROMA AND DESMOPLASTIC FIBROBLASTOMA

Clinical Features

Nuchal-type fibroma is a benign, ill-defined neoplasm, usually occurring in the subcutaneous tissues of the posterior neck of middle aged to older males, often with diabetes mellitus. Extra-nuchal sites include the upper back and extremities.

Pathologic Features

GROSS FINDINGS

Firm white, ill-defined nodule, between 2 and 5 cm is usually observed.

MICROSCOPIC FINDINGS

Nuchal-type fibromas are paucicellular and poorly circumscribed lesions, composed of monomorphic spindled cells, within a densely collagenous background stroma, entrapping fat and peripheral nerve bundles (Fig. 8.31).

Ancillary Studies

The spindled fibroblasts are positive for CD34 negative, variably positive for SMA, but negative for desmin and β-catenin.

Differential Diagnosis

Gardner fibroma, histologically indistinguishable from nuchal type fibroma, but is associated with familial

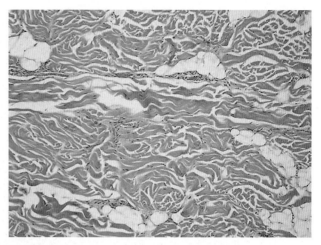

FIG. 8.31
Nuchal-type fibroma forms a poorly circumscribed, hypocellular lesion, composed of monomorphic spindled cells, within a background composed of thick collagenous bundles, often entrapping fat and small peripheral nerves.

adenomatous polyposis and germline *APC* mutations. They are most commonly seen in children < 10 years of age. The spindled cells are positive for CD34 but typically negative for SMA.

Desmoplastic fibroblastoma (collagenous fibroma) is a relatively circumscribed, benign, hypocellular neoplasm with an abundantly collagenous to lightly myxoid stroma, composed of bland stellate to spindled fibroblasts (Fig. 8.32). Most arise in the subcutaneous tissues of the extremities of adults. SMA is variably expressed, but S100, EMA, and CD34 are usually negative. Simple excision is curative.

Prognosis and Therapy

Nuchal-type fibroma is a benign tumor with potential for local recurrence.

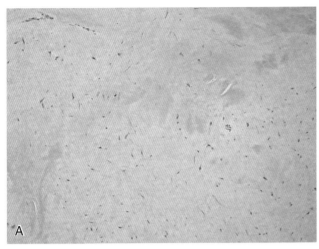
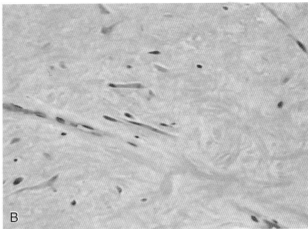

FIG. 8.32

Desmoplastic fibroblastomas are relatively circumscribed, hypocellular neoplasms composed of bland stellate to spindled fibroblasts with an abundantly and uniformly collagenous to lightly myxoid stroma (**A,** low power; **B,** high power).

NUCHAL-TYPE FIBROMA – PATHOLOGIC FEATURES

Gross Findings

▸▸ Poorly circumscribed, firm white soft tissue nodule

Microscopic Findings

▸▸ Paucicellular, poorly defined soft tissue neoplasm composed of bland spindled cells and abundant and thick collagenous fibers, entrapping adipose tissue

Pathologic Differential Diagnoses

▸▸ Gardner fibroma and desmoplastic fibroblastoma

DERMATOFIBROSARCOMA PROTUBERANS

DIFFERENTIAL DIAGNOSIS: DEEP FIBROUS HISTIOCYTOMA

Clinical Features

DFSP is a locally aggressive and rarely metastasizing neoplasm, arising as a solitary to multinodular, painless, and superficial mass of the trunk and proximal extremities/limb girdle, in young to middle-aged adults. It is rarely seen involving the head and neck, acral distal extremities, or genital area.

Pathologic Features

GROSS FINDINGS

DFSP displays a nodular to indurated plaque-like appearance with overlying skin, with ill-defined margins and extensive involvement of the subcutis.

MICROSCOPIC FINDINGS

DFSP is characteristically hypercellular and diffusely infiltrates the dermis and subcutis (Fig. 8.33), often associated with trails of adipocytes even up into the superficial dermis. The spindled neoplastic cells are remarkably monotonous, arranged in tight storiform patterns and short fascicles. Infiltration within the subcutaneous tissue often creates a characteristic honeycomb-like appearance (Fig. 8.33C). Mitotic activity tends to be low, not exceeding 5 mitoses/10 HPF. Admixed inflammatory cells are not a feature of DFPS. Myxoid stromal changes rarely occurs.

In fibrosarcomatous transformation, the cells exhibit a morphologic progression toward greater cytologic atypia, forming intersecting fascicles, often with a herringbone appearance (Fig. 8.33D). Mitotic activity inherently becomes more prominent, frequently exceeding 10 mitoses/10 HPF.

Ancillary Studies

The neoplastic cells are diffusely and strongly positive for CD34, sometimes express EMA, but are typically negative for desmin, SMA, STAT6, and S100. Loss of CD34 expression commonly occurs in areas of fibrosarcomatous transformation. DFSP has a recurrent t(17;22) (q22;q13), with the COL1A1-PDGFB gene fusion; however, establishing the diagnosis of DFSP rarely requires confirmation of this gene fusion.

Differential Diagnosis

Deep fibrous histiocytoma represents the most common tumor in the differential diagnosis. It is typically a subcutaneous lesion, often well circumscribed and heterogeneous, being composed of a mixture of benign-appearing

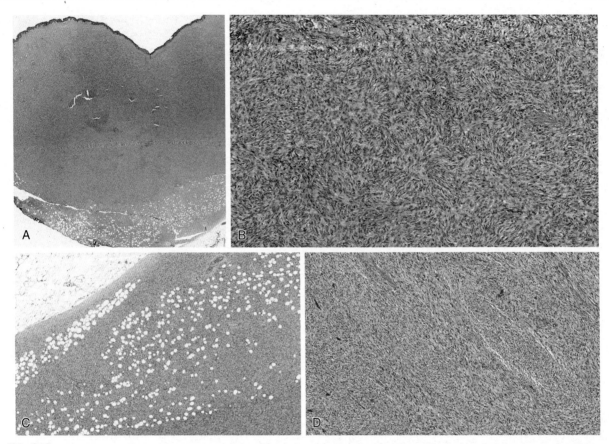

FIG. 8.33

Dermatofibrosarcoma protuberans is a hypercellular spindle cell neoplasm, occupying the dermis and subcutis **(A)**, composed of remarkably monotonous spindled cells, arranged in tight storiform patterns and short fascicles **(B)**, extensively infiltrating the underlying subcutaneous fat, creating a characteristic honeycomb-like appearance **(C)**. Fibrosarcomatous transformation is defined by the presence of intersecting fascicles, often with a herringbone appearance, with increased mitotic activity and cytologic atypia **(D)**.

spindled cells, arranged in short fascicles and storiform patterns, inflammatory cells, usually lymphocytes, and histiocytes (xanthomatous change). The periphery may show the lesional cells interdigitating with keloidal collagen. The overlying epidermis often is hyperplastic, but this tends to be more common in superficial fibrous histiocytomas occurring in the dermis. Diffuse CD34 positivity is not a feature and helps confirm the diagnosis.

Diffuse neurofibromas may resemble DFSP at low power. At high power, they lack the characteristic storiform pattern, exhibit tactoid structures or other features of neural differentiation, and always show diffuse S100 positivity. Most examples arise in the head and neck region of children and young adults, sometimes in association with neurofibromatosis, type 1.

Prognosis and Therapy

Locally aggressive neoplasm with propensity for local recurrences if incompletely excised. With the fibrosarcomatous transformation, the tumor acquires more aggressive course, including distant metastatic potential, most commonly involving the lungs.

DERMATOFIBROSARCOMA PROTUBERANS – DISEASE FACT SHEET

Definition
▸▸ Locally aggressive, superficial, diffusely CD34 positive and monotonous spindle cell neoplasm, arranged in tight storiform patterns, typically involving the trunk and proximal extremities, characterized by a *COL1A1-PDGFB* gene fusion

Incidence and Location
▸▸ Rare, subcutis of trunk and proximal extremities/limb girdles

Age Distribution
▸▸ Young to middle-aged adults

Clinical Features
▸▸ Elevated and indurated plaque-like to multinodular superficial painless lesion

Prognosis and Therapy
▸▸ Repeated local recurrences require wide excision with negative margins
▸▸ Fibrosarcomatous transformation results in increased risk of metastasis

SOLITARY FIBROUS TUMOR

DIFFERENTIAL DIAGNOSIS: SYNOVIAL SARCOMA

Clinical Features

Solitary fibrous tumor (SFT) is a slowly growing and painless mass that may occur at virtually any anatomical site; the most common anatomic locations include superficial and deep soft tissues of the extremities, abdominal cavity, pelvis, and head and neck regions. Additional symptoms may be related to anatomic site and relationship to viscera.

Pathologic Features

GROSS FINDINGS

SFT forms well-circumscribed and lobulated masses, often quite large, appearing heterogeneous, with dark red to brown cut surface, occasionally exhibiting hemorrhage, cystic degeneration, and/or necrosis.

MICROSCOPIC FINDINGS

Histologic features demonstrate a well-circumscribed, non-encapsulated spindled cell neoplasm with variable cellularity, fibrous to myxoid stroma, and prominent vasculature (Fig. 8.34); the spindled cells may be arranged haphazardly, as sheets, or in storiform patterns. There is usually no significant cytologic atypia/pleomorphism or increased mitotic activity (usually <4 mitoses/10 HPF). Rarely, admixed adipose tissue is prominent, mimicking a lipomatous neoplasm. Giant cell–rich examples have

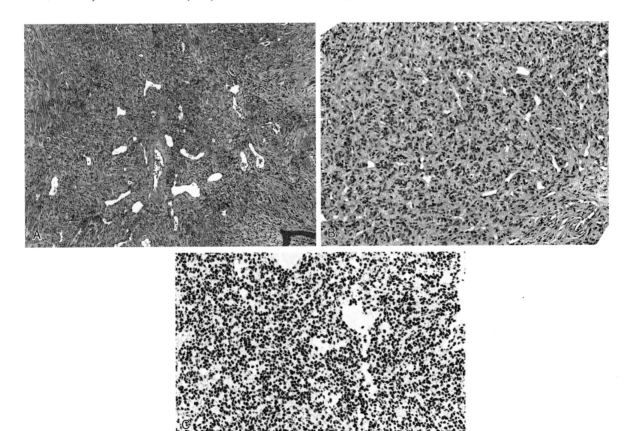

FIG. 8.34

Solitary fibrous tumors are generally hypercellular spindle cell lesions composed of mostly uniform spindled cells arranged haphazardly, in sheets, and short fascicles, often associated with a prominent hemangiopericytoma-like vascular pattern (**A**, low power; **B**, high power). Diffuse nuclear positivity for STAT6 confirms the diagnosis (**C**).

abundant multinucleated giant cells (formerly known as giant cell angiofibroma). Dilated and branching "hemangiopericytoma-like" blood vessels are at least focally observed, and such blood vessels may have densely, hyalinized walls. Dedifferentiation of SFT is characterized by anaplastic transition to a high-grade sarcoma, which may be associated with heterologous elements.

Ancillary Studies

STAT6 nuclear positivity represents a highly sensitive and specific immunohistochemical feature (Fig. 8.34C). In the vast majority of cases, CD34 is also strongly expressed; however, negative examples have been well documented. Like fibrosarcomatous change in DFSP, expression of CD34 may be lost in dedifferentiated SFT.

A distinctive molecular trait is inversion of the 12q13 chromosomal locus, resulting in the *NAB2-STAT6* intrachromosomal gene fusion.

Differential Diagnosis

Synovial sarcoma (SS), monophasic fibrous subtype, the most important differential diagnosis, is a fully malignant tumor that may exhibit significant morphologic overlap with SFT, including the characteristic hemangiopericytoma-like vascular pattern. However, it is classically positive for cytokeratin and EMA, but uniformly negative for STAT6 and CD34. SS is discussed in greater detail in a separate section later in this chapter.

Prognosis and Therapy

Histology is an imperfect predictor of prognosis in SFT. Traditionally, a mitotic rate exceeding 4 mitoses/10 HPF classified cases as "malignant." More recent risk stratification models (Demicco et al. 2017, Risk assessment in solitary fibrous tumors: validation and refinement of a risk stratification model), based on the patient's age, tumor size, mitotic index, and presence or absence of tumor necrosis, have attempted to better address this issue, identifying tumors more likely to display aggressive behavior. Regardless, surgical excision with negative margins should be the goal of therapy.

SOLITARY FIBROUS TUMOR – DISEASE FACT SHEET

Definition
▶▶ Cellular spindle cell neoplasm composed of uniform spindled cells, arranged haphazardly and in fascicles, within a variably fibrous to myxoid stroma with branching and hyalinizing vasculature, and associated with diffuse and strong STAT6 nuclear expression

---

Incidence and Location
▶▶ Rare, superficial, and deep soft tissues of the extremities, trunk, pelvis, and intra-abdominal cavity

Age Distribution
▶▶ Wide age range, but peak incidence is after the fifth decade

Clinical Features
▶▶ Painless, soft tissue mass
▶▶ Symptoms also are dependent on the anatomic location relative to viscera

Prognosis and Therapy
▶▶ Histology is an imperfect predictor of prognosis
▶▶ Risk stratification models based on patient's age, tumor size, mitotic rate, and presence or absence of tumor necrosis may be utilized to predict more aggressive behavior

---

SOLITARY FIBROUS TUMOR – PATHOLOGIC FEATURES

Gross Findings
▶▶ Well-circumscribed heterogeneous mass, variably hemorrhage, necrosis and/or cystic changes

Microscopic Findings
▶▶ Monotonous spindled cells arranged "patternless" and within fascicles, within a variably collagenous to myxoid stroma, associated with a prominent branching to angulated vascular pattern

Pathologic Differential Diagnoses
▶▶ Synovial sarcoma

INFLAMMATORY MYOFIBROBLASTIC TUMOR

DIFFERENTIAL DIAGNOSIS: NODULAR FASCIITIS AND DESMOID FIBROMATOSIS

Clinical Features

Inflammatory myofibroblastic tumor (IMT) is a distinctive soft tissue lesion primarily arising in the viscera and soft tissues of children and young adults (average age around 10 years). It may occur in virtually any anatomic site, but it is most frequently seen in the abdominal cavity, especially the mesentery and omentum, thorax, and mediastinum, followed by the head and neck. The anatomic location determines the symptoms and presentation but occasionally includes systemic signs, such as fever, malaise, night sweats, and weight loss. Most present as solitary masses, but multicentric disease may be seen in up to one third of cases.

Pathologic Features

GROSS FINDINGS

Nodular to multinodular mass with whorled cut surface and variable amount of hemorrhage, necrosis, and calcifications.

MICROSCOPIC FINDINGS

IMTs are composed of plump, uniform spindled cells, arranged in a variety of patterns, loosely, sheets, fascicles, and/or whorls, admixed with an inflammatory infiltrate, typically lymphoplasmacytic, within a variably collagenous to myxoid stroma (Fig. 8.35). A densely collagenous stroma with a sparse inflammatory infiltrate is characteristic of the "hypocellular" fibrous pattern. Mitotic figures in more cellular examples may be numerous but are not atypical.

Some examples of IMT exhibit substantial nuclear atypia, epithelioid to histiocytoid features, with vesicular nuclei, and prominent nucleoli; such tumors have been designated as "epithelioid" IMT.

Ancillary Studies

By definition, IMTs are myofibroblastic and therefore virtually always positive for SMA, MSA, and/or calponin, but usually negative for desmin. Focal keratin positivity may be observed in up to 30% of the tumors. An ALK immunohistochemical stain is often positive in *ALK*-rearranged tumors (Fig. 8.35C), but the immunohistochemical stain does not correlate perfectly with *ALK* mutations.

A majority of IMT are characterized by genetic translocations involving the *ALK* gene (2p23), resulting in fusion of the 3' kinase region of the *ALK* gene with various partner genes, including *TPM3/4*, *CLTC*, *CARS*, *EML4*, among others. Epithelioid inflammatory myofibroblastic sarcoma may be associated with *RANBP2-ALK* or *RRBP1-ALK* gene rearrangements.

Differential Diagnosis

The differential diagnosis may vary depending upon the anatomic site. In the head and neck and extremities, nodular fasciitis may enter the differential diagnosis. Nodular fasciitis are superficial lesions, with a tissue culture-like growth pattern and SMA positivity but lack ALK immunoreactivity and harbor a classic *USP6* gene rearrangement.

For retroperitoneal, pelvic, and intra-abdominal tumors, desmoid fibromatosis should be considered. Desmoid fibromatosis are infiltrative tumors, associated with long sweeping fascicles of spindled cells, within a

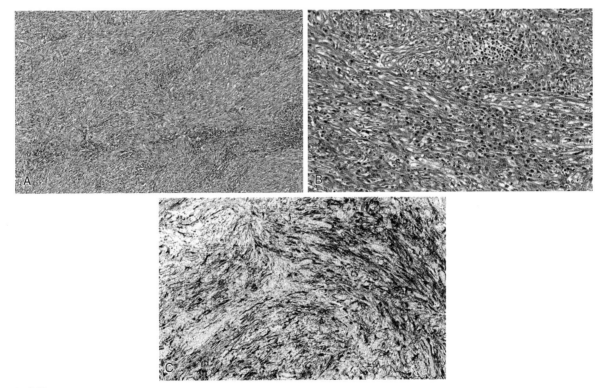

FIG. 8.35

Inflammatory myofibroblastic tumor is composed of plump, uniform spindled cells, arranged in a variety of patterns, including sheets, fascicles, and/or whorls, admixed with an inflammatory infiltrate, typically lymphoplasmacytic, within a variably collagenous to myxoid stroma (**A,** low power; **B,** high power). The neoplastic cells are commonly positive for ALK (**C**).

generally uniformly collagenous stroma that, with the exception of peripheral lymphoid aggregates, lacks significant intermingled inflammation. ALK immunopositivity is not observed.

Prognosis and Therapy

Local recurrences are seen in approximately 25% of abdominal and retroperitoneal tumors, but distant metastasis has tended to be uncommon. Epithelioid IMT behave more aggressively clinically, but otherwise, histologic features have not consistently been shown to correlate with clinical outcome. The mainstay of therapy remains surgical resection and attempts to achieve negative margins. Chemotherapy, including tyrosine kinase inhibitors, has proven effective in some tumors.

INFLAMMATORY MYOFIBROBLASTIC TUMOR – DISEASE FACT SHEET

Definition
▸▸ Rarely metastasizing myofibroblastic neoplasm with a variable mixed inflammatory infiltrate, collagenous to myxoid stroma, usually arising in the mesentery and omentum of children and young adults

Incidence and Location
▸▸ Rare tumor, potentially any location, but most commonly intra-abdominal, especially mesentery/omentum, and retroperitoneum

Age Distribution
▸▸ Children and young adults

Clinical Features
▸▸ Well-circumscribed mass presenting with symptoms related to tumor location

Prognosis and Therapy
▸▸ Local recurrences are seen up to 25% of abdominal/retroperitoneal tumors
▸▸ Epithelioid IMTs tend to behave more aggressively
▸▸ Surgical resection with negative margins remains the mainstay of therapy

---

INFLAMMATORY MYOFIBROBLASTIC TUMOR – PATHOLOGIC FEATURES

Gross Findings
▸▸ Nodular mass with whorled cut surface and variable amounts of hemorrhage, necrosis, and calcifications

Microscopic Findings
▸▸ Plump oval to spindled cells embedded in myxoid to collagenous stroma accompanied by a significant mixed inflammatory cell infiltrate, usually lymphoplasmacytic

Pathologic Differential Diagnoses
▸▸ Nodular fasciitis and desmoid fibromatosis

MYXOID TUMORS

MYXOINFLAMMATORY FIBROBLASTIC SARCOMA

DIFFERENTIAL DIAGNOSIS: MYXOFIBROSARCOMA

Clinical Features

Myxoinflammatory fibroblastic sarcoma (MFS) is a locally aggressive and infiltrative tumor predominantly involving the distal extremities in middle-aged adults. Majority of cases involve the wrists and hands, primarily the fingers, with most patients complaining of slowly growing, painless soft tissue swelling.

Pathologic Features

GROSS FINDINGS

Most are multinodular, variably fibrous to myxoid with ill-defined margins.

MICROSCOPIC FINDINGS

MFS classically manifests as an infiltrative spindle cell neoplasm associated with large, epithelioid fibroblasts with inclusion-like nucleoli (described as virocyte-like or Reed-Sternberg-like), accompanied by a prominent mixed inflammatory infiltrate and a variably myxoid to hyalinized stroma (Fig. 8.36). Within the latter, the lesional cells often appear vacuolated (pseudolipoblasts). Mitotic activity tends to be minimal despite significant cytologic atypia.

Ancillary Studies

Ancillary studies are generally not required or helpful for this diagnosis. MFS shows variable positivity for CD34 and SMA. Focal keratin positivity may be seen. Molecular events likewise have been inconsistent, with abnormalities involving *TGFBR3*, *VGLL3*, and *BRAF* documented. Hybrid examples with hemosiderotic fibrolipomatous tumor-like areas have been found to have *TGFBR3* gene rearrangements, most notably t(1;10)(p22;q24), leading to some to postulate that a subset of MFS may occupy a spectrum with hemosiderotic lipomatous tumor (HLT) and possibly pleomorphic hyalinizing angiectatic tumor (PHAT).

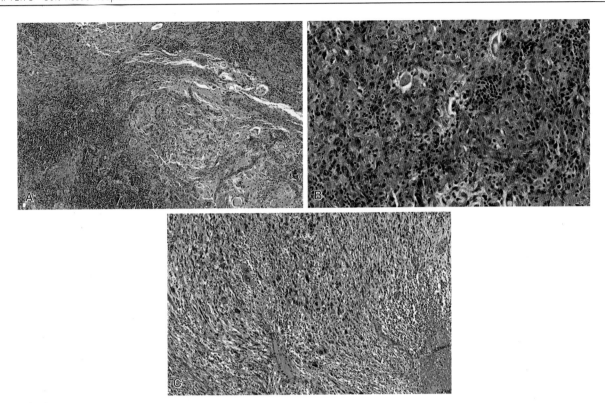

FIG. 8.36

Myxoinflammatory fibroblastic sarcoma appears as a fibroinflammatory process often associated with a myxoid to hyalinized stroma at low power **(A)**. Closer inspection uncovers an infiltrative spindle cell neoplasm composed of large, epithelioid fibroblasts with inclusion-like nucleoli **(B)**.

Differential Diagnosis

The main differential diagnosis relates to an infectious process. Attention to the clinical presentation and the presence of the markedly atypical and enlarged epithelioid fibroblasts with the inclusion-like nucleoli establishes the diagnosis of MFS. Myxofibrosarcoma may also enter the differential, but it tends to lack a significant inflammatory component, a more prominent myxoid stroma, greater mitotic activity, and more often arises in the proximal extremities.

Prognosis and Therapy

Local recurrences are relatively common, leading to amputation in up to one third of cases. Regional metastases to lymph nodes and invasion of underlying bone may occur, but distant metastases are very rare. Excision with negative margins remains the mainstay of treatment.

MYXOINFLAMMATORY FIBROBLASTIC TUMOR – DISEASE FACT SHEET

Definition
▸▸ Infiltrative neoplasm of the distal extremity characterized by markedly atypical fibroblastic cells with virocyte-like macronucleoli, a mixed inflammatory component, and a myxoid to hyalinized stroma

Incidence and Location
▸▸ Very rare, distal acral locations, especially the wrist, hands, and fingers

Age Distribution
▸▸ Wide age range, most young to middle-aged adults

Clinical Features
▸▸ Solitary, painless mass/soft tissue swelling

Prognosis and Therapy
▸▸ Excision with negative margins is the goal of treatment
▸▸ Multiple local recurrences are common

MYXOINFLAMMATORY FIBROBLASTIC TUMOR – PATHOLOGIC FEATURES

Gross Findings
▸▸ Multinodular and infiltrative, variably myxoid

Microscopic Findings
▸▸ Infiltrative, prominent mixed inflammatory infiltrative, myxoid to hyalinized stroma, and a population of markedly atypical fibroblastic cells with inclusion-like macronucleoli
▸▸ Mitotic activity is minimal

Pathologic Differential Diagnoses
▸▸ Infectious process and myxofibrosarcoma

MYXOFIBROSARCOMA

DIFFERENTIAL DIAGNOSIS: MYXOMA

Clinical Features

Mxyofibrosarcomas typically arise as superficial subcutaneous and painless masses in the extremities of older adults, between 50 and 80 years of age. Pediatric involvement is very rare, but intramuscular and/or subfascial lesions occasionally occur. Myxofibrosarcoma-like lesions arising in intra-abdominal and retroperitoneal regions almost always represent ALT/WDL and/or, when high grade, DLs.

Pathologic Features

GROSS FINDINGS

Most are superficial, multinodular but infiltrative firm fibrous to mucinous lesions. Deep-seated lesions more often form a solitary, infiltrative mass.

MICROSCOPIC FINDINGS

Histologic features of myxofibrosarcoma are variable, largely reflecting the histologic grade of the neoplasm; however, regardless of grade, these tumors, especially when superficial, tend to be significantly pleomorphic, multinodular, and infiltrative. Low-grade lesions are relatively hypocellular, closely resembling myxoma, with scattered atypical, sometimes multinucleated hyperchromatic cells accompanied by arborizing to curvilinear blood vessels (Fig. 8.37A). Mitotic figures are not easily found. High-grade examples also have solid areas, largely devoid of myxoid stroma, consisting entirely of the pleomorphic spindled cells, arranged in cellular fascicles and compact sheets, with numerous mitoses. As expected, intermediate-grade tumors lack the solid sheets, instead showing at least moderate cellularity with clearly evident background myxoid stroma (Fig. 8.37B). Histologic grade may vary from one field to the next, with nodules of low-grade tumor immediately adjacent to higher-grade areas. Sampling is therefore critical to establish the correct diagnosis and provide data for prognostication. On occasion, multivacuolated cells, so-called pseudolipoblasts, are associated with mucin.

Rarely, myxofibrosarcoma may be composed of predominantly epithelioid cells, with round vesicular nuclei and abundant eosinophilic cytoplasm, resembling carcinoma or melanoma.

Ancillary Studies

Immunohistochemical studies are not generally helpful nor needed to establish the diagnosis. Myxofibrosarcomas may show focal SMA and CD34 expression but are negative for S100, desmin, myogenin, and MDM2. There is no recurrent gene fusion/rearrangement, characteristic of myxofibrosarcoma.

Differential Diagnosis

For lower-grade lesions, the most important differential diagnosis is intramuscular myxoma. Myxofibrosarcomas are less often intramuscular, more often multinodular and infiltrative, and always, regardless of grade, exhibit significantly more nuclear atypia than should ever be observed in myxomas. Conversely, myxomas are by definition intramuscular neoplasms, often entrapping skeletal muscle in their myxoid matrix (Fig. 8.38). On occasion, myxomas may be more cellular and vascularity

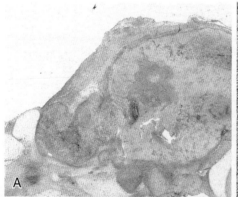
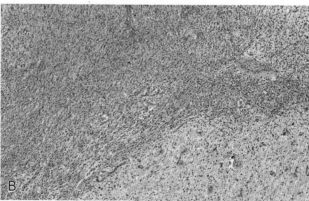

FIG. 8.37

Myxofibrosarcoma is a highly infiltrative, nodular, and variably cellular to myxoid neoplasm with exhibiting significant cytologic atypia (**A,** low power; **B,** high power). Lower-grade areas may resemble myxoma, while the highest grade more cellular foci resemble undifferentiated pleomorphic sarcomas with minimal evident myxoid stroma (**C**).

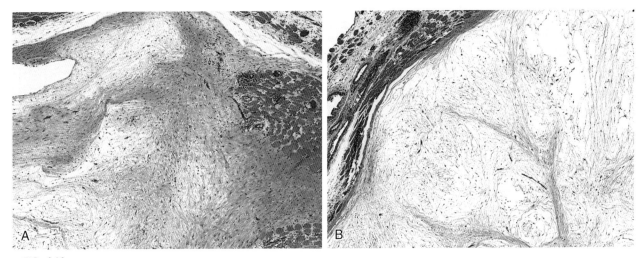

FIG. 8.38

A and **B,** Intramuscular myxomas are usually hypocellular and hypovascular neoplasms with prominent myxoid matrix, often entrapping skeletal muscle.

more prominent, but nuclear atypia/pleomorphism, significant mitotic activity, and tumor necrosis always are absent. When necessary, GNAS mutation analysis may help confirm the diagnosis of intramuscular myxoma. Higher-grade forms of myxofibrosarcoma may raise the possibility of UPS. However, the presence of a minor myxoid component with the classic vascular (at least 10% of the tumor volume) helps establish the diagnosis of high-grade myxofibrosarcoma.

Prognosis and Therapy

Regardless of grade, local recurrences are frequent, affecting up to 50% of cases, largely the result of incomplete excision. To be fair, obtaining negative margins can be difficult. Histologic grade correlates with risk of metastases and overall survival. Local control generally requires aggressive surgery, and radiation therapy also may be employed. A worse prognosis is associated with epithelioid variant.

MYXOFIBROSARCOMA – DISEASE FACT SHEET

Definition
▸▸ A pleomorphic myxoid mesenchymal neoplasm ranging from low-grade lesions resembling myxoma to more solid, less myxoid lesions, with features of undifferentiated pleomorphic sarcoma

Incidence and Location
▸▸ A common sarcoma of elderly patients, extremities and limb girdles, subcutis more common than intramuscular

Age Distribution
▸▸ Elderly patients, majority 50–80 years of age

Clinical Features
▸▸ Slowly growing, painless superficial mass

Prognosis and Therapy
▸▸ Local recurrences are common, up to 50% of cases
▸▸ Distant metastases are more likely in higher grade, larger tumors and the epithelioid subtype

---

MYXOFIBROSARCOMA – PATHOLOGIC FEATURES

Gross Findings
▸▸ Superficial, multinodular, and infiltrative solid fleshy to mucinous and gelatinous masses

Microscopic Findings
▸▸ Multinodular and infiltrative, pleomorphic spindled to less commonly epithelioid neoplasm, with variable cellularity and myxoid change, ranging from myxoma-like nodules to solid sheets reminiscent of undifferentiated pleomorphic sarcoma
▸▸ Arborizing and curvilinear vascular pattern, especially prominent in more myxoid zones

Pathologic Differential Diagnoses
▸▸ Myxoma, if low grade, and undifferentiated pleomorphic sarcoma, for high-grade lesions

---

EXTRASKELETAL MYXOID CHONDROSARCOMA

DIFFERENTIAL DIAGNOSIS: MYOEPITHELIOMA/MYOEPITHELIAL CARCINOMA

Clinical Features

Most patients are middle-aged to older adults and present with a painless, deep-seated soft tissue mass, typically

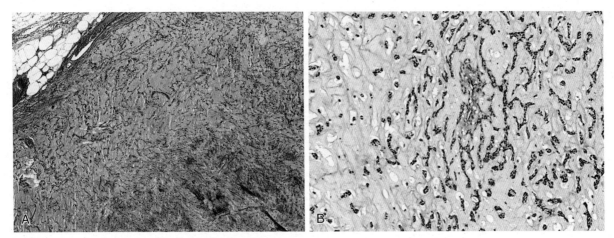

FIG. 8.39

Extraskeletal myxoid chondrosarcoma is a deceptively circumscribed, multinodular neoplasm **(A)**, composed of uniform, round to spindled cells, organized in nests, rings, chains, cords, and/or anastomosing strands **(B)**.

involving the proximal extremities, especially the thigh. Less common anatomic sites include the trunk, abdomen, pelvis, paraspinal tissues, and very rarely, as a primary bone tumor.

Pathologic Features

GROSS FINDINGS

Extraskeletal myxoid chondrosarcoma (EMC) form well-defined, multinodular tumors, with a glistening mucoid cut surface dissected by fibrous septa, accompanied by variable amounts of hemorrhage and necrosis.

MICROSCOPIC FINDINGS

EMC appear deceptively circumscribed and multinodular, dissected into variably sized myxoid nodules by fibrous septa. The neoplastic cells are uniform, round to spindled, often organized in nests, rings, chains, cords, and/or anastomosing strands (Fig. 8.39). The cellularity is variable but often increased toward the periphery of individual nodules. Importantly, some cases exhibit hypercellularity throughout the tumor, accompanied by epithelioid features and a less conspicuous myxoid stroma. Rhabdoid features, with eccentrically placed round nuclei and abundant eosinophilic cytoplasm with hyaline globules, is a well-described phenomenon in a minority of tumors. Despite the name, true hyaline cartilage differentiation is virtually never seen. Mitotic figures tend to be low, with fewer than 1 to 2 mitoses/10 HPF. Significant nuclear atypia/pleomorphism is not a feature of EMC.

Ancillary Studies

Immunohistochemically, S100 and CD117 are positive in only a minority of tumors, while GFAP and broad-spectrum cytokeratin expression is very rare. INI-1

(SMARCB1) nuclear loss is characteristic of tumors with rhabdoid features. *NR4A3* (9q22) gene rearrangements are a defining feature of EMC, usually involving the *EWSR1* gene (22q12); less often, the *TAF15* (17q12) gene is the partner.

Differential Diagnosis

EMC may be virtually indistinguishable from myoepithelial neoplasms, especially myoepithelial carcinoma. Co-expression of S100 and keratins, a defining feature of myoepithelial tumors, is rarely observed in EMC. Both may share *EWSR1* gene rearrangements, but EMC alone has a *NR4A3* gene fusion. The curvilinear and arborizing vasculature, typical of other myxoid neoplasms, such as ML or myxofibrosarcoma, are not present. Significant nuclear pleomorphism and atypia is not observed in EMC.

Prognosis and Therapy

Prolonged survival is characteristic of EMC; however, long-term follow-up reveals high rates of local recurrence and metastatic disease, indicative of a higher-grade neoplasm than morphologic features suggest. Adverse prognostic indicators include older age of the patient, tumor size >10 cm, and proximal anatomic location. Wide surgical resection with negative margins is the treatment of choice, but prolonged close clinical follow-up is necessary.

EXTRASKELETAL MYXOID CHONDROSARCOMA – DISEASE FACT SHEET

Definition

▸▸ Malignant mesenchymal neoplasm characterized by a multinodular growth pattern, abundant myxoid changes, and mostly uniform round to spindled cells arranged in cords, chains and rings, and anastomosing strands

Incidence and Location
▶▶ Rare tumor, proximal extremities, especially the thigh

Age Distribution
▶▶ Middle-aged to older patients, 40–60 years of age

Clinical Features
▶▶ Painless, deep-seated soft tissue mass

Prognosis and Therapy
▶▶ Long-term follow-up reveals higher rates of aggressive behavior than would be expected by analysis of morphology alone
▶▶ Wide surgical excision with negative margins is the primary goal of therapy

EXTRASKELETAL MYXOID CHONDROSARCOMA – PATHOLOGIC FEATURES

Gross Findings
▶▶ Well-defined, multilobulated, gelatinous to mucinous nodules separated by fibrous septa, variably hemorrhage and necrosis

Microscopic Findings
▶▶ Deceptively circumscribed, multinodular abundantly myxoid neoplasm traversed by fibrous septa, variably cellularity, uniform round to spindled cells arranged in cords, rings, nests, and anastomosing strands
▶▶ Significant nuclear atypia/pleomorphism is not observed
▶▶ Rhabdoid features in a minority of cases
▶▶ True hyaline cartilage differentiation is virtually never seen

Pathologic Differential Diagnoses
▶▶ Most commonly myoepithelioma/myoepithelial carcinoma, less often myxofibrosarcoma and myxoid liposarcoma

LOW-GRADE FIBROMYXOID SARCOMA

DIFFERENTIAL DIAGNOSIS: SCLEROSING EPITHELIOID FIBROSARCOMA AND NODULAR FASCIITIS

Clinical Features

LGFS typically presents a painless mass, usually involving the deep soft tissues of proximal extremities and trunk, in young adult patients, affecting males and females equally. Superficial lesions appear to be more common in children.

Pathologic Features

GROSS FINDINGS

Usually relatively well-circumscribed, densely fibrous to mucoid lesions, ranging from 1 to >20 cm.

MICROSCOPIC FINDINGS

LGFS are well-circumscribed to infiltrative lesions composed of deceptively bland-appearing spindled cells, arranged in sheets and fascicles, associated with moderately cellular collagenized zones alternating with more myxoid regions (Fig. 8.40). In the latter, arcades of blood vessels are common. Mitotic figures tend to be scarce. Less often, large collagenized rosettes surrounded by a layer of more epithelioid fibroblasts occur (Fig. 8.40C), a lesion formally known as hyalinizing spindle cell tumor with giant rosettes. Rarely, LGFS may exhibit round cell areas indistinguishable from sclerosing epithelioid fibrosarcoma (SEF).

Ancillary Studies

MUC-4 is expressed in the cytoplasm of virtually all cases (Fig. 8.40D), being highly sensitive and specific for LGFS. EMA is commonly positive, and focal reactivity for SMA is sometimes seen. S100, cytokeratin, and desmin are negative. *FUS* gene rearrangements are the defining molecular abnormality, most often manifesting as the t(7;16)(q33;p11), *FUS-CREBL2* gene fusion, and, less often, (11;16)(p11;p11), *FUS-CREB3L1*.

Differential Diagnosis

Given its deceptively bland appearance, benign lesions, such as nodular fasciitis, may be confused with LGFS. Nodular fasciitis is typically more superficial and smaller and exhibits bland spindled cells in a loose tissue culture-like stroma. Immunohistochemically, nodular fasciitis is diffusely positive for SMA and always negative for MUC-4.

SEF is a rare sarcoma characterized by epithelioid fibroblasts arranged in distinct cords and nest in a densely sclerotic collagenized stroma (Fig. 8.41). The majority also appear positive for MUC-4 (Fig. 8.41B). A subset has areas indistinguishable from LGFS, and these tumors typically contain the same *FUS* gene rearrangements, likely within the spectrum of LGFS. The majority of SEF have *EWSR1* gene rearrangements, likely indicating a separate distinct neoplasm. The prognosis of SEF is very similar to that seen with LGFS, with local recurrence and metastatic rates approaching 50%.

Prognosis and Therapy

Despite its bland appearance, long-term follow-up reveals local recurrences in approximately 60% to 70% of

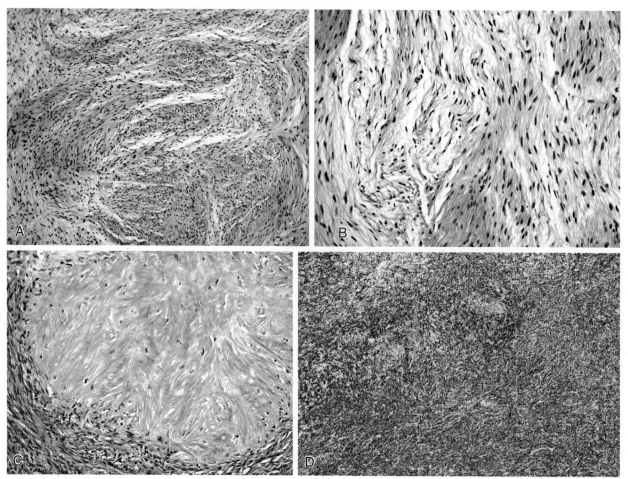

FIG. 8. 40

Low-grade fibromyxoid sarcoma is composed of bland spindled cells, arranged in sheets and fascicles, associated with moderately cellular collagenized zones alternating with more myxoid regions (**A,** low power; **B,** high power). Occasionally, large collagenized rosettes can be seen, as part of a spectrum originally designated as hyalinizing spindle cell tumor with giant rosettes (**C**). The spindled cells are diffusely and strongly positive for MUC4 (**D**).

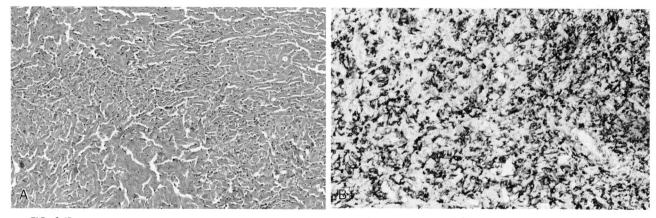

FIG. 8.41

Sclerosing epithelioid fibrosarcoma (SEF) is characterized by epithelioid fibroblasts arranged in distinct to vague cords and nest in a densely sclerotic and collagenized stroma (**A**). A subset of these tumors likely represents a spectrum with low-grade fibromyxoid sarcoma and also are positive for MUC4 (**B**).

patients, with distant metastases and death in approximately 40% to 50%. Surgical resection with negative margins is recommended. There is no specific histologic feature that correlates with prognosis.

LOW-GRADE FIBROMYXOID SARCOMA – DISEASE FACT SHEET

Definition
▶▶ A bland-appearing fibromyxoid sarcoma characterized by alternating more cellular collagenous zones and myxoid areas, composed of uniform spindled cells arranged in short fascicles and whorls

Incidence and Location
▶▶ Rare sarcoma, deep subfascial tissues of the proximal extremities and trunk

Age Distribution
▶▶ Wide age range, but most commonly young adults

Clinical Features
▶▶ Painless soft tissue mass, deep seated

Prognosis and Therapy
▶▶ Long-term close clinical follow-up is indicated, as local recurrence and metastatic rates ultimately range higher than would be expected based on the morphologic features alone

---

LOW-GRADE FIBROMYXOID SARCOMA – PATHOLOGIC FEATURES

Gross Findings
▶▶ Usually well-circumscribed, firm to focally mucinous lesions

Microscopic Findings
▶▶ Deceptively bland spindled cells, arranged in fascicles and whorls, associated with alternating more cellular collagenous zones and less cellular myxoid areas

Pathologic Differential Diagnoses
▶▶ Nodular fasciitis and a subset of sclerosing epithelioid fibrosarcomas represent a spectrum

---

OSSIFYING FIBROMYXOID TUMOR

DIFFERENTIAL DIAGNOSIS: LOW-GRADE FIBROMYXOID SARCOMA

Clinical Features

Frequently, patients complain of superficial soft tissue swelling, involving the extremities, particularly the lower limb. There is a wide age range, but most affected patients are middle-aged to older adults. Lesions typically arise in the subcutis; intramuscular localization tends to be rare.

Pathologic Features

GROSS FINDINGS

Ossifying fibromyxoid tumors (OFMTs) are well-circumscribed, lobulated and firm, white-tan to slightly myxoid masses, without significant hemorrhage or necrosis.

MICROSCOPIC FINDINGS

The tumors are classically well circumscribed with fibrous capsule/pseudocapsule associated with septa, lobulation, and at least a partial peripheral woven to lamellar bone shell. Individual tumor cells are relatively uniform, ovoid to slightly spindled, arranged in cellular sheets, nests, and anastomosing cords, within a variably fibrous to myxoid stroma (see Fig. 8.42). Mitotic activity tends to be inconspicuous. Some have proposed a "malignant" subtype, with high cellularity, nuclear atypia, mitotic activity >2 mitoses/50 HPF, and more centrally located osteoid/bone deposition.

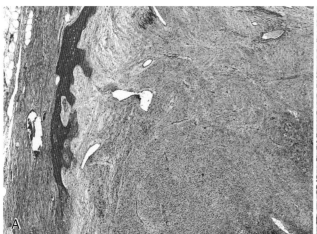
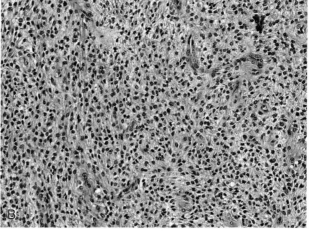

FIG. 8.42

Ossifying fibromyxoid tumor is a well-circumscribed neoplasm with usually with a peripheral woven to lamellar bone shell **(A)** and composed of uniform, ovoid to slightly spindled cells, arranged in cellular sheets, nests, and anastomosing cords, within a variably fibrous to myxoid stroma **(B)**.

Ancillary Studies

Classic examples co-express desmin and S100, but some may be positive for MUC4, EMA, SMA, and cytokeratins. The majority, whether typical or malignant, exhibit a gene fusion, usually involving the *PHF1* gene.

Differential Diagnosis

Given the fact that OFMT may occasionally express MUC4, an important differential diagnosis is LGFS. The latter does not express desmin or S100, and molecular studies show a consistent, reliable, and recurrent *FUS* gene rearrangement. Myoepithelioma may be difficult to distinguish from OFMT, especially given the frequent co-expression of S100 and myoid markers, but, unlike OFMT, these tumors tend to lack desmin positivity. A subset of myoepithelial carcinomas has *EWSR1* gene rearrangements.

Prognosis and Therapy

Long-term clinical follow-up is recommended, as even cases without obvious "atypical" or "malignant" features may locally recur or metastasize a decade or more after the initial diagnosis. Those with "malignant" features are significantly more likely to develop distant metastases. Surgical excision with negative margins is recommended.

OSSIFYING FIBROMYXOID TUMOR – DISEASE FACT SHEET

Definition
- ▸▸ Circumscribed and lobulated mesenchymal neoplasm with at least a partial bony capsule and a population of uniform ovoid cells arranged in nests and cords, within a fibromyxoid stroma

Incidence and Location
- ▸▸ Rare mesenchymal tumor, most commonly subcutis of the extremities

Age Distribution
- ▸▸ Wide age range, but most are adults

Clinical Features
- ▸▸ Painless, slow-growing mass

Prognosis and Therapy
- ▸▸ Histology is an imperfect predictor of prognosis, although most appear indolent
- ▸▸ Those with "malignant features," including high cellularity and mitotic figures, are more likely to exhibit distant metastases
- ▸▸ Surgical excision with negative margins

OSSIFYING FIBROMYXOID TUMOR – PATHOLOGIC FEATURES

Gross Findings
- ▸▸ Well circumscribed, often encapsulated, fibrous white-tan to slightly myxoid

Microscopic Findings
- ▸▸ Well circumscribed, variably encapsulated, nodular, with a partial to complete peripheral bone shell, composed of mostly uniform ovoid cells, arranged in sheets, nests, and cords, within a fibrous to myxoid stroma

Pathologic Differential Diagnoses
- ▸▸ Low-grade fibromyxoid sarcoma and myoepithelioma

MYOEPITHELIOMA/MIXED TUMOR

DIFFERENTIAL DIAGNOSIS: MYOEPITHELIAL CARCINOMA

Clinical Features

Myoepithelial neoplasms of soft tissue usually arise in subcutaneous tissues of the extremities, particularly the lower limb. Less commonly, the trunk and/or intramuscular tissues are involved. The age range is wide, but peak incidence is between 30 and 50 years of age. Most patients complain of a palpable, painless mass/swelling.

Pathologic Features

GROSS FINDINGS

Myoepitheliomas tend to be well-circumscribed, nodular, and variably myxoid to fleshy lesions. Myoepithelial carcinomas more often exhibit infiltrative margins and tend to be larger.

MICROSCOPIC FINDINGS

Similar to those seen in the salivary glands, myoepithelial neoplasms are generally circumscribed, lobular neoplasms, typically composed of epithelioid to spindled cells, with uniform nuclei and eosinophilic to clear cytoplasm, arranged in cords, nests, trabecula, and sheets, within a myxoid to hyalinized stroma (Fig. 8.43). Extensive cytoplasmic vacuolation is a feature described in the past as "parachordoma," representing a spectrum of myoepithelial tumors. The presence of true ductal differentiation defines the "mixed tumor" spectrum. Foci of osteoid/bone and/or hyaline cartilaginous differentiation

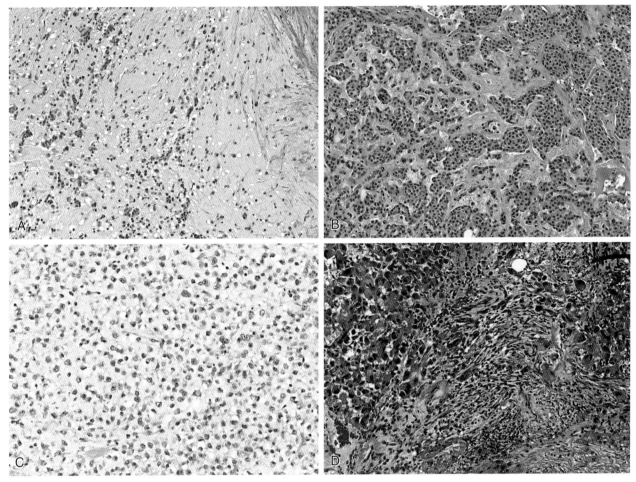

FIG. 8.43

Myoepitheliomas are generally circumscribed, lobular tumors, typically composed of epithelioid to spindled cells, with uniform nuclei and eosinophilic to clear cytoplasm, arranged in cords **(A)**, nests **(B)**, trabecula, and sheets **(C)**, within a myxoid to hyalinized stroma. Myoepithelial carcinomas exhibit greater nuclear atypia with prominent nucleoli, a higher mitotic index, and/or tumor necrosis **(D)**.

is seen in a minority of cases. Myoepithelial carcinomas share many of the above features of their benign counterparts but tend to show greater nuclear atypia with prominent nucleoli, a higher mitotic index, and/or tumor necrosis (Fig. 8.43D). An undifferentiated small round cell component may be prominent, especially in pediatric cases.

Ancillary Studies

In the absence of ductal differentiation, confirmation of myoepithelial differentiation usually requires the use of immunohistochemistry. Co-expression of broad-spectrum cytokeratin and S100 is observed in the virtually all cases, helping define this group of tumors. EMA, SMA, and/or calponin also are positive in the majority of tumors. Desmin is infrequently seen, but myogenin and Myo-D1 are negative. In our experience, Sox10 is only rarely expressed. INI-1 (SMARCB1) nuclear loss is detected in a minority of myoepithelial carcinomas.

EWSR1 (less often *FUS*) gene rearrangements are observed in about 50% of cases, with a variety of partners including *POU5F1*, *PBX1*, *ZNF444*, *ATF1*, and others. *EWSR1-POU5F1* tumors are typically seen in the deep soft tissues of pediatric patients and may be mistaken for Ewing sarcoma-like round cell lesions. Like their salivary gland counterparts, tumors with ductal differentiation (mixed tumors) usually have *PLAG1* gene fusions.

Differential Diagnosis

The most important differential diagnosis is recognizing myoepithelial neoplasms that are more likely to behave aggressively, namely "carcinomas." The presence of moderate to severe nuclear atypia, with prominent nucleoli, is the only reliable criteria for this separation. Myoepitheliomas and, especially, myoepithelial carcinoma may be virtually indistinguishable from EMC. Immunohistochemically, most examples of the latter are negative for S100, and keratin, SMA, and calponin are virtually always negative. Both myoepithelioma/myoepithelial carcinoma and EMC can have *EWSR1* gene rearrangements. Identification of the *NR4A3* gene rearrangement in EMC may be helpful in difficult cases.

Prognosis and Therapy

Most myoepithelial neoplasms exhibit benign clinical behavior. However, histology is an imperfect predictor of prognosis in myoepithelial tumors of soft tissue, and even tumors without any obvious "malignant features" may locally recur and rarely metastasize. Moderate to severe nuclear atypia is the only reliable criteria, defining "carcinoma," capable of predicting a higher risk of metastatic disease, in up to 50% of cases. Surgical excision with negative margins is the recommended therapy.

MIXED TUMOR/MYOEPITHELIOMA – DISEASE FACT SHEET

Definition
▸▸ A mesenchymal neoplasm of soft tissues with morphologic and immunohistochemical features closely resembling those seen in the salivary gland

Incidence and Location
▸▸ Rare, extremities, especially lower limb, subcutis more common than intramuscular

Age Distribution
▸▸ Wide age range, but most common in young to middle-aged adults

Clinical Features
▸▸ Soft tissue mass/swelling, painless

Prognosis and Therapy
▸▸ Histology is an imperfect predictor of prognosis, although most behave in a benign fashion
▸▸ Most important criteria of aggressive behavior are nuclear atypia and prominent nucleoli, helping define "carcinomas"

MIXED TUMOR/MYOEPITHELIOMA – PATHOLOGIC FEATURES

Gross Findings
▸▸ Most circumscribed, lobulated and variably myxoid
▸▸ Malignant (carcinomas) lesions more commonly have infiltrative margins

Microscopic Findings
▸▸ Well demarcated, lobulated neoplasm, composed of mostly uniform epithelioid to plasmacytoid to spindled cells, arranged in cords, nests, and sheets within a variably myxoid to hyalinized stroma
▸▸ Osseous and/or cartilaginous metaplasia is present in a minority of cases
▸▸ "Carcinomas" defined by moderate to severe nuclear atypia and prominent nucleoli

Pathologic Differential Diagnoses
▸▸ Myoepithelial carcinoma and extraskeletal myxoid chondrosarcoma

---

GIANT CELL–RICH TUMORS

TENOSYNOVIAL GIANT CELL TUMOR

DIFFERENTIAL DIAGNOSIS: GIANT CELL TUMOR OF SOFT TISSUE, PLEXIFORM FIBROHISTIOCYTIC TUMOR

Clinical Features

TGCTs are a group of lesions defined by evidence of "synovial differentiation" and a localized to diffuse growth pattern, associated with extremity tendon sheaths and the synovium bursae and joint capsules. The localized form, also known as giant cell tumor of tendon sheath, occurs predominantly in the hands (and feet), typically the tendon sheaths of the fingers, as a painless soft tissue mass. The diffuse form, also known as pigmented villonodular synovitis, may be intra-articular, commonly affecting the knee and hip, or extra-articular, adjacent to the knee, thigh, and ankle/foot. Intra-articular involvement often leads to hemorrhagic joint effusions, pain, swelling, and limitation of movement.

Pathologic Features

GROSS FINDINGS

Localized TGCT forms well-circumscribed and nodular lesions, white-yellow to brown, and usually small. Diffuse TGCT is larger, multinodular and, when intra-articular, expands synovial fronds creating a villous appearance.

MICROSCOPIC FINDINGS

Localized lesions are well-circumscribed, lobulated lesions, characterized by fibrous septa separating the tumor into variably sized nodules and nests, containing mixtures of histiocytoid cells, inflammatory cells, xanthomatous changes, and hemosiderin pigment (Fig. 8.44). The characteristic lesional cells range from the predominant, smaller histiocytoid cells, with pale cytoplasm and round to reniform nuclei, to larger epithelioid cells with mostly round nuclei, often associated with a cytoplasmic rim of hemosiderin pigment. Osteoclast-type giant cells are randomly distributed. The stroma ranges from minimal collagenous to hyalinized. Aggregates of foamy histiocytes (xanthomatous change) are variable but virtually always seen.

Virtually identical cytologic and histologic features are observed in the "diffuse" form, but these tumors are infiltrative and, if intra-articular, show a villous appearance, with variably expansion of synovial fronds (Fig. 8.45). Osteoclast-type giant cells may be less conspicuous, and

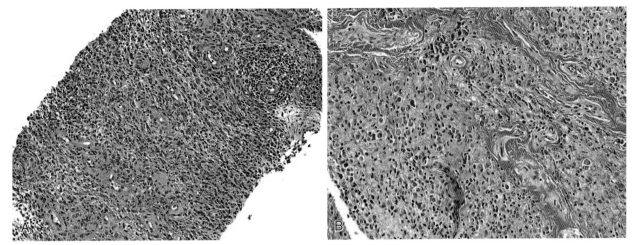

FIG. 8.44

A and **B**, Tenosynovial giant cell tumor, localized type is a well-circumscribed, lobulated lesion, characterized by fibrous septa separating the tumor into variably sized nodules and nests, containing mixtures of histiocytoid cells, inflammatory cells, xanthomatous changes, and hemosiderin pigment.

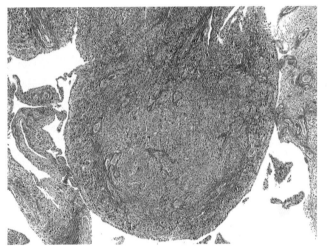

FIG. 8.45

Tenosynovial giant cell tumor, diffuse type has similar cytologic features as the localized type, but is infiltrative, can be intra-articular with villous appearance, and variably expansion of synovial fronds.

pseudosynovial clefts and blood-filled pseudoalveolar spaces may be present. Hemosiderin deposits always are at least focally present. Mitotic activity may be brisk, and necrosis can be present.

Ancillary Studies

The lesional cells are positive for histiocytic markers CD68 and CD163. Clusterin and, sometimes, desmin are expressed by the larger histiocytoid to epithelioid cells. S100, Sox10, and SMA are negative. Gene rearrangements of the *CSF1* gene characterize all forms of TGCT.

Differential Diagnosis

The development of malignant transformation of TGCT is an extremely rare and somewhat controversial event. Generally, it is heralded by the development of a more obvious malignant component, with large cells, atypical mitoses, necrosis, and spindling; the pre-existing benign-appearing TGCT often remains at least focally evident.

Giant cell tumor of soft tissue is a rare tumor that shows morphologic overlap with the more common giant cell tumor of bone. These tumors arise as superficial masses in the extremities and, less frequently, in the trunk, in adults. Histologically, they are well circumscribed with cellular nodules composed of mononuclear histiocytoid cells and abundant osteoclast-type giant cells (Fig. 8.46). Most display evidence of osseous metaplasia, often existing as at least a partial peripheral shell. Aneurysmal bone cyst-like changes are less often present.

Plexiform fibrohistiocytic tumor is a very rare multinodular to plexiform tumor, arising in the dermis and subcutis (Fig. 8.47) of the extremities in children and young adults. Bland-appearing and infiltrative, often SMA-positive spindled cells are arranged in fascicles and accompany the classic nodules of more epithelioid cells and osteoclast-type giant cells. The characteristic morphologic features and anatomic location should easily distinguish this tumor from TGCT.

Prognosis and Therapy

Simple excision is usually curative for the localized form, with local, but non-destructive, recurrence in about 20% of cases. Given its large size and growth pattern, diffuse TGCT is more difficult to eradicate, and

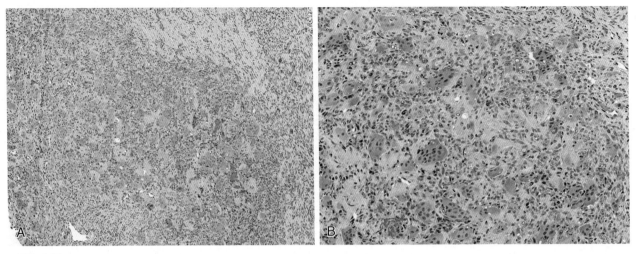

FIG. 8.46

A and **B,** Giant cell tumor of soft tissue is a well-circumscribed lesion composed of uniform mononuclear cells admixed with abundant osteoclast-type giant cells, closely resembling giant cell tumor of bone.

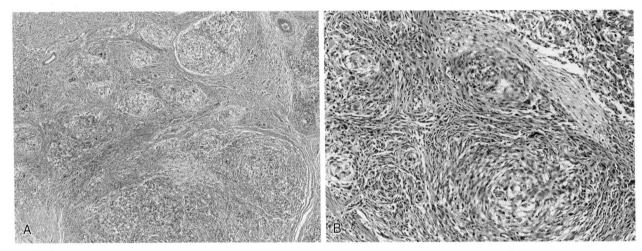

FIG. 8.47

Plexiform fibrohistiocytic tumor is a bland, infiltrative and "plexiform" neoplasm **(A)**, composed of spindled cells arranged in fascicles and accompanied by nodules of more epithelioid cells admixed with osteoclast-type giant cells **(B)**.

locally recurs in up to 50% of cases. Malignant transformation results in an aggressive clinical course with distant metastases and a frequently fatal outcome.

TENOSYNOVIAL GIANT CELL TUMOR – DISEASE FACT SHEET

Definition

▶▶ An intra- or extra-articular histiocytoid-appearing neoplasm with synovial differentiation, most commonly arising in tendon sheaths of the hands and fingers (localized form) and, less often, diffusely affecting large joints, usually the knee (diffuse form)

Incidence and Location

▶▶ Localized form is one of the most common tumors of the hand
▶▶ Diffuse form commonly affects larger joints, especially the knee, less commonly the hips

Age Distribution

▶▶ Young to middle-aged adults

Clinical Features

▶▶ Superficial painless mass for localized form
▶▶ Diffuse form may be associated with swelling, limitation of movement, pain, and joint effusions

Prognosis and Therapy

▶▶ Localized form generally easily managed by surgery
▶▶ Diffuse form, locally recurs in up to 50% of cases

TENOSYNOVIAL GIANT CELL TUMOR – PATHOLOGIC FEATURES

Gross Findings

▶▶ Circumscribed and nodular to diffuse and villous, variably firm white to yellow to brown cut surface

Microscopic Findings

▶▶ Localized to diffuse growth pattern, characteristic small to larger histiocytoid cells, admixed with foamy histiocytes, hemosiderin pigment, and osteoclast-type giant cells, within a variably collagenous stroma

VASCULAR TUMORS

HEMANGIOMA AND VARIANTS

DIFFERENTIAL DIAGNOSIS: ANGIOSARCOMA

Clinical Features

Hemangiomas are benign vascular proliferations. Based on specific histologic features and clinical presentation, the hemangiomas may be further classified into a variety of subtypes, some of which are prognostically relevant.

The most common form of hemangioma, infantile (juvenile or capillary) hemangioma is seen in infancy and children, usually involving the head and neck. The natural history is one of rapid growth, often beginning shortly after birth, followed by gradual involution over months to years. Lobular capillary hemangioma, also known as pyogenic granuloma, presents as a rapidly growing, often ulcerated superficial vascular proliferation, most commonly seen in the skin and oral mucosa of the head and neck and fingers, affecting patients over a wide age range. Intramuscular angiomas are benign vascular lesions specifically occurring within skeletal muscle, associated with slow growth and often pain, especially when localized to the extremities and following exercise. Most cases present in adolescents and young adults, representing one of the most common deep-seated soft tissue tumors of adults. When involving multiple tissue planes or forming extremely large lesions, it may be referred to as "angiomatosis." Anastomosing hemangiomas typically occur in the viscera of adults, most often kidney and retroperitoneum, and symptoms are related to the specific anatomic site but may be incidental. Spindle cell hemangioma, originally referred to as "hemangioendotheliomas," commonly presents as solitary to multiple cutaneous nodules on the extremity, is rarely associated with Maffucci syndrome (with enchondromatosis), often mimics Kaposi sarcoma, and usually arises in middle-aged adults.

Pathologic Features

GROSS FINDINGS

Infantile hemangiomas typically resemble a birth mark, being superficial and forming flat, red lesions. Lobular capillary hemangiomas are superficial, polypoid, and exophytic, and commonly ulcerated and hemorrhagic lesions. Intramuscular angiomas are typically large, intramuscular lesions which infiltrate the surrounding tissue. Thrombi may be grossly visible in the largest vessels, but admixed adipose tissue is always present. Anastomosing hemangiomas form a hemorrhagic and ill-defined, red-brown vascular neoplasm, often multifocal. Spindle cell hemangioma exhibit solitary to multiple, cutaneous dark red to blue nodules.

MICROSCOPIC FINDINGS

Infantile hemangiomas are characteristic lobulated lesions composed of compact, often uniform capillary-sized blood vessels, often associated with a central feeder blood vessel (Fig. 8.48). Older lesions exhibit more dilated and canalized blood vessels. Endothelial cells appear benign and flattened.

Lobular capillary hemangioma represents an exophytic to polypoid vascular proliferation, at least partially surrounded by an epidermal collaret and more centrally ulcerated. The tumor is composed of capillaries of variable caliber, arranged in lobules, often with a more central feeding vessel (Fig. 8.49). The endothelial cells lack any significant cytologic atypia. The background stroma is edematous and commonly shows significant neutrophilic infiltration. Mitotic activity is seen.

Intramuscular angiomas exhibit a heterogeneous appearance, being composed of a mixture of small, capillary sized, medium to large thin-walled and ectatic, and muscular-walled blood vessels, admixed with variable amounts of adipose tissue.

Anastomosing hemangiomas are characteristically lobulated and composed of thin-walled, anastomosing vascular channels, lined by single layer of endothelial cells with prominent protuberant (hobnail) nuclei. Thrombi with areas of necrosis and hyalinization are common (Fig. 8.50). Extramedullary hematopoiesis and hyaline globules may be striking.

Spindle cell hemangioma are well circumscribed, often intravascular, and composed of endothelial cells with spindled to epithelioid morphology, forming vascular spaces, some cavernous and ectatic (Fig. 8.51). The low-power view has often been described as looking like a combination of Kaposi sarcoma and cavernous hemangioma. Scattered vacuolated cells with abundant clear cytoplasm and thrombi with or without calcifications (also known as phleboliths) also are characteristic.

Ancillary Studies

Vascular endothelial Immunohistochemical markers obviously are positive in the endothelial cells (CD31, CD34 and ERG) of hemangiomas, but ancillary studies

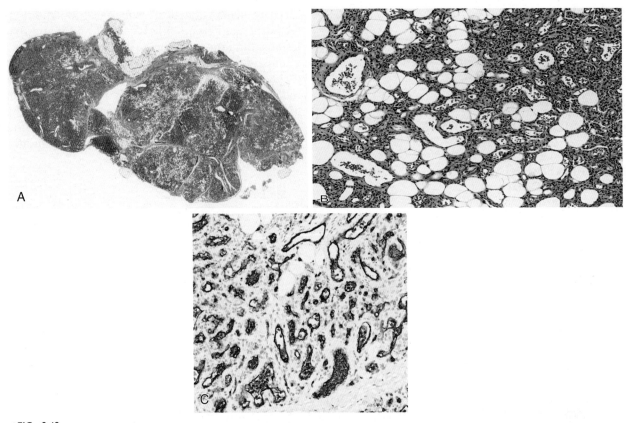

FIG. 8.48

Infantile hemangioma is lobulated vascular neoplasm **(A)**, usually composed of compact, often uniform capillary-sized blood vessels with a pericyte layer **(B)**. They are characteristically positive for GLUT-1 **(C)**.

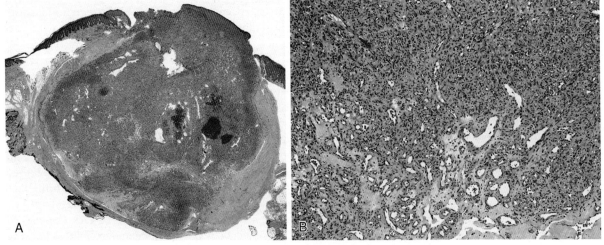

FIG. 8.49

Lobular capillary hemangioma, also known as pyogenic granuloma, are polypoid, lobulated, and often ulcerated hypervascular neoplasms composed of capillaries of variable caliber, often with a more central feeding vessel **(A,** low power; **B,** high power).

are generally not needed, as the vascular differentiation is obvious based on morphology alone. A prominent pericyte layer, which is SMA positive, may be helpful in separating benign vascular tumors from malignant ones. The endothelial cells in juvenile hemangioma also express Glut-1 (see Fig. 8.48C), which may be helpful in separating it from other similar capillary-type hemangiomas.

Differential Diagnosis

Because of its unique clinical course and tendency to spontaneous regress, it is important to distinguish juvenile hemangioma from other hemangioma variants. The young age, the presence of a lobular capillary sized vascular proliferation, and GLUT1 positivity helps aid in this distinction.

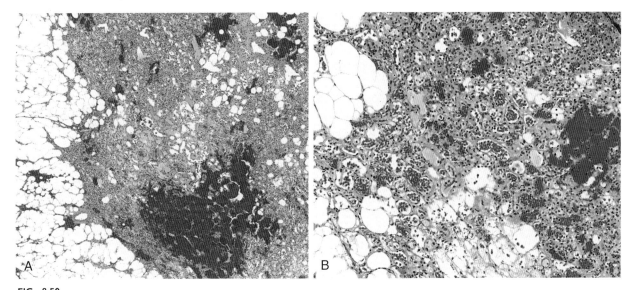

FIG. 8.50

Anastomosing hemangiomas are ill-circumscribed, commonly retroperitoneal vascular neoplasms, composed of thin-walled, anastomosing vascular channels **(A)**, lined by single layer of endothelial cells with prominent protuberant (hobnail) nuclei **(B)**.

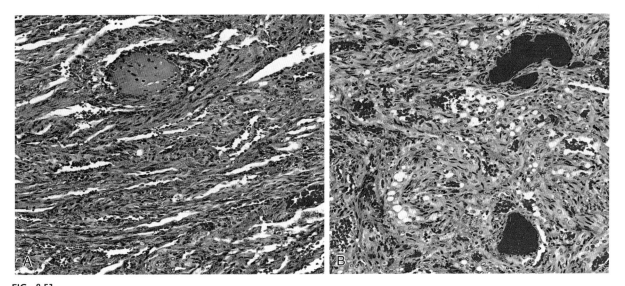

FIG. 8.51

A and **B,** Spindle cell hemangioma are often intravascular, composed of a mixture of cavernous spaces and spindled endothelial cells, forming slit-like vascular spaces, resembling Kaposi sarcoma. A second population of more epithelioid cells, some vacuolated, also are present.

Spindle cell hemangioma may be mistaken for Kaposi sarcoma, but the presence of epithelioid endothelial cells, cavernous vascular spaces, and absence of human herpesvirus 8 (HHV8) immunopositivity confirms the diagnosis.

Angiosarcomas are high-grade and infiltrative malignant vascular neoplasms, associated with variably sized and anastomosing vascular channels, generally with complex arrangements, including multilayering, and at least some cytologic atypia, features not seen in usual hemangiomas.

Prognosis and Therapy

Most juvenile hemangiomas do not require treatment, as involution and regression are the rule. Propranolol is the treatment of choice during the early proliferative phase of the disease. Surgery and/or laser treatment can be helpful, especially as a final treatment of residual skin changes in involuted lesions.

Most pyogenic granulomas are cured by local excision, but spontaneous regression also may occur.

It is often difficult to obtain a negative margin with intramuscular angiomas, and local recurrences occur in up to 50% of cases.

Anastomosing hemangiomas are benign, but persistence may occur, particularly in multicentric lesions.

Spindle cell hemangioma also are benign but may locally recur following excision, presumably related to contiguous or multifocal vascular involvement.

Prognosis and Therapy

▸▸ Infantile hemangioma: spontaneous regression/involution
▸▸ Lobular capillary hemangioma: benign, local excision curative, spontaneous regression can occur
▸▸ Intramuscular angioma: local recurrence occurs frequently if incompletely excised
▸ Anastomosing hemangioma: benign but may be multifocal
▸ Spindle cell hemangioma: benign, local recurrence may be related to multicentric disease

---

HEMANGIOMAS AND VARIANTS – DISEASE FACT SHEET

Definition

▸▸ Infantile hemangioma: superficial benign capillary sized vascular proliferations with a lobular growth pattern, arising in infants and children and associated with involution and regression
▸▸ Lobular capillary hemangioma: benign exophytic and polypod, superficial vascular proliferation, often associated with ulceration, composed of lobules of capillaries embedded in edematous stroma, arising in adults, commonly fingers, lips, oral mucosa
▸▸ Intramuscular angioma: heterogeneous vascular lesion, ill-defined, variable amounts of adipose tissue, within skeletal muscle of adults
▸▸ Anastomosing hemangioma: benign, ill-defined vascular neoplasm, composed of thin-walled anastomosing vessels lined by endothelial cells with somewhat protuberant/hobnail nuclei, arising in viscera of adults
▸▸ Spindle cell hemangioma: benign solitary to multifocal vascular neoplasm, composed of cellular areas resembling Kaposi sarcoma coupled with cavernous spaces, spindled to epithelioid endothelial cells, and scattered vacuolated endothelial cells

Incidence and Location

▸▸ Infantile hemangioma: most common vascular neoplasm, skin, head and neck
▸▸ Lobular capillary hemangioma: relatively common, finger and head and neck area, including oral mucosa and lips
▸▸ Intramuscular angioma: one of the most common deep-seated tumors, intramuscular, extremities, especially lower limb
▸▸ Anastomosing hemangioma: rare lesion, viscera, especially kidney
▸▸ Spindle cell hemangioma: rare, cutaneous, distal extremities

Age Distribution

▸▸ Infantile hemangioma: infancy and young children
▸▸ Lobular capillary hemangioma: wide age range
▸▸ Intramuscular angioma: adolescents and young adults
▸▸ Anastomosing hemangioma: middle-aged adults
▸ Spindle cell hemangioma: second and third decades of life

Clinical Features

▸▸ Infantile hemangioma: rapidly growing followed by involution, birth mark-like, flat and red cutaneous lesion
▸▸ Lobular capillary hemangioma: exophytic, commonly ulcerated and hemorrhagic cutaneous nodule
▸▸ Intramuscular angioma: infiltrative, large hemorrhagic lesion, deeply seated in skeletal muscle
▸▸ Anastomosing hemangioma: viscera, particularly kidney, symptoms vary but may be incidental
▸ Spindle cell hemangioma: asymptomatic dark red to blue, solitary to multicentric cutaneous nodules, rarely associated with Maffucci syndrome

---

HEMANGIOMAS AND VARIANTS – PATHOLOGIC FEATURES

Gross Findings

▸▸ Infantile hemangioma: birth mark-like, flat red cutaneous lesion
▸▸ Lobular capillary hemangioma: exophytic mass of the skin and mucosal surfaces, ulcerations and hemorrhage
▸▸ Intramuscular angioma: infiltrative and intramuscular, variable yellow fat, hemorrhage and thrombi
▸ Anastomosing hemangioma: ill-defined, slightly lobulated, and hemorrhagic
▸▸ Spindle cell hemangioma: red to blue nodule, well defined

Microscopic Findings

▸▸ Infantile hemangioma: lobulated, compact capillary sized blood vessels, with central feeder vessel
▸▸ Lobular capillary hemangioma: exophytic lesion with epidermal collarettes, lobules of capillary sized blood vessels with variable sized lumens, edematous stroma, ulceration and neutrophilic infiltration
▸▸ Intramuscular angioma: infiltrative heterogeneous lesion composed of variable sized, small capillary to large, muscular-walled blood vessels, admixed with adipose tissue
▸▸ Anastomosing hemangioma: lobulated but ill-circumscribed vascular neoplasm composed of thin walled, anastomosing blood vessels lined by single layer of endothelial cells with hobnail morphology, with stromal fibrosis/sclerosis and extramedullary hematopoiesis.
▸▸ Spindle cell hemangioma: low-power cavernous hemangioma and Kaposi sarcoma appearance, mixture of spindled and epithelioid cells, vascular channels with scattered vacuolated ("blister") cells, thrombi, with/without calcifications (phleboliths)

Pathologic Differential Diagnoses

▸▸ Kaposi sarcoma, angiosarcoma

EPITHELIOID HEMANGIOMA

DIFFERENTIAL DIAGNOSIS: EPITHELIOID ANGIOSARCOMA

Clinical Features

Epithelioid hemangioma presents as an asymptomatic, erythematous cutaneous plaque or nodule, rarely multifocal, arising in the head and neck, especially the scalp and forehead, distal extremities, and trunk. Peak incidence is in young adulthood, but the age range is wide.

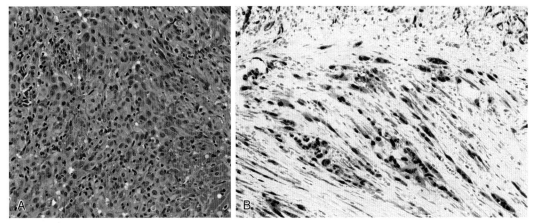

FIG. 8.52

Epithelioid hemangiomas form generally well-circumscribed vascular neoplasms composed of plump, epithelioid endothelial cells **(A)** with abundant eosinophilic cytoplasm lining compact to well-defined vascular channels. The loose background stroma often has scattered eosinophils **(A)**. The neoplastic cells may be positive for FOSB **(B)**.

Pathologic Features

GROSS FINDINGS

Grossly, they form well-circumscribed, superficial erythematous papules/nodules.

MICROSCOPIC FINDINGS

Epithelioid hemangiomas are well circumscribed and lobulated, composed of well-formed vascular channels lined by plump epithelioid endothelial cells with abundant eosinophilic cytoplasm (Fig. 8.52). Solid, more compact areas may obscure the vascular pattern. The background stroma is loose, often with abundant eosinophils and variable lymphocytes. Mitotic figures tend to be rare.

Ancillary Studies

The endothelial cells are diffusely and strongly positive for CD31 and ERG, less frequently express CD34, but often show keratin and EMA positivity. SMA decorates the pericytic lining. Recurrent *FOS* and *FOSB* gene rearrangements are detected in up to 50% of cases. Consequently, FOSB immunohistochemical stain is often positive but usually not needed to establish the diagnosis (Fig. 8.52B).

Differential Diagnosis

Epithelioid hemangioendothelioma (EHE) is infiltrative, exhibits less obviously vasoformative features, and has a chondromyxoid stroma, devoid of eosinophils. Epithelioid angiosarcomas are more obviously malignant, typically deeply seated, highly infiltrative lesions with significant cytologic atypia, increased mitotic activity, and necrosis.

Prognosis and Therapy

Epithelioid hemangioma is a benign vascular neoplasm, but local recurrences may occur in up to one third of cases, sometimes related to multicentricity and anatomic location. Regional lymph node metastases rarely occur, but distant metastases have not been reported.

EPITHELIOID HEMANGIOMA – DISEASE FACT SHEET

Definition
▸▸ Vasoformative and epithelioid vascular neoplasm, often with increased number of eosinophils, within a loose hemorrhagic stroma, typically involving the head and neck region of young adults

Incidence and Location
▸▸ Head and neck, less commonly distal extremities and trunk

Age Distribution
▸▸ Wide age range, but peak incidence in the fourth decade of life

Clinical Features
▸▸ Erythematous-violaceous nodule or papule, usually asymptomatic

Prognosis and Therapy
▸▸ Benign but increased risk for local recurrence
▸▸ Occasionally multifocal
▸▸ Surgical resection with negative margins recommended

EPITHELIOID HEMANGIOMA – PATHOLOGIC FEATURES

Gross Findings
▸▸ Well-circumscribed hemorrhagic nodular lesion, cutaneous

Microscopic Findings
▸▸ Epithelioid endothelial cells with abundant eosinophilic cytoplasm forming well-formed vascular channels, accompanied by eosinophils, within a loose background stroma

Continued

EPITHELIOID HEMANGIOMA – PATHOLOGIC FEATURES—cont'd

Pathologic Differential Diagnoses
▸▸ Epithelioid angiosarcoma, epithelioid hemangioendothelioma

KAPOSI SARCOMA

DIFFERENTIAL DIAGNOSIS: ANGIOSARCOMA

Clinical Features

Kaposi sarcoma is a locally aggressive, HHV8-induced endothelial cell proliferation, usually presenting as cutaneous lesions in the form of solitary to multiple, red purple to dark brown patches, plaques, and/or nodules. Mucosal membranes, lymph nodes, and visceral organs are sometimes affected. There are four main types of Kaposi sarcoma: classic indolent Kaposi sarcoma in the distal extremities, endemic African Kaposi sarcoma, AIDS-associated Kaposi sarcoma, and iatrogenic Kaposi sarcoma.

Pathologic Features

GROSS FINDINGS

Reddish-purple/dark-brown skin macules, plaques, and nodules that may ulcerate are typical for Kaposi sarcoma.

MICROSCOPIC FINDINGS

Histologic findings vary based on the stage of the disease but not the clinical group/type. The patch stage consists of a subtle but slightly increased vascular proliferation, lined by bland, flat endothelial cells, accompanied by variable numbers of lymphocytes and plasma cells and hemosiderin pigment. The plaque stage reveals a more extensive vascular proliferation with jagged vascular spaces, lined by spindled endothelial cells, accompanied by a dense lymphoplasmacytic infiltrate, extravascular erythrocytes, and hyaline globules. In the nodular stage, the tumor assumes the appearance of cellular nodules, composed of fascicles of mostly uniform spindled cells with hyaline globules and slit-like vascular spaces (Fig. 8.53). Mitoses may be identified.

Ancillary Studies

In addition to the usual vascular immunohistochemical markers, CD31 and CD34, HHV8 also is positive in the spindled and endothelial cells (Fig. 8.53B).

Differential Diagnosis

Early stages of Kaposi sarcoma may be difficult to distinguish from a well-differentiated angiosarcoma. A high level of suspicion, correlation with the clinical setting, and use of HHV8 immunostain resolves most such cases. The presence of cavernous spaces and more epithelioid cells help distinguish spindle cell hemangioma. More advanced stages of Kaposi sarcoma show more characteristic and diagnostic features including the presence of hyaline globules.

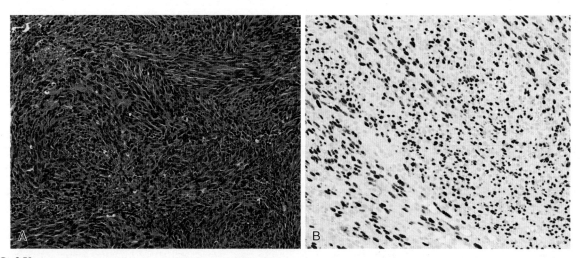

FIG. 8.53

Kaposi sarcoma, nodular stage, is characterized by hypercellular nodules, composed of fascicles of mostly uniform spindled cells with hyaline globules and slit-like vascular spaces **(A)**. The nuclei of the neoplastic cells are classically positive for human herpesvirus 8 **(B)**.

Prognosis and Therapy

Prognosis correlates with the clinical type of disease. When applicable, the degree of immunosuppression at the time of diagnosis represents the most important predictor of clinical outcome. Treatment may include surgery, radiotherapy, and chemotherapy, including antiretroviral therapy. For iatrogenically induced cases, withdrawal of immunosuppression usually results in resolution of the disease. Widespread visceral involvement is associated with a poor prognosis.

KAPOSI SARCOMA – DISEASE FACT SHEET

Definition
- ▸▸ A locally aggressive, HHV8-related vascular proliferation, usually involving the skin and often associated with immunosuppression
- ▸▸ Exists as four types: classic indolent, endemic African, AIDS-associated, and iatrogenic

Incidence and Location
- ▸▸ Rare, location and extent based on specific type
- ▸▸ Skin, less commonly mucosal membranes, lymph nodes, and viscera

Age Distribution
- ▸▸ Wide age range

Clinical Features
- ▸▸ Reddish-purple/dark-brown macules, plaques, and nodules that can ulcerate, are particularly frequent in distal extremities, and may be accompanied by lymphedema

Prognosis and Therapy
- ▸▸ Primarily dependent on clinical type of disease and the extent of the disease
- ▸▸ For iatrogenic and AIDS-related cases, prognosis may depend on the degree of immunosuppression
- ▸▸ Treatment is variable, also based on the clinical type of disease, but may include surgery, radiation therapy, and chemotherapy, including antiretroviral drugs

---

KAPOSI SARCOMA – PATHOLOGIC FEATURES

Gross Findings
- ▸▸ Reddish-purple/dark-brown macules, plaques, and nodules

Microscopic Findings
- ▸▸ Depends upon the stage of the disease, ranging from an infiltrative vascular proliferation (patch stage) to a more advanced nodular stage, accompanied by nodules of mostly uniform spindled cells arranged in fascicles with slit-like vascular spaces and hyaline globules.
- ▸▸ Lymphoplasmacytic infiltrate is present but variable

Pathologic Differential Diagnoses
- ▸▸ Angiosarcoma, hemangioma (especially spindle cell type)

PSEUDOMYOGENIC HEMANGIOENDOTHELIOMA

DIFFERENTIAL DIAGNOSIS: EPITHELIOID SARCOMA

Clinical Features

Pseudomyogenic hemangioendothelioma (PHE) is a vascular tumor of intermediate malignancy, also known as epithelioid sarcoma (ES)-like hemangioendothelioma, which usually presents with solitary to multiple superficial to deep, variably painful nodules of the lower extremities (and occasionally bone), typically in young adult males. It is most commonly seen in the lower extremities, followed by the upper extremities and trunk, and the head/neck. A majority of patients have multifocal disease.

Pathologic Features

GROSS FINDINGS

PHE demonstrates ill-defined margins and appear firm to gray-white, often multicentric.

MICROSCOPIC FINDINGS

Most cases exhibit a multinodular growth pattern composed of mostly uniform epithelioid to spindled cells with glassy, eosinophilic cytoplasm, arranged in sheets and fascicles (Fig. 8.54). Vascular differentiation is mostly not apparent morphologically, making the diagnosis potentially difficult. Mitoses tend to be scarce.

Ancillary Studies

Cytokeratin, ERG, and CD31 are generally strongly expressed, while CD34 is negative. FOSB positivity is helpful when present but tends to be inconsistent (Fig. 8.54B–F). INI-1 is retained by the nuclei.

The most common molecular abnormality associated with PHE is t(7;19)(q22;q13), with a *SERPINE1-FOSB* gene fusion. Alternative *FOSB* fusion involves the *ACTB* gene has been described as well.

Differential Diagnosis

ES often has a pseudogranulomatous appearance, the cells are negative for CD31, and nuclear INI-1 is commonly lost.

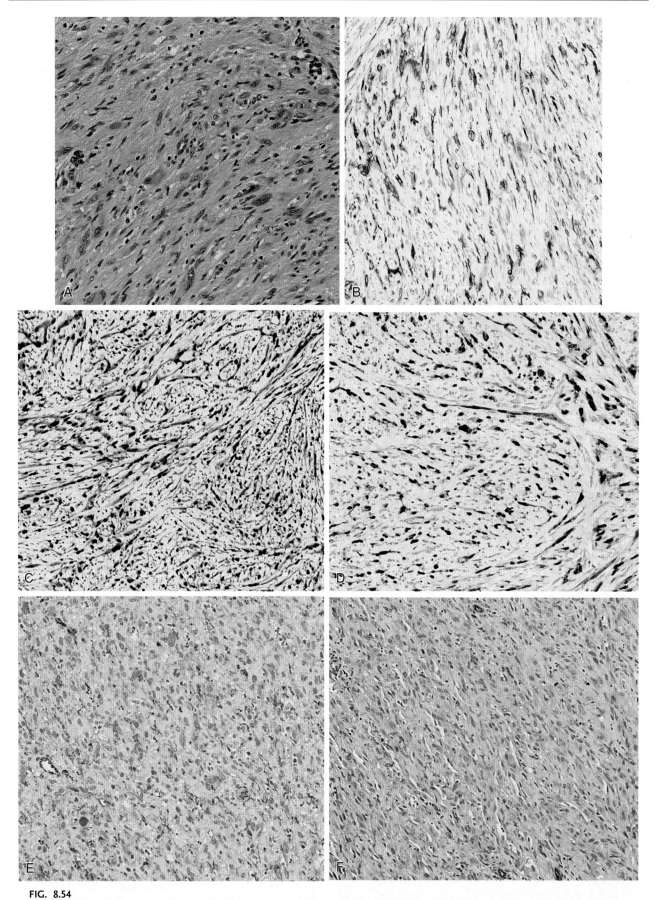

FIG. 8.54

Pseudomyogenic hemangioendothelioma is composed of relatively uniform epithelioid to spindled cells with glassy, eosinophilic cytoplasm, arranged in vague sheets and fascicles, without obvious vascular differentiation **(A)**. By immunohistochemistry, the cells express cytokeratins **(B)**, ERG **(C)**, FOSB **(D)**, and CD31 **(E)** but are negative for CD34 **(F)**.

EHE is characterized by epithelioid cells arranged in cords and nests, associated with primitive vascular lumina, and a chondromyxoid stroma. By immunohistochemistry, they are positive for CAMTA1.

Prognosis and Therapy

Local recurrences (often multiple) are commonly seen, up to 60% of cases. Additional nodules arising within the same anatomical region within short interval period is a common occurrence as well. A minority of cases (<5%) develop regional lymph node and distant metastases, rarely years or decades after the initial presentation.

PSEUDOMYOGENIC HEMANGIOENDOTHELIOMA – DISEASE FACT SHEET

Definition
▸▸ Vascular tumor of intermediate malignancy, characterized by epithelioid to spindled cells with glassy, eosinophilic cytoplasm, arranged in sheets and fascicles, lacking obvious vascular differentiation, commonly presenting as multifocal disease, within soft tissues and bone, in young adults

Incidence and Location
▸▸ Very rare, superficial soft tissues of the lower limbs, followed by the upper limbs, and trunk

Age Distribution
▸▸ Young adults, but wide age range

Clinical Features
▸▸ Variably painful, superficial nodules, often multifocal and involving multiple tissue planes

Prognosis and Therapy
▸▸ Local recurrences and multifocality are commonly seen, but metastases tend to be rare
▸▸ Surgical resection with negative margins is the goal of therapy

---

PSEUDOMYOGENIC HEMANGIOENDOTHELIOMA – PATHOLOGIC FEATURES

Gross Findings
▸▸ Superficial, ill-defined nodular lesions, grayish white

Microscopic Findings
▸▸ Superficial nodular, relatively uniform epithelioid to spindled cells with glassy, eosinophilic cytoplasm, arranged in sheets and fascicles, without obvious vascular differentiation

Pathologic Differential Diagnoses
▸▸ Epithelioid hemangioendothelioma, epithelioid sarcoma

EPITHELIOID HEMANGIOENDOTHELIOMA

DIFFERENTIAL DIAGNOSIS: METASTATIC CARCINOMA

Clinical Features

EHE most commonly arises as a solitary painful mass in deep somatic soft tissues, and less commonly arises as multifocal disease in visceral organs, such as the lung and the liver. Vascular involvement may result in edema and/or thrombophlebitis. There is a wide age range, but adults are more often afflicted than children.

Pathologic Features

GROSS FINDINGS

Gross findings typically show a firm white-tan and large soft tissue mass, sometimes associated with a vascular structure.

MICROSCOPIC FINDINGS

EHE is composed of infiltrative cords and/or nests of mostly uniform epithelioid cells with abundant pale eosinophilic cytoplasm and occasional cytoplasmic vacuolization, sometimes containing erythrocytes indicative of primitive vascular differentiation, embedded within a myxochondroid to hyalinized stroma (Fig. 8.55). When associated with a blood vessel, the epithelioid cells appear to obliterate the lumen and expand the blood vessel wall, concentrically. Most exhibit minimal atypia, and mitotic figures tend to be scarce.

YAP1-TFE3 gene fusion EHE is characterized by a distinct morphology, displaying a nested pattern and/or well-formed vessels, lined by plump epithelioid endothelial cells with abundant eosinophilic cytoplasm (Fig. 8.55C).

Ancillary Studies

Immunohistochemically, markers of classic endothelial differentiation, such as CD34, CD31, and ERG, are diffusely and strongly positive. Keratins and SMA may be expressed in up to 50% of cases. CAMTA1 nuclear expression (Fig. 8.55D) as well as TFE3 nuclear expression are positive in tumors with their respective genetic fusions.

A t(1;3)(p36;q23-q25), *WWTR1-CAMTA1* gene fusion characterizes over 90% of cases of EHE. A minority,

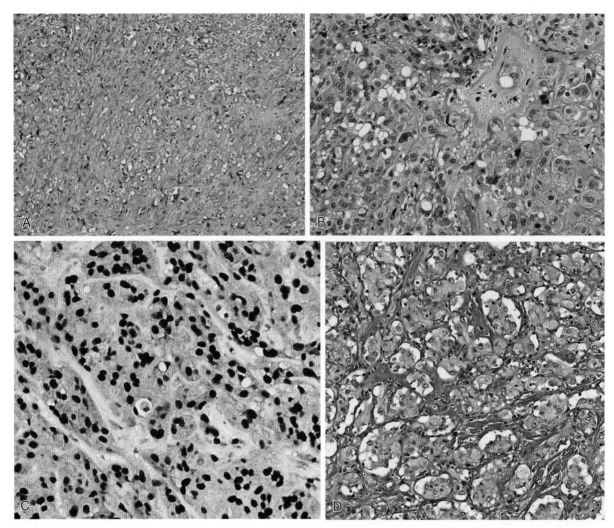

FIG. 8.55

Epithelioid hemangioendothelioma is an infiltrative tumor composed of nests and cords of mostly uniform epithelioid cells, some with vacuolation and red blood cells, embedded in a chondromyxoid to hyaline background matrix (**A,** low power; **B,** high power). CAMTA1 is strongly positive in the more common *CAMTA1* rearranged epithelioid hemangioendothelioma **(C)**. Epithelioid hemangioendothelioma with a *YAP1-TFE3* gene fusion also has plump epithelioid endothelial cells with abundant eosinophilic cytoplasm but display a more obvious nested pattern and/or well-formed blood vessels **(D)**.

with rather distinctive morphologic features as described above, display an alternative molecular event, namely a t(X;11)(p11;q22), *YAP1-TFE3* gene fusion.

Differential Diagnosis

As it was originally described, poorly differentiated carcinomas, especially lobular carcinoma of the breast, represented a common diagnostic challenge. However, carcinomas, while positive for keratins, are negative for the spectrum of endothelial markers, including ERG, CD34, and CD31. CAMTA1 is expressed by the vast majority of EHE.

ESs are always positive for keratins and may express CD34 and ERG but are negative for CAMTA1 and CD31. In the vast majority of cases, INI-1 nuclear expression is lost.

Prognosis and Therapy

Some forms of EHEs (like cutaneous) can be indolent. However, up to 21% will metastasize and have an aggressive clinical course, resulting in death in approximately 17%. Risk stratification can be used to stratify EHE into high- and low-risk categories, based on the mitotic activity (>3 mitoses/50 HPF) and tumor size (>3 cm). This risk stratification has shown that the high-risk versus low-risk tumors have 5-year survival rate of 59% and 100%, respectively. Severe cytologic atypia, spindled morphology, and necrosis are poor indicators. Patients with *CAMTA1* gene fusions appear to behave more aggressively than those with *YAP1*.

EPITHELIOID HEMANGIOENDOTHELIOMA – DISEASE FACT SHEET

Definition

▸▸ Intermediate to malignant vascular neoplasm composed of epithelioid endothelial cells within a distinctive myxohyaline stroma and t(1;3)(p36;q23-q25), resulting in *WWTR1-CAMTA1* gene fusion or more rarely, usually in young patients t(X;11)(p11;q22) resulting in *YAP1-TFE3* gene fusion

Incidence and Location

▸▸ Somatic soft tissues, followed by the visceral organs

Age Distribution

▸▸ Wide age distribution
▸▸ *YAP1-TFE3* gene fusions are commonly seen in younger population

Clinical Features

▸▸ Skin and subcutaneous tumors are solitary, whereas visceral tumors are commonly multifocal
▸▸ Can be associated with large vessels

Prognosis and Therapy

▸▸ Cutaneous EHE has favorable course
▸▸ Visceral and bone EHE have high risk for local recurrences and metastasis

---

EPITHELIOID HEMANGIOENDOTHELIOMA – PATHOLOGIC FEATURES

Gross Findings

▸▸ White firm soft tissue mass

Microscopic Findings

▸▸ Nests and cords of epithelioid cells embedded in myxoid to hyaline background matrix

Pathologic Differential Diagnoses

▸▸ Epithelioid sarcoma, carcinoma

ANGIOSARCOMA

DIFFERENTIAL DIAGNOSIS: HEMANGIOMA, HEMANGIOENDOTHELIOMA

Clinical Features

Angiosarcomas are rare, high-grade sarcomas that may arise at any location or viscera but tend to have a predilection for sun-damaged skin, especially the head and neck in elderly patients. When occurring in deep soft tissues, the extremities are more commonly involved. In the skin, most begin as ill-defined, contusion-like areas rapidly progress to ulcerated nodular regions, while in deep soft tissues, angiosarcomas form poorly defined, rapidly growing, and sometimes painful masses, associated with hemorrhage (persistent hematoma). Chronic lymphedema is a predisposing risk factor for angiosarcoma; consequently, it represents a potentially rare complication in post-mastectomy patients.

Pathologic Features

GROSS FINDINGS

Hemorrhagic, multinodular or diffuse masses with sometimes spongy cut surface. Overlying skin may appear as an ill-defined bruise.

MICROSCOPIC FINDINGS

Angiosarcomas form ill-defined and infiltrative lesions, with variably degrees of vascular differentiation and cytologic atypia. They range from well-differentiated but often complex and anastomosing vascular channels with variably atypical endothelial cells (Fig. 8.56), to more complex vascular formations with multilayering/intraluminal budding of endothelial cells, to solid sheet-like growth of spindled or epithelioid cells, lacking obvious vascular differentiation. Epithelioid angiosarcomas are more likely to display a solid growth pattern (Fig. 8.56D). Likewise, endothelial cytologic atypia ranges from mild, even flattened to marked and pleomorphic. Mitotic activity and tumor necrosis are often present, most obvious in deeply seated tumor. Extensive hemorrhage may obscure the underlying neoplasm and suggest hematoma.

Ancillary Studies

Immunohistochemically, nuclear positivity with ERG and membranous expression of CD31 are typical, while CD34 may be negative (Fig. 8.56E and F). Keratin positivity is most commonly observed in epithelioid forms. An outer layer of SMA-positive cells, likely pericytes, is usually absent but can be difficult to interpret if a significant desmoplastic reaction is present. High-level *MYC* gene amplifications (8q24) are present in almost all post-radiation and chronic lymphedema-associated angiosarcomas. Consequently, these latter tumors are immunopositive for MYC (Fig. 8.56G and H). Otherwise, there is no reproducible genetic fusion and/or mutation diagnostic of angiosarcoma.

Differential Diagnosis

Compared with cutaneous hemangiomas, angiosarcomas are infiltrative lesions, exhibiting more irregular, complex to anastomosing vascular spaces, often with

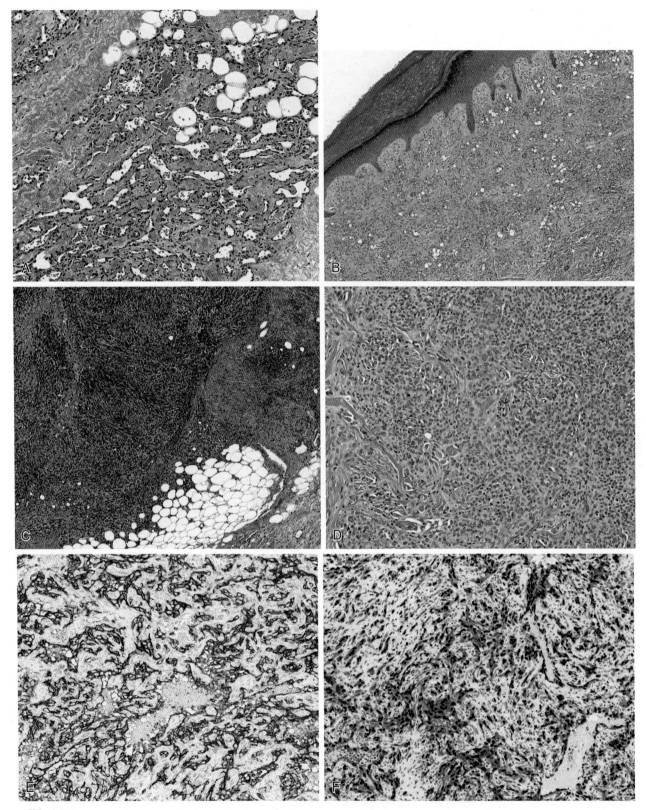

FIG. 8.56

Angiosarcoma are infiltrative, usually cutaneous lesions but have variable morphology, ranging from anastomosing vascular channels with "hobnailing" endothelial cells and multilayering **(A, B)**, to more solid, non-vasoformative, densely packed high-grade spindled cells **(C)** or even epithelioid morphology **(D)**. The neoplastic cells are typically positive for most vascular markers, including CD34 **(E)** and ERG **(F)**.

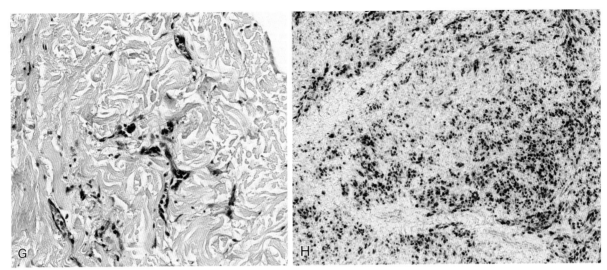

FIG. 8.56, cont'd

Angiosarcoma arising secondary to lymphedema can present as scattered atypical vessels in the dense collagenous background stroma with prominent cytologic atypia **(G)**. Such tumors usually exhibit *cMYC* amplification and are positive for the cMYC immunohistochemical stain **(H)**.

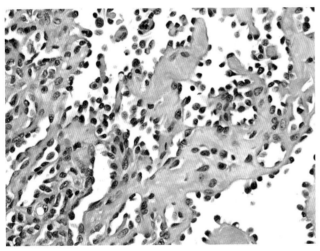

FIG. 8.57

Retiform hemangioendothelioma is characterized by variably sized, branching vessels, lined by endothelial cells with hobnail morphology without significant atypia, associated with a sclerotic stroma.

multilayering and papillary configurations. Retiform hemangioendothelioma is a locally aggressive, rarely metastasizing vascular lesion, most commonly seen in the skin and subcutaneous tissues of the distal extremities in young adults and children without sex predilection. Histologically, it is characterized by branching vessels lined by endothelial cells with hobnail morphology (Fig. 8.57). Mitotic activity is not significant.

Prognosis and Therapy

Regardless of anatomic site of origin, angiosarcomas are highly aggressive malignancies with 5-year survival rates ranging between 30% and 50%. Death is most often attributed to metastases, often to regional lymph nodes, bone, liver, and/or lungs. Surgical excision with negative margins is the first-line therapeutic goal and may be combined with adjuvant radiation therapy. Adverse prognostic indicators include older age, large tumor size, and margin status. Histologic grade has not consistently proven to predict clinical behavior.

ANGIOSARCOMA – DISEASE FACT SHEET

Definition

▸▸ High-grade infiltrative sarcoma of endothelial cells with variable morphology and vascular differentiation, ranging from dissecting to anastomosing vascular channels, with multilayering, to solid sheets, usually involving the skin of the head and neck in elderly patients

Incidence and Location

▸▸ Rare sarcoma, most commonly cutaneous, arising in the sun-exposed skin of the head and neck
▸▸ Deep soft tissue angiosarcoma more common in the extremities

Age Distribution

▸▸ Wide age range, peak incidence in elderly population

Clinical Features

▸▸ Ill-defined contusion-like area on skin progressing to nodular and ulcerated
▸▸ In deep soft tissues, poorly defined, rapidly growing, sometimes painful lesions, occasionally associated with hemorrhage/hematoma

Prognosis and Therapy

▸▸ Highly aggressive sarcoma with poor prognosis, especially when deep seated
▸▸ Surgical resection with negative margins

ANGIOSARCOMA – PATHOLOGIC FEATURES

Gross Findings

▸▸ Deep soft tissues, poorly defined hemorrhagic mass
▸▸ Skin, ill-defined bruise-like to nodular and ulcerated

Microscopic Findings

▸▸ Highly infiltrative sarcoma of endothelial cells with variable morphology and vascular differentiation, ranging from dissecting to anastomosing vascular channels, with multilayering, to solid sheets, without obvious morphologic evidence of vascular differentiation
▸▸ Epithelioid variant more often encountered in deep soft tissues

Pathologic Differential Diagnoses

▸▸ Hemangioma, hemangioendothelioma

PERICYTIC (PERIVASCULAR) TUMORS
GLOMUS TUMOR

DIFFERENTIAL DIAGNOSIS: HEMANGIOMA

Clinical Features

Glomus tumors generally arise as small (<1 cm), cutaneous red-blue painful papules/nodules in the distal acral extremities of young adults, but the age range is wide. Common, more specific locations include subungual regions, hand, foot, and wrist, but bone and visceral involvement, most notably gastric, have been documented. Deep-seated locations are more often seen in "malignant" examples. Multiple glomus tumors (10% of cases) may represent a familial syndrome with autosomal dominant inheritance.

Pathologic Features

GROSS FINDINGS

Most appear as well-circumscribed, sometimes lobulated cutaneous nodules, variably cystic to hemorrhagic.

MICROSCOPIC FINDINGS

Glomus tumors are composed of remarkably uniform round cells, with round nuclei, arranged in sheets and nests, distinctly forming collars around pre-existing capillary-sized blood vessels (Fig. 8.58). Tumors with prominent cavernous-like vascular spaces may be designated as glomangiomas (glomuvenous malformations), while those that show a transition to areas of mature smooth muscle differentiation represent glomangiopericytomas. The updated definition of "malignancy" in glomus tumors requires the presence of marked nuclear atypia (with any level of mitotic activity) or atypical mitotic figures. Malignant glomus tumors may exhibit morphologic patterns resembling a small round cell sarcoma or leiomyosarcoma; they also are more often deep seated and larger (>2 cm).

Ancillary Studies

Immunohistochemically, classic glomus tumors always exhibit strong and diffuse positivity for SMA (Fig. 8.58B) and caldesmon. CD34 may be focally expressed, but desmin and myogenin are negative. Immunohistochemical confirmation is generally not required for benign glomus tumors but may be necessary in malignant ones. *NOTCH* gene rearrangements represent the most common molecular abnormality, being present most commonly in malignant glomus tumors. *BRAF* mutations

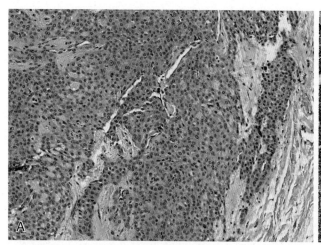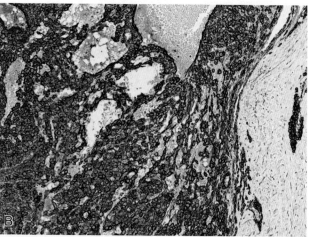

FIG. 8.58

Glomus tumors are composed of remarkably uniform, round tumor cells arranged in sheets and nests, often forming collars around pre-existing blood vessels, within a variably myxoid stroma **(A)**. Immunohistochemically, they are strongly and diffusely positive for SMA **(B)**.

may be detected in a subset of glomus tumors, usually malignant ones as well.

Differential Diagnosis

Glomus tumors are usually easily recognized with routine light microscopy. Glomangiomas are most likely to be mistaken for cavernous hemangiomas if the characteristic glomus cells surrounding the cavernous vascular spaces are not recognized. Malignant glomus tumors may resemble a small round cell sarcoma or leiomyosarcoma, especially if a benign precursor is absent. Immunohistochemistry and/or molecular testing may be required to establish the correct diagnosis.

Prognosis and Therapy

Classic solid glomus tumors and its variants (glomangioma/glomuvenous malformation, glomangiopericytomas) are benign. Surgical excision is curative. Malignant glomus tumors, especially those arising in deep soft tissues, tend to be aggressive and frequently metastasize.

GLOMUS TUMOR – DISEASE FACT SHEET

Definition
▸▸ Mesenchymal neoplasm composed of perivascular modified smooth muscle cells typical of the normal glomus body

Incidence and Location
▸▸ Rare tumors, typically arise in the distal, acral areas of the extremities, particularly the subungual regions, but may rarely occur in visceral locations

Age Distribution
▸▸ Wide age range, peak in young adults

Clinical Features
▸▸ Small, cutaneous, often painful red-blue nodules

Prognosis and Therapy
▸▸ Overwhelming majority are benign
▸▸ Rare malignant forms may exhibit aggressive behavior
▸▸ Surgical excision

GLOMUS TUMOR – PATHOLOGIC FEATURES

Gross Findings
▸▸ Small, well-circumscribed nodules, solid to cystic, hemorrhagic

Microscopic Findings
▸▸ Majority composed of remarkably uniform, round tumor cells arranged in sheets and nests, often forming collars around pre-existing blood vessels, within a variably myxoid stroma

---

▸▸ Minority also show cavernous-like vascular spaces (glomangioma/glomuvenous malformation) and/or transition to smooth muscle (glomangiopericytoma)
▸▸ Malignant examples show marked nuclear atypia and/or atypical mitoses

Pathologic Differential Diagnoses
▸▸ Hemangioma, especially cavernous type

MYOFIBROMA/MYOPERICYTOMA

DIFFERENTIAL DIAGNOSIS: ANGIOLEIOMYOMA

Clinical Features

Myopericytomas/myofibroma generally arise as solitary and painless cutaneous nodules, dermal or subcutis, in the extremities and head and neck region. Myopericytomas usually afflict young adults, whereas myofibromas are common in children and adolescents. Myofibromas also may be multicentric (myofibromatosis) and, when occurring in infants or at birth (congenital), can involve viscera and bone. A familial form of myofibromatosis shows autosomal dominant inheritance, with variably penetrance.

Pathologic Features

GROSS FINDINGS

Most are well-circumscribed, small (<2 cm) cutaneous lesions with a variably firm fibrous cut surface.

MICROSCOPIC FINDINGS

Myopericytomas are typically well-circumscribed, lobular and variably cellular neoplasms, composed of uniform and benign-appearing spindled cells, arranged in short fascicles, whorls, and characteristic collars around muscular-walled blood vessels. The stroma may be myxoid and rarely hyalinized (Fig. 8.59). Like myopericytoma, solitary examples of myofibroma also are well-circumscribed nodular lesions but characteristically display a biphasic growth pattern, with a periphery of nodules and fascicles of myoid to chondroid cells surrounding a central hypercellular region with a prominent hemangiopericytoma-like vascular pattern (Fig. 8.60). The neoplastic cells in the hypercellular central areas appear more primitive, but remain uniform without cytologic atypia, and may be associated with mitotic activity. The stroma is variably myxoid to chondroid and may have areas of necrosis and calcifications.

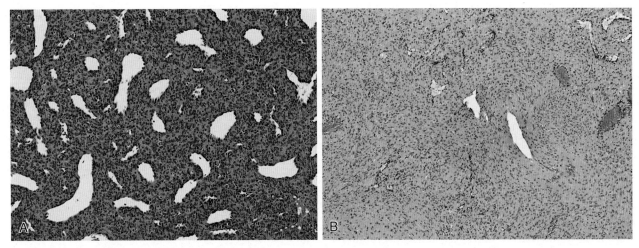

FIG. 8.59

Myopericytoma is well circumscribed, lobular and variably cellular, composed of uniform and benign-appearing ovoid to spindled cells, arranged in short fascicles and whorls, often forming characteristic collars around muscular-walled blood vessels **(A)**. The stroma may be myxoid and rarely hyalinized **(B)**.

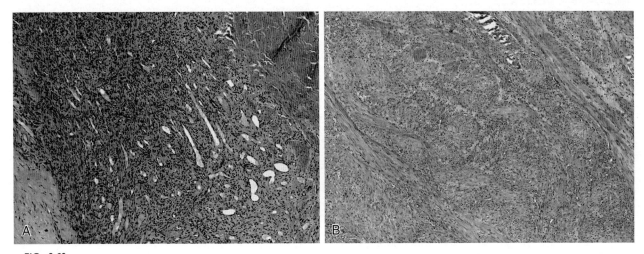

FIG. 8.60

Myofibromas are classically biphasic benign spindle cell lesions, most commonly displaying a central hypercellular zone with hemangiopericytoma-like vascular pattern **(A)** surrounded by a peripheral myoid to hyalinized zone, with short fascicles **(B)**.

Intravascular growth may be seen but has no prognostic relevance. Rarely do "cellular" forms of myofibroma display intersecting fascicles, infiltrative growth, and perineural invasion. However, nuclear atypia and tumor necrosis are absent, and foci with more typical features of myofibroma are present, albeit sometimes may be difficult to find.

Ancillary Studies

Myopericytomas/myofibromas are characteristically diffusely positive for SMA and caldesmon but negative for S100 and myogenin. Desmin may be focal expressed in myopericytoma but is generally absent in myofibroma. *PDGFRB* mutations are found among tumors within the spectrum of myopericytoma/myofibroma, and similar

germline mutations are typical of the autosomal dominant familial forms of infantile myofibromatosis. An *SRF-RELA* gene fusion appears relatively specific for the cellular form of myofibroma.

Differential Diagnosis

Angioleiomyoma shows a morphologic and immunohistochemical continuum with myopericytoma and myofibroma but does not share their distinctive molecular events. Angioleiomyomas are benign, well-circumscribed, variably painful lesions, arising in the dermis and subcutis of the extremities, most often the lower limb, often in association with a blood vessel (Fig. 8.61), predominantly in adults between 30 and 50 years of age. Microscopically, these tumors are usually solid, composed of

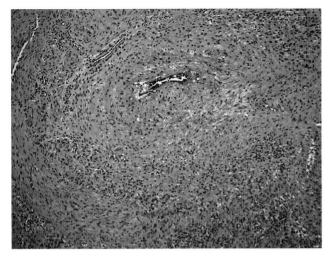

FIG. 8.61

Angioleiomyomas, occupying a morphologic spectrum with myopericytomas, are composed of mature smooth muscles arranged in fascicles and admixed with large muscular-walled blood vessels, often appearing as slit-like vascular spaces.

mature smooth muscles arranged in fascicles admixed with a prominent vasculature, ranging from slit-like spaces to dilated and thick, muscular-walled forms. Less frequently, it may appear cavernous or display adipocytic metaplasia.

Prognosis and Therapy

Most do not locally recur even if incompletely surgically excised. A worse clinical outcome is expected for infants with multicentric myofibromatosis, especially with visceral involvement.

MYOFIBROMA/MYOPERICYTOMA – DISEASE FACT SHEET

Definition
▶▶ Myopericytoma represents a spectrum of largely benign, perivascular myoid mesenchymal neoplasms, including myofibroma/myofibromatosis and angioleiomyoma

Incidence and Location
▶▶ Rare, dermis and subcutis of extremities, followed by head and neck
▶▶ Infantile myofibromatosis is multicentric and may have involvement of bone and viscera

Age Distribution
▶▶ Wide age range, myopericytoma mostly afflicts adults, whereas myofibroma/myofibromatosis is more common in infants, children, and adolescents

Clinical Features
▶▶ Painless, slow-growing superficial nodule/mass
▶▶ Myofibromatosis may have symptoms related to multicentric localization in bone or viscera

---

Prognosis and Therapy
▶▶ Surgical excision is curative
▶▶ Infantile myofibromatosis with visceral involvement has a worse clinical outcome

---

MYOFIBROMA/MYOPERICYTOMA – PATHOLOGIC FEATURES

Gross Findings
▶▶ Well-circumscribed superficial nodules, <2 cm

Microscopic Findings
▶▶ Well-circumscribed superficial nodules, dermis or subcutis
▶▶ Myopericytoma, myoid but bland spindled cells forming peripheral cuffs around thick-walled blood vessels
▶▶ Myofibroma, biphasic benign spindle cell lesion with central hypercellular zone with hemangiopericytoma-like vascular pattern, necrosis and calcifications, surrounded by a peripheral myoid to hyalinized zone

Pathologic Differential Diagnoses
▶▶ Angioleiomyoma

MYOID TUMORS

LEIOMYOSARCOMA

DIFFERENTIAL DIAGNOSIS: LEIOMYOMA

Clinical Features

Leiomyosarcoma of deep soft tissues generally manifests as one of two forms: one involving the subcutaneous and intramuscular tissues of the extremities, retroperitoneal, and intra-abdominal regions and another subgroup arising specifically from muscular-walled blood vessels, usually veins. Regardless of the specific site of origin, most examples arise in middle-aged to older adults, although they may occur at any age. Overall, the most common anatomic location is the retroperitoneum. Many intra-abdominal forms appear to arise from large blood vessels, principally the inferior vena cava and its tributaries. Clinical symptoms are related to the anatomic site of origin but generally include soft tissue swelling or mass-effect, with or without displacement of adjacent structures.

Pathologic Features

GROSS FINDINGS

Gross features of leiomyosarcoma largely depend upon the grade and size of the neoplasm but generally include an infiltrative to circumscribed, nodular mass

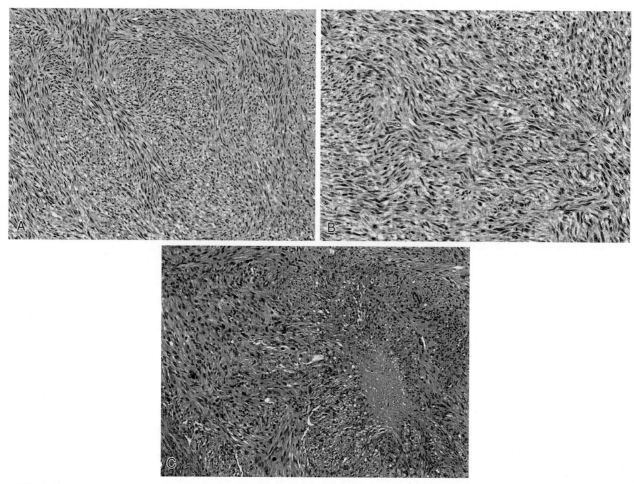

FIG. 8.62

Leiomyosarcoma are composed of intersecting fascicles and bundles of spindled cells with cigar-shaped nuclei and abundant eosinophilic cytoplasm (**A,** low power; **B,** high power). Higher-grade forms exhibit significant cytologic atypia and pleomorphism, increased mitotic activity, and necrosis **(C)**.

with whorls of white-tan tissue and variable amounts of hemorrhage, cystic change, and/or necrosis.

MICROSCOPIC FINDINGS

At low power, leiomyosarcomas may appear deceptively circumscribed, with the whorled appearance (Fig. 8.62). Intersecting fascicles and bundles of spindled cells with cigar-shaped nuclei and abundant eosinophilic cytoplasm are characteristic. Large lesions may display extensive hyalinization, coagulative tumor necrosis (Fig. 8.62C), and dystrophic microcalcifications. Nuclear pleomorphism is variable but, in high-grade tumors, may be significant. Myxoid stroma is infrequent, but epithelioid change is extremely rare in soft tissue leiomyosarcomas. By definition, even in low-grade lesions, mitotic figures should be evident.

Ancillary Studies

Leiomyosarcomas routinely express one or more of the typical smooth muscle markers, including desmin, smooth muscle actin, and caldesmon but are classically negative for myogenin and Myo-D1. EMA, keratin, and CD34 are rarely positive. There are no specific molecular markers or gene fusions characteristic of leiomyosarcoma.

Differential Diagnosis

For low-grade lesions, the differential diagnosis primarily includes deep soft tissue leiomyoma, an even rarer tumor in deep soft tissues than leiomyosarcoma. Based on current data and biologic outcome, the presence of nuclear atypia and any level of mitotic activity should be considered diagnostic of leiomyosarcoma. Deep soft tissue leiomyomas are even rarer than their malignant counterpart (Fig. 8.63). The absence of ER positivity, especially in women, can help separate intra-abdominal leiomyosarcoma from leiomyomas, which are virtually always ER positive (Fig. 8.62B). For high-grade lesions, the differential diagnosis is mainly UPS. To establish the diagnosis of pleomorphic leiomyosarcoma, clearly separating it from UPS requires the presence, at least focally, of definite "leiomyosarcomatous" fascicles and

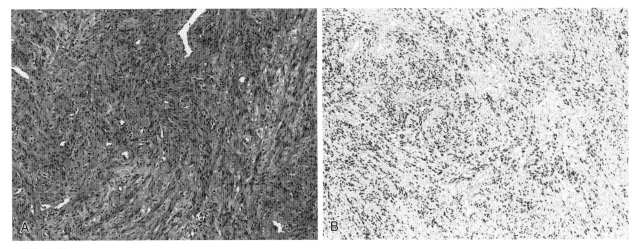

FIG. 8.63
Leiomyomas of soft tissue are extraordinarily rare, composed of intersecting bundles and fascicles of mature smooth muscle, lacking virtually any degree of mitotic activity **(A)**. Intra-abdominal and retroperitoneal forms are usually diffusely and strongly positive for estrogen receptors **(B)**.

positivity for one or more myoid immunohistochemical markers, namely actin, SMA, and/or desmin.

DL may have areas of heterologous smooth muscle differentiation. The finding of a low-grade adipocytic component helps confirm the diagnosis. For abdominal and retroperitoneal lesions without an obvious WDL component, FISH analysis or immunohistochemical confirmation of *MDM2* gene amplification characterizes DL.

Prognosis and Therapy

Adverse prognostic indicators for soft tissue leiomyosarcoma include mainly localization within the retroperitoneum and large tumor size (>10 cm). Retroperitoneal tumors are often fatal. For extremity tumors, older age, FNCLCC (Fédération Nationale des Centres de Lutte Contre le Cancer) grade 3, and localization within deep soft tissues portend a worse clinical outcome. Wide surgical resection is the therapy of choice. The role of chemotherapy has not been well established.

LEIOMYOSARCOMA – DISEASE FACT SHEET

Definition
▶▶ A generally spindled cell neoplasm exhibiting intersecting fascicles and bundles of variably pleomorphic spindled cells, with mitotic activity and at least focal positivity for one of the following SMA, desmin, and/or caldesmon

Incidence and Location
▶▶ Relatively common sarcoma, usually arising within the deep tissues of the extremities, retroperitoneum, and intra-abdominal regions, sometimes associated with large muscular-walled blood vessels

Age Distribution
▶▶ Wide age range, but primarily middle-aged to older adults

Clinical Features
▶▶ Soft tissue mass/swelling, sometimes with symptoms related to site of origin and/or organ displacement

Prognosis and Therapy
▶▶ Usually an aggressive tumor, especially when intra-abdominal or retroperitoneal and large
▶▶ Surgical excision is the primary treatment with chemotherapy reserved for cases with metastatic disease

ENTITY – PATHOLOGIC FEATURES

Gross Findings
▶▶ Circumscribed to infiltrative, fleshy white-tan to whorled/nodular mass, variably hemorrhagic, cystic, and necrotic

Microscopic Findings
▶▶ At least focally infiltrative, mostly spindled cell neoplasm, composed of variably atypical nuclei and abundant eosinophilic cytoplasm, arranged in intersecting fascicles and bundles, at least focally reminiscent of smooth muscle

Pathologic Differential Diagnoses
▶▶ Leiomyoma if low grade, and undifferentiated pleomorphic sarcoma for high grade lesions, and, for both circumstances, dedifferentiated liposarcoma should be considered, especially for intra-abdominal and retroperitoneal lesions

EMBRYONAL RHABDOMYOSARCOMA

DIFFERENTIAL DIAGNOSIS: RHABDOMYOMA

Clinical Features

Embryonal rhabdomyosarcoma accounts for the vast majority of all childhood rhabdomyosarcomas, often affecting children <10 years of age. Common sites of involvement in decreasing order frequency are the head neck region, including parameningeal and orbit, genito-urinary tract, and deep soft tissues of the extremities/pelvis/retroperitoneum. Clinical symptoms are most often related to the site of origin but most commonly manifest as a soft tissue mass/swelling with or without mass effect. Head and neck lesions may cause diplopia and proptosis. Jaundice can occur with involvement of the biliary tract.

Pathologic Features

GROSS FINDINGS

The gross appearance varies depending upon the degree of cellularity, myxoid stroma, and anatomic site of origin. Most examples display a gray-white to gelatinous and myxoid cut surface, with variable amounts of hemorrhage and necrosis. Intramuscular lesions within

the extremities are usually infiltrative and gray-white to tan.

MICROSCOPIC FINDINGS

Most conventional or classic embryonal rhabdomyosarcomas consist of poorly differentiated round to spindled tumor cells arranged in diffuse aggregates and nests, often within alternating hypocellular and hypercellular regions, creating a pulmonary edema-like pattern. The stroma ranges from myxoid to hyalinized, individual tumor cells are ovoid to slightly spindled and, less commonly, have abundant eosinophilic cytoplasm with diagnostic cross striations (Fig. 8.64). Large, polygonal-shaped rhabdomyoblasts may be scattered among the undifferentiated cells but tend to be more common in post-chemotherapy specimens. Rare examples may have heterologous cartilage differentiation or an alveolar-like component.

The botryoid subtype of embryonal rhabdomyosarcoma is characterized by a polyploid/grape-like growth

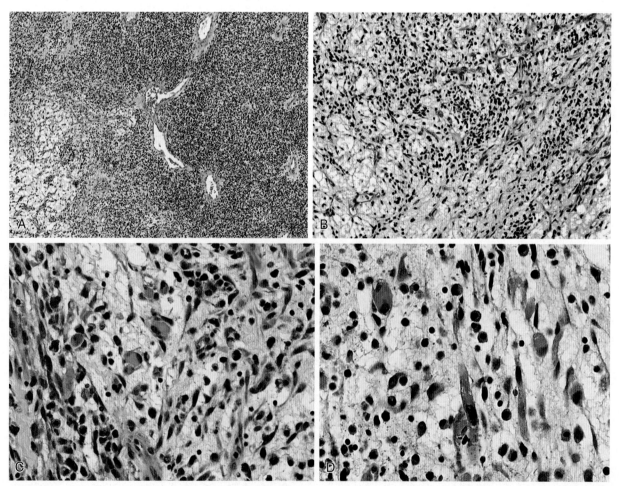

FIG. 8.64

Embryonal rhabdomyosarcoma is an undifferentiated round to spindled cell neoplasm (A), with variable morphologic evidence of skeletal muscle differentiation (rhabdomyoblasts), alternating hypercellular and hypocellular zones, and variable myxoid stroma (B). High power shows the characteristic variably morphology (C), including cells with abundant cytoplasm and striations (D).

pattern, largely due to its origin with thin mucosal lined, hollow organs, most notably the genitourinary tract and the sinonasal regions. Within viscera, an overlying intact epithelial layer is associated with a condensed hypercellular tumor layer of spindled cells and rhabdomyoblasts, sometimes referred to as the cambium layer, accompanied by an abundant myxoid stroma and randomly distributed undifferentiated round to spindled cells.

Ancillary Studies

Immunohistochemically, embryonal rhabdomyosarcoma, including the botryoid subtype, are usually diffusely and strongly positive for desmin but focally express myogenin and Myo-D1 (Fig. 8.64C and D). Expression of SMA and keratin is infrequent, and CD99 is negative. There is no specific gene fusion characteristic of embryonal rhabdomyosarcoma. Chromosome gains, particularly chromosomes 2, 8, 11, 12, 13, and 20, are frequently observed, as are chromosome losses, especially monosomy 10 and 15.

Differential Diagnosis

The differential diagnoses include other rhabdomyosarcoma subtypes, especially alveolar and spindle cell/sclerosing forms, and rarely, rhabdomyoma. Rhabdomyomas usually form non-encapsulated, slow-growing, and painless masses and, with the exception of the fetal type, are mainly seen in middle-aged to older adults. The most common form of extracardiac rhabdomyoma is the adult form, typically arising in the head neck region of middle-aged to older adults. The lesions are generally well circumscribed, usually <5 cm, and exhibit sheets of polyclonal eosinophilic cells with granular cytoplasm, frequent cross striations, and round to ovoid peripherally placed nuclei (Fig. 8.65). Fetal rhabdomyomas, an exceedingly rare neoplasm, also predominantly arise in the head and neck, particularly the postauricular region, in infants around 2 years of age. Spindled cells typically alternate with mature rhabdomyoblasts within a variably myxoid stroma. Mitoses may be present, but fetal rhabdomyomas are well demarcated and lack significant nuclear atypia and necrosis. Genital rhabdomyomas originate from genitalia, most commonly the vagina, of middle-aged to older adult females.

Absence of *FOXO1* gene rearrangements help separate embryonal rhabdomyosarcoma from most but not all alveolar rhabdomyosarcomas, which is generally more likely to be mistaken for Ewing sarcoma, morphologically.

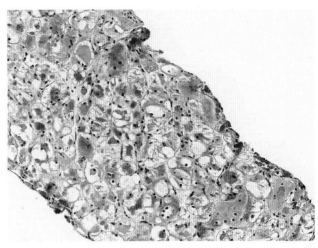

FIG. 8.65
Adult rhabdomyoma presents as sheets of polyclonal eosinophilic cells with granular to vacuolated cytoplasm, frequent cross striations, and round to ovoid peripherally placed nuclei. No significant atypia or mitotic activity is present.

Prognosis and Therapy

Adverse prognostic factors include high tumor stage or clinical grouping, older age, and histologic subtype and fusion status. Multimodality therapy, including surgery, chemotherapy, and, depending upon the location and stage, often radiation therapy, is the preferred form of treatment.

EMBRYONAL RHABDOMYOSARCOMA – DISEASE FACT SHEET

Definition
- ▶▶ A predominantly spindled malignant mesenchymal neoplasm associated with evidence of skeletal muscle differentiation, variable myxoid stroma and rhabdomyoblasts, and positivity for desmin and at least one more specific marker of skeletal muscle differentiation, myogenin or Myo-D1

Incidence and Location
- ▶▶ Rhabdomyosarcoma is most common soft tissue sarcoma in children and adolescents, and embryonal rhabdomyosarcoma represents the most common subtype.
- ▶▶ Head and neck and genitourinary tract

Age Distribution
- ▶▶ Children and adolescents, less commonly young adults

Clinical Features
- ▶▶ Soft tissue mass/swelling, but symptoms vary depending upon anatomic location

Prognosis and Therapy
- ▶▶ Aggressive neoplasm, associated with local recurrences and distant metastases
- ▶▶ Most important risk factors are age, with children having a better prognosis than adults, and tumor stage
- ▶▶ Multimodality therapy with surgery, chemotherapy, and radiation often employed

EMBRYONAL RHABDOMYOSARCOMA – PATHOLOGIC FEATURES

Gross Findings

▸▸ Most are poorly demarcated, fleshy white-tan infiltrative masses
▸▸ Botryoid variant exhibits a polypoid, grape-like growth pattern emanating from a mucosal surface

Microscopic Findings

▸▸ Undifferentiated round to spindled cell neoplasm, with variable morphologic evidence of skeletal muscle differentiation (rhabdomyoblasts), alternating hypercellular and hypocellular zones, and variable myxoid stroma
▸▸ Botryoid variant is characterized by a submucosal, hypercellular cambium layer composed of the same primitive cells, admixed rhabdomyoblasts, and an underlying myxoid stroma

Pathologic Differential Diagnoses

▸▸ Extracardiac rhabdomyomas and alveolar rhabdomyosarcoma

ALVEOLAR RHABDOMYOSARCOMA

DIFFERENTIAL DIAGNOSIS: EWING SARCOMA

Clinical Features

Alveolar rhabdomyosarcoma is a rapidly growing soft tissue malignancy with signs and symptoms often related to the anatomic site of origin. Most examples arise in the extremities of adolescents and young adults, between 10 and 25 years of age. Head and neck, pelvic, or paraspinal localization is less often seen.

Pathologic Features

GROSS FINDINGS

An infiltrative, fleshy gray-tan mass with occasional necrosis and hemorrhage is typical of alveolar rhabdomyosarcoma.

MICROSCOPIC FINDINGS

Hypercellular, primitive, and relatively uniform round cells, with high nuclear-to-cytoplasmic ratios, resembling Ewing sarcoma, are characteristic. These cells may be arranged in cords, solid sheets, and/or nests, often surrounded by fibrovascular septa. When the cells exhibit significant central dyscohesiveness, the nested pattern may appear "alveolar"-like (Fig. 8.66). Multinucleated tumor giant cells are frequently observed, a feature not seen in Ewing sarcoma. Some cells may exhibit more abundant eosinophilic cytoplasm, rhabdomyoblasts. Cytoplasmic clear cell change is rarely observed. Mitotic activity is significant and brisk.

Ancillary Studies

The primitive round cells are generally diffusely positive for desmin and myogenin, often display focal Myo-D1 expression, and occasional positivity with keratin, CD56, and synaptophysin. Approximately 75% to 85% of cases have a *FOXO1* (13q14) gene rearrangement, most commonly associated with *PAX3* (2q36) gene, with a minority involving the *PAX7* (1p36) gene. Interestingly, MUC4 is often variably expressed in fusion positive examples.

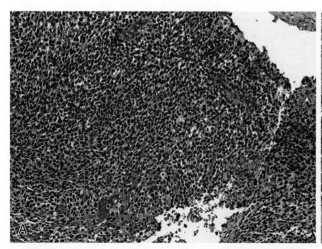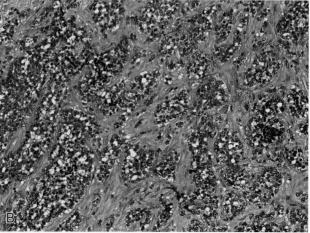

FIG. 8.66

Alveolar rhabdomyosarcoma is essentially a small round cell sarcoma, resembling Ewing sarcoma, with evidence of skeletal muscle differentiation. The cells may display a variety of growth including solid sheets **(A)** and nests **(B)**. Dyscohesiveness may result in an "alveolar-like" appearance.

Differential Diagnosis

Both Ewing sarcoma and desmoplastic small round cell tumor (DSRT) consistently lack myogenin and Myo-D1 immunopositivity and have an *EWSR1* gene rearrangement. Ewing sarcoma and related entities are discussed in greater detail in Chapter 7, regarding bone tumors. Embryonal rhabdomyosarcoma always has at least focal spindled areas and more morphologic variability.

Prognosis and Therapy

The prognosis for alveolar rhabdomyosarcoma is worse than that seen with embryonal rhabdomyosarcoma. Local lymph node and distant metastases are common. *FOXO1* fusion positive tumors behave worse than those without the fusion. *PAX7* (1p36) gene rearrangements predict a better prognosis than tumors with *PAX3* (2q36).

ALVEOLAR RHABDOMYOSARCOMA – DISEASE FACT SHEET

Definition
- ▸▸ Malignant round cell neoplasm with evidence of skeletal muscle differentiation
- ▸▸ May be *FOXO1* fusion positive or negative

Incidence and Location
- ▸▸ Second most common form of rhabdomyosarcoma, after embryonal
- ▸▸ Deep soft tissues of extremities, less often head and neck, trunk, and paraspinal

Age Distribution
- ▸▸ 10 to 25 years of age

Clinical Features
- ▸▸ Rapidly growing soft tissue mass, frequently with local regional lymph node spread or distant metastases

Prognosis and Therapy
- ▸▸ Highly aggressive and rapidly growing neoplasm, frequently associated with distant metastases and worse prognosis than embryonal rhabdomyosarcoma
- ▸▸ *FOXO1* fusion positive examples have a worse prognosis than fusion negative tumors
- ▸▸ Patients with *PAX7-FOXO1* gene fusions have a better prognosis than those with *PAX3-FOXO1* rearrangements

---

ALVEOLAR RHABDOMYOSARCOMA – PATHOLOGIC FEATURES

Gross Findings
- ▸▸ Infiltrative, fleshy tan to gray soft tissue mass, sometimes with hemorrhage and necrosis

Microscopic Findings
- ▸▸ Primitive round cell neoplasm, arranged in solid sheets, cords, and/or nests, with the latter separated by fibrovascular septa

---

- ▸▸ Loss of cellular cohesion creates the characteristic "alveolar" pattern
- ▸▸ Multinucleated tumor giant cells are a common feature

Pathologic Differential Diagnoses
- ▸▸ Ewing sarcoma and other round cell sarcomas, desmoplastic small round cell tumor, embryonal rhabdomyosarcoma

---

PLEOMORPHIC RHABDOMYOSARCOMA

DIFFERENTIAL DIAGNOSIS: DEDIFFERENTIATED LIPOSARCOMA

Clinical Features

Pleomorphic rhabdomyosarcoma is a highly aggressive, rapidly growing neoplasm, generally arising in elderly adults in the extremities, especially the lower limb. Localization to the head and neck, trunk, and intra-abdominal/retroperitoneal regions is less frequent. Most present as painless soft tissue masses.

Pathologic Features

GROSS FINDINGS

The tumors are generally large, infiltrative white-gray and fleshy masses, with variable amounts of hemorrhage and necrosis.

MICROSCOPIC FINDINGS

Pleomorphic spindled cells are organized as sheets, fascicles, or variably sized nests, associated with markedly atypical, often multi-nucleated cells with abundant eosinophilic cytoplasm (Fig. 8.67). Cross striations tend to be uncommon.

Ancillary Studies

Immunohistochemically, these tumors typically display strong and diffuse desmin positivity and at least focal myogenin and/or Myo-D1 expression. There are no recurrent gene fusions or rearrangements characteristic of pleomorphic rhabdomyosarcoma.

Differential Diagnosis

DL should be considered, especially for tumors arising in intra-abdominal/retroperitoneum. The presence of a

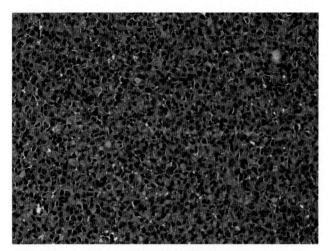

FIG. 8.67

Pleomorphic rhabdomyosarcoma are composed of sheets, fascicles, or variably sized nests, associated with markedly atypical, often multi-nucleated cells with abundant eosinophilic cytoplasm. Immunohistochemical evidence of skeletal muscle differentiation is generally required to separate it from undifferentiated pleomorphic sarcoma.

concomitant low-grade lipomatous component and/or evidence of *MDM2* amplification supports the diagnosis of DL. The morphologic features of pleomorphic rhabdomyosarcoma show significant overlap with UPS. However, the latter is a diagnosis of exclusion, lacking desmin and myogenin expression.

Prognosis and Therapy

Pleomorphic rhabdomyosarcomas are highly aggressive neoplasm, often with distant metastases at the time of initial diagnosis. Most patients die of their disease within the first year following the diagnosis.

PLEOMORPHIC RHABDOMYOSARCOMA – DISEASE FACT SHEET

Definition
▶▶ High-grade adult pleomorphic sarcoma with evidence of skeletal muscle differentiation

Incidence and Location
▶▶ Rare, deep soft tissues of the lower extremities, less often trunk and head and neck

Age Distribution
▶▶ Adults, elderly

Clinical Features
▶▶ Rapidly growing, deep soft tissue mass

Prognosis and Therapy
▶▶ Highly aggressive and usually lethal sarcoma
▶▶ Distant metastases common at initial diagnosis
▶▶ Surgical resection is the treatment of choice if disease is localized to the primary site

---

PLEOMORPHIC RHABDOMYOSARCOMA – PATHOLOGIC FEATURES

Gross Findings
▶▶ Large, infiltrative tumors, white to fleshy, often with hemorrhage and necrosis

Microscopic Findings
▶▶ Sheets, fascicles, and variable sized nests of spindled to rhabdoid cells, the latter with enlarged nuclei and abundant eosinophilic cytoplasm

Pathologic Differential Diagnoses
▶▶ Undifferentiated pleomorphic sarcoma and dedifferentiated liposarcoma

---

SPINDLE CELL/SCLEROSING RHABDOMYOSARCOMA

DIFFERENTIAL DIAGNOSIS: LEIOMYOSARCOMA

Clinical Features

Spindle cell/sclerosing rhabdomyosarcoma (SSR) generally presents as a rapidly growing, painless mass, most commonly involving the head and neck region. The age range is wide, being seen in infants to older adults. Paratesticular involvement represents the most common anatomic site in children.

Pathologic Features

GROSS FINDINGS

SSRs present as well-demarcated to infiltrative, variably fibrous, and whorled masses, occasionally displaying necrosis.

MICROSCOPIC FINDINGS

Classic examples of the spindle cell variant are hypercellular neoplasms, composed of mostly uniform spindled cells arranged in intersecting fascicles and bundles, often resembling a leiomyosarcoma (Fig. 8.68). Strap cell rhabdomyoblasts, with identifiable cross striations, indicative of skeletal muscle differentiation, occasionally are observed. The sclerosing variant displays a prominent hyalinized and sclerotic stroma, with entrapped tumor cells arranged in variably sized cords, nests, and pseudoalveolar patterns. Significant nuclear pleomorphism is not a feature of SSR, but mitotic figures may be abundant.

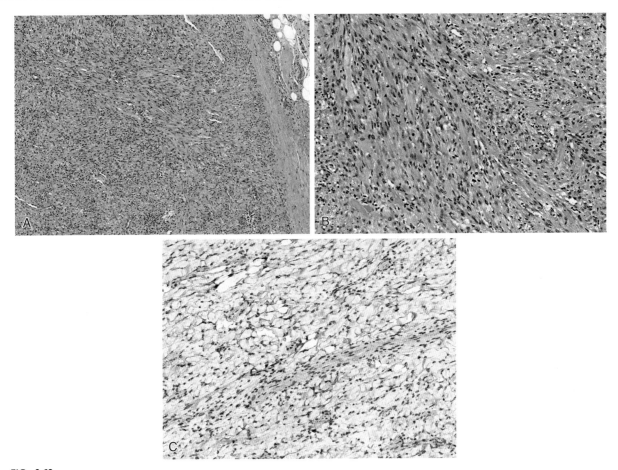

FIG. 8.68
Spindle cell sclerosing rhabdomyosarcomas are hypercellular spindle cell neoplasms, arranged in intersecting fascicles and bundles **(A)**. Strap cell rhabdomyoblasts, with abundant eosinophilic cytoplasm and occasionally identifiable cross striations, are often observed **(B)**. The cells exhibit variable MyoD1 immunoexpression **(C)**.

Ancillary Studies

Immunohistochemically, virtually all show diffuse and strong desmin expression and focal myogenin positivity. Myo-D1 expression is variable (Fig. 8.68C), but SMA is negative. The type of molecular abnormalities seen often vary based on the age of the patient. Most cases of SSR, arising in adolescents and young adults, exhibit *MYOD1* gene mutations. Infantile and congenital SSR usually show gene fusions primarily involving *SRF*, *TEAD1*, *NCOA2*, and *VGLL2* genes. However, another subset of patients lacks any discernible gene rearrangement.

Differential Diagnosis

The cellular variant is most likely to be mistaken for leiomyosarcoma. The combination of SMA positivity and myogenin negativity is typical of leiomyosarcoma. When SSR has a prominent "sclerosing" pattern, extraskeletal osteosarcoma or SEF may enter the differential. In this setting, myogenin positivity coupled with the absence of MUC4 expression is essentially diagnostic of SSR.

Prognosis and Therapy

MYOD1-mutant SSR are high-grade and aggressive neoplasms with a poor prognosis; the vast majority of patients succumb to their disease within 5 years of the initial diagnosis. Conversely, congenital and infantile SSR with the characteristic gene fusions have a favorable clinical outcome. Multimodality therapy is generally employed.

**SPINDLE CELL/SCLEROSING RHABDOMYOSARCOMA –
DISEASE FACT SHEET**

Definition
▶▶ A malignant spindle cell lesion, arranged in cellular fascicles, variably collagenized stroma, and evidence of skeletal muscle differentiation

---

Incidence and Location
▶▶ Rapidly growing, painless mass, most commonly the head and neck region

Continued

PERIPHERAL NERVE SHEATH TUMORS

NEUROFIBROMA

DIFFERENTIAL DIAGNOSIS: MALIGNANT PERIPHERAL NERVE SHEATH TUMOR

Clinical Features

Neurofibromas are the most common peripheral nerve
sheath tumors, arising as fusiform expansions of a peripheral nerve. In deep-seated lesions, this association
with nerve is easily identified, but in the more common
superficial forms, it is usually not clinically demonstrable. Most occur as solitary lesions, but multiple tumors, particularly specific forms, occur in individuals
with neurofibromatosis type 1. Neurofibromas exist as
one of three forms: solitary (localized), diffuse, and
plexiform. The solitary form is the most common, typically a sporadic, cutaneous/subcutaneous circumscribed nodule/papule in young adults. Plaque-like,
infiltrative skin lesions, especially in the head and neck,
characterize the diffuse form. A minority of such cases
are associated with neurofibromatosis type 1. Plexiform

neurofibromas are pathognomonic for neurofibromatosis type 1, growing as tortuous, worm-like extensions
of peripheral nerve, producing a multicentric nodular
superficial and/or deep masses.

Pathologic Features

GROSS FINDINGS

Solitary and circumscribed, cutaneous papule or nodule, with firm white-tan cut surface, is typical of the
solitary form. Diffuse neurofibromas are larger, more
extensive lesions, have ill-defined borders, and extend
from the dermis to subcutis. Plexiform neurofibromas
form tortuous, multifocal masses and appear as multicentric lesions on the skin. When gross enlargement of
an extremity occurs, it is referred to as elephantiasis
neuromatosa. The cut surface of plexiform neurofibromas is frequently at least partly mucoid.

MICROSCOPIC FINDINGS

Neurofibromas produce expansions of peripheral nerve,
often circumscribed, non-encapsulated, and composed
of a mixture of Schwann cells, perineurial cells, fibroblasts, and mast cells, within a lightly myxocollagenous
stroma with scattered, variably thick collagenous fibers.
Cytologically, the lesional cells appear elongated, with
spindled to wavy nuclei (see Fig. 8.69). Diffuse neurofibromas grow as dermal to subcutis masses, entrapping
but not destroying adnexal structures. The stroma consists of fine fibrillary collagen, and pseudomeissnerian
corpuscles are a common feature. The lesional cells are
remarkably uniform, with stubby to ovoid nuclei, arranged in short fascicles and sheets. Plexiform neurofibromas display tortuous expansion of multiple nerve
branches, ranging from simply an increase in endoneu-
rial contents to solitary neurofibroma-like with more
prominent myxoid changes. Combinations of diffuse
and plexiform neurofibroma are common in neurofibromatosis type 1. Occasionally, scattered atypical/bi-
zarre nuclei with smudged chromatin can be seen, and
without a significant increase in cellularity, mitotic activity, and absence of necrosis; these features are known
as "ancient change." Overall, mitotic figures are rarely
seen in usual neurofibromas.

Ancillary Studies

Immunohistochemically, neurofibromas are diffusely
positive for S100, highlighting the Schwann cells; CD34
also is expressed by supporting fibroblasts, admixed
with the Schwann cells. EMA often decorates perineurial
cells, peripherally.

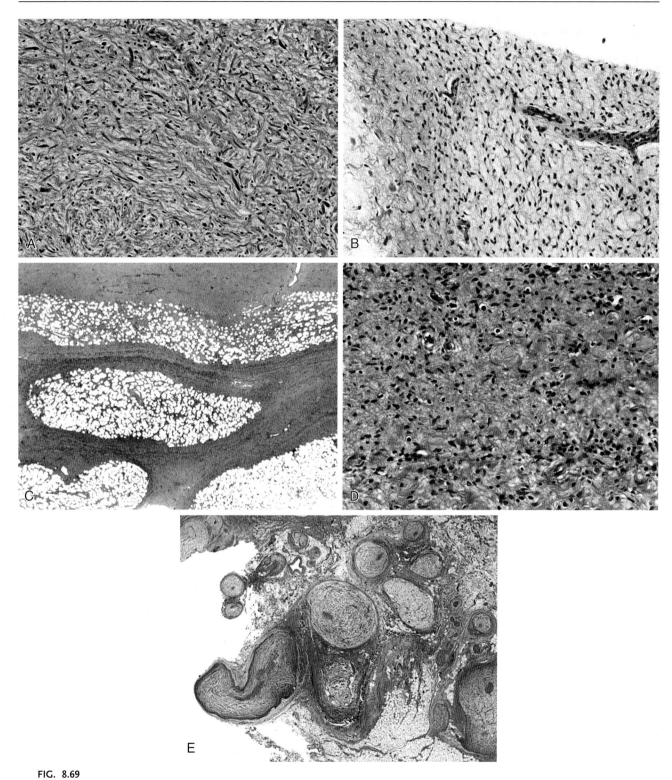

FIG. 8.69

Neurofibroma are generally circumscribed, unencapsulated mixture of S100-positive Schwann cells, perineurial cells, fibroblasts, and mast cells, within a variably myxocollagenous stroma **(A, B)**. Diffuse neurofibromas appear highly infiltrative and are composed of mostly stubby appearing spindled cells, often forming pseudomeissnerian structures **(C,** low power; **D,** high power). Plexiform neurofibromas show tortuous expansions of peripheral nerve **(E)**.

Differential Diagnosis

The most important differential diagnoses include atypical neurofibroma, also known as atypical neurofibromatous neoplasm of uncertain biologic potential, and malignant peripheral nerve sheath tumor (MPNST). The classification of neurofibroma subtypes and MPNST are summarized in the pathologic features section below. Criteria for diagnosis atypical neurofibroma are as follows: two or more of the following four features: cytological atypia, loss of neurofibroma architecture, hypercellularity, but <3 mitotic figures/10 HPF.

MPNST is a well-known complication of neurofibroma and neurofibromatosis type 1. MPNST may arise from a pre-existing peripheral nerve sheath tumor, and most are clearly identifiable as high-grade sarcomas. When associated with neurofibromas or in patients with neurofibromatosis, the histologic criteria for diagnosis of low-grade MPNST represent essentially an "atypical neurofibroma" with a mitotic count of between 3 and 9 mitotic figures/10 HPF, but no necrosis. High-grade forms of MPNST essentially have the features of a high-grade sarcoma, namely mitotic activity exceeding 10 mitotic figures/10 HPF combined with at least focal tumor necrosis (Fig. 8.70). Most examples of MPNSTs are high-grade spindle cell lesions with a fascicular growth pattern, often displaying perivascular accentuation, and rarely heterologous differentiation (e.g., rhabdomyosarcoma, osteosarcoma). Progression to malignancy in neurofibroma is heralded by loss of S100/Sox10 immunoexpression. In fact, spindle cell MPNST is entirely negative for S100/Sox10 in up to 50% of cases and, when positive, typically focal and patchy. Complete loss of H3K27me (Fig. 8.70D) in MPNST may be helpful but tends to be inconsistent in our experience. Most cases of MPNSTs arising in neurofibromas have nuclear immunoreactivity for p53, but this expression is rare in neurofibromas without malignant change.

Prognosis and Therapy

Solitary neurofibromas are benign lesions cured by local excision. Diffuse neurofibromas rarely undergo malignant

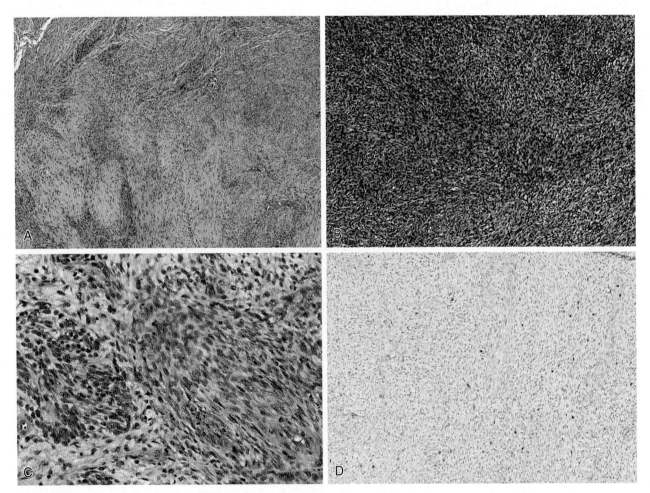

FIG. 8.70
Malignant peripheral nerve sheath tumors (MPNSTs) exhibit variably cellularity, sometimes creating a "marble-like" low-power appearance **(A)**. Hypercellular regions are generally composed of spindled cells with variably atypia, arranged in fascicles and storiform patterns, associated with significantly increased mitotic activity and frequent necrosis **(B)**. Heterologous differentiation, including rhabdomyosarcoma, is rarely observed **(C)**. Immunohistochemically, although not entirely reliable, nuclear loss of H3k27me3 is typical of most examples of MPNST **(D)**.

transformation. Atypical neurofibromas have increased risk of malignant transformation, highest in patients with neurofibromatosis type 1. MPNSTs are generally aggressive, high-grade lesions with a poor prognosis. Those arising in association with neurofibromatosis have a worse clinical outcome than sporadic forms.

NEUROFIBROMA – DISEASE FACT SHEET

Definition
▶▶ Neurofibromas are benign nerve sheath tumors, producing fusiform expansion of the nerve of origin, histologically composed of mixture of S100-positive Schwann cells, perineurial/perineurial-like cells, fibroblasts, mast cells, and residual interspersed myelinated and unmyelinated axons embedded in a myxoid background with thick collagenous fibers

Incidence and Location
▶▶ Solitary form relatively common, cutaneous, most any anatomic site
▶▶ Diffuse form is rare, typically head and neck
▶▶ Plexiform rare, seen in neurofibromatosis type 1, multiple, cutaneous and deep

Age Distribution
▶▶ Wide age range

Clinical Features
▶▶ Most are solitary, sporadic, and cutaneous, well-circumscribed, painless papules and nodules
▶▶ Diffuse form plaque-like skin lesions
▶▶ Neurofibromatosis is associated multiple lesions, typically plexiform neurofibromas, tortuous lesions

Prognosis and Therapy
▶▶ Localized cutaneous neurofibromas and diffuse neurofibromas entirely benign
▶▶ Plexiform neurofibromas are diagnostic for NF1 and have increased risk of malignant transformation

---

NEUROFIBROMA – PATHOLOGIC FEATURES

Gross Findings
▶▶ Cutaneous localized to plaque-like, diffuse firm white-tan
▶▶ Deeper lesions show more obvious fusiform expansion of existing peripheral nerve
▶▶ Plexiform neurofibromas form tortuous expansile to mucoid, multifocal lesions

Microscopic Findings
▶▶ Cutaneous and circumscribed, unencapsulated mixture of S100-positive Schwann cells, perineurial cells, fibroblasts, and mast cells, within a myxocollagenous stroma
▶▶ Diffuse form, cutaneous/subcutaneous, infiltration around and entrapping pre-existing adnexal structures, pseudomeissnerian bodies, mitotic activity absent
▶▶ Plexiform, features of solitary neurofibroma but expansion of multiple nerve branches, often more myoid

Pathologic Differential Diagnoses
▶▶ Atypical neurofibroma, schwannoma, and malignant peripheral nerve sheath tumor

---

SCHWANNOMA

DIFFERENTIAL DIAGNOSIS: MALIGNANT PERIPHERAL NERVE SHEATH TUMOR

Clinical Features

Schwannomas are slow-growing benign tumors, arising as peripheral expansions of peripheral nerves, often associated with pain and neurologic symptoms. Although they may occur at any location, most are solitary, deep seated, well circumscribed, and encapsulated and arise from the extremities and head and neck. When these tumors arise in the latter, symptoms such as headache, nasal obstruction, and otitis media may occur. There is a wide age range, but most occur between 20 and 50 years. Multiple schwannomas may be associated with neurofibromatosis type 2 and schwannomatosis. Patients with neurofibromatosis type 2 usually present due to loss of hearing and/or tinnitus, secondary to bilateral acoustic (vestibular) schwannomas, during adolescence or young adulthood.

Pathologic Features

GROSS FINDINGS

Grossly, schwannomas form well-circumscribed and encapsulated masses with firm, tan-white to yellowish cut surfaces that may have areas of hemorrhage or cystic change.

MICROSCOPIC FINDINGS

Schwannomas (Fig. 8.71) are well-circumscribed and encapsulated neoplasms that usually arise as eccentric, sometimes dumbbell-shaped lesions of peripheral nerve. Encapsulation may be less evident in tumors arising in the sinonasal tract and nasopharynx. The histologic hallmark of schwannomas is the presence of alternating Antoni A (hypercellular with compactly arranged spindled cells arranged in bundles and fascicles) and Antoni B (hypocellular spindle cell proliferation arranged haphazardly in a loose matrix). In Antoni A areas, cells will often align in a linear fashion, producing Verocay bodies. Microcystic changes and inflammatory cells often are seen in the Antoni B zones. Additional helpful diagnostic features include hyalinized blood vessels and variable numbers of lipid-laden macrophages. Cytologically, the tumor is entirely composed of Schwann cells, which have eosinophilic cytoplasm and wavy spindled nuclei with tapering ends and finely granular chromatin. The vessels commonly have thick

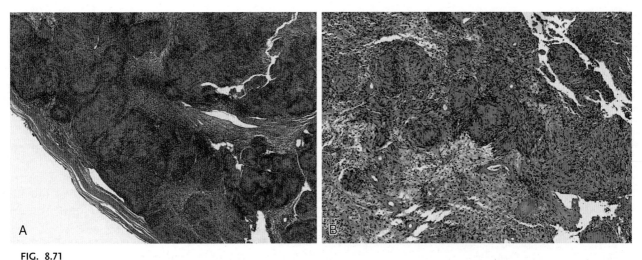

FIG. 8.71

Schwannomas are well circumscribed and encapsulated, variably cellular spindle cell neoplasms, composed of hypercellular, Antoni A regions alternating with less cellular Antoni B areas **(A)** The hypercellular regions often show aggregates of cells with nuclear palisading (Verocay bodies) **(A,** low power; **B,** high power).

hyalinized walls. Schwannomas composed almost exclusively of Antoni A are designated "cellular" schwannomas but remain well circumscribed and have the characteristic hyalinized blood vessels.

Some tumors may display scattered atypical cells with enlarged and bizarre nuclei with dense chromatin (Schwannoma with ancient changes). Such changes may also be widespread, but the degree of atypia exceeds the expected mitotic activity. Degenerative cystic changes and hyalinization rarely dominates.

Ancillary Studies

Immunohistochemically, S100 and Sox10 are strongly and diffusely positive. EMA may be expressed by the cells in and around the capsule, and CD34 often decorates a population of non-schwannian cells, mostly in Antoni A regions. Melanocytic markers are negative; H3K27me3 is retained by the nuclei.

Differential Diagnosis

The most important differential diagnosis is MPNST. These tumors are infiltrative (not circumscribed) and most exhibit significant cytologic atypia, accompanied by mitotic activity and tumor necrosis. Among spindled MPNSTs, S100 and Sox10 are negative in up to 50% of cases and, when positive, are focal and patchy. The epithelioid variant of MPNST should be mentioned given its association with malignant transformation in schwannoma. It is typically a deep-seated, obviously high-grade malignant neoplasm composed of variably

sized nests of epithelioid cells, often associated with a myxoid stroma. Unlike its spindled cell counterpart, epithelioid MPNST is strongly and diffusely positive for S100/Sox10, negative for melanocytic markers, and frequently shows nuclear loss of IN—1.

Prognosis and Therapy

Schwannomas are benign and surgical excision is curative. Malignant transformation is an exceedingly less common event than that seen in neurofibromas, and most commonly manifests as an epithelioid MPNST, less frequently, angiosarcoma.

SCHWANNOMA – DISEASE FACT SHEET

Definition
▸▸ Benign, well-circumscribed and encapsulated peripheral nerve sheath tumors, associated with a nerve and composed of Schwann cells

Incidence and Location
▸▸ Common peripheral nerve sheath tumor that can occur at any location, most commonly seen in the head and neck and extremities

Age Distribution
▸▸ Any age group

Clinical Features
▸▸ Slow-growing neoplasm, associated with a nerve with symptomatology related to the involved nerve

Prognosis and Therapy
▸▸ Benign, simple excision is curative

SCHWANNOMA – PATHOLOGIC FEATURES

Gross Findings

▸▸ Well-circumscribed and encapsulated tan, firm mass

Microscopic Findings

▸▸ Encapsulated, variably cellular neoplasm (Antony A and Antony B areas) composed of spindled cells with wavy nuclei, focally palisading (Verocay bodies)

Pathologic Differential Diagnoses

▸▸ MPNST

PERINEURIOMA

DIFFERENTIAL DIAGNOSIS: DERMATOFI-BROSARCOMA PROTUBERANS

Clinical Features

Perineuriomas present as painless, usually subcutaneous masses, occurring over a wide age range, but usually arising on the extremities, especially the lower limb, and trunk.

Pathologic Features

GROSS FINDINGS

Grossly, these lesions are well circumscribed, unencapsulated with white to tan-yellow and firm cut surfaces.

MICROSCOPIC FINDINGS

Perineuriomas form well-circumscribed spindle cell neoplasms, composed of bland spindled cells with elongated to wavy nuclei with delicate bipolar cytoplasmic processes, arranged most commonly in distant whorls, often perivascular, and storiform growth patterns (Fig. 8.72). Some areas can be more cellular, exhibiting fascicular growth. The stroma is variably myxoid to collagenous, but there is no significant increase in mitotic activity or necrosis. Sclerosing perineuriomas are defined as having a dense, collagenous and sclerotic background stroma, with a population of uniform epithelioid to spindled cells.

Ancillary Studies

The perineurial cells consistently express EMA, which may be focal to diffuse; Glut-1 and CD34 also are frequently positive, but S100 and Sox10 are negative.

Differential Diagnosis

The storiform pattern of perineurioma may mimic DFSP. However, the latter is more obviously infiltrative, typically more cellular, and lacks EMA expression.

Deep forms of perineuriomas, especially if a myxoid stroma is present, may be confused with LGFS. MUC4 immunoexpression confirms the latter diagnosis.

Prognosis and Therapy

Perineuriomas are benign; local recurrences are rare following simple excision.

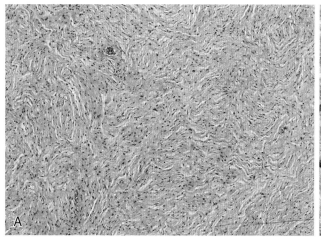
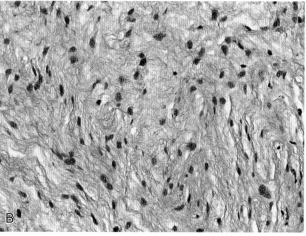

FIG. 8.72

Perineuriomas are unencapsulated neoplasms composed of monotonous spindled cells, with whorled to storiform growth patterns, within a myxocollagenous stroma (**A,** low power; **B,** high power). Immunohistochemical evidence of EMA positivity coupled with S100 negativity is required for definitive diagnosis.

GRANULAR CELL TUMOR

DIFFERENTIAL DIAGNOSIS: CUTANEOUS SQUAMOUS CELL CARCINOMA

Clinical Features

Granular cell tumors are rare soft tissue neoplasms, usually arising as cutaneous painless masses, particularly involving the head and neck and tongue of young to middle-aged adults. Less commonly, the lesion may be painful to pruritic. Multiple lesions are more often associated with African Americans.

Pathologic Features

GROSS FINDINGS

Nodular firm to slightly granular, fleshy to red-brown cutaneous to submucosal soft tissue mass, with overlying epithelial hyperplasia, is typical of the gross features.

MICROSCOPIC FINDINGS

Granular cell tumors are ill-defined lesions, composed of invasive sheets, nests, and trabeculae of epithelioid to polygonal-shaped cells with abundant granular cytoplasm and round, centrally placed nuclei, often with prominent nucleoli. Mitoses can be seen, and overlying pseudoepitheliomatous hyperplasia may be marked (Fig. 8.73).

Increased cellularity, prominent spindling, cytologic atypia, and/or increased mitotic activity with tumor necrosis suggests a greater potential for aggressive behavior and has resulted in a rare subset of granular cell tumors being designated "malignant."

Ancillary Studies

The granular cells are diffusely and strongly positive for S100 (Fig. 8.73C), Sox10, CD68, and calretinin, but negative for HMB45 and SMA.

Differential Diagnosis

Marked pseudoepitheliomatous hyperplasia overlying the tumor may result in a mistaken diagnosis of squamous cell carcinoma.

The cells of granular cell tumor may be confused with those in adult rhabdomyoma. The coarsely granular cytoplasm and absence of cross striations is typical of granular cell tumor. Desmin positivity and S100 negativity is expected in rhabdomyoma.

Prognosis and Therapy

Although the majority of these tumors are benign, local recurrences are common due to the nodular architecture of the tumor, which makes it difficult to be completely excised.

For malignant granular cell tumors, adverse prognostic factors include local recurrence, metastasis (seen in 50% of malignant granular cell tumors), larger tumor size, and older age.

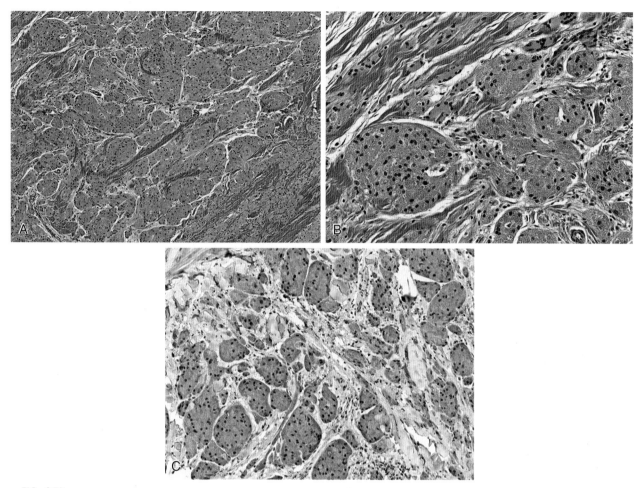

FIG. 8.73
Granular cell tumors are composed of epithelioid to polygonal-shaped cells with abundant granular cytoplasm, round, centrally placed nuclei, and often prominent nucleoli, forming infiltrative nests and trabeculae (**A,** low power; **B,** high power). The cells are diffusely positive for S100 (**C**).

Age Distribution
▶▶ Young to middle-aged adults

Clinical Features
▶▶ Skin and subcutaneous, firm painless nodule, occasionally pruritic

Prognosis and Therapy
▶▶ Benign but may locally recur if incompletely excised
▶▶ Malignant granular cell tumors, usually deep seated, have a significant risk of metastases

▶▶ Malignant granular cell tumors are more often deep seated, associated with increased cellularity, prominent spindling, marked atypia, increased mitotic activity, and necrosis

Pathologic Differential Diagnoses
▶▶ Squamous cell carcinoma, rhabdomyoma

TUMORS OF UNCERTAIN DIFFERENTIATION

ANGIOMATOID FIBROUS HISTIOCYTOMA

DIFFERENTIAL DIAGNOSIS: CELLULAR AND ATYPICAL FIBROUS HISTIOCYTOMAS

Clinical Features

Angiomatoid fibrous histiocytoma (AFH), a tumor of intermediate malignancy, is a distinctive, slowly growing, nodular to cystic soft tissue neoplasm, usually arising in

GRANULAR CELL TUMOR – PATHOLOGIC FEATURES

Gross Findings
▶▶ Unencapsulated firm nodule, pale gray to yellow, dermal to subcutis

Microscopic Findings
▶▶ Infiltrative sheets, nests and trabeculae of polygonal cells with abundant granular cytoplasm, round, centrally placed nuclei, occasionally prominent nucleoli, dermal/subcutaneous, often associated with overlying epidermal/mucosal hyperplasia

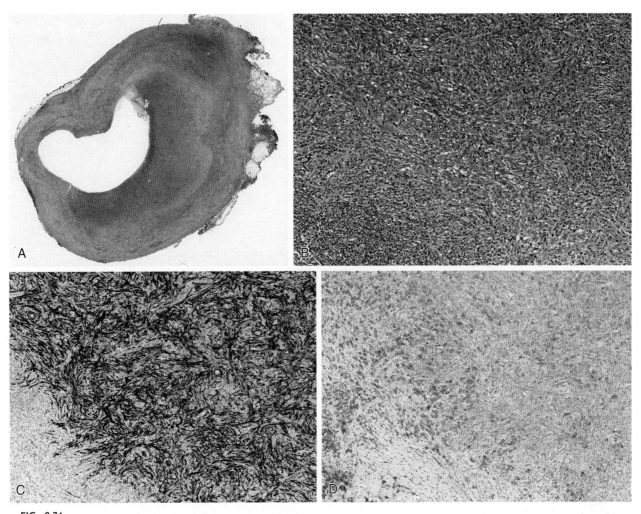

FIG. 8.74

Angiomatoid fibrous histiocytoma is a circumscribed, lobulated neoplasm, usually with a peripheral capsular lymphoid cuff, characterized by an epithelioid to spindled cell population arranged in fascicles, whorls, and sheets. Pseudoangiomatous spaces and hemosiderin pigment deposition are common (**A,** low power; **B,** high power). Co-expression of desmin (**C**) and EMA (**D**) is characteristic.

the subcutis of the extremities, particularly popliteal fossa, antecubital fossa, or inguinal regions, in children and young adults. Head and neck localization is less commonly observed.

Pathologic Features

GROSS FINDINGS

AFH present as subcutaneous, small (<3 cm) and nodular, generally well circumscribed masses with variable amounts of hemorrhage and cystic change.

MICROSCOPIC FINDINGS

At low power, these tumors are circumscribed, lobulated, and characterized by an epithelioid to spindled cell population arranged in fascicles, whorls, and sheets,

pseudoangiomatous spaces, hemosiderin pigment deposition, and a peripheral capsular lymphoid cuff. Nuclear pleomorphism may be significant, but mitotic figures are not prominent (Fig. 8.74). Rarely, AFH may contain a small round cell population or exhibit a myxoid stroma.

Ancillary Studies

The majority of cases express desmin (Fig. 8.74C), CD99, and/or EMA (Fig. 8.74D) but are consistently negative for myogenin and Myo-D1. Like clear cell sarcoma (CCS), which may exhibit identical gene rearrangements, AFH is associated with an *EWSR1* gene rearrangement, namely a t(2;22)(q32.3;q12), with an *EWSR1-CREB1* gene fusion and, less commonly, a t(11;22)(q13;q12), *EWSR1-ATF1* gene fusion.

Differential Diagnosis

Given its classic location within the subcutis, cellular and deep fibrous histiocytomas may show some morphologic overlap with AFH. However, the characteristic peripheral capsular lymphoid cuff and co-expression of desmin and EMA (and absence of myogenin expression) is diagnostic of AFH. In difficult cases, confirmation of an *EWSR1* gene rearrangement may be necessary.

Prognosis and Therapy

Surgical resection with negative margins is the therapy of choice. Local recurrences occur in 10% to 15% of patients and metastatic disease, almost always to regional lymph nodes, is seen in 5% of cases.

ANGIOMATOID FIBROUS HISTIOCYTOMA – DISEASE FACT SHEET

Definition
▶▶ Subcutis well demarcated, spindled to epithelioid lesion, variably pleomorphic, with a peripheral lymphoid cuff, immunoexpression of CD99, EMA, and/or desmin, characterized by an *EWSR1* gene rearrangement

Incidence and Location
▶▶ Rare neoplasm, usually subcutis, extremities, particularly inguinal, antecubital, and popliteal regions

Age Distribution
▶▶ Wide age range, but usually children and young adults

Clinical Features
▶▶ Slowly growing, superficial/subcutis painless mass

Prognosis and Therapy
▶▶ Mostly an indolent course with rare metastases to lymph nodes and lungs
▶▶ Surgical excision with negative margins

ANGIOMATOID FIBROUS HISTIOCYTOMA– PATHOLOGIC FEATURES

Gross Findings
▶▶ Subcutis, small nodular to partially cystic lesions

Microscopic Findings
▶▶ Lobulated and circumscribed, epithelioid to spindled cell neoplasms, variably pleomorphic and cystic, with a peripheral lymphoid cuff

Pathologic Differential Diagnoses
▶▶ Cellular and deep fibrous histiocytomas

PLEOMORPHIC HYALINIZING ANGIECTATIC TUMOR OF SOFT PARTS

DIFFERENTIAL DIAGNOSIS: HEMOSIDEROTIC FIBROLIPOMATOUS TUMOR

Clinical Features

PHAT most often presents as a slowly growing, painless, and longstanding subcutaneous mass, usually occurring in the lower extremities, especially the ankle and foot, of middle-aged to older adults.

Pathologic Features

GROSS FINDINGS

Most examples appear infiltrative, subcutaneous, white-tan to hemorrhagic. Myxoid stromal changes and cysts may be evident.

MICROSCOPIC FINDINGS

Classically, PHAT is an infiltrative, subcutaneous neoplasm composed of clusters of variably sized, thin-walled, hyaline to fibrinous blood vessels, sometimes associated with fibrin thrombi. The lesional cells are spindled to epithelioid, often exhibiting significant pleomorphism, nuclear pseudoinclusions, but little to no mitotic activity (Fig. 8.75). Hemosiderin pigment deposition is common, and the stroma may be myxoid.

Ancillary Studies

Immunohistochemically, the neoplastic cells express CD34 but are negative for S100, CD31, EMA, SMA, and desmin. A subset of cases may exhibit *TGFBR3* and/or *OGA* (*MGEA5*) gene rearrangements, particularly t(1;10) (p22;q24).

Differential Diagnosis

The main differential diagnosis is HLT (Fig. 8.76), which may show significant overlap with PHAT. In fact, some believe that HLT and PHAT represent a spectrum of a similar entity, since HLT-like areas may exist in PHAT and similar gene rearrangements may occur. The hyalinized blood vessels raise the possibility of schwannoma; however, PHAT is infiltrative and uniformly S100 negative. UPS lacks the characteristic blood vessels of PHAT and exhibits significantly greater mitotic activity.

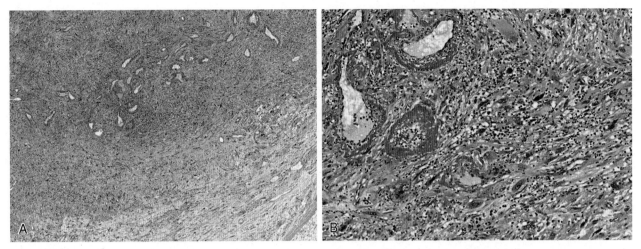

FIG. 8.75

Pleomorphic hyalinizing angiectatic tumor of soft parts forms an infiltrative mass composed of clusters of variably sized, ectatic blood vessels, often hyalinized with fibrin-like material, and surrounded by pleomorphic cells with nuclear pseudoinclusions and hemosiderin pigment deposition (**A,** low power; **B,** high power).

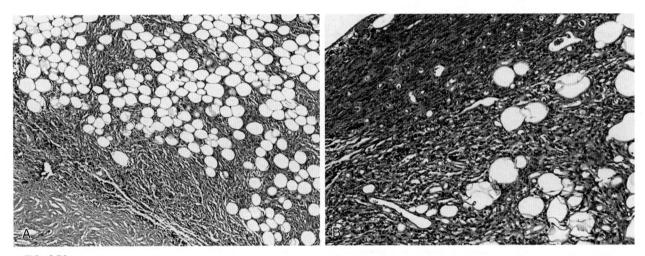

FIG. 8.76

Hemosiderotic fibrolipomatous tumor is an infiltrative neoplasm composed of uniform atypical spindled to ovoid cells with abundant background hemosiderin-laden macrophages and prominent vasculature (**A,** low power; **B,** high power).

Prognosis and Therapy

Up to 50% of cases may locally recur, but PHAT does not metastasize. Re-excision of local recurrences generally is curative.

**PLEOMORPHIC HYALINIZING ANGIECTATIC TUMOR OF SOFT PARTS –
DISEASE FACT SHEET**

Definition

▶▶ Locally recurring but non-metastasizing neoplasm, composed of ectatic blood vessels, lined with fibrin-like hyaline material, surrounded by pleomorphic spindled cells with nuclear pseudoinclusions and hemosiderin pigment

Incidence and Location

▶▶ Very rare, subcutis of distal lower extremities

Age Distribution

▶▶ Wide range, from older children to elderly

Clinical Features

▶▶ Slowly growing and longstanding subcutis mass, often resembling a hemangioma

Prognosis and Therapy

▶▶ Up to 50% locally recur if not complete resected initially
▶▶ Re-excision of recurrences generally curative

**PLEOMORPHIC HYALINIZING ANGIECTATIC TUMOR OF SOFT PARTS –
PATHOLOGIC FEATURES**

Gross Findings

▶▶ Infiltrative, lobulated, white-tan to hemorrhagic, subcutis mass

Microscopic Findings

▸▸ An infiltrative subcutis mass composed of clusters of variably sized, ectatic blood vessels, often hyalinized with fibrin-like material, and surrounded by pleomorphic cells with nuclear pseudoinclusions and hemosiderin pigment deposition

Pathologic Differential Diagnoses

▸▸ Hemosiderotic fibrolipomatous tumor

SYNOVIAL SARCOMA

DIFFERENTIAL DIAGNOSIS: SOLITARY FIBROUS TUMOR

Clinical Features

Although it may arise at any age, most examples occur in adolescents and young to middle-aged adults, usually involving the deep soft tissues of the lower extremities, often in close proximity to a joint. Rarely, SS arises within the head and neck, bone, or viscera. Despite the name, SS virtually never arises in intra-articular locations but has been described in the lungs, heart, kidney, and adrenal glands. The majority are slow growing and may exhibit calcifications on imaging studies.

Pathologic Features

GROSS FINDINGS

SS are typically tan-white to yellow and partially myxoid, <10 cm in greatest dimensions. In the hands or feet, the tumors may be very small, <1 cm.

MICROSCOPIC FINDINGS

SS are usually monophasic, being composed of a mostly uniform population of ovoid cells with high N:C ratios, without significant nuclear atypia, arranged in cellular sheets and fascicles, often interspersed with wiry strands and bands of collagen. Occasional myxoid stromal change may be prominent (Fig. 8.77). Biphasic SS has

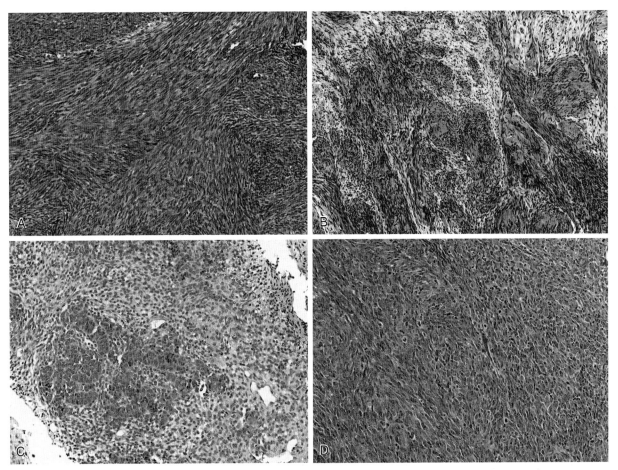

FIG. 8.77

Synovial sarcoma is characterized by largely uniform ovoid cells, without significant nuclear atypia, arranged in cellular sheets and fascicles **(A)**, often interspersed with wiry strands and bands of collagen **(B)**. Biphasic synovial sarcoma has an additional component of distinct epithelial cells, with more abundant cytoplasm, arranged as glands, nests, and/or cords **(C)**. High-grade synovial sarcoma has increased cellularity, hyperchromasia, and increased mitotic activity; some examples may appear more "round cell," mimicking Ewing sarcoma **(D)**.

an additional component of distinct epithelial cells, with more abundant cytoplasm, arranged as glands, nests, and/or cords (Fig. 8.77C). The glandular lumina contain mucin. Staghorn-shaped hemangiopericytoma-like vascular areas may cause diagnostic confusion with SFT. Poorly differentiated areas, frequently resembling Ewing sarcoma, are associated with greater cellularity, hyperchromasia, and increased mitotic activity, exceeding 10 mitoses/10 HPF (Fig. 8.77D).

Ancillary Studies

The monophasic and poorly differentiated forms of SS consistently express, at least focally, EMA and, less often, cytokeratins. Both are expressed in the epithelial cells of biphasic SS. CD99, TLE1, and Bcl-2 positivity are observed in the majority of SS, regardless of subtype. Focal S100 expression is not uncommon, but SMA, desmin, and CD34 are typically negative. At the molecular level, SS is characterized by a unique and specific t(X;18) (p11;q11), resulting in a *SS18-SSX1/2/4* gene fusion.

Differential Diagnosis

SFT is perhaps the most frequent tumor in the differential diagnosis. SFT are consistently positive for CD34 and, more specifically, STAT6, and generally negative for EMA and cytokeratins. SFT also harbors characteristic *STAT6* gene fusions.

Prognosis and Therapy

SS requires long-term follow-up, as 5- and 10-year survival rates, 70%–80% and 50%–60%, respectively, reflect not uncommon late recurrences and metastases. Regional lymph nodes, bone, and lungs represent the more common sites of metastases. A better prognosis can be expected for those without a poorly differentiated component, absence of tumor necrosis, young age (<19 years), and tumor size <5 cm. Surgical resection remains the therapy of choice, with chemotherapy often reserved for those with metastatic spread.

SYNOVIAL SARCOMA – DISEASE FACT SHEET

Definition
- ▶▶ Classically a monotonous ovoid to spindle cell sarcoma with variable epithelial differentiation, diffuse and strong nuclear TLE1 positivity, and a characteristic *SS18-SSX1/2/4* gene fusion

Incidence and Location
- ▶▶ Rare sarcoma, typically arising in the deep soft tissues of the extremities, less commonly trunk, viscera, and head and neck regions

Age Distribution
- ▶▶ Adolescents and young adults, rarely seen >50 years of age

Clinical Features
- ▶▶ Slowly growing, often painless soft tissue swelling/mass

Prognosis and Therapy
- ▶▶ Long-term follow-up is necessitated as distant metastases and local recurrences may be seen a decade or more after the initial diagnosis
- ▶▶ Surgery remains the treatment of choice

SYNOVIAL SARCOMA – PATHOLOGIC FEATURES

Gross Findings
- ▶▶ Solitary, tan-white to yellow masses, occasionally glistening and, at least focally, myxoid

Microscopic Findings
- ▶▶ Monomorphic spindle cell sarcoma composed of mostly uniform ovoid cells, arranged in sheets and fascicles, associated with variable amounts of epithelial differentiation and collagen stroma

Pathologic Differential Diagnoses
- ▶▶ Solitary fibrous tumor

EPITHELIOID SARCOMA

DIFFERENTIAL DIAGNOSIS: NECROTIZING GRANULOMATOUS INFLAMMATION

Clinical Features

ES is a sarcoma, typically afflicting children and young adults, which may exist as a classical "distal" extremity form or a proximal extremity/trunk, less common "large cell" variant. The vast majority of classic ES involves the flexor surfaces of the forearm, hand, or fingers, as one or more, slowly growing but painless skin nodules. Conversely, the large cell variant is more often seen in the truncal, pelvic/inguinal, and lower extremity regions, often in middle-aged to elderly patients.

Pathologic Features

GROSS FINDINGS

The classical distal form demonstrates one or more indurated and poorly defined, dermal to subcutaneous nodules, usually <5 cm. The proximal, large cell variant is generally deep seated, grayish-white, multinodular, with areas of hemorrhage and necrosis.

MICROSCOPIC FINDINGS

Classic ES forms cellular nodules of mostly uniform epithelioid to slightly spindled cells, often with a central area of necrosis/degeneration, sometimes mimicking a granulomatous process. Individual cells have generally round to ovoid nuclei, eosinophilic cytoplasm, and inconspicuous nucleoli (Fig. 8.78). Mitotic activity is low. Dystrophic calcifications may be present, sometimes being seen radiologically. The proximal, large cell variant is characterized by a multinodular to sheet-like growth pattern of large, often pleomorphic epithelioid cells with round, vesicular nuclei, abundant cytoplasm, and prominent nucleoli. Background inflammation is common, and rhabdoid changes are more commonly observed with this variant.

Ancillary Studies

All forms of ES display strong and diffuse keratin positivity, including AE1/3 (Fig. 8.78B) and Cam5.2. Expression of CK5/6 is less consistent. Approximately 50% of cases also express CD34, and nuclear ERG positivity also may occur. However, ES is negative for CD31 and CAMTA1. Loss of nuclear SMARCB1 (INI-1) is seen in approximately 90% of cases (Fig. 8.78C).

Differential Diagnosis

For the classic form, the differential diagnosis includes necrotizing granulomatous processes, including rheumatoid arthritis (nodules) and granuloma annulare. Careful correlation with clinical history and judicious use of immunostains, including cytokeratins, help

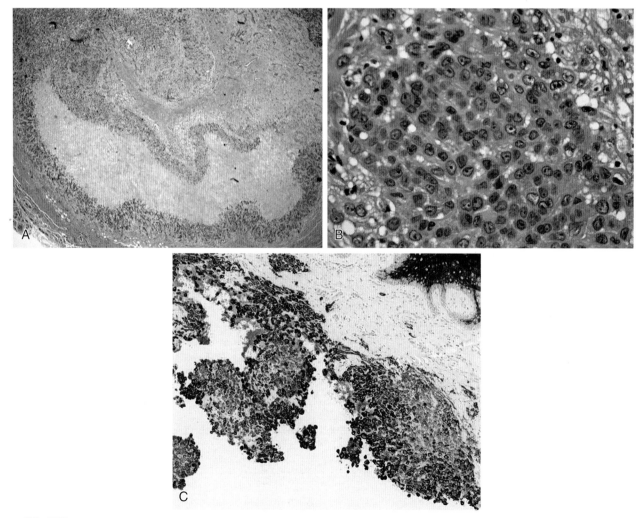

FIG. 8.78

Epithelioid sarcoma is composed of nodules of mostly uniform epithelioid to slightly spindled cells, often with a central area of necrosis/degeneration (**A,** low power; **B,** high power). The neoplastic cells are always positive for keratin (**C**).

establish the correct diagnosis. Vascular tumors, primarily EHE and PHE, may be mistaken for ES. CAMTA1 and CD31 immunostains can help confirm these tumors, respectively. For the proximal type of ES, metastatic carcinoma is the most likely alternative diagnosis.

Prognosis and Therapy

Like SS, long-term follow-up is essential in ES. The 5- and 10-year survival rates range up to 70% and 60%, respectively. The proximal form tends to have a worse prognosis, perhaps also related to its deeper location and the older ages of the patients afflicted. Common sites of metastases include regional lymph nodes and lungs. Surgical resection with negative margins remains the treatment of choice.

EPITHELIOID SARCOMA – DISEASE FACT SHEET

Definition
▸▸ Distinctive keratin positive epithelioid to spindled cell sarcoma, with a predilection for the upper extremities, usually associated with loss of SMARCB1 (INI-1)

Incidence and Location
▸▸ All forms of ES are rare
▸▸ Classic ES involves the hands and fingers commonly
▸▸ Proximal ES arises in the proximal extremities and trunk

Age Distribution
▸▸ Older children to young adults for classic ES
▸▸ The proximal form of ES is usually seen in middle-aged to older adults

Clinical Features
▸▸ Classic ES may exhibit multiple, firm and painless superficial nodules
▸▸ Proximal ES produces deep-seated and more infiltrative tumors

Prognosis and Therapy
▸▸ Long-term follow-up is necessary as classic ES may locally recur and develop metastases a decade or more after initial diagnosis
▸▸ Metastases to lymph nodes and lungs are common
▸▸ Proximal ES has a worse survival
▸▸ Surgery with negative margins is recommended

EPITHELIOID SARCOMA – PATHOLOGIC FEATURES

Gross Findings
▸▸ One or more nodules, less than 5.0 cm, usually dermal to subcutaneous with variably central necrosis
▸▸ Deep-seated tumors may be larger, associated with hemorrhage and necrosis

Microscopic Findings
▸▸ Uniform epithelioid cells forming sheets and a pseudogranulomatous pattern typical of classic ES

▸▸ The proximal large cell variant may be associated with significant nuclear atypia and pleomorphism, accompanied by necrosis

Pathologic Differential Diagnoses
▸▸ Necrotizing granulomatous inflammation, malignant vascular tumors, including hemangioendothelioma and angiosarcoma, cutaneous squamous cell carcinoma and metastatic carcinomas

---

ALVEOLAR SOFT PART SARCOMA

DIFFERENTIAL DIAGNOSIS: RENAL CELL CARCINOMA

Clinical Features

Alveolar soft part sarcoma (ASPS) is a rare but very distinctive sarcoma, usually seen in teenagers and young adults, between 15 and 35 years of age, involving the lower extremity, particularly the buttock and thigh. Usually manifests a slowly growing, painless soft tissue mass.

Pathologic Features

GROSS FINDINGS

ASPS are poorly circumscribed, pale gray to slightly yellow, frequently containing areas of hemorrhage and necrosis.

MICROSCOPIC FINDINGS

Most commonly, the neoplastic cells are arranged in well-defined nests separated by thin fibrovascular partitions/septa. Although the nests usually appear uniform, solid or pseudoalveolar growth patterns may occur (Fig. 8.79). Individual cells are large but relatively uniform in size, round to polygonal, with abundant clear to eosinophilic, well-defined cytoplasmic borders, round vesicular nuclei, and one or more prominent nucleoli. Mitotic figures are uncommon. Intracytoplasmic, eosinophilic rod-shaped crystals are rarely observed on routine hematoxylin and eosin staining but are more easily confirmed with periodic acid–Schiff (PAS) stain.

Ancillary Studies

Strong nuclear immunohistochemical expression of TFE3 is consistently present (Fig. 8.79C). Approximately 50% to 70% of cases show focal desmin positivity. However, myogenin, MYOD1, keratins, and EMA are negative. The tumor is defined by the t(X;17)(p11;q25), resulting in the *TFE3-ASPCR1(ASPL)* gene fusion.

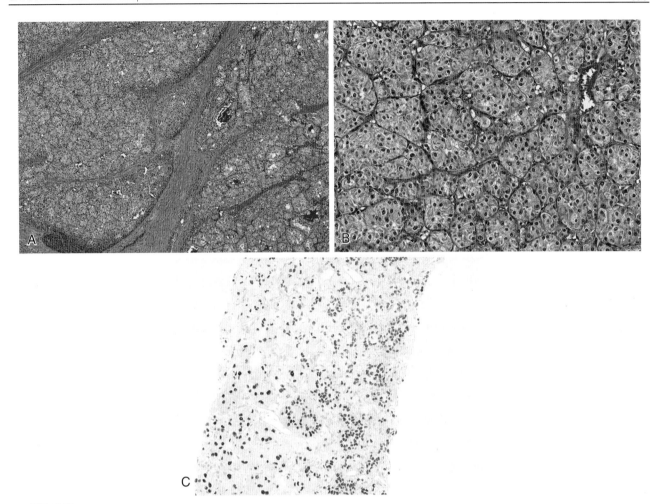

FIG. 8.79

Alveolar soft part sarcoma is characterized by well-defined nests and pseudoalveolar patterns, separated by thin fibrovascular partitions/septa. The cells have abundant amount of granular cytoplasm with round to oval, central nuclei, and often prominent nucleoli (**A,** low power; **B,** high power). TFE3 immunopositivity is consistently present (**C**).

Differential Diagnosis

In adults the main differential diagnosis, depending upon location, is clear cell renal cell carcinoma. Clinico-pathologic correlation and absence of staining with Pax8 and keratins help to exclude this diagnosis. In children, ASPS may be confused with "rhabdomyosarcoma," especially when associated with desmin positivity. But the absence of myogenin and Myo-D1 positivity also excludes the diagnosis of rhabdomyosarcoma. Importantly, the *TF3-ASPCR1* gene fusion may also be found in subset of renal cell carcinomas, mainly found in young patients.

Prognosis and Therapy

Although 5-year survival rates approach 60% to 70%, longer-term follow-up, 10 to 20 years, shows death in the vast majority of cases. Local recurrence rarely occurs following complete excision, but distant metastases, especially lung, bone, and brain, are common, sometimes decades following the initial presentation. Favorable prognostic indicators include young age at presentation, size <5 cm, and absence of metastases at diagnosis.

ALVEOLAR SOFT PART SARCOMA – DISEASE FACT SHEET

Definition
▶▶ Distinctive sarcoma composed of large eosinophilic polygonal cells, arranged in an organoid pattern, with TFE3 nuclear expression and gene rearrangement

Incidence and Location
▶▶ Extremely rare, typically buttock and thigh

Age Distribution
▶▶ Usually adolescents to young adults, 15–35 years of age

Clinical Features
▶▶ Deep-seated painless soft tissue swelling

Continued

CLEAR CELL SARCOMA

DIFFERENTIAL DIAGNOSIS: CUTANEOUS MALIGNANT MELANOMA

Clinical Features

CCS, also known as malignant melanoma of soft parts, is a rare soft tissue malignancy, most commonly involving the deep soft tissues of the extremities of young adults, aged 20 to 40 years. The majority of cases affect the lower limb and foot, often in close proximity to tendons and aponeurotic structures. Most patients complain of a painless palpable mass.

Pathologic Features

GROSS FINDINGS

The tumors are deceptively circumscribed, generally less than 5 cm with a gray-white cut surface. Pigmentation, cystic changes, and necrosis are uncommon.

MICROSCOPIC FINDINGS

At low power, CCS appear as variably sized nests and clusters of mostly uniform ovoid to epithelioid cells, separated by fibrous septa. Individual cells display abundant clear to slightly basophilic cytoplasm, vesicular nuclear chromatin, and prominent nucleoli (Fig. 8.80). The mitotic rate is generally less than 5 mitoses/10 HPF.

Multinucleated cells, resembling Touton giant cells, are frequently present. Melanin pigment is only rarely seen.

Ancillary Studies

CCS demonstrates strong and diffuse positivity for S100 and Sox10 (Fig. 8.80C), and HMB45 positivity also is typically encountered. The genetic hallmark of CCS is an *EWSR1* gene rearrangement, namely a t(11;22)(q13;q12), with the resulting *EWSR1-ATF1* gene fusion and, less commonly, a t(2;22)(q32.3;q12), *EWSR1-CREB1* gene fusion is seen.

Differential Diagnosis

The main differential diagnosis is malignant melanoma. The deeper anatomic location, absence of an epidermal junctional *in situ* component, and the younger age of the patient help exclude cutaneous melanoma. Malignant melanoma lacks the *EWSR1* gene rearrangement.

Prognosis and Therapy

Prognosis is generally poor, with 5-year survival rates ranging from 50% to 70%, declining at 10 and 20 years to 33% and 10%, respectively. In contrast to most sarcomas, CCS frequently metastasizes to lymph nodes in up to 50% of patients. Adverse prognostic indicators include tumor size >5 cm, tumor necrosis, and metastases at initial presentation. Optimal treatment is complete resection with the role of chemotherapy less certain.

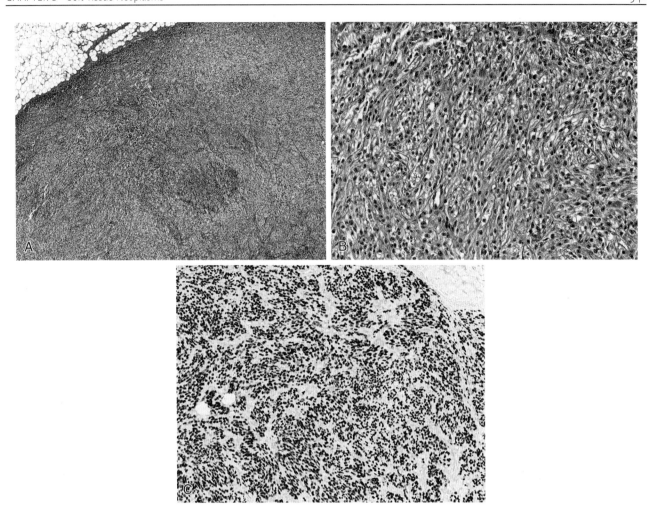

FIG. 8.80

Clear cell sarcoma is composed of variably sized nests and clusters of mostly uniform ovoid to epithelioid cells, separated by variably thick fibrous septa. Individual cells display abundant clear to slightly basophilic cytoplasm, vesicular nuclear chromatin, and prominent nucleoli (**A**, low power; **B**, high power). Like cutaneous melanoma, these cells are positive for melanocytic markers, including Sox10 **(C)**.

Prognosis and Therapy

▸▸ Prognosis is poor with most patients succumbing to the disease, sometimes decades after the initial diagnosis

▸▸ Lymph node metastases are common

▸▸ Complete surgical resection is the mainstay of treatment

CLEAR CELL SARCOMA – PATHOLOGIC FEATURES

Gross Findings

▸▸ Small, <5 cm, deceptively circumscribed, gray-white mass

Microscopic Findings

▸▸ Uniform, ovoid to epithelioid cells, with clear to slightly basophilic cytoplasm, vesicular nuclei, prominent nucleoli, arranged in variably sized nests and clusters, separated by fibrous septa.

▸▸ Wreath-like multinucleated giant cells are common, but melanin pigment is rarely seen

Pathologic Differential Diagnoses

▸▸ Cutaneous malignant melanoma

DESMOPLASTIC SMALL ROUND CELL TUMOR

DIFFERENTIAL DIAGNOSIS: EWING SARCOMA

Clinical Features

DSRT typically arises in children and young adults, most frequently males, within the abdomen, pelvis, and retroperitoneum. Symptoms largely depend upon relationship of the tumor to surrounding viscera, but it may include a palpable mass, abdominal distention, serosal implants, and ascites. Rarely, DSRT may arise in the thoracic cavity, paratesticular region, head and neck, or extremities.

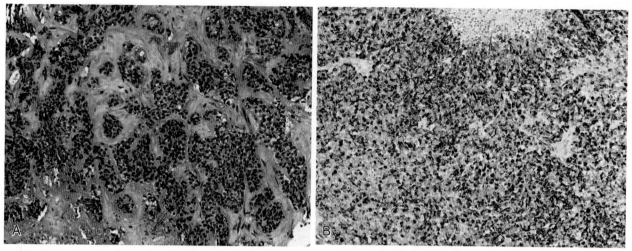

FIG. 8.81

Desmoplastic small round cell tumor is composed of variably sized nests of mostly uniform round to slightly spindled cells surrounded by a prominent desmoplastic stroma **(A)**. Immunohistochemically, the neoplastic cells are commonly at least focally express keratins, desmin **(B)**, and neuroendocrine markers.

Pathologic Features

GROSS FINDINGS

DSRT most frequently displays multiple abdominal and serosal firm, white-gray implants, with occasional foci of necrosis.

MICROSCOPIC FINDINGS

Classically, the tumor is composed of variably sized nests of mostly round to slightly spindled cells, with high nuclear-to-cytoplastic ratios, surrounded by a dense and prominent desmoplastic stroma (Fig. 8.80). Rosette formation and glandular differentiation, with mucin, may occur. Tumor necrosis is common.

Ancillary Studies

As initially descried, DSRT is immunoreactive to keratins, EMA, desmin (dot-like cytoplasmic positivity) (Fig. 8.81B), and neural markers, such as neuron-specific enolase, but more specific markers of skeletal muscle differentiation, myogenin and Myo-D1, are negative. WT-1 nuclear positivity, specifically related to antibodies to the C-terminus, is usually observed. DSRT consistently harbors a characteristic t(11;22)(p13;q22), resulting in a *EWSR1-WT1* gene fusion.

Differential Diagnosis

The most common differential diagnosis is Ewing sarcoma. Most examples of Ewing sarcoma lack a desmoplastic stroma, arise within bony sites (unusual in DSRT), and have *EWSR1* gene rearrangements with different fusion partners, most commonly FLI-1 and *ERG*. Absence of myogenin positivity reliably separates DSRT from alveolar rhabdomyosarcoma.

Prognosis and Therapy

Unfortunately, DSRT is usually disseminated at the time of initial diagnosis, necessitating multimodality therapy. Despite the latter, the overall prognosis remains poor, with 85% to 90% of patients dying of their disease within 5 years of the diagnosis.

DESMOPLASTIC SMALL ROUND CELL TUMOR – DISEASE FACT SHEET

Definition
- ▶▶ Desmoplastic small round cell tumor is an aggressive small round cell mesenchymal neoplasm with polyphenotypic differentiation, desmoplastic stroma, and a characteristic *EWSR1-WT1* gene fusion

Incidence and Location
- ▶▶ Very rare tumor, typically involving the abdominal cavity, pelvis, and retroperitoneum

Age Distribution
- ▶▶ Primarily children and young adults

Clinical Features
- ▶▶ Symptoms relate to anatomic location, possibly including soft tissue mass, abdominal distention and ascites, and acute abdomen

Prognosis and Therapy
- ▶▶ Multimodality therapy, including surgery and chemotherapy, are indicated
- ▶▶ Prognosis remains poor with 5-year survival rates approaching only 15%

DESMOPLASTIC SMALL ROUND CELL TUMOR – PATHOLOGIC FEATURES

Gross Findings

▶▶ Multiple, variably sized firm nodules/serosal implants, gray-white

Microscopic Findings

▶▶ Variably sized nests of mostly uniform round to slightly spindled cells surrounded by a prominent desmoplastic stroma

Pathologic Differential Diagnoses

▶▶ Ewing sarcoma and potentially other small round cell neoplasms, alveolar rhabdomyosarcoma

---

SUGGESTED READINGS

Lipoma

Fletcher CD, Martin-Bates E. Intramuscular and intermuscular lipoma: neglected diagnoses. *Histopathology.* 1988;12(3):275-287.

Dixon AY, McGregor DH, Lee SH. Angiolipomas: an ultrastructural and clinicopathological study. *Hum Pathol.* 1981;12(8):739-747.

Fukushima M, Schaefer IM, Fletcher CD. Myolipoma of soft tissue: clinicopathologic analysis of 34 cases. *Am J Surg Pathol.* 2017;41(2):153-160.

Meis JM, Enzinger FM. Myolipoma of soft tissue. *Am J Surg Pathol.* 1991;15(2):121-125.

Meis JM, Enzinger FM. Chondroid lipoma. A unique tumor simulating liposarcoma and myxoid chondrosarcoma. *Am J Surg Pathol.* 1993;17(11):1103-1112.

Huang D, Sumegi J, Dal Cin P, et al. C11orf95-MKL2 is the resulting fusion oncogene of t(11;16)(q13;p13) in chondroid lipoma. *Genes Chromosomes Cancer.* 2010;49(9):810-818.

Lipoblastoma

Bartuma H, Domanski HA, Von Steyern FV, Kullendorff CM, Mandahl N, Mertens F. Cytogenetic and molecular cytogenetic findings in lipoblastoma. *Cancer Genet Cytogenet.* 2008;183(1):60-63.

Coffin CM, Lowichik A, Putnam A. Lipoblastoma (LPB): a clinicopathologic and immunohistochemical analysis of 59 cases. *Am J Surg Pathol.* 2009;33(11):1705-1712.

Fritchie K, Wang Lu, Yin Z, et al. Lipoblastomas presenting in older children and adults; analysis of 22 cases with identification of novel PLAG1 fusion partners. *Mod Pathol.* 2021;34(3):584-591.

Hibernoma

Furlong MA, Fanburg-Smith JC, Miettinen M. The morphologic spectrum of hibernoma: a clinicopathologic study of 170 cases. *Am J Surg Pathol.* 2001;25(6):809-814.

Gisselsson D, Höglund M, Mertens F, Dal Cin P, Mandahl N. Hibernomas are characterized by homozygous deletions in the multiple endocrine neoplasia type I region. Metaphase fluorescence in situ hybridization reveals complex rearrangements not detected by conventional cytogenetics. *Am J Pathol.* 1999;155(1):61-66.

Gjorgova-Gjeorgjievski S, Fritchie K, Folpe AL. CD10 (neprilysin) expression: a potential adjunct in the distinction of hibernoma from morphologic mimics. *Hum Pathol.* 2021;110:12-19.

Al Hmada Y, Schaefer IM, Fletcher CDM. Hibernoma mimicking atypical lipomatous tumor: 64 cases of a morphologically distinct subset. *Am J Surg Pathol.* 2018;42(7):951-957.

Spindle Cell/Pleomorphic Lipoma

Enzinger FM, Harvey DA. Spindle cell lipoma. *Cancer.* 1975;36(5):1852-1859.

Shmookler BM, Enzinger FM. Pleomorphic lipoma: a benign tumor simulating liposarcoma. A clinicopathologic analysis of 48 cases. *Cancer.* 1981;47(1):126-133.

Ko JS, Daniels B, Emanuel PO, et al. Spindle cell lipomas in women: a report of 53 cases. *Am J Surg Pathol.* 2017;41(9):1267-1274.

Hawley IC, Krausz T, Evans DJ, Fletcher CD. Spindle cell lipoma—a pseudoangiomatous variant. *Histopathology.* 1994;24(6):565-569.

Mariño-Enriquez A, Nascimento AF, Ligon AH, Liang C, Fletcher CD. Atypical spindle cell lipomatous tumor: clinicopathologic characterization of 232 cases demonstrating a morphologic spectrum. *Am J Surg Pathol.* 2017;41(2):234-244.

Atypical Lipomatous Tumor/Well-differentiated Liposarcoma

Evans HL. Atypical lipomatous tumor, its variants, and its combined forms: a study of 61 cases, with a minimum follow-up of 10 years. *Am J Surg Pathol.* 2007;31(1):1-14.

Weiss SW, Rao VK. Well-differentiated liposarcoma (atypical lipoma) of deep soft tissue of the extremities, retroperitoneum, and miscellaneous sites. A follow-up study of 92 cases with analysis of the incidence of "dedifferentiation." *Am J Surg Pathol.* 1992;16(11):1051-1058.

Sirvent N, Coindre JM, Maire G, et al. Detection of MDM2-CDK4 amplification by fluorescence in situ hybridization in 200 paraffin-embedded tumor samples: utility in diagnosing adipocytic lesions and comparison with immunohistochemistry and real-time PCR. *Am J Surg Pathol.* 2007;31(10):1476-1489.

Lucas DR, Nascimento AG, Sanjay BK, Rock MG. Well-differentiated liposarcoma. The Mayo Clinic experience with 58 cases. *Am J Clin Pathol.* 1994;102(5):677-683.

Bonvalot S, Miceli R, Berselli M, et al. Aggressive surgery in retroperitoneal soft tissue sarcoma carried out at high-volume centers is safe and is associated with improved local control. *Ann Surg Oncol.* 2010;17(6):1507-1514.

Creytens D, Van Gorp J, Speel EJ, Ferdinande L. Characterization of the 12q amplicons in lipomatous soft tissue tumors by multiplex ligation-dependent probe amplification-based copy number analysis. *Anticancer Res.* 2015;35(4):1835-1842.

Dedifferentiated Liposarcoma

Tap WD, Eilber FC, Ginther C, et al. Evaluation of well-differentiated/de-differentiated liposarcomas by high-resolution oligonucleotide array-based comparative genomic hybridization. *Genes Chromosomes Cancer.* 2011;50(2):95-112.

Kilpatrick SE. Dedifferentiated liposarcoma: a comprehensive historical review with proposed evidence-based guidelines regarding a diagnosis in need of further clarification. *Adv Anat Pathol.* 2021;28(6):426-438.

Elgar F, Goldblum JR. Well-differentiated liposarcoma of the retroperitoneum: a clinicopathologic analysis of 20 cases, with particular attention to the extent of low-grade dedifferentiation. *Mod Pathol.* 1997;10(2):113-120.

McCormick D, Mentzel T, Beham A, Fletcher CD. Dedifferentiated liposarcoma. Clinicopathologic analysis of 32 cases suggesting a better prognostic subgroup among pleomorphic sarcomas. *Am J Surg Pathol.* 1994;18(12):1213-1223.

Weiss SW, Rao VK. Well-differentiated liposarcoma (atypical lipoma) of deep soft tissue of the extremities, retroperitoneum, and miscellaneous sites. A follow-up study of 92 cases with analysis of the incidence of "dedifferentiation." *Am J Surg Pathol.* 1992;16(11):1051-1058.

Henricks WH, Chu YC, Goldblum JR, Weiss SW. Dedifferentiated liposarcoma: a clinicopathological analysis of 155 cases with a proposal for an expanded definition of dedifferentiation. *Am J Surg Pathol.* 1997;21(3):271-281.

Thway K. Well-differentiated liposarcoma and dedifferentiated liposarcoma: an updated review. *Semin Diagn Pathol.* 2019;36(2):112-121.

Myxoid Liposarcoma

Kilpatrick SE, Doyon J, Choong PF, Sim FH, Nascimento AG. The clinicopathologic spectrum of myxoid and round cell liposarcoma. A study of 95 cases. *Cancer.* 1996;77(8):1450-1458.

Smith TA, Easley KA, Goldblum JR. Myxoid/round cell liposarcoma of the extremities: a clinicopathologic study of 29 cases with particular attention to extent of round cell liposarcoma. *Am J Surg Pathol.* 1996;20(2):171-180.

Fiore M, Grosso F, Lo Vullo S, et al. Myxoid/round cell and pleomorphic liposarcomas: prognostic factors and survival in a series of patients treated at a single institution. *Cancer.* 2007;109(12):2522-2531.

Tallini G, Akerman M, Dal Cin P, et al. Combined morphologic and karyotypic study of 28 myxoid liposarcomas: an implication of revised morphologic typing (a report from the CHAMP Group). *Am J Surg Pathol.* 1996;20(9):1047-1055.

Orvieto E, Furlanetto A, Laurino L, Dei Tos AP. Myxoid and round cell liposarcoma: a spectrum of myxoid adipocytic neoplasia. *Semin Diagn Pathol.* 2001;18(4):267-273.

Baxter KJ, Govsyeyev N, Namm JP, Gonzalez RJ, Roggin KK, Cardona K. Is multimodality therapy necessary for the management of pure myxoid liposarcomas? A multi-institutional series of pure myxoid liposarcomas of the extremities and torso. *J Surg Oncol.* 2015; 111(2):146-151.

Pleomorphic Liposarcoma

Downes KA, Goldblum JR, Montgomery EA, Fisher C. Pleomorphic liposarcoma: a clinicopathologic analysis of 19 cases. *Mod Pathol.* 2001;14(3):179-184.

Hornick JL, Bosenberg MW, Mentzel T, McMenamin ME, Oliveira AM, Fletcher CD. Pleomorphic liposarcoma: clinicopathologic analysis of 57 cases. *Am J Surg Pathol.* 2004;28(10):1257-1267.

Gebhard S, Coindre JM, Michels JJ, et al. Pleomorphic liposarcoma: clinicopathologic, immunohistochemical, and follow-up analysis of 63 cases: a study from the French Federation of Cancer Centers Sarcoma Group. *Am J Surg Pathol.* 2002;26(5):601-616.

Nodular Fasciitis

de Feraudy S, Fletcher CD. Intradermal nodular fasciitis: a rare lesion analyzed in a series of 24 cases. *Am J Surg Pathol.* 2010;34(9): 1377-1381.

Kumar E, Patel NR, Demicco EG, et al. Cutaneous nodular fasciitis with genetic analysis: a case series. *J Cutan Pathol.* 2016;43(12):1143-1149. doi:10.1111/cup.12828. [Erratum in: J Cutan Pathol. 2017;44(5):512].

Meister P, Bückmann FW, Konrad E. Extent and level of fascial involvement in 100 cases with nodular fasciitis. *Virchows Arch A Pathol Anat Histol.* 1978;380(2):177-185.

Erickson-Johnson MR, Chou MM, Evers BR, et al. Nodular fasciitis: a novel model of transient neoplasia induced by MYH9-USP6 gene fusion. *Lab Invest.* 2011;91(10):1427-1433.

Bernstein KE, Lattes R. Nodular (pseudosarcomatous) fasciitis, a nonrecurrent lesion: clinicopathologic study of 134 cases. *Cancer.* 1982;49(8):1668-1678.

Ischemic Fasciitis (Atypical Decubital Fibroplasia)

Montgomery EA, Meis JM, Mitchell MS, Enzinger FM. Atypical decubital fibroplasia. A distinctive fibroblastic pseudotumor occurring in debilitated patients. *Am J Surg Pathol.* 1992;16(7):708-715.

Perosio PM, Weiss SW. Ischemic fasciitis: a juxta-skeletal fibroblastic proliferation with a predilection for elderly patients. *Mod Pathol.* 1993;6(1):69-72.

Liegl B, Fletcher CD. Ischemic fasciitis: analysis of 44 cases indicating an inconsistent association with immobility or debilitation. *Am J Surg Pathol.* 2008;32(10):1546-1552.

Chung EB, Enzinger FM. Proliferative fasciitis. *Cancer.* 1975;36:1450-1458.

Enzinger FM, Dulcey F. Proliferative myositis: report of thirty-three cases. *Cancer.* 1967;20:2213-2223.

Myositis Ossificans and Fibro-Osseous Pseudotumor of Digits

Kilpatrick SE, Koplyay P, Pope Jr TL, Ward WG. Clinical, radiologic, and pathologic spectrum of myositis ossificans and related lesions: a unifying concept. *Adv Anat Pathol.* 1997;4(5):277-286.

Dupree WB, Enzinger FM. Fibro-osseous pseudotumor of the digits. *Cancer.* 1986;58(9):2103-2109.

Marián Švajdler, Michael Michal, Petr Martínek, et al. Fibro-osseous pseudotumor of digits and myositis ossificans show consistent COL1A1-USP6 rearrangement: a clinicopathological and genetic study of 27 cases. *Hum Pathol.* 2019;88:39-47.

Bekers EM, Eijkelenboom A, Grunberg K, et al. Myositis ossificans – Another condition with USP6 rearrangement, providing evidence of a

relationship with nodular fasciitis and aneurysmal bone cyst. *Ann Diagn Pathol.* 2018;34:56-59.

Fetsch JF, Miettinen M. Calcifying aponeurotic fibroma: a clinicopathologic study of 22 cases arising in uncommon sites. *Hum Pathol.* 1998;29(12):1504-1510.

Murphy BA, Kilpatrick SE, Panella MJ, White WL. Extra-acral calcifying aponeurotic fibroma: a distinctive case with 23-year follow-up. *J Cutan Pathol.* 1996;23(4):369-372.

Elastofibroma

Giebel GD, Bierhoff E, Vogel J. Elastofibroma and pre-elastofibroma – a biopsy and autopsy study. *Eur J Surg Oncol.* 1996;22(1):93-96.

Nagamine N, Nohara Y, Ito E. Elastofibroma in Okinawa: a clinicopathologic study of 170 cases. *Cancer.* 1982;50(9):1794-1805.

Naylor MF, Nascimento AG, Sherrick AD, et al. Elastofibroma dorsi: radiologic findings in 12 patients. *AJR Am J Roentgenol.* 1996;167(3): 683-687.

Kransdorf MJ, Meis JM, Montgomery E. Elastofibroma: MR and CT appearance with radiologic-pathologic correlation. *AJR Am J Roentgenol.* 1992;159(3):575-579.

Fibrous Hamartoma of Infancy

Enzinger FM. Fibrous hamartoma of infancy. *Cancer.* 1965;18:241-248.

Fletcher CDM, Powell G, Van Noorden S, et al. Fibrous hamartoma of infancy: a histochemical and immunohistochemical study. *Histopathology.* 1988;12(1):65-74.

Greco MA, Schinella RA, Vuletin JC. Fibrous hamartoma of infancy: an ultrastructural study. *Hum Pathol.* 1984;15(8):717-723.

Groisman G, Lichtig C. Fibrous hamartoma of infancy: an immunohis-tochemical and ultrastructural study. *Hum Pathol.* 1991;22(9):914-918.

Fetsch JF, Miettinen M, Laskin WB, et al. A clinicopathologic study of 45 pediatric soft tissue tumors with an admixture of adipose tissue and fibroblastic elements, and a proposal for classification as lipofibromatosis. *Am J Surg Pathol.* 2000;24(11):1491-1500.

Desmoid Fibromatosis

Mikkelsen OA. Dupuytren's disease: initial symptoms, age of onset and spontaneous course. *Hand.* 1977;9(1):11-15.

Allen RA, Woolner LB, Ghormley RK. Soft tissue tumors of the sole with special reference to plantar fibromatosis. *J Bone Joint Surg Am.* 1955;37-A(1):14-26.

Wever ID, Dal Cin P, Fletcher CDM, et al. Cytogenetic, clinical, and morphologic correlations in 78 cases of fibromatosis: a report from the CHAMP Study Group. *Mod Pathol.* 2000;13(10):1080-1085.

Merchant NB, Lewis JJ, Woodruff JM, et al. Extremity and trunk desmoid tumors: a multifactorial analysis of outcome. *Cancer.* 1999;86(10): 2045-2052.

Yantiss RK, Spiro IJ, Compton CC, et al. Gastrointestinal stromal tumor versus intra-abdominal fibromatosis of the bowel wall: a clinically important differential diagnosis. *Am J Surg Pathol.* 2000;24(7): 947-957.

Huss S, Nehles J, Binot E, et al. β-catenin (CTNNB1) mutations and clinicopathological features of mesenteric desmoid-type fibromatosis. *Histopathology.* 2013;62(2):294-304.

Fibroma of Tendon Sheath

Chung EB, Enzinger FM. Fibroma of tendon sheath. *Cancer.* 1979;44: 1945-1954.

Pulitzer DR, Martin PC, Reed RJ. Fibroma of tendon sheath: a clinico-pathologic study of 32 cases. *Am J Surg Pathol.* 1989;13:472-479.

Dal Cin P, Sciot R, De Smet L, et al. Translocation 2;11 in a fibroma of tendon sheath. *Histopathology.* 1998;332:433-435.

Carter JM, Wang X, Dong J, et al. USP6 genetic rearrangements in cellular fibroma of tendon sheath. *Mod Pathol.* 2016;29(8):865-869.

Myofibroblastoma

Chen BJ, Mariño-Enríquez A, Fletcher CD, Hornick JL. Loss of retino-blastoma protein expression in spindle cell/pleomorphic lipomas and cytogenetically related tumors: an immunohistochemical study with diagnostic implications. *Am J Surg Pathol.* 2012;36(8):1119-1128.

Howitt BE, Fletcher CD. Mammary-type myofibroblastoma: clinicopathologic characterization in a series of 143 cases. *Am J Surg Pathol*. 2016;40(3):361-367.

Angiomyofibroblastoma

Nielsen GP, Rosenberg AE, Young RH, Dickersin GR, Clement PB, Scully RE. Angiomyofibroblastoma of the vulva and vagina. *Mod Pathol*. 1996;9(3):284-291.

Schoolmeester JK, Fritchie KJ. Genital soft tissue tumors. *J Cutan Pathol*. 2015;42(7):441-451.

Fetsch JF, Laskin WB, Lefkowitz M, et al. Aggressive angiomyxoma: a clinicopathologic study of 29 female patients. *Cancer*. 1996;78:79-90.

Steeper TA, Rosai J. Aggressive angiomyxoma of the female pelvis and perineum: report of nine cases of a distinctive type of gynecologic soft-tissue neoplasm. *Am J Surg Pathol*. 1983;7:463-475.

Iezzoni JC, Fechner RE, Wong LS, et al. Aggressive angiomyxoma in males: a report of four cases. *Am J Clin Pathol*. 1995;104:391-396.

Michal M, Fetsch JF, Hes O, et al. Nuchal-type fibroma: a clinicopathologic study of 52 cases. *Cancer*. 1999;85:156-163.

Nuchal-Type Fibroma

Balachandran K, Allen PW, MacCormac LB. Nuchal fibroma: a clinicopathologic study of nine cases. *Am J Surg Pathol*. 1995;19(3):313-317.

Shek TWH. Extranuchal nuchal fibroma. *Am J Surg Pathol*. 1996;20(7):902-903.

Zamecnik M, Michal M. Nuchal-type fibroma is positive for CD34 and CD99. *Am J Surg Pathol*. 2001;25(7):970.

Evans HL. Desmoplastic fibroma: a report of seven cases. *Am J Surg Pathol*. 1995;19(9):1077-1081.

Nielsen GP, O'Connell JX, Dickersin R, et al. Collagenous fibroma (desmoplastic fibroblastoma): a report of seven cases. *Mod Pathol*. 1996;9(7):781-785.

Hasegawa T, Shimoda T, Hiroshashi S, et al. Collagenous fibroma (desmoplastic fibroblastoma): report of four cases and review of the literature. *Arch Pathol Lab Med*. 1998;122(5):455-460.

Dermatofibrosarcoma Protuberans

Harvell J, Kilpatrick SE, White WL. The giant cell patterns in giant cell fibroblastoma and dermtofibrosarcoma protuberans: CD34 staining showing the spectrum and a simulator. *Am J Dermatopathol*. 1998;20(4):339-345.

Browne WB, Antonescu CR, Leung DHY, et al. Dermatofibrosarcoma protuberans: a clinicopathologic analysis of patients treated and followed at a single institution. *Cancer*. 2000;88(12):2711-2720.

McKee PH, Fletcher CDM. Dermatofibrosarcoma protuberans presenting in infancy and childhood. *J Cutan Pathol*. 1991;18(4):241-246.

Mentzel T, Beham A, Katenkamp D, et al. Fibrosarcomatous ("high-grade") dermatofibrosarcoma protuberans: clinicopathologic and immunohistochemical study of a series of 41 cases with emphasis on prognostic significance. *Am J Surg Pathol*. 1998;22(5):576-587.

Goldblum JR, Reith JD, Weiss SW. Sarcomas arising in dermatofibrosarcoma protuberans: a reappraisal of biologic behavior in eighteen cases treated by wide local excision with extended clinical follow up. *Am J Surg Pathol*. 2000;24(8):1125-1130.

Fletcher CDM. Benign fibrous histiocytoma of subcutaneous and deep soft tissue: a clinicopathologic analysis of 21 cases. *Am J Surg Pathol*. 1990;14(9):801-809.

Maire G, Pedeutour F, Mrózek K, et al. COLIA1-PDGFB gene fusion in dermatofibrosarcoma protuberans. Molecular analysis of a case with an unusual large marker containing sequences from chromosomes 7, 8, 17, 21, and 22. *Cancer Genet Cytogenet*. 2002;135(2):197-199.

Solitary Fibrous Tumor

Dermawan JK, Rubin BP, Kilpatrick SE, et al. CD34-negative solitary fibrous tumor: a clinicopathologic study of 25 cases and comparison to their CD34-positive counterparts. *Am J Surg Pathol*. 2021;45(12):1616-1625.

Suster S, Nascimento AG, Miettinen M, et al. Solitary fibrous tumors of soft tissue: a clinicopathologic and immunohistochemical study of 12 cases. *Am J Surg Pathol*. 1995;19(11):1257-1266.

Nielsen GP, O'Connell JX, Dickersin R, et al. Solitary fibrous tumor of soft tissue: a report of 15 cases, including 5 malignant examples with light microscopic, immunohistochemical, and ultrastructural data. *Mod Pathol*. 1997;10(10):1028-1037.

Demicco EG, Wagner MJ, Maki RG, Gupta V, Iofin I, Lazar AJ, Wang WL. Risk assessment in solitary fibrous tumors: validation and refinement of a risk stratification model. *Mod Pathol*. 2017 Oct;30(10):1433-1442. doi: 10.1038/modpathol.2017.54. Epub 2017 Jul 21. PMID: 28731041.

Tai HC, Chuang IC, Chen TC, et al. NAB2-STAT6 fusion types account for clinicopathological variations in solitary fibrous tumors. *Mod Pathol*. 2015;28(10):1324-1335.

Inflammatory Myofibroblastic Tumor

Meis JM, Enzinger FM. Inflammatory fibrosarcoma of the mesentery and retroperitoneum. *Am J Surg Pathol*. 1991;15(12):1146-1156.

Coffin CM, Watterson J, Priest JR, et al. Extrapulmonary inflammatory myofibroblastic tumor (inflammatory pseudotumor): a clinicopathologic and immunohistochemical study of 84 cases. *Am J Surg Pathol*. 1995;19(8):859-872.

Chan JKC, Cheuk W, Shimizu M. Anaplastic lymphoma kinase expression in inflammatory pseudotumors. *Am J Surg Pathol*. 2001;25(6):761-768.

Coffin CM, Patel A, Perkins S, et al. ALK1 and p80 expression and chromosomal rearrangements involving 2p23 in inflammatory myofibroblastic tumor. *Mod Pathol*. 2001;14(6):569-576.

Myxoinflammatory Fibroblastic Tumor

Montgomery EA, Devaney KO, Giordano T, et al. Inflammatory myxohyaline tumor of distal extremities with virocyte or Reed-Sternberg-like cells: a distinctive lesion with features simulating inflammatory conditions, Hodgkin's disease, and various sarcomas. *Mod Pathol*. 1998;11(4):384-391.

Meis-Kindblom JM, Kindblom LG. Acral myxoinflammatory fibroblastic sarcoma: a low-grade tumor of the hands and feet. *Am J Surg Pathol*. 1998;22(8):911-924.

Laskin WB, Fetsch JF, Miettinen M. Myxoinflammatory fibroblastic sarcoma: a clinicopathologic analysis of 104 cases, with emphasis on predictors of outcome. *Am J Surg Pathol*. 2014;38(1):1-12.

Suster D, Michal M, Huang H, et al. Myxoinflammatory fibroblastic sarcoma: an immunohistochemical and molecular genetic study of 73 cases. *Mod Pathol*. 2020;33(12):2520-2533.

Myxofibrosarcoma

Mentzel T, Calonje E, Wadden C, et al. Myxofibrosarcoma: clinicopathologic analysis of 75 cases with emphasis on the low-grade variant. *Am J Surg Pathol*. 1996;20(4):391-405.

Tjarks BJ, Ko JS, Billings SD. Myxofibrosarcoma of unusual sites. *J Cutan Pathol*. 2018;45(2):104-110.

Yoshimoto M, Yamada Y, Ishinara S, et al. Comparative study of myxofibrosarcoma with undifferentiated pleomorphic sarcoma: histopathologic and clinicopathologic review. *Am J Surg Pathol*. 2020;44:87-97.

Nascimento AF, Bertoni F, Fletcher CDM. Epithelioid variant of myxofibrosarcoma: expanding the clinicomorphologic spectrum of myxofibrosarcoma in a series of 17 cases. *Am J Surg Pathol*. 2007;31(1):99-105.

Nielsen GP, O'Connell JX, Rosenberg AE. Intramuscular myxoma: a clinicopathologic study of 51 cases with emphasis on hypercellular and hypervascular variants. *Am J Surg Pathol*. 1998;22(10):1222-1227.

Enzinger FM. Intramuscular myxoma: a review and follow-up study of 34 cases. *Am J Clin Pathol*. 1965;43:104-113.

Extraskeletal Myxoid Chondrosarcoma

Kilpatrick SE, Inwards CY, Fletcher CDM, Smith MA, Gitelis S. Myxoid chondrosarcoma (chordoid sarcoma) of bone: a report of two cases and review of the literature. *Cancer*. 1997;79(10):1903-1910.

Meis-Kindblom JM, Bergh P, Gunterberg B, et al. Extraskeletal myxoid chondrosarcoma: a reappraisal of its morphological spectrum and prognostic factors based on 117 cases. *Am J Surg Pathol*. 1999;23(6):636-650.

Oliveira AM, Sebo TJ, McGrory JE, et al. Extraskeletal myxoid chondrosarcoma: a clinicopathologic, immunohistochemical, and ploidy analysis of 23 cases. *Mod Pathol*. 2000;13(8):900-908.

Goh YW, Spagnolo DV, Platten M, et al. Extraskeletal myxoid chondrosarcoma: a light microscopic, immunohistochemical, ultrastructural and immuno-ultrastructural study indicating neuroendocrine differentiation. *Histopathology*. 2001;39(5):514-524.

Antonescu C, Argani P, Erlandson R, et al. Skeletal and extraskeletal myxoid chondrosarcoma: a comparative clinicopathologic, ultrastructural, and molecular study. *Cancer*. 1998;83(8):1504-1521.

Low-Grade Fibromyxoid Sarcoma

Evans HL. Low-grade fibromyxoid sarcoma: a report of 12 cases. *Am J Surg Pathol*. 1993;17(6):595-600.

Folpe AL, Lane KL, Paull G, et al. Low-grade fibromyxoid sarcoma and hyalinizing spindle cell tumor with giant rosettes: a clinicopathologic study of 73 cases supporting their identity and assessing the impact of high grade areas. *Am J Surg Pathol*. 2000;24(10):1353-1360.

Lane KL, Shannon RJ, Weiss SW. Hyalinizing spindle cell tumor with giant rosettes: a distinctive tumor closely resembling low-grade fibromyxoid sarcoma. *Am J Surg Pathol*. 1997;21(12):1481-1488.

Mezzelani A, Sozzi G, Nessling M, et al. Low grade fibromyxoid sarcoma: a further low-grade soft tissue malignancy characterized by a ring chromosome. *Cancer Genet Cytogenet*. 2000;122(2):144-148.

Mohamed M, Fisher C, Thway K. Low-grade fibromyxoid sarcoma: clinical, morphologic and genetic features. *Ann Diagn Pathol*. 2017;28:60-67.

Guillou L, Benhattar J, Gengler C, et al. Translocation-positive low-grade fibromyxoid sarcoma: clinicopathologic and molecular analysis of a series expanding the morphologic spectrum and suggesting potential relationship to sclerosing epithelioid fibrosarcoma: a study from the French Sarcoma Group. *Am J Surg Pathol*. 2007;31(9):1387-1402.

Kosemehmetoglu K, Michal M, Ardic F, Kilpatrick SE, Sumathi VP. Sclerosing epithelioid fibrosarcoma of bone: morphological, immunophenotypical, and molecular findings in 9 cases. *Virchows Archiv*. 2021;478(4):767-777.

Ossifying Fibromyxoid Tumor

Enzinger FM, Weiss SW, Liang CY. Ossifying fibromyxoid tumor of soft parts: a clinicopathological analysis of 59 cases. *Am J Surg Pathol*. 1989;13(10):817-827.

Kilpatrick SE, Ward WG, Mozes M, Miettinen M, Fukunaga M, Fletcher CDM. Atypical and malignant variants of ossifying fibromyxoid tumor of soft parts: a clinicopathologic analysis of six cases. *Am J Surg Pathol*. 1995;19(9):1039-1046.

Gebre-Medhin S, Nord KH, Möller E, et al. Recurrent rearrangement of the PHF1 gene in ossifying fibromyxoid tumors. *Am J Pathol*. 2012;181(3):1069-1077.

Nishio J, Iwasaki H, Ohjimi Y, et al. Ossifying fibromyxoid tumor of soft parts. Cytogenetic findings. *Cancer Genet Cytogenet*. 2002;133(2):124-128.

Folpe AL, Weiss SW. Ossifying fibromyxoid tumor of soft parts: a clinicopathologic study of 70 cases with emphasis on atypical and malignant variants. *Am J Surg Pathol*. 2003;27(4):421-431.

Myoepithelioma/Mixed Tumor

Kilpatrick SE, Hitchcock MG, Kraus MD, Calojne E, Fletcher CDM. Mixed tumors and myoepitheliomas of soft tissue: a clinicopathologic study of 19 cases with a unifying concept. *Am J Surg Pathol*. 1997;21(1):13-22.

Folpe AL, Agoff SN, Willis J, et al. Parachordoma is immunohistochemically and cytogenetically distinct from axial chordoma and extraskeletal myxoid chondrosarcoma. *Am J Surg Pathol*. 1999;23(9):1059-1067.

Dabska M. Parachordoma: a new clinicopathologic entity. *Cancer*. 1977;40(4):1586-1592.

Jo VY, Fletcher CD. Myoepithelial neoplasms of soft tissue: an updated review of the clinicopathologic, immunophenotypic, and genetic features. *Head Neck Pathol*. 2015;9(1):32-38.

Tenosynovial Giant Cell Tumor

Abdul-Karim FW, El-Naggar AK, Joyce MJ, et al. Diffuse and localized tenosynovial giant cell tumor and pigmented villonodular synovitis: a clinicopathologic and flow cytometric DNA analysis. *Hum Pathol*. 1992;23(7):729-735.

Schwartz HS, Unni KK, Pritchard DJ. Pigmented villonodular synovitis: a retrospective review of large affected joints. *Clin Orthop*. 1989;247:243-255.

De Saint Aubain Somerhausen, Fletcher CD. Diffuse-type giant cell tumor: clinicopathologic and immunohistochemical analysis of 50 cases with extraarticular disease. *Am J Surg Pathol*. 2000;24(4):479-492.

O'Connell JX, Fanburg JC, Rosenberg AE. Giant cell tumor of tendon sheath and pigmented villonodular synovitis: immunophenotype suggests a synovial origin. *Hum Pathol*. 1995;26(7):771-775.

Sciot R, Rosai J, Dal Cin P, et al. Analysis of 35 cases of localized and diffuse tenosynovial giant cell tumor: a report from the Chromosomes and Morphology (CHAMP) study group. *Mod Pathol*. 1999;12(6):576-579.

Enzinger FM, Zhang R. Plexiform fibrohistiocytic tumor presenting in children and young adults: an analysis of 65 cases. *Am J Surg Pathol*. 1988;12(11):818-826.

Remstein ED, Arndt CAS, Nascimento AG. Plexiform fibrohistiocytic tumor: clinicopathologic analysis of 22 cases. *Am J Surg Pathol*. 1999;23(6):662-670.

Folpe AL, Morris RJ, Weiss SW. Soft tissue giant cell tumor of low malignant potential: a proposal for the reclassification of malignant giant cell tumor of soft parts. *Mod Pathol*. 1999;12:894-902.

Lee JC, Liang CW, Fletcher CD. Giant cell tumor of soft tissue is genetically distinct from its bone counterpart. *Mod Pathol*. 2017;30(5):728-733.

Hemangioma

North PE, Waner M, Mizeracki A, et al. GLUT1: a newly discovered immunohistochemical marker for juvenile hemangioendotheliomas. *Hum Pathol*. 2000;31(1):11-22.

Beham A, Fletcher CDM. Intramuscular angioma: a clinicopathologic analysis of 74 cases. *Histopathology*. 1991;18(1):53-59.

Allen PW, Enzinger FM. Hemangioma of skeletal muscle: an analysis of 89 cases. *Cancer*. 1972;29(1):8-22.

Kerr DA. Granuloma pyogenicum. *Oral Surg Oral Med Oral Pathol*. 1951;4(2):158-176.

Dermawan JK, Kilpatrick SE. Ossifying pyogenic granuloma: a rare variant usually not recognized. *J Cutan Pathol*. 2021;48(7):954-957.

Lappa E, Drakos E. Anastomosing hemangioma: short review of a benign mimicker of angiosarcoma. *Arch Pathol Lab Med*. 2020;144(2):240-244.

Perkins P, Weiss SW. Spindle cell hemangioendothelioma: an analysis of 78 cases with reassessment of its pathogenesis and biologic behavior. *Am J Surg Pathol*. 1996;20(10):1196-1204.

Fanburg JC, Meis-Kindblom JM, Rosenberg AE. Multiple enchondromas associated with spindle-cell hemangioendotheliomas: an overlooked variant of Maffucci's syndrome. *Am J Surg Pathol*. 1995;19(9):1029-1038.

Epithelioid Hemangioma

Fetsch JF, Weiss SW. Observations concerning the pathogenesis of epithelioid hemangiomas (angiolymphoid hyperplasia). *Mod Pathol*. 1991;4:449-455.

Huang SC, Zhang L, Sung YS, et al. Frequent FOS gene rearrangements in epithelioid hemangioma: a molecular study of 58 cases with morphologic reappraisal. *Am J Surg Pathol*. 2015;39(10):1313-1321.

Hung YP, Fletcher CD, Hornick JL. FOSB is a useful diagnostic marker for pseudomyogenic hemangioendothelioma. *Am J Surg Pathol*. 2017;41(5):596-606.

Kaposi Sarcoma

Gottlieb GJ, Ackerman AB. Kaposi's sarcoma: an extensively disseminated form in young homosexual men. *Hum Pathol*. 1982;13(10):882-892.

Brenner B, Weissman-Brenner A, Rakowsky E, et al. Classical Kaposi sarcoma: prognostic factor analysis of 248 patients. *Cancer*. 2002;95(9):1982-1987.

Chang Y, Cesarman E, Pessin MS, et al. Identification of herpesvirus-like DNA sequences in AIDS-associated Kaposi's sarcoma. *Science*. 1994;266(5192):1865-1869.

Moore PS, Chang Y. Detection of herpesvirus-like DNA sequences in Kaposi's sarcoma in patients with and those without HIV infection. *N Engl J Med*. 1995;332(18):1181-1185.

Radu O, Pantanowitz L. Kaposi sarcoma. *Arch Pathol Lab Med.* 2013; 137(2):289-294.

Pseudomyogenic Hemangioendothelioma

Billings SD, Folpe AL, Weiss SW. Epithelioid sarcoma-like hemangioendothelioma. *Am J Surg Pathol.* 2003;27(1):48-57.

Caballero GA, Roitman PD. Pseudomyogenic hemangioendothelioma (epithelioid sarcoma-like hemangioendothelioma). *Arch Pathol Lab Med.* 2020;144(4):529-533.

Ko JS, Billings SD. Diagnostically challenging epithelioid vascular tumors. *Surg Pathol Clin.* 2015;8(3):331-351.

Epithelioid Hemangioendothelioma

Weiss SW, Enzinger FM. Epithelioid hemangioendothelioma: a vascular tumor often mistaken for a carcinoma. *Cancer.* 1982;50(5):970-981.

Mentzel T, Beham A, Calonje E, et al. Epithelioid hemangioendothelioma of skin and soft tissues: clinicopathologic and immunohistochemical study of 30 cases. *Am J Surg Pathol.* 1997;21(4):363-374.

Makhlouf HR, Ishak KG, Goodman ZD. Epithelioid hemangioendothelioma of the liver: a clinicopathologic study of 137 cases. *Cancer.* 1999; 85(3):562-582.

Mendlick MR, Nelson M, Pickering D, et al. Translocation t(1;3) (p36.3;q25) is a nonrandom aberration in epithelioid hemangioendothelioma. *Am J Surg Pathol.* 2001;25(5):684-687.

Antonescu CR, Le Loarer F, Mosquera JM, et al. Novel YAP1-TFE3 fusion defines a distinct subset of epithelioid hemangioendothelioma. *Genes Chromosomes Cancer.* 2013;52(8):775-784.

Rosenbaum E, Jadeja B, Xu B, et al. Prognostic stratification of clinical and molecular epithelioid hemangioendothelioma subsets. *Mod Pathol.* 2020;33(4):591-602.

Angiosarcoma

Meis-Kindblom JM, Kindblom LG. Angiosarcoma of soft tissue: a study of 80 cases. *Am J Surg Pathol.* 1998;22(6):683-697.

Mark RJ, Poen JC, Tran LM, et al. Angiosarcoma: a report of 67 patients. *Cancer.* 1996;77(11):2400-2406.

Yan M, Gilmore H, Bomeisl P, Harbhajanka A. Clinicopathologic and immunohistochemical study of breast angiosarcoma. *Ann Diagn Pathol.* 2021;54:151795.

Feller JK, Mahalingam M. C-myc and cutaneous vascular neoplasms. *Am J Dermatopathol.* 2013;35(3):364-369.

Calonje E, Fletcher CDM, Wilson-Jones E, et al. Retiform hemangioendothelioma: a distinctive form of low-grade angiosarcoma delineated in a series of 15 cases. *Am J Surg Pathol.* 1994;18(2):115-125.

Glomus Tumor

Van Geertruyden J, Lorea P, Goldschmidt D, et al. Glomus tumours of the hand. A retrospective study of 51 cases. *J Hand Surg Br.* 1996; 21(2):257-260.

Folpe AL, Fanburg-Smith JC, Miettinen M, Weiss SW. Atypical and malignant glomus tumors: analysis of 52 cases, with a proposal for the reclassification of glomus tumors. *Am J Surg Pathol.* 2001;25(1):1-12.

Robinson JC, Kilpatrick SE, Kelly Jr DL. Intraosseous glomus tumor of the spine. Case report and review of the literature. *J Neurosurg.* 1996;85(2):344-347.

Agaram NP, Zhang L, Jungbluth AA, et al. A molecular reappraisal of glomus tumors and related pericytic neoplasms with emphasis on NOTCH-gene fusions. *Am J Surg Pathol.* 2020;44(11):1556-1562.

Myofibroma/Myopericytoma

Chung EB, Enzinger FM. Infantile myofibromatosis. *Cancer.* 1981;48(8):1807-1818.

Inwards CY, Unni KK, Beabout JW, Shives TC. Solitary congenital fibromatosis (infantile myofibromatosis) of bone. *Am J Surg Pathol.* 1991;15(10):935-941.

Mentzel T, Calonje E, Nascimento AG, Fletcher CD. Infantile hemangiopericytoma versus infantile myofibromatosis. Study of a series suggesting a continuous spectrum of infantile myofibroblastic lesions. *Am J Surg Pathol.* 1994;18(9):922-930.

Granter SR, Badizadegan K, Fletcher CD. Myofibromatosis in adults, glomangiopericytoma, and myopericytoma: a spectrum of tumors showing perivascular myoid differentiation. *Am J Surg Pathol.* 1998;22(5):513-525.

Hachisuga T, Hashimoto H, Enjoji M. Angioleiomyoma. A clinicopathologic reappraisal of 562 cases. *Cancer.* 1984;54(1):126-130.

Leiomyosarcoma

Kilpatrick SE, Mentzel T, Fletcher CDM. Leiomyoma of deep soft tissue: clinicopathologic analysis of a series. *Am J Surg Pathol.* 1994; 18(6):576-582.

Billings SD, Folpe AL, Weiss SW. Do leiomyomas of deep soft tissue exist? An analysis of highly differentiated smooth muscle tumors of deep soft tissue supporting two distinct subtypes. *Am J Surg Pathol.* 2001;25:1134-1142.

Paal E, Miettinen M. Retroperitoneal leiomyomas: a clinicopathologic and immunohistochemical study of 56 cases with a comparison to retroperitoneal leiomyosarcomas. *Am J Surg Pathol.* 2001;25(11): 1355-1363.

Farshid G, Pradhan M, Goldblum J, Weiss SW. Leiomyosarcoma of somatic soft tissues: a tumor of vascular origin with multivariate analysis of outcome in 42 cases. *Am J Surg Pathol.* 2002;26(1):14-24.

Hines OJ, Nelson S, Quinones-Baldrich WJ, Eilber FR. Leiomyosarcoma of the inferior vena cava: prognosis and comparison with leiomyosarcoma of other anatomic sites. *Cancer.* 1999;85(5):1077-1083.

de Saint Aubain Somerhausen N, Fletcher CD. Leiomyosarcoma of soft tissue in children: clinicopathologic analysis of 20 cases. *Am J Surg Pathol.* 1999;23(7):755-763.

Embryonal Rhabdomyosarcoma

Newton Jr WA, Gehan EA, Webber BL, et al. Classification of rhabdomyosarcomas and related sarcomas, pathologic aspects and proposal for a new classification – An Intergroup Rhabdomyosarcoma Study. *Cancer.* 1995;76(6):1073-1085.

Horn RC, Enterline HT. Rhabdomyosarcoma: a clinicopathologic study and classification of 39 cases. *Cancer.* 1958;11(1):181-199.

Kumar S, Perlman E, Harris CA, Rafield M, Tsokos M. Myogenin is a specific marker for rhabdomyosarcoma: an immunohistochemical study in paraffin-embedded tissues. *Mod Pathol.* 2000;13(9):988-993.

Leiner J, Le Loarer F. The current landscape of rhabdomyosarcomas: an update. *Virchows Arch.* 2020;476(1):97-108.

Coffin CM, Rulon J, Smith L, et al. Pathologic features of rhabdomyosarcoma before and after treatment: a clinicopathologic and immunohistochemical analysis. *Mod Pathol.* 1997;10(12):1175-1187.

Kapadia SB, Meis JM, Frisman DM, Ellis GL, Heffner DK, Hyams VJ. Adult rhabdomyoma of the head and neck: a clinicopathologic and immunophenotypic study. *Hum Pathol.* 1993;24(6):608-617.

Willis J, Abdul-Karim FW, di Sant'Agnese PA. Extracardiac rhabdomyomas. *Semin Diagn Pathol.* 1994;11(1):15-25.

Alveolar Rhabdomyosarcoma

Parham DM, Shapiro DN, Downing JR, et al. Solid alveolar rhabdomyosarcomas with the t(2;13): report of two cases with diagnostic implications. *Am J Surg Pathol.* 1994;18(5):474-478.

Parham DM, Barr FG. Classification of rhabdomyosarcoma and its molecular basis. *Adv Anat Pathol.* 2013;20(6):387-397.

Williamson D, Missiaglia E, de Reyniès A, et al. Fusion gene-negative alveolar rhabdomyosarcoma is clinically and molecularly indistinguishable from embryonal rhabdomyosarcoma. *J Clin Oncol.* 2010;28(13):2151-2158.

Forgó E, Hornick JL, Charville GW. MUC4 is expressed in alveolar rhabdomyosarcoma. *Histopathology.* 2021;78(6):905-908.

Hostein I, Andraud-Fregeville M, Guillou L, et al. Rhabdomyosarcoma: value of myogenin expression analysis and molecular testing in diagnosing the alveolar subtype: an analysis of 109 paraffin-embedded specimens. *Cancer.* 2004;101(12):2817-2824.

Pleomorphic Rhabdomyosarcoma

Gaffney EF, Dervan PA, Fletcher CDM. Pleomorphic rhabdomyosarcoma in adulthood: analysis of 11 cases with definition of diagnostic criteria. *Am J Surg Pathol.* 1993;17(6):601-609.

Furlong MA, Mentzel T, Fanburg-Smith JC. Pleomorphic rhabdomyosar-coma in adults: a clinicopathologic study of 38 cases with emphasis on morphologic variants and recent skeletal muscle-markers. *Mod Pathol.* 2001;14(6):595-603.

Agaram NP. Evolving classification of rhabdomyosarcoma. *Histopathology.* 2022;80(1):98-108.

Spindle Cell/Sclerosing Rhabdomyosarcoma

Nascimento AF, Fletcher CD. Spindle cell rhabdomyosarcoma in adults. *Am J Surg Pathol.* 2005;29(8):1106-1113.

Rekhi B, Upadhyay P, Ramteke MP, Dutt A. MYOD1 (L122R) mutations are associated with spindle cell and sclerosing rhabdomyosarcomas with aggressive clinical outcomes. *Mod Pathol.* 2016;29(12):1532-1540.

Leuschner I, Newton WA, Schmidt D, et al. Spindle cell variants of embryonal rhabdomyosarcoma in the paratesticular region: a report of the Intergroup Rhabdomyosarcoma Study. *Am J Surg Pathol.* 1993; 17(3):221-230.

Rubin BP, Hasserjian RP, Singer S, et al. Spindle cell rhabdomyosar-coma (so-called) in adults: report of two cases with emphasis on differential diagnosis. *Am J Surg Pathol.* 1998;22(4):459-464.

Neurofibroma

Sorensen SA, Mulvihill JJ, Nielsen A. A long term follow-up of von Recklinghausen neurofibromatosis: survival and malignant neoplasms. *N Engl J Med.* 1986;314(16):1010-1015.

Zoller MET, Rembeck B, Oden A. Malignant and benign tumors in patients with neurofibromatosis type 1 in a defined Swedish population. *Cancer.* 1997;79(11):2125-2131.

Lin BTY, Weiss LM, Medeiros LJ. Neurofibroma and cellular neurofibroma with atypia: a report of 14 tumors. *Am J Surg Pathol.* 1997;21(12):1443-1449.

McCarron KF, Goldblum JR. Plexiform neurofibroma with and without associated malignant peripheral nerve sheath tumor: a clinicopathologic and immunohistochemical analysis of 54 cases. *Mod Pathol.* 1998;11(7):612-617.

Halling KC, Scheithauer BW, Halling AC, et al. p53 expression in neurofibroma and malignant peripheral nerve sheath tumor: an immunohistochemical study of sporadic and NF1-associated tumors. *Am J Clin Pathol.* 1996;106(3):282-288.

Schwannoma

White W, Shiu MH, Rosenblum MK, et al. Cellular schwannoma: a clinicopathologic study of 57 patients and 58 tumors. *Cancer.* 1990;66(6):1266-1275.

Antinheimo J, Sankila R, Carpen O, et al. Population based analysis of sporadic and type 2 neurofibromatosis-associated meningiomas and schwannomas. *Neurology.* 2000;54(1):71-76.

Hasegawa SL, Mentzel T, Fletcher CDM. Schwannomas of the sinonasal tract and nasopharynx. *Mod Pathol.* 1997;10(8):777-784.

McMenamin ME, Fletcher CDM. Expanding the spectrum of malignant change in schwannomas: epithelioid malignant change, epithelioid malignant peripheral nerve sheath tumor, and epithelioid angiosarcoma: a study of 17 cases. *Am J Surg Pathol.* 2001;25(1):13-25.

Woodruff JM, Selig AM, Crowley K, et al. Schwannoma (neurilemoma) with malignant transformation: a rare, distinctive peripheral nerve sheath tumor. *Am J Surg Pathol.* 1994;18(9):882-895.

Weiss SW, Langloss JM, Enzinger FM. Value of S-100 protein in the diagnosis of soft tissue tumors with particular reference to benign and malignant Schwann cell tumors. *Lab Invest.* 1983;49(3):299-308.

Khalifa MA, Montgomery EA, Ismiil N, et al. What are the CD34+ cells in benign peripheral nerve sheath tumors? Double immunostaining study of CD34 and S-100 protein. *Am J Clin Pathol.* 2000;114(1): 123-126.

Laskin WB, Weiss SW, Bratthauer GL. Epithelioid variant of malignant peripheral nerve sheath tumor (malignant epithelioid schwannoma). *Am J Surg Pathol.* 1991;15(12):1136-1145.

Perineurioma

Hornick JL, Fletcher CD. Soft tissue perineurioma: clinicopathologic analysis of 81 cases including those with atypical histologic features. *Am J Surg Pathol.* 2005;29(7):845-858.

Fox MD, Gleason BC, Thomas AB, Victor TA, Cibull TL. Extra-acral cutaneous/soft tissue sclerosing perineurioma: an under-recognized entity in the differential of CD34-positive cutaneous neoplasms. *J Cutan Pathol.* 2010;37(10):1053-1056.

Carter JM, Wu Y, Blessing MM, et al. Recurrent genomic alterations in soft tissue perineuriomas. *Am J Surg Pathol.* 2018;42(12):1708-1714.

Granular Cell Tumor

Ordonez NG. Granular cell tumor: a review and update. *Adv Anat Pathol.* 1999;6(4):186-203.

Fanburg-Smith JC, Meis-Kindblom JM, Fante R, Kindblom LG. Malignant granular cell tumor of soft tissue: diagnostic criteria and clinicopathologic correlation. *Am J Surg Pathol.* 1998;22(7):779-794.

Mazur MT, Shultz JJ, Myers JL. Granular cell tumor. Immunohistochemical analysis of 21 benign tumors and one malignant tumor. *Arch Pathol Lab Med.* 1990;114(7):692-696.

Angiomatoid Fibrous Histiocytoma

Costa MJ, Weiss SW. Angiomatoid fibrous histiocytoma: a follow-up study of 108 cases with evaluation of possible histologic predictors of outcome. *Am J Surg Pathol.* 1990;14(12):1126-1132.

Fletcher CDM. Angiomatoid "malignant fibrous histiocytoma": an immunohistochemical study indicative of myoid differentiation. *Hum Pathol.* 1991;22(6):563-568.

Hasegawa T, Seki K, Ono K, et al. Angiomatoid (malignant) fibrous histiocytoma: a peculiar low grade tumor showing immunophenotypic heterogeneity and ultrastructural variations. *Pathol Int.* 2000;50(9):731-738.

Fanburg-Smith JC, Miettinen M. Angiomatoid "malignant" fibrous histiocytoma: a clinicopathologic study of 158 cases and further exploration of the myoid phenotype. *Hum Pathol.* 1999;30(11): 1336-1343.

Waters BL, Panagopoulos I, Allen EF. Genetic characterization of angiomatoid fibrous histiocytoma identifies fusion of the FUS and ATF-1 genes induced by a chromosomal translocation involving bands 12q13 and 16p11. *Cancer Genet Cytogenet.* 2000;121(2):109-116.

Pleomorphic Hyalinizing Angiectatic Tumor of Soft Parts

Smith ME, Fisher C, Weiss SW. Pleomorphic hyalinizing angiectatic tumor of soft parts: a low-grade neoplasm resembling neurilemoma. *Am J Surg Pathol.* 1996;20:21-29.

Marshall-Taylor C, Fanburg-Smith JC. Hemosiderotic fibrohistiocytic lipomatous lesion: ten cases of a previously undescribed fatty lesion of the foot/ankle. *Mod Pathol.* 2000;13(11):1192-1199.

Synovial Sarcoma

Bergh P, Meis-Kindblom JM, Gherlinzoni F, Berlin O, et al. Synovial sarcoma: identification of low and high risk groups. *Cancer.* 1999;85:2596-2607.

Oda Y, Hashimoto H, Tsuneyoshi M, Takeshita S. Survival in synovial sarcoma: a multivariate study of prognostic factors with special emphasis on the comparison between early death and long-term survival. *Am J Surg Pathol.* 1993;17:35-44.

Krane JF, Bertoni F, Fletcher CDM. Myxoid synovial sarcoma: an underappreciated morphologic subset. *Mod Pathol.* 1999;12:456-462.

Folpe AL, Schmidt RA, Chapman D, Gown AM. Poorly differentiated synovial sarcoma: immunohistochemical distinction from primitive neuroectodermal tumors and high-grade malignant peripheral nerve sheath tumors. *Am J Surg Pathol.* 1998;22:673-682.

Dei Tos AP, Wadden C, Calonje E, et al. Immunohistochemical demonstration of glycoprotein p30/32mic2 (CD99) in synovial sarcoma: a potential cause of diagnostic confusion. *Appl Immunohistochem.* 1995;3:168-173.

Smith TA, Machen SK, Fisher C, Goldblum JR. Usefulness of cytokeratin subsets for distinguishing monophasic synovial sarcoma from malignant peripheral nerve sheath tumor. *Am J Clin Pathol.* 1999;112:641-648.

De Leeuw B, Balemans M, Olde Weghuis D, Geurts van Kessel A. Identification of two alternative fusion genes, SYT-SSX1 and SYT-SSX2, in t(X;18)(p11.2;q11.2)-positive synovial sarcoma. *Hum Mol Genet.* 1995;4:1097-1099.

Kawai A, Woodruff J, Healey JH, et al. SYT-SSX gene fusion as a determinant of morphology and prognosis in synovial sarcoma. *N Engl J Med*. 1998;338:153-160.

Epithelioid Sarcoma

Chase DR, Enzinger FM. Epithelioid sarcoma: diagnosis, prognostic indicators, and treatment. *Am J Surg Pathol*. 1985;9:241-263.

Evans HL, Baer SC. Epithelioid sarcoma: a clinicopathologic and prognostic study of 26 cases. *Semin Diagn Pathol*. 1993;10:286-291.

Guillou L, Wadden C, Coindre JM, et al. "Proximal-type" epithelioid sarcoma, a distinctive aggressive neoplasm showing rhabdoid features. *Am J Surg Pathol*. 1997;21:130-146.

Arber DA, Kandalaft PL, Mehta P, Battifora H. Vimentin-negative epithelioid sarcoma: the value of an immunohistochemical panel that includes CD34. *Am J Surg Pathol*. 1993;17:302-307.

Alveolar Soft Part Sarcoma

Auerbach HE, Brooks JJ. Alveolar soft-part sarcoma: a clinicopathologic and immunohistochemical study. *Cancer*. 1987;60(1):66-73.

Evans HL. Alveolar soft-pat sarcoma. A study of 13 typical examples and one with a histologically atypical component. *Cancer*. 1985;55(4):912-917.

Portera Jr CA, Ho CA, Patel SR, et al. Alveolar soft part sarcoma: clinical course and patterns of metastasis in 70 patients treated at a single institution. *Cancer*. 2001;91(3):585-591.

Ladanyi M, Lui MY, Antonescu CR, et al. The der(17)t(X;17)(p11;q25) of human alveolar soft part sarcoma fuses the TFE3 transcription factor gene to ASPL, a novel gene at 17q25. *Oncogene*. 2001;20(1):48-57.

Clear Cell Sarcoma

Chung EB, Enzinger FM. Malignant melanoma of soft parts: a reassessment of clear cell sarcoma. *Am J Surg Pathol*. 1983;7(5):405-413.

Lucas DR, Nascimento AG, Sim FH. Clear cell sarcoma of soft tissues: Mayo Clinic experience with 35 cases. *Am J Surg Pathol*. 1992;16(12):1197-1204.

Deenik W, Mooi WJ, Rutgers EJ, et al. Clear cell sarcoma (malignant melanoma) of soft parts: a clinicopathologic study of 30 cases. *Cancer*. 1999;86(6):969-975.

Zucman J, Delattre O, Desmaze C, et al. EWS and ATF-1 gene fusion induced by t(12;22) translocation in malignant melanoma of soft parts. *Nature Genet*. 1993;4(4):341-345.

Desmoplastic Small Round Cell Tumor

Ordonez NG. Desmoplastic small round cell tumor: a histopathologic study of 39 cases with emphasis on unusual histological patterns. *Am J Surg Pathol*. 1998;22(11):1303-1313.

Cummings OW, Ulbright TM, Young RH, et al. Desmoplastic small round cell tumors of the paratesticular region: a report of six cases. *Am J Surg Pathol*. 1997;21(2):219-225.

Adsay V, Cheng J, Athanasian E, et al. Primary desmoplastic small cell tumor of soft tissues and bone of the hand. *Am J Surg Pathol*. 1999;23(11):1408-1413.

Hill DA, Pfeifer JD, Marley EF, et al. WT1 staining reliably differentiates desmoplastic small round cell tumor from Ewing sarcoma/primitive neuroectodermal tumor: an immunohistochemical and molecular diagnostic study. *Am J Clin Pathol*. 2000;114(3):345-353.

Kilpatrick SE, Reith JD, Rubin B. Ewing sarcoma and the history of similar and possibly related small round cell tumors. From whence have we come and where are we going? *Adv Anat Pathol*. 2018;25(5):314-326.

Christopher Griffith • Mobeen Rahman

PLEOMORPHIC ADENOMA

DIFFERENTIAL DIAGNOSES: POLYMORPHOUS ADENOCARCINOMA & EPITHELIAL-MYOEPITHELIAL CARCINOMA

Clinical Features

Pleomorphic adenoma (PA), also called benign mixed tumor, is a benign tumor of the salivary glands. PAs are the most common salivary gland neoplasm and the vast majority occur in the parotid glands (~80%) with lower incidence in submandibular glands (~10%). PAs also arise in minor salivary glands of the upper aerodigestive tract (~10%) with oral sites (particularly palate, lip, and buccal) being most common. As with many salivary gland tumor types, PAs occur more commonly in women than in men with a female-to-male ratio of ~2:1. On average, PAs are most commonly diagnosed in middle-aged adults (average age is 46 years), but they also arise in children. The most common clinical presentation of PA is that of a nonspecific slowly growing, painless mass. The overall consistency of PA can be variable depending on the cellular composition, but a firm mass is most common.

Pathologic Features

GROSS FINDINGS

A well-circumscribed nodule is a characteristic gross feature of PA. Smaller tumors will have an entirely round contour and those arising in major glands can show evidence of encapsulation. In larger tumors, the borders can have a more multinodular, bosselated appearance. A solitary tumor is most common but in cases of recurrent PA, multiple nodules of various sizes are scattered throughout the prior surgical bed. PA nodules are usually white to tan in color but may show areas of hemorrhage, especially following prior aspiration. Cystic change can also be seen, sometimes to include larger cystic structures. PA consistency is also variable depending on the cellular composition. Tumors containing prominent chondroid matrix or sclerosis are firm, whereas those that are more myxoid or cellular tend to be softer.

MICROSCOPIC FINDINGS

The cellular composition of PA includes luminal ductal epithelium surrounded by abluminal myoepithelial cells. Myoepithelial cells are also present in the stroma and classically have the appearance of "spinning off" ductal structures (Fig. 9.1). Classic PAs show a fairly even mixture of cellular and stromal elements, but composition varies from more myxoid/stroma rich to more cellular stroma poor examples. True chondroid differentiation is also common and can be seen in approximately half of cases. The cellular components are typically bland with low mitotic activity. Focal changes that can be seen in the ductal cells include squamous, sebaceous, and apocrine metaplasia. Psammomatous calcifications and tyrosine crystalloids can also be seen in small numbers of cases but are not specific for PA. As with the gross appearance, most PAs are well circumscribed and can show a surrounding fibrous capsule; however, minor gland tumors commonly lack a capsule. One unusual feature that is seen in PA is the occurrence of pseudopods extending beyond the capsule or border of the PA. Pseudopods can raise concern for invasion (i.e., carcinoma ex PA) but in comparison with true invasion, pseudopods tend to be mostly myxoid and lack destruction of surrounding structures. Carcinoma ex PAs represent malignant transformation of a PA and are diagnosed based on malignant cytologic features and/or true invasion.

Ancillary Studies

Immunostains can be most helpful for confirming the biphasic nature of the cellular components. Depending on the laboratory, most pan-keratins and cytokeratin 7 will stain the luminal ductal cells strongly and demonstrate weaker reactivity in the surrounding myoepithelial cells.

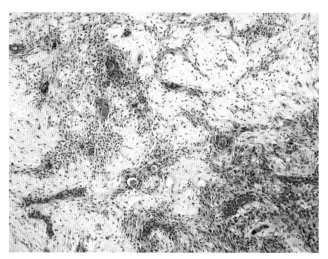

FIG. 9.1

Pleomorphic adenoma. Pleomorphic adenomas are composed of a biphasic population of bland myoepithelial cells and ducts in a chondromyxoid stroma. Myoepithelial cells surround the ducts and are present in the stroma.

Conversely, immunostains for myoepithelial cells (p63/p40, S100, smooth muscle actin [SMA], calponin) will only be positive in these abluminal and stromal cells.

PAs frequently show cytogenetic abnormalities with the most common being rearrangements of *PLAG1* (50%–60%) and *HMGA2* (10%–20%) with a variety of partner genes. While fluorescence *in situ* hybridization (FISH) or sequencing assays are able to detect these rearrangements, these tests are not commonly used clinically for diagnosis. Immunohistochemistry for PLAG1 and HMGA2 is also possible and can indicate overexpression of these proteins even in cases that lack the specific rearrangement. These immunostains are less specific than molecular tests to confirm such rearrangements.

Differential Diagnosis

While the diagnosis of PA is straightforward in many cases, the variable composition and overall appearance of PA results in a diagnostic challenge in some cases. Two entities that may commonly enter into the differential diagnosis with PA are polymorphous adenocarcinoma (PAC; formerly polymorphous low-grade adenocarcinoma [PLGA]) and epithelial-myoepithelial carcinoma (EMCA).

The distinction between PA and PAC can be particularly challenging in biopsy specimens from oral minor salivary gland sites where both entities occur. Both tumor entities can show similar architectural patterns and myxoid type stroma at low power (Fig. 9.2A). An important distinction between PAC and PA is that PAC is composed of tumor cells with almost purely ductal differentiation, whereas PAs show both ductal and myoepithelial cell components (Table 9.1). Perineural invasion is also common in PAC (Fig. 9.2B) and does not occur in benign PA. Immunostains can be very helpful to highlight myoepithelial differentiation in most cases. PACs are characteristically strongly and diffusely S100 positive. Abluminal myoepithelial cells in PA generally show strong expression of several specific myoepithelial markers (SMA, calponin, smooth muscle myosin, etc), but some cases of PAC may also show focal weak reactivity with these markers also. A common finding in PAC is a p63-positive/p40-negative phenotype.

EMCA is a low-grade biphasic salivary gland malignancy. The overall similarity in differentiation with luminal ductal and abluminal myoepithelial cells and the common low-grade nodular invasive growth can

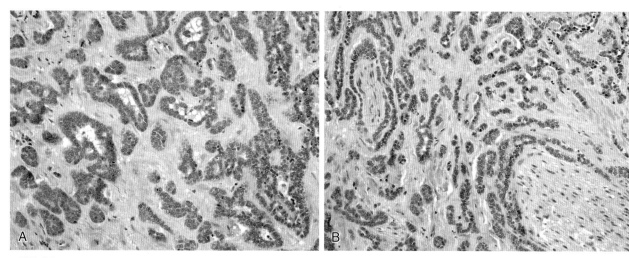

FIG. 9.2

Polymorphous adenocarcinoma. Polymorphous adenocarcinoma can mimic a pleomorphic adenoma of the palate as it frequently shows bland ductal structures and can have focal myxoid stroma as seen in this case (**A**). The key diagnostic distinction is the lack of biphasic differentiation in polymorphous adenocarcinoma with no overt myoepithelial differentiation. Here it can be seen that there is only a single population of tumor cells and this can be confirmed with immunohistochemistry. Polymorphous adenocarcinoma also frequently shows perineural invasion (**B**).

TABLE 9.1

Features of Pleomorphic Adenoma Versus Polymorphous Adenocarcinoma

Pleomorphic Adenoma	Polymorphous Adenocarcinoma
• Biphasic growth with definitive myoepithelial differentiation of abluminal and stromal cells	• Purely ductal without overt myoepithelial cell differentiation (focal myoepithelial marker expression may be seen)
• Myoepithelial cells co-express p40 and p63 as well as other myoepithelial markers	• Ductal cells commonly express p63 but are negative for p40
• Chondromyxoid stroma with embedded myoepithelial cells	• Myxoid stroma may be present but lacks chondroid differentiation and embedded myoepithelial cells
• No evidence of invasion	• Invasive including common perineural invasion

TABLE 9.2

Features of Pleomorphic Adenoma Versus Epithelial-Myoepithelial Carcinoma

Pleomorphic Adenoma	Epithelial-Myoepithelial Carcinoma
• Biphasic with luminal ductal cells and abluminal myoepithelial cells	• Biphasic with luminal ductal cells and abluminal myoepithelial cells
• Myoepithelial cells show various morphologies including spindle, stellate, plasmacytoid and epithelioid	• Myoepithelial cells are most commonly enlarged with prominent clear cytoplasm (i.e., activated myoepithelial cells)
• No evidence of invasion	• Invasion is present and may represent a minor invasive component of a carcinoma ex pleomorphic adenoma

make the distinctions between EMCA and PA challenging, particularly in cases of EMCA ex PA (Table 9.2). EMCA is characterized by an "activated" myoepithelial phenotype that is commonly manifested by myoepithelial cells with prominent clear cytoplasm (Fig. 9.3). Unfortunately, similar areas can be seen within benign PA, and EMCA ex PA frequently show areas of residual PA. Increased cytologic atypia (including mitotic activity) can be a helpful sign of EMCA, but the most important feature to distinguish these entities is the presence of invasion in EMCA. Immunostains offer very little help in this differential diagnosis as both tumors show similar immunophenotypes. In some cases, S100 may be helpful to highlight foci of perineural invasion which does not occur in PA. When there is a concern for invasion, additional sampling and/or deeper histologic sections from tissue blocks are helpful in some cases.

Prognosis and Therapy

Recurrence is reported to occur in the 4% to 7% range, with some authors suggesting a higher risk of recurrence association with stroma-rich (i.e., myxoid) PA. Following an initial recurrence of PA, patients continued to suffer

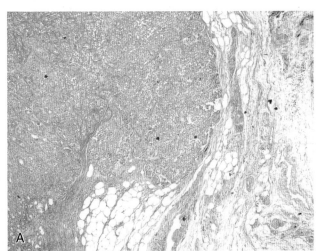
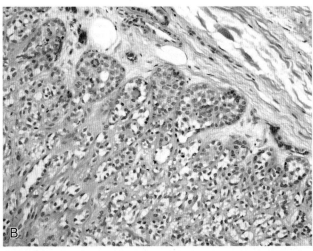

FIG. 9.3

Epithelial-myoepithelial carcinoma (EMCA) ex pleomorphic adenoma (PA). Invasion beyond the original PA capsule is evident with invasion into surrounding fibroadipose (**A**). Compared with benign pseudopodia which are not evidence of invasion, this focus shows characteristic EMCA morphology with so-called "activated" myoepithelial cells having abundant clear cytoplasm surrounding smaller ductal structures and a lack of stroma (**B**).

from higher rates of additional recurrences due to seeding of the area. Malignant transformation (i.e., carcinoma ex PA) can occur and is generally reported in up to 5% to 15%. Some studies report the rate of malignant transformation is higher in cases of recurrent PA. In general, complete surgical excision is the treatment of choice but radiation therapy is used in some patients, particularly for management of challenging recurrent disease.

PLEOMORPHIC ADENOMA – DISEASE FACT SHEET

Definition
- ▸▸ Pleomorphic adenoma is a benign salivary gland tumor showing biphasic ductal and myoepithelial cell differentiation in chondromyxoid stroma

Incidence and Location
- ▸▸ Pleomorphic adenoma is the most common salivary gland tumor
- ▸▸ Pleomorphic adenomas are most common in the parotid gland

Age and Sex Distribution
- ▸▸ Most commonly diagnosed in middle age (average age 46 years)
- ▸▸ More common in women with a female-to-male ratio of 2:1

Clinical Features
- ▸▸ Slow-growing painless mass

Prognosis and Therapy
- ▸▸ Most have benign behavior
- ▸▸ Recurrence occurs in 4%–7%, possibly more common in myxoid tumors
- ▸▸ Malignant transformation (i.e., carcinoma ex PA) occurs in 5%–15%
- ▸▸ Complete surgical excision

PLEOMORPHIC ADENOMA – PATHOLOGIC FEATURES

Gross Findings
- ▸▸ Well circumscribed
- ▸▸ Usually solitary
- ▸▸ May be cystic, myxoid, or firm

Microscopic Findings
- ▸▸ Bland luminal ductal cells surrounded by abluminal myoepithelial cells, stromal myoepithelial cells, and chondromyxoid stroma
- ▸▸ Cellularity can range from very myoepithelial cell-rich to very stroma-rich
- ▸▸ Lack of invasion
- ▸▸ Cystic change and fibrosis/sclerosis possible
- ▸▸ May contain apocrine, squamous, or adipocytic metaplasia
- ▸▸ Malignant transformation indicated by cytologic atypia and/or invasion

Pathologic Differential Diagnoses
- ▸▸ Polymorphous adenocarcinoma
- ▸▸ Epithelial-myoepithelial carcinoma

WARTHIN TUMOR

DIFFERENTIAL DIAGNOSES: LOW-GRADE MUCOEPIDERMOID CARCINOMA AND SQUAMOUS CELL CARCINOMA

Clinical Features

Warthin tumor (WT) is a benign tumor of the salivary glands. WTs have historically been the second most common salivary gland tumor, but some studies have shown a higher incidence of WT in some regions of the world where smoking is highly prevalent. Although some extraparotid examples can be found in the literature, it is thought that WT occurs in the parotid gland and periparotid regions as it is theorized to arise from ductal inclusions found only in intra- and periparotid lymph nodes. WTs have a strong association with tobacco smoking or significant secondhand smoke exposure. WTs are most common in older men, but the incidence in women has increased over time with the rate of smoking. WTs are extremely rare in patients aged less than 40 years. When WT becomes clinically apparent, it is typically as a slow-growing painless mass. Incidental WTs are also identified by imaging, particularly for patients receiving staging images for treatment of other smoking-related malignancies such as lung and upper aerodigestive tract carcinoma.

Pathologic Features

GROSS FINDINGS

WTs are circumscribed cystic tumors with complex internal papillary growth. The cystic fluid is often gray to brown and commonly described as oil-like. WT is also the most common salivary gland tumor to be multifocal with multiple lesions possible in the same gland or bilateral parotid glands.

MICROSCOPIC FINDINGS

The classic histologic feature of WT is a bilayered epithelium growing along papillary fronds surrounded by lymphoid stroma (Fig. 9.4). The bilayered epithelium has a specific appearance with an oncocytic ductal layer toward the cystic space with an underlying layer of cuboidal basal cells. An important diagnostic feature is the unusual nuclear orientation in the luminal oncocytic ductal cells in that the nuclei line up at approximately the one third apical area of the cell. The diagnosis of WT is generally straight forward when these diagnostic features are prominent, but in some cases these classical

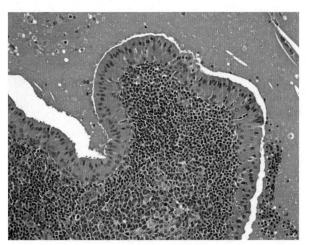

FIG. 9.4

Warthin tumor. The characteristic bilayered epithelium of Warthin tumor is a key morphologic feature that helps differentiate this diagnosis from mimics such as low-grade mucoepidermoid carcinoma. Warthin tumors show at least focal areas with columnar oncocytic luminal epithelial cells with nuclei lined up at the one third apical aspect. Basal cells are also present.

architectural changes may only be identified focally. Minor areas with mucinous metaplasia are common in WT and have been reported in up to 83% of cases. However, particularly following aspiration or other trauma, there can be extensive squamous and/or mucinous metaplasia in WT. These metaplastic changes can obscure the diagnostic features of WT, but in most cases diagnostic morphologic features are still focally identifiable. Infarcted WT after aspiration can show extensive squamous metaplasia and fibrosis potentially mimicking squamous cell carcinoma (SCC).

The overall amount of lymphoid stroma can vary with some authors referring to lymphoid-poor and lymphoid-rich WT. The lymphoid stroma can show germinal centers.

Ancillary Studies

In general, immunostains are not helpful in confirming the diagnosis of WT versus many of the tumors that may fall into the differential diagnosis. This is because a similar staining pattern can be seen in most of these tumors. Specifically, the basal layer in WT stains positively for p63/p40, whereas luminal ductal cells are negative. Unfortunately, a common entity included in the differential diagnosis of WT is low-grade mucoepidermoid carcinoma (MEC), and these tumors will show a similar pattern. Additionally, when there is extensive squamous metaplasia causing concern for SCC, there is also more diffuse reactivity with squamous markers in WT and therefore the diagnosis may rely on morphology and clinical history.

FISH can be helpful in cases of WT with extensive mucinous metaplasia raising concern for MEC. In these cases, the finding of a *MAML2* rearrangement is

diagnostic of MEC, whereas the lack of such a rearrangement argues against MEC.

Differential Diagnosis

As noted, most cases of WT are straightforward on morphologic features but unusual morphologic changes can raise differential considerations for other tumors. MEC, particularly low-grade forms, have a prominent cystic component, "oncocytoid" tumor cells, and may have a prominent tumor-associated lymphoid response (Table 9.3). Such tumors can closely mimic a WT and have been termed the Warthin-like variant of MEC by many authors (Fig. 9.5). Clinical features can be very helpful in such cases as WTs are far more likely to occur in patients over 40 years of age while MEC are more common in younger patients. On a morphologic basis, the most important feature to look for is the very classic and characteristic bilayered epithelium of WT with apical columnar oncocytic tumor cells having nuclei oriented at approximately one third position from the apical membrane and underlying basal cells. When this feature is seen, even focally, the diagnosis of WT is strongly favored over that of MEC. In contrast, the lack of this appearance after extensive and thorough examination would argue for the diagnosis of MEC. As noted above, FISH for the *MAML2* rearrangement is helpful to confirm the diagnosis of MEC when detected in these cases.

Following aspiration or other trauma, WT can show extensive squamous metaplasia, infarction, and fibrosis. In these cases, the degree of cytologic atypia and pattern of squamous nests can cause considerable concern for SCC (Fig. 9.6) (Table 9.4). While a thorough examination for any features diagnostic of WT can be helpful, it

---

TABLE 9.3

Features of Warthin Tumor Versus Low-Grade Mucoepidermoid Carcinoma

Warthin Tumor (WT)	Low-Grade Mucoepidermoid Carcinoma
• Characteristic bilayered epithelium is at least focally present	• Lacks the characteristic bilayered epithelial lining of WT
• Mucinous and/or squamous metaplasia is common	• Mucinous and epidermoid differentiation is an important diagnostic feature
• Lymphoid stroma is present	• A tumor-associated lymphoid response can mimic the lymphoid stroma of WT
• Lacks invasion	• Invasion is usually present but may not be obvious
• Negative for *MAML2* rearrangement	• *MAML2* rearrangements are very common

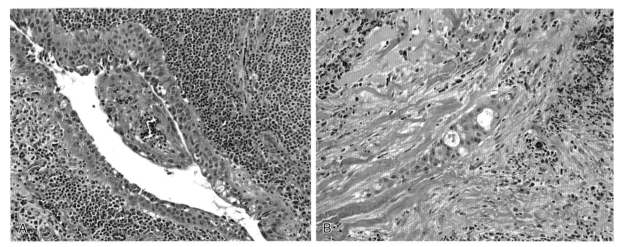

FIG. 9.5

Mucoepidermoid carcinoma (MEC), Warthin-like. A tumor-associated lymphoid response when combined with the fairly bland epithelial lining of a low-grade MEC can closely mimic a benign Warthin tumor (WT) (**A**). This is especially true given the abundant eosinophilic cytoplasm the MEC tumor cells and the fact that WT may show extensive squamous and mucinous metaplasia. A helpful feature to alert one to the possibility of MEC is that the very characteristic bilayered epithelium of WT is not even focally present in the tumor. Additionally, MEC often times have some morphologic evidence of invasion as seen in (**B**) with an infiltrative tumor nest composed of epidermoid and mucinous cells. The case shown was confirmed to be positive for a *MAML2* gene rearrangement which would not be present in WT.

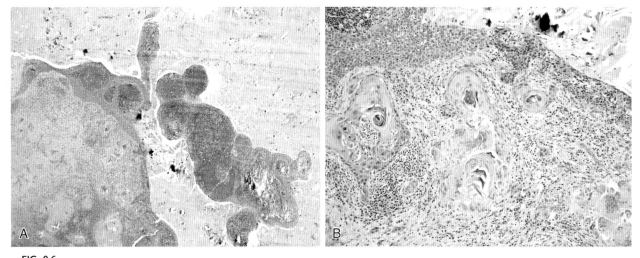

FIG. 9.6

Cystic metastatic squamous cell carcinoma. Occasionally cystic metastatic squamous cell carcinoma to an intraparotid lymph node may have a pattern similar to Warthin tumor at low power (**A**). However, the presence of significant cytologic atypia and invasive nests are diagnostic of squamous cell carcinoma (**B**).

is also important to correlate the findings with any history of prior fine-needle aspiration (FNA; and the cytology results of such an FNA) and history of other cancers. Many of these patients are smokers and therefore at risk for SCC making this an even more challenging endeavor.

Prognosis and Therapy

WT is a benign tumor and therefore surgical excision is generally the treatment of choice. Malignant transformation is uncommon in WT and is most often a lymphoma which has been reported in up to approximately

3% of cases. Due to the low risk of malignancy, the possibility of observation can be offered to patients in which the tumor is asymptomatic and a cytologic and clinical diagnosis of WT is quite certain. WT may recur if incompletely excised, but the multifocality of WT can also lead to patients having apparent "recurrence."

WARTHIN TUMOR – DISEASE FACT SHEET

Definition

▸▸ Warthin tumors are benign tumors characterized by a bilayered epithelial proliferation with oncocytic luminal cells and basal cells with a lymphoid stroma

Continued

TABLE 9.4

Features of Infarcted Warthin Tumor Versus Squamous Cell Carcinoma

Infarcted Warthin Tumor	Squamous Cell Carcinoma
• Focal residual bilayered epithelial lining may be identified on extensive sampling	• Bilayered oncocytic epithelial lining is not identified
• Frequently shows areas of necrosis and squamous metaplasia	• Squamous differentiation is present but may require immunostains for confirmation
• Sclerotic stroma surrounding angulated nests of atypical squamous cells may be present	• Desmoplastic stroma surrounding invasive nests of carcinoma
• Periphery of lesion is overall very well circumscribed (i.e., at the edge of the fibrosis)	• Infiltrative nests usually extend into surrounding tissue
• A history of prior trauma, particularly FNA	• May or may not have a history of prior trauma/FNA

FNA, Fine-needle aspiration.

WARTHIN TUMOR – DISEASE FACT SHEET—cont'd

Incidence and Location
▸▸ Warthin tumors are the second most common salivary gland tumor
▸▸ Highly associated with tobacco smoking or secondhand smoke exposure
▸▸ Occur only in parotid and periparotid lymph nodes

Age and Sex Distribution
▸▸ Warthin tumors almost never occur in patients less than 40 years of age
▸▸ Men are more commonly affected historically, but this is highly related to the prevalence of smoking

Clinical Features
▸▸ Slow-growing painless mass of the parotid gland in a smoker

Prognosis and Therapy
▸▸ Benign
▸▸ Malignant transformation is very rare, most commonly a lymphoproliferative neoplasm
▸▸ Surgical excision is curative

WARTHIN TUMOR – PATHOLOGIC FEATURES

Gross Findings
▸▸ Well circumscribed and usually cystic mass in the parotid gland
▸▸ Cystic fluid is usually thick and brown ("motor oil-like")

Microscopic Findings
▸▸ Bilayered epithelium with luminal columnar oncocytic cells and basal cells

---

▸▸ Nuclei of oncocytic cells have nuclear polarization at about one third apical portion of the cell
▸▸ Cystic with broad papillary architecture into the cystic space
▸▸ Lymphoid stroma is usually prominent but can be scant
▸▸ Lacks invasion

Pathologic Differential Diagnoses
▸▸ Low-grade mucoepidermoid carcinoma
▸▸ Infarcted Warthin tumor can mimic squamous cell carcinoma

SCLEROSING POLYCYSTIC ADENOSIS/ADENOMA

DIFFERENTIAL DIAGNOSES: SALIVARY DUCT CARCINOMA AND PLEOMORPHIC ADENOMA

Clinical Features

Sclerosing polycystic adenosis (SPA) is a rare salivary gland tumor with fewer than 100 cases reported in the literature. SPA most commonly involves the parotid gland and much less frequently the submandibular gland and minor salivary glands of the oral cavity. SPA shows a slight female predilection and occurs over a wide age range including children and older adults (range 7–84 years), but on average they occur between 40 and 50 years. Similar to other benign salivary gland tumors, SPA presents as a slow-growing, usually painless mass. This tumor was initially thought to be non-neoplastic reactive process, but increasing evidence (X-chromosome inactivation studies and the findings of mutations of the PI3K pathway) indicates clonality and thus a true neoplasm. Based on the emerging neoplastic nature of this tumor, some authors now prefer the term sclerosing polycystic *adenoma*.

Pathologic Features

GROSS FINDINGS

SPA are grossly firm and well circumscribed to multinodular. Many cases are reported to lack a capsule but occasional encapsulation can be found. Small cystic spaces are commonly visible grossly. SPA are usually solitary but multifocality has been reported in rare cases. Tumors range from 0.7 to 12 cm, but most are small (3 cm or less).

MICROSCOPIC FINDINGS

SPA are circumscribed with fibrotic stroma containing cysts, ducts, and acinar cells with myoepithelial cells surrounding each ductal/acinar structure (Fig. 9.7A).

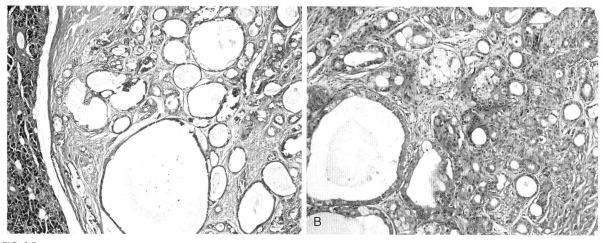

FIG. 9.7

Sclerosing polycystic adenoma (SPA). SPA is a well-circumscribed noninvasive tumor characterized by ductal structures in a fibrocellular to sclerotic stroma (**A**). The ductal structures are frequently at least focally cystic and show evidence of variable differentiation including apocrine, serous, and mucinous (**B**).

Sclerotic stroma is most common, but focal myxoid stroma can be seen as can stromal adipose. The epithelial components of SPA show a variety of differentiation (Fig. 9.7B). Lining ductal cells frequently show a variety of changes including vacuolization (sebaceous-like), apocrine differentiation, and squamous differentiation. Acinar cells are common and frequently show characteristic bright eosinophilic cytoplasmic granules that have been theorized to represent modified zymogen granules by some authors. However, similar eosinophilic cytoplasmic granules can be seen in a variety of tumors with apocrine differentiation. Ducts range from small fairly normal caliber to large cystically dilated structures. Cystic ductal spaces commonly contain mucoid material and foamy macrophages. An important diagnostic feature for SPA is that the pattern of ducts maintains a lobular growth pattern. Apocrine intraductal proliferations are common in SPA, ranging from features similar to atypical ductal hyperplasia to those of ductal carcinoma *in situ* of breast.

Ancillary Studies

Tumor cells are positive for keratins. Ductal cells can show immunohistochemical evidence of apocrine differentiation with positive staining for GCDFP-15 and androgen receptor. All the ductal structures represent an *in situ* component and therefore are lined by a myoepithelial layer that can be highlighted with various markers including p63, SMA, and calponin. S100 also highlights the myoepithelial layer and frequently also stains ductal epithelium.

Likely related to molecular alterations of *PTEN* and other elements of the PI3K pathway, SPA have been reported to show PTEN loss only in the ductal population by immunohistochemistry.

Differential Diagnosis

Although the histologic features of SPA can be variable, common histologic features make it possible to diagnosis most cases based solely on H&E morphology when one is aware of this rare tumor entity but, due to the rarity of this tumor, it can commonly be misdiagnosed as another salivary gland neoplasm. Some of the most helpful clues to the diagnosis of SPA are the lobular ductal growth pattern, variability of ductal cell differentiation, and prominent sclerotic fibrosis. Although SPA show apocrine differentiation and commonly intraductal proliferations similar to salivary duct carcinoma (SDC), SPA usually lack overtly malignant cytologic features that are common in SDC (Fig. 9.8;

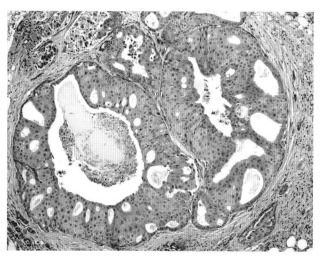

FIG. 9.8

Salivary duct carcinoma. Similarly, to sclerosing polycystic adenoma, salivary duct carcinoma has extensive apocrine differentiation. Areas of intraductal proliferation in sclerosing polycystic adenoma may also be seen and mimic the ductal carcinoma *in situ*–like appearance that is also seen in salivary duct carcinoma. The presence of a widely invasive tumor is indicative of salivary duct carcinoma, whereas sclerosing polycystic adenomas are only rarely associated with invasive carcinoma.

TABLE 9.5

Features of Sclerosing Polycystic Adenoma Versus Salivary Duct Carcinoma

Sclerosing Polycystic Adenosis/Adenoma	Salivary Duct Carcinoma
• Apocrine differentiation is seen in almost all cases	• Apocrine differentiation is seen in almost all cases
• May show intraductal proliferations approaching ductal carcinoma in situ	• Invasive tumor nests commonly have the appearance of ductal carcinoma *in situ*
• Tumor is well circumscribed and lacks invasion	• Aggressive invasive pattern with common perineural and angiolymphatic invasion
• Ductal structures are surrounded by basal layer of myoepithelial cells	• May have a residual basal layer of myoepithelial cells within an *in situ* component of a carcinoma ex pleomorphic adenoma

TABLE 9.6

Features of Sclerosing Polycystic Adenoma Versus Pleomorphic Adenoma

Sclerosing Polycystic Adenosis/Adenoma	Pleomorphic Adenoma
• Apocrine differentiation is seen in almost all cases	• Apocrine differentiation can be seen but is usually focal
• Sclerotic stroma	• Chondromyxoid stroma
• Malignant transformation is extremely rare	• Malignant transformation in 5%–15%

Table 9.5). In comparison to PA, SPA lack significant chondromyxoid stroma and preponderance of myoepithelial cells (Fig. 9.9; Table 9.6). While the focal acinar differentiation in SPA may raise the possibility of acinic cell carcinoma (AciCC), the lobular growth pattern and surrounding myoepithelial cell layer of SPA are not seen in AciCC. MEC can also be distinguished from SPA for the same reasons as AciCC. Several features of SPA also overlap with features of intraductal carcinoma including surrounding myoepithelial cells and *in situ* ductal hyperplasia/carcinoma *in situ*. Both entities can also show similar immunophenotypic features as intraductal carcinoma may be S100 positive while others having apocrine differentiation are androgen receptor positive. Helpful features in this differential diagnosis include the overall more circumscribed nature of SPA, the lobular ductal growth pattern, and the variability of ductal cell differentiation.

Prognosis and Therapy

Most SPA are benign but can show a low rate of recurrence (~10%–30%). Malignant transformation (i.e., carcinoma ex SPA) has been reported in a single case following multiple recurrences, but metastases and death have not been seen. Complete surgical excision is recommended.

SCLEROSING POLYCYSTIC ADENOSIS/ADENOMA – DISEASE FACT SHEET

Definition
▶▶ Sclerosing polycystic adenosis/adenoma is a benign, most likely neoplastic salivary gland tumor

Incidence and Location
▶▶ SPA is very rare
▶▶ Most commonly occurs in the parotid gland

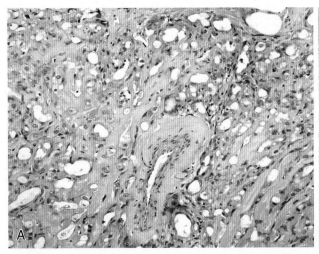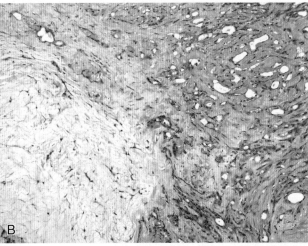

FIG. 9.9

Pleomorphic adenoma. This example of a pleomorphic adenoma had extensive stromal sclerosis and apocrine metaplasia of the ductal epithelium mimicking some features of sclerosing polycystic adenoma in many areas (**A**). However, the tumor lacked an overall lobular pattern and there were also prominent areas of myxoid stroma containing spindle myoepithelial cells diagnostic of pleomorphic adenoma (**B**).

Age Distribution
▸▸ Wide age range (7–84 years)
▸▸ Average age is 40–50 years

Clinical Features
▸▸ Slow-growing painless mass

Prognosis and Therapy
▸▸ Most have benign behavior
▸▸ Recurrence is rare
▸▸ Malignant transformation is reported in a single case
▸▸ Surgical excision is usually curative

**SCLEROSING POLYCYSTIC ADENOSIS/ADENOMA –
PATHOLOGIC FEATURES**

Gross Findings
▸▸ Well circumscribed
▸▸ Usually small to large cysts
▸▸ Firm
▸▸ Usually solitary

Microscopic Findings
▸▸ Cystically dilated ductal structures with variable differentiation
▸▸ All ductal structures lined by abluminal myoepithelial layer
▸▸ Ductal cells with large eosinophilic granules
▸▸ Sclerotic stroma
▸▸ Lacks invasion
▸▸ Commonly shows ductal proliferations with a range similar to atypical ductal hyperplasia and ductal carcinoma *in situ* of the breast

Pathologic Differential Diagnoses
▸▸ Pleomorphic adenoma
▸▸ Salivary duct carcinoma
▸▸ Mucoepidermoid carcinoma
▸▸ Acinic cell carcinoma

MUCOEPIDERMOID CARCINOMA

**DIFFERENTIAL DIAGNOSES:
ADENOSQUAMOUS CARCINOMA
AND ACANTHOLYTIC SQUAMOUS
CELL CARCINOMA**

Clinical Features

MEC is a common salivary gland malignancy, comprising 25% of all malignant diagnoses. It occurs in patients at a wide variety of ages (ranging from 35 to 65 years) and is the most common pediatric malignancy of the salivary glands. There is a predilection toward female patients (3:2). The parotid gland is commonly affected, followed by the minor salivary glands of the palate, submandibular gland, and other intraoral sites (floor of the mouth, buccal mucosa, lip, and tongue). Patients will experience a painless swelling of varying duration at

these aforementioned sites. On physical examination, some may impart a bluish-red and fluctuant appearance if submucosal in location, quite similarly to mucoceles or vascular lesions. Prior radiation exposure is a risk factor for the development of MEC (up to 44% by some authors), with reported latency of 7 to 32 years.

Pathologic Features

GROSS FINDINGS

Most tumors are smaller than 4 cm in size. If a tumor is circumscribed or variably encapsulated with areas of cystic change, it would be suggestive of a lower-grade tumor. However, on the other hand, if the tumor is infiltrative and fixed, it would be suggestive of a higher-grade MEC.

MICROSCOPIC FINDINGS

MEC classically comprise a three-cell population: squamous/epidermoid, intermediate, and mucinous cells. Solid, cystic, or infiltrative growth architecture can be appreciated or a combination of the three (Figs. 9.10 and 9.11). Origin from overlying epithelium is not appreciated, a distinction that is critical to note when differentiating it from other epithelial malignancies (see Differential Diagnosis). Keratinization or keratin pearls are not a typical feature of this malignancy. The intermediate cells can be larger and have a basal-like appearance. Variant morphologic patterns with an oncocytic or clear cell appearance are rarely encountered (Fig. 9.12). A surrounding dense lymphoid stroma may be identified with MEC.

MEC can be graded according to several systems: Armed Forces Institute of Pathology (AFIP) system, Brandwein system, Katabi system, and the Healey system (see Suggested Readings). In general, parameters such as cystic architecture, circumscription, necrosis,

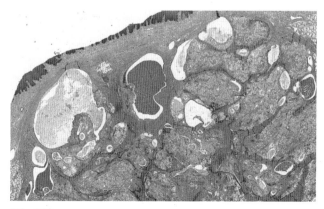

FIG. 9.10

Mucoepidermoid carcinoma. The tumor is submucosal with association with the surface mucosa. In this example, there is a combination of both cystic and solid architectural growth patterns.

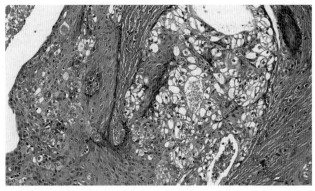

FIG. 9.11

Mucoepidermoid carcinoma. An area of the tumor where there are pre-dominantly squamoid/epidermoid cells. The cells demonstrate mild nuclear atypia with ample cytoplasmic material. In the center of this micrograph the tumor cells have clear cytoplasm, a feature that can be occasionally noted in mucoepidermoid carcinomas.

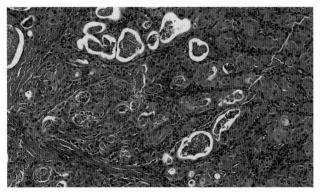

FIG. 9.12

Mucoepidermoid carcinoma. An example of an oncocytic variant of mucoepidermoid carcinoma. There is focal cystic change, but most of the tumor grows in a nested pattern. Mucocytes are readily identified in this field.

cellular anaplasia, perineural/lymphovascular invasion, and bone invasion should be noted when applying these grading schemes. The grade of the tumor is important as it carries therapeutic and prognostic significance.

Ancillary Studies

MEC is immunohistochemically positive for cytokeratins, epithelial membrane antigen (EMA), carcinoembryonic antigen (CEA), and p63. A mucin stain will be positive in the mucocytes. MEC is typically negative for S100, CK20, SMA, and muscle-specific actin (MSA).

From a molecular standpoint, lower- to intermediate-grade MEC are likely to harbor specific translocations. The most common translocation is t(11;19)(q21:p13) with a *CRTC1-MAML2* fusion. A less common fusion is a translocation involving t(11;15)(q21;q26) with a *CRTC3-MAML2* fusion. The absence of a rearrangement may occur in high-grade MEC.

Differential Diagnosis

The differential diagnosis for MEC includes adenosquamous carcinoma (ASC), acantholytic squamous cell carcinoma (aSCC), and sialometaplasia (Table 9.7).

ASC is an aggressive epithelial malignancy with combined squamous and glandular phenotype. Adequate sampling may show a "transition" between these two components. ASC may present as a polypoid or exophytic mass with mucosal induration or ulceration. Mucin will be appreciated, either luminally or rarely intracytoplasmically. High-grade features of perineural and lymphovascular invasion are often present. The squamous component will be immunohistochemically positive for CK5/6 and p63, and the adenocarcinoma component will be CK7 and CEA positive. CK20 is negative.

Although there may be some morphologic similarities between ASC and MEC, it is important to keep in mind that MEC is a tumor that is derived from salivary gland tissue, and that ASC is a malignant tumor with mucosal origin. The presence of invasive carcinoma arising from surface dysplasia excludes a diagnosis of MEC. Keratinization and keratin pearl formation is consistent with ASC and is not compatible with MEC. The pattern of invasion is critical, where in ASC the tumor invades into submucosal glands due to its derivation from the surface epithelium, whereas in MEC the tumor originates from the submucosal glands. Furthermore, the presence of intermediate cells would favor a MEC.

In histologically challenging cases, rearrangement studies for *MAML2* via FISH can be performed. A potential pitfall is that high-grade MEC is less likely to harbor

---

TABLE 9.7

Histologic Features of Mucoepidermoid Carcinoma (MEC) compared with Adenosquamous Carcinoma (ASC) and Acantholytic Squamous Cell Carcinoma (aSCC)

MEC	ASC	aSCC
• Three cell population: Squamous/epidermoid, intermediate, and mucinous cells	• Malignant squamous and glandular cells	• Malignant squamous cells only
• No keratinization	• Keratinization present	• +/− Keratinization
• No association with dysplasia	• May be associated with dysplasia	• May be associated with dysplasia
• Intracytoplasmic mucin present	• Luminal mucin and/or rarely intracytoplasmically	• No intracytoplasmic mucin
• *MAML2* rearrangement	• No *MAML2* rearrangement	• No *MAML2* rearrangement

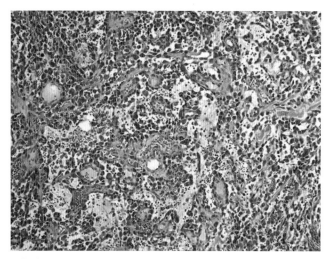

FIG. 9.13
Acantholytic squamous cell carcinoma with a papillary-like and pseudo-glandular appearance.

a *MAML2* rearrangement. Compared with MEC, ASC has a worse prognosis (5-year-survival rates of 15%–25%) and are aggressively treated with surgery.

aSCC is an uncommon variant of a poorly differentiated SCC. On low power, it may impart a "pseudoglandular," pseudoacinar-like, angiosarcoma-like appearance (Fig. 9.13). A point of distinction is that the pseudoglandular spaces in aSCC do not contain mucin. However, surface epithelial dysplasia or a frank SCC is helpful for distinction from MEC. The unusual appearance of this SCC is partly due to the loss or loosening of cell to cell adhesion proteins.

Sialometaplasia is an important distinction as the clinical management drastically differs. In sialometaplasia, there will be necrosis of the acini with squamous metaplasia of ductular elements. However, this process retains a "lobular" architecture reminiscent of the affected salivary glands. Occasionally, the overlying epithelium over the areas of sialometaplasia will demonstrate features of pseudoepitheliomatous hyperplasia (PEH).

Finally, as a practical point, in small biopsies where the classification of a specific carcinoma is challenging, a descriptive diagnosis (i.e., "carcinoma with squamous and glandular features") can be provided with a definitive diagnosis deferred to a resection specimen.

Treatment and Prognosis

The reported 5-year survival rates depend on the grade of the MEC. Low-grade MEC have a 5-year-survival rate of 92% to 100%, intermediate-grade tumors have 62% to 92%, and high-grade tumors have 0% to 43%. The management will depend on the grade of the tumor, where surgical excision will be adequate for lower-grade tumors. Higher-grade tumors will require surgical excision with adjuvant radiation and neck dissection.

MUCOEPIDERMOID CARCINOMA – DISEASE FACT SHEET

Definition
▸▸ Malignant salivary gland neoplasm composed of squamous/epidermoid, intermediate, and mucinous cells

Incidence
▸▸ 0.44 per 100,000
▸▸ 12%–30% of malignancy salivary gland tumors

Morbidity and Mortality
▸▸ 5-year survival rate: low grade 92%–100%; intermediate grade 62%–92%; high grade 0%–43%

Sex and Age Distribution
▸▸ Middle-age patients, although MEC is the most common pediatric salivary gland tumor
▸▸ Females > males (3:2)

Clinical Features
▸▸ Swelling or mass of varying duration

Treatment and Prognosis
▸▸ Survival rate depends on the grade of the tumor
▸▸ Surgical excision for lower-grade tumors and adjuvant radiation and neck dissection of higher-grade tumors

---

MUCOEPIDERMOID CARCINOMA – PATHOLOGIC FEATURES

Gross Findings
▸▸ May be solid or cystic in appearance
▸▸ Cystic and well-circumscribed nature is found in lower-grade tumors
▸▸ Solid and infiltrative tumors are suggestive of a higher grade

Microscopic Findings
▸▸ Squamoid/epidermoid, intermediate, and mucinous cells
▸▸ Cystic or solid areas, or a combination of both
▸▸ No associated surface dysplasia
▸▸ No keratinization or keratin pearls
▸▸ May have oncocytic or clear cell appearance

Pathologic Differential Diagnosis
▸▸ Adenosquamous carcinoma, acantholytic squamous cell carcinoma, sialometaplasia

POLYMORPHOUS ADENOCARCINOMA

DIFFERENTIAL DIAGNOSES: ADENOID CYSTIC CARCINOMA AND CRIBRIFORM ADENOCARCINOMA OF SALIVARY GLANDS

Clinical Features

PAC is low- to intermediate-grade salivary gland malignancy. Majority of PAC will arise in the region and interface of the posterior hard and soft palate (60%), although it can be found in the oral and sinus/nasal cavity sites. There is a notable female predilection (2:1) and is usually encountered in the sixth decade of life, although rarely can be encountered in children. PACs are typically slow growing with accompanying pain, bleeding, and ulceration.

PAC was historically classified as polymorphous *low-grade* adenocarcinoma (PLGA). However, in the 2017 edition of the WHO Tumors of the Head and Neck, it has been recognized that a subset of PACs have a non-negligible risk of local recurrence and metastatic potential. Potentially in these cases, an elective neck dissection and postoperative long-term surveillance may be required.

Pathologic Features

GROSS FINDINGS

The tumor is a firm, solid, and circumscribed tan to yellowish mass that is unencapsulated. The average size is 2.1 ± 1.3 cm. The mass lies in close proximity to the overlying surface epithelium. In cases involving the hard palate and sinuses, bone invasion can often be appreciated.

MICROSCOPIC FINDINGS

PAC is a monophasic salivary gland tumor that demonstrates cellular *uniformity* with architectural and growth pattern *diversity*. Growth patterns include cords, trabeculae, solid nests, and/or tubules (Fig. 9.14). Occasionally in areas of tubular architecture, one- to two-cell layer thick growth pattern can be identified; however, these are all ductal cells in lineage and no myoepithelial differentiation is present. Targetoid growth pattern around nerves and lymphovascular spaces is a strongly suggestive feature in PAC ("eye of the storm" pattern) (Fig. 9.15). PAC can produce slate blue to gray extracellular matrix, microcalcifications, and tyrosine-rich crystalloids (Fig. 9.16). The tumor cells are small to ovoid in shape with vesicular and dispersed chromatin in otherwise bland nuclei. Nucleoli are inconspicuous (Fig. 9.17). Occasionally oncocytic, mucinous, clear, and squamous metaplastic alteration can be appreciated.

Ancillary Studies

PACs demonstrate cytokeratin expression, especially CK7. They will also stain positive for S100 and SOX10 and can demonstrate expression for DOG1 and mammaglobin. However, as myoepithelial cells are not a component of

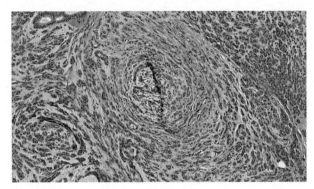

FIG. 9.15

"Eye of the storm" pattern of growth in polymorphous adenocarcinoma. Scattered within this type of growth pattern are small tubules and cords of tumors cells. Although different (polymorphous) patterns of architectural growth are expected, the constituent cells are themselves monotonous.

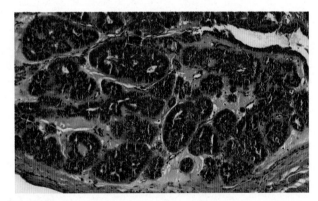

FIG. 9.16

Polymorphous adenocarcinoma with extracellular slate blue-gray matrix material. The tumor cells maintain a monotonous appearance and do not exhibit a two-cell population as seen in adenoid cystic carcinoma. Note the absence of the "crenated" myoepithelial cells.

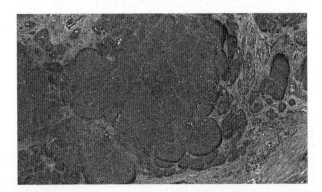

FIG. 9.14

Solid nests architecture in polymorphous adenocarcinoma in a fibrous stroma. In the top left, there is a focal area of cribriform pattern.

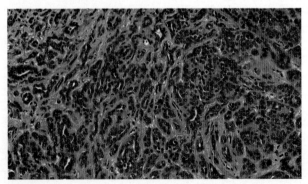

FIG. 9.17

Monotonous appearing cells in an infiltrative tubular architecture in polymorphous adenocarcinoma.

this malignancy, SMA has aberrant or negative expression. Furthermore, in comparing adenoid cystic carcinoma (AdCC) with PAC, p63 is positive in PAC and AdCC; however, p40 will be positive in AdCC but negative in PAC (PAC: p63+/p40−; AdCC: p63+/p40+).

Differential Diagnosis

PAC needs to be separated from AdCC due to management and prognostic implications. In the 2017 edition of the WHO Tumors of the Head and Neck, cribriform adenocarcinoma of (minor) salivary glands (CASG/CAMSG) was considered as a subtype of PAC. There is new molecular evidence to question whether this entity falls within the spectrum of PAC. Regardless, it should be noted that CASG/CAMSG differs in its potential biological course compared with PAC.

AdCC is similar to PAC in that it is derived from an intercalated duct lineage; however, a key distinguishing feature between these two tumors is that adenoid cystic is a biphasic salivary gland tumor composed of ductal and myoepithelial cells (Table 9.8). Architecturally, these two entities can be difficult to separate based off of growth pattern alone, as they can demonstrate a tubular, cribriform, or solid growth pattern. In AdCC, tumor nests will be surrounded by myoepithelial cells with ductal elements as well as additional lumina lined by myoepithelial cells producing a myxohyaline matrix. In AdCC, the tumor nests demonstrate a "clefting" phenomenon with the tissue stroma. An additional feature in AdCC is that the myoepithelial cells have hyperchromatic nuclei in a peg or angulated shape intermixed with the bland-appearing ductular elements.

SOX10 and S100 can identify myoepithelial cells in AdCC; however, they may also be positive in PAC. SMA is helpful in identifying the myoepithelial cells in AdCC, although as noted above, aberrant SMA positivity can be seen in PAC. A panel of p63 and p40 is helpful, as the immunophenotype in AdCC is p63+/p40+ and in PAC it is p63+/p40−. Majority of AdCC also have recurrent chromosomal translocations characterized by a *MYB-NFIB* gene fusion (80%–85%), although other gene fusions can be seen as well.

The biological behavior of AdCC is markedly different from PAC. Recurrence rates are high for AdCC (up to 67%) with metastases in half of the cases. Although AdCC is considered a slow-growing tumor, in some cases it still has clinical progression and higher mortality rates. A particular challenge should be noted in cases where there is high-grade transformation of AdCC, where there is loss of biphasic nature of the tumor. However, to distinguish this from a PAC, in these high-grade transformation cases there is significant cellular atypia in AdCC with areas of increased mitoses and necrosis.

CASG/CAMSG is currently considered a clinically aggressive variant of PAC. CASG/CAMSG was historically identified in the minor salivary glands and tongue; however, these tumors have been identified in the major salivary glands.

CASG/CAMSG demonstrates a cellular proliferation with variable proportion of cribriform, tubular, lobules, glomeruloid, and solid areas. The tumor lobules and nests are separated by fibrous septae. In areas of glomeruloid architecture, peripheral palisading of tumor cells is appreciated. The characteristic feature is that there are pale and vesicular nuclei with ground glass appearance, similar to that seen in papillary thyroid carcinoma. Interestingly, psammoma bodies may also be identified in CASG/CAMSG. The tumor often invades into adjacent muscular tissue if found in the tongue or adjacent tissues with lymphatic and vascular invasion.

It is debatable if CASG falls under the umbrella of PAC as it is considered as an emerging entity by the WHO – it is currently considered as a "cribriform" variant of PAC. Regardless, it does have higher incidence of cervical lymph nodes metastases (72% vs. 10%–17% in PAC) than PAC and should be reported.

Prognosis and Therapy

PAC recurs in 10% to 33% of the cases, with half the cases occurring within the first 5 years of diagnosis. Furthermore, regional metastases are noted in 9% to 17% and distant metastases are rare. Surgery is the treatment of choice for PAC; however, radiotherapy can be utilized in cases with extensive spread, positive margins, perineural invasion, or vascular spread. In cases where it has metastasized, the lungs are the most common site, although abdominal, skin, and orbital metastases have been reported. Deaths are reported in cases after prolonged periods.

TABLE 9.8

Histologic Features of Polymorphous Adenocarcinoma Versus Adenoid Cystic Carcinoma

Polymorphous Adenocarcinoma	Adenoid Cystic Carcinoma
• Composed of one cell population in mixed growth pattern	• Composed of ductal and myoepithelial cell population in tubular, cribriform, or solid pattern
• No myoepithelial cells	• Myoepithelial cells with a crenated appearance
• Clefting typically not appreciated	• Stromal to tumor nest clefting
• P63+/P40−	• P63+, P40+

SECRETORY CARCINOMA

DIFFERENTIAL DIAGNOSES: ACINIC CELL CARCINOMA AND INTRADUCTAL CARCINOMA

Clinical Features

Secretory carcinoma (SC) of salivary glands (originally designated mammary analog secretory carcinoma [MASC]) is a low-grade adenocarcinoma with morphologic, immunophenotypic, and molecular features essentially identical to those seen in SC of the breast. This entity was first clearly characterized in 2010 and many retrospective reviews have identified SC from cases previously diagnosed as AciCC, adenocarcinoma, not otherwise specified (NOS),

and MEC. There is a slight male predominance. A wide age range is reported for SC with patients including children and older adults, but the mean age is in the 40s and 50s. Most patients with SC present with a slow-growing, painless mass. These lesions may be either cystic or solid.

Pathologic Features

GROSS FINDINGS

SCs are usually solitary and represent a well-circumscribed nodule most commonly arising in the parotid gland. SCs can also arise in other salivary glands and have been reported in the submandibular gland, minor salivary glands of various sites, and even in the thyroid gland. Cystic change is also a common finding.

MICROSCOPIC FINDINGS

SCs are low grade and many of the morphologic findings are consistent with a fairly indolent tumor. As with the gross appearance, most SCs have a very circumscribed appearance with some lacking definitive evidence of invasion but others having overt evidence of invasive growth. Tumor cell nuclei are monotonous with only rare mitotic activity. The most characteristic feature of SC is the abundant eosinophilic, multivacuolated ("bubbly") cytoplasm of SC tumor cells (Fig. 9.18). Extracellular mucus is also common and is frequently present as dense eosinophilic mucus between glandular structures giving a similar appearance to that of colloid in thyroid. Architecturally, SC shows a variety of growth patterns (including solid, cribriform, papillary, and intracystic) similar to those of AciCC. Rare examples of high-grade SC occur and these show high mitotic activity, necrosis, and prominent nuclear pleomorphism.

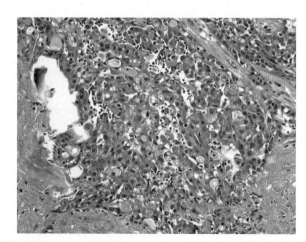

FIG. 9.18

Secretory carcinoma. Secretory carcinoma is characterized by monotonous tumor cells having abundant eosinopahilic cytoplasm. This cytoplasm characteristically shows multiple small vacuoles. In the setting of characteristic morphology, immunostains showing diffuse and strong S100 and mammaglobin expression are helpful to support the diagnosis. In more challenging cases, fluorescence *in situ* hybridization for an *ETV6* gene rearrangement is diagnostic.

Ancillary Studies

An immunophenotypic hallmark of SC is strong and diffuse reactivity for both S100 and mammaglobin. SOX10 is also usually positive. Similar to other salivary gland tumors, SCs are positive for CK7, and GATA-3 can also be expressed. SCs can show focal p63 reactivity but this is usually limited to areas at the periphery and has been theorized by some to possibly represent evidence for an area of intraductal growth.

ETV6 rearrangements are present in almost all cases with the most common partner gene being *NTRK3* as a result of t(12;15)(p13;q25). Less common genes may also partner with *ETV6* including *RET*, *MAML3*, and *MET*. Very rare cases have been shown to contain rearrangements of genes other than *ETV6*.

Differential Diagnosis

There can be considerable morphologic overlap between SC and AciCC which is supported by the fact that many archival cases of SC have been culled from files of AciCC following the description of SC in 2010 (Table 9.9). Both these tumors show similar variable architectural patterns

TABLE 9.9	
Features of Secretory Carcinoma Versus Acinic Cell Carcinoma	
Secretory Carcinoma	Acinic Cell Carcinoma
• Invasive, cytologically low-grade carcinoma	• Invasive, cytologically low-grade carcinoma
• Lacks serous acinar differentiation	• Serous acinar differentiation is required for diagnosis
• Tumor cells have abundant cytoplasm with multiple small vacuoles	• Tumor cells have abundant cytoplasm containing basophilic zymogen granules
• Mucus production is present	• Mucus production is absent to rare
• SOX10 positive	• SOX10 positive
• Strongly and diffusely positive for S100 and mammaglobin	• Strong, diffuse, complete membranous reactivity with DOG-1
• Rearrangement of *ETV6* present	• Negative for *ETV6* rearrangement

and are generally well circumscribed or have a nodular pattern of invasion. For many cases of AciCC, the diagnosis is straight forward due to the presence of prominent cytoplasmic zymogen granules (Fig. 9.19C) in tumor cells which can be highlighted by periodic acid-Schiff

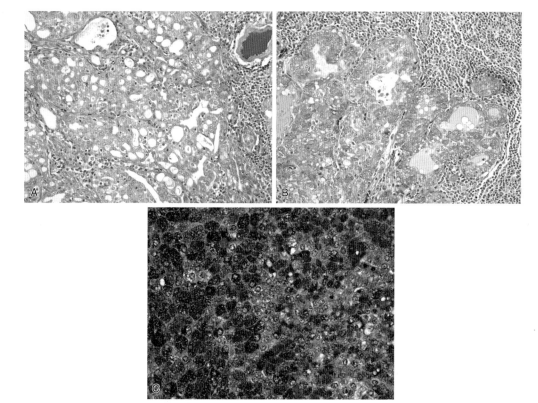

FIG. 9.19

Acinic cell carcinoma. Acinic cell carcinoma may occasionally show prominent intercalated duct phenotype and the lack of obvious zymogen granules causes very close overlap with secretory carcinoma (**A**). The tumor in A had scattered areas in which no cytoplasmic zymogen granules could be identified but other areas did have subtle zymogen granules (**B**) allowing for the diagnosis of acinic cell carcinoma. Many cases of acinic cell carcinoma will show obvious serous acinar differentiation as seen in (**C**). Immunostains can be very helpful in this differential diagnosis as well.

with diastase (PASD). However, occasional cases of AciCC show more prominent intercalated duct type differentiation and cells with zymogen granules may be rarer (i.e., intercalated duct-rich AciCC) (Figs. 9.19A and 9.19B) – immunostains and/or FISH can be helpful in such cases. SCs are usually strongly and diffusely positive for both S100 and mammaglobin, whereas AciCC is usually negative for both markers but commonly shows complete membranous reactivity for DOG-1. DOG-1 can show focal weak apical staining in SC. SOX10 is usually positive in both entities.

Intraductal carcinoma is a rare low-grade salivary gland tumor with several variant forms. Salivary intraductal carcinoma shares many similarities with ductal carcinoma *in situ* of the breast and can also be associated with an invasive component. Several forms can be seen including those with apocrine or intercalated duct-like differentiation of the intraductal proliferation. Low-grade and high-grade cytologic features may also be seen. Low-grade intercalated duct-like intraductal carcinoma can show striking morphologic similarity to SC and also shares strong reactivity for S100 and mammaglobin (Fig. 9.20; Table 9.10). The most helpful feature in distinguishing

TABLE 9.10
Features of Secretory Carcinoma Versus Intraductal Carcinoma

Secretory Carcinoma	Intercalated Duct-Like Intraductal Carcinoma
• Tumor cells with abundant eosinophilic cytoplasm	• Tumor cells with abundant eosinophilic cytoplasm
• Tumor cells are strongly and diffusely S100 positive	• Tumor cells are strongly and diffusely S100 positive
• Lacks an apocrine component	• May be mixed time with an apocrine component
• Invasive tumor	• Predominantly an *in situ* carcinoma with or without invasion
• Rare possible residual basal cell layer can be highlighted by p63	• All or most of the tumor usually shows a p63 positive myoepithelial cell layer
• Rearrangement of *ETV6* present	• Negative for *ETV6* rearrangement

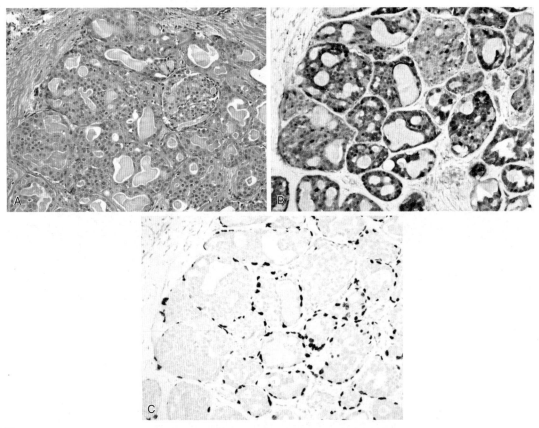

FIG. 9.20

Intraductal carcinoma. Intraductal carcinoma may show an intercalated duct-like phenotype that can closely mimic the morphology and immunophenotype of secretory carcinoma (**A**). S100 is usually diffusely positive in this form of intraductal carcinoma (**B**). An important distinguishing finding is the presence of a myoepithelial cell lining the tumor cell nests that can be highlighted with various myoepithelial cell markers (**C**).

these two entities is the finding of a prominent layer of p63/p40 myoepithelial cells surrounding tumor nests in intraductal carcinoma (Fig. 9.20C). In contrast, only very focal residual myoepithelial cells are identified when staining SC for p63, p40, or other myoepithelial markers.

When immunostains are unable to confirm the diagnosis, FISH showing breakapart of *ETV6* supports the diagnosis of SC (most commonly partnered with *NTRK3*). In contrast, AciCC commonly show rearrangement of *NR4A3* and intraductal carcinoma show rearrangement of the *RET* gene in almost half of cases. *RET* rearrangements can also rarely be found in SC partnered with *ETV6*, whereas *RET* partners in intraductal carcinoma are usually *NCOA4* or *TRIM27*.

Prognosis and Therapy

In general, SC is an indolent tumor with most studies reporting 5- and 10-year overall survival rates close to or greater than 90%. Lymph node and distant metastases can be seen in a minority of patients. In general, most patients are treated with surgical excision with or without elective neck lymph node dissection. Some centers also include adjuvant chemotherapy and/or radiation in cases with higher-risk features such as lymph node metastasis. High-grade transformation is reported in occasional cases and may show a more aggressive disease course. Rare cases with a more aggressive course may see a benefit from a TRK inhibitor when *NTRK3* rearrangement is present.

SECRETORY CARCINOMA – DISEASE FACT SHEET

Definition
- ▸▸ Low-grade adenocarcinoma of the salivary gland with multiple small cytoplasmic vacuoles

Incidence and Location
- ▸▸ Uncommon
- ▸▸ Mostly in parotid gland but also occurs in minor salivary glands at various sites

Age and Sex Distribution
- ▸▸ Wide age range but most cases occur between 40 and 50 years of age
- ▸▸ Slight male predominance

Clinical Features
- ▸▸ Slow-growing, usually painless mass

Prognosis and Therapy
- ▸▸ Most cases are cured by surgical excision
- ▸▸ Occasional high-grade or aggressive tumors may occur with metastatic disease
- ▸▸ Aggressive tumors with *NTRK3* rearrangements may benefit from targeted therapy

---

SECRETORY CARCINOMA – PATHOLOGIC FEATURES

Gross Findings
- ▸▸ Usually fairly well circumscribed
- ▸▸ Cystic change is common

Microscopic Findings
- ▸▸ Low-grade uniform tumor cells with round nuclei
- ▸▸ Tumor cells have abundant eosinophilic cytoplasm containing microvacuoles
- ▸▸ Dense extracellular cytoplasm may have a colloid-like appearance
- ▸▸ Mitotic activity and necrosis are rare
- ▸▸ Variable growth patterns including cribriform, papillary, solid, and cystic

Pathologic Differential Diagnoses
- ▸▸ Acinic cell carcinoma
- ▸▸ Intraductal carcinoma
- ▸▸ Mucoepidermoid carcinoma
- ▸▸ Adenocarcinoma, not otherwise specified

SALIVARY DUCT CARCINOMA

DIFFERENTIAL DIAGNOSES: HIGH-GRADE MUCOEPIDERMOID CARCINOMA AND METASTATIC CARCINOMA

Clinical Features

SDC is a high-grade carcinoma of the salivary glands defined by apocrine differentiation and a resemblance to ductal carcinoma of the breast. SDC represents up to 10% of all salivary gland carcinomas and is most common in elderly men with a peak incidence in the sixth to seventh decade. The parotid gland is the most common site, but any salivary gland can give rise to SDC. At least half (and possibly up to 80%) of all SDC are thought to arise from a pre-existing PA.

Pathologic Features

GROSS FINDINGS

SDC is an aggressive malignancy and commonly shows gross evidence of invasion into surrounding salivary gland and adjacent structures including skin. Multiple regional lymph node metastases are also usually evident grossly when lymph node dissection is performed. Tumors may be firm or soft depending on the degree of cellularity, fibrosis, and necrosis. A gritty cut surface is described in some cases as a result of calcifications. In examples arising from a PA, it

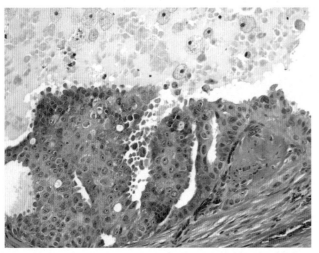

FIG. 9.21

Salivary duct carcinoma (SDC). SDC is a high-grade adenocarcinoma and is defined by its apocrine phenotype. Morphologic evidence of apocrine differentiation in this tumor includes abundant eosinophilic cytoplasm, prominent nucleoli, and apocrine snouts with decapitation secretions as seen in this image. Positive nuclear reactivity for androgen receptor is also good immunophenotypic evidence of apocrine differentiation.

may be possible to grossly appreciate the pre-existing circumscribed PA depending on the extent of SDC invasion.

MICROSCOPIC FINDINGS

SDCs characteristically show high-grade features with tumor cells having abundant eosinophilic cytoplasm. This prominent eosinophilic cytoplasm is likely related to the apocrine phenotype of SDC and many tumors also show at least focal tumor cells with apocrine snouts (Fig. 9.21). Mucus cells can be identified occasionally but more prominent mucinous differentiation is rare. Most SDCs have clearly high-grade features with high mitotic activity, comedonecrosis and nuclear enlargement, and pleomorphism. Angiolymphatic and perineural invasion are common. In cases of SDC ex PA, residual areas of PA, or more commonly a hyalinized nodule, may be identified.

Rare variants of SDC include those with sarcomatoid differentiation, mucinous differentiation, micropapillary architecture, and oncocytic cells.

Ancillary Studies

SDCs are cytokeratin 7 positive and show considerable immunophenotypic overlap with breast ductal carcinoma, particularly apocrine breast carcinoma. Mammaglobin is positive in some cases of SDC. Androgen receptor positivity is very common (in more than 90% of cases in some reports) as this marker is

indicative of apocrine differentiation. SDCs are generally positive for GCDFP-15 also. Her2 amplification is seen in approximately a quarter to a third of cases and immunohistochemistry for Her2 is usually 3+ in these cases.

Differential Diagnosis

SDC is a high-grade carcinoma and therefore the differential diagnosis includes other similar high-grade carcinomas including high-grade MEC and metastatic carcinoma.

Although nuclear atypia, mitotic activity, and necrosis can lead to grading of MEC as high grade, these findings remain uncommon in this diagnosis as most high-grade MEC achieve this grade as a result of invasive growth patterns (Table 9.11). However, rare cases of high-grade MEC will show considerable nuclear atypia, mitotic activity, and/or necrosis (Fig. 9.22). Additionally, although overt mucinous differentiation is uncommon in SDC, it can occur in some case. In such situations, the morphologic distinction between high-grade MEC and SDC can be nearly impossible and may require ancillary testing. Androgen receptor is almost always positive in SDC but rarely expressed in MEC. In contrast, MEC usually express squamous markers such as p63 which are only rarely positive in SDC. Identification of a *MAML2* rearrangement is diagnostic of MEC.

Metastatic carcinoma is common to intraparotid lymph nodes with head and neck cutaneous and upper aerodigestive tract primaries representing the majority of cases. In these situations, metastatic poorly differentiated SCC can show high-grade features as well as

---

TABLE 9.11

Features of Salivary Duct Carcinoma Versus High-Grade Mucoepidermoid Carcinoma

Salivary Duct Carcinoma	High-Grade Mucoepidermoid Carcinoma
• Apocrine differentiation almost always present	• Lacks apocrine differentiation
• Epidermoid (squamous) differentiation is very uncommon	• Epidermoid differentiation is an important diagnostic feature but keratinization is extremely rare
• Pronounced nuclear pleomorphism is very common	• Nuclei are usually more uniform and pleomorphism is rare
• Mucinous differentiation is uncommon	• Mucus cells are an important diagnostic feature but may be rare
• *MAML2* rearrangements are not identified	• *MAML2* rearrangements are common

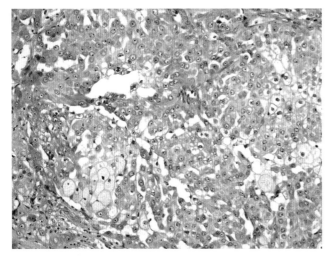

FIG. 9.22

High-grade mucoepidermoid carcinoma (MEC). Occasional cases of high-grade MEC can show nuclear atypia and solid nests of tumor cells with abundant eosinophilic cytoplasm that mimics salivary duct carcinoma (SDC). The example shown also has prominent nucleoli. Most cases of SDC are more pleomorphic, whereas MEC usually has more uniform nuclei. Also, mucus cell differentiation is required for the diagnosis of MEC but is fairly uncommon in SDC.

being positive in SCC and androgen receptor being positive in SDC.

Prognosis and Therapy

SDC is aggressive and many patients present at an advanced stage with approximately half of patients having regional lymph node metastases. Median survival rates are in the 3- to 4-year range and 5-year overall survival rates are less than 50%. Locoregional recurrence is not uncommon and distant metastases are the main reason or failure and death occurring in about 30% to 60% of patients. Wide surgical resection with lymph node dissection continues to be the main treatment option. Postoperative adjuvant chemotherapy and/or radiation are also common. Ongoing research is examining the role of Her2 blockade, androgen deprivation therapy, and molecular targets in SDC. Of note, National Comprehensive Cancer Network guidelines specifically recommend testing for androgen receptor and HER2 prior to treatment of metastatic disease in SDC.

TABLE 9.12

Histologic Features of Salivary Duct Carcinoma Versus Metastatic Carcinoma

Salivary Duct Carcinoma	Metastatic Squamous Cell Carcinoma
• Apocrine differentiation is almost always present	• Apocrine differentiation is not present
• Squamoid differentiation is rare	• Squamous differentiation is present but may require immunostains to confirm
• Arises in parotid parenchyma	• Present in intra- or periparotid lymph nodes but residual lymph node may not be evident
• May have evidence of pre-existing pleomorphic adenoma	• No precursor lesion is present in the parotid gland

---

SALIVARY DUCT CARCINOMA – DISEASE FACT SHEET

Definition
▶▶ Salivary duct carcinoma is an aggressive salivary gland adenocarcinoma with apocrine differentiation

Incidence and Location
▶▶ SDC is rare and accounts for approximately 10% of all primary salivary gland carcinomas
▶▶ Most common in the parotid gland

Age and Sex Distribution
▶▶ Most common in older men with a peak in the sixth to seventh decade

Clinical Features
▶▶ Usually a larger symptomatic mass with paralysis and possibly facial nerve paralysis
▶▶ Associated lymph node metastases may also be appreciated clinically

Prognosis and Therapy
▶▶ Aggressive malignancy
▶▶ Metastases are common at presentation
▶▶ Death due to metastatic disease remains common despite aggressive surgery and adjuvant chemoradiation

---

SALIVARY DUCT CARCINOMA – PATHOLOGIC FEATURES

Gross Findings
▶▶ Large infiltrative and destructive mass
▶▶ Invasion of nearby structures
▶▶ May be cystic and necrotic
▶▶ Gritty texture
▶▶ Grossly positive lymph nodes may be present if sampled

abundant eosinophilic cytoplasm. In such cases, histologic examination can be helpful in identifying the tumor within a lymph node which supports the diagnosis of metastasis over primary SDC (Table 9.12). Similarly, the finding of a precursor PA or hyalinized nodule supports the diagnosis of a primary salivary gland carcinoma such as SDC over a metastasis. Clinical history can also be helpful, particularly for patients with known history of cutaneous malignancy. In cases in which the differential is unresolved, immunostains can help with p63 (and other squamous markers)

Continued

SALIVARY DUCT CARCINOMA – PATHOLOGIC FEATURES—cont'd

Microscopic Findings

▶▶ High-grade adenocarcinoma with abundant eosinophilic cytoplasm
▶▶ Increased mitotic activity, atypical mitoses, nuclear pleomorphism, and comedonecrosis
▶▶ Apocrine snouts reflect apocrine differentiation
▶▶ Various growth patterns including solid and cribriform architecture
▶▶ Large invasive nests with the appearance of ductal carcinoma *in situ* of the breast
▶▶ Variant morphologies include sarcomatoid, micropapillary, and mucinous
▶▶ Perineural and angiolymphatic invasion are common

Pathologic Differential Diagnoses

▶▶ High-grade mucoepidermoid carcinoma
▶▶ Metastatic carcinoma

BIPHENOTYPIC SINONASAL SARCOMA

DIFFERENTIAL DIAGNOSES: SOLITARY FIBROUS TUMOR, LEIMYOSARCOMA, SYNOVIAL SARCOMA, SINONASAL GLOMANGIOPERICYTOMA, AND SCHWANNOMA

Clinical Features

Biphenotypic sinonasal sarcoma (BPSS) is a recently described disease entity and was formally introduced into the 2017 edition of the WHO Classification of Head and Neck Tumors. It is a low-grade malignant neoplasm that is exclusive to the sinonasal tract, specifically occurring in the superior aspects of the nasal cavity and the ethmoid sinuses (Fig. 9.23). This sarcoma demonstrates concomitant neural and smooth muscle phenotype and differentiation. There is a strong predilection for this malignancy to occur in women (2:1). Although it can occur over a wide range of ages, most are identified in the fifth decade of life. Patients will present with nonspecific symptoms such as difficulty in nasal breathing, epistaxis, nasal/sinus pain, and congestion. Where there is more extensive spread, cranial nerve palsies and ocular-related symptoms such as proptosis and blurry vision may occur. It is characterized by a slow and progressive growth.

Pathologic Features

GROSS FINDINGS

There are no specific gross features that are unique to BPSS. The tissue fragments may impart a polypoid

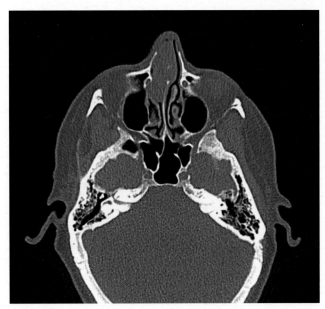

FIG. 9.23

A computed tomography scan will demonstrate a mass that is typically located in anterior-superior aspect of the nasal cavity. The tumor can also be found in the ethmoid sinuses.

appearance and are reportedly firmer than sinonasal inflammatory polyps. The tumor size can be large (~4 cm) with local destruction and invasion into bone.

MICROSCOPIC FINDINGS

BPSS is an infiltrative, poorly circumscribed, and unencapsulated tumor. It is a cellular tumor composed of uniform/monotonous spindle cells arranged in medium to long fascicles with areas of herringbone growth pattern (Fig. 9.24). Tumor nuclei are wavy with tapered ends. The nuclei are hyperchromatic, contain finely granular chromatin, and often overlap. Mitotic

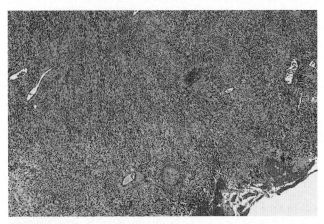

FIG. 9.24

Biphenotypic sinonasal sarcoma is a cellular spindle cell neoplasm with tumor cells arranged in medium to long fascicles in a herringbone pattern.

figures are typically rare. Intercellular collagen is scant or rarely present (Fig. 9.25). Hemangiopericytoma-like vascular spaces may also be appreciated. What is characteristic of this entity is the presence of entrapped benign epithelial elements/glands of respiratory epithelial origin with mucinous metaplasia (Fig. 9.26). In some cases, the entrapped epithelial elements may impart a cystic appearance. Bone invasion can be appreciated (25% have orbital extension and 10% have cribriform plate extension). In approximately 10% of the cases, rhabdomyoblastic elements may be identified. Ulceration, hemorrhage, and necrosis are not appreciated.

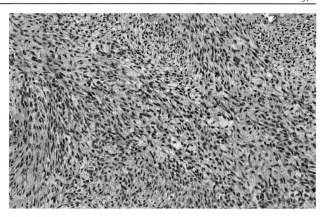

FIG. 9.27

The tumor cells are notably monotonous and bland. The nuclei have wavy or tapered ends. Notably elevated mitotic activity is not typically appreciated in these tumors.

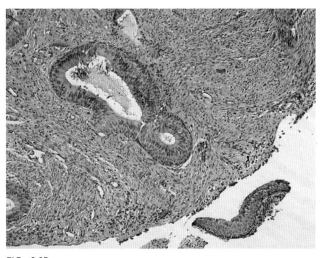

FIG. 9.25

Entrapped glands with respiratory-type mucosa are a helpful feature in biphenotypic sinonasal sarcoma.

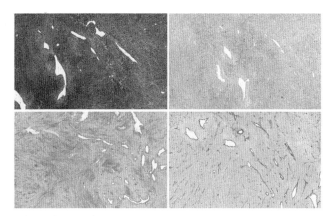

FIG. 9.26

(*Top left*) Example of a biphenotypic sinonasal sarcoma with staghorn-like blood vessels. (*Top right* and *bottom left*) Immunohistochemical studies show that the tumor is positive for S100 and smooth muscle actin. (*Bottom right*) CD34 expression is restricted to the blood vessels.

Ancillary Studies

BPSS has a dual neural and smooth muscle phenotype: (1) S100 is positive in all cases, even focally, and (2) calponin and/or SMA are positive at least focally (Fig. 9.27). In a series review by Rooper et al. a majority of BPSS demonstrated consistent nuclear expression of beta-catenin, an additional marker that can be helpful in panel. Focally, factor XIIIa staining may be positive. Occasionally, aberrant expression for cytokeratin/epithelial markers is present. SOX10 is consistently negative. If rhabdomyoblastic differentiation is present, desmin, myoD1, and myogenin positivity may be appreciated. As the differential diagnosis is broad, a panel of S100, SOX10, SMA, calponin, desmin, myogenin, beta-catenin, factor XIIIa, and pan cytokeratin is helpful.

From a molecular standpoint, this malignancy is characterized by a translocation of t(2;4)(q35; q31.1) – *PAX3-MAML3* fusion, although other fusions such as *PAX3-FOX01* and *PAX3-NCOA1* are reported. A potential pitfall may be that BPSS may demonstrate immunohistochemical positivity for TLE1, a stain utilized for the diagnosis of synovial sarcoma. In these cases, re-arrangement studies for *SS18* (*SYT*) will be helpful to exclude a BPSS (see Differential Diagnosis section below).

In the cases with rhabdomyoblastic differentiation, a *PAX3-NCOA1* fusion is present.

Differential Diagnosis

The differential diagnoses for BPSS include any spindle cell neoplasm that occurs in the sinonasal tract, such as solitary fibrous tumor (SFT), leiomyosarcoma, synovial sarcoma, sinonasal glomangiopericytoma, and schwannoma. Of these differential diagnoses, differentiating BPSS from monophasic synovial sarcomas may prove to be the most challenging and requires ancillary molecular studies.

SFT, quite similarly to BPSS, has bland neoplastic spindle cells. The key difference, however, is that in SFT the spindle cells will have a haphazard arrangement with areas that are hyper and hypocellular (Table 9.13). SFT lacks the fascicular and herringbone pattern as seen in BPSS. Both tumors may have hemangiopericytoma-like blood vessels. The stroma is different from BPSS as there is a collagenous stroma in SFT. In terms of immunohistochemistry, SFTs are positive for CD34 and nuclear STAT6 (Fig. 9.28). STAT6 staining can be seen in BPSS; however, it is reported to be cytoplasmically restricted and not nuclear. Rarely S100 and SMA can be expressed in SFT.

At low power, leiomyosarcomas may demonstrate a similar growth architecture, but the tumor nuclei have blunted ends, "box car nuclei", and not the wavy or

TABLE 9.13

Histologic Features of Biphenotypic Sinonasal Sarcoma Versus Solitary Fibrous Tumor

Biphenotypic Sinonasal Sarcoma	Solitary Fibrous Tumor
• Uniform and monotonous spindle cells with tapered and/or wavy nuclei	• Bland spindle cells in a collagenous stroma
• Tumor cells arranged in herringbone or fasicular growth pattern	• Haphazard architecture with hypo- and hypercellular areas
• Entrapped glandular/surface epithelial elements	• Entrapped epithelial or glandular elements are typically not appreciated
• May have blood vessels in a staghorn pattern arrangement	• Staghorn-type blood vessel pattern
• Occasional cytoplasmic STAT6 positivity, no nuclear STAT6	• Nuclear STAT6 positivity
• S100 positive with positive calponin and/or smooth muscle actin	• Expresses CD34, bcl-2, CD99, and nuclear STAT6; negative for S100 and actins

TABLE 9.14

Histologic Features of Biphenotypic Sinonasal Sarcoma versus Leiomyosarcoma

Biphenotypic Sinonasal Sarcoma (BPSS)	Leiomyosarcoma
• Uniform and monotonous spindle cells with tapered and/or wavy nuclei	• Classically have blunted ends ("box-car" type nuclei); variant leiomyosarcomas may have different nuclear features
• Mitotic figures are limited	• Mitotically active
• Tumor cells arranged in herringbone or fasicular growth pattern	• May show similar growth architecture to BPSS
• Entrapped glandular/surface epithelial elements	• Entrapped epithelial elements are not typically appreciated
• S100 positive with positive calponin and/or smooth muscle actin	• Express smooth muscle markers; negative for S100 and beta catenin

tapered end like in BPSS (Table 9.14). Immunohistochemically, S100 and beta-catenin staining is not seen.

Although synovial sarcomas are diagnostically challenging to separate from BPSS, they rarely occur in the sinonasal tract. Biphasic synovial sarcomas may appear similar to BPSS in that the epithelial elements in synovial sarcomas may appear like entrapped glandular elements in BPSS. However, the key difference is that in biphasic synovial sarcomas the epithelial elements comprise polygonal cells rather than the squamous- or respiratory-type sinonasal epithelium entrapped in BPSS. In larger series reviewing synovial sarcomas, a markedly higher mitotic rate (>10/10 HPF) has been noted than that identified in BPSS (0–4/10 HPF). Furthermore, synovial sarcomas will have scattered areas of thick ("ropey") collagen bundles and calcification. Immunohistochemical studies are of limited use as there can be significant overlap in staining patterns such as S100, SMA, nuclear beta-catenin, and myogenin. As a side note, TLE1 is a specific and sensitive marker for synovial sarcoma; however, a single case of BPSS with a *PAX3-FOX01* fusion has reportedly demonstrated diffuse expression. Ultimately, the correct diagnosis may depend on molecular testing.

Other differential diagnoses to consider are sinonasal glomangiopericytoma, which may demonstrate similar immunohistochemical profile like BPSS, such as positive SMA, nuclear beta-catenin, and factor XIIIa. However, it lacks S100 staining as seen in BPSS. Schwannoma is also a possibility; however, differentiation from BPPS is straightforward as SOX10 will be positive in schwannomas. Furthermore, compared with BPSS, S100 has a more diffuse pattern in schwannomas. Smooth muscle markers will be negative in schwannoma, a finding seen in BPSS. Beta-catenin is negative in schwannomas.

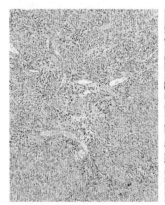 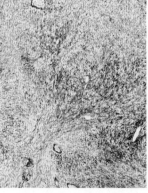

FIG. 9.28

Immunohistochemical studies. S100 (*left*) will be heterogeneously positive as well as the SMA (*right*).

Prognosis and Treatment

BPSS is treated by local excision with or without adjuvant radiation therapy. A recurrence rate of 40% to 50% with a varying disease recurrence-free interval (1 to 9 years) is noted. The data on the efficacy of neoadjuvant radiation and chemotherapy for these tumors is limited only to a few cases. However, some authors have recommended these additional modalities in cases with close or positive margins, high-grade features, or imaging evidence of perineural spread. No regional metastasis or distant metastases have been reported, and only one case of death due to BPSS has been reported due to cranial vault involvement.

BIPHENOTYPIC SINONASAL SARCOMA – DISEASE FACT SHEET

Definition
▸▸ Low-grade sarcoma exclusive to the sinonasal cavity with dual neural and smooth muscle phenotype

Incidence
▸▸ Rare
▸▸ Superior aspect of nasal cavity or ethmoid sinuses

Morbidity and Mortality
▸▸ Death from this disease has only rarely been reported

Sex and Age Distribution
▸▸ 2:1 female-to-male ratio
▸▸ Wide range of ages, commonly in the fifth decade

Clinical Features
▸▸ Slow and progressive growth – Locoregional symptoms such as epistaxis, nasal/sinus pain, and congestion

Treatment and Prognosis
▸▸ Surgical excision is the treatment of choice
▸▸ Approximately half of cases will recur
▸▸ Limited data of chemotherapy and radiation, at discretion of clinician

---

BIPHENOTYPIC SINONASAL SARCOMA – PATHOLOGIC FEATURES

Gross Findings
▸▸ Nonspecific

Microscopic Findings
▸▸ Uniform/monotonous spindle cells with tapered/wavy nuclei
▸▸ Overt atypia not present
▸▸ Arranged in medium to long fascicles in herringbone pattern
▸▸ Entrapped glandular/surface epithelial elements
▸▸ Mitotically inactive or low activity
▸▸ Necrosis not appreciated

Differential Diagnosis
▸▸ Solitary fibrous tumor, leiomyosarcoma, synovial sarcoma, sinonasal glomangiopericytoma, schwannoma

---

SINONASAL UNDIFFERENTIATED CARCINOMA

DIFFERENTIAL DIAGNOSES: SMARCB1-DEFICIENT SINONASAL CARCINOMA AND NUT CARCINOMA

Clinical Features

Sinonasal undifferentiated carcinoma (SNUC) is a rare tumor of the sinonasal tract that lacks glandular, squamous, and neuroendocrine features and is not further classifiable. In reported series, SNUC occurs over a wide age range from adolescents to elderly adults. The most common site for SNUC is the nasal cavity and ethmoid sinuses, but SNUC can arise in any sinonasal site and commonly the tumor is so large at the initial presentation that defining a precise subsite of origin is often not possible. Patients present with complaints that are nonspecific and common to other large sinonasal tumors including nasal obstruction and epistaxis. More advanced tumors can also result in diplopia and other vision abnormalities.

Pathologic Features

GROSS FINDINGS

SNUCs are usually large fungating masses with extensive invasion of surrounding structures and poorly defined borders.

MICROSCOPIC FINDINGS

The defining histomorphologic feature of SNUC is a lack of identifiable differentiation, and these tumors are composed of sheets or lobules of large malignant cells. The overall morphologic features are those of a high-grade undifferentiated carcinoma (Fig. 9.29) but are otherwise nonspecific. Tumor cells have large round nuclei and variable amounts of cytoplasm. Nuclear chromatin can be vesicular or hyperchromatic and a prominent nucleolus is common. High-grade features including apoptosis, necrosis, and prominent mitotic activity are common. Keratinization and mucus cells are not identified.

Ancillary Studies

SNUC is essentially a diagnosis of exclusion and therefore the main purpose of ancillary testing in the setting of possible SNUC is to exclude the possibility of a better

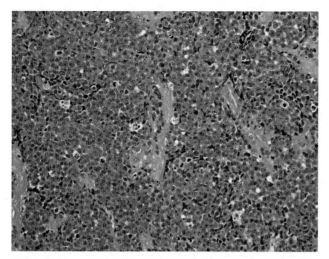

FIG. 9.29

Sinonasal undifferentiated carcinoma (SNUC). The morphologic features of SNUC are not specific but are those of a high-grade undifferentiated carcinoma. This image shows the common morphologic finding of sheets of undifferentiated tumor cells that have enlarged nuclei, high nuclear-to-cytoplasmic ratios, and prominent nucleoli. The diagnosis of SNUC requires exclusion of other tumors in the sinonasal tract with similar morphology and this example was negative for NUT and showed retained expression of SMARCB1.

defined tumor type. SNUC should be positive for a variety of keratins to confirm a carcinoma but negative for CK5/6 specifically as this is indicative of squamous cell differentiation. p63 may be seen in some cases but p40, a more specific marker of squamous differentiation, should be negative. Focal reactivity with neuroendocrine markers synaptophysin and chromogranin may be seen but should only be accepted in the diagnosis of SNUC if morphologic evidence of neuroendocrine differentiation is lacking. p16 is very commonly positive in SNUC but does not correlate with human papillomavirus (HPV) infection; however, up to 20% of SNUCs may show evidence of high-risk HPV by direct

testing methods such as *in situ* hybridization. *IDH2* mutations have also been shown to occur in approximately a third of SNUC.

Differential Diagnosis

SNUC is likely not a specific disease entity and molecular and morphologic discoveries have begun to better define some tumors that may have once been categorized as SNUC. SMARCB1 (INI-1)–deficient tumors have recently been described in the sinonasal cavity and therefore this entity should be excluded in cases in which SNUC is being considered (Table 9.15). Tumors with loss of SMARB1 by immunohistochemistry commonly show a basaloid morphology with high nuclear-to-cytoplasmic ratios (Fig. 9.30A). The finding

TABLE 9.15

Features of Sinonasal Undifferentiated Carcinoma Versus SMARCB1-Deficient Carcinoma

Sinonasal Undifferentiated Carcinoma	INI-1-Deficient Carcinoma
• Undifferentiated high-grade carcinoma	• Most tumors are composed predominantly of basaloid tumor cells
• Lacks morphologic and immunophenotypic evidence of differentiation	• At least rare rhabdoid tumor cells are seen in most cases
	• Some examples show diffuse to focal glandular differentiation
• Retains expression of SMARB1 (INI1)	• Loss of SMARB1 (INI1) expression by immunohistochemistry

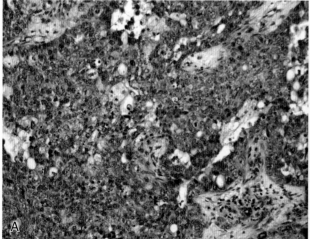 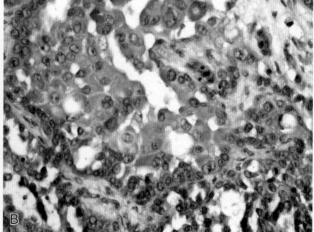

FIG. 9.30

SMARCB1-deficient sinonasal carcinoma. **(A)** SMARCB1-deficient sinonasal carcinoma most commonly show a predominance of undifferentiated appearing basaloid tumor cells. High-grade features are usually obvious with increased mitotic activity, apoptotic cells, and necrosis. **(B)** One morphologic clue to the diagnosis of SMARB1-deficient sinonasal carcinoma is the presence of rhabdoid tumor cells having an eccentric nucleus and dense eosinophilic cytoplasm. An immunostain showing loss of SMARB1 is important for diagnosis.

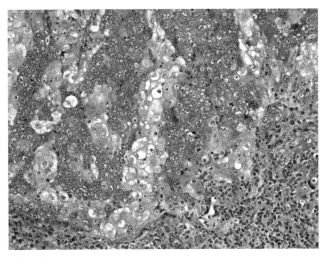

FIG. 9.31

NUT carcinoma. NUT carcinoma arising in the sinonasal tract has a similar appearance to those in other sites and is characterized by undifferentiated tumor cells. Abrupt squamous differentiation as seen in this example is also a helpful clue but can result in a misdiagnosis of squamous cell carcinoma if the possibility of NUT carcinoma is not excluded by immunohistochemistry or molecular testing.

of at least focal rhabdoid cells with dense eccentric cytoplasm is also a very helpful feature to suggest the possibility of a SMARCB1 (INI-1)–deficient sinonasal carcinoma (Fig. 9.30B).

NUT carcinoma can also occur in the sinonasal tract and should be excluded prior to the diagnosis of SNUC. NUT carcinoma is mostly composed of undifferentiated tumor cells but can show focal areas of abrupt squamous differentiation (Fig. 9.31) and is defined by rearrangement of the *NUT* gene (Table 9.16). Immunophenotypically, NUT carcinoma shows diffuse p63 reactivity but only focal p40 reactivity in a majority of cases; however, it can be negative for both these markers. When a carcinoma is encountered having predominantly undifferentiated or poorly differentiated tumor cells and abrupt squamous differentiation, NUT carcinoma should be considered as the differential diagnosis in such cases include poorly differentiated SCC which is less aggressive. In cases of NUT carcinoma lacking evidence of squamous differentiation morphologically and immunophenotypically, the differential diagnosis is more likely to include SNUC. In these cases, consideration of NUT carcinoma is also important. Immunohistochemistry for NUT is useful diagnostically and is considered positive when at least 50% of tumor cell nuclei are positive. Alternatively or in indeterminate cases, FISH and other molecular methods can be used to confirm or exclude a *NUT* gene rearrangement.

Prognosis and Therapy

SNUC is aggressive and patients with this diagnosis have a poor prognosis. Patients usually present with T4 disease. Despite the common finding of a large aggressive primary tumor, lymph node metastases are only identified in approximately 10% to 15% of patients and distant metastasis is less common. Most patients are treated with a multimodality approach using a combination of induction chemotherapy, surgery, adjuvant chemoradiation, and/or definitive chemoradiation. Despite the better prognosis of HPV association in other tumors, limited data available for SNUC has not suggested an improved prognosis for those associated with high-risk HPV infection. Interestingly, tumors with *IDH2* mutations appear to have a better prognosis than wild-type tumors and may represent a distinct entity.

TABLE 9.16

Features of Sinonasal Undifferentiated Carcinoma Versus NUT Carcinoma

Sinonasal Undifferentiated Carcinoma	NUT Carcinoma
• Undifferentiated high-grade carcinoma	• Undifferentiated high-grade carcinoma
• Lacks morphologic and immunophenotypic evidence of differentiation (including a lack of squamous and neuroendocrine differentiation)	• Frequently shows squamous differentiation
• p40 negative	• p40 is commonly positive
• Lacks rearrangement of *NUT* gene	• *NUT* gene rearrangement present
• Negative for NUT by immunohistochemistry	• Positive for NUT by immunohistochemistry (>50% nuclear staining)

SINONASAL UNDIFFERENTIATED CARCINOMA – DISEASE FACT SHEET

Definition

▸▸ Aggressive, undifferentiated carcinoma of the sinonasal tract not meeting criteria for another more definitive diagnosis

Incidence and Location

▸▸ Rare
▸▸ Most common in nasal cavity and ethmoid sinus but can occur in any sinonasal location

Age Distribution

▸▸ Wide age range from adolescents to elderly

Clinical Features

▸▸ Usually present with nonspecific symptoms of epistaxis and nasal obstruction
▸▸ More advanced tumors may cause diplopia

Prognosis and Therapy

▸▸ SNUC is aggressive and is often treated with multimodality therapy including surgery and adjuvant chemoradiation

HUMAN PAPILLOMAVIRUS–RELATED MULTIPHENOTYPIC SINONASAL CARCINOMA

DIFFERENTIAL DIAGNOSES: ADENOID CYSTIC CARCINOMA AND SQUAMOUS CELL CARCINOMA

Clinical Features

HPV-related multiphenotypic sinonasal carcinoma (HMSC) is a recently described tumor with characteristic morphology showing evidence of salivary-type differentiation (specifically AdCC) and squamous differentiation. Due to the morphologic similarity with AdCC, this tumor was initially designated as HPV-related sinonasal carcinoma with adenoid cystic-like features. The nasal cavity is the most common site and paranasal sinuses can also be involved, either in isolation or in combination with nasal involvement. In the limited number of cases reported, there is a slight female predominance and patients range from 28 to 90 years (average 50–60 years). Patients present with nonspecific symptoms of nasal obstruction, epistaxis, and nasal discharge. Pain and ocular symptoms may occur but are uncommon.

Pathologic Features

HMSC is composed of basaloid tumor cells most commonly in sheets and lobules having considerable morphologic similarity to solid-type AdCC. Cribriform architecture is also common, but a tubular pattern is seen in only a minority of cases (Figs. 9.32A and 9.32B). Biphasic differentiation with ductal and myoepithelial

components is seen in most cases. Squamous differentiation is most commonly present in the form of surface squamous dysplasia (Fig. 9.32C) and may extend further into the tumor in rare cases. Increased mitotic activity, necrosis, and nuclear pleomorphism are also common (Fig. 9.32D). Perineural invasion can occur but is not common.

Ancillary Studies

Immunostains are useful to confirm the multiphenotypic nature of this tumor. The myoepithelial component frequently stains with a variety of sensitive and specific myoepithelial markers including p63, S100, SOX10, calponin, and actin. In contrast, when ductal differentiation is present, these cells will stain with CK7 and frequently c-kit. HMSC is associated with high-risk HPV, and this must be confirmed to make the diagnosis. While p16 is strongly and diffusely positive in almost all cases, this finding does not correlate with the presence of HPV in the sinonasal tract as closely as it does in oropharynx and therefore cannot be used as surrogate marker for HPV in this setting. *In situ* hybridization or other direct testing method for high-risk HPV is therefore required. When using such testing for this diagnosis, it is important to ensure the testing method includes a variety of high-risk HPV types. HPV 16 has been found in some cases but the most common HPV type found in HMSC is HPV 33. HPV 35 and 56 have also been reported in small numbers of cases.

Rearrangement of the *MYB* gene which can be seen in AdCC is not identified in HMSC. However, it has been shown that MYB overexpression is detectable by immunohistochemistry in many cases and this could be a potential pitfall in the diagnosis.

Differential Diagnosis

As has been noted, there is considerable morphologic overlap between HMSC and AdCC, but several features can be helpful to favor the diagnosis of one entity over the other. HMSC commonly shows surface squamous dysplasia which argues against salivary gland tumor such as AdCC in which surface dysplasia is typically not present. AdCC is also much more infiltrative and almost always has small infiltrative nests or tubules and perineural invasion. Compared with HMSC, solid AdCC (Fig. 9.33A) usually lacks profound nuclear atypia and pleomorphism (i.e., anaplasia) that is common in HMSC (Table 9.17). HMSC has a more pushing pattern of invasion with large tumor nests and perineural invasion is rare. In contrast, perineural invasion is common in AdCC (Fig. 9.33B). Unfortunately, this difference in

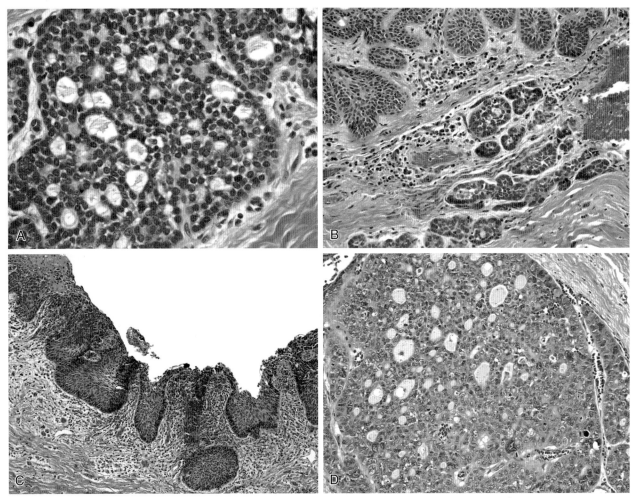

FIG. 9.32

Human papillomavirus (HPV) – related multiphenotypic sinonasal carcinoma (HMSC). Many cases of HMSC show extensive morphologic overlap with adenoid cystic carcinoma (AdCC) as seen in this case with cribriform architecture with hyaline stromal spheres and scattered ductal structures surrounded by myoepithelial cells with very high nuclear-to-cytoplasmic ratios (**A**). The presence of myoepithelial and squamous differentiation are important diagnostic features of HMSC. In (**B**) there is a focus with more squamoid appearance adjacent to an area with a myoepithelial appearance. Surface squamous dysplasia is also common in HMSC but rare to nonexistent in true AdCC (**C**). HMSC can also show more atypical tumor cells including overt nuclear anaplasia (**D**). These images are all from the same case which was confirmed to contain transcriptionally active high-risk HPV.

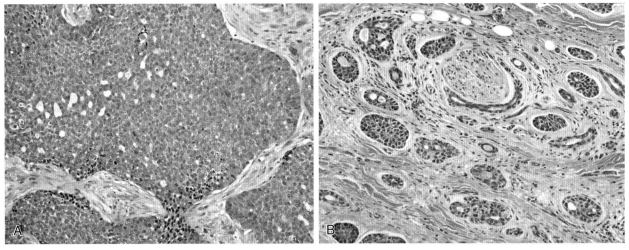

FIG. 9.33

Adenoid cystic carcinoma (AdCC). The solid variant of AdCC grows in large nests of basaloid tumor cells (**A**). Occasional ductal structures can also usually be seen and this appearance significantly overlaps with that of human papillomavirus (HPV)-related multiphenotypic sinonasal carcinoma (HMSC). Perineural invasion is very common in AdCC (**B**) and uncommon in HMSC. AdCC lack transcriptionally active high-risk HPV.

TABLE 9.17

Features of HPV-Related Multiphenotypic Sinonasal Carcinoma Versus Adenoid Cystic Carcinoma

HPV-Related Multiphenotypic Sinonasal Carcinoma	Adenoid Cystic Carcinoma
• Basaloid tumor cells	• Basaloid tumor cells
• Surface squamous dysplasia is common	• None to rare surface squamous dysplasia
• Myoepithelial and squamous differentiation, many also show at least focal ductal differentiation	• Biphasic myoepithelial and ductal differentiation
• Most with solid and cribriform, tubules are rare	• Solid, cribriform, and tubular growth are common in most examples
• Areas of pronounced pleomorphic are common	• Pronounced pleomorphism is uncommon except in those with high-grade transformation
• Perineural invasion is rare	• Perineural invasion is common
• Positive for high-risk HPV (especially type 33)	• Negative for high-risk HPV
• Negative for *MYB* rearrangement	• Many examples have an *MYB* rearrangement

HPV, Human papillomavirus.

TABLE 9.18

Histologic Features of HPV-Related Multiphenotypic Sinonasal Carcinoma Versus Squamous Cell Carcinoma

HPV-Related Multiphenotypic Sinonasal Carcinoma	Squamous Cell Carcinoma
• Basaloid tumor cells	• Basaloid tumor cells are common for HPV-associated tumors
• Surface squamous dysplasia with limited to no squamous differentiation deeper in the tumor	• Squamous differentiation is diffuse throughout the tumor
• Myoepithelial differentiation is present	• Lacks myoepithelial differentiation
• Ductal differentiation is common	• Adenosquamous carcinoma will have focal glandular differentiation
• Positive for high-risk HPV	• Positive for high-risk HPV

HPV, Human papillomavirus.

---

invasion is not completely specific and may not be identifiable on a biopsy specimen and therefore immunostains may be needed. While p16 is not specific, it is less likely to be strongly positive in AdCC. The most useful diagnostic test, however, is identification of high-risk HPV in HMSC.

Nonkeratinizing SCC of the sinonasal tract can also occur and in some cases is also associated with high-risk HPV infection. HPV-positive SCC of the sinonasal tract can have very similar growth pattern and basaloid appearance to HMSC and the identification of high-risk HPV is not useful in this distinction (Table 9.18). Therefore, the distinction between HPV-associated SCC of the sinonasal tract and HMSC is dependent on the identification of biphasic growth and/or areas with a myoepithelial phenotype and immunostains are helpful in this regard. HPV-associated SCC usually shows more overt squamous differentiation throughout the invasive tumor (Fig. 9.34) which is only rarely seen in HMSC.

Prognosis and Therapy

Patients frequently present at high pT3 or pT4 stage. While the morphologic findings of HMSC suggest an

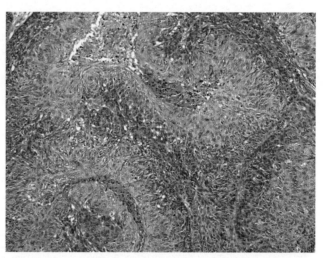

FIG. 9.34

Human papillomavirus (HPV)-associated sinonasal squamous cell carcinoma. Sinonasal squamous cell carcinomas can be associated with high-risk HPV and morphologically are composed of more basaloid tumor cells with large invasive nests. In contrast to HPV-related multiphenotypic sinonasal carcinoma, these squamous cell carcinomas lack evidence of ductal and myoepithelial differentiation and have more pronounced squamous differentiation deep into the invasive tumor.

aggressive phenotype, this tumor appears to have very limited metastatic potential with only rare reports of distant metastatic disease and no known deaths at this time. Recurrence is not uncommon and occurs in at least a third of patients, including some with late recurrence over 10 years later. Most patients have been treated with surgical resection with some receiving adjuvant chemotherapy or radiation.

HPV-RELATED MULTIPHENOTYPIC SINONASAL CARCINOMA – DISEASE FACT SHEET

Definition

- High-risk HPV-associated carcinoma of the sinonasal tract showing squamous and myoepithelial differentiation

Incidence and Location

- Rare
- Unique to the sinonasal tract with nasal cavity involvement most common

Age and Sex Distribution

- Wide age range with an average age range of 50–60 years
- Slight female predominance

Clinical Features

- Locally aggressive with most patients presenting with nonspecific symptoms of a sinonasal mass

Prognosis and Therapy

- Recurrences occur in about a third of patients
- Lymph node and distant metastases are rare
- No reported deaths to date
- Surgical excision is the primary treatment modality

HPV-RELATED MULTIPHENOTYPIC SINONASAL CARCINOMA – PATHOLOGIC FEATURES

Gross Findings

- Locally destructive mass of the sinonasal tract

Microscopic Findings

- Sheets and lobules of basaloid tumor cells
- Surface squamous dysplasia is common
- Cribriform architecture is also common
- Biphasic growth may also be evident morphologically but evidence of myoepithelial differentiation is required for the diagnosis

Pathologic Differential Diagnoses

- Adenoid cystic carcinoma
- Squamous cell carcinoma

BRANCHIAL CLEFT CYST

DIFFERENTIAL DIAGNOSIS: METASTATIC CYSTIC SQUAMOUS CELL CARCINOMA

Clinical Features

Branchial cleft anomalies are attributed to the failure of embryological branchial apparatus to improperly develop or involute in the head and neck region. As a result, patients will present with cysts, sinuses, fistulas, or a combination of these aberrations. Defects in the second branchial cleft are a common cause (approximately 90%) of lateral neck cysts. Although patients can present at any age, branchial cleft cysts are more frequently encountered in a bimodal distribution in children and adults (third to fourth decade of life). Imaging studies will show homogenous attenuation throughout the cyst with a thick wall. Infections of the cyst may show worrisome radiographic features similar to those found in nodal metastasis of SCC.

Depending on the type of branchial cleft, the presentation can vary. Classically, patients will present with a cyst in the lateral neck near the angle of the mandible, along the anterior border of the sternocleidomastoid muscle, which is characteristic of second branchial cleft anomalies (>90% of all cases). First branchial cleft anomalies occur in the preauricular region, either periauricular or periparotid in location. Third branchial cleft cysts involve the posterior neck triangle area, and fourth branchial apparatus anomalies present as recurrent suppurative thyroiditis.

Pathologic Features

GROSS FINDINGS

A smooth-walled cystic mass with mucoid or watery content.

MICROSCOPIC FINDINGS

The majority of branchial cleft anomalies present as cysts (75%) that are characterized by a uniform, smooth, and unilocular space, lined by stratified squamous epithelium (90%), respiratory epithelium (8%), or a combination of both (Fig. 9.35). Atypical cellular features or mitoses should not be present. Occasionally goblet cells, sebaceous glands, salivary tissue, and/or cholesterol clefts with foreign body giant cell reaction may be concomitantly appreciated. The epithelial lining is surrounded by a rich lymphoid stroma that contains

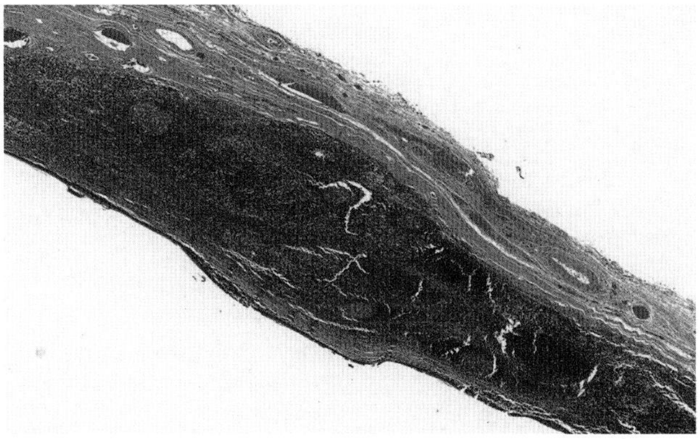

FIG. 9.35
Branchial cleft cyst presenting as a unilocular cyst with a thin epithelial lining associated with lymphoid stroma.

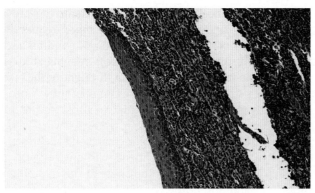

FIG. 9.36
Bland stratified squamous epithelium with maturation and no evidence of atypia.

germinal centers (Fig. 9.36). The cyst contents are composed of keratin debris.

Ancillary Studies

Immunohistochemical studies may show focal positivity for p16 and does not demonstrate the unequivocally strong and diffuse pattern as found in HPV-associated SCCs. In biopsies or in cases with equivocal p16 immunohistochemistry, additional studies with high-risk HPV chromogenic *in situ* hybridization (CiSH) will be negative, as these cysts are not HPV associated.

Differential Diagnosis

The most important differential diagnosis for a branchial cleft cyst is the exclusion of a cystic metastatic HPV-associated SCC (Table 9.19). Clinically, although

TABLE 9.19

Histologic Features of Branchial Cleft Cyst Versus Squamous Cell Carcinoma

Branchial Cleft Cyst	Metastatic Cystic HPV-Associated Squamous Cell Carcinoma
• Younger patients (pediatric and young adults)	• Older patients, typically male patients above the age of 40
• Stratified squamous epithelium demonstrates maturity and no atypia	• Epithelial atypia with no maturation
• Mitoses are rare or absent	• Frequent mitoses are readily identified
• May have rare or focal p16 positivity; however, HPV-CiSH is negative	• Cyst lining is diffusely positive for p16 (strong nuclear and cytoplasmic) with positive HPV-CiSH

CiSH, Chromogenic *in situ* hybridization; *HPV,* human papillomavirus.

branchial cleft cysts can be identified over a wide range of ages, they have a bimodal predilection toward pediatric populations or patients in third to fourth decade of life. Compared with branchial cleft cysts, metastatic cystic SCCs usually occur in male patients that are in their sixth decade of life. Overall, 11% to 21% of lateral neck cysts presumed to be branchial cleft anomalies are found to be actually metastatic cystic SCCs. In patients over the age of 40, 44% of these cysts are found to be malignant on histopathologic examination. From a radiographic perspective, cystic neck masses with internal vascularization, intracystic solid components, and irregular wall outlines are suspected to be malignant. Septations within the cyst should be viewed as a suspicious feature for malignancy. Thus, clinical and radiographic correlation is essential.

The most common head and neck SCC that presents as a metastatic unknown primary are those with an origin from the oropharynx (90% of cases). These are typically nonkeratinizing SCCs that are HPV associated. To a lesser degree, another set of metastatic SCCs that present from an "unknown site" with an undifferentiated or nonkeratinizing appearance are those with an origin in the nasopharynx or hypopharynx, which furthermore may be Epstein-Barr virus (EBV) associated. However, as the current discussion pertains to branchial cleft cysts, it should be noted that the presence of a cystic cervical lymph node metastasis is strongly associated with HPV-related SCCs.

Metastatic cystic SCCs can present either as a unilocular or multilocular mass. The growth architecture demonstrates ribbons of epithelium associated with a lymphoid stroma. The squamous lining is nonkeratinizing (although occasional abrupt keratinization can be seen) with a transitional or basaloid appearance. The epithelium is markedly atypical with an increased nuclear-to-cytoplasmic ratio with no evidence of maturation. The atypia in these cases and the lack of maturation help differentiate them from branchial cleft cysts. Furthermore, mitotic activity is an exceptional feature in a branchial cleft cyst, which are readily identified in a metastatic SCC. Although focal expression of p16 can be identified in branchial cleft cysts, they do not demonstrate the degree of positivity identified in HPV-associated SCCs (>70% tumor cells, strong and diffuse with nuclear and cytoplasmic staining). Furthermore, high-risk HPV CiSH will be negative in a branchial cleft cyst.

The phenomenon of a malignant transformation of a branchial cleft cyst into a *bronchiogenic carcinoma* either does not exist or is exceedingly rare.

Prognosis

Branchial cleft cysts are cured by surgical excision, with rare recurrence.

MIDDLE EAR ADENOMA

DIFFERENTIAL DIAGNOSES: PARAGANGLIOMA, SCHWANNOMA, MENINGIOMA, CERUMINOUS ADENOMA, AND PAPILLARY ADENOCARCINOMA

Clinical Features

Middle ear adenomas (MEAs) or neuroendocrine adenomas of middle ear (NAME) are rare and benign neoplasms of the middle ear with indolent biological behavior. Middle ear tumors are generally rare overall (with an incidence of 1:40,000 to 1:200,000) and MEAs are reported as the most common type of middle ear tumor. They have an exocrine/epithelial phenotype with or without concomitant neuroendocrine differentiation.

There is no sex predilection and these neoplasms occur in a wide range of ages (13–84 years; mean of 45 years). The most common symptom is unilateral hearing loss, especially conductive hearing loss if the tumor involves the ossicles. Other reported symptoms may include pain, tinnitus, pressure, or "feeling" of a mass.

Radiographically, these tumors will be avascular soft tissue densities without notable destructive, invasive, or erosive properties. Surgically, these tumors will peel off the bones of the middle ear unless they involve or entrap other middle ear structures. Uncommonly, tumors may perforate the tympanic membrane and extend into the external auditory canal, involve the eustachian tube, or the chorda tympani.

Pathologic Features

GROSS FINDINGS

White-gray or a reddish-brown appearance. Grossly vascular and well circumscribed. Generally are unencapsulated and measure around 1 cm in size.

MICROSCOPIC FINDINGS

The tumor is composed of monotonous tumor cells arranged often in solid, trabecular, lobular, glandular, or insular growth patterns (Figs. 9.37 and 9.38). Papillary growth architecture is not a typical feature of this neoplasm. In some cases, bilayering may be noted in a luminal-abluminal arrangement; however, there is no myoepithelial differentiation. The tumor cells are uniform with acidophilic cytoplasm and may impart a plasmacytoid appearance or even have mucin production. The tumor nuclei will be hyperchromatic or impart a "salt-and-pepper"–like chromatin pattern of distribution with an inconspicuous nucleolus. Increased mitotic activity or necrosis is not appreciated.

Although the tumor nests may be embedded in a fibrotic or desmoplastic stroma, invasion into adjacent

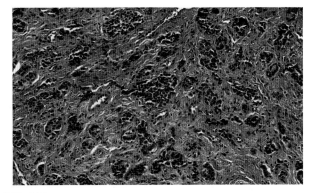

FIG. 9.37

Middle ear adenoma where the nest and clusters of tumor cells are monotonous. Note that in some instances due to the nature of the specimen, the nests have a crushed appearance (see top right).

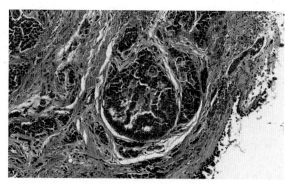

FIG. 9.38
Example of a middle ear adenoma with a glomeruloid-like/glandular architecture. Papillary architecture is not a feature of middle ear adenomas.

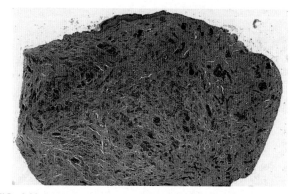

FIG. 9.39
Example of a middle ear adenoma where the tumor nests are embedded in a fibrotic stroma.

structures is not typically appreciated (Fig. 9.39). Perineural or lymphovascular invasion is not typically appreciated, although in occasional cases it may entrap these structures. From a practical point, a concurrent cholesteatoma or cholesterol granuloma may be identified. Tissue from the middle ear may have significant crush artifact which may prove to be challenging to characterize diagnostically.

Ancillary Studies

Tumors demonstrate evidence of epithelial differentiation (pan-keratin, CK7, and EMA) and most cases will show at least focal expression of CK7. Neuroendocrine differentiation may also be appreciated with chromogranin, synaptophysin, or neurospecific enolase (NSE). As noted prior, true myoepithelial differentiation is not present as S100 and SMA expression is not present. These tumors are negative for TTF1, CDX2, and PAX8. A low Ki-67/MiB (~1%) is found.

Differential Diagnosis

Different types of primary neoplasms can occur in the middle ear and in rare instances, consideration to metastases may be given.

Paragangliomas (*glomus jugulare/glomus tympanicum*) are richly vascularized neoplasms arising from paraganglia. The tumor will typically have clusters (*zellballen*) of epithelioid or spindled cells that are surrounded and supported by sustentacular cells. Unlike MEAs, paragangliomas will not typically have evidence of epithelial differentiation by immunohistochemistry (negative for cytokeratin markers), however, can express neuroendocrine differentiation (Table 9.20). Additionally, the sustentacular cell network can be highlighted with S100 or SOX10, stains that are not positive in an MEA.

Schwannomas are benign spindle cell neoplasms of nerve sheath origin. Tumors are composed of hypercellular (Antoni A) and hypocellular (Antoni B). Palisading tumor cells separated by areas of hypocellularity are characteristic of *Verocay bodies*. Unlike MEAs, strong S100 and SOX10 expression will be found in schwannomas (Table 9.21). Cytokeratin expression is not present in typical schwannomas.

TABLE 9.20	
Histologic Features of Middle Ear Adenoma Versus Paraganglioma	
Middle Ear Adenoma	Paraganglioma
• Monotonous tumor cells arranged often in solid, trabecular, lobular, glandular, or insular growth patterns	• Tumor cells arranged in nests (*zellballen* arrangement)
• Uniform with acidophilic cytoplasm and may impart a plasmacytoid appearance or even have mucin production	• Tumor cells have an epithelioid or spindled appearance
• No sustentacular cells (S100 and SOX10 negative)	• Sustentacular cells are present (S100 and SOX10 positive)
• CK7 and EMA positive; chromogranin, synaptophysin, NSE negative	• Cytokeratin negative but will have chromogranin and synaptophysin positivity

TABLE 9.21	
Histologic Features of Middle Ear Adenoma Versus Squamous Cell Carcinoma	
Middle Ear Adenoma	Schwannoma
• Monotonous tumor cells arranged often in solid, trabecular, lobular, glandular, or insular growth patterns	• Tumor cells are arranged in hypercellular (*Antoni A*) and hypocellular areas (*Antoni B*). Palisading tumor cells in hypocellular areas (*Verocay bodies*)
• Uniform with acidophilic cytoplasm and may impart a plasmacytoid appearance or even have mucin production	• Spindle cell neoplasm
• SOX10 and S100 are negative; tumor is positive for cytokeratins	• S100 and SOX10 are positive; cytokeratins are negative

Meningiomas in the middle ear are relatively uncommon, but may represent extension from an intracranial tumor or an origin from ectopic arachnoid cells in the middle ear. Morphological patterns are diverse; however, the most common variant reported at this site is the meningothelial variant (WHO grade I), which demonstrates lobular growth of tumor nests in variable fibrous stroma. The tumor nests will consist of cells with pale cytoplasm and indistinct borders with round- or oval-shaped tumor nuclei. Intranuclear inclusions may be appreciated. Typically, most meningiomas demonstrate EMA expression and in some cases, variable cytokeratin positivity. Progesterone receptor positivity is helpful, however, if negative, does not exclude the diagnosis of meningioma. S100 expression is variable and neuroendocrine markers are typically negative, a feature helpful for distinction from MEA (Table 9.22).

Ceruminous adenoma is of consideration given that it has a glandular appearance that may be similar to MEA. However, the difference is that ceruminous adenomas are neoplasms of the external auditory canal. Furthermore, ceruminous adenomas will demonstrate true gland formation with eosinophilic luminal secretions. Cytoplasmic yellow-brown cerumen pigment will be appreciated. Unlike MEAs, a myoepithelial component may also be found that is SMA and S100 positive.

Papillary adenocarcinomas are rare low-grade malignant tumors that although are histologically benign appearing, however, have clinically aggressive behavior with bone invasion, cranial nerve involvement, and posterior cranial fossa invasion. Tumors are arranged in interdigitating papillae with a single layer of cuboidal to low columnar cells without any overt atypia or mitoses. Colloid-like substance similar to what is seen in the thyroid may also be identified. These tumors may be difficult to differentiate from MEAs as they may also express epithelial/cytokeratin markers. Furthermore, rarely they have been reported to express neuroendocrine markers.

However, although EMA and cytokeratin expression is shared between these two tumors, papillary adenocarcinomas will often demonstrate S100 positivity. Furthermore, clinically these tumors are aggressive with bone and nerve invasion. An additional point of consideration is differentiation from a metastatic thyroid carcinoma when encountering a papillary adenocarcinoma.

Prognosis and Therapy

Tumors are treated successfully with surgery. If recurrences do occur after surgery, a re-excision will be warranted. These tumors have not been associated with a paraneoplastic syndrome.

MIDDLE EAR ADENOMA – DISEASE FACT SHEET

Definition
▸▸ Benign neoplasm of the middle ear with indolent biological behavior

Incidence
▸▸ Rare

Morbidity and Mortality
▸▸ No significant morbidity or mortality

Sex and Age Distribution
▸▸ No sex predilection
▸▸ 13 to 84 years; mean of 45 years

Clinical Features
▸▸ Unilateral hearing loss, especially conductive hearing loss if the tumor involves the ossicles Other reported symptoms may include pain, tinnitus, pressure, or "feeling" of a mass

Treatment and Prognosis
▸▸ Treat with surgery
▸▸ Most recurrences treated successfully with re-excision

MIDDLE EAR ADNEOMA – PATHOLOGIC FEATURES

Gross Findings
▸▸ Grossly vascular, well circumscribed, and unencapsulated

Microscopic Findings
▸▸ Solid, trabecular, lobular, glandular, or insular growth patterns; papillary growth not present
▸▸ Monotonous and uniform tumor cells with acidophilic cytoplasm which may impart a plasmacytoid appearance
▸▸ Hyperchromatic nucleus or "salt-and-pepper"–like chromatin pattern of distribution
▸▸ Inconspicuous nucleolus

Pathologic Differential Diagnosis
▸▸ Paraganglioma, meningioma, schwannoma, ceruminous adenoma, papillary adenocarcinoma

---

TABLE 9.22

Histologic Features of Middle Ear Adenoma Versus Squamous Cell Carcinoma

Middle Ear Adenoma	Meningioma
• Monotonous tumor cells arranged often in solid, trabecular, lobular, glandular, or insular growth patterns	• Variable growth pattern depending on WHO type; however, meningothelial variant is common at this location
• Uniform with acidophilic cytoplasm and may impart a plasmacytoid appearance or even have mucin production	• Cells with pale cytoplasm and indistinct borders with round- or oval-shaped tumor nuclei. Intranuclear inclusions may be appreciated
• At least focal CK7 and EMA positivity. May or may not demonstrate neuroendocrine marker positivity	• EMA and variable cytokeratin positivity; variable progesterone receptor positivity; Neuroendocrine markers are negative

PSEUDOEPITHELIOMATOUS HYPERPLASIA

DIFFERENTIAL DIAGNOSES: SQUAMOUS CELL CARCINOMA AND GRANULAR CELL TUMOR

Clinical Features

PEH is an exaggerated reactive or reparative process that occurs on mucocutaneous surfaces. It is uncertain if this process is driven by surface epithelium or underlying adnexa, or a combination of both. PEH is not a specific disease entity, but rather describes a histopathological pattern within a number of disease processes, including adjacent to areas of malignancy.

On the skin, PEH has varied clinical presentations depending on the underlying etiology. For example, causes of PEH commonly may be infection, neoplasm, or inflammatory conditions (*see reference by El-Khoury et al. in Suggested Readings*). Generally speaking, the lesion presents as a nodule or plaque that has scaling and/or crusting. When pigmentation is present in PEH, an underlying melanocytic process has to be excluded. In reactive contexts, PEH may be associated with an ulcer, burn scar, or a colostomy site. When associated with a fungal infection, for example like blastomycosis, the lesion may have a plaque-like appearance with central scarring and serpiginous borders at the lesional edge. Often a deeper biopsy will be required if a nodule is deeper to the PEH identified to exclude the possibility of a malignancy.

In the oral cavity, several lesions are associated with PEH. Half of all granular cell tumors occur in the head and neck region and the tongue is the most common site. In a third of these cases, the overlying squamous epithelium will demonstrate marked PEH. In terms of inflammatory conditions, chronic hyperplastic candidosis presents with an adherent white and/or red patch on mucosal surfaces. It commonly occurs at the commissure of the lips and is often bilateral. Median rhomboid glossitis can also have PEH. It is typically found on the dorsum of the tongue, between the posterior third and anterior two third tongue. Sialometaplasia is typically found on the hard palate and has a crater-like ulcer. The overlying epithelium often shows marked PEH. Papillary hyperplasia is found on the palate of patients who wear ill-fitting dentures and is associated with numerous erythematous papillary nodules.

Pathologic Features

GROSS FINDINGS

PEH can be ulcerated, exophytic, or dome-shaped swellings with smooth/warty surfaces depending on the underlying etiology.

MICROSCOPIC FINDINGS

The growth pattern of PEH demonstrates acanthotic surface epithelium with downward projections that have jagged borders and sharply pointed bases. The surface has ortho- or parakeratosis with often hypergranulosis present (Fig. 9.40). Scattered areas of keratinization within the epithelium can also be appreciated. However, cytologic atypia is usually confined at the basal level of the epithelium and is not full thickness. Few mitotic figures and dyskeratotic cells can be appreciated. The underlying connective tissue may demonstrate squamous metaplasia of supporting adnexal structures or salivary glands. There is no perineural, lymphatic, or vascular invasion. If associated with an infection, acute inflammation and multinucleated giant cells can be found (Fig. 9.41).

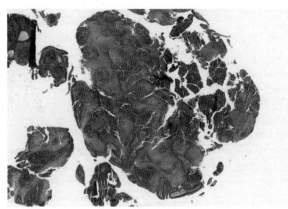

FIG. 9.40
Pseudoepitheliomatous hyperplasia in the larynx. There is complexity to the squamous architecture; however, it is connected to the surface in an anastomosing fashion. There is concomitant inflammation in the submucosal fibrous tissue. Even at this low power, the epithelial surface appears to demonstrate a degree of maturation in that the basal layer is prominent with increasing pallor to the surface of the mucosa.

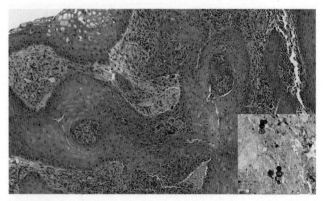

FIG. 9.41
Laryngeal pseudoepitheliomatous hyperplasia secondary to blastomycosis infection. Some degree of architectural complexity is noted; however, there is extensive acute inflammation without atypical mitosis or cellular atypia. Glassy change in the cytoplasm is appreciated in some areas of this picture. The inset in the bottom right demonstrates organisms consistent with blastomycosis by Grocott methenamine silver (GMS) stain.

Ancillary Studies

The gold standard is an adequately processed and oriented H&E slide. Deeper level sections may be required in many instances. Special stain studies for fungal and mycobacterial organisms are often necessary especially if there is significant inflammation.

Differential Diagnosis

PEH is commonly mistaken for a well-differentiated squamous cell carcinoma (WD-SCC), leading to inappropriate clinical management and intervention. Such a distinction is challenging on small biopsy specimens. Both processes may demonstrate complex growth patterns; however, the presence of overt cytologic atypia, numerous mitotic figures, and necrotic keratinocytes would favor the diagnosis of SCC (Table 9.23). The presence of an infection, inflammatory process, or an underlying malignancy (i.e., granular cell tumor) would favor the diagnosis of PEH. Some authors suggest that p53 may be helpful in separating PEH from SCC; however, others have noted that p53 is a marker of immaturity and proliferative capacity of the cells, rather than one for malignancy. The results are mixed for the utility of immunohistochemical studies in this context. In the cases where it was noted to be helpful, p53 staining in a WD-SCC is intense and diffuse, whereas in PEH it is localized to the basal layer of nests. From a practical standpoint, multiple histological sections with deeper sections are the gold standard along with correlating the results with clinical findings. Special stains should be performed in cases where microorganisms are suspected.

A pitfall to be aware of is that a PEH may mimic SCC in patients who were previously radiated.

Granular cell tumors can be associated with an overlying PEH. Carefully examining the base of the hyperplasia will show sheets of large polyhedral cells with acidophilic cytoplasm and round/pyknotic nucleus. S100 immunohistochemical will stain the tumor cells.

Necrotizing sialometaplasia is a self-limiting condition with a probable etiology rooted in ischemia that commonly presents as an ulcerative lesion on the palate. The mucoserous glands will show coagulation necrosis of glandular acini and squamous metaplasia of the salivary ductal epithelium. In these instances, PEH can be identified of the overlying squamous epithelium. Reactive stromal fibrosis can be identified. Most lesions are self-limiting and will heal.

Prognosis and Therapy

The treatment of PEH depends on the underlying inciting cause, however, if conservative medical treatment is warranted. However, at most, only local conservative excision should be utilized.

PSEUDOEPITHELIOMATOUS HYPERPLASIA – PATHOLOGIC FEATURES

Gross Findings
▶▶ Varied clinical appearance depending on the context and underlying etiology

Microscopic Findings
▶▶ Downward projections with jagged borders and sharply pointed bases
▶▶ Ortho- or parakeratosis with hypergranulosis present
▶▶ Scattered areas of keratinization within the epithelium can also be appreciated
▶▶ Cytologic atypia is usually confined at the basal level of the epithelium and is not full thickness
▶▶ Few mitotic figures and dyskeratotic cells
▶▶ No perineural, lymphatic, or vascular invasion

Pathologic Differential Diagnosis
▶▶ Well-differentiated squamous cell carcinoma and granular cell tumor

---

SPINDLE CELL SQUAMOUS CELL CARCINOMA

DIFFERENTIAL DIAGNOSES: MUCOSAL MELANOMA AND SARCOMAS

Clinical Features

Spindle cell squamous cell carcinoma (SC-SCC) is an aggressive variant of SCC that demonstrates sarcomatoid differentiation. From a molecular standpoint, the conventional epithelial and sarcomatoid components are monoclonal in origin. These tumors affect men more than women, and there is an etiologic link to cigarette smoking, chewing tobacco, and alcohol. Prior exposure to

---

TABLE 9.23

Histologic Features of Pseudoepitheliomatous Hyperplasia Versus Squamous Cell Carcinoma

Pseudoepitheliomatous Hyperplasia	Squamous Cell Carcinoma
• Cytologic atypia may be present but is not full thickness	• Surface epithelium if present is dysplastic
• Keratinization is scattered	• Keratinization is present throughout tumor
• No perineural or lymphovascular invasion present	• Perineural or lymphovascular invasion may be present
• Histopathologic pattern in association with a disease entity	• Specific disease entity

radiation may also potentially be a risk factor. Within the head and neck, the two most common sites for SC-SCC are the oral cavity and larynx. In the larynx, SC-SCC is commonly found on the glottis. Other uncommon head and neck sites also include the oropharynx, hypopharynx, and sinonasal tract. Patients will classically present with a polypoid mass that has an ulcerated surface or will complain of voice quality changes if involving the larynx.

Pathologic Features

GROSS FINDINGS

About 90% of the tumors have an ulcerated surface with or without a polypoid shape.

MICROSCOPIC FINDINGS

Surface epithelial dysplasia or frank carcinomatous component in association with the malignant spindle cell proliferation is found in half of cases. If the surface epithelium is ulcerated and precludes the assessment of dysplasia, squamous differentiation may be found at the advancing edge at the base of the lesion or in areas of invaginations of the surface epithelium (Fig. 9.42).

The sarcomatoid spindle cell proliferation may be arranged in intersecting fascicles, storiform configuration, whorled pattern, and/or demonstrate herringbone pattern (Fig. 9.43). Cellularity is often variable between tumors and within the same tumor. Cellular pleomorphism may be present; however, in most cases cellular anaplasia is appreciated. Majority of cases will have a significant number of atypical mitotic figures (>10 figures/

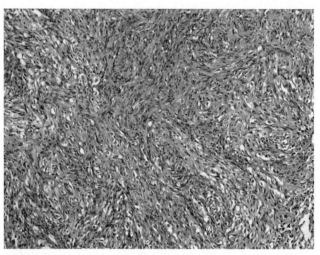

FIG. 9.43

Biopsy of a sarcomatoid squamous cell carcinoma from the larynx arranged in a storiform pattern. The cells impart an epithelioid and spindled appearance with mild to moderate cellular pleomorphism. Differential diagnoses in this context may include melanoma or other sarcomas or spindle cell tumors with an epithelioid and spindled appearance. Note, this is a different field of the same tumor as shown in Fig. 9.42.

10 HPF). Multinucleated tumor cells may be identified in some cases. In one fifth of cases there will not be any evidence of squamous differentiation by light microscopy and immunohistochemical studies. Heterologous mesenchymal differentiation can be present in 10% to 15% of cases in the form of malignant bone, cartilage, or skeletal muscle formation.

Ancillary Studies

A panel of a pan-keratin, EMA, p63, cytokeratin 5/6, and cytokeratin AE1/A3 has shown that at least one of these markers are expressed in slightly more than half of SC-SCC. However, aberrant expression of calponin, SMA, and S100 may also be expressed in around half of cases and is a diagnostic pitfall.

The presence of a negative epithelial immunohistochemical reactivity should not dissuade the diagnosis of SC-SCC, given that there is appropriate clinical context and history.

Differential Diagnosis

Commonly encountered spindle cell malignancies in the head and neck include SC-SCC, mesenchymal malignancies, and melanoma; SC-SCC is most frequently encountered in the head and neck region.

For a malignant spindle cell neoplasm of the head and neck, correlating tissue findings with the radiographic appearance is critical. For example, a

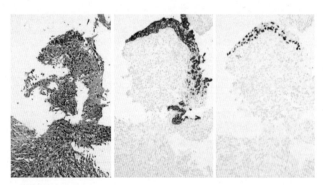

FIG. 9.42

Biopsy from the larynx. The H&E (*left picture*) shows a minute focus of dysplastic surface in this biopsy with the underlying sarcomatoid carcinoma. The presence of overlying dysplasia is helpful in the context of high-grade spindle cell malignancies. The CK 5/6 immunohistochemistry (*center picture*) shows cytokeratin positivity restricted only to the overlying areas of dysplasia. The p40 immunohistochemistry (*right picture*) shows a similar pattern only limited to the surface. In small biopsy cases, additional deeper level sections may be warranted to identify areas of dysplasia or a frank carcinomatous component. Although the immunohistochemical studies in this specific example could not support the diagnosis of a sarcomatoid squamous cell carcinoma, the presence of overlying dysplasia and prior clinical history is sufficient for the diagnosis.

TABLE 9.24

Features of Spindle Cell Squamous Cell Carcinoma Versus Mucosal Melanoma

Spindle Cell Squamous Cell Carcinoma	Mucosal Melanoma
May have either overlying epithelial dysplasia or frank squamous cell carcinoma	*In situ* component in the overlying mucosa or in adjacent salivary ducts
Can present as a polypoid mass and pigmentation would be an unusual feature	May have gross pigmentation
Slightly more than half of cases will express p63, cytokeratins, and EMA	S100, MelanA, HMB45, SOX10, and MiTF positive

radiographic intraosseous epicenter would favor an osteosarcoma. However, for a tumor to have a radiographic mucosal epicenter, consideration should be given to sarcomatoid carcinoma, melanoma, myoepithelial carcinoma, and other mesenchymal malignancies. However, the presence of dysplasia or frank carcinomatous components is consistent with SC-SCC, as opposed to a mesenchymal malignancy or melanoma. Due to spatial limitations, only two select differential diagnoses to SC-SCC are discussed below.

Mucosal melanoma: The two major sites of mucosal melanomas in the head and neck are in the sinonasal and oral cavity. In 30% to 50% of oral cavity cases, there will be antecedent mucosal pigmentation that occurs months to years in duration. Although in some cases the cellular morphology can be polytypic, the identification of an *in situ* or a junctional component is helpful (Table 9.24). Attention should be drawn to the salivary ducts, as an incipient *in situ* component can spread along the length of the duct. Tumor cells are pleomorphic and may demonstrate polyhedral, round, fusiform, epithelioid, spindle, or a mixture of these cytoarchitectural patterns. The finding of a prominent nucleolus is also helpful. The finding of pigmentation is advantageous to reaching a conclusive diagnosis of melanoma, although 15% to 50% mucosal melanomas are amelanotic. Unusual findings may even include focal osteocartilagenous differentiation. A potential pitfall in utilizing immunohistochemistry is that mucosal melanomas can occasionally express cytokeratin. Finally, a broad panel of melanoma-specific markers such as S100, MelanA, HMB45, SOX10, and MiTF will be supportive of diagnosis of a mucosal melanoma over SC-SCC.

Osteosarcoma: As SC-SCC may have elements of divergent differentiation consisting of either bone or cartilage, consideration to osteosarcoma should be given. This challenge is further compounded by osteosarcomas that have submucosal extension. The identification of osteoid production by malignant cells and the exclusion of surface epithelial dysplasia will be most diagnostic of osteosarcoma. Correlation with radiographic studies is essential to determine if the tumor epicenter is within bone. The use of immunohistochemical studies is often limited in this context.

Finally, utilizing a systemic approach for an accurate diagnosis in this context is driven by histologic findings supported by clinical and radiographic considerations.

Prognosis and Therapy

The tumor location and stage are the two most important factors for influencing management and outcome of SC-SCC. SC-SCC of the larynx will have a better prognosis than oral cavity SC-SCC. In fact, stage for stage, SC-SCC and SCC have similar prognosis in the larynx. Furthermore, SC-SCC exhibits a lower tendency toward locoregional spread than conventional SCC. Exophytic tumors are easily resectable and will have a better prognosis (80% 5-year survival rate), but local recurrences are seen in 20% of cases. In these situations, radiation therapy may be indicated or in cases where there is extensive stromal invasion. The presence of heterologous elements is not associated with significant differences in prognosis.

Lymph node metastasis are seen in 42% of cases and distant metastasis in the lung is common. A mortality rate of 14% to 32% has been noted in the literature.

SARCOMATOID CARCINOMA – DISEASE FACT SHEET

Definition
- ▸▸ An aggressive variant of squamous cell carcinoma with sarcomatoid features

Incidence
- ▸▸ Rare

Morbidity and Mortality
- ▸▸ Varies based on the site of the tumor
- ▸▸ Larynx: outcomes of SC-SCC are similar to that of a conventional SC-SCC, stage for stage
- ▸▸ Oral cavity: SC-SCC outcomes are worse than laryngeal SC-SCC

Sex and Age Distribution
- ▸▸ Men > women
- ▸▸ Elderly patients

Clinical Features
- ▸▸ Polypoid mass with ulceration
- ▸▸ Laryngeal cases may have change in quality of voice
- ▸▸ May be associated with smoking, chewing tobacco, or alcohol use

Treatment and Prognosis
- ▸▸ Excision +/− radiation therapy

SARCOMATOID CARCINOMA – PATHOLOGIC FEATURES

Gross Findings

▶▶ Polypoid mass with ulceration

Microscopic Findings

▶▶ Half of cases will have either dysplasia or a conventional squamous cell carcinoma

▶▶ Varied cytologic features, some cases can lack frank anaplasia

▶▶ May have scattered multinucleated cells

▶▶ May have heterologous mesenchymal differentiation (bone, cartilage, or skeletal muscle)

▶▶ Absence of some of the above findings should not exclude the diagnosis of a sarcomatoid squamous cell carcinoma

Pathologic Differential Diagnosis

▶▶ Mucosal melanoma and mesenchymal malignancies

SUGGESTED READINGS

Pleomorphic Adenoma

O'Dwyer PJ, Farrar WB, Finkelmeier WR, McCabe DP, James AG. Facial nerve sacrifice and tumor recurrence in primary and recurrent benign parotid tumors. *Am J Surg.* 1986;152(4):442-445.

Schapher M, Koch M, Agaimy A, Goncalves M, Mantsopoulos K, Iro H. Parotid pleomorphic adenomas: factors influencing surgical techniques, morbidity, and long-term outcome relative to the new ESGS classification in a retrospective study. *J Craniomaxillofac Surg.* 2019;47(9):1356-1362.

Valstar MH, de Ridder M, van den Broek EC, et al. Salivary gland pleomorphic adenoma in the Netherlands: a nationwide observational study of primary tumor incidence, malignant transformation, recurrence, and risk factors for recurrence. *Oral Oncol.* 2017;66:93-99.

Andreasen S, Therkildsen MH, Bjørndal K, Homøe P. Pleomorphic adenoma of the parotid gland 1985–2010: a Danish nationwide study of incidence, recurrence rate, and malignant transformation. *Head Neck.* 2016;38(suppl 1):E1364-E1369.

Jo VY, Krane JF. Ancillary testing in salivary gland cytology: a practical guide. *Cancer Cytopathol.* 2018;126(suppl 8):627-642.

Warthin Tumor

Zhang X, Baloch ZW, Cooper K, Zhang PJ, Puthiyaveettil R, LiVolsi VA. The significance of mucinous metaplasia in Warthin tumor: a frequent occurrence and potential pitfall. *Hum Pathol.* 2020;99:13-26.

Bieńkowski M, Kunc M, Iliszko M, Kuźniacka A, Studniarek M, Biernat W. MAML2 rearrangement as a useful diagnostic marker discriminating between Warthin tumour and Warthin-like mucoepidermoid carcinoma. *Virchows Arch.* 2020;477:393-400. doi:10.1007/s00428-020-02798-5.

Li S, Baloch ZW, Tomaszewski JE, LiVolsi VA. Worrisome histologic alterations following fine-needle aspiration of benign parotid lesions. *Arch Pathol Lab Med.* 2000;124(1):87-91.

Psychogios G, Vlastos I, Thölken R, Zenk J. Warthin's tumour seems to be the most common benign neoplasm of the parotid gland in Germany. *Eur Arch Otorhinolaryngol.* 2020;277(7):2081-2084.

Tan Y, Kryvenko ON, Kerr DA, et al. Diagnostic pitfalls of infarcted Warthin tumor in frozen section evaluation. *Ann Diagn Pathol.* 2016;25:26-30.

Sclerosing Polycystic Adenosis

Bishop JA, Gagan J, Baumhoer D, et al. Sclerosing polycystic "adenosis" of salivary glands: a neoplasm characterized by PI3K pathway alterations more correctly named sclerosing polycystic adenoma. *Head Neck Pathol.* 2020;14:630-636. doi:10.1007/s12105-019-01088-0.

Skálová A, Gnepp DR, Simpson RH, et al. Clonal nature of sclerosing polycystic adenosis of salivary glands demonstrated by using the polymorphism of the human androgen receptor (HUMARA) locus as a marker. *Am J Surg Pathol.* 2006;30(8):939-944.

Petersson F. Sclerosing polycystic adenosis of salivary glands: a review with some emphasis on intraductal epithelial proliferations. *Head Neck Pathol.* 2013;7(suppl 1):S97-S106.

Canas Marques R, Félix A. Invasive carcinoma arising from sclerosing polycystic adenosis of the salivary gland. *Virchows Arch.* 2014;464(5):621-625.

Perottino F, Barnoud R, Ambrun A, Poupart M, Pignat JC, Merrot O. Sclerosing polycystic adenosis of the parotid gland: diagnosis and management. *Eur Ann Otorhinolaryngol Head Neck Dis.* 2010;127(1):20-22.

Gnepp DR, Wang LJ, Brandwein-Gensler M, Slootweg P, Gill M, Hille J. Sclerosing polycystic adenosis of the salivary gland: a report of 16 cases. *Am J Surg Pathol.* 2006;30(2):154-164.

Smith BC, Ellis GL, Slater LJ, Foss RD. Sclerosing polycystic adenosis of major salivary glands. A clinicopathologic analysis of nine cases. *Am J Surg Pathol.* 1996;20(2):161-170.

Mucoepidermoid Carcinoma

Seethala R. An update on grading of salivary gland carcinomas. *Head Neck Pathol.* 2009;3(1):69-77. Available at: http://link.springer.com/10.1007/s12105-009-0102-9.

Bai S, Clubwala R, Adler E, et al. Salivary mucoepidermoid carcinoma: a multi-institutional review of 76 Patients. *Head Neck Pathol.* 2013;7(2):105-112. Available at: http://link.springer.com/10.1007/s12105-012-0405-0.

Auclair PL, Goode RK, Ellis GL. Mucoepidermoid carcinoma of intraoral salivary glands evaluation and application of grading criteria in 143 cases. *Cancer.* 1992;69(8):2021-2030.

Hicks MJ, el-Naggar AK, Flaitz CM, Luna MA, Batsakis JG. Histocytologic grading of mucoepidermoid carcinoma of major salivary glands in prognosis and survival: a clinicopathologic and flow cytometric investigation. *Head Neck.* 1995;17(2):89-95. Available at: http://doi.wiley.com/10.1002/hed.2880170203.

Katabi N, Ghossein R, Ali S, et al. Prognostic features in mucoepidermoid carcinoma of major salivary glands with emphasis on tumour histologic grading. *Histopathology.* 2014;65(6):793-804. Available at: http://doi.wiley.com/10.1111/his.12488.

Cipriani NA, Lusardi JJ, McElherne J, et al. Mucoepidermoid carcinoma. *Am J Surg Pathol.* 2019;43(7):885-897. Available at: http://journals.lww.com/00000478-201907000-00002.

WHO Classification of Head and Neck Tumours; El-Naggar AK, Chan JKC, Grandis JR, Takata T, Slootweg PJ, eds. *WHO Classification of Head and Neck Tumors.* 4th ed. Lyon: International Agency for Research on Cancer; 2017.

Gnepp DR, Bishop JR. *Gnepp's Diagnostic Surgical Pathology of the Head and Neck.* Open WorldCat; 2021. Available at: https://www.sciencedirect.com/science/book/9780323531146.

Griffin JR, Wriston CC, Peters MS, Lehman JS. Decreased expression of intercellular adhesion molecules in acantholytic squamous cell carcinoma compared with invasive well-differentiated squamous cell carcinoma of the skin. *Am J Clin Pathol.* 2013;139(4):442-447.

Prabhakar M, Sabarinath B, Sivapathasundharam B, Vasanthakumar V. Adenosquamous carcinoma of the tongue: a case report and an overview of histogenetic concepts. *J Oral Maxillofac Pathol.* 2020;24(suppl 1):S110-S114. Available at: http://www.jomfp.in/text.asp?2020/24/4/110/279761.

Yeshwant BR, Anderson KM. Adenosquamous carcinoma of the tongue. *Head Neck Pathol.* 2018;12(4):576-579. Available at: http://link.springer.com/10.1007/s12105-017-0877-z.

Skálová A, Stenman G, Simpson RHW, et al. The role of molecular testing in the differential diagnosis of salivary gland carcinomas. *Am J Surg Pathol.* 2018;42(2):e11-e27. Available at: http://journals.lww.com/00000478-201802000-00001.

Thompson LD. Mucoepidermoid carcinoma. *Ear Nose Throat J.* 2005;84(12):762-763. Available at: http://www.ncbi.nlm.nih.gov/pubmed/16408550.

Zhu S, Schuerch C, Hunt J. Review and updates of immunohistochemistry in selected salivary gland and head and neck tumors. *Arch Pathol Lab Med.* 2015;139(1):55-66. Available at: http://www.archivesofpathology.org/doi/abs/10.5858/arpa.2014-0167-RA.

Polymorphous Adenocarcinoma

Adkins BD, Geromes A, Zhang LY, et al. SOX10 and GATA3 in adenoid cystic carcinoma and polymorphous adenocarcinoma. *Head Neck*

Pathol. 2020;14(2):406-411. Available at: https://doi.org/10.1007/s12105-019-01046-w.

Castle JT, Thompson LDR, Frommelt RA, Wenig BM, Kessler HP. Polymorphous low grade adenocarcinoma. *Cancer.* 1999;86(2): 207-219. Available at: https://doi.org/10.1002/(SICI)1097-0142(19990715)86:2<207::AID-CNCR4>3.0.CO;2-Q.

García JJ. Polymorphous adenocarcinoma. In: *Atlas of Salivary Gland Pathology.* Springer; 2019:171-177. Available at: https://doi.org/10.1007/978-3-319-09021-4_24.

Hernandez-Prera JC. Historical evolution of the polymorphous adenocarcinoma. *Head Neck Pathol.* 2019;13(3):415-422. Available at: https://doi.org/10.1007/s12105-018-0964-9.

Uraizee I, Cipriani NA, Ginat DT. Adenoid cystic carcinoma of the oral cavity: radiology–pathology correlation. *Head Neck Pathol.* 2018;12(4):562-566. Available at: https://doi.org/10.1007/s12105-017-0849-3.

Vander Poorten V, Triantafyllou A, Skálová A, et al. Polymorphous adenocarcinoma of the salivary glands: reappraisal and update. *Eur Arch Otorhinolaryngol.* 2018;275(7):1681-1695. Available at: https://doi.org/10.1007/s00405-018-4985-5.

WHO Classification of Head and Neck Tumours; El-Naggar AK, Chan JKC, Grandis JR, Takata T, Slootweg PJ, eds. *WHO Classification of Head and Neck Tumors.* 4th ed. Lyon: International Agency for Research on Cancer; 2017.

Xu B, Barbieri AL, Bishop JA, et al. Histologic classification and molecular signature of polymorphous adenocarcinoma (PAC) and cribriform adenocarcinoma of salivary gland (CASG). *Am J Surg Pathol.* 2020;44(4):545-552. Available at: https://doi.org/10.1097/PAS.0000000000001431.

Secretory Carcinoma

Skálová A, Vanecek T, Sima R, et al. Mammary analogue secretory carcinoma of salivary glands, containing the ETV6-NTRK3 fusion gene: a hitherto undescribed salivary gland tumor entity. *Am J Surg Pathol.* 2010;34(5):599-608.

Skalova A. Mammary analogue secretory carcinoma of salivary gland origin: an update and expanded morphologic and immunohisto-chemical spectrum of recently described entity. *Head Neck Pathol.* 2013;7 (Suppl 1):S30-S36.

Skálová A, Vanecek T, Majewska H, et al. Mammary analogue secretory carcinoma of salivary glands with high-grade transformation: report of 3 cases with the ETV6-NTRK3 gene fusion and analysis of TP53, β-catenin, EGFR, and CCND1 genes. *Am J Surg Pathol.* 2014;38(1):23-33.

Skalova A, Vanecek T, Martinek P, et al. Molecular profiling of mammary analog secretory carcinoma revealed a subset of tumors harboring a novel ETV6-RET translocation: report of 10 cases. *Am J Surg Pathol.* 2018;42(2):234-246.

Chiosea SI, Griffith C, Assaad A, Seethala RR. Clinicopathological characterization of mammary analogue secretory carcinoma of salivary glands. *Histopathology.* 2012;61(3):387-394.

Skálová A, BaneČkova M, Thompson LDR, et al. Expanding the molecular spectrum of secretory carcinoma of salivary glands with a novel VIM-RET fusion. *Am J Surg Pathol.* 2020;44(10):1295-1307. doi:10.1097/PAS.0000000000001535.

Salivary Duct Carcinoma

Soares CD, de Lima Morais TM, Carlos R, et al. Immunohistochemical expression of mammaglobin in salivary duct carcinomas de novo and salivary duct carcinoma ex pleomorphic adenoma. *Hum Pathol.* 2019;92:59-66.

Boon E, Bel M, van Boxtel W, et al. A clinicopathological study and prognostic factor analysis of 177 salivary duct carcinoma patients from The Netherlands. *Int J Cancer.* 2018;143(4):758-766.

D'heygere E, Meulemans J, Vander Poorten V. Salivary duct carcinoma. *Curr Opin Otolaryngol Head Neck Surg.* 2018; 26(2):142-151.

Udager AM, Chiosea SI. Salivary duct carcinoma: an update on morphologic mimics and diagnostic use of androgen receptor immunohistochemistry. *Head Neck Pathol.* 2017;11(3):288-294.

Chiosea SI, Thompson LD, Weinreb I, et al. Subsets of salivary duct carcinoma defined by morphologic evidence of pleomorphic adenoma, PLAG1 or HMGA2 rearrangements, and common genetic alterations. *Cancer.* 2016;122(20):3136-3144.

Gilbert MR, Sharma A, Schmitt NC, et al. A 20-year review of 75 cases of salivary duct carcinoma. *JAMA Otolaryngol Head Neck Surg.* 2016;142(5):489-495.

Williams L, Thompson LD, Seethala RR, et al. Salivary duct carcinoma: the predominance of apocrine morphology, prevalence of histologic variants, and androgen receptor expression. *Am J Surg Pathol.* 2015;39(5):705-713.

Chiosea SI, Williams L, Griffith CC, et al. Molecular characterization of apocrine salivary duct carcinoma. *Am J Surg Pathol.* 2015;39(6): 744-752.

Bahrami A, Perez-Ordonez B, Dalton JD, Weinreb I. An analysis of PLAG1 and HMGA2 rearrangements in salivary duct carcinoma and examination of the role of precursor lesions. *Histopathology.* 2013; 63(2):250-262.

Fan CY, Melhem MF, Hosal AS, Grandis JR, Barnes EL. Expression of androgen receptor, epidermal growth factor receptor, and transforming growth factor alpha in salivary duct carcinoma. *Arch Otolaryngol Head Neck Surg.* 2001;127(9):1075-1079.

Biphenotypic Sinonasal Sarcoma

Andreasen S, Bishop JA, Hellquist H, et al. Biphenotypic sinonasal sarcoma: demographics, clinicopathological characteristics, molecular features, and prognosis of a recently described entity. *Virchows Archiv.* 2018;473(5):615-626. Available at: https://doi.org/10.1007/s00428-018-2426-x.

Bishop JA. Newly described tumor entities in sinonasal tract pathology. *Head Neck Pathol.* 2016;10(1):23-31. Available at: https://doi.org/10.1007/s12105-016-0688-7.

Carter CS, East EG, McHugh JB. Biphenotypic sinonasal sarcoma: a review and update. *Arch Pathol Lab Med.* 2018;142(10):1196-1201. Available at: https://doi.org/10.5858/arpa.2018-0207-RA.

Contrera KJ, Woody NM, Rahman M, Sindwani R, Burkey BB. Clinical management of emerging sinonasal malignancies. *Head Neck.* 2020;42(8):2202-2212. Available at: https://doi.org/10.1002/hed.26150.

Huang SC, Ghossein RA, Bishop JA, et al. Novel PAX3-NCOA1 fusions in biphenotypic sinonasal sarcoma with focal rhabdomyoblastic differentiation. *Am J Surg Pathol.* 2016;40(1):51-59. Available at: https://doi.org/10.1097/PAS.0000000000000492.

Kühn AL, Jalisi S, Nishino M, Ivanovic V. Biphenotypic sinonasal sarcoma – description of radiologic, intraoperative and pathologic findings. *Otolaryngol Case Rep.* 2019;11:100113. Available at: https://doi.org/10.1016/j.xocr.2019.100113.

Le Loarer F, Laffont S, Lesluyes T, et al. Clinicopathologic and molecular features of a series of 41 biphenotypic sinonasal sarcomas expanding their molecular spectrum. *Am J Surg Pathol.* 2019;43(6):747-754. Available at: https://doi.org/10.1097/PAS.0000000000001238.

Lewis JT, Oliveira AM, Nascimento AG, et al. Low-grade sinonasal sarcoma with neural and myogenic features. *Am J Surg Pathol.* 2012;36(4):517-525. Available at: https://doi.org/10.1097/PAS.0b013e3182426886.

Rooper LM, Huang SC, Antonescu CR, Westra WH, Bishop JA. Biphenotypic sinonasal sarcoma: an expanded immunoprofile including consistent nuclear β-catenin positivity and absence of SOX10 expression. *Human Pathol.* 2016;55:44-50. Available at: https://doi.org/10.1016/j.humpath.2016.04.009.

Thompson LDR, Lau SK. Sinonasal tract solitary fibrous tumor: a clinicopathologic study of six cases with a comprehensive review of the literature. *Head Neck Pathol.* 2018;12(4):471-480. doi:10.1007/s12105-017-0878-y.

Sinonasal Undifferentiated Carcinoma

Agaimy A, Franchi A, Lund VJ, et al. Sinonasal undifferentiated carcinoma (SNUC): from an entity to morphologic pattern and back again-a historical perspective. *Adv Anat Pathol.* 2020;27(2):51-60.

Agaimy A, Hartmann A, Antonescu CR, et al. SMARCB1 (INI-1)-deficient sinonasal carcinoma: a series of 39 cases expanding the morphologic and clinicopathologic spectrum of a recently described entity. *Am J Surg Pathol.* 2017;41(4):458-471.

Baraban E, Tong CCL, Adappa ND, Cooper K. A subset of sinonasal undifferentiated carcinoma is associated with transcriptionally active high-risk human papillomavirus by in situ hybridization: a clinical and pathologic analysis. *Hum Pathol.* 2020;101:64-69.

Guilmette J, Sadow PM. High-grade sinonasal carcinoma: classification through molecular profiling. *Arch Pathol Lab Med.* 2019;143(11): 1416-1419.

Riobello C, López-Hernández A, Cabal VN, et al. IDH2 mutation analysis in undifferentiated and poorly differentiated sinonasal carcinomas for diagnosis and clinical management. *Am J Surg Pathol.* 2020;44(3):396-405.

Shah AA, Jain D, Ababneh E, et al. SMARCB1 (INI-1)-deficient adenocarcinoma of the sinonasal tract: a potentially under-recognized form of sinonasal adenocarcinoma with occasional yolk sac tumor-like features. *Head Neck Pathol.* 2020;14(2): 465-472.

Tilson MP, Bishop JA. Utility of p40 in the differential diagnosis of small round blue cell tumors of the sinonasal tract. *Head Neck Pathol.* 2014;8(2):141-145.

HPV-Related Mulitphenotypic Sinonasal Carcinoma

Bishop JA, Andreasen S, Hang JF, et al. HPV-related multiphenotypic sinonasal carcinoma: an expanded series of 49 cases of the tumor formerly known as HPV-related carcinoma with adenoid cystic carcinoma-like features. *Am J Surg Pathol.* 2017;41(12):1690-1701.

Bishop JA, Guo TW, Smith DF, et al. Human papillomavirus-related carcinomas of the sinonasal tract. *Am J Surg Pathol.* 2013;37(2): 185-192.

Bishop JA, Ogawa T, Stelow EB, et al. Human papillomavirus-related carcinoma with adenoid cystic-like features: a peculiar variant of head and neck cancer restricted to the sinonasal tract. *Am J Surg Pathol.* 2013;37(6):836-844.

Bishop JA, Westra WH. Human papillomavirus-related multiphenotypic sinonasal carcinoma: an emerging tumor type with a unique microscopic appearance and a paradoxical clinical behaviour. *Oral Oncol.* 2018;87:17-20.

Shah AA, Oliai BR, Bishop JA. Consistent LEF-1 and MYB Immunohistochemical expression in human papillomavirus-related multiphenotypic sinonasal carcinoma: a potential diagnostic pitfall. *Head Neck Pathol.* 2019;13(2):220-224.

Branchial Cleft Cyst

Bradley PT, Bradley PJ. Branchial cleft cyst carcinoma. *Curr Opin Otolaryngol Head Neck Surg.* 2013;21(2):118-123. Available at: https://doi.org/10.1097/MOO.0b013e32835cebde.

Chavan S, Deshmukh R, Karande P, Ingale Y. Branchial cleft cyst: a case report and review of literature. *J Oral Maxillofac Pathol.* 2014; 18(1):150. Available at: https://doi.org/10.4103/0973-029X.131950.

Chernock RD, Lewis JS. Approach to metastatic carcinoma of unknown primary in the head and neck: squamous cell carcinoma and beyond. *Head Neck Pathol.* 2015;9(1):6-15. Available at: https://doi.org/10.1007/s12105-015-0616-2.

Gaddikeri S, Vattoth S, Gaddikeri RS, et al. Congenital cystic neck masses: embryology and imaging appearances, with clinicopathological correlation. *Curr Probl Diagn Radiol.* 2014;43(2):55-67. Available at: https://doi.org/10.1067/j.cpradiol.2013.12.001.

Goldenberg D, Begum S, Westra WH, et al. Cystic lymph node metastasis in patients with head and neck cancer: an HPV-associated phenomenon. *Head Neck.* 2008;30(7):898-903. Available at: https://doi.org/10.1002/hed.20796.

Liang HH, Chen CY, Chen WY, Chen TM, Chan WP. Solitary cystic metastatic lymph node of occult human papillomavirus-related oropharyngeal cancer mimicking second branchial cleft cyst. *Medicine.* 2019;98(44):e17800. Available at: https://doi.org/10.1097/MD.0000000000017800.

McHugh JB. Association of cystic neck metastases and human papillomavirus-positive oropharyngeal squamous cell carcinoma. *Arch Pathol Lab Med.* 2009;133(11):1798-1803. Available at: https://doi.org/10.1043/1543-2165-133.11.1798.

Veivers D, Dent J. Lateral cervical cysts: an Australian perspective. *ANZ J Surg.* 2012;82(11):799-802. Available at: https://doi.org/10.1111/j.1445-2197.2012.06187.x.

WHO Classification of Head and Neck Tumours; El-Naggar AK, Chan JKC, Grandis JR, Takata T, Slootweg PJ, eds. *WHO Classification of Head and Neck Tumors.* 4th ed. Lyon: International Agency for Research on Cancer; 2017.

Wratten C, Anne S, Tieu MT, Kumar B, Eisenberg R. The dangers of diagnosing cystic neck masses as benign in the era of HPV-associated oropharyngeal cancer. *Med J Aust.* 2015;203(9):371-372. Available at: https://doi.org/10.5694/mja15.00697.

Coste AH, Lofgren DH, Shermetaro C. Branchial Cleft Cyst. [Updated 2020 Apr 22]. In: *StatPearls* [Internet]. Treasure Island (FL): StatPearls Publishing; 2020. Available at: https://www.ncbi.nlm.nih.gov/books/NBK499914/.

Middle Ear Adenoma

Bell D, El-Naggar AK, Gidley PW. Middle ear adenomatous neuroendocrine tumors: a 25-year experience at MD Anderson Cancer Center. *Virchows Archiv.* 2017;471(5):667-672. Available at: https://doi.org/10.1007/s00428-017-2155-6.

Berns S, Pearl G. Middle ear adenoma. *Arch Pathol Lab Med.* 2006;130(7):1067-1069. Available at: https://doi.org/10.1043/1543-2165(2006)130[1067:MEA]2.0.CO;2.

Duderstadt M, Förster C, Welkoborsky HJ, Ostertag H. Adenomatous tumors of the middle ear and temporal bone: clinical, morphological and tumor biological characteristics of challenging neoplastic lesions. *Eur Arch Otorhinolaryngol.* 2012;269(3):823-831. Available at: https://doi.org/10.1007/s00405-011-1729-1.

Hernandez-Prera JC, Wenig BM. Tumors of the ear and temporal bone. In: Moran CA, Kalhor N, Weissferdt A, eds. *Oncological Surgical Pathology.* Springer; 2020:471-495. Available at: https://doi.org/10.1007/978-3-319-96681-6_5.

Lott Limbach AA, Hoschar AP, Thompson LDR, Stelow EB, Chute DJ. Middle ear adenomas stain for two cell populations and lack myoepithelial cell differentiation. *Head Neck Pathol.* 2012;6(3):345-353. Available at: https://doi.org/10.1007/s12105-012-0365-4.

WHO Classification of Head and Neck Tumours; El-Naggar AK, Chan JKC, Grandis JR, Takata T, Slootweg PJ, eds. *WHO Classification of Head and Neck Tumors.* 4th ed. Lyon: International Agency for Research on Cancer; 2017.

Pseudoepitheliomatous Hyperplasia

El-Khoury J, Kibbi AG, Abbas O. Mucocutaneous pseudoepitheliomatous hyperplasia. *Am J Dermatopathol.* 2012;34(2):165-175. Available at: https://doi.org/10.1097/DAD.0b013e31821816ab.

Farthing PM, Speight PM. Problems and pitfalls in oral mucosal pathology. *Curr Diagn Pathol.* 2006;12(1):66-74. Available at: https://doi.org/10.1016/j.cdip.2005.10.004.

Ferlito A, Devaney KO, Woolgar JA, et al. Squamous epithelial changes of the larynx: diagnosis and therapy. *Head Neck.* 2012;34(12):1810-1816. Available at: https://doi.org/10.1002/hed.21862.

Imbery TA, Edwards PA. Necroticizing sialometaplasia: literature review and case reports. *J Am Dent Assoc.* 1996;127(7):1087-1092. Available at: https://doi.org/10.14219/jada.archive.1996.0334.

Kaplan I, Alterman M, Kleinman S, et al. The clinical, histologic, and treatment spectrum in necrotizing sialometaplasia. *Oral Surg Oral Med Oral Pathol Oral Radiol.* 2012;114(5):577-585. Available at: https://doi.org/10.1016/j.oooo.2012.02.020.

Sandmeier D, Bouzourene H. Necrotizing sialometaplasia: a potential diagnostic pitfall. *Histopathology.* 2002;40(2):200-201. Available at: https://doi.org/10.1046/j.1365-2559.2002.1179a.x.

Sarangarajan R, Vedam VKV, Sivadas G, Krishnaraj R, Sarangarajan A, Shanmugam KT. Pseudoepitheliomatous hyperplasia: relevance in oral pathology. *J Int Oral Health.* 2015;7(7):132-136. Available at: http://wSww.ncbi.nlm.nih.gov/pubmed/26229388.

Sarcomatoid Squamous Cell Carcinoma

Anderson CE, Al-Nafussi A. Spindle cell lesions of the head and neck: an overview and diagnostic approach. *Diagn Histopathol.* 2009;15(5): 264-272. Available at: https://doi.org/10.1016/j.mpdhp.2009.02.009.

Femiano F, Lanza A, Buonaiuto C, Gombos F, Di Spirito F, Cirillo N. Oral malignant melanoma: a review of the literature. *J Oral Pathol Med.* 2008;37(7):383-388. Available at: https://doi.org/10.1111/j.1600-0714.2008.00660.x.

Gerry D, Fritsch VA, Lentsch EJ. Spindle cell carcinoma of the upper aerodigestive tract. *Ann Otol Rhinol Laryngol.* 2014;123(8):576-583. Available at: https://doi.org/10.1177/0003489414525337.

López F, Rodrigo JP, Cardesa A, et al. Update on primary head and neck mucosal melanoma. *Head Neck*. 2016;38(1):147-155. Available at: https://doi.org/10.1002/hed.23872.

Marioni G, Altavilla G, Marino F, Marchese-Garona R, Lelli-Mami G, Staffers A. Squamous cell carcinoma of the larynx with osteosarcoma-like stromal metaplasia. *Acta Otolaryngol*. 2004;124(7):870-873. Available at: https://doi.org/10.1080/00016480410017288.

McLean N, Tighiouart M, Muller S. Primary mucosal melanoma of the head and neck. Comparison of clinical presentation and histopathologic features of oral and sinonasal melanoma. *Oral Oncol*. 2008;44(11):1039-1046. Available at: https://doi.org/10.1016/j.oraloncology.2008.01.014.

Roy S, Purgina B, Seethala RR. Spindle cell carcinoma of the larynx with rhabdomyoblastic heterologous element: a rare form of divergent differentiation. *Head Neck Pathol*. 2013;7(3):263-267. Available at: https://doi.org/10.1007/s12105-012-0402-3.

Smith SM, Schmitt AC, Carrau RL, Iwenofu OH. Primary sinonasal mucosal melanoma with aberrant diffuse and strong desmin reactivity: a potential diagnostic pitfall! *Head Neck Pathol*. 2015;9(1):165-171. Available at: https://doi.org/10.1007/s12105-014-0553-5.

Takata T, Ito H, Ogawa I, Miyauchi M, Ijuhin N, Nikai H. Spindle cell squamous carcinoma of the oral region. *Virchows Archiv A Pathol Anat Histopathol*. 1991;419(3):177-182. Available at: https://doi.org/10.1007/BF01626345.

Thompson LDR. Squamous cell carcinoma variants of the head and neck. *Curr Diagn Pathol*. 2003;9(6):384-396. Available at: https://doi.org/10.1016/S0968-6053(03)00069-3.

Thompson, Lester DR, Wieneke JA, Miettinen M, Heffner DK. Spindle cell (sarcomatoid) carcinomas of the larynx. *Am J Surg Pathol*. 2002;26(2):153-170. Available at: https://doi.org/10.1097/00000478-200202000-00002.

Viswanathan S, Rahman K, Pallavi S, et al. Sarcomatoid (spindle cell) carcinoma of the head and neck mucosal region: a clinicopathologic review of 103 cases from a Tertiary Referral Cancer Centre. *Head Neck Pathol*. 2010;4(4):265-275. Available at: https://doi.org/10.1007/s12105-010-0204-4.

WHO Classification of Head and Neck Tumours; El-Naggar AK, Chan JKC, Grandis JR, Takata T, Slootweg PJ, eds. *WHO Classification of Head and Neck Tumors*. 4th ed. Lyon: International Agency for Research on Cancer; 2017.

Yi CH, Jim Zhai Q, Wang BY. Updates on immunohistochemical and molecular markers in selected head and neck diagnostic problems. *Arch Pathol Lab Med*. 2017;141(9):1214-1235. Available at: https://doi.org/10.5858/arpa.2016-0245-RA.

DIFFUSE SCLEROSING VARIANT OF PAPILLARY THYROID CARCINOMA

DIFFERENTIAL DIAGNOSIS: METASTATIC CARCINOMA

Clinical Features

The diffuse sclerosing variant of papillary thyroid carcinoma (PTC) is recognized to exhibit specific clinical characteristics including female predominance and younger age at presentation (mean age, 18–29 years). Compared with classical PTC, this variant tends to be characterized by more aggressive biological behavior as evidenced by involvement of both thyroid lobes, extrathyroidal extension, higher rates of lymph node metastasis, and greater incidence of pulmonary involvement.

Pathologic Features

GROSS FINDINGS

Due to the infiltrative nature of the tumor, involvement of both thyroid lobes is common. In some cases, a dominant tumor nodule can be found; however, diffuse glandular enlargement can also be seen simulating chronic lymphocytic thyroiditis (CLT). The tumors are typically white and firm due to the presence of dense fibrosis.

MICROSCOPIC FINDINGS

The tumor background exhibits dense fibrosis and marked lymphoplasmacytic infiltrate similar to that seen in CLT. In this setting, there are scattered islands and clusters of epithelial cells that demonstrate cytologic and architectural features typical of classical PTC (Fig. 10.1). Multifocal lymphovascular invasion along with abundant psammoma bodies are typical features as well. Squamous morular metaplasia is also a common finding in these tumors.

Ancillary Studies

The diffuse sclerosing variant of PTC demonstrates the typical immunophenotype characteristic of PTC in general. Specifically, the tumor cells should be positive for thyroid transcription factor-1 (TTF1), paired box gene 8 (*PAX8*), and thyroglobulin. The most common molecular alteration seen in these tumors is the *RET/PTC* rearrangement.

Differential Diagnosis

While the diffuse sclerosing variant of PTC may mimic multinodular goiter and CLT on gross examination, histologic studies will confirm the malignant nature of the neoplasm. Microscopically, the tumor demonstrates abundant evidence of lymphovascular space invasion and due to this appearance, the differential diagnosis can include metastatic carcinoma. This differential diagnostic consideration is more likely to be entertained in the setting of a thyroid tissue biopsy. In Fig. 10.2, a case of metastatic breast carcinoma is illustrated in which an inflammatory background is appreciable and tumor clusters are seen within lymphovascular spaces. Morphologic assessment is often sufficient in distinguishing the diffuse sclerosing variant of PTC as this tumor is often associated with psammoma bodies and demonstrates nuclear features in keeping with PTC. In more challenging cases, immunohistochemistry can be helpful in distinguishing metastasis from a PTC. Immunoreactivity for PAX8, TTF1, and thyroglobulin would favor the diagnosis of PTC. Absence of staining for all three markers would lend support for metastasis. As a cautionary note, it should be noted that carcinomas of renal and female genital tract origin are often positive for PAX8 and pulmonary adenocarcinomas are often TTF1 positive (Table 10.1).

Prognosis and Therapy

Patients with diffuse sclerosing variant of PTC are often treated with aggressive surgical intervention. Specifically, surgical treatment consists of total thyroidectomy, central

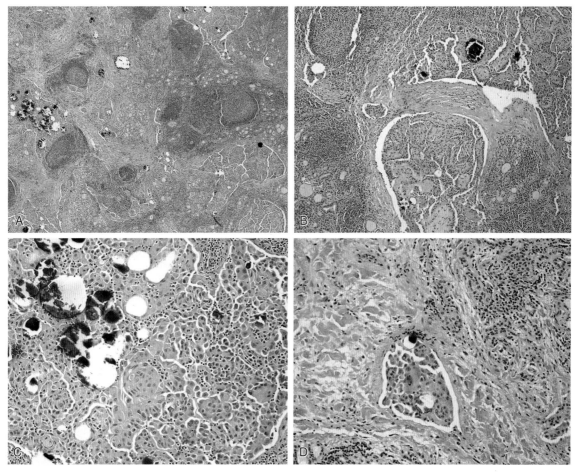

FIG. 10.1

Diffuse sclerosing variant of papillary thyroid carcinoma. **A,** On low-power magnification, a sclerotic, inflammatory background is appreciable, and islands of epithelial tumor cells are scattered throughout. **B,** Islands and clusters of tumor cells within lymphovascular spaces adopting a papillary architecture are seen on higher magnification. **C,** Clusters of tumor cells associated with psammoma bodies are seen. A squamous morule is seen near the center of the photomicrograph. **D,** A small cluster of tumor cells within a lymphovascular space is present in the background of dense fibrosis and chronic inflammatory infiltrate.

compartment lymph node dissection, and bilateral cervical lymph node dissections. Although the incidence of pulmonary metastasis is higher in these patients, the mortality associated with this tumor is lower than expected. Long-term survival and prognosis remain very good, with a mortality rate of less than 2%. Postoperative radioiodine treatment improves disease-free survival.

DIFFUSE SCLEROSING VARIANT OF PAPILLARY THYROID CARCINOMA (PTC) – DISEASE FACT SHEET

Definition

▸▸ Aggressive variant of PTC characterized by diffuse involvement of the thyroid parenchyma, abundant evidence of lymphovascular invasion, numerous psammoma bodies, and associated marked inflammatory infiltrate

Incidence and Location

▸▸ Rare subtype of PTC representing approximately 2% of PTC cases overall

▸▸ Can involve one or both thyroid lobes with bilateral involvement being more common

Age Distribution

▸▸ Younger patients with a mean age of 18–29 years at presentation

Clinical Features

▸▸ More aggressive biological behavior than classical PTC as evidenced by higher rates of cervical lymph node involvement, extrathyroidal extension, and metastases to the lung

Radiologic Features

▸▸ Hyperechogenic thyroid gland with diffuse scattered microcalcifications and ill-defined margins on ultrasound

▸▸ Evidence of cervical lymph node involvement is not uncommon

Prognosis and Therapy

▸▸ Despite aggressive biological behavior, the prognosis is generally good

▸▸ Aggressive surgical intervention (total thyroidectomy, central and bilateral neck dissection) with postoperative radioiodine treatment represents the mainstay of treatment

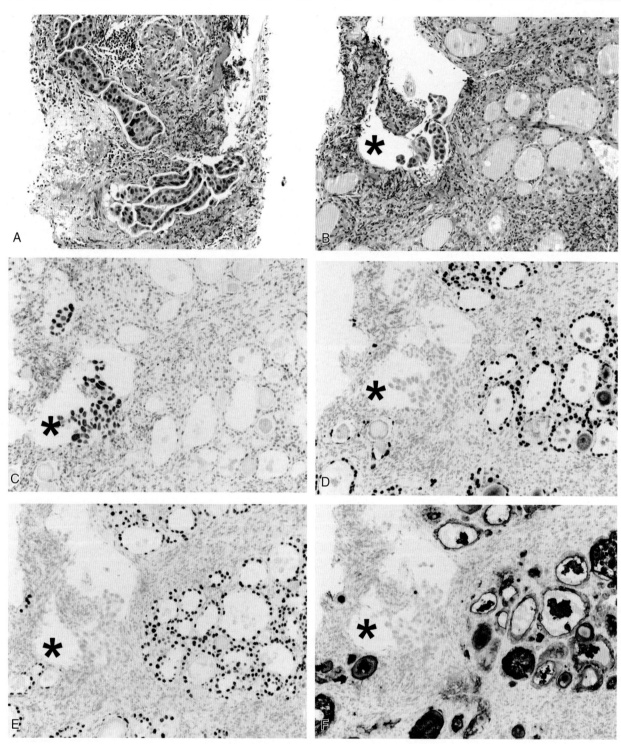

FIG. 10.2

Metastatic breast carcinoma to the thyroid. **A,** Tumor clusters are present within lymphovascular spaces. The background parenchyma in this photomicrograph exhibits a prominent inflammatory infiltrate. **B,** In this photomicrograph, the tumor clusters, in a space indicated by an *asterisk*, are cytologically distinct from the thyroid follicles in the background. Immunostains for GATA3 (**C**), TTF1 (**D**), PAX8 (**E**), and thyroglobulin (**F**) are shown. The tumor clusters, in the spaces marked with *asterisks*, demonstrate strong positivity for GATA3 and are negative for TTF1, PAX8, and thyroglobulin. In contrast, the surrounding thyroid follicular epithelium demonstrates the inverse immunophenotype, confirming metastasis to the thyroid.

TABLE 10.1

Histologic and Immunohistochemical Features of Diffuse sclerosing Variant of Papillary Thyroid Carcinoma (PTC) and Metastatic Carcinomas

Diffuse Sclerosing Variant of PTC	Metastatic Carcinoma
• Nuclear features in keeping with PTC (nuclear membrane irregularities, chromatin clearing, nuclear grooves, and intranuclear pseudoinclusions) • Lymphovascular space involvement • Psammoma bodies • Immunoreactive for TTF1, PAX8, and thyroglobulin	• Nuclear cytologic features variable, but PTC-like nuclear features are less commonly seen • Lymphovascular space involvement • Psammoma bodies uncommon • Not immunoreactive for thyroglobulin • Typically not immunoreactive for TTF1 (lung primary adenocarcinoma being an exception) • Typically not immunoreactive for PAX8 (primary female genital tract and renal carcinomas being exceptions)

DIFFUSE SCLEROSING VARIANT OF PAPILLARY THYROID CARCINOMA (PTC) – PATHOLOGIC FEATURES

Gross Findings
▸▸ Firm tumors that diffusely involve and replace the thyroid parenchyma. Occasionally a dominant tumor nodule can be identified.

Microscopic Findings
▸▸ Diffuse involvement of one or both thyroid lobes
▸▸ Numerous papillary tumor clusters located within lymphovascular channels
▸▸ Squamous metaplasia
▸▸ Numerous psammoma bodies
▸▸ Marked inflammatory infiltrate
▸▸ Prominent fibrosis

Pathologic Differential Diagnoses
▸▸ Metastatic carcinoma

SECRETORY CARCINOMA OF THYROID

DIFFERENTIAL DIAGNOSIS: PAPILLARY THYROID CARCINOMA

Clinical Features

Secretory carcinoma (also known as mammary analogue secretory carcinoma) presents as a thyroid mass with a reported age range of 36–74 years of age. Extrathyroidal extension and lymph node metastases at presentation have been reported.

Pathologic Features

GROSS FINDINGS

Reported tumors have ranged from 2.4 to 7.0 cm in size. The tumors have a solid white appearance.

MICROSCOPIC FINDINGS

Secretory carcinoma is an infiltrative tumor showing tubular, papillary, solid, microcystic, and cribriform growth in variable proportions. The tumor cells contain abundant eosinophilic cytoplasm, which may appear coarsely vacuolated. The nuclei of the tumor cells contain vesicular-appearing chromatin and conspicuous nuclei. Nuclear grooves can be seen. Pink luminal secretions mimicking colloid may be seen. Most reported cases appear low grade. However, high-grade features, such as increased mitotic activity, may be seen.

Ancillary Studies

The tumor cells of secretory carcinoma may express mammaglobin, GCDFP-15, and S100. Expression of PAX8 and TTF1 may be seen but is usually weak or focal. Immunostaining for thyroglobulin is negative. Molecular analysis reveals the presence of an *ETV6-NTRK3* gene fusion.

Differential Diagnosis

The architectural and cytologic features of secretory carcinoma share some similarities with conventional PTC (Table 10.2). Both tumors can show papillary architecture, nuclear clearing, and nuclear membrane irregularities. Rare nuclear pseudoinclusions may be seen in secretory carcinoma. Despite these similarities, a few distinguishing differences can be seen. Coarsely vacuolated cytoplasm imparting a microcystic appearance is a common feature of secretory carcinoma and is unusual to see in conventional PTC (Fig. 10.3). While vesicular chromatin imparting nuclear clearing can be seen in secretory carcinoma, the chromatin is usually coarser than conventional PTC. In addition, conspicuous central nucleoli are frequently present in secretory carcinoma. PTC typically has a fine powdery chromatin distribution and nucleoli are sparse to absent. It should be noted that secretory carcinoma is not always mutually exclusive from conventional PTC. Cases of secretory carcinoma arising in conjunction with PTC have been described. Immunostains are helpful to distinguish secretory carcinoma from conventional PTC. Thyroglobulin positivity is characteristic of conventional PTC, while negative in secretory carcinoma. While some cases of

TABLE 10.2
Histologic and Immunohistochemical Features of Secretory Carcinoma and Conventional Papillary Thyroid Carcinoma

Secretory Carcinoma	Papillary Thyroid Carcinoma
• Shows solid cribriform, microcystic, papillary, and tubular growth patterns	• Typically shows papillary or follicular growth
• Tumor cells contain abundant eosinophilic cytoplasm	• May contain abundant eosinophilic cytoplasm (especially tall cell and oncocytic variants)
• Tumor nuclei contain vesicular chromatin with grooves and possibly rare pseudoinclusions. Prominent nucleoli are present.	• Tumor nuclei show fine chromatin with nuclear clearing, grooves, and pseudoinclusions. Prominent nucleoli usually not present.
• Positive for S100, mammaglobin, and GCDFP-15	• Positive for TTF1 and thyroglobulin
• *ETV6* gene rearrangement characteristic	• *ETV6* gene rearrangement uncommon

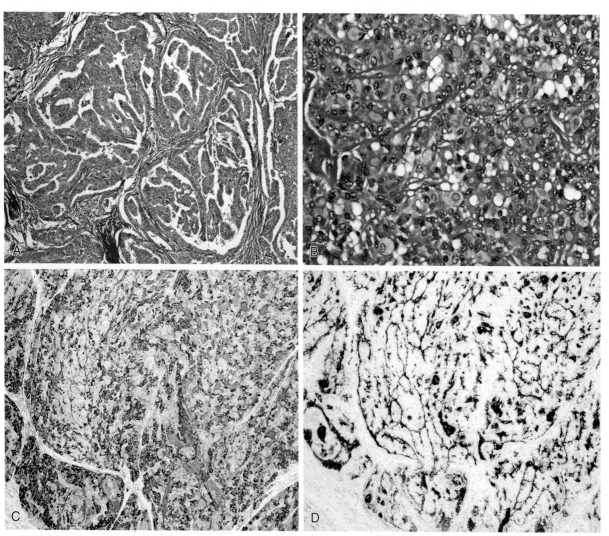

FIG. 10.3

Secretory carcinoma. **A,** Secretory carcinoma showing papillary architecture and tumor cells with abundant eosinophilic cytoplasm. **B,** Tumor cells showing coarsely vacuolated cytoplasm; nuclei, vesicular chromatin, and prominent nucleoli. **C,** Positive mammaglobin staining in secretory carcinoma. **D,** Positive GCDFP-15 staining in secretory carcinoma.

secretory carcinoma express TTF1 and PAX8, the staining is usually weak and focal. In contrast, conventional PTC is strongly positive for both TTF1 and PAX8. *ETV6-NTRK3* gene fusion is present in secretory carcinoma. Since secretory carcinoma can arise at other sites, such as the breast or salivary glands, correlation with clinical and imaging findings is needed to exclude a metastasis.

Prognosis and Therapy

As only a small number of case reports have been documented, the overall prognosis of secretory carcinoma is not well elucidated. Local regional lymph node metastases and extrathyroidal extension can be seen. Some tumors show frequent recurrences but favorable long-term survival. However, rare fatal cases with distant metastases have been reported. The primary treatment is surgical excision.

SECRETORY CARCINOMA – DISEASE FACT SHEET

Definition
▶▶ Invasive carcinoma associated with ETV6-NTRK3 fusion

Incidence and Location
▶▶ True incidence is unknown. Can occur in any location of thyroid

Age Distribution
▶▶ Age range of 36–74 years reported

Clinical Features
▶▶ Presents with thyroid mass which may be associated with extrathyroidal extension and local regional lymph node metastases

Radiologic Features
▶▶ Heterogeneous tumor visualized by CT scan

Prognosis and Therapy
▶▶ Limited information available on prognosis. May be subject to recurrences with favorable long-term survival. Rare clinically aggressive with high-grade features cases described.
▶▶ Treatment primarily is surgical

SECRETORY CARCINOMA– PATHOLOGIC FEATURES

Gross Findings
▶▶ Firm tumor with white cut surface

Microscopic Findings
▶▶ Invasive carcinoma showing solid, papillary, cribriform, microcystic, tubular growth
▶▶ Tumor cells contain abundant pink cytoplasm and conspicuous central nucleoli

Pathologic Differential Diagnoses
▶▶ Conventional papillary thyroid carcinoma

CRIBRIFORM-MORULAR VARIANT OF PAPILLARY THYROID CARCINOMA

DIFFERENTIAL DIAGNOSIS: CONVENTIONAL PAPILLARY THYROID CARCINOMA; COLUMNAR CELL VARIANT OF PAPILLARY THYROID CARCINOMA; TALL CELL VARIANT OF PAPILLARY THYROID CARCINOMA (TCV-PTC)

Clinical Features

The cribriform-morular variant of papillary thyroid carcinoma (CMV-PTC) occurs mostly in females, with only rare cases reported in male patients. The tumor usually occurs in the third decade of life, presenting as an incidental nodule or mass detected by palpation or imaging. Multiple nodules may be seen, especially in syndromic cases. The CMV-PTC is associated with familial adenomatous polyposis (FAP) in about half of the cases.

Pathologic Features

GROSS FINDINGS

The CMV-PTC usually forms a white to tan mass with a circumscribed or encapsulated appearance. The cut surface is usually not gritty due to the absence of calcifications.

MICROSCOPIC FINDINGS

The tumor is frequently encapsulated, showing of a combination of cribriform, follicular, papillary, trabecular, and solid growth patterns. While follicular and cystic growth is frequently present, colloid secretions are sparse to absent. The follicles and papillae are lined by columnar-appearing cells, which may show some nuclear stratification. Variable nuclear clearing, nuclear grooves, and pseudoinclusions can be identified. A characteristic feature is the presence of morules, which may appear squamoid, containing optically clear nuclei or nuclear pseudoinclusion-like bodies that result from biotin accumulation (Fig. 10.4).

Ancillary Studies

Immunohistochemical expression of TTF1 is a consistent feature in CMV-PTC, while staining for thyroglobulin is frequently weak or focal. β-catenin immunohistochemistry shows strong nuclear staining reflecting abnormalities in the Wnt signaling pathway. APC mutations have been reported in 64% of cases and CTNNB1

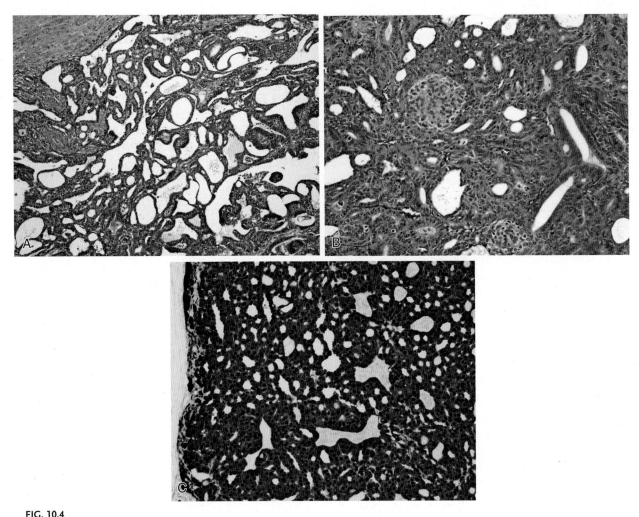

FIG. 10.4
Cribriform-morular variant of papillary thyroid carcinoma (CMV-PTC). **A,** CMV-PTC showing cribriform growth. Note spaces are devoid of colloid. **B,** Squamoid morules. **C,** Nuclear expression of β-catenin.

mutations in 32% of cases. While BRAFV600E mutations are not seen, RET/PTC rearrangements may be present. Rare cases showing immunohistochemical expression of neuroendocrine markers have been reported.

Differential Diagnosis

The differential diagnosis of CMV-PTC includes variants of PTC. The most common considerations include classical PTC, the tall cell variant of papillary thyroid carcinoma (TCV-PTC), and the columnar cell variant of papillary thyroid carcinoma (CCV-PTC) (Fig. 10.5 and Table 10.3). CMV-PTC shows similar cytologic features to conventional PTC including nuclear grooves and pseudoinclusions. In general, the degree of nuclear clearing is more pronounced in classical PTC. The CMV-PTC frequently contains back-to-back follicular spaces that impart a cribriform appearance. The presence of squamoid morules, containing cells with nuclear incisions

from biotin accumulation, is characteristic of CMV-PTC. In addition, the conspicuous near-total absence of colloid seen in CMV-PTC is usually quite striking, serving as a clue for the diagnosis of CMV-PTC.

The CMV-PTC may contain columnar-shaped tumor cells lining the follicles and papillae, which shows morphologic overlap with the CCV-PTC and TCV-PTC. In addition, CCV-PTC can also have solid areas of growth causing further confusion with CMV-PTC. In contrast to CMV-PTC, CCV-PTC is composed of tumor cells containing relatively dark nuclei with a stratified appearance. Typical features of PTC, including pseudoinclusions, are generally not seen. In addition, subnuclear vacuolization is a frequent feature of CCV-PTC, imparting an endometrioid appearance. TCV-PTC usually shows conspicuous nuclear features of PTC, including marked nuclear clearing and easily identifiable pseudoinclusions. The classic nuclear features of PTC are more difficult to appreciate in CMV-PTC. An abundance of granular oncocytic cytoplasm is identified in TCV-PTC, causing the tumor cells to appear two to three

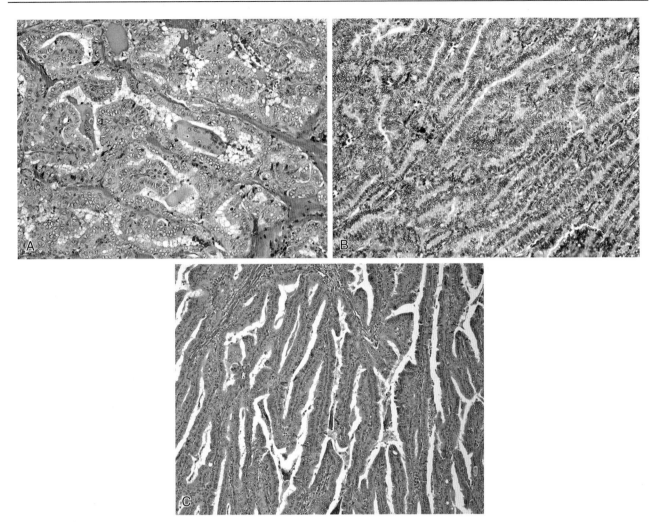

FIG. 10.5

A, Conventional papillary thyroid carcinoma (PTC) showing characteristic nuclear features. **B,** Columnar cell variant of PTC showing dark stratified nuclei. **C,** Tall cell variant of PTC showing elongated follicles composed of cells containing abundant eosinophilic cytoplasm and classic PTC nuclear features.

TABLE 10.3

Histologic and Immunohistochemical Features of Cribriform-Morular Variant of Papillary Thyroid Carcinoma (CMV-PTC) Versus Conventional PTC, Tall Cell Variant of PTC (TCV-PTC), and Columnar Cell Variant of PTC (CCV-PTC)

CMV-PTC	Conventional PTC	TCV-PTC	CCV-PTC
• Cribriform, papillary, follicular, solid growth patterns • Morular structures present • Colloid sparse to absent • Nuclear features somewhat diminished from conventional PTC • Nuclear staining for β-catenin present	• Papillary and follicular growth • Morular structures usually absent • Colloid present • Classic nuclear features of PTC present • Membranous staining for β-catenin only	• Papillary and follicular growth (follicles frequently elongated) • Morular structures absent • Colloid present • Classic nuclear features of PTC present • Membranous staining for β-catenin only	• Papillary, follicular, and solid growth • Morular structures absent • Colloid sparse to absent • Dark stratified nuclei, classic nuclear features of PTC absent • Membranous staining for β-catenin only

times tall as they are wide. In addition, many of the infiltrating tumor follicles comprising TCV-PTC have elongated and sometimes serpiginous contours. This is accompanied by a more conspicuous pattern of infiltration seen with TCV-PTC. These features impart a distinctive low-power appearance to TCV-PTC compared with CMV-PTC, appearing as a tumor with a radial infiltrative growth pattern composed of elongated follicular structures containing abundant oncocytic cytoplasm and conspicuous nuclear features of PTC.

Immunohistochemically, CMV-PTC shows nuclear β-catenin staining reflecting abnormalities of the Wnt signaling pathway. In conjunction with the histologic features, this excludes other variants of PTC. Investigation of the clinical history, to determine if the patient has FAP, can also be useful to corroborate the diagnosis.

Prognosis and Therapy

Patients diagnosed with CMV-PTC have a favorable prognosis. Approximately 10% of patients recur in the form of regional neck lymph node metastases. Distant metastases have been reported but are uncommon. Rare reports of aggressive behavior have been identified with tumors showing neuroendocrine differentiation. Patients are treated with total thyroidectomy and may be treated with radioactive iodine. External beam radiation has been used in patients with locally advanced disease.

CRIBRIFORM-MORULAR VARIANT OF PAPILLARY THYROID CARCINOMA – DISEASE FACT SHEET

Definition
▶▶ Malignant thyroid tumor of follicular cell origin frequently associated with FAP

Incidence and Location
▶▶ Rare tumor with a relative prevalence of approximately 0.2% of all PTC variants. May be solitary or multifocal. Tumors associated with FAP are frequently multifocal.

Age Distribution
▶▶ Age range of 8 to 69 years, with most cases occurring in the third decade of life

Clinical Features
▶▶ Occurs mostly in females (31:1 female-to-male ratio). Frequently associated with FAP.

Radiologic Features
▶▶ Usually shows low-risk features by ultrasound imaging

Prognosis and Therapy
▶▶ Favorable prognosis with lower incidence of lymph node metastasis compared with conventional PTC

CRIBRIFORM-MORULAR VARIANT OF PAPILLARY THYROID CARCINOMA – PATHOLOGIC FEATURES

Gross Findings
▶▶ Circumscribed or encapsulated appearance grossly

Microscopic Findings
▶▶ Shows combination of cribriform, follicular, papillary, trabecular, and solid growth patterns
▶▶ Morular structures are present
▶▶ Nuclear staining for β-catenin is present

Pathologic Differential Diagnoses
▶▶ Conventional PTC; CC-PTC; TCV-PTC

NONINVASIVE FOLLICULAR VARIANT OF PAPILLARY THYROID CARCINOMA

DIFFERENTIAL DIAGNOSIS: ENCAPSULATED FOLLICULAR VARIANT OF PAPILLARY THYROID CARCINOMA, FOLLICULAR ADENOMA, ENCAPSULATED CONVENTIONAL PAPILLARY THYROID CARCINOMA

Clinical Features

NIFTP, formerly classified as noninvasive encapsulated follicular variant of PTC, usually presents as solitary painless nodule. In some cases, when presenting as a large mass, may cause compressive symptoms.

Pathologic Features

GROSS FINDINGS

NIFTP is a well-circumscribed mass typically surrounded by a thin uniform capsule. Tumors with a thickened capsule can also be seen. The cut surface of the tumor appears white-tan to brown. Cystic changes are uncommon but may be observed as a consequence of infarction or prior fine-needle aspiration (FNA).

MICROSCOPIC FINDINGS

NIFTP is either well demarcated from the surrounding thyroid tissue or surrounded by capsule. Capsule irregularities may be present in some cases. However, no capsular or vascular invasion is identified. The tumor shows a follicular growth pattern which usually includes some combination of microfollicular, macrofollicular, and normofollicular growth. Colloid is typically present within the follicles. When microfollicular growth predominates, caution should be exercised to not misinterpret packed microfollicular growth as solid growth, as small lumens will still be discernable. NIFTP should not have any true papillary structures as evidenced by the presence of fibrovascular cores. However, abortive papillae may be seen. The cytologic features are central to the diagnosis of NIFTP. Nuclear features resembling PTC are encompassed within three categories including: nuclear size and shape alternations, nuclear membrane irregularities, and chromatin characteristics. Stated another way, NIFTP contains tumor cells showing clear, enlarged, and overlapping nuclei with nuclear membrane irregularities such as irregular contours or grooves. The extent to which these changes are present within NIFTP is variable, and frequently less pronounced than seen in classical PTC. To help improve consistency in the diagnosis of NIFTP, a three-point scoring system assessing the cytologic features has been established as a guide in the consensus paper published by the Endocrine Pathology Society working group.

Ancillary Studies

Molecular analysis has revealed NIFTP to share similar genetic abnormalities to follicular neoplasia including RAS mutations. RET fusions and BRAFV660E mutations are absent. CK19, HBME-1, and Galectin-3 can be positive in NIFTP. However, as these stains can also be positive in classical PTC and sometimes in follicular neoplasia, interpretation for classification should not be done independently from the morphologic features.

Differential Diagnosis

The main differential diagnosis is with the invasive encapsulated follicular variant of papillary thyroid carcinoma (EN-FVPTC), encapsulated papillary thyroid carcinoma (EN-PTC), and follicular adenoma (FA) as seen in Fig. 10.6 and listed in Table 10.4. FAs are typically

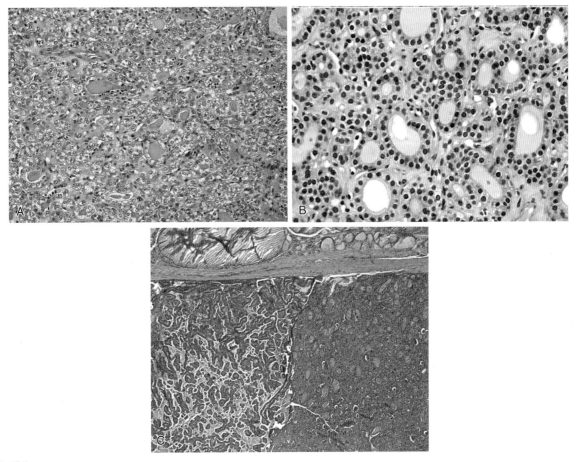

FIG. 10.6

A, Noninvasive encapsulated follicular variant of papillary thyroid carcinoma (PTC) showing enlarged overlapping clear nuclei with nuclear membrane irregularities. **B,** Follicular adenoma with uniform round nuclei. **C,** Encapsulated PTC showing a combination of papillary and follicular growth.

TABLE 10.4

Histologic and Molecular Features of Non-Invasive Encapsulated Follicular Variant of Papillary Thyroid Carcinoma (NIFTP), Encapsulated Follicular Variant of Papillary Thyroid Carcinoma (EN-FVPTC), Encapsulated Papillary Thyroid Carcinoma (EN-PTC), and Follicular adenoma (FA)

NIFTP	EN-FVPTC	EN-PTC	FA
• Completely noninvasive • Follicular growth pattern • Nuclear features resembling classic PTC present • RAS mutations most common	• Capsular or vascular invasion present • Follicular growth pattern • Nuclear features resembling classic PTC present • RAS mutations most common	• Capsular or vascular invasion may be present • Follicular and variable papillary growth • Classic nuclear features present • RET fusions or BRAFV600E mutation most common	• Completely noninvasive • Follicular growth. Rare cases may have papillary growth • Nuclear features of PTC not present • RAS mutations most common

composed of tumor cells containing uniform round nuclei without significant nuclear enlargement, clearing, or nuclear membrane irregularities. The presence of papillary architecture or psammoma bodies excludes the diagnosis of NIFTP and instead indicates the diagnosis of EN-PTC. Caution should be exercised in cases showing conspicuous cytologic features of PTC including intranuclear pseudoinclusions and marked nuclear clearing. Such cases often show papillary architecture, in keeping with PTC. Therefore, tumors should be generously sampled to exclude conventional PTC with a predominant follicular growth pattern. If features typical of other variants of PTC are present, then NIFTP is also excluded. Any invasive features exclude the possibility of NIFTP, and the diagnosis of invasive EN-FVPTC (or other thyroid carcinoma) should be rendered. This underscores the need for generous or complete sampling of the tumor capsule to ensure that invasion has been unequivocally excluded. Regarding invasion, keep in mind that papillary microcarcinomas can have circumscribed, noninfiltrative appearance. Therefore, the diagnosis of NIFTP should be rendered cautiously in tumors less than 1.1 cm in size, especially when multifocal lesions are present. Other features which can exclude the diagnosis of NIFTP include increased mitotic activity (>3 mitoses/10 HPF), solid/trabecular/insular growth (>30% of the tumor area), and tumor necrosis (excluding FNA-induced necrosis) as these are features more frequently observed with higher-grade thyroid carcinomas.

Prognosis and Therapy

NIFTP is a clinically indolent tumor which rarely causes metastatic disease. Indeed, according to some studies, no metastatic cases were reported. Since the tumor behaves in a clinically benign fashion in most cases, NIFTP is generally treated in a similar fashion to FA, with lobectomy alone sufficing in the majority of cases.

NONINVASIVE FOLLICULAR VARIANT OF PAPILLARY THYROID CARCINOMA – DISEASE FACT SHEET

Definition
▶▶ Encapsulated noninvasive follicular patterned neoplasm sharing some cytologic similarities with conventional PTC

Incidence and Location
▶▶ True incidence of NIFTP is unknown. May involve any region of thyroid gland.

Age Distribution
▶▶ Most patients present in sixth decade of life, but wide age range observed

Clinical Features
▶▶ Usually presents as painless asymptomatic nodule

Radiologic Features
▶▶ Well-circumscribed mass appearing homogenous and hypoechoic by ultrasound imaging

Prognosis and Therapy
▶▶ Excellent prognosis with extremely low risk of adverse events. Can be treated by lobectomy alone without need for radioactive iodine.

NONINVASIVE FOLLICULAR VARIANT OF PAPILLARY THYROID CARCINOMA - PATHOLOGIC FEATURES

Gross Findings
▶▶ Circumscribed or encapsulated, usually solitary, nodule, with homogenous white-tan to brown cut surface

Microscopic Findings
▶▶ Follicular growth pattern with no true papillae seen
▶▶ Cytologic atypia resembling classical PTC is present scored in three categories: nuclear size and shape alternations; nuclear membrane irregularities; and chromatin characteristics

Pathologic Differential Diagnoses
▶▶ EN-FVPTC, EN-PTC, FA

FOLLICULAR THYROID NEOPLASMS WITH CLEAR CELL CHANGE

DIFFERENTIAL DIAGNOSIS: METASTATIC RENAL CELL CARCINOMA

Clinical Features

Follicular neoplasms can occasionally demonstrate cytoplasmic clear cell change. Clear cell change, in isolation, does not necessarily equate to malignancy as this can be seen to varying degrees in both benign and malignant follicular neoplasms. Clear cell change can be seen in up to 3% of primary thyroid carcinomas including follicular carcinoma and PTC.

Pathologic Features

GROSS FINDINGS

On gross examination, follicular neoplasms exhibiting clear cell change demonstrate similarities to conventional follicular neoplasms.

MICROSCOPIC FINDINGS

Clear cell change can occur in both FAs as well as malignant follicular epithelial-derived tumors (Fig. 10.7 and Table 10.5). This can be seen to varying degrees within the tumor. Ultrastructurally, the cytoplasmic clearing has been attributed to a variety of etiologies such as intracellular accumulation of glycogen, lipid, or colloid vacuoles. Diagnostic criteria for distinguishing between FAs and

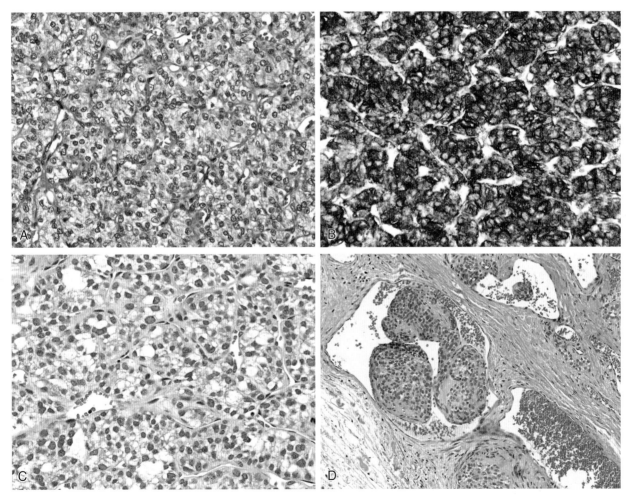

FIG. 10.7

Two cases of follicular neoplasms with clear cell change. **A,** This photomicrograph was obtained from a case of a papillary thyroid carcinoma (PTC) in which cytoplasmic clear cell change was present. **B,** Immunohistochemistry for HBME1 diffusely highlights the tumor cells supporting the diagnosis of PTC. **C,** This photomicrograph was obtained from a case of follicular carcinoma in which cytoplasmic clearing is seen in the tumor cells. **D,** The diagnosis of follicular carcinoma was made based on the presence of vascular invasion; in this focus, clear cell change is less evident in the tumor cells.

TABLE 10.5

Histologic and Immunohistochemical Features of Follicular Neoplasms With Clear Cell Change Versus Metastatic Renal Cell Carcinoma

Follicular Neoplasms With Clear Cell Change	Metastatic Renal Cell Carcinoma
• Chromatin can vary from granular to vesicular depending on tumor type	• In low-grade tumors, the nuclei are small and hyperchromatic. In higher-grade tumors, prominent nucleoli are visible.
• Immunoreactive for TTF1 and PAX8	• Immunoreactive for PAX8 but negative for TTF1
• Immunoreactive for thyroglobulin	• Negative for thyroglobulin

follicular carcinomas with clear cell change are identical to those for their counterparts without clear cell change; the presence of capsular and/or vascular invasion is necessary for diagnosis of malignancy in this context. If nuclear features in keeping with PTC are seen in a follicular epithelial tumor with clear cell change that fulfills criteria for PTC, then a diagnosis of PTC is rendered.

Ancillary Studies

Follicular neoplasms of the thyroid gland that demonstrate clear cell change should exhibit the typical immunophenotype as conventional follicular neoplasms. Specifically, they should demonstrate nuclear immunoreactivity for TTF1 and PAX8 as well as cytoplasmic immunoreactivity for thyroglobulin.

Differential Diagnosis

Metastatic carcinoma to the thyroid gland is a rare phenomenon; however, renal cell carcinoma (RCC) represents one of the more common neoplasms to involve the thyroid gland (Fig. 10.8). The clearing of cytoplasm in occasional thyroid follicular neoplasms, especially if the clear cell changes are diffusely present throughout the nodule, can occasionally raise the possibility of metastatic RCC to the thyroid gland. Nonetheless, the presence of follicular architecture would argue against metastatic RCC. Metastatic RCC typically demonstrates a more packeted, nested pattern associated with delicate capillary vasculature. In case of PTCs that demonstrate clear cell change, the chromatin clearing can lead to easier visualization of nucleoli. Thus, the nuclear features in this context can overlap with the nuclear features of metastatic RCC. Immunohistochemical distinction between follicular neoplasms with

clear cell change from metastatic RCC should be straightforward. The former should demonstrate immunoreactivity for TTF1, PAX8, and thyroglobulin. In contrast, the latter should immunostain only for PAX8 and be negative for TTF1 and thyroglobulin.

Prognosis and Therapy

Surgical excision represents the mainstay of treatment of these tumors. The prognosis of follicular neoplasms that exhibit clear cell change is similar to follicular neoplasms for which clear cell change is absent.

FOLLICULAR NEOPLASMS WITH CLEAR CELL CHANGE – DISEASE FACT SHEET

Definition
▸▸ Prominent cytoplasmic clearing and vacuolization in the epithelial cells within a follicular derived epithelial neoplasm

Incidence and Location
▸▸ Uncommon but can be seen in up to 3% of thyroid neoplasms

Age Distribution
▸▸ No known age predilection

Clinical Features
▸▸ Clear cell change does not equate to malignancy as both benign and malignant follicular neoplasms can demonstrate varying degrees of clear cell change

Radiologic Features
▸▸ Discrete nodule seen on imaging, indistinct from follicular neoplasms without clear cell change

Prognosis and Therapy
▸▸ Dependent on whether the thyroid follicular neoplasm is diagnosed as benign or malignant rather than if clear cell change is present or absent
▸▸ Surgical excision represents the mainstay of treatment

FOLLICULAR NEOPLASM WITH CLEAR CELL CHANGE – PATHOLOGIC FEATURES

Gross Findings
▸▸ Can manifest as discrete thyroid nodules, similar to conventional follicular neoplasms

Microscopic Findings
▸▸ Prominent cytoplasmic clearing within a subset of follicular epithelial cells within a follicular neoplasm; can be a diffuse feature within the nodule
▸▸ Diagnosis of malignancy is based on known criteria such as presence of capsular and/or vascular invasion along with features that would justify a diagnosis of PTC

Pathologic Differential Diagnoses
▸▸ Metastatic RCC to the thyroid gland

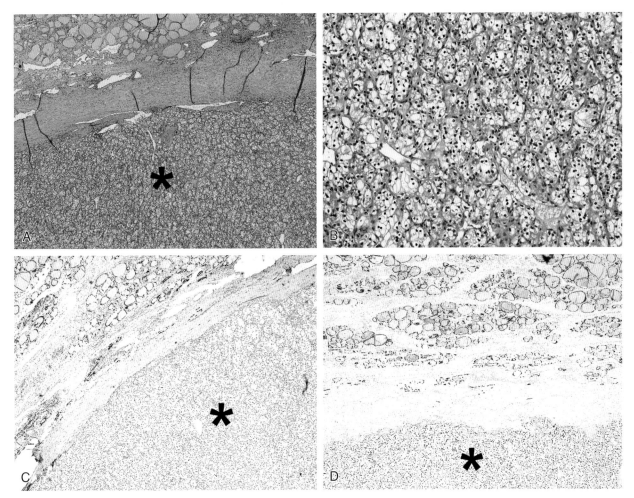

FIG. 10.8

Metastatic renal cell carcinoma to the thyroid. **A,** The *asterisk* demonstrates an array of neoplastic cells that are morphologically distinct from the thyroid follicles seen in the upper aspect of the image. **B,** On higher magnification, nests of epithelial cells that demonstrate prominent cytoplasmic vacuolization are seen. **C** and **D,** The tumor in the area indicated by the *asterisk* is negative for TTF1 (**C**) in contrast to the thyroid follicles, which stain positively for this marker. The nuclei of both the tumor cells and thyroid follicles demonstrate immunoreactivity for PAX8 (**D**).

HYALINIZING TRABECULAR TUMOR OF THYROID

DIFFERENTIAL DIAGNOSES: FOLLICULAR VARIANT OF PAPILLARY THYROID CARCINOMA, PARAGANGLIOMA, MEDULLARY THYROID CARCINOMA

Clinical Features

Hyalinizing trabecular tumor (HTT) is a rare neoplasm derived from thyroid follicular cells. HTT can raise suspicion for PTC preoperatively on FNA due to overlapping cytomorphologic features that exist between HTT and PTC. This rare tumor was initially described by Carney et al. in 1987 and was initially termed "hyalinizing trabecular adenoma." This tumor has also been described as "paraganglioma-like adenoma of the thyroid."

Pathologic Features

GROSS FINDINGS

On gross examination, HTTs are well circumscribed and can be encapsulated. These tumors are yellow to tan in complexion and are grossly similar to FAs and adenomatoid nodules.

MICROSCOPIC FINDINGS

The cells within HTTs demonstrate a prominent trabecular architectural pattern with intervening hyalinized stroma (Fig. 10.9). The trabeculae form straight to curved ribbons, but the tumor cells can also form compact, nested clusters or follicles. The cells are elongated in shape and oriented perpendicular to the trabeculae. The nuclei are oval in shape and features typically seen in PTC, especially intranuclear pseudoinclusions, are often encountered. These tumors are

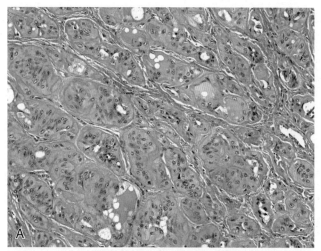

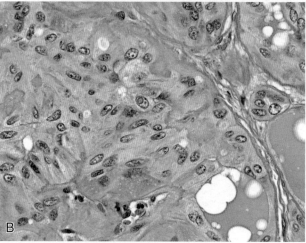

FIG. 10.9

Hyalinizing trabecular tumor. **A,** Trabecular cords of neoplastic cells are present in a hyalinized stromal background. **B,** On higher magnification, the cells are elongated and an intranuclear pseudoinclusion can be seen.

histologically well circumscribed, sometimes encapsulated, and invasion is absent.

Ancillary Studies

Immunohistochemistry demonstrates a similar immunophenotype to conventional thyroid nodules as HTTs demonstrate immunoreactivity for thyroglobulin and TTF1. Cytoplasmic and membrane staining on MIB-1 immunohistochemistry can be observed; the degree to which this is observed appears to be dependent on the method of antigen retrieval. The expression of neuroendocrine markers, such as chromogranin and synaptophysin, is typically negative in these tumors. Recently, rearrangements involving *GLIS family zinc finger gene 1 (GLIS1)* and *GLIS family zinc finger gene 3 (GLIS3)* have been observed in these tumors by Nikiforova et al.; thus, GLIS rearrangements could represent a genomic hallmark of HTTs. These rearrangements were not observed

in PTC, suggesting that HTTs are genetically distinct tumors from PTC.

Differential Diagnosis

The cytologic features of HTTs may mimic that of FVPTC, especially when the crowded microfollicular architecture in the latter is seen in association with intervening hyalinized stroma (Fig. 10.10C). The distinction between these two entities is still often possible based on morphologic grounds due to the elongated nature of the neoplastic cells in HTTs along with the configuration of the tumor cells within the linear to curved trabeculae. In addition, HTT usually contains many more pseudoinclusions than any other variant of PTC. In fact, it is not uncommon to find multiple nuclear pseudoinclusions in each high-power field examined in a typical HTT. In contrast, nuclear pseudoinclusions can be difficult to find in EN-FVPTC. Immunohistochemistry can be helpful given the peculiar aforementioned MIB-1 staining pattern in some HTTs and the tendency of FVPTC to overexpress HBME-1 (Fig. 10.10B). As a cautionary note, not every case of PTC overexpresses HBME-1 and a small subset of HTTs can express HBME-1. Furthermore, as the MIB-1 positivity in HTTs appears to be dependent on antigen retrieval methodology, a negative MIB-1 immunophenotype does not necessarily exclude the diagnosis of HTT.

Sometimes the tumor cells in HTTs can form compact, nested clusters reminiscent of the "zellballen" architectural pattern seen in paragangliomas. The organoid nests of tumor cells in paragangliomas can also be separated by intervening hyalinized stroma (Fig. 10.11). Both tumors can also demonstrate intranuclear pseudoinclusions. Due to the overlapping morphologic features of these tumors, HTTs were also previously described as "paraganglioma-like adenomas of the thyroid." Immunohistochemical distinction between these two tumors is straightforward as paragangliomas typically are immunoreactive for neuroendocrine markers, chromogranin, and synaptophysin, and are typically negative for TTF-1 and thyroglobulin. In contrast, the inverse immunophenotype is expected in HTTs. Furthermore, immunohistochemistry for S100 should highlight sustentacular cells in paragangliomas, whereas these cells are absent in HTTs.

Finally, HTT can occasionally share morphologic overlap with medullary thyroid carcinoma (MTC), especially when a spindled morphology is seen in the latter (Fig. 10.12). Intranuclear pseudoinclusions along with extracellular hyaline material can be seen in both. Nonetheless, with respect to the latter, the tumor cells in MTC are more haphazardly arranged in relation to the extracellular hyaline material, which represents amyloid. Congo red staining can be useful

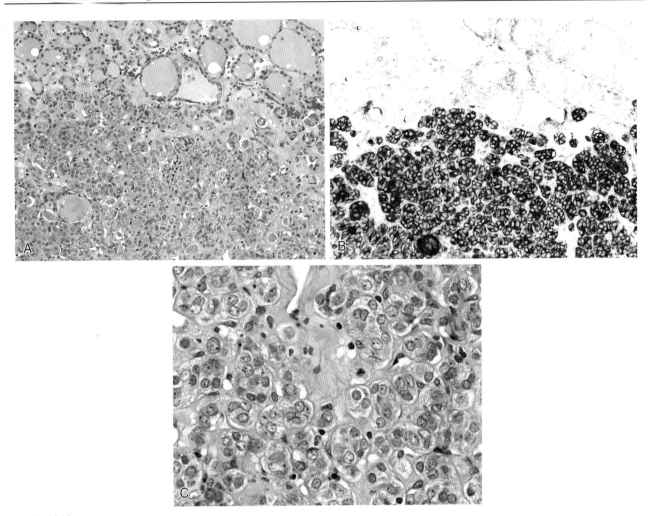

FIG. 10.10

Follicular variant of papillary thyroid carcinoma. **A,** The tumor cells are arranged in a packed microfollicular pattern and admixed with cyto-logically benign macrofollicles at the top aspect of the image. **B,** Immunohistochemistry for HBME-1 demonstrates strong overexpression in the tumor cells, whereas the adjacent benign thyroid follicles are negative. **C,** On higher magnification, the tumor cells demonstrate nuclear enlargement, chromatin clearing, and nuclear membrane irregularities along with occasional nuclear grooves. The intervening stroma between the microfollicles demonstrates foci of hyalinized change.

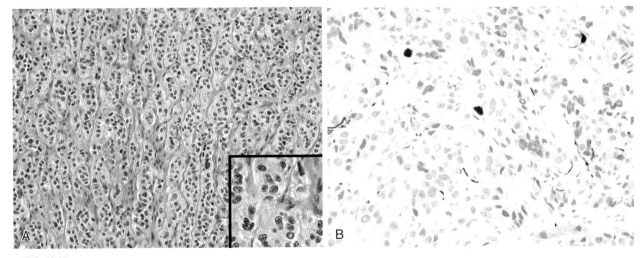

FIG. 10.11

Paraganglioma. **A,** Trabecular cords of neoplastic cells are present in a hyalinized stromal background. The inset at the lower right highlights the presence of intranuclear pseudoinclusions. **B,** Immunohistochemistry for S100 demonstrates the presence of sustentacular cells along with their delicate cytoplasmic processes.

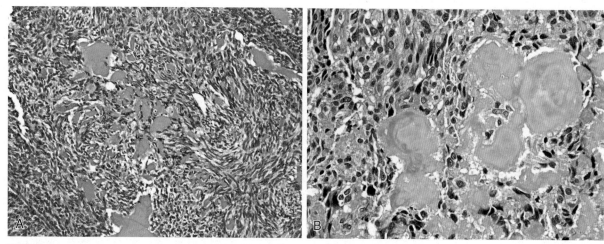

FIG. 10.12

Medullary thyroid carcinoma (MTC). **A,** In this example of MTC, the tumor cells adopt an elongated spindled morphology. The spindled tumor cells are more haphazardly arranged and amorphous hyaline-like areas are present. **B,** On higher magnification, the tumor cells are distributed more haphazardly with respect to the hyaline-like areas, which exhibit a texture consistent with extracellular amyloid deposits.

TABLE 10.6

Histologic and Immunohistochemical Features of Hyalinizing Trabecular Tumor (HTT) Versus Follicular Variant of Papillary Thyroid Carcinoma (FVPTC), Paraganglioma, and Medullary Thyroid Carcinoma (MTC)

HTT	FVPTC	Paraganglioma	MTC
• Small trabecular nests in a prominent hyalinized stromal background • Elongated tumor cells	• Packed array of microfollicles can sometimes resemble trabeculae • Hyalinized stroma can be present in areas	• Small organoid nests in a "zell-ballen" architecture • Variable degrees of stromal hyalinization can be present	• Elongated cells can be present similar to those seen in HTT • Amyloid can mimic stromal hyalinization; however, the distribution of tumor cells relative to amyloid is more haphazard
• Nuclear pseudoinclusions frequently seen	• Nuclear pseudoinclusions can be present to varying degrees	• Nuclear pseudoinclusions can be present to varying degrees	• Nuclear pseudoinclusions can be present to varying degrees
• Immunoreactive for TTF1 and thyroglobulin • HBME1 expression can be observed in a subset of cases • Typically negative for neuroendocrine markers (chromogranin and synaptophysin) • Cell membrane and cytoplasmic staining for MIB-1 can be observed	• Immunoreactive for TTF1 and thyroglobulin • HBME1 expression more frequently observed than in HTT • Typically negative for neuroendocrine markers (chromogranin and synaptophysin)	• Immunoreactive for neuroendocrine markers (chromogranin and synaptophysin) • Negative for TTF1, calcitonin, and thyroglobulin • S100 positive sustentacular cells present	• Immunoreactive for TTF1 and neuroendocrine markers (chromogranin and synaptophysin) • Negative for thyroglobulin • Amyloid highlighted by Congo red stain • Positive for calcitonin

in demonstrating apple green birefringence of the amyloid under polarized light in MTC. Immunohistochemical adjuncts are also helpful as MTCs are positive for chromogranin, synaptophysin, and calcitonin, whereas HTTs should be negative for all three markers (Table 10.6).

Prognosis and Therapy

HTTs typically behave in a benign fashion and should be treated conservatively. These are often diagnosed in lobectomy or total thyroidectomy specimens, and surgical excision represents sufficient treatment.

HYALINIZING TRABECULAR TUMOR – DISEASE FACT SHEET

Definition
▸▸ Rare neoplasm derived from thyroid follicular cells that does not exhibit invasion

Incidence and Location
▸▸ True incidence unknown due to the rarity of these tumors
▸▸ Present as a well-circumscribed nodule in the thyroid gland

HYALINIZING TRABECULAR TUMOR – DISEASE FACT SHEET—cont'd

Age Distribution

▸▸ Can occur at any age

Clinical Features

▸▸ Occasionally interpreted as PTC on fine-needle aspiration

Radiologic Features

▸▸ Present similarly to typical thyroid nodules on radiologic examination

▸▸ Ultrasonographic features of hyalinizing trabecular tumor are similar to that of follicular adenomas

Prognosis and Therapy

▸▸ Generally exhibit a benign clinical course

HYALINIZING TRABECULAR TUMOR – PATHOLOGIC FEATURES

Gross Findings

▸▸ Well-circumscribed thyroid nodules that grossly resemble prototypical adenomatoid nodules or follicular adenomas

Microscopic Findings

▸▸ Elongated cells arranged in straight to curved trabeculae
▸▸ Intervening hyalinized stroma separating the trabeculae
▸▸ Nuclear features seen in PTC, especially intranuclear pseudoinclusions, are often observed
▸▸ Can be encapsulated
▸▸ Lack of invasion

Pathologic Differential Diagnoses

▸▸ Follicular variant of papillary thyroid carcinoma
▸▸ Paraganglioma
▸▸ Medullary thyroid carcinoma

MEDULLARY THYROID CARCINOMA

DIFFERENTIAL DIAGNOSES: POORLY DIFFERENTIATED THYROID CARCINOMA AND SOLID CELL NESTS

Clinical Features

MTC is an uncommon thyroid malignancy that accounts for approximately 2% of thyroid cancers. These tumors are composed of cells that demonstrate evidence of C-cell differentiation. Most MTCs arise sporadically, but up to 30% of tumors represent a component of heritable multiple endocrine neoplasia type 2 syndromes. Patients with MTCs often exhibit elevated serum carcinoembryonic antigen (CEA) and calcitonin levels.

Pathologic Features

GROSS FINDINGS

These tumors can vary grossly from circumscribed, nonencapsulated, solitary nodules of tan to yellow complexion to widely infiltrative tumors that diffusely involve a thyroid lobe. Microscopic tumors measuring less than 1 cm have been termed micro-MTCs.

MICROSCOPIC FINDINGS

MTCs demonstrate a broad range of architectural and cytologic features. With respect to the former, these tumors can demonstrate a mixture of solid, insular, and trabecular architectural patterns. Cytologically, the tumor cells can be epithelioid, plasmacytoid, or spindled. The degree of anisonucleosis is typically mild to moderate and the chromatin is often granular and stippled. Although nuclear features associated with PTC are not typical in these tumors, intranuclear pseudoinclusions can be observed in occasional tumor cell nuclei. The cytoplasm can vary from amphophilic to oxyphilic. Extracellular amyloid deposits are often present and can be present in up to 90% of cases (Fig. 10.13A).

Ancillary Studies

MTCs are typically positive for TTF1 (Fig. 10.13B), similar to follicular epithelial-derived neoplasms. However, unlike follicular neoplasms, MTCs are usually negative for thyroglobulin on immunohistochemistry. Focal immunostaining for thyroglobulin should be interpreted with caution as this could result from staining of adjacent or admixed follicular cells. Although a subset of MTCs can demonstrate immunoreactivity for PAX8, the majority of these tumors are negative for this marker (Fig. 10.13C). Neuroendocrine markers, such as chromogranin and synaptophysin, are certainly helpful in highlighting these tumors (Fig. 10.13D and E). Calcitonin immunohistochemistry is expected to stain positively in these tumors (Fig. 10.13F); nonetheless, occasional cases show only focal staining or can even be negative for calcitonin. Finally, immunohistochemistry for CEA is often positive in MTCs. The most common mutation identified in MTC is activating mutations of the RET proto-oncogene, which encodes the RET receptor tyrosine kinase.

Differential Diagnosis

Due to the sheet-like, trabecular, and/or insular architectural patterns that manifest in MTCs, these tumors

TABLE 10.7

Histologic and Immunohistochemical Features of Medullary Thyroid Carcinoma (MTC) Versus Poorly Differentiated Thyroid Carcinoma (PDTC)

MTC	PDTC
• Often adopts a mixture of solid, trabecular, and/or insular architecture	• Defined by solid, trabecular, and/or insular architecture
• Granular, stippled chromatin	• Granular, stippled chromatin typically not a defining feature
• Immunoreactive for TTF1, variable expression of PAX8, and negative for thyroglobulin	• Immunoreactive for TTF1, PAX8, and thyroglobulin
• Immunoreactive for chromogranin, synaptophysin, and calcitonin	• Negative for chromogranin, synaptophysin, and calcitonin

can occasionally be confused with poorly differentiated thyroid carcinomas (PDTCs) (Table 10.7). Both tumors can demonstrate evidence of tumor necrosis. The chromatin pattern tends to be more stippled in MTCs than in PDTCs. Furthermore, the presence of amyloid can aid in the diagnosis of MTCs. The immunohistochemical distinction between these two tumors is generally straightforward. MTCs should immunostain positively for chromogranin, synaptophysin, and calcitonin (Fig. 10.13), whereas PDTCs should not (Fig. 10.14). Thyroglobulin immunoreactivity may be present to varying degrees in PDTC but not expected in MTC. Both tumors would expect to immunostain positively for TTF1 and can demonstrate immunoreactivity for PAX8. With respect to PAX8, PDTCs are often diffusely positive for PAX8, whereas the degree of PAX8 positivity varies in MTCs. A subset of MTCs do not exhibit expression of PAX8 and this can be helpful in arguing against a PDTC.

When MTCs are small and measure <1 cm, these tumors are regarded as micro-MTCs. When the tumor is quite microscopic in size, this can occasionally mimic the morphology of solid cell nests (SCNs; Table 10.8). SCNs often demonstrate a vaguely squamoid and/or transitional cell appearance. The chromatin is hyperchromatic but not typically stippled. Immunohistochemistry can aid in the distinction of SCNs from micro-MTCs. The former should immunostain positively for p63 and not exhibit immunoreactivity for the neuroendocrine markers, chromogranin, and synaptophysin (Fig. 10.15).

Prognosis and Therapy

It is not uncommon for MTC to demonstrate evidence of nodal metastases at the time of presentation. The 10-year survival rates range from 45% to 85% depending on the stage of the tumor. MTCs are optimally treated by total thyroidectomy with central compartment lymph node dissection as these tumors often metastasize to locoregional cervical lymph nodes. More advanced-stage cases

are treated via a multimodal approach that includes surgery, radiation, and/or chemotherapy. Recently, targeted agents which inhibit mutated RET-receptor tyrosine kinase activity have become available. Postoperative monitoring of serum CEA and calcitonin levels can determine whether there is evidence of residual or recurrent disease on clinical follow-up.

MEDULLARY THYROID CARCINOMA – DISEASE FACT SHEET

Definition
▸▸ Rare malignant neoplasm derived from cells with C-cell differentiation

Incidence and Location
▸▸ Uncommon and represent approximately 2% of all thyroid malignancies
▸▸ Can involve one or both lobes of the thyroid gland

Age Distribution
▸▸ Sporadic tumors occur in fourth to sixth decades of life
▸▸ Younger age at presentation for patients with multiple endocrine neoplasia type 2 syndrome

Clinical Features
▸▸ Approximately 70% of cases are sporadic and approximately 30% are heritable cases
▸▸ Patients often present with painless palpable thyroid nodules
▸▸ Elevated CEA and calcitonin levels are observed in patients with MTC

Radiologic Features
▸▸ MTCs can present with solitary, circumscribed nodules that are cold on radioiodide scans
▸▸ For cases in which there is a more diffuse involvement of the thyroid lobe, the mass lesion may be more subtle on imaging

Prognosis and Therapy
▸▸ Tumors often involve locoregional cervical lymph nodes at presentation. Ten-year survival rates range from 45% to 85%
▸▸ Optimal treatment is typically surgical and involves total thyroidectomy with central component lymph node dissection
▸▸ Patients with advanced stage tumors can also be treated with radiation therapy and/or chemotherapy

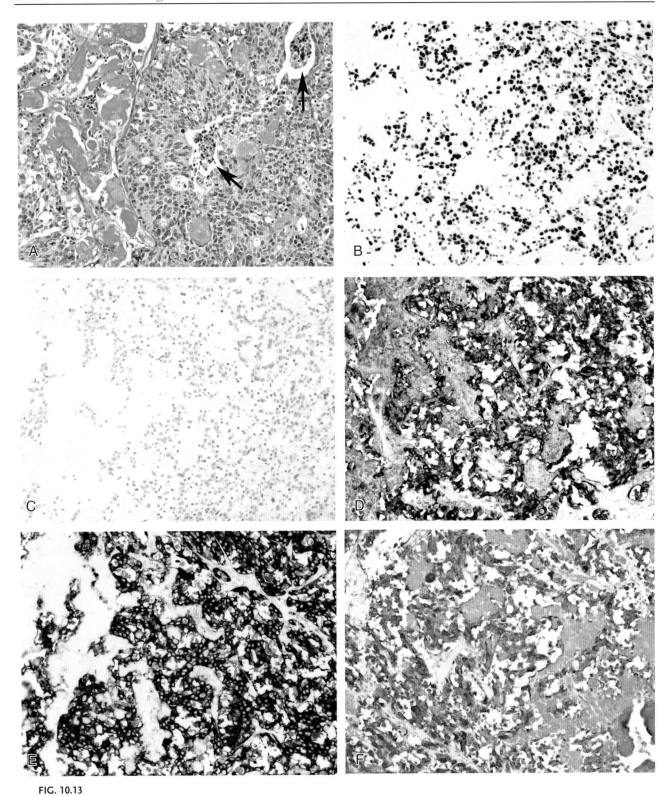

FIG. 10.13

Medullary thyroid carcinoma. **A,** In this photomicrograph, the tumor adopts a solid, sheet-like architecture and demonstrates amyloid deposition as well as microscopic foci of tumor necrosis *(arrows)*. **B,** Immunohistochemistry for TTF1 highlights the nuclei of the tumor cells. **C,** Immunohistochemistry for PAX8 is negative in this tumor. **D–F,** The tumor demonstrates immunoreactivity for chromogranin (**D**), synaptophysin (**E**), and calcitonin (**F**).

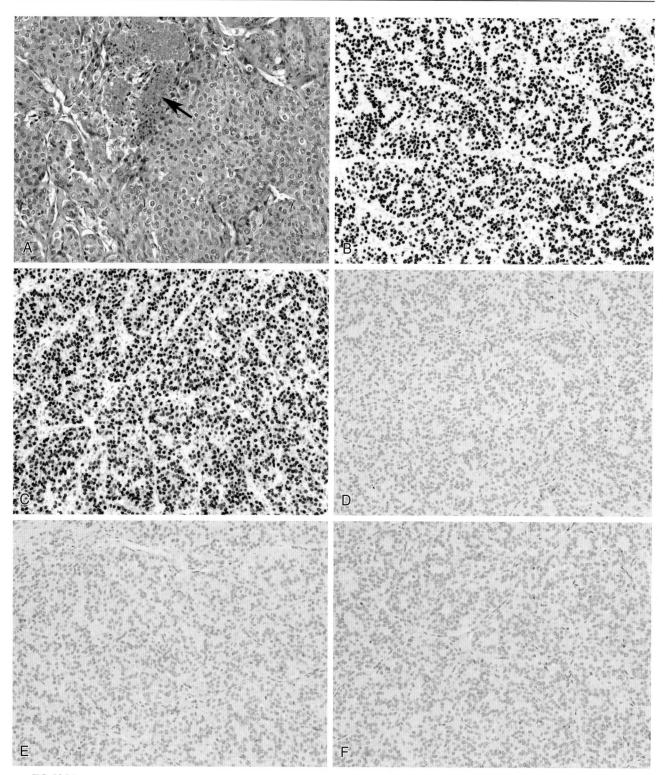

FIG. 10.14

Poorly differentiated thyroid carcinoma. The tumor demonstrates an insular architecture (**A**); geographic tumor necrosis is indicated by the *arrow*. The tumor cells demonstrate diffuse nuclear immunoreactivity for TTF1 (**B**) and PAX8 (**C**). The tumor cells do not exhibit immunoreactivity for chromogranin (**D**), synaptophysin (**E**), or calcitonin (**F**).

TABLE 10.8

Histologic and Immunohistochemical Features of Micromedullary Thyroid Carcinoma Versus Solid Cell Nests

Micromedullary Thyroid Carcinoma	Solid Cell Nests
• Nuclei with granular, stippled chromatin	• Uniformly hyperchromatic nuclei
• Immunoreactive for chromogranin and synaptophysin	• Negative for chromogranin or synaptophysin on immunohistochemistry
• Negative for p63 on immunohistochemistry	• Immunoreactive for p63

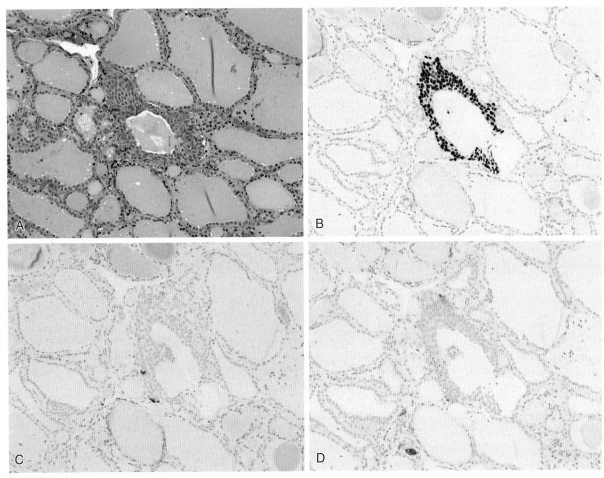

FIG. 10.15

Solid cell nest (SCN). **A,** The center of the photomicrograph contains a nest of cytologically bland cells with a squamoid, transitional cell–like morphology. **B,** Immunohistochemistry for p63 highlights the nuclei of the cells within the SCN. **C and D,** The cells within the SCN are negative for chromogranin and synaptophysin, respectively.

MEDULLARY THYROID CARCINOMA – PATHOLOGIC FEATURES

Gross Findings
▶▶ MTCs can vary from well-circumscribed, nonencapsulated tan to yellow tumors to demonstrating more infiltrative behavior to involve a thyroid lobe diffusely

Microscopic Findings
▶▶ MTCs can demonstrate a mixture of solid, insular, and trabecular architectural patterns

▶▶ Cytologically, the tumor cells can be epithelioid, plasmacytoid, and/or spindled and demonstrate amphophilic to oxyphilic cytoplasm
▶▶ Nuclei with granular and stippled chromatin. Intranuclear pseudoinclusions can be observed.
▶▶ Extracellular amyloid deposits are often present

Pathologic Differential Diagnoses
▶▶ Poorly differentiated thyroid carcinoma
▶▶ Solid cell nests

UNDIFFERENTIATED (ANAPLASTIC) THYROID CARCINOMA

DIFFERENTIAL DIAGNOSIS: SARCOMA, SQUAMOUS CELL CARCINOMA, AND METASTATIC HIGH-GRADE MALIGNANCIES

Clinical Features

Undifferentiated (anaplastic) carcinoma of the thyroid represents a relatively rare form of malignancy, comprising up to 5% of thyroid carcinomas in general. Anaplastic thyroid carcinoma (ATC) is more commonly encountered in elderly patients (mean age of 70 years) and typically presents as a rapidly enlarging thyroid mass. This can be seen in the setting of long-standing multinodular goiter. ATC can also manifest in the setting of a recurrence of a previously known well-differentiated thyroid carcinoma. Hoarseness, dysphagia, and/or dyspnea secondary to the rapidly growing neck mass lesion are common symptoms.

Pathologic Features

GROSS FINDINGS

Grossly, ATCs often manifest as widely infiltrative tumors that extensively replace one or both thyroid lobes and invade adjacent anatomic structures such as the larynx, trachea, and/or esophagus. ATCs are firm to fleshy and tan/white in complexion; necrosis and hemorrhage are common findings on gross examination.

MICROSCOPIC FINDINGS

The histologic appearance of ATC is variable but typically demonstrates high-grade cytologic atypia, nuclear pleomorphism, and prominent nucleoli. The shape of the cells can be epithelioid, sarcomatoid, or a mixture thereof (Fig. 10.16A and B). Varying degrees of background fibrosis and inflammation can be seen in association with the tumor cells. For paucicellular tumors, there is abundant dense fibrosis in association with the tumor cells. Vascular invasion, necrosis, and mitotic activity, including atypical mitotic figures, are

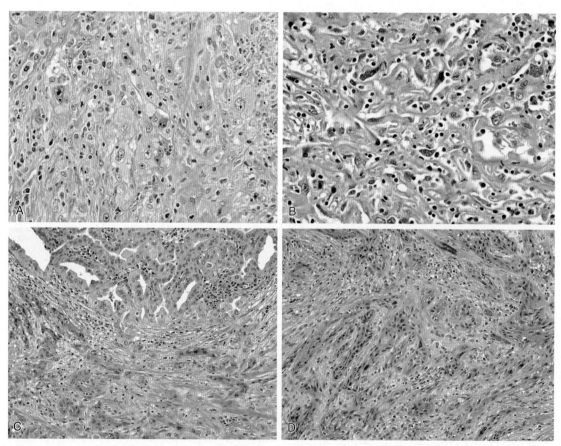

FIG. 10.16

Anaplastic thyroid carcinoma. **A,** Large epithelioid tumor cells exhibiting severe anisonucleosis and macronucleoli are present. **B,** A sarcomatoid population of tumor cells exhibiting hyperchromasia and severe nuclear pleomorphism is present. **C,** The upper aspect of the photomicrograph demonstrates a well-differentiated papillary thyroid carcinoma adjacent to the undifferentiated component in the lower aspect. **D,** Squamoid morphology is seen in this field.

often identifiable. A component of well-differentiated thyroid carcinoma, such as PTC (Fig. 10.16C), can be seen in approximately half of cases lending credence to the notion that ATC often arises through dedifferentiation of more conventional, differentiated thyroid carcinomas. Squamoid morphology may be present (Fig. 10.16D).

Ancillary Studies

The immunophenotype of ATC is variable and often nonspecific. Proof of epithelial differentiation, for instance, via immunohistochemistry for cytokeratins, is not always confirmatory positive in these tumors. Thyroglobulin and TTF1 are often negative in these tumors. However, PAX8 has been reported to be positive in 76% of cases and this can be a useful marker in helping to confirm the diagnosis.

Differential Diagnosis

Given the variable morphology of the tumor cells along with the high-grade cytologic features exhibited by ATC, the differential diagnosis includes sarcoma, squamous cell carcinoma, and metastatic high-grade malignancies (Table 10.9). With respect to the first two entities in the differential diagnosis, primary sarcomas and squamous cell carcinomas of the thyroid gland are exceedingly rare. Sarcomatoid-appearing tumors of the thyroid gland most likely represents ATC, in the absence of strong evidence to suggest otherwise. Molecular genetic studies can be helpful in identifying unique sarcomas that involve the thyroid gland, whether as a primary tumor or as a metachronous event. Squamous cell carcinoma of the thyroid gland demonstrates a purely squamous morphology and demonstrates a similar degree of lethality to ATC. In general, primary squamous cell carcinoma of the thyroid gland is currently best regarded as a variant of ATC. In this setting, a metastatic squamous cell carcinoma must be excluded as well as direct involvement of the thyroid from an adjacent site such as the larynx. Finally, metastatic high-grade malignancies can mimic the appearance of ATC. For this diagnosis to be made, there should ideally be strong documented evidence of an extrathyroidal primary. If possible, morphologic comparison with the primary tumor is helpful in establishing the diagnosis. An example of a metastatic carcinosarcoma to the thyroid gland is shown in Fig. 10.17. Comparison with the morphology of the uterine primary tumor (not shown) aided in clinching the diagnosis.

Prognosis and Therapy

Often times, ATCs are so widely invasive at presentation that they are inoperable. The prognosis is generally poor with most patients succumbing to the disease within 1 year of initial presentation. For patients with surgically operable tumors, radical resection along with chemotherapy and/or radiotherapy is the treatment of choice.

UNDIFFERENTIATED (ANAPLASTIC) CARCINOMA – DISEASE FACT SHEET

Definition
▶▶ Infiltrative, aggressive thyroid malignancy that demonstrates high-grade, anaplastic cytologic features

Incidence and Location
▶▶ Uncommon but represents up to 5% of thyroid malignancies

Continued

TABLE 10.9

Features of Anaplastic Thyroid Carcinoma (ATC) Versus Sarcoma, Squamous Cell Carcinoma, and Metastatic High-Grade Malignancies

ATC	Sarcoma	Squamous Cell Carcinoma	Metastatic High-Grade Malignancies
• High-grade epithelioid and/or sarcomatoid tumor cell morphology • Squamoid morphology can be observed • Vascular and/or lymphatic space invasion is commonly encountered • Presence of an associated differentiated thyroid carcinoma component argues in favor of ATC	• Can mimic the histologic appearance of ATC • Sarcomatoid neoplasms involving the thyroid should be considered as ATC in the absence of strong evidence to suggest otherwise • Molecular genetic studies can be helpful in the identification of certain sarcomas that rarely involve the thyroid gland	• Tumor cells demonstrate a pure squamous morphology • Considered as a variant of ATC in the absence of strong evidence to suggest otherwise • Metastatic squamous cell carcinoma should be excluded • Direct involvement of the thyroid by an extrathyroidal squamous cell carcinoma from an adjacent anatomic site (e.g., larynx) should be excluded	• Can mimic the histologic appearance of ATC • Involvement of vascular and/or lymphatic spaces can be seen • Strong documented evidence of an extrathyroidal primary is helpful • Comparison of the suspected metastatic tumor to the thyroid and the primary tumor is particularly helpful

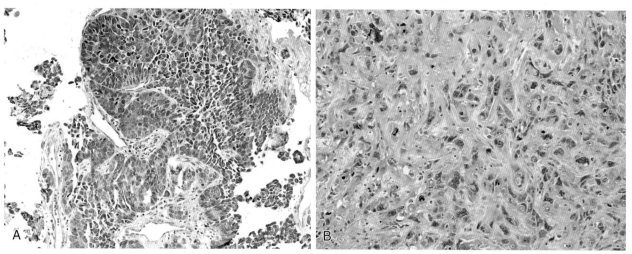

FIG. 10.17
Metastatic carcinosarcoma to the thyroid in a patient with a known history of uterine carcinosarcoma. **A,** A cohesive focus of epithelial cells consistent with a high-grade carcinomatous component to the tumor is seen in this photomicrograph. **B,** In contrast, the sarcomatoid component in this case demonstrated a less cohesive, haphazard arrangement to the cells along with a high degree of nuclear hyperchromasia and pleomorphism.

Age Distribution
▸▸ Typically presents in elderly patients (mean age of 70 years)

Clinical Features
▸▸ Rapidly enlarging neck mass with frequent involvement of anatomic structures adjacent to the thyroid such as the larynx, trachea, and esophagus
▸▸ Can be seen in the setting of long-standing multinodular goiter as well as in the setting of recurrence of a differentiated thyroid carcinoma

Radiologic Features
▸▸ Large neck mass that is seen to infiltrate and replace the thyroid parenchyma
▸▸ Involvement of adjacent anatomic structures and/or tracheal deviation can be detected radiologically

Prognosis and Therapy
▸▸ Poor prognosis in general. Most patients die within 1 year of presentation.
▸▸ Due to widely invasive behavior seen at presentation, these tumors are often inoperable
▸▸ For surgically resectable tumors, radical surgery with radiation and/or chemotherapy is an option

UNDIFFERENTIATED (ANAPLASTIC) CARCINOMA – PATHOLOGIC FEATURES

Gross Findings
▸▸ Often manifests as widely infiltrative tumors that replaces the thyroid parenchyma with involvement of adjacent extrathyroidal anatomic structures

Microscopic Findings
▸▸ High-grade, anaplastic cytologic atypia
▸▸ Tumor cells can adopt either an epithelioid or sarcomatoid morphology or a mixture thereof

▸▸ In approximately 50% of well sampled tumors, a well-differentiated thyroid carcinoma component can be seen in association with the undifferentiated carcinoma

Pathologic Differential Diagnoses
▸▸ Sarcoma
▸▸ Squamous cell carcinoma
▸▸ Metastatic high-grade malignancies

SPINDLE AND EPITHELIAL TUMOR WITH THYMUS-LIKE DIFFERENTIATION

DIFFERENTIAL DIAGNOSIS: SYNOVIAL SARCOMA

Clinical Features

Spindle and epithelial tumor with thymus-like differentiation (SETTLE) most commonly presents as a thyroid mass in children or young adults with mean age of presentation of about 15 years. A painless enlarging neck mass is the most common reported presentation.

Pathologic Features

GROSS FINDINGS

The tumor may appear grossly circumscribed or infiltrative with an average size of approximately 4.0 cm. However, tumor sizes as small as 0.5 cm and as large 12 cm have been reported. The cut surface is grayish-white and may have a whorled or nodular appearance. Small cystic areas may be present.

MICROSCOPIC FINDINGS

On low-power examination, SETTLE has a nodular or bosselated appearance associated with irregular thick fibrous bands. The tumor comprises a cellular biphasic proliferation of spindled and epithelial cell growth (Fig. 10.18). The spindle cell component of the tumor shows a mixture of fascicular, reticular, and microcystic growth patterns. The spindle cells have a relatively monotonous appearance, containing elongated nuclei with a fine chromatin distribution. The spindled areas merge imperceptibly with epithelium-forming tubules, papillae, and complex or glomeruloid structures. The epithelial component of the tumor can show mucinous or squamous differentiation. Only sparse mitotic activity is identified and necrosis is typically absent.

Ancillary Studies

The spindled and glandular cell components of the tumor are diffusely positive for high-molecular-weight cytokeratin and CK7, including the spindle cell component of the tumor. Immunostains are negative for markers of thyroid differentiation including TTF1 and thyroglobulin. Immunostains for neuroendocrine differentiation are negative.

Differential Diagnosis

The primary differential diagnosis for SETTLE is synovial sarcoma (Table 10.10). The spindle cells of synovial sarcoma tend to show a higher nuclear grade than SETTLE. Mast cells are usually easily identified in synovial sarcoma but are usually absent in SETTLE. The glandular

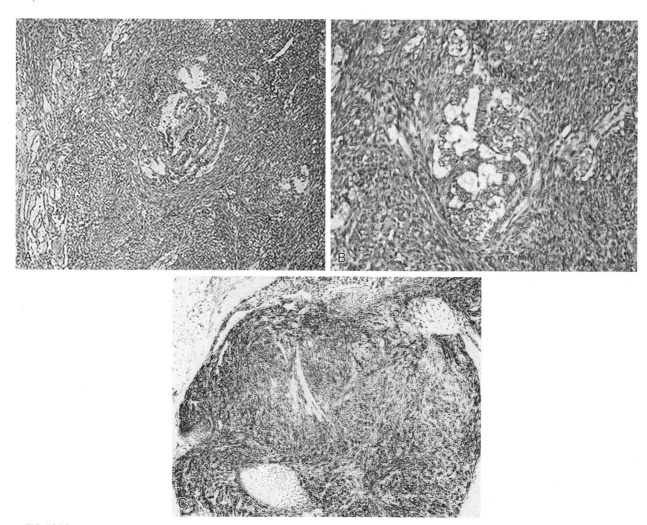

FIG. 10.18

A, spindle and epithelial tumor with thymus-like differentiation showing cellular spindle cell areas that merge with glandular growth. **B,** Glandular structure with complex appearance. **C,** Diffuse CK5/6 positivity in spindle cell component of the tumor.

TABLE 10.10

Histologic, Molecular and Immunohistochemical Features of Spindle and Epithelial Tumor With Thymus-like Differentiation (SETTLE) Versus Synovial Sarcoma

SETTLE	Synovial Sarcoma
• Cells show less nuclear atypia, crowding, and overlap	• Hyeprchromatic nuclei which frequently overlap
• Complex glandular structures with papillary formations or glomeruloid structures	• Less complex glandular structures present
• No necrotic debris seen in glands	• Necrotic debris common in glands
• Mast cells rare or absent	• Frequent mast cells can be seen
• Diffuse staining for high-molecular-weight cytokeratins present	• Only focal staining for high-molecular-weight cytokeratins present
• *SS18* gene translocation absent	• *SS18* gene translocation present

structures in SETTLE show more complex arrangements, including papillary projections, glomeruloid structures, and elongated glandular spaces which may contain mucin. Such structures are uncommon in synovial sarcoma. Necrotic debris is frequently identified in the glands of synovial sarcoma, which is typically absent in SETTLE. Immunohistochemically, high-molecular-weight cytokeratin is frequently diffusely expressed in the stromal cells of SETTLE, whereas only scattered spindle cells are positive for high-molecular-weight cytokeratin in synovial sarcoma. To resolve diagnostically difficult cases, molecular analysis for synovial sarcoma–associated fusions may be necessary, which are absent in SETTLE.

Prognosis and Therapy

SETTLE can show an unpredictable long-term course. While many cases behave in a low-grade malignant fashion, metastasis to local lymph nodes and distant sites such as lung, vertebrae, and kidney have been reported. The median time interval between diagnosis and presentation of metastatic disease is approximately 10 years. However, metastases have been reported even 20 years after initial diagnosis. Complete surgical excision is the standard treatment for SETTLE.

SPINDLE AND EPITHELIAL TUMOR WITH THYMUS-LIKE DIFFERENTIATION – DISEASE FACT SHEET

Definition
▸▸ Biphasic malignant tumor composed of spindle cells that merge with epithelial structures

Incidence and Location
▸▸ Very rare tumor mostly represented in cases reports or small series
▸▸ Tumor can involve any portion of the thyroid gland

Age Distribution
▸▸ Mean age of diagnosis is approximately 15 years, with a reported range of 2–59 years

Clinical Features
▸▸ Presents mostly as painless enlarging mass. May present as rapid enlarging mass rarely.

Radiologic Features
▸▸ Solid mass with heterogeneous appearance on ultrasound

Prognosis and Therapy
▸▸ Overall survival of 86% (median follow-up 6.3 years)
▸▸ Metastasis in up to 41% of cases after 5 years. Late metastasis after 20 years reported.

SPINDLE AND EPITHELIAL TUMOR WITH THYMUS-LIKE DIFFERENTIATION – PATHOLOGIC FEATURES

Gross Findings
▸▸ Vaguely lobulated mass with circumscribed or invasive appearance and a gray to whit-tan cut surface

Microscopic Findings
▸▸ Cellular neoplasm comprising spindled cells with low-grade nuclear features that merge with areas of glandular differentiation
▸▸ Microcystic and reticular areas are present. Glomeruloid structures are seen.
▸▸ Diffuse staining with high-molecular-weight cytokeratin is present

Pathologic Differential Diagnoses
▸▸ Synovial sarcoma

SCLEROSING MUCOEPIDERMOID CARCINOMA OF THYROID WITH EOSINOPHILIA

DIFFERENTIAL DIAGNOSIS: REACTIVE CHANGES IN CHRONIC LYMPHOCYTIC THYROIDITIS, SOLID CELL NESTS, MUCOEPIDERMOID CARCINOMA OF THE THYROID

Clinical Features

Sclerosing mucoepidermoid carcinoma of thyroid with eosinophilia (SMECE) most often presents as a slow-growing painless mass. Large tumors can cause symptoms related to compression such as dysphagia or airway compromise. Occasionally, rapid tumor growth has been reported. Patients may present with cervical lymph node metastasis.

Pathologic Features

GROSS FINDINGS

SMECE forms tumors that are usually firm with irregular borders. The cut surface is white-tan in appearance.

MICROSCOPIC FINDINGS

SMECE almost always occurs in a background of CLT, usually the fibrosing type. The tumor is formed by squamoid cells forming infiltrative short cords, small nests, and glandular cysts in a background of dense fibrosis (Fig. 10.19A–D). Mucus-containing cells are present,

scattered among the nests or cyst-lining cells. Foci of keratinization and mucin pools are frequently seen. Characteristically, eosinophils are scattered throughout the fibrous stroma. In addition, abundant plasma cells and lymphocytes are also identified. Cytologically, the tumor cells contain mild to moderately enlarged nuclei and may contain conspicuous central nuclei. Perineural invasion may be observed.

Ancillary Studies

Immunostains for pan and high-molecular-weight cytokeratins are positive in the tumor cells. About half SMECE cases are positive for TTF-1, frequently in a patchy distribution. Immunostaining for thyroglobulin is typically negative; however, focal positive staining may be seen.

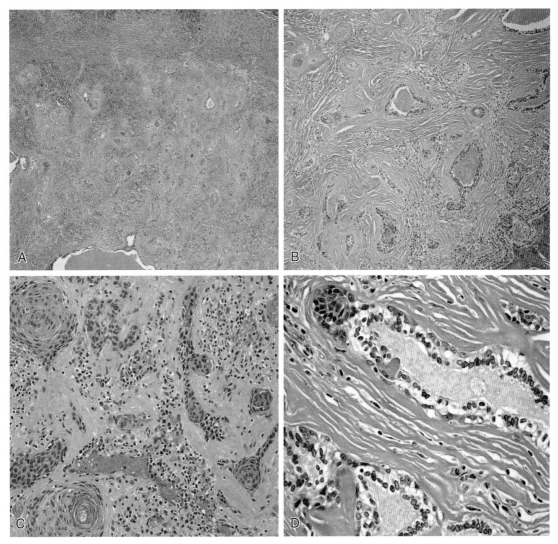

FIG. 10.19

A, Sclerosing mucoepidermoid carcinoma of thyroid with eosinophilia showing infiltrative growth pattern in the background of dense fibrosis. **B,** A combination of infiltrative thin cords of tumor and cysts are seen. **C,** Tumor nest with keratin whorl is seen in the lower portion of the photomicrograph. Note the presence of numerous eosinophils in the background. **D,** Mucicarmine stain highlights mucin-containing tumor cells.

TABLE 10.11

Histologic Features of Sclerosing Mucoepidermoid Carcinoma of Thyroid With Eosinophilia (SMECE) Versus Chronic Lymphocytic Thyroiditis (CLT), Solid Cell Nest (SCN), and Mucoepidermoid Carcinoma (MEC)

SMECE	CLT	SCN	MEC
• Infiltrative tumor	• Noninfiltrative	• Noninfiltrative	• Infiltrative tumor
• Epidermoid, glandular, and mucous cells present	• Squamous and oncocytic meta-plasia may be seen	• Squamoid or transitional appearing nests	• Epidermoid, glandular, and mucous cells present
• Small nests and thin cords of tumor	• Small metaplastic nests with squa-moid appearance may be present	• Small nests	• Large epithelial sheets or confluent nests present
• Fibosclerotic stroma present	• Fibroscerlotic stroma present	• Mild fibrosis may be seen	• Fibrosclertoic stroma may be present
• Numerous eosinophils present	• A moderate number of eosino-phils can be seen in some cases	• Eosinophils usually not seen	• Eosinophils usually not seen in abundance

Unlike conventional mucoepidermoid carcinoma (MEC), SMECE is negative for *MAML2* gene rearrangement.

Differential Diagnosis

While SMECE has a distinctive appearance, its rarity may cause diagnostic confusion with CLT, SCNs, or conventional MEC (Table 10.11). As the tumor occurs in a background of lymphocytic thyroiditis, confusion with reactive metaplastic changes in benign CLT may occur. In contrast to reactive changes in chronic lymphocytic reactive thyroiditis, SMECE is an infiltrative carcinoma which may show extrathyroidal invasion and perineural invasion. In addition, SMECE has a tumefactive appearance both grossly and microscopically. SCNs may have a squamoid appearance and may show cystic changes similar to SMECE. However, SCNs typically consist of small islands of squamoid or transitional epithelium and are not infiltrative. Distinction of SMECE from conventional mucoepidermoid involving the thyroid is difficult since they share similar cellular compositions. Conventional MEC involving the thyroid usually consists of larger sheets of squamoid-appearing cells (epidermoid cells) than SMECE and forms larger and more numerous cystic spaces than SMECE. The dense fibrous stroma rich with eosinophils, so characteristic of SMECE, is not usually observed in conventional MEC. *MAML2* gene rearrangement has been reported in some cases of primary MEC of the thyroid, which appears to be absent in SMECE.

Prognosis and Therapy

Initial reports suggested that SMECE was a low-grade malignant tumor. More recently, reports showing aggressive potential have emerged showing extrathyroidal extension and distant metastases to the lung, liver, or bone. The mainstay of treatment is surgical excision of the primary tumor with close observation. Additional adjuvant treatment may be administered in cases of recurrent or metastatic disease.

SCLEROSING MUCOEPIDERMOID CARCINOMA OF THYROID WITH EOSINOPHILIA – DISEASE FACT SHEET

Definition
▸▸ Malignant epithelial tumor showing epidermoid and glandular differentiation in a background of sclerotic stroma with numerous eosinophils, plasma cells, and lymphocytes

Incidence and Location
▸▸ Very rare tumor with mostly individual case reports documented

Age Distribution
▸▸ Most cases reported between approximately 30 and 80 years of age

Clinical Features
▸▸ Most commonly presents as slowly growing painless mass

Radiologic Features
▸▸ May present as cold nodule on thyroid scan or incidentally discovered nodule

Prognosis and Therapy
▸▸ Potential for aggressive behavior has been reported, with distant metastases reported in 20% of cases

---

SCLEROSING MUCOEPIDERMOID CARCINOMA OF THYROID WITH EOSINOPHILIA – PATHOLOGIC FEATURES

Gross Findings
▸▸ Tumors range from 1 to 13 cm
▸▸ Most tumors have poorly defined borders
▸▸ Firm white-tan cut surface

PARATHYROID CARCINOMA

DIFFERENTIAL DIAGNOSES: ATYPICAL PARATHYROID ADENOMA AND ONCOCYTIC FOLLICULAR NEOPLASMS

Clinical Features

Parathyroid carcinomas are rare and account for approximately 1% of cases of primary hyperparathyroidism. Compared to patients with parathyroid adenomas, those with parathyroid carcinomas are more likely to present with symptoms associated with hypercalcemia (e.g., weakness, polyuria, bone pain and/or fractures, and pancreatitis). Furthermore, the degree of hypercalcemia and symptoms tend to be more severe in patients with parathyroid carcinomas. These patients also are more likely to present with palpable neck mass than patients with parathyroid adenomas. There appears to be no sex predilection in patients with parathyroid carcinomas.

Pathologic Features

GROSS FINDINGS

Patients with parathyroid carcinomas tend to present with larger tumors (average weight of 12 g) than patients with parathyroid adenomas (average weight, <1 g). Parathyroid carcinomas tend to be firm and can either demonstrate overt gross evidence of invasion or can appear circumscribed. In the latter scenario, it is possible for these to be misdiagnosed as parathyroid adenomas on initial pathologic review.

MICROSCOPIC FINDINGS

The tumor cells in parathyroid carcinoma are generally polygonal and typically arranged in a trabecular architecture and/or solid sheets. Nuclei can range from being monotonously uniform and cytologically bland to

exhibiting severe pleomorphism. In fact, anisonucleosis is unreliable in distinguishing parathyroid carcinomas from parathyroid adenomas as both can demonstrate varying degrees of nuclear pleomorphism. Macronucleoli can be present especially when severe nuclear atypia is present. Mitotic activity is often evident but unreliable as a sole indicator in the diagnosis of malignancy. The cytoplasmic texture can range from vacuolated to oxyphilic in nature. Ultimately, gross and histologic evidence of invasive behavior is required for an absolute diagnosis of parathyroid carcinoma including: invasion of surrounding soft tissues, organs, and vital structures such as the thyroid gland, esophagus, and larynx; vascular invasion (Fig. 10.20); lymphovascular invasion; perineural invasion; and distant metastasis (Fig. 10.21).

Ancillary Studies

Immunohistochemistry for parathyroid hormone (PTH) can be helpful for confirming parathyroid origin for parathyroid carcinomas (Fig. 10.21B and C). About 60% to 70% of parathyroid carcinomas demonstrate loss of expression for parafibromin (Fig. 10.21D), the gene product of the HRPT2 gene that is implicated in the hyperparathyroidism-jaw tumor syndrome, as a result of inactivating mutations. In contrast, parathyroid adenomas should demonstrate retention of parafibromin gene expression. This is not a perfect marker, however, as approximately one-third of parathyroid carcinomas demonstrate normal parafibromin expression and rare parathyroid adenomas can exhibit aberrant loss of parafibromin expression. Immunohistochemistry for protein gene product 9.5 (PGP9.5) may also have utility in diagnosing parathyroid carcinomas, as overexpression would favor the diagnosis. Next, galectin-3 expression on immunohistochemistry tends to be expressed more frequently in parathyroid carcinomas. However, the utility of this marker is limited due to low sensitivity and the possibility that a small subset of parathyroid adenomas can also be positive for this marker. Finally, Ki67 immunohistochemistry tends to show a higher proliferation index in parathyroid carcinomas than in parathyroid adenomas (0.4%–26% vs. 0.5%–5.1%, respectively). A Ki67 proliferation index of greater than 5% appears to correlate with the diagnosis of parathyroid carcinoma; nonetheless, given the overlap in these Ki67 proliferation indices, a low proliferation index does not exclude the diagnosis of parathyroid carcinoma.

Differential Diagnosis

Definitive diagnosis of parathyroid carcinomas and accordingly, distinction from atypical parathyroid neoplasms

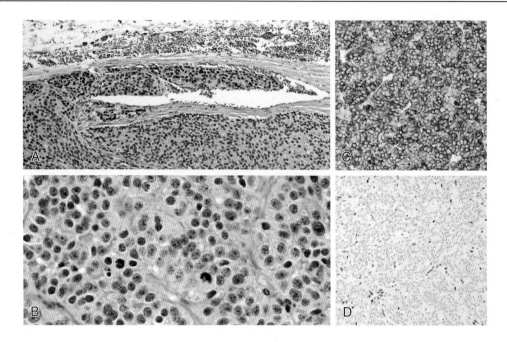

FIG. 10.20

Parathyroid carcinoma. **A,** Vascular invasion is present at the top aspect of the photomicrograph. **B,** Increased nuclear atypia and mitotic activity is evident on higher magnification. **C,** Immunohistochemistry for parathyroid hormone diffusely highlights the tumor cells. **D,** Loss of nuclear parafibromin expression is observed in the tumor cells. Endothelial cell nuclei retain expression (internal positive control).

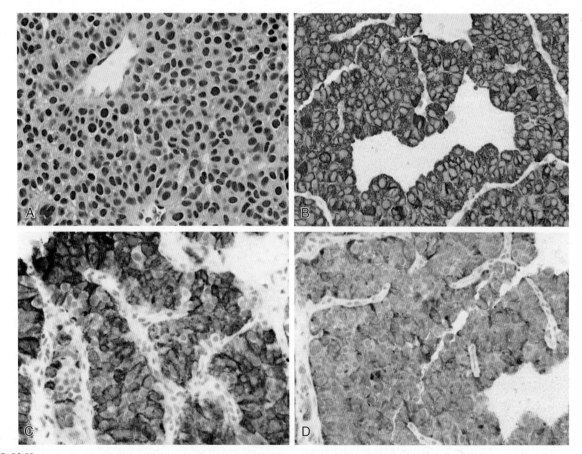

FIG. 10.21

The photomicrographs were obtained from a case of metastatic parathyroid carcinoma. **A,** Anisonucleosis and oxyphilic cytoplasm is evident in the tumor cells. A mitotic figure can be seen near the center of the image. **B,** Immunostain for parathyroid hormone highlights the tumor cells. The tumor cells are immunoreactive for the neuroendocrine markers chromogranin (**C**) and synaptophysin (**D**).

that fall short of a malignant diagnosis can be challenging (Table 10.12). Atypical parathyroid adenoma is a diagnosis that is rendered when a parathyroid neoplasm demonstrating some worrisome histologic features is encountered. Worrisome features that raise concern for malignancy but do not fulfill absolute pathologic criteria that justify the diagnosis of parathyroid carcinoma include: capsular invasion without unequivocal evidence of invasion into surrounding tissues; mitotic activity exceeding 5 per 10 HPF; dense fibrous banding within the neoplasm (Fig. 10.22); coagulative tumor necrosis; nuclear pleomorphism; or prominent macronucleoli. Typically, the management of atypical parathyroid adenomas consists of close clinical observation and follow-up with regular monitoring of serum calcium

and PTH levels. The role of immunohistochemical panels to distinguish between parathyroid carcinomas and atypical parathyroid adenomas continues to be investigated. The challenge lies in the rarity of parathyroid carcinomas and insufficient validation, especially with regard to whether a loss of parafibromin expression and positive expression of PGP9.5 can allow for a definitive reclassification of atypical parathyroid adenomas to parathyroid carcinomas.

Next, when parathyroid carcinomas present in close association with and invade the thyroid parenchyma, they can occasionally mimic oncocytic follicular cell neoplasms of the thyroid gland, particularly follicular carcinoma, oncocytic variant (Table 10.13). This malignant follicular neoplasm is encapsulated and demonstrates capsular invasion and/or vascular invasion (Fig. 10.23A), features that can be observed in parathyroid carcinomas. Morphologically, parathyroid carcinomas would not be expected to exhibit follicular architecture; hence, the presence of follicles (Fig. 10.23B) would help differentiate oncocytic follicular neoplasms from parathyroid carcinomas. Nonetheless, there are occasions where follicle formation is not readily evident in oncocytic follicular neoplasms (Fig. 10.23C), which could lead to morphologic overlap with parathyroid carcinomas. Especially when a widely invasive oncocytic variant of follicular carcinoma is encountered (Fig. 10.24), this can mimic a parathyroid carcinoma that invades and infiltrates the thyroid gland. Immunohistochemistry can be helpful in the distinction between parathyroid carcinomas and oncocytic follicular neoplasms. The latter would be expected to be positive for TTF1 and thyroglobulin while negative for PTH and neuroendocrine markers (chromogranin and synaptophysin); the former should exhibit the inverse immunophenotype.

TABLE 10.12

Histologic Features of Parathyroid Carcinomas Versus Atypical Parathyroid Adenomas

Parathyroid Carcinoma	Atypical Parathyroid Adenoma
• Invasion into surrounding soft tissues, organs, and vital structures	• Capsular invasion without unequivocal histologic evidence of invasion into surrounding tissues, organs, and vital structures
• Perineural invasion	• Dense fibrous banding
• Vascular invasion	• Nuclear pleomorphism
• Lymphovascular invasion	• Prominent macronucleoli
• Distant metastasis	• Elevated mitotic activity (>5 per 10 HPF)
	• Coagulative tumor necrosis
	• Absence of any of the criteria displayed on the left column

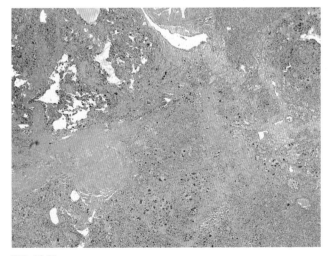

FIG. 10.22

Atypical parathyroid adenoma. Dense fibrotic bands are seen coursing throughout this parathyroid neoplasm. Even at this lower-magnification image, severe anisonucleosis is evident.

TABLE 10.13

Histologic and Immunohistochemical Features of Parathyroid Carcinoma Versus Oncocytic Thyroid Follicular Neoplasms

Parathyroid Carcinoma	Oncocytic Thyroid Follicular Neoplasms
• Follicular architecture is typically absent	• Follicular architecture present to varying degrees
• Immunoreactive for PTH	• Negative for PTH on immunohistochemistry
• Negative for TTF1 and thyroglobulin on immunohistochemistry	• Immunoreactive for TTF1 and thyroglobulin
• Immunoreactive for neuroendocrine markers (chromogranin and synaptophysin)	• Negative for chromogranin and synaptophysin on immunohistochemistry

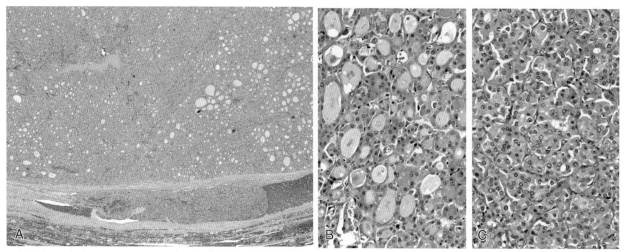

FIG. 10.23

Follicular carcinoma, oncocytic variant. **A,** The encapsulated nature of this oncocytic follicular neoplasm is evident. Furthermore, a focus of angioinvasion is present at the bottom aspect of the tumor. **B,** Some areas of the tumor clearly demonstrated a follicular architecture. **C,** In other areas of the tumor, follicle formation was not readily evident.

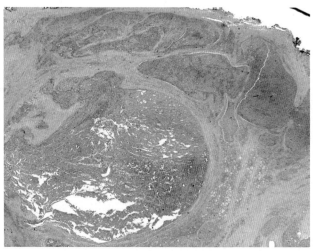

FIG. 10.24

Widely invasive oncocytic follicular carcinoma. In this low-magnification image, the clearly infiltrative nature of the tumor within the thyroid parenchyma can be appreciated. This appearance can mimic parathyroid carcinoma in cases where the tumor invades and infiltrates the thyroid parenchyma.

Prognosis and Therapy

Parathyroid carcinomas are usually treated by surgical excision. Despite their generally indolent nature, local recurrence and metastasis can be seen in up to one third to half of patients. Radiation therapy contributes to reducing the frequency of local recurrences. The value of chemotherapy is questionable. Complications secondary to hypercalcemia is more likely to contribute to death rather than tumor burden late in the course of the disease.

PARATHYROID CARCINOMA – DISEASE FACT SHEET

Definition

▸▸ Invasive carcinoma composed epithelial cells of parathyroid origin
▸▸ Demonstrates invasion of surrounding soft tissues, organs, and vital structures (e.g., thyroid gland, larynx, trachea, esophagus, and/or carotid artery)
▸▸ Presence of vascular, lymphovascular, perineural invasion, and/or distant metastasis

Incidence and Location

▸▸ Can present as a palpable neck mass due to the relatively large size of the tumor (average weight, 12 g)

Age Distribution

▸▸ Patients with parathyroid carcinomas are typically diagnosed in their 40s or 50s
▸▸ Patients with parathyroid carcinomas tend to be younger by approximately one decade on average than patients with parathyroid adenomas

Clinical Features

▸▸ The vast majority of tumors are functional and it is common for patients to exhibit symptoms related to hypercalcemia

Radiologic Features

▸▸ Depending on the degree of invasion into adjacent tissues, organs, and vital structures, the invasive nature of the tumor may be evident on radiologic imaging

Prognosis and Therapy

▸▸ Surgical excision of the tumor and adjacent affected tissue(s) represents the mainstay of treatment
▸▸ Postoperative radiation therapy can reduce local recurrences. The benefit of chemotherapy is inconclusive.
▸▸ Complications related to hypercalcemia contribute significantly to morbidity and mortality

---

PARATHYROID CARCINOMA – PATHOLOGIC FEATURES

Gross Findings

▸▸ Parathyroid carcinomas, on average, are larger at presentation than parathyroid adenomas

▸▸ Tumors are firm with a tan to gray complexion

▸▸ Overt evidence of invasion into adjacent tissues and organs may be grossly evident

Microscopic Findings

▸▸ Polygonal cells arranged in trabeculae and/or solid sheets

▸▸ Nuclear pleomorphism is common but occasional tumors can be more cytologically bland and monotonous

▸▸ Cytoplasm can be clear to oxyphilic in nature

▸▸ Invasion into adjacent soft tissues, organs, and vital structures

▸▸ The presence of perineural invasion, vascular invasion, lymphovascular invasion, and/or distant metastasis allows for the diagnosis of malignancy

▸▸ Macronucleoli and mitotic activity can be evident

Pathologic Differential Diagnoses

▸▸ Atypical parathyroid adenoma

▸▸ Oncocytic follicular neoplasms of the thyroid

ADRENAL CORTICAL CARCINOMA

DIFFERENTIAL DIAGNOSES: METASTATIC RENAL CELL CARCINOMA, METASTATIC HEPATOCELLULAR CARCINOMA, EPITHELIOID ANGIOSARCOMA

Clinical Features

Adrenal cortical carcinoma (ACC) affects approximately 1 to 2 patients per million in the population. These tumors can occur at any age; however, they are more frequently encountered in patients in the fourth and fifth decades of life. There is a slight female predilection and the left adrenal gland is slightly more often involved than the right adrenal gland. Metastasis is common at the time of presentation and in one series by van Slooten et al., 93% of patients exhibited metastases within 10 years of initial diagnosis. The lung and liver represent the most common sites of metastasis. The mortality rate overall exceeds 70%.

Pathologic Features

GROSS FINDINGS

ACCs are bulky tumors and can range in weight from approximately 500 to 1200 g; cases of tumors exceeding 4500 g have been reported. They are often coarsely lobulated and variegated with a tan to yellow complexion and admixed areas of hemorrhage and necrosis.

MICROSCOPIC FINDINGS

ACCs can exhibit a variety and combination of architectural patterns including nested, solid, and trabecular with anastomosing cords. The cytoplasm of the tumor cells can range from a vacuolated to a lipid-depleted, eosinophilic texture. Anisonucleosis can often be appreciated; however, this feature alone does not equate to malignancy. The Weiss system is commonly utilized to assess the malignant potential of adrenal cortical neoplasms. Histologic criteria evaluated in this system include the presence of high nuclear grade, mitotic rate of greater than 5 per 50 HPF, presence of atypical mitotic figures, clear cells comprising ≤25% of the tumor, diffuse architecture in greater than one third of the tumor, tumor necrosis, invasion of venous structures, invasion of sinusoidal structures, and capsular invasion. The most specific features of ACCs include mitotic rate of greater than 5 per 50 HPF, atypical mitoses, and invasion of venous structures. This system was subsequently modified in order to eliminate criteria that were considered more subjective and prone to higher interobserver variability. The modified Weiss system evaluates only five histologic criteria: mitotic rate (>5 per 50 HPF); cytoplasm (clear cells comprising ≤25% of the tumor volume); atypical mitotic figures; necrosis; and capsular invasion. A score is given based on the presence of any of these five parameters and equates to $2 \times$ mitotic rate $+ 2 \times$ cytoplasm $+$ atypical mitotic figures $+$ necrosis $+$ capsular invasion. A score of 3 or greater correlates with malignant biologic behavior and therefore permits the diagnosis of ACC. The histologic findings of one example of ACC are illustrated in Fig. 10.25A–C.

Ancillary Studies

Immunohistochemistry is often utilized to distinguish ACCs from other malignancies, especially metastases (Fig. 10.25D–G). The vast majority of these tumors demonstrate nuclear immunoreactivity for steroidogenic factor-1 (SF-1). Variable degrees of Melan-A, inhibin, and calretinin expression are also observed in ACCs. Although cytokeratin immunoreactivity can range from none to focal or patchy, diffuse immunoreactivity for cytokeratins is not a characteristic feature in these tumors. Furthermore, immunohistochemistry for synaptophysin is also often positive in these tumors. The immunostain chromogranin is typically negative in ACC. Although ACCs tend to demonstrate a higher Ki67 proliferative index, the extent of Ki67 positivity ranges widely in these tumors and sometimes overlaps with the Ki67 labeling indices of adrenocortical adenomas.

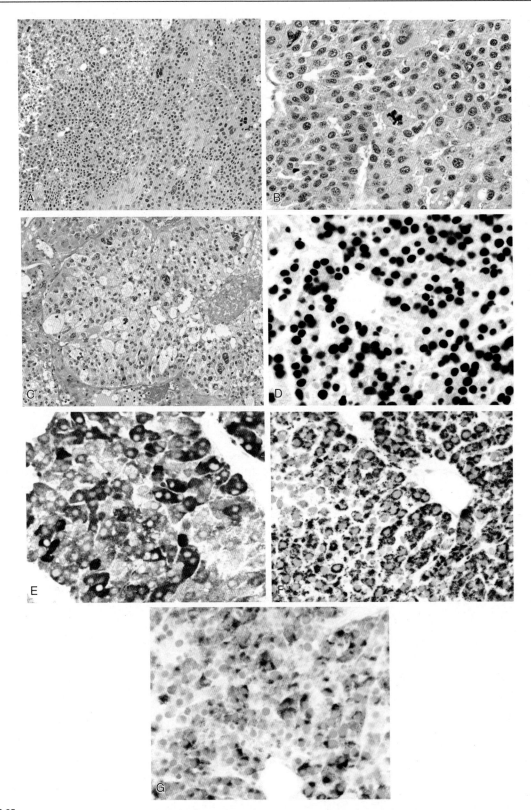

FIG. 10.25

Adrenal cortical carcinoma. **A,** At low magnification, sheets and vague trabecular arrays of malignant-appearing epithelial cells with eosinophilic and focally vacuolated cytoplasm are appreciable. Anisonucleosis is evident and a tripolar mitotic figure is present at the right edge of the photomicrograph. **B,** In this higher-magnification image, an atypical mitosis is evident in the center. **C,** In other areas of the tumor, marked nuclear pleomorphism and vacuolization of the cytoplasm were present. **D,** Immunohistochemistry for SF-1 highlights the nuclei of the tumor cells. Cytoplasmic immunoreactivity for inhibin (**E**), Melan A (**F**), and synaptophysin (**G**) was observed.

Differential Diagnosis

The morphologic features of ACCs can be similar to those of a variety of malignant epithelioid neoplasms. For the purposes of this section, the discussion will center around three particular entities in the differential diagnosis: metastatic RCC, metastatic hepatocellular carcinoma (HCC), and epithelioid angiosarcoma (Table 10.14). It is not uncommon for RCCs to involve the adjacent, ipsilateral adrenal gland. Both ACCs and RCCs can demonstrate clear to eosinophilic cytoplasm and high-grade nuclei with prominent nucleoli. Clear cell RCCs are most likely to be encountered in the adrenal gland and tend to demonstrate a nested architecture associated with a delicate capillary network (Fig. 10.26). Immunohistochemistry is helpful in distinguishing between metastatic RCC and

ACC in challenging instances. Unlike ACCs, metastatic RCCs would be expected to be positive for PAX8 and RCC antigen while negative for SF-1, inhibin, and Melan A.

Next, metastatic HCC can exhibit varying degrees of clear to granular cytoplasm (Fig. 10.27). As these tumors often demonstrate widened cords of malignant epithelial cells, this architectural pattern can mimic the trabecular architecture of some ACCs. Again, immunohistochemistry can be of value in distinguishing between these two entities. HCCs should demonstrate positivity for HepPar1 and/or arginase and not demonstrate immunoreactivity for SF-1, inhibin, or Melan A.

Finally, epithelioid angiosarcomas have been known to occasionally arise in the adrenal gland. These tumors can demonstrate varying degrees of nuclear atypia and pleomorphism similar to ACCs. They can be distinguished from ACCs based on their peculiar architectural

TABLE 10.14

Histologic and Immunohistochemical Features of Adrenal Cortical Carcinoma (ACC) Versus Metastatic Renal Cell Carcinoma (RCC), Metastatic Hepatocellular Carcinoma (HCC), and Epithelioid Angiosarcoma

ACC	Metastatic RCC	Metastatic HCC	Epithelioid Angiosarcoma
• Nested, diffuse sheet-like, and/or trabecular architecture	• Nested architecture associated with delicate capillary network	• Widened trabecular cords of malignant epithelial cells	• Tumor cells line vascular spaces and can demonstrate intracytoplasmic lumina filled with red blood cells
• Clear to eosinophilic cytoplasm	• Clear to eosinophilic cytoplasm	• Cytoplasm usually granular but can be vacuolated	• Delicate cytoplasm
• Variable degrees of nuclear pleomorphism	• Variable degree of nuclear atypia depending on grade	• Variable degrees of nuclear atypia	• Variable degrees of nuclear atypia
• Immunoreactive for SF1, synaptophysin, inhibin, and Melan A	• Immunoreactive for PAX8 and RCC antigen	• Immunoreactive for HepPar1 and arginase	• Immunoreactive for CD31, CD34, ERG, and Fli-1

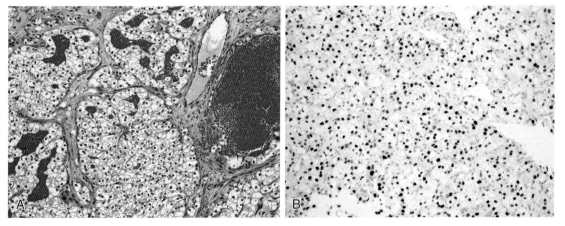

FIG. 10.26

Metastatic renal cell carcinoma to the adrenal gland. **A,** Nests of neoplastic epithelial cells with vacuolization of the cytoplasm are intimately associated with delicate vasculature. **B,** Immunohistochemistry for PAX8 highlights the tumor cell nuclei.

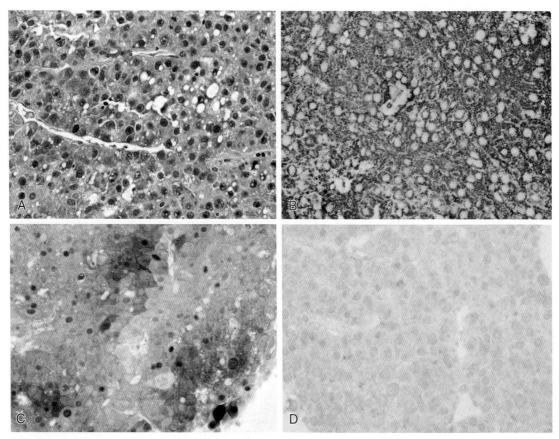

FIG. 10.27

Metastatic hepatocellular carcinoma to the adrenal gland. **A,** Widened cords and trabeculae of neoplastic epithelial cells with vacuolated to granular cytoplasm are present. Immunohistochemistry for arginase (**B**) and HepPar1 (**C**) demonstrate cytoplasmic immunoreactivity in the tumor cells. **D,** Immunohistochemistry for SF-1 is negative in the tumor cells.

pattern. Specifically, the tumor cells in epithelioid angiosarcoma tend to line vascular spaces and can demonstrate intracytoplasmic lumina. These spaces and lumina are occupied by erythrocytes, a distinctive feature of this tumor. Immunohistochemical staining for vascular markers (CD31, CD34, ERG, and Fli-1) can be of aid in confirming the diagnosis of epithelioid angiosarcoma (Fig. 10.28).

Prognosis and Therapy

The prognosis of ACC is poor, with an overall mortality rate of at least 70%. Survival depends mostly on the degree to which the tumor is surgically removed; incompletely resected tumors are uniformly associated with poor outcomes. The presence of metastasis at the time of presentation, predictably, would render surgical intervention less effective of an option. With respect to metastasis, the lung and liver represent two most common sites of metastatic involvement. Chemotherapy is often utilized in patients with ACCs.

ADRENAL CORTICAL CARCINOMA – DISEASE FACT SHEET

Definition
▸▸ Malignant tumor derived from the adrenal cortex
▸▸ Weiss criteria or the modified Weiss system is utilized to assess for malignancy

Incidence and Location
▸▸ Affects 1–2 patients per million in the population
▸▸ Either adrenal gland can be involved but the left adrenal gland is slightly more affected

Age Distribution
▸▸ ACCs are frequently encountered in patients in the fourth and fifth decades of life

Clinical Features
▸▸ These tumors are generally biologically aggressive tumors; metastasis at the time of presentation is common
▸▸ The liver and lung represent most common sites of metastatic involvement

Radiologic Features
▸▸ Large retroperitoneal tumors in the suprarenal region can be appreciated on imaging

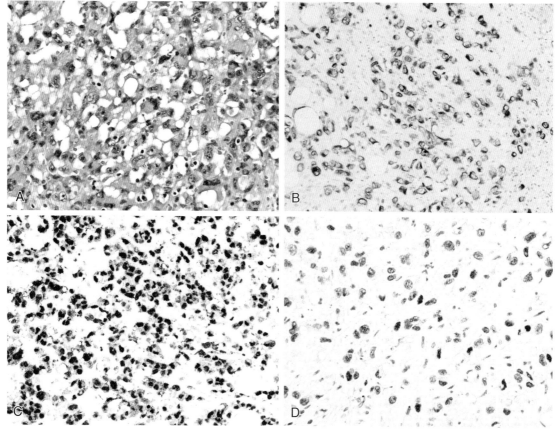

FIG. 10.28

Epithelioid angiosarcoma of the adrenal gland. **A,** Neoplastic epithelioid tumor cells are associated with delicate vascular spaces and demonstrate intracytoplasmic lumina containing erythrocytes. **B,** Immunoreactivity for cytokeratin OSCAR was observed in this tumor. Immunohistochemistry for ERG (**C**) and Fli-1 (**D**) highlight the nuclei of the tumor cells.

▸▸ Imaging can also reveal whether the tumor has metastasized which can preoperatively support the impression of a malignant adrenal cortical tumor

Prognosis and Therapy

▸▸ Prognosis is generally poor with an overall mortality rate of 70% or more
▸▸ Surgical resection of localized tumors; chemotherapy often utilized especially in the context of metastases

---

ADRENAL CORTICAL CARCINOMA – PATHOLOGIC FEATURES

Gross Findings

▸▸ ACCs tend to be large tumors and can range in weight from 500 to 1200 g; tumors exceeding 4500 g have been reported
▸▸ Coarsely lobulated and variegated with tan to yellow complexion
▸▸ Admixed areas of hemorrhage and necrosis

Microscopic Findings

▸▸ Epithelial cells arranged in a nested, trabecular, and/or solid, sheet-like architecture
▸▸ Nuclear pleomorphism is common
▸▸ Cytoplasm can be clear to eosinophilic

▸▸ Mitotic activity is appreciable; atypical mitotic figures can be seen
▸▸ Capsular, vascular, and/or sinusoidal invasion present
▸▸ Geographic tumor necrosis can be variably present

Pathologic Differential Diagnoses

▸▸ Metastatic carcinomas (e.g., RCC and HCC)
▸▸ Epithelioid angiosarcoma

ADENOMATOID TUMOR

DIFFERENTIAL DIAGNOSIS: ADRENAL CORTICAL NEOPLASMS, VASCULAR NEOPLASMS, METASTATIC ADENOCARCINOMA, MESOTHELIOMA

Clinical Features

The majority of adenomatoid tumors are incidentally discovered, producing no clinical symptoms. Rare cases may cause symptoms related to mass effect on the adjacent adrenal tissue, such as hypertension. The tumor has a male-to-female ratio of 10:1.

Pathologic features

GROSS FINDINGS

The usual tumor size is 1 to 3.0 cm, but a wide size range has been reported. Adenomatoid tumors are usually circumscribed with a yellow-tan cut surface. Cystic changes may be present.

MICROSCOPIC FINDINGS

Adenomatoid tumor shows solid, adenoidal, and cystic growth patterns formed by variously sized tubular structures. The growth pattern can impart an angiomatoid or glandular appearance. A variable amount of fibrous tissue is present in the background. The tubular spaces are lined by epithelial cells containing pink cytoplasm, which varies in abundance, from flattened endothelial-like cells to polygonal cells with abundant cytoplasm.

Cytoplasmic vacuolization may create signet-ring–like cells. The nuclei may show some size variability and contain dark chromatin. Mitotic activity is usually sparse to absent.

Ancillary Studies

Adenomatoid tumors are positive for WT-1, D2-40, and calretinin indicating the tumor is derived from mesothelial cells. Immunostaining for Melan-A, SF-1, inhibin, CD31, CD34, and CK5/6 are negative.

Differential Diagnosis

The tubular growth pattern and angiomatoid appearance of adenomatoid tumor overlap with vascular tumors and metastatic adenocarcinoma (Fig. 10.29 and Table 10.15). The absence of staining with CD31 and CD34, and positivity for mesothelial markers should exclude vascular

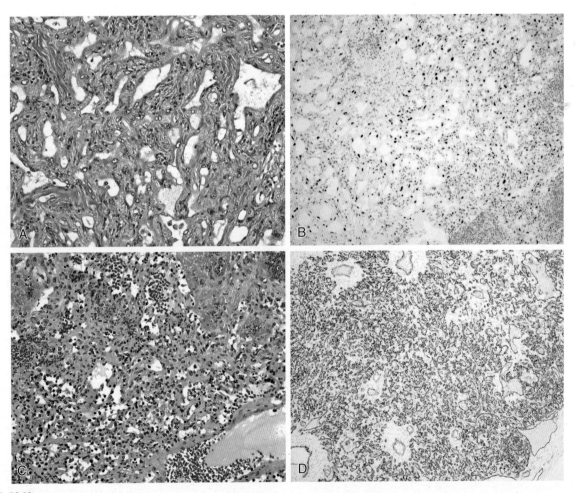

FIG. 10.29

A, Adenomatoid tumor showing a packed tubular growth pattern. **B,** WT-1 positivity in adenomatoid tumor. **C,** Hemangioma involving adrenal gland showing vascular spaces containing erythrocytes. **D,** CD31 highlighting endothelial cells of hemangioma.

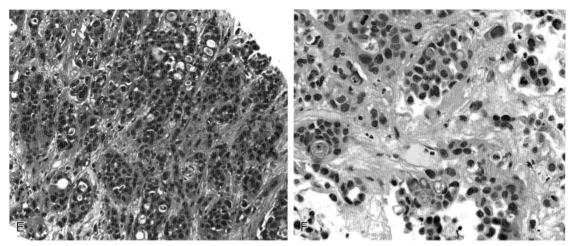

FIG. 10.29, cont'd

E, Metastatic adenocarcinoma involving adrenal gland with marked cytologic atypia. **F,** Mucicarmine-positive cells highlight secretions in metastatic adenocarcinoma.

TABLE 10.15

Histologic and Immunohistochemical Features of Adenomatoid Tumor Versus Metastatic Adenocarcinoma, Vascular Neoplasms, and Mesothelioma

Adenomatoid Tumor	Metastatic Adenocarcinoma	Vascular Neoplasms	Mesothelioma
• Usually tightly packed tubular growth pattern present with a sieve-like appearance	• Tubular or solid growth patterns common	• Varies from well-formed vessels to poorly formed vascular channels	• Nested, solid, corded and papillary patterns observed. Tubular structures may be seen.
• Usually circumscribed, noninvasive	• Usually appears infiltrative	• Benign hemangioma appears noninvasive. Malignant vascular tumor appears infiltrative.	• Appears infiltrative
• Benign cytology	• Malignant cytologic appearance. Mucin may be present.	• Benign cytologic features in hemangioma. Malignant vascular tumors usually show marked atypia.	• Marked cytologic atypia usually present.
• Immunoreactive for WT-1, calretinin, and D2-40	• Negative for WT-1, calretinin, and D2-40. May be positive for lineage-specific markers according to site of origin.	• Negative for WT-1, calretinin, and D2-40. Immunoreactive for vascular markers.	• Immunoreactive for WT-1, calretinin, and D2-40

neoplasms. Overall, adenomatoid tumor is cytologically bland, not showing significant nuclear pleomorphism, coarse chromatin, or conspicuous mitotic activity seen in metastatic adenocarcinomas. In addition, staining of adenomatoid tumor for markers of mesothelial differentiation excludes the possibility of metastatic adenocarcinoma. Adrenal cortical neoplasms may enter into the differential diagnosis with adenomatoid tumor. However, the extensive tubular architecture seen in adenomatoid tumor is not typically observed in adrenal cortical neoplasms. In addition, adenomatoid tumor is negative for markers of adrenal cortical differentiation such as SF-1. Mesothelioma and adenomatoid tumor are both positive for markers of mesothelial differentiation. However, the circumscribed appearance of adenomatoid tumor, innocuous cytologic features, and lack of infiltrative growth excludes the possibility of mesothelioma.

Prognosis and Therapy

Adenomatoid tumor is a clinically benign tumor. Surgical excision is curative.

ADENOMATOID TUMOR – DISEASE FACT SHEET

Definition
▸▸ Benign tumor of mesothelial cell origin

Incidence and Location
▸▸ Rare tumor, true incidence is not known
▸▸ Left adrenal gland is involved more frequently than right

Continued

PHEOCHROMOCYTOMA

DIFFERENTIAL DIAGNOSIS: ADRENAL CORTICAL NEOPLASMS, METASTATIC NEUROENDOCRINE TUMOR/CARCINOMA

Clinical Features

Pheochromocytoma affects approximately equal numbers of males and females, with most occurring between the fourth and fifth decades of life. However, the age range is wide. Syndromic cases tend to present at younger ages. Genetic predisposition for pheochromocytoma occurs in several syndromes such as multiple endocrine neoplasia type 1, von Hippel-Lindau syndrome, and neurofibromatosis type 2. Germline mutations involving the succinate dehydrogenase complex are the most common cause of hereditary pheochromocytoma/paraganglioma. Clinical signs and symptoms of catecholamine excess are seen in many patients, most commonly signaled by hypertension. Other symptoms include headache, tachycardia, sweating, and palpitations. Pheochromocytomas can also rarely cause Cushing syndrome by ACTH or CRH secretion.

Pathologic Features

GROSS FINDINGS

Pheochromocytomas are circumscribed tumors usually measuring about 3 to 5 cm, centered in the adrenal medulla. Larger tumors can compress and thin the surrounding cortex. The tumor is not encapsulated; however, a pseudocapsule may be identified, separating the mass from the adjacent adrenal cortex.

MICROSCOPIC FINDINGS

Pheochromocytomas are composed of chromaffin cells, which are usually arranged as rounded nests referred to as "zellballen" (Fig. 10.30A). The tumor nests are segregated by a delicate capillary network and also surrounded by a variable number of sustentacular cells (Fig. 10.30B). Larger organoid nests, trabecular cords, and diffuse growth patterns may also be seen. Cytologically, the tumor cells usually contain granular cytoplasm that appears basophilic or amphophilic. The tumor cells contain variably sized nuclei, including scattered large nuclei with open chromatin and prominent nucleoli. Intranuclear pseudoinclusions and cytoplasmic hyaline globules are common. Mitoses are typically few in number. Ganglion cells may be present in some cases.

Ancillary Studies

Pheochromocytoma is positive for markers of neuroendocrine differentiation such as chromogranin and synaptophysin. Immunostaining for S-100 and Sox-10 can highlight sustentacular cells. Pheochromocytoma also shows immunohistochemical expression of tyrosine hydroxylase and dopamine beta-hydroxylase, enzymes involved in the synthesis of catecholamines.

Differential Diagnosis

The primary differential considerations with pheochromocytoma include adrenal cortical neoplasms and metastatic neuroendocrine tumors or neuroendocrine carcinomas (Fig. 10.31 and Table 10.16). Adrenal cortical neoplasms can show a nested growth pattern similar to pheochromocytoma and can share some degree of cytologic overlap. However, other growth patterns, such as solid or trabecular growth, are usually more common in adrenal cortical neoplasms. In challenging cases where morphologic overlap is present, use of immunostains is helpful in separating these two entities. Pheochromocytoma does not express markers of adrenal cortical cells

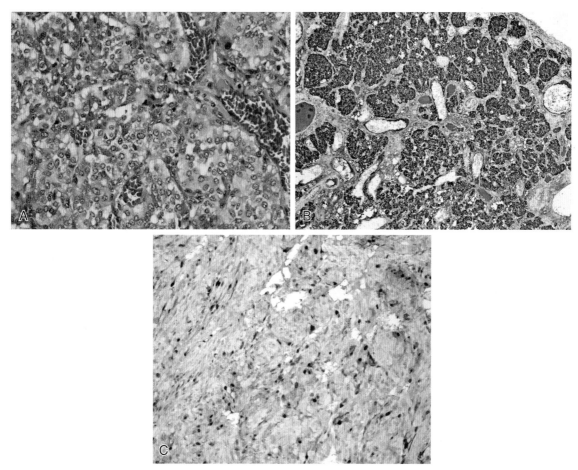

FIG. 10.30
Pheochromocytoma. **A,** Typical "zellballen" growth pattern. **B,** Strong staining for chromogranin. **C,** S-100 positive sustentacular cells.

including SF-1 and Melan-A. Pheochromocytoma is positive for neuroendocrine markers and S-100 usually highlights sustentacular cells. In addition, pheochromocytoma is negative for cytokeratin stains, whereas adrenal cortical neoplasms can show variable positivity for cytokeratins such as Oscar, AE1/AE3, and Cam5.2. Caution should be exercised with synaptophysin staining, as both adrenal cortical neoplasms and pheochromocytoma are positive for synaptophysin. However, pheochromocytoma is usually diffusely positive chromogranin, which is usually negative in adrenal cortical neoplasms.

Metastatic neuroendocrine tumors and carcinomas involving the adrenal gland are relatively common, especially in the case of small cell carcinoma. These tumors can show an organoid or nested growth pattern, which may create diagnostic difficulty in some cases. The nests seen in metastatic neuroendocrine tumors or carcinomas usually show greater variability ins size and shape and may be associated with a greater degree of fibrosis. On a clinical level, if the tumor produces excessive catecholamines, this usually correlates with the diagnosis of pheochromocytoma. As overt malignant cytological features are uncommon in the usual pheochromocytoma, if marked cytologic atypia is present, consideration should be given to the possibility of metastatic neuroendocrine carcinoma. Metastatic neuroendocrine tumors and carcinomas are frequently cytokeratin positive. In contrast, pheochromocytoma is usually negative for all cytokeratin immunostains or, at most, shows focal weak immunoreactivity. In small-cell carcinoma, a dot-like para-nuclear pattern of staining may be seen with pancytokeratins. In addition, TTF-1 and CDX-2 immunostains are negative in pheochromocytoma and may be expressed in metastatic neuroendocrine tumors or carcinomas. Furthermore, staining for S-100 can be useful to highlight the sustentacular cells surrounding the tumor nests of pheochromocytoma.

Prognosis and Therapy

All pheochromocytomas are thought to have some metastatic potential. Malignancy is most reliably diagnosed when extensive local invasion is identified, or when metastatic disease is identified at a site where normal chromaffin tissue is absent. Two proposed risk assessment systems are the Pheochromocytoma of the Adrenal gland Scale Score (PASS) and Grading System

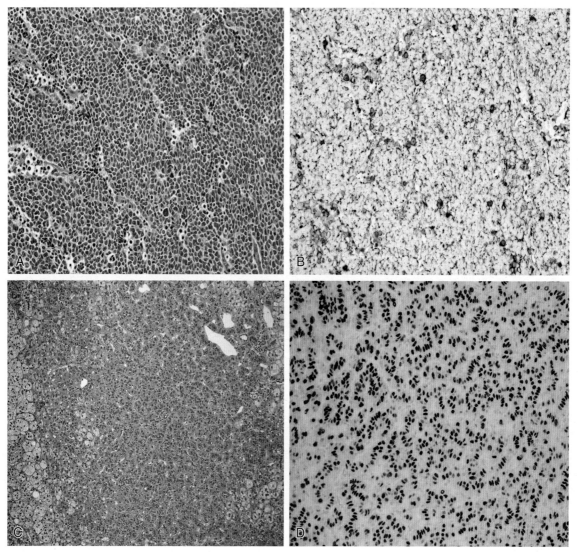

FIG. 10.31

A, Metastatic small cell carcinoma showing nested/organoid growth pattern and high-grade features. **B,** Dot-like paranuclear staining pattern with cytokeratin staining in small cell carcinoma. **C,** Adrenal cortical adenoma showing nested growth composed of eosinophilic to clear cells. **D,** SF-1 positivity of adrenal cortical adenoma.

TABLE 10.16

Histologic and Immunohistochemical Features of Pheochromocytoma Versus Adrenal Cortical Neoplasms and Metastatic Neuroendocrine Tumors or Carcinoma

Pheochromocytoma	Adrenal Cortical Neoplasms	Metastatic Neuroendocrine Tumor or Carcinoma
• Nested (zellballen) architecture is typical	• May show nested growth pattern, but other patterns (such as solid or trabecular) are usually also present.	• Tumor nests are usually more variable in size and shape compared to pheochromocytoma.
• Negative for cytokeratin stains and positive for markers of neuroendocrine differentiation • S-100 positive sustentacular cells are present	• Variable expression for cytokeratin stains • Synaptophysin positivity can be seen; however, chromogranin is negative • S-100 positive sustentacular cells absent	• Frequently positive for cytokeratin stains • Positive for neuroendocrine markers • S-100 positive sustentacular-like cells usually absent

for Adrenal Pheochromocytoma and Paraganglioma (GAPP). Both systems take into account several histologic parameters such as vascular or invasion, necrosis, and the histologic growth pattern. The GAPP score also includes Ki-67 labeling index and type of catecholamine produced to stratify risk. The prognosis is also dependent on the genetic profile of the tumor. Inherited SDHB mutations are associated with a higher risk of metastasis. The overall 5-year survival rate of metastatic pheochromocytoma is 34% to 60%. Complete surgical excision is the primary treatment of choice for pheochromocytoma. For metastatic disease, various adjuvant therapies may be employed including chemotherapy and peptide receptor radionuclide therapy.

PHEOCHROMOCYTOMA – PATHOLOGIC FEATURES

Gross Findings

▸▸ Circumscribed, usually unencapsulated tumor with a pink-gray to tan surface. Hemorrhage, degenerative changes, and fibrosis may be present.

Microscopic Findings

▸▸ Nested growth pattern supported by delicate fibrovascular network is the most common pattern seen

Pathologic Differential Diagnoses

▸▸ Adrenal cortical neoplasms, metastatic neuroendocrine tumor, metastatic neuroendocrine carcinoma

---

PHEOCHROMOCYTOMA – DISEASE FACT SHEET

Definition

▸▸ Neoplasm composed of chromaffin cells arising from the adrenal medulla

Incidence and Location

▸▸ Arise in the adrenal glands with an incidence of approximately 0.95 per 100,000 person-years

Age Distribution

▸▸ Most tumors present in the fourth to fifth decade of life

Clinical Features

▸▸ Signs and symptoms attributable to excess catecholamine secretion seen in many cases. 24% of cases present with a triad of headache, tachycardia, and sweating. 51% of reported cases were discovered by blood pressure anomalies.

Radiologic Features

▸▸ MRI shows a hyperintense mass with T2-weighted imaging

Prognosis and Therapy

▸▸ Malignancy rate historically cited to be approximately 10%; however, lower or higher rates have been reported depending on how malignancy is defined or mutation status. Surgery is usually the primary treatment modality. Greater than 90% of patients with nonmetastatic disease at presentation are alive 5 years after surgery.

SUGGESTED READINGS

Diffuse Sclerosing Variant of Papillary Thyroid Carcinoma

Carcangiu ML, Bianchi S. Diffuse sclerosing variant of papillary thyroid carcinoma: clinicopathologic study of 15 cases. *Am J Surg Pathol.* 1989;13(12):1041-1049.

Chan JK, Tsui MS, Tse CH. Diffuse sclerosing variant of papillary carcinoma of the thyroid: a histological and immunohistochemical study of three cases. *Histopathology.* 1987;11(2):191-201.

Fujimoto Y, Obara T, Ito Y, Kodama T, Aiba M, Yamaguchi K. Diffuse sclerosing variant of papillary carcinoma of the thyroid: clinical importance, surgical treatment, and follow-up study. *Cancer.* 1990;66(11):2306-2312.

Jung HK, Hong SW, Kim EK, Yoon JH, Kwak JY. Diffuse sclerosing variant of papillary thyroid carcinoma: sonography and specimen radiography. *J Ultrasound Med.* 2013;32(2):347-354.

Lee JY, Shin JH, Han BK, et al. Diffuse sclerosing variant of papillary carcinoma of the thyroid: imaging and cytologic findings. *Thyroid.* 2007;17(6):567-573.

Marshall CB. Diffuse sclerosing variant of papillary thyroid carcinoma preoperative diagnosis through imaging and cytology allows for optimal patient care. *Pathol Case Rev.* 2015;20:125-128.

Rossi ED, Faquin WC, Pantanowitz L. Aggressive variants of follicular- and parafollicular-derived thyroid carcinoma. *AJSP: Reviews & Reports.* 2019;24(2):61-71.

Soares J, Limbert E, Sobrinho-Simões M. Diffuse sclerosing variant of papillary thyroid carcinoma: a clinicopathologic study of 10 cases. *Pathol Res Pract.* 1989;185(2):200-206.

Thompson LDR, Wieneke JA, Heffess CS. Diffuse sclerosing variant of papillary thyroid carcinoma: a clinicopathologic and immunophenotypic analysis of 22 cases. *Endocr Pathol.* 2005;16(4):331-348.

Vickery AL Jr, Carcangiu ML, Johannessen JV, Sobrinho-Simoes M. Papillary carcinoma. *Semin Diagn Pathol.* 1985;2(2):90-100.

Hyalinizing Trabecular Tumor of Thyroid

Carney JA, Ryan J, Goellner JR. Hyalinizing trabecular adenoma of the thyroid gland. *Am J Surg Pathol.* 1987;11(8):583-591.

Nikiforova MN, Nikitski AV, Panebianco F, et al. GLIS rearrangement is a genomic hallmark of hyalinizing trabecular tumor of the thyroid gland. *Thyroid.* 2019;29(2):161-173.

Adrenal Cortical Carcinoma

van Slooten H, Schaberg A, Smeenk D, Moolenaar AJ. Morphologic characteristics of benign and malignant adrenocortical tumors. *Cancer.* 1985;55(4):766-773.

11 Lung

Grace Lin • Vera Vavinskaya

SQUAMOUS PAPILLOMA

> **DIFFERENTIAL DIAGNOSES: GLANDULAR PAPILLOMA, MIXED SQUAMOUS CELL AND GLANDULAR PAPILLOMA, AND SQUAMOUS CELL CARCINOMA**

Clinical Features

Squamous cell papillomas account for less than 1% of lung neoplasms and are much less common compared with their incidence in the upper aerodigestive tract. However, they are the most common type of papilloma in the lung. Patients typically present with cough, wheezing, or hemoptysis. Up to 25% of patients are asymptomatic, and papillomas are discovered as incidental radiographic findings. Squamous cell papillomas may be either solitary or multiple.

Solitary squamous papillomas are more commonly found in men than in women (3:1) and occur in the fifth to sixth decade of life. Most patients with solitary lesions are smokers. About half of the cases are associated with human papillomavirus (HPV), most commonly low-risk serotypes 6 and 11.

Multiple squamous papillomas are associated with recurrent respiratory papillomatosis and involvement of the upper aerodigestive tract. Recurrent respiratory papillomatosis occurs in children (<20 years of age) and adults (30–40 years of age). Between 2% and 8% of patients show involvement of the lower respiratory tract, and less than 5% of cases show extension into the alveolar parenchyma. Bronchial or pulmonary involvement may be associated with either reflux disease or prior therapy. Virtually all cases of recurrent respiratory papillomatosis are associated with HPV, most commonly low-risk serotypes 6 and 11. High-risk HPV serotypes 16, 18, 31, 33, and 35 have been found in some squamous papillomas and are associated with malignant transformation.

Pathologic Features

GROSS FINDINGS

Solitary squamous papillomas arise from the wall of the mainstem, secondary or tertiary bronchi. They range from 0.7 to >9 cm, with a median size of 1.5 cm. Almost all are exophytic, polypoid, friable, tan-white lesions protruding into airway lumens. The distal lung may show secondary obstructive effects, such as atelectasis, consolidation, or interstitial fibrosis.

Multiple squamous papillomas may lead to a velvety appearance of the bronchial mucosa. The involved lung may show bronchiectasis, with dilated airways filled with white-tan friable papillary fronds.

MICROSCOPIC FINDINGS

Squamous cell papilloma is a papillary tumor that consists of delicate connective tissue fronds lined by stratified squamous epithelium. They may be either solitary or multiple. They may be exophytic or inverted.

Exophytic tumors have orderly epithelial maturation (Fig. 11.1). The surface may be keratinized. Acanthosis, parakeratosis, and intraepithelial neutrophils are common. Less than 25% of solitary cases will have HPV viral cytopathic effect (perinuclear haloes, enlarged hyperchromatic nuclei with wrinkled nuclear contours).

Inverted papillomas usually also have an exophytic component but have invaginations into seromucinous glands (Fig. 11.2). Cells are usually nonkeratinizing and show orderly maturation. Nests are surrounded by intact basement membrane.

Parenchymal involvement may show two main patterns. There may be solid intra-alveolar nests of cytologically bland nonkeratinizing cells (Fig. 11.3). Reactive type II pneumocytes may be prominent. Alternatively, there may be large cysts lined by cytologically bland nonkeratinizing cells.

Malignant transformation of squamous papillomas may occur in up to 2% of cases. Neoplastic progression of squamous papillomas can range from mild dysplasia

636

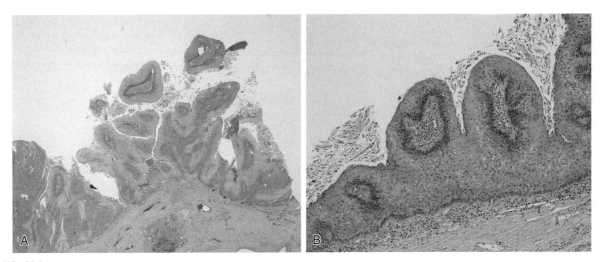

FIG. 11.1

A and **B,** Exophytic squamous papilloma with fibrovascular cores lined by bland squamous epithelium showing orderly maturation and no high-grade dysplasia. Intraepithelial neutrophils are present **(B).**

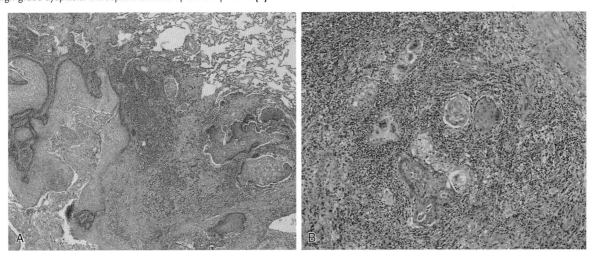

FIG. 11.2

Squamous papilloma with inverted/endophytic growth pattern. **A,** Low power shows nests of bland squamous cells involving the surrounding stroma (center). **B,** The nests show normal squamous maturation. Some of the nests (bottom center) still show a few mucinous cells. Inflammatory cells, including foreign body-type giant cells, and fibrosis may be present due to obstruction. There is no significant atypia or desmoplastic stromal response for a diagnosis of invasive squamous cell carcinoma.

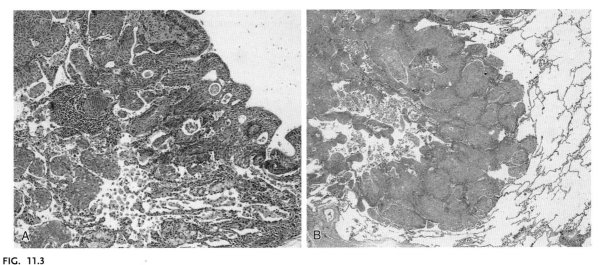

FIG. 11.3

A and **B,** Squamous papillomas extending into surrounding alveolar lung parenchyma showing solid intra-alveolar nests of cytologically bland nonkeratinizing cells. The architecture of the surrounding alveolar lung parenchyma is intact, and there is no evidence of desmoplastic stromal response or destruction of the lung parenchyma, unlike in invasive squamous cell carcinoma.

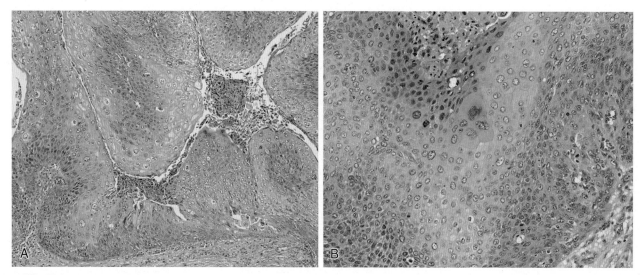

FIG. 11.4

A and **B,** Exophytic squamous papilloma with severe dysplasia/carcinoma *in situ*. These images are from the same case as Fig. 11.1, demonstrating that squamous papillomas may show varying degrees of dysplasia. There is loss of orderly maturation with areas of multinucleation and coarse chromatin.

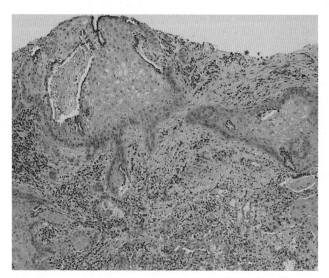

FIG. 11.5

Focal well-differentiated squamous cell carcinoma arising in a squamous papilloma. Differentiating between inverted squamous papilloma and well-differentiated squamous cell carcinoma may be difficult. There is desmoplastic stromal response and a few small irregular nests, so focal invasive squamous cell carcinoma was favored.

to carcinoma *in situ* (Fig. 11.4) to invasive squamous cell carcinoma (Fig. 11.5). Dysplasia within the squamous epithelium is graded similarly to other sites.

Ancillary Studies

Typically, immunochemical studies are not necessarily for diagnosis. Recurrent respiratory papillomatosis without dysplasia or invasive carcinoma may be positive for p16 and p53 by immunostaining. Some but not all cases of invasive carcinoma arising out of recurrent respiratory

papillomatosis are positive for p53. Neither p53 nor p16 immunostaining has been shown in small studies to be helpful for predicting malignant transformation.

Differential Diagnosis

The differential diagnosis for endobronchial, papillary tumors includes glandular papillomas and invasive squamous cell carcinoma. Glandular papillomas (Table 11.1) are typically endobronchial tumors but they may extend into the surrounding lung parenchyma. Histologically, glandular papillomas are lined by ciliated or nonciliated columnar cells with varying numbers of cuboidal and

TABLE 11.1

Histologic Features of Squamous Cell Papilloma Versus Glandular Papilloma

Squamous Cell Papilloma	Glandular Papilloma
• Lined by stratified squamous epithelium	• Lined by ciliated or nonciliated columnar cells with varying numbers of cuboidal and goblet cells
• Arise from the wall of the mainstem, secondary or tertiary bronchi	• Arise from the central lobar or segmental bronchi, but peripheral endobronchiolar lesion may occur
• Solitary or multiple	• Solitary
• Exophytic or inverted (growth into underlying seromucinous glands)	• Exophytic
• May extend into the surrounding lung parenchyma	• May extend into the surrounding lung parenchyma

goblet cells. Pure glandular papillomas do not show any squamous lining. However, mixed squamous cell and glandular papillomas show fibrovascular cores lined by a mixture of predominantly pseudostratified ciliated and nonciliated cuboidal-to-columnar cells with scattered mucin–filled cells and interspersed squamous islands.

Differentiating the squamous papillomas with inverted pattern or extension into the underlying lung parenchyma from squamous cell carcinoma may be quite difficult. Squamous cell carcinomas may show an exophytic, papillary growth pattern with involvement of the lumen of the bronchi (Fig. 11.6). In the 2004 WHO Classification of Tumours of the Lung, Pleura, Thymus and Heart, these tumors were classified as papillary squamous cell carcinomas; however, subtyping of squamous cell carcinomas based on architectural or cytologic features is no longer recommended in the 2015 WHO Classification. Squamous cell carcinoma with a papillary growth pattern shows malignant cytologic features and may show desmoplastic stromal invasion or destruction of the surrounding parenchyma (Table 11.2). In contrast, inverted squamous papillomas have nests of nonkeratinizing cells with orderly maturation surrounded by intact basement membrane (Table 11.3). Invasive squamous cell carcinomas commonly show areas with destruction of the normal alveolar architecture, whereas squamous papillomas with intra-alveolar growth show intact architecture of the alveolar lung parenchyma (Table 11.4).

Prognosis and Therapy

Surgically resected solitary squamous cell papillomas do not recur, but endoscopically removed tumors have up to 20% tumor recurrence. It is unclear whether

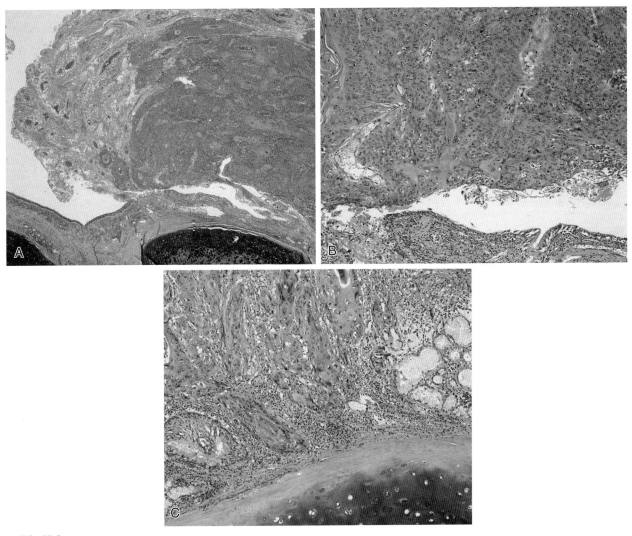

FIG. 11.6

A, Low magnification showing papillary endobronchial growth by squamous cell carcinoma. **B,** High magnification showing disordered maturation and atypia. **C,** An area with irregular invasive nests and cords of tumor cells with keratinization.

TABLE 11.2

Histologic Features of Exophytic Squamous Cell Papilloma Versus Squamous Cell Carcinoma

Squamous Cell Papilloma	Squamous Cell Carcinoma
• Papillary tumor that consists of delicate connective tissue fronds lined by stratified squamous epithelium	• Papillary endobronchial growth may occur • Complex architecture
• Squamous papillomas *without* high-grade dysplasia have orderly epithelial maturation. The surface may be keratinized. • Acanthosis, parakeratosis, and intraepithelial neutrophils are common	• Disordered maturation
• Squamous papillomas *with* high-grade dysplasia/carcinoma *in situ* show increased cytologic atypia, atypical mitotic figures, superficial mitotic figures	• Increased cytologic atypia • Atypical mitotic figures • Surface mitotic figures
• No invasion	• Desmoplastic stromal invasion

TABLE 11.3

Histologic Features of Inverted Squamous Cell Papilloma Versus Squamous Cell Carcinoma

Inverted Squamous Cell Papilloma	Squamous Cell Carcinoma
• Inverted papillomas show extension into seromucinous glands	• Complex architecture
• Cells are usually nonkeratinizing and show orderly maturation	• Disordered maturation • Increased cytologic atypia • Atypical mitotic figures • Surface mitotic figures
• Nests should be surrounded by intact basement membrane	• Desmoplastic stromal invasion • Destruction of surrounding lung architecture

TABLE 11.4

Histologic Features of Squamous Cell Papilloma Extending Into Lung Parenchyma Versus Squamous Cell Carcinoma

Squamous Cell Papilloma With Extension into Surrounding Alveoli	Squamous Cell Carcinoma
• Intra-alveolar nests of cytologically bland nonkeratinizing cells or large cysts lined by similar cells	• Complex architecture • Increased cytologic atypia • Atypical mitotic figures • Surface mitotic figures
• Cells are usually nonkeratinizing and show orderly maturation	• Disordered maturation
• Architecture of the alveolar lung parenchyma should be intact	• Desmoplastic stromal invasion • Destruction of surrounding lung architecture

SQUAMOUS CELL PAPILLOMAS – DISEASE FACT SHEET

Definition

▸▸ Papillary tumor that consists of delicate connective tissue fronds lined by stratified squamous epithelium

▸▸ They may be either solitary or multiple

▸▸ They may be exophytic or inverted

Incidence and Location

▸▸ Represent less than 1% of lung neoplasms and are much less common compared with their incidence in the upper aerodigestive tract

▸▸ May be solitary or multiple

Age Distribution

▸▸ Solitary squamous papillomas are more commonly found in men than in women (3:1) and occur in the fifth to sixth decade of life

▸▸ Multiple squamous papillomas are associated with recurrent respiratory papillomatosis and involvement of the upper aerodigestive tract. Recurrent respiratory papillomatosis occurs in children (<20 years of age) and in adults (30–40 years of age).

Clinical Features

▸▸ Patients typically present with cough, wheezing, or hemoptysis, but up to 25% are asymptomatic and are incidental radiographic findings

Radiologic Features

▸▸ High-resolution CT scans demonstrate endobronchial plaques, nodules, or airway thickening. Distal to the lesions, CT scans may show obstructive findings such as air trapping, atelectasis, consolidation, and/or bronchiectasis.

▸▸ Lung involvement with papillomatosis demonstrates diffuse, poorly defined, noncalcified parenchymal centrilobular opacities, and cavitated thick-walled nodules

Prognosis and Therapy

▸▸ Surgically resected solitary squamous cell papillomas do not recur, but up to 20% of patients with endoscopic removal have tumor recurrence

▸▸ Multiple squamous cell papillomas which are associated with recurrent respiratory papillomatosis may undergo malignant transformation in up to 2% of cases

solitary squamous papillomas transform into carcinoma, and it is possible that reported cases may represent misdiagnosed squamous cell carcinoma due to lack of sampling of the tumor stromal interface.

Multiple squamous cell papillomas, which are associated with recurrent respiratory papillomatosis, may undergo malignant transformation in up to 2% of cases, typically in the setting of high-risk HPV-associated papillomas (subtypes 16 and 18). However, malignant transformation has been described with low-risk HPV subtypes 6 and 11 as well. Malignant transformation is more common in adults with recurrent respiratory papillomatosis, and risk factors for transformation include multiple recurrences, smoking, alcohol consumption, radiation, immunosuppression, and chemotherapy.

SQUAMOUS CELL PAPILLOMA – PATHOLOGIC FEATURES

Gross Findings

▸▸ Solitary squamous papillomas arise from the wall of the main-stem, secondary or tertiary bronchi
  ▸▸ They range from 0.7 to >9 cm, with a median size of 1.5 cm
  ▸▸ Almost all are exophytic, polypoid, friable, tan-white lesions protruding into airway lumens. The distal lung may show secondary obstructive effects such as atelectasis, consolidation, or honeycomb change.
▸▸ Multiple squamous papillomas may lead to a velvety appearance of the bronchial mucosa. The involved lung may show bronchiectasis, with dilated airways filled with white-tan friable papillary fronds.

Microscopic Findings

▸▸ Papillary tumor that consists of delicate connective tissue fronds lined by stratified squamous epithelium
▸▸ May be either solitary or multiple
▸▸ May be exophytic or inverted
▸▸ Exophytic tumors have orderly epithelial maturation
  ▸▸ The surface may be keratinized
  ▸▸ Acanthosis, parakeratosis, and intraepithelial neutrophils are common
  ▸▸ Less than 25% of solitary cases will have HPV viral cytopathic effect
▸▸ Inverted papillomas usually also have an exophytic component but have invaginations into seromucinous glands
  ▸▸ Cells are usually nonkeratinizing and show orderly maturation
  ▸▸ Nests should be surrounded by intact basement membrane
  ▸▸ Reactive type II pneumocytes lining alveolar walls may be prominent
  ▸▸ Inflammation and fibrosis may be present (secondary to obstruction)

Pathologic Differential Diagnoses

▸▸ Glandular papilloma
▸▸ Mixed squamous cell and glandular papilloma
▸▸ Squamous cell carcinoma with papillary architecture

CARCINOID TUMOR (ATYPICAL AND TYPICAL)

DIFFERENTIAL DIAGNOSES: TUMORLETS, PARAGANGLIOMA, METASTATIC WELL-DIFFERENTIATED NEUROENDOCRINE TUMOR, DIFFUSE IDIOPATHIC PULMONARY NEUROENDOCRINE CELL HYPERPLASIA, LARGE CELL NEUROENDOCRINE CARCINOMA, SMALL CELL CARCINOMA

Clinical Features

Carcinoid tumor is a low- to intermediate-grade neuroendocrine epithelial malignancy. This malignancy accounts for <1% of lung cancers. Typical carcinoids are neuroendocrine tumors with <2 mitoses per 2 mm² without necrosis (Table 11.5). Atypical carcinoids are intermediate-grade neuroendocrine epithelial tumors

TABLE 11.5
Comparison of Typical Carcinoid and Atypical Carcinoid

	Typical Carcinoid	Atypical Carcinoid
Mitoses	<2 per 2 mm²	2–10 per 2 mm²
Necrosis	–	+/– (focal)

with 2 to 10 mitoses per 2 mm² and/or foci of necrosis. Carcinoid tumors occur more often in females younger than 60 years old. These tumors are not related to tobacco smoking. Risk factors include family history of carcinoid tumors and *MEN1* gene carriers. The majority of carcinoids arise in central airways; however, approximately one third of tumors occur at the periphery of the lung. Given that the tumors arise in airways and may cause airway obstruction, the presenting symptoms may include wheezing, cough, or pneumonia.

Pathologic Features

GROSS FINDINGS

Tumors are well circumscribed, may be sessile or pedunculated and may fill an airway.

MICROSCOPIC FINDINGS

On low power, carcinoid tumors are characterized by neuroendocrine growth pattern (organoid, trabecular, rosette-like, pseudoglandular). The neoplastic cells are uniform in appearance with round to oval nuclei and moderate amount of cytoplasm (Fig. 11.7). Peripheral tumors may have spindle cell morphology (Fig. 11.8). Nuclear pleomorphism is not one of the criteria to diagnose an atypical carcinoid. The defining feature of atypical carcinoid tumor is the number of mitoses per 2 mm² and/or the presence of necrosis. The mitoses should be counted in the area of the highest mitotic activity. Nodular neuroendocrine proliferations measuring less than 0.5 cm are classified as carcinoid tumorlets.

Ancillary Studies

The vast majority of carcinoid tumors show expression of pankeratin and at least one of the neuroendocrine markers (chromogranin, synaptophysin, CD56, INSM1). Some tumors may stain for TTF-1 (up to 50%, however, the expression may be focal and weak) with peripheral carcinoid tumors being more frequently positive than central tumors.

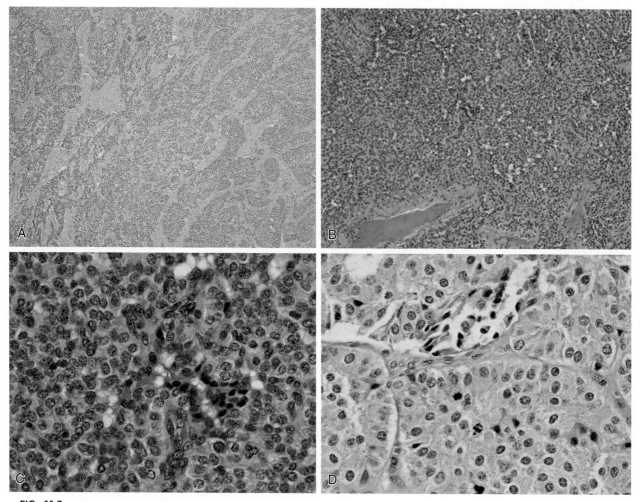

FIG. 11.7

Low-power **(A and B)** and high-power **(C and D)** views of carcinoid tumor showing organoid growth pattern and typical neuroendocrine cytomorphology. Note the easily identifiable mitotic figure **(D)** of atypical carcinoid tumor.

Differential Diagnosis

The histologic differential diagnosis includes tumorlets, paragangliomas, metastatic neuroendocrine tumors, in some cases diffuse idiopathic pulmonary neuroendocrine cell hyperplasia (DIPNECH), and high-grade neuroendocrine carcinomas.

Tumorlets are separated from carcinoid tumors based on the size of the lesion. Nodular epithelial neuroendocrine proliferations measuring less than 0.5 cm are classified as tumorlets.

Paragangliomas are rare neuroendocrine neoplasms that have been described to involve the lung. Paragangliomas have a similar morphology to carcinoid tumors (Fig. 11.9). Like carcinoid tumors, paragangliomas may show nested architecture and will express neuroendocrine markers, such as chromogranin and synaptophysin. In this case, documenting expression of epithelial markers (keratins) helps in separating carcinoid tumors from paragangliomas, as carcinoids are epithelial neoplasms and should show keratin expression by immunohistochemistry.

Differentiating primary lung carcinoid tumor from metastatic well-differentiated neuroendocrine tumor can be challenging (Table 11.6). Several studies suggest that the presence of TTF-1 staining favors lung or thyroid origin, whereas PAX8 staining suggests the possibility of well-differentiated neuroendocrine tumor of pancreatic origin. Strong *CDX-2* expression in combination with negative TTF-1 staining favors gastrointestinal origin. Of note, TTF-1 expression is seen only in half of the cases of pulmonary carcinoid tumors. In addition, the expression may be weak and focal.

DIPNECH is a generalized preinvasive proliferation of neuroendocrine cells in the lung (Fig. 11.10). This condition is typically seen in middle-aged females and tends to present with obstructive symptoms, such as cough and dyspnea. Histologically, it can appear as scattered clusters of neuroendocrine cells, linear proliferations, or small nodules in the small terminal bronchioles.

However, by definition, the neuroendocrine cells in DIPNECH should not extend beyond the basement membrane. If the neuroendocrine cells extend beyond

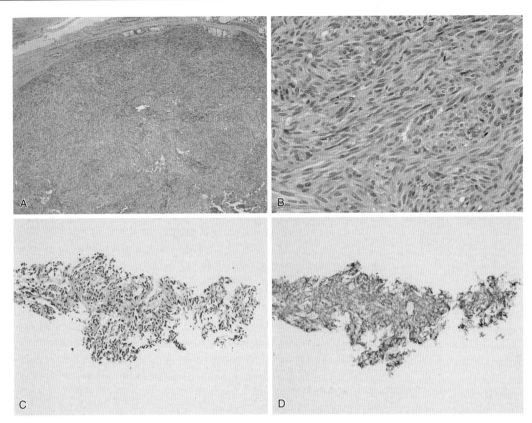

FIG. 11.8
Low-power view **(A)** and high-power view **(B)** of paraganglioma. Negative pancytokeratin immunostain **(C)** and positive synaptophysin immunostain **(D)**.

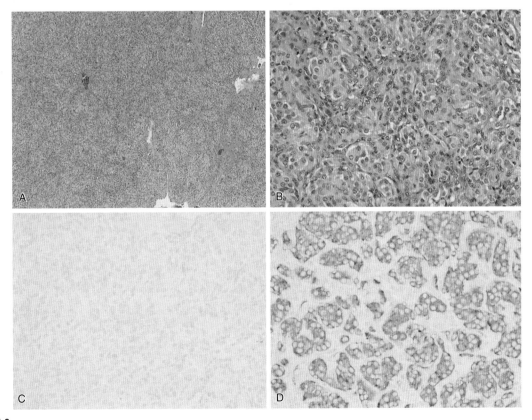

FIG. 11.9
Low-power view **(A)** and high-power view **(B)** of a carcinoid tumor with spindle cell morphology **(A)**. Carcinoid tumor with spindle cell morphology in a biopsy specimen **(C)** with positive synaptophysin immunostain **(D)**.

the basement membrane and form lesions less than 5 mm, they are classified as carcinoid tumorlets. If the nodules are greater than 5 mm, they are classified as carcinoid tumors.

While typical and atypical carcinoid tumors represent low- and intermediate-grade neuroendocrine tumors, the high-grade neuroendocrine epithelial malignancies include small cell and large cell neuroendocrine carcinoma (LCNC) (Fig. 11.11). Neuroendocrine carcinomas are separated based on mitotic count, >10 mitoses per 2 mm². Small cell carcinomas show scant cytoplasm, prominent apoptotic bodies, and brisk mitotic activity. When comparing biopsies with resection specimens, the biopsies tend to demonstrate more prominent nuclear molding and crush artifact. While currently Ki-67 proliferation index is not routinely utilized in discriminating atypical and typical carcinoid tumors, it is incredibly valuable when evaluating small biopsies with marked crush artifact. Small cell carcinoma has a proliferation index that is greater than 50%, whereas carcinoid tumors tend to show a proliferation index of less than 20%. In general, LCNCs show extensive necrosis, which is evident on low-power examination, large cells with prominent nucleoli, moderate to abundant cytoplasm, and >10 mitoses per 2 mm² (Table 11.7). On occasion, a tumor with carcinoid-like morphology has a mitotic index of more >10 mitoses per 2 mm². It is more likely to be aggressive and currently is best classified as LCNC.

TABLE 11.6

Comparison of Lung Carcinoid and Metastatic Neuroendocrine Tumor

	Lung Carcinoid	Metastatic Neuroendocrine Tumor
Glandular structures	Unusual	Often present
TTF-1	Positive in one third to one half cases	Usually negative
PAX-8 or CDX2	Usually negative	May suggest pancreatic or gastrointestinal origin

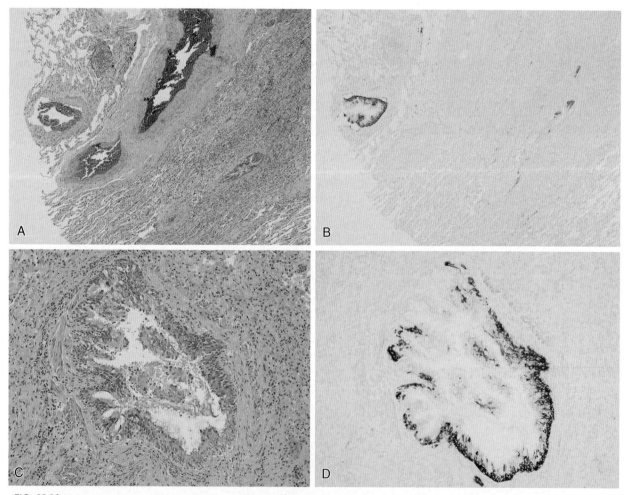

FIG. 11.10

Low power-view of diffuse idiopathic pulmonary neuroendocrine cell hyperplasia **(A)** with synaptophysin immunostain highlighting neuroendocrine cell hyperplasia around the airways **(B)**. High-power view of an airway with neuroendocrine cell hyperplasia **(C)** with synaptophysin immunostain **(D)**.

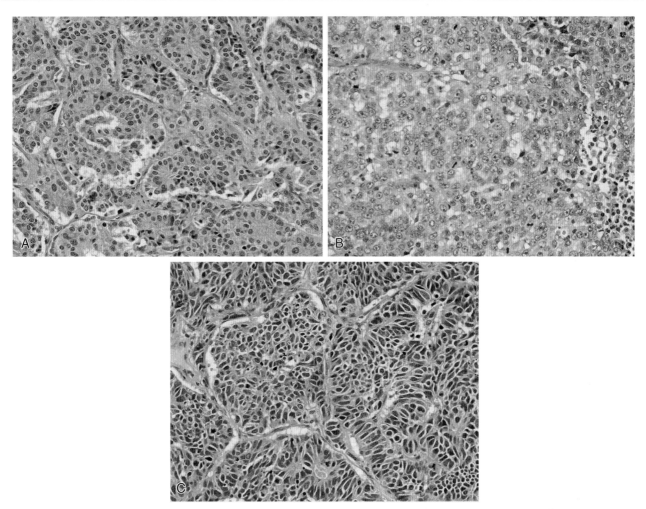

FIG. 11.11
High power view of carcinoid tumor **(A)**, large cell neuroendocrine carcinoma **(B)**, and small cell carcinoma **(C)**.

TABLE 11.7

Comparison of Carcinoid Tumor (Typical and Atypical) and Large Cell Neuroendocrine Carcinoma (LCNC)

	Carcinoid Tumor	LCNC
Smoking	Unrelated	Related
Location	Central airways	Peripheral lung
Necrosis	Focal, punctate	Extensive
Mitoses	$\leq$10 per 2 mm^2	>10 per 2 mm^2 Usually >30 per 2 mm^2

Prognosis and Therapy

Distinction between typical carcinoid and atypical carcinoid is the most important prognostic factor because the 5-year survival rate for patients with typical carcinoid tumors is 90% which drops to 60% for the patients with atypical carcinoid.

CARCINOID TUMORS – DISEASE FACT SHEET

Definition
▶▶ Neuroendocrine epithelial malignancy
▶▶ Less than 10 mitoses per 2 mm^2

Incidence and Location
▶▶ <1% of lung cancers

Age Distribution
▶▶ <60 years

Clinical Features
▶▶ Arise in central airways (approximately one third at the periphery)
▶▶ More common in females
▶▶ Not related to tobacco smoking

Radiologic Features
▶▶ Lobulated mass involving airways

Prognosis and Therapy
▶▶ Important to distinguish typical carcinoids from atypical carcinoids
▶▶ Atypical carcinoid tumors are more likely to metastasize and have a lower 5-year survival rate

---

CARCINOID TUMOR – PATHOLOGIC FEATURES

Gross Findings
▸▸ Lobulated mass filling the airway
▸▸ Well circumscribed

Microscopic Findings
▸▸ Neuroendocrine growth pattern
▸▸ Round to oval nuclei and moderate cytoplasm
▸▸ Peripheral tumors may have spindle cell morphology
▸▸ <10 mitoses per 2 mm²
▸▸ Positive neuroendocrine markers
▸▸ Positive pancytokeratin

Pathologic Differential Diagnoses
▸▸ Tumorlets, paraganglioma, metastatic well-differentiated neuro-endocrine tumor, diffuse idiopathic pulmonary neuroendocrine cell hyperplasia (DIPNECH), large cell neuroendocrine carcinoma, small cell carcinoma

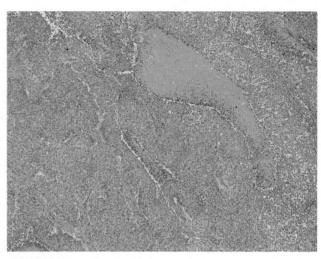

FIG. 11.12
Low-power view of large cell neuroendocrine carcinoma showing ribbons of tumor cells and zones of necrosis. No keratinization or gland formation is present.

LARGE CELL NEUROENDOCRINE CARCINOMA

DIFFERENTIAL DIAGNOSES: CARCINOID TUMOR, NON–SMALL CELL CARCINOMA, SMALL CELL CARCINOMA, NUT MIDLINE CARCINOMA

Clinical Features

LCNC is a non–small cell lung carcinoma that shows histologic features of neuroendocrine morphology (including rosettes and peripheral palisading) and expresses immunohistochemical neuroendocrine markers. It is associated with smoking. The majority of the tumors are peripheral, but pleural effusions are rare. The tumor is centrally located in approximately 20% of cases. Paraneoplastic syndromes are uncommon.

Pathologic Features

GROSS FINDINGS

The tumors present as large peripheral masses (1–10 cm), frequently with central necrosis. Cavitation and effusions are rare.

MICROSCOPIC FINDINGS

Tumor shows neuroendocrine morphology (rosette-like structures, peripheral palisading) and frequently extensive necrosis (Figs. 11.12–11.14). Tumor cells have abundant cytoplasm, prominent nucleoli, and high mitotic count (>10 mitoses per 2 mm²). The Ki-67 proliferation index ranges between 40% and 80%.

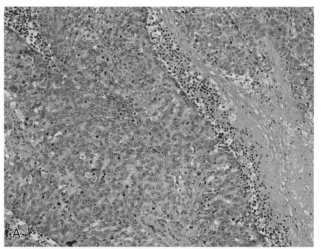

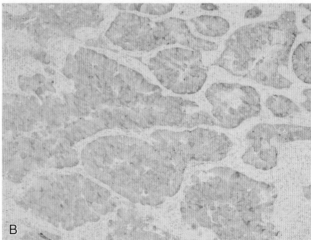

FIG. 11.13
A, Large cell neuroendocrine carcinoma showing characteristic morphology. **B,** Synaptophysin immunostain demonstrating positive staining in tumor cells.

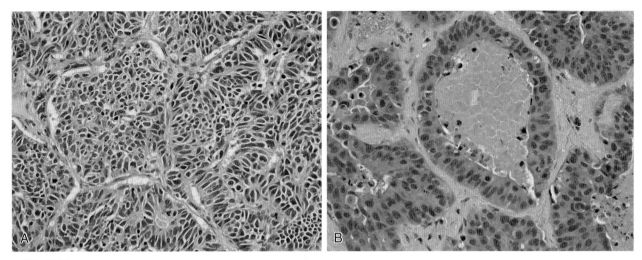

FIG. 11.14

A, Small cell neuroendocrine carcinoma showing molding and speckled chromatin. **B,** Large cell neuroendocrine carcinoma demonstrating more abundant cytoplasm and prominent nucleoli.

TABLE 11.8

Comparison of Immunohistochemical Staining in Large Cell Neuroendocrine Carcinoma, Small Cell Carcinoma, NUT Carcinoma, and Other Non–Small Cell Lung Carcinomas

	Large Cell Neuroendocrine Carcinoma	Small Cell Carcinoma	Squamous Cell Carcinoma	Adenocarcinoma	NUT Carcinoma
Neuroendocrine markers (chromogranin, synaptophysin, CD56)	+	+	−	−	<10%
p40	−	−	+	Up to 30%	+
TTF-1	50%	+	−	+	Occasionally
Napsin	−	−	−	+	Not enough data
NUT	−	−	−	−	+

Ancillary Studies

Confirmation of neuroendocrine differentiation is required (see Fig. 11.13, Table 11.8). Chromogranin is positive in 80% to 85% of cases. Synaptophysin is positive in 50% to 60%. CD56 is the most sensitive marker; however, it is not specific. Approximately 50% of LCNCs express TTF-1. The expression of markers of squamous differentiation is usually absent.

Differential Diagnosis

The differential diagnosis for LCNC includes carcinoid tumors, small cell carcinoma, and other non–small cell carcinomas. LCNC is differentiated from carcinoid tumors largely on the basis of mitotic count (>10 mitoses per 2 mm²) (Fig. 11.15, Table 11.9).

Compared with small cell carcinoma, LCNC shows polygonal rather than fusiform cells, more abundant cytoplasm, prominent nucleoli, and vesicular to clumped chromatin (see Fig. 11.14, Table 11.10).

To differentiate LCNC from other non–small cell carcinomas, a documentation of neuroendocrine marker expression is essential (see Table 11.8). It is important to remember that about half of LCNC express TTF-1 and if neuroendocrine markers are not performed, these tumors can be inappropriately classified as adenocarcinomas. Low-power recognition of organoid growth and zonal necrosis are very helpful features.

NUT midline carcinomas are rare tumors of unknown etiology. They are typically associated with pleural effusion and present as a large mass extending into hilar structures. Using monoclonal nuclear NUT antibody, the tumor consistently shows speckled nuclear positivity in more than 50% of tumor cells. In addition, NUT midline carcinomas are typically positive for squamous markers, indicating squamous lineage. Occasionally these tumors may express neuroendocrine markers and even TTF-1.

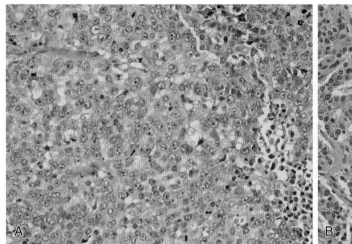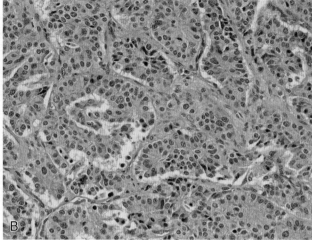

FIG. 11.15

A, Large cell neuroendocrine carcinoma showing large nuclei, prominent nucleoli, and numerous mitotic figures. **B,** Atypical carcinoid tumor demonstrating small eccentric nuclei and rare mitotic figures. Necrosis and nuclear pleomorphism are not prominent.

TABLE 11.9

Comparison of Large Cell Neuroendocrine Carcinoma and Carcinoid Tumor

	Large Cell Neuroendocrine Carcinoma	Carcinoid Tumor
Nuclei	Vesicular	Granular
Nucleoli	Prominent	Small
Nucleocytoplasmic ratio	Lower	High
Necrosis	Infarct-like	Punctate, if present
Mitotic activity	>10 (typically >50) per 2 mm²	<10 per 2 mm²

TABLE 11.10

Comparison of Large Cell Neuroendocrine Carcinoma and Small Cell Carcinoma

	Large Cell Neuroendocrine Carcinoma	Small Cell Carcinoma
Incidence	3%	20%
Location	Peripheral	Central
Clinical features	Smoking/male/older	Smoking/male/older
Nuclear/cytoplasmic ration	Low	High
Cell shape	Polygonal	Fusiform
Nuclear molding	+	+++
Prognosis	Poor	Poor

Prognosis and Therapy

Survival is worse than similarly staged non–small cell lung carcinomas. Some studies show that patient may benefit from chemotherapy for small cell lung cancer.

LARGE CELL NEUROENDOCRINE CARCINOMA – DISEASE FACT SHEET

Definition
▸▸ Non–small cell lung carcinomas that show histologic features of neuroendocrine morphology (including rosettes and peripheral palisading) and express immunohistochemical neuroendocrine markers

Incidence and Location
▸▸ Approximately 3%
▸▸ Majority of tumors are located peripherally (80%)

Age Distribution
▸▸ Median age 65 years

Clinical Features
▸▸ Associated with smoking (>90% of these tumors occur in heavy smokers)
▸▸ More common in men

Radiologic Features
▸▸ Usually peripheral (>80%) and upper lobes (>60%)
▸▸ Effusion is rare
▸▸ Cavitation may occur but is uncommon

Prognosis and Therapy
▸▸ More likely to recur than other non–small cell lung carcinomas
▸▸ Poor overall survival

PULMONARY SALIVARY GLAND-TYPE NEOPLASMS

DIFFERENTIAL DIAGNOSES: LUNG ADENOCARCINOMA, SQUAMOUS CELL CARCINOMA, MIXED ADENOSQUAMOUS CARCINOMA, NEUROENDOCRINE NEOPLASMS

Clinical Features

Pulmonary salivary gland-type neoplasms are rare, representing less than 1% of lung carcinomas; however, it is important to recognize these tumors and differentiate from lung adenocarcinoma, squamous cell carcinoma, and adenosquamous carcinoma due to different treatment options and outcomes. They arise from the seromucinous glands in the submucosa of the trachea and bronchi. The most common salivary gland-type neoplasms include mucoepidermoid carcinoma and adenoid cystic carcinoma. In a review of the National Cancer Database of cases between 2004 and 2014, Resio et al. identified over 1100 salivary gland-type neoplasms, about two third of which were mucoepidermoid carcinoma and one third adenoid cystic carcinoma. Other salivary gland neoplasms such as epithelial-myoepithelial carcinoma or pleomorphic adenoma are even more rare.

Salivary gland-type neoplasms occur in a wide age range. Resio et al. found that the median age of presentation for mucoepidermoid carcinoma was 54 years (range 18–88 years) and that for adenoid cystic carcinoma was 60 years (range 22–90 years) with a nearly equal sex distribution. There is no association with smoking.

Salivary gland-type tumors may present with wheezing, cough, hemoptysis, and obstructive pneumonia. Some patients may be asymptomatic. Imaging typically shows a centrally located mass. Mediastinal lymph node metastases are rare in low-grade mucoepidermoid carcinoma but have been described in 16% of high-grade mucoepidermoid carcinoma and 39% of adenoid cystic carcinomas. Distant metastasis is rare.

Pathologic Features

GROSS FINDINGS

Salivary gland-type neoplasms typically arise in an endobronchial location in the central airways. Resio et al. reported that the mean size of mucoepidermoid carcinoma is 3.1 cm and that of adenoid cystic carcinoma is 3.8 cm. Low-grade mucoepidermoid carcinomas show a gray-white to pink-tan, variably mucinous and cystic cut surface. High-grade tumors are more infiltrative. Adenoid cystic carcinomas may be well defined or infiltrative and show a gray-white homogenous cut surface. Adenoid cystic carcinomas are frequently highly microscopically infiltrative beyond the grossly identified mass because of perineural invasion, so careful sampling of the surrounding soft tissue is recommended.

MICROSCOPIC FINDINGS

Microscopically, mucoepidermoid carcinoma and adenoid cystic carcinoma are similar in appearance to those described in the salivary glands. It has been proposed that pulmonary mucoepidermoid carcinoma be classified into two tiers rather than three or four: low grade and high grade. Of the mucoepidermoid carcinomas, Resio et al. reported that two third were low grade and one third were high grade. Mucoepidermoid carcinoma is composed of three cell types: mucin-secreting, squamous, and intermediate cells. Low-grade mucoepidermoid carcinoma shows a cystic predominant pattern with tumor islands containing both cystic and solid patterns (Fig. 11.16). The cystic component is lined by cytologically bland columnar cells with apical mucin. The solid components typically surround the cysts and are composed of the squamous and/or intermediate cells. Mitotic activity is low and necrosis is rare.

High-grade mucoepidermoid carcinoma typically shows predominantly solid growth pattern with less cystic growth (Fig. 11.17). It is mainly composed of atypical squamous and intermediate cells with frequent mitosis and necrosis. Variable numbers of mucin-secreting cells are present.

Adenoid cystic carcinoma is a biphasic tumor composed of luminal cells and abluminal (outer) myoepithelial cells growing in cribriform, tubular and solid patterns. The classic cribriform pattern shows cells

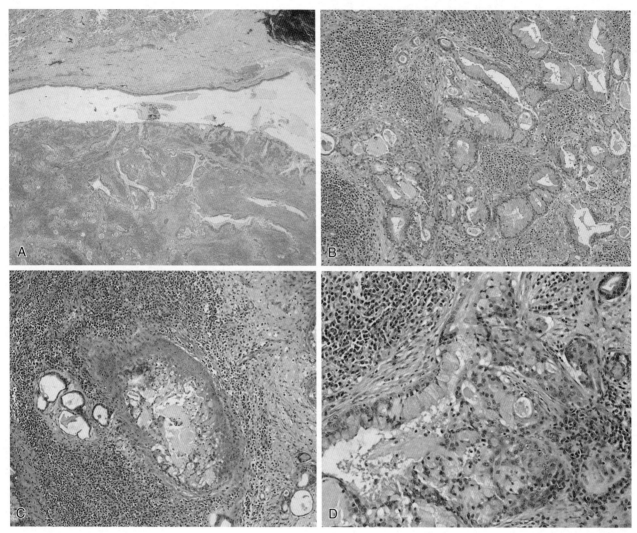

FIG. 11.16

Low-grade mucoepidermoid carcinoma. **A,** Low-power view of an endobronchial mass filling the lumen of the airway. The mass is composed predominantly of mucin-secreting cells **(B)** with focal epidermoid (squamous) cells **(C)** and intermediate cells **(D)**.

surrounding connective tissue cylinders containing myxoid or hyalinized basement membrane-like material (Fig. 11.18A). Perineural invasion is common (Fig. 11.18B). While grading of pulmonary adenoid cystic carcinomas is not described in the 2015 WHO Classification, salivary gland adenoid cystic carcinomas have been graded with either a two- or three-tier system. In a two-tier system, the presence of any solid component is compatible with high grade (Fig. 11.19A–C). In a three-tier system, a solid component of 1% to 29% is intermediate grade, whereas solid component of 30% or greater is high grade.

Ancillary Studies

Mucoepidermoid carcinomas are typically CK7 positive in the glandular component with intracellular mucin which is positive on mucicarmine stain. Mucoepidermoid carcinomas are negative for TTF-1 and Napsin A.

The squamous and intermediate cells are typically positive for CK5/6, p40, and p63. *MAML2* gene rearrangements have been reported in 67% to 100% of cases.

The abluminal cells in adenoid cystic carcinomas typically are positive for myoepithelial markers such as SMA, S100, calponin, p40, p63, and GFAP. The luminal component of the tumor is typically more strongly positive than the abluminal component for CK7 and CAM5.2. C-kit immunostain may be positive. *MYB* gene rearrangements have been described in 41% to 100% of pulmonary adenoid cystic carcinoma, and MYB1 immunostaining is frequently positive (Fig. 11.19D).

Differential Diagnosis

Primary salivary gland-type neoplasms in the lung must be differentiated from metastases of salivary gland neoplasms. Clinical history, imaging studies of the salivary

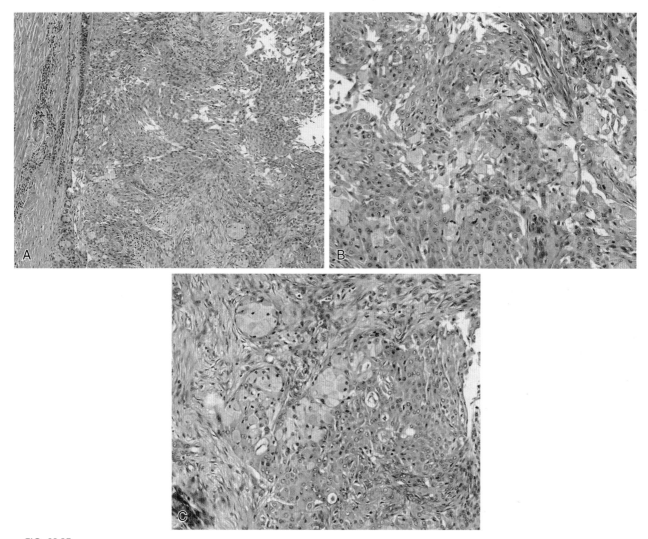

FIG. 11.17

A and **B**, High-grade mucoepidermoid carcinoma with predominantly solid growth with interspersed mucin-secreting cells. **C**, Small cystic structures are identified which are lined by bland columnar cells with abundant intracellular mucin. No overt keratinization or squamous pearls are identified.

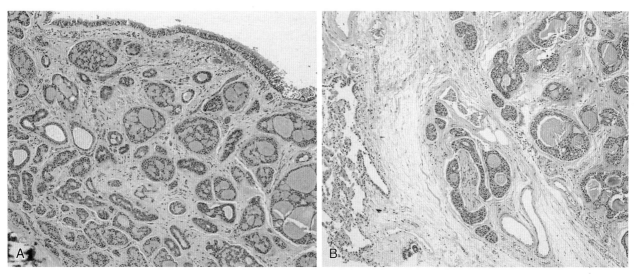

FIG. 11.18

A and **B**, Low-grade adenoid cystic carcinoma with classic cribriform pattern showing cells surrounding connective tissue cylinders containing myxoid or hyalinized basement membrane–like material. Perineural invasion is present **(B)**.

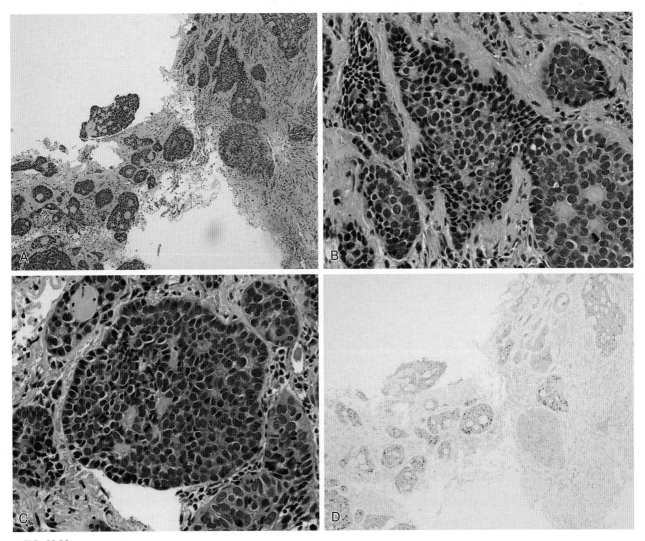

FIG. 11.19

Endobronchial excision of high-grade adenoid cystic carcinoma. **A,** There is a mixture of tubular, cribriform and solid architecture (left). **B,** Solid areas may morphologically resemble carcinoid tumor with fine chromatin. The cribriform areas could be mistaken for neuroendocrine rosettes particularly on small biopsies. **C,** High-grade adenoid cystic carcinoma may show peripheral palisading, as seen in basaloid squamous carcinoma. **D,** MYB immunostain may be positive in adenoid cystic carcinoma.

glands, and multifocality of the pulmonary lesions may be helpful to differentiate between a primary tumor and metastatic disease.

Mucoepidermoid carcinoma can be confused with invasive mucinous adenocarcinoma, squamous cell carcinoma, or adenosquamous carcinomas particularly on small biopsies or fine-needle aspiration specimens. In particular, differentiating low-grade mucoepidermoid carcinoma from mucinous adenocarcinoma may be difficult but important due to the significant difference in prognosis with a 5-year survival of 95% for low-grade mucoepidermoid carcinoma versus 5-year survival of 69% for mucinous adenocarcinoma. Clues to differentiate low-grade mucoepidermoid carcinoma from invasive mucinous adenocarcinoma include: (1) central, endobronchial location; (2) identification of the squamous component (which may be scant); and (3) transitional or intermediate areas between the squamous and the mucinous component (Table 11.11). While TTF-1

and Napsin A are negative in the glandular component of mucoepidermoid carcinoma, TTF-1 and Napsin A are also frequently negative in invasive mucinous adenocarcinoma. Identification of the squamous component by CK5/6, p40, or p63 immunostaining may be helpful. Mucoepidermoid carcinoma may show *MAML2* gene rearrangements, whereas invasive mucinous adenocarcinomas may show *KRAS, NRG1, NTRK1, BRAF*, and *ALK* mutations.

High-grade mucoepidermoid carcinomas are most likely to be confused with adenosquamous carcinoma or squamous cell carcinoma (Table 11.12). Unlike squamous carcinomas or adenosquamous carcinomas, the squamous component of mucoepidermoid carcinoma typically does not show keratinization or overt keratin pearls (Fig. 11.20). Mucoepidermoid carcinoma also does not have a component of squamous carcinoma *in situ*. Both high-grade mucoepidermoid carcinoma and squamous cell carcinomas are typically centrally

TABLE 11.11

Histologic, Immunohistochemical, and Molecular Features of Low-Grade Mucoepidermoid Carcinoma Versus Invasive Mucinous Adenocarcinoma

Low-Grade Mucoepidermoid Carcinoma	Invasive Mucinous Adenocarcinoma
• Central, endobronchial location	• Usually located in the periphery of the lung
• Cystic components are lined by cytologically bland columnar cells with apical mucin	• Histologic subtype of invasive lung adenocarcinoma that shows tumor cells with goblet or columnar morphology with abundant intracytoplasmic mucin
• Should have a squamous component (which may be scant)	• No squamous component
• Should also have transitional or intermediate areas between the squamous and the mucinous component	• No transitional or intermediate areas
• Negative for TTF-1 and Napsin A	• Invasive mucinous adenocarcinomas are positive for TTF-1 in 27.5%–42% of cases and Napsin A in one third of cases
• Squamous component should be CK5/6, p63, and/or p40 positive	• CK5/6, p63, and p40 are negative
• *MAML2* gene rearrangements	• *KRAS, NRG1, NTRK1, BRAF,* and *ALK* mutations

TABLE 11.12

Histologic, Immunohistochemical, and Molecular Features of High-Grade Mucoepidermoid Carcinoma Versus Squamous Cell Carcinoma and Adenosquamous Carcinoma

High-Grade Mucoepidermoid Carcinoma	Squamous Cell Carcinoma	Adenosquamous Carcinoma
• Central, endobronchial location	• Arising in the main or lobar bronchus • Two third are central • One third are peripheral	• Usually located in the periphery of the lung
• Predominantly solid growth pattern • Cystic components are lined by cytologically bland columnar cells with apical mucin	• No glandular component and no cells with intracytoplasmic mucin	• Adenocarcinoma component should be evident by light microscopy and account for at least 10% of the tumor • Adenocarcinoma component may be separate from the squamous component or may be intermingled with the squamous component
• Should have a squamous component	• Only squamous component	• Squamous cell carcinoma component should be evident by light microscopy and account for at least 10% of the tumor
• No squamous carcinoma *in situ*	• Squamous carcinoma *in situ* may be present	• Squamous carcinoma *in situ* may be present
• No overt keratinization or squamous pearls	• May show overt keratinization or squamous pearls	• May show overt keratinization or squamous pearls
• Should also have transitional or intermediate areas between the squamous and the mucinous component.	• No transitional or intermediate areas	• No transitional or intermediate areas
• Negative for TTF-1 and Napsin A	• Negative for TTF-1 and Napsin A	• Adenocarcinoma component may be positive for TTF-1 and Napsin A
• Squamous component should be CK5/6, p63, and/or p40 positive	• CK5/6, p63, and p40 positive	• Squamous component should be CK5/6, p63, and/or p40 positive
• *MAML2* gene rearrangements	• Gene copy number alterations including gains/amplifications • Deletion of 9p *(CDKN2A)* • Most common gene mutation *TP53*	• *EGFR, KRAS, ALK, HER2, LKB1, ROS1,* or *RET* mutations or rearrangements or *FGFR1* amplification

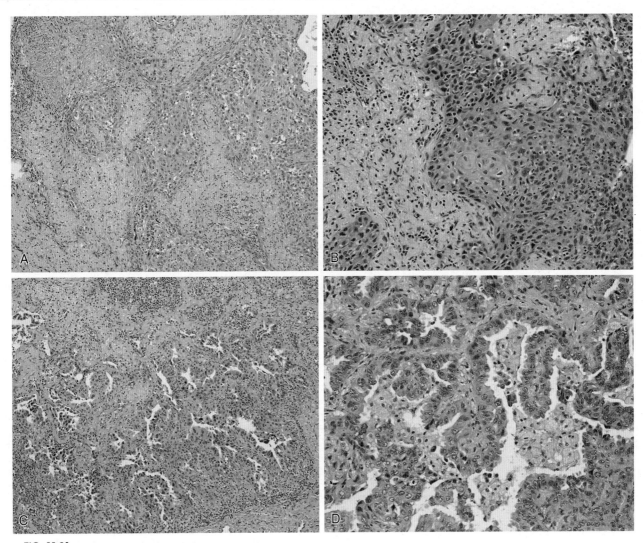

FIG. 11.20

Adenosquamous carcinoma. **A** and **B,** The majority of this tumor was squamous cell carcinoma with keratinization and no mucin-secreting cells. **C,** Parts of this tumor showed micropapillary pattern of adenocarcinoma. **D,** Other areas in this tumor showed papillary pattern of adenocarcinoma.

located; however, identification of interspersed cells containing intracellular mucin may suggest that the tumor is not squamous cell carcinoma. High-grade mucoepidermoid carcinomas frequently show central location with exophytic growth, whereas adenosquamous carcinomas typically are peripherally located. More extensive sampling to identify a low-grade mucoepidermoid carcinoma component may be helpful. The adenocarcinoma component of adenosquamous carcinomas may be positive for TTF-1 and Napsin A, both of which are negative in mucoepidermoid carcinoma. Mucoepidermoid carcinoma may show *MAML2* gene rearrangements, whereas adenosquamous carcinomas may show *EGFR, KRAS, ALK, HER2, LKB1, ROS1,* or *RET* mutations or rearrangements or *FGFR1* amplification.

While low-grade adenoid cystic carcinoma with tubular and cribriform architecture may be easily recognizable, high-grade (predominantly solid) adenoid cystic carcinomas may be more difficult to recognize. The differential diagnosis for adenoid cystic carcinoma includes nonmucinous adenocarcinoma (acinar or solid patterns), neuroendocrine neoplasms, and basaloid squamous carcinomas. Adenoid cystic carcinoma can be differentiated from nonmucinous lung adenocarcinoma by recognition of the biphasic pattern with the presence of abluminal myoepithelial cells either histologically or by immunohistochemical stains such as SMA, S100, calponin, p40, p63, and GFAP (Table 11.13). Adenoid cystic carcinomas are also typically negative for TTF-1 and Napsin A. Adenoid cystic carcinomas and neuroendocrine neoplasms such as carcinoid tumors and small cell carcinomas are all typically centrally located tumors, and the glandular structure of adenoid cystic carcinoma and neuroendocrine rosettes may show some morphologic resemblance (see Table 11.13). However, immunohistochemical staining for neuroendocrine markers such as chromogranin, synaptophysin, and CD56 should differentiate these tumors. High-grade adenoid

TABLE 11.13

Histologic, Immunohistochemical, and Molecular Features of Adenoid Cystic Carcinoma Versus Lung Adenocarcinoma Versus Neuroendocrine Neoplasms

Adenoid Cystic Carcinoma	Adenocarcinoma (Acinar or Solid)	Neuroendocrine Neoplasms (Carcinoid Tumors or Small Cell)
• Central, endobronchial location	• Peripheral	• Central • Carcinoid tumors may be endobronchial
• Biphasic tumor composed of luminal cells and abluminal (outer) myoepithelial cells growing in cribriform, tubular and solid patterns	• No myoepithelial cells	• May show neuroendocrine rosettes
• High-grade tumors may show nested growth with few or no obvious gland-like areas	• Solid growth pattern may have only scattered cells with intracytoplasmic mucin (at least 2 high-power fields should have ≥5 cells with intracellular mucin)	• Carcinoid tumors frequently have an organoid, nested appearance (zellballen architecture) or trabecular growth
• Luminal cells typically more strongly positive for keratins, including CK7 • Luminal cells c-Kit positive	• Typically CK7 positive • Infrequently positive for c-Kit	• May be positive for CK7 • Infrequently positive for c-Kit
• Abluminal myoepithelial cells positive for SMA, S100, calponin, p40, p63, and/or GFAP	• Negative for SMA, S100, calponin, p40, p63, and/or GFAP	• Negative for SMA, S100, calponin, p40, p63, and/or GFAP
• Negative for TTF-1, Napsin A, chromogranin, synaptophysin, CD56	• Frequently TTF-1 or Napsin positive	• Usually positive for chromogranin, synaptophysin, or CD56 • Up to 10% of small cell lung carcinoma may be negative for all neuroendocrine markers • TTF-1 is usually negative in carcinoid tumors, but positive in small cell lung carcinoma

cystic carcinoma may also mimic basaloid squamous cell carcinomas (Fig. 11.21, Table 11.14); however, myoepithelial markers such as SMA, S100, and calponin may be helpful to recognize the biphasic pattern. MYB immunostain or *MYB* gene rearrangement assays may also be helpful to differentiate these tumors.

Prognosis and Therapy

Surgically resected low-grade mucoepidermoid carcinoma has a 5-year survival of 95%, whereas surgically resected high-grade mucoepidermoid carcinoma has a 5-year survival of 48%. Surgically resected adenoid cystic carcinoma has a 5-year survival of 90%; however, due to the infiltrative nature of adenoid cystic carcinoma with frequent perineural invasion, positive margins and recurrence are common.

PULMONARY SALIVARY GLAND-TYPE NEOPLASMS – DISEASE FACT SHEET

Definition

▸▸ Arise from the seromucinous glands in the submucosa of the trachea and bronchi

▸▸ Of the salivary gland-type neoplasms, around two third are mucoepidermoid carcinoma and around one third are adenoid cystic carcinoma

Incidence and Location

▸▸ Pulmonary salivary gland-type neoplasms are rare, representing less than 1% of lung carcinomas

▸▸ Salivary gland-type neoplasms typically arise in an endobronchial location in the central airways

Age Distribution

▸▸ Median age of presentation for mucoepidermoid carcinoma: 54 years (range 18–88 years)

▸▸ Median age of presentation for adenoid cystic carcinoma: 60 years (range 22–90 years)

▸▸ Nearly equal sex distribution

Clinical Features

▸▸ May present with wheezing, cough, hemoptysis, and obstructive pneumonia

▸▸ Some patients may be asymptomatic

Radiologic Features

▸▸ Imaging typically shows a centrally located mass

Prognosis and Therapy

▸▸ Surgically resected low-grade mucoepidermoid carcinoma has a 5-year survival of 95%

▸▸ Surgically resected high-grade mucoepidermoid carcinoma has a 5-year survival of 48%

▸▸ Surgically resected adenoid cystic carcinoma has a 5-year survival of 90%; however, positive margins and recurrence are common

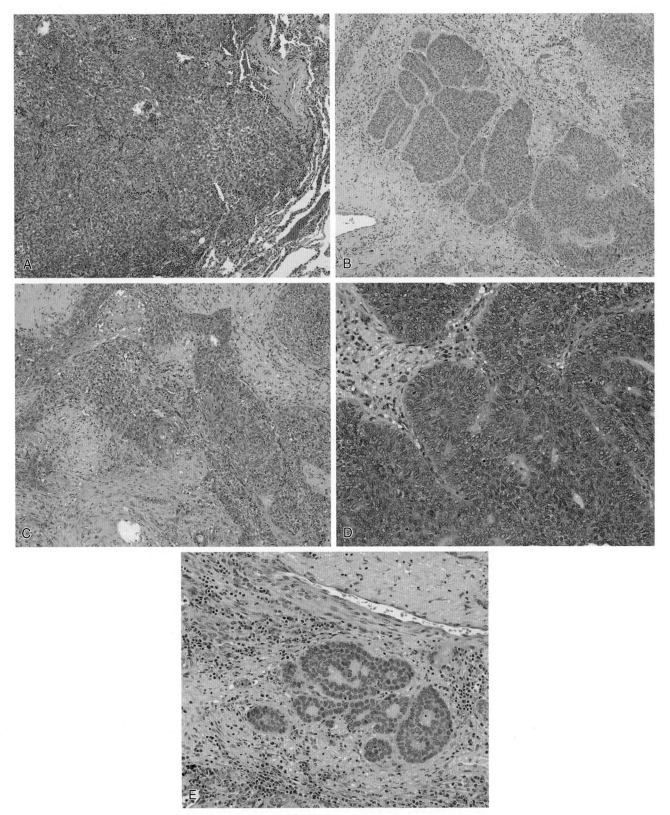

FIG. 11.21

A and **B,** Low-power view of basaloid squamous carcinoma with predominantly nodular appearance. **C,** The tumor may show areas of central keratinization and comedonecrosis (top). **D,** Higher-power view showing peripheral palisading and cribriform-like areas containing mucoid or hyalinized basement membrane material. **E,** Basaloid squamous cell carcinoma may show foci with tubular or cribriform architecture containing mucoid or hyalinized basement membrane material.

TABLE 11.14

Histologic, Immunohistochemical, and Molecular Features of Adenoid Cystic Carcinoma Versus Basaloid Squamous Cell Carcinoma

Adenoid Cystic Carcinoma	Basaloid Squamous Cell Carcinoma
• Central, endobronchial location	• Central, endobronchial location
• Biphasic tumor composed of luminal cells and abluminal (outer) myoepithelial cells growing in cribriform, tubular and solid patterns	• No glandular component and no cells with intracytoplasmic mucin • Rosettes may be present • Peripheral palisading • Comedonecrosis may be present
• The classic cribriform pattern shows cells surrounding the connective tissue cylinders containing myxoid or hyalinized basement membrane-like material	• Most have hyaline or mucoid stroma
• High-grade tumors may show nested growth with few or no obvious gland-like areas	• Solid, nodular or trabecular growth patterns
• No squamous carcinoma *in situ*	• Squamous carcinoma *in situ* may be present and extensive
• No overt keratinization or squamous pearls	• May show squamous pearls
• Abluminal myoepithelial cells positive for SMA, S100, calponin, p40, p63, and/or GFAP.	• CK5/6, p63, and p40 are positive • Negative for SMA, S100, calponin, GFAP
• *MYB* gene rearrangements	• *TP53* mutations • Many gene alterations, similar to conventional squamous cell carcinoma

PULMONARY SALIVARY GLAND-TYPE NEOPLASMS – PATHOLOGIC FEATURES

Gross Findings

▶▶ Arise in an endobronchial location in the central airways
▶▶ Mean size of mucoepidermoid carcinoma is 3.1 cm and that of adenoid cystic carcinoma is 3.8 cm
▶▶ Low-grade mucoepidermoid carcinomas show a gray-white to pink-tan, variably mucinous and cystic cut surface
▶▶ High-grade mucoepidermoid carcinomas are more infiltrative
▶▶ Adenoid cystic carcinomas may be well defined or infiltrative and show a gray-white homogenous cut surface
▶▶ Adenoid cystic carcinomas are frequently highly microscopically infiltrative beyond the grossly identified mass due the presence of perineural invasion, so careful sampling of the surrounding soft tissue is recommended

Microscopic Findings

▶▶ Mucoepidermoid carcinoma is composed of three cell types: mucin-secreting, squamous, and intermediate cells
▶▶ Low-grade mucoepidermoid carcinoma shows a cystic predominant pattern with tumor islands containing both cystic and solid patterns
 ▶▶ Cystic components are lined by cytologically bland columnar cells with apical mucin
 ▶▶ The solid components typically surround the cysts and are composed of the squamous and/or intermediate cells
 ▶▶ Mitotic activity is low and necrosis is rare
▶▶ High-grade mucoepidermoid carcinoma typically shows predominantly solid growth pattern with less cystic growth
 ▶▶ Mainly composed of atypical squamous and intermediate cells with frequent mitosis and necrosis
 ▶▶ Variable numbers of mucin-secreting cells are present
▶▶ Adenoid cystic carcinoma is a biphasic tumor composed of luminal cells and abluminal (outer) myoepithelial cells growing in cribriform, tubular and solid patterns
 ▶▶ The classic cribriform pattern shows cells surrounding connective tissue cylinders containing myxoid or hyalinized basement membrane-like material
 ▶▶ Perineural invasion is common

Pathologic Differential Diagnoses

▶▶ The main differential diagnosis for low-grade mucoepidermoid carcinoma is invasive mucinous adenocarcinoma
▶▶ The differential diagnosis for high-grade mucoepidermoid carcinoma includes squamous cell carcinoma and adenosquamous carcinoma
▶▶ The differential diagnosis for adenoid cystic carcinoma includes nonmucinous adenocarcinoma (acinar or solid patterns), neuroendocrine neoplasms, and basaloid squamous carcinomas

ATYPICAL ADENOMATOUS HYPERPLASIA

DIFFERENTIAL DIAGNOSES: REACTIVE TYPE II PNEUMOCYTE HYPERPLASIA, ADENOCARCINOMA *IN SITU*, ADENOCARCINOMA

Clinical Features

Atypical adenomatous hyperplasia (AAH) is defined in the 2015 WHO Classification as a small (usually less than or equal to 0.5 cm) localized proliferation of mildly to moderately atypical type II pneumocytes and/or Clara cells lining the alveolar walls and sometimes respiratory bronchioles. AAH is a preinvasive dysplastic lesion. By definition, there should be no evidence of stromal, lymphatic or vascular invasion or distant metastasis.

AAH is not detectable on chest x-rays but may sometimes be seen as a faint, nonsolid, focal ground glass nodule on CT scans. AAH typically occurs in the periphery of the lung. Most often AAH is an incidental finding which is seen in up to 30% of surgical lung resections for carcinoma, particularly in female patients with adenocarcinoma. In autopsy studies, AAH has been reported in 2% to 4% patients without lung cancer.

Pathologic Features

GROSS FINDINGS

AAH is usually an incidental microscopic finding, but rarely may be seen grossly as a small, poorly defined, tan-yellow nodule.

MICROSCOPIC FINDINGS

AAH is a small localized lesion (usually less than or equal to 0.5 cm) often arising in the centriacinar region, near respiratory bronchioles (Fig. 11.22). Either mildly to moderately atypical type II pneumocytes and/or Clara cells line the alveolar walls and sometimes respiratory bronchioles. Typically, AAH is not a confluent proliferation of cells, and there are gaps remaining between the atypical cells along the surface of the basement membranes of the alveolar septa.

The atypical type II pneumocytes are cuboidal or dome-shaped with fine cytoplasmic vacuoles or clear to foamy cytoplasm. Eosinophilic intranuclear inclusions may be present. The atypical Clara cells are columnar with cytoplasmic snouts and pale eosinophilic cytoplasm. The cells may show varying degrees of cytologic atypia. Mitotic figures are rare.

Ancillary Studies

The dysplastic cells in AAH are positive for TTF-1.

In studies of Asian populations, EGFR, BRAF, and KRAS mutations have been identified in AAH. However, the relative proportion of cells with EGFR mutation and the number of other nondriver mutations was found to be less in AAH than in nonmucinous adenocarcinoma *in situ* (AIS) or adenocarcinoma.

Differential Diagnosis

Distinguishing AAH from reactive type II pneumocyte hyperplasia may be challenging (Table 11.15). The presence of clinical or histologic evidence of injury such as diffuse alveolar damage, acute or organizing pneumonia, or interstitial fibrosis typically favor reactive type II pneumocyte hyperplasia (Fig. 11.23). On larger specimens, more diffuse involvement of scattered atypical cells which are not confluent also favors reactive type II pneumocyte hyperplasia.

The differential diagnosis for AAH includes nonmucinous AIS (Table 11.16). AAH and nonmucinous AIS represent a continuum from preinvasive dysplasia to *in situ* carcinoma. The cytologic features of AAH and nonmucinous AIS are similar, and both show type II pneumocyte or Clara cell differentiation. However, nonmucinous AIS is usually larger (>0.5 cm) and more cellular and crowded than AAH (Fig. 11.24). AIS is also typically better circumscribed with an abrupt transition to surrounding normal lung than AAH. AAH is not as well circumscribed with gradual transition to surrounding normal lung. Neither AAH nor AIS should show features diagnostic of adenocarcinoma such as tufting of tumor cells into the airspaces (micropapillary architecture), papillary structures, stromal invasion, or lymphatic or

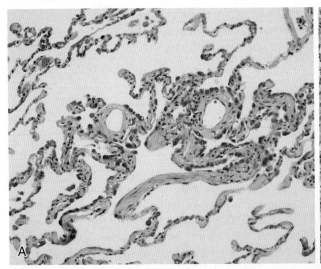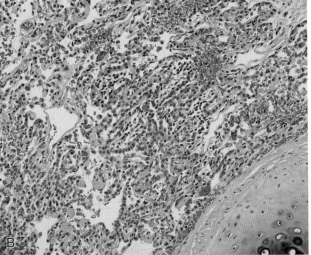

FIG. 11.22

Atypical adenomatous hyperplasia. **A,** Mildly atypical cells line alveolar septa but are not confluent (i.e., small gaps are present between some of the tumor cells). **B,** 1.5 mm focus of bland cuboidal cells lining some of the alveolar septa which is more confluent than in panel **A**; however, around the periphery it is not fully confluent. This lesion borders on adenocarcinoma *in situ*.

TABLE 11.15

Histologic Features of Atypical Adenomatous Hyperplasia Versus Reactive Type II Pneumocyte Hyperplasia

Atypical Adenomatous Hyperplasia	Reactive Type II Pneumocyte Hyperplasia
• Either mildly to moderately atypical type II pneumocytes and/or Clara cells line alveolar walls and sometimes respiratory bronchioles • Not confluent growth, gaps between cells	• May vary between mildly to severely atypical type II pneumocytes • May have gaps between cells, but may also have confluent growth
• No inflammation	• Inflammation such as acute or organizing pneumonia • Foreign material, vegetable matter, or foreign body giant cell reaction in aspiration pneumonia • Granulomas • Interstitial inflammation in viral pneumonia
• No associated tissue injury	• Underlying tissue injury such as hyaline membranes in acute or organizing diffuse alveolar damage
• No to minimal interstitial fibrosis	• Moderate to severe interstitial fibrosis raises the possibility of scar or underlying interstitial lung disease with reactive epithelial changes
• Localized involvement, typically less than or equal to 0.5 cm	• Diffuse involvement

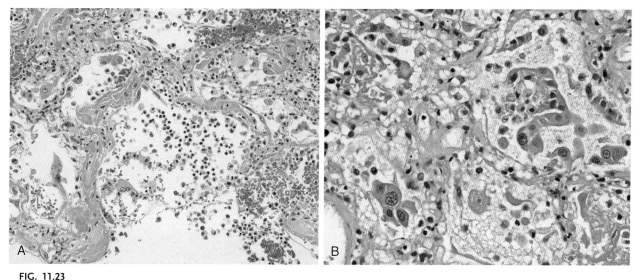

FIG. 11.23

A and **B,** Very atypical reactive type II pneumocytes in the setting of diffuse alveolar damage and acute pneumonia.

TABLE 11.16

Histologic Features of Atypical Adenomatous Hyperplasia Versus Nonmucinous Adenocarcinoma *In Situ*

Atypical Adenomatous Hyperplasia	Nonmucinous Adenocarcinoma *In Situ*
• Less than or equal to 0.5 cm	• Greater than 0.5 cm
• Either mildly to moderately atypical type II pneumocytes and/or Clara cells line alveolar walls and sometimes respiratory bronchioles	• Either mildly to moderately atypical type II pneumocytes and/or Clara cells line alveolar walls and sometimes respiratory bronchioles
• Lower cellularity • Gaps between cells • Not confluent growth	• More cellular and crowded with confluent growth
• Not as well circumscribed with gradual transition to surrounding normal lung	• Better circumscribed with more abrupt transition to surrounding normal lung

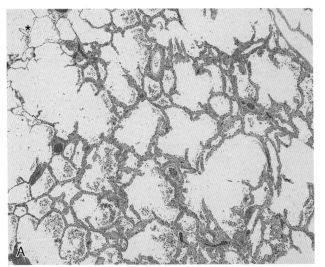

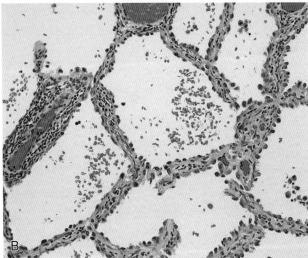

FIG. 11.24

A, Low-power view of 7 mm focus of nonmucinous adenocarcinoma *in situ* showing an abrupt transition to the background emphysematous lung (*). **B,** While cytologic features of tumor cells are similar to those seen in atypical adenomatous hyperplasia, higher magnification of AIS shows a more confluent proliferation involving all the adjacent alveolar septa. Disrupted alveolar septa similar to the background emphysematous lung are present; however, no definitive papillary or micropapillary structures are identified.

vascular invasion (Table 11.17). It should be noted that on small biopsies, a diagnosis of AIS cannot be rendered because the biopsy may not be representative of the entire lesion.

Prognosis and Therapy

Patients with resected AAH are cured. However, as these lesions are usually found incidentally in surgical resections in patients with adenocarcinoma, it is unclear how frequently or rapidly nonresected AAH could progress to nonmucinous AIS or invasive adenocarcinoma. Prognosis for patients with adenocarcinoma with or without AAH is not significantly different.

TABLE 11.17

Histologic Features of Atypical Adenomatous Hyperplasia Versus Adenocarcinoma

Atypical Adenomatous Hyperplasia	Adenocarcinoma
• Either mildly to moderately atypical type II pneumocytes and/or Clara cells line alveolar walls and sometimes respiratory bronchioles	• Malignant epithelial tumor with glandular differentiation, mucin production, or pneumocyte marker expression
• Lower cellularity • Gaps between cells • Not confluent growth	• More cellular and crowded with confluent growth
• No tufting of tumor cells into the airspaces (micropapillary architecture) • No papillary structures • No stromal invasion • No lymphatic or vascular invasion	• May have tufting of tumor cells into the airspaces (micropapillary architecture) • May have papillary structures • May have stromal invasion • May have lymphatic or vascular invasion

---

ATYPICAL ADENOMATOUS HYPERPLASIA – DISEASE FACT SHEET

Definition
▸▸ Preinvasive dysplastic lesion
▸▸ Small (usually less than or equal to 0.5 cm) and localized proliferation of mildly to moderately atypical type II pneumocytes and/or Clara cells lining alveolar walls and sometimes respiratory bronchioles

Incidence and Location
▸▸ Incidental finding
▸▸ Present in 30% of resections for carcinoma
▸▸ In autopsy studies, present in 2%–4% of patients without lung cancer

Age Distribution
▸▸ Most often incidentally discovered

Clinical Features
▸▸ Most often incidentally discovered

Radiologic Features
▸▸ Most often incidentally discovered
▸▸ May sometimes be seen as a faint, nonsolid, focal ground glass nodule on CT scans

Prognosis and Therapy
▸▸ Patients with resected AAH are cured
▸▸ Prognosis for patients with adenocarcinoma with or without AAH is not significantly different

---

ATYPICAL ADENOMATOUS HYPERPLASIA – PATHOLOGIC FEATURES

Gross Findings
▸▸ AAH is usually an incidental microscopic finding
▸▸ Rarely may be seen grossly as a small, poorly defined, tan-yellow nodule

MICROPAPILLARY ADENOCARCINOMA

DIFFERENTIAL DIAGNOSES: ADENOCARCINOMA *IN SITU*, LEPIDIC ADENOCARCINOMA, PAPILLARY ADENOCARCINOMA

Clinical Features

Micropapillary adenocarcinoma is a histologic subtype of invasive lung adenocarcinoma that shows tumor cells growing in tufts lacking fibrovascular cores. Micropapillary adenocarcinoma was added to the 2011 IASLC/ATS/ERS Classification of Lung Adenocarcinoma and subsequent 2015 WHO Classification of Tumours of the Lung but was not in prior editions of the WHO Classification. In prior classifications, micropapillary subtype would have been considered part of nonmucinous bronchioloalveolar carcinoma (BAC). Per the current guidelines, the lesions that were previously classified as BAC would be classified currently as AIS, minimally invasive adenocarcinoma (MIA), lepidic predominant adenocarcinoma (LPA), adenocarcinoma, or invasive mucinous adenocarcinoma. The current WHO recommendation is to give the predominant subtype of adenocarcinoma because of prognostic significance (discussed below) and to report all subtypes present in 5% increments. In particular, it is important to recognize micropapillary components of adenocarcinomas because even small amounts of micropapillary subtype have been found to predict worse clinical outcome in several studies. Thus, micropapillary adenocarcinoma is considered one of the high-grade subtypes of adenocarcinoma.

The overall lung adenocarcinoma incidence from 2006 to 2010 was 33.6 per 100,000 population. In a large meta-analysis of lung adenocarcinoma, in stage I–III patients, the overall incidence of micropapillary predominant adenocarcinoma was 10%. In patients with distant metastases, the incidence of micropapillary predominant adenocarcinoma was 15%.

In a large study including 207 adenocarcinomas containing micropapillary histologic subtype, adenocarcinomas with micropapillary subtype showed a slight male predominance with patient age ranging from 42 to 86 years (median age 61 years). Micropapillary pattern has been found in both smokers and nonsmokers.

There are no known specific clinical presenting features to differentiate micropapillary subtype from other subtypes of adenocarcinoma. Patients with lung adenocarcinoma may be asymptomatic or may have progressive shortness of breath, cough, chest pain, or hemoptysis. Like other patterns of invasive adenocarcinoma of the lung, on CT, micropapillary predominant adenocarcinomas typically present as semi-solid or solid nodules, typically in the periphery of the lung.

Pathologic Features

GROSS FINDINGS

The micropapillary subtype of adenocarcinoma like other invasive adenocarcinomas are typically peripheral lesions. Tumor size varies between 0.5 and 6.5 cm. As seen with other invasive adenocarcinomas, tumors are typically gray-white nodules. Pleural puckering may be present.

MICROSCOPIC FINDINGS

The micropapillary subtype of lung adenocarcinoma is similar to the micropapillary pattern described in other organ systems including breast and ovary. Micropapillary adenocarcinomas show tumor cells growing in tufts or florets that lack fibrovascular cores (Fig. 11.25). These structures may be connected to alveolar walls or may be detached. Ring-like glandular structures may float within alveolar spaces. The tumor cells are usually small and cuboidal with variable nuclear atypia. Psammoma bodies may be seen. Vascular and stromal invasion is common; however, stromal invasion is not required for a diagnosis of micropapillary subtype.

Micropapillary adenocarcinomas may show spread through airspaces (STAS) where micropapillary clusters of tumor cells are thought to detach from alveolar walls and are found in alveolar spaces away from the main tumor mass. Identification of STAS is significantly associated with the presence of micropapillary pattern.

Even small adenocarcinomas which show micropapillary pattern are more likely to have lymph node,

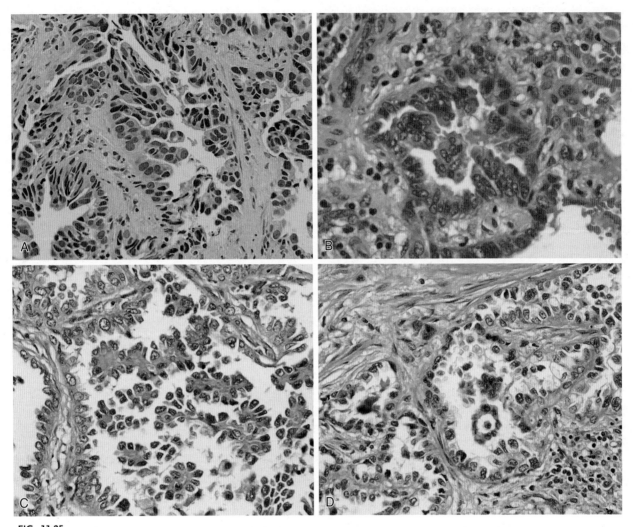

FIG. 11.25

Examples of micropapillary adenocarcinoma. **A** and **B,** Tufting of tumor cells into the alveolar lumen. Tufts of tumor cells lack fibrovascular cores. **C,** Tufts appearing to be "detached" and floating in the alveolar lumen. **D,** Micropapillary area forming "ring-like" structure in the alveolar lumen.

intrapulmonary, brain, and bone metastases. Regardless of the predominant pattern of adenocarcinoma present (acinar, papillary, etc.), when even small amounts of micropapillary pattern are present, micropapillary adenocarcinoma has been found to be over represented in the metastases. Tumors with micropapillary subtype have also been found to more likely have micrometastases in the lymph nodes.

Ancillary Studies

Micropapillary adenocarcinomas are typically positive for cytokeratin (CK) 7 (90%), TTF-1 (80%–90%), Napsin A (89%), and MUC1. Infrequently, CK20 (13%) may be positive. Surfactant apoprotein A (SP-A) may be lost. MUC4 and CEA are typically negative.

Molecular studies have shown that micropapillary predominant adenocarcinomas harbor a mix of mutually exclusive driver mutations including EGFR in 20% to 86% of cases, BRAF in 20%, ALK in 10%, KRAS in 12% to 33%. Other mutations found in micropapillary adenocarcinomas include RET and Her2.

Differential Diagnosis

The differential diagnosis for micropapillary adenocarcinoma includes some of the current histologic subtypes that formerly were classified as BAC including nonmucinous AIS, MIA, and LPA. Nonmucinous AIS is small (less than or equal to 3 cm), localized adenocarcinoma with growth restricted to single layer of neoplastic cells along the pre-existing alveolar structures (see Fig. 11.24A and B, Table 11.18). The diagnosis of nonmucinous AIS is not allowed to contain areas of intra-alveolar tufting or the ring-like glandular structures seen in micropapillary adenocarcinoma. AIS is

TABLE 11.18

Histologic Features of Micropapillary Adenocarcinoma Versus Nonmucinous Adenocarcinoma *In Situ*

Micropapillary Adenocarcinoma	Nonmucinous Adenocarcinoma *In Situ*
• Tumor cells growing in tufts or florets that lack fibrovascular cores	• Either mildly to moderately atypical type II pneumocytes and/or Clara cells line alveolar walls and sometimes respiratory bronchioles
• Tufts or florets may be connected to alveolar walls or may be detached	• No tufting or intra-alveolar tumor cells
• Ring-like glandular structures may float within alveolar spaces	
• Vascular and stromal invasion is common	• No stromal, pleural, or vascular invasion
• May show spread through air-spaces	• Better circumscribed with more abrupt transition to surrounding normal lung

TABLE 11.19

Histologic Features of Micropapillary Adenocarcinoma Versus Minimally Invasive Adenocarcinoma (MIA) or Lepidic Predominant Adenocarcinoma (LPA)

Micropapillary Adenocarcinoma	MIA or LPA
• Histologic subtype of invasive lung adenocarcinoma that shows tumor cells growing in tufts or florets lacking fibrovascular cores	• Both MIA and LPA are defined as tumors which shows predominantly bland type II pneumocyte or Clara type cells growing along the alveolar walls with an invasive component
• Tufts or florets may be connected to alveolar walls or may be detached	• For both MIA and LPA, the invasive component of the tumor could include the micropapillary histologic subtype or other subtypes such as acinar, papillary, or solid
• Ring-like glandular structures may float within alveolar spaces	
• Micropapillary predominant adenocarcinoma should have micropapillary pattern as the predominant pattern	• For MIA, the invasive component is less than or equal to 5 mm in greatest dimension
	• For LPA, the invasive component is greater than 5 mm in greatest dimension

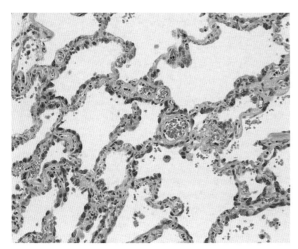

FIG. 11.26
Lepidic growth pattern at the periphery of an invasive adenocarcinoma shows minimally atypical cuboidal tumor cells lining the alveolar walls in a single layer. No tufting of tumor cells into the alveolar spaces is identified.

TABLE 11.20

Histologic Features of Micropapillary Adenocarcinoma Versus Papillary Adenocarcinoma

Micropapillary Adenocarcinoma	Papillary Adenocarcinoma
• Tumor cells growing in tufts or florets that lack fibrovascular cores	• Neoplastic glandular cells growing along the central fibrovascular cores

also not allowed to contain areas of stromal, pleural, or vascular invasion. It should be noted that on small biopsies, a diagnosis of AIS cannot be rendered because the biopsy may not be representative of the entire lesion.

Both MIA and LPA are defined by the 2015 WHO Classification as tumors which shows predominantly bland type II pneumocyte or Clara type cells growing along alveolar walls with an invasive component (Fig. 11.26, Table 11.19). For MIA, the invasive component is less than or equal to 5 mm in greatest dimension; whereas, for LPA, the invasive component is greater than 5 mm in greatest dimension. For both MIA and LPA, the invasive component of the tumor could include the micropapillary histologic subtype or other subtypes such as acinar, papillary, or solid. LPA rather than MIA should also be used for

the diagnosis when there is: (1) lymphatic, blood vascular, or pleural invasion; (2) tumor necrosis; or (3) STAS.

Micropapillary adenocarcinoma may also be confused with papillary adenocarcinoma, another subtype of invasive adenocarcinoma (Table 11.20). For micropapillary adenocarcinoma, the tufts of tumor cells or floating intra-alveolar tumor cells do not contain fibrovascular cores; whereas, for papillary adenocarcinoma, the intra-alveolar component shows growth of neoplastic glandular cells along the central fibrovascular cores (Fig. 11.27).

Prognosis and Therapy

Utilizing the prior 2004 WHO Classification, 80% to 90% of cases of adenocarcinoma fell under the category of "Adenocarcinoma, mixed subtype," a diagnosis that had little prognostic significance. In addition, grading of the tumor into well (grade 1), moderately (grade 2), and poorly (grade 3) differentiated had limited prognostic significance. Because numerous studies were

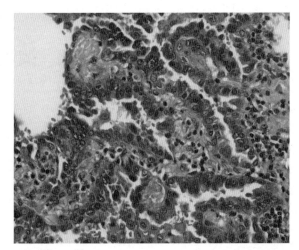

FIG. 11.27

Papillary adenocarcinoma. Tumor cells are growing along the central fibrovascular cores which are protruding into the alveolar lumens.

being published indicating that certain histologic subtypes (including micropapillary) do have prognostic significance, the 2011 IASLC/ATS/ERS and 2015 WHO Classification of Lung Adenocarcinomas made a recommendation to give predominant subtype and other histologic subtypes in 5% increments (e.g., 45% acinar, 35% lepidic, and 20% papillary).

After micropapillary adenocarcinoma was added to the 2011 IASLC/ATS/ERS Classification of Lung Adenocarcinomas, numerous studies have been published verifying that micropapillary adenocarcinoma tends to have a worse prognosis. Even for stage I tumors, patients with micropapillary predominant adenocarcinoma have 65% to 67% 5-year disease-free survival, and for stage I, II, and III tumors, patients with micropapillary predominant adenocarcinomas have 38% to 47% 5-year overall survival. In addition, there have been studies indicating that even for tumors ≤2 cm, small amounts of micropapillary pattern in a lung adenocarcinoma may have a worse prognosis.

In patients with stage IA micropapillary predominant adenocarcinoma with EGFR mutations, there is a study indicating that EGFR tyrosine kinase inhibitors can improve the 5-year disease-free survival, although they did not improve overall survival. In patients with stage IB micropapillary predominant adenocarcinoma, there is a study indicating that there is a survival benefit to adjuvant chemotherapy.

MICROPAPILLARY ADENOCARCINOMA – DISEASE FACT SHEET

Definition

▸▸ Histologic subtype of invasive lung adenocarcinoma that shows tumor cells growing in tufts lacking fibrovascular cores

Incidence and Location

▸▸ In patients with stage I–III lung adenocarcinoma, the overall incidence of micropapillary predominant adenocarcinoma was 10%
▸▸ In patients with stage IV lung adenocarcinoma, the incidence of micropapillary predominant adenocarcinoma was 15%

Age Distribution

▸▸ Slight male predominance with patient age ranging from 42 to 86 years (median age 61 years)

Clinical Features

▸▸ Asymptomatic or may have progressive shortness of breath, cough, chest pain, or hemoptysis

Radiologic Features

▸▸ Semisolid or solid nodules
▸▸ Typically in the periphery of the lung

Prognosis and Therapy

▸▸ Patients with stage I, II, and III micropapillary predominant adenocarcinomas have a 38%–47% 5-year overall survival
▸▸ Even for tumors ≤2 cm, small amounts of micropapillary pattern in a lung adenocarcinoma may have a worse prognosis

---

MICROPAPILLARY ADENOCARCINOMA – PATHOLOGIC FEATURES

Gross Findings

▸▸ Typically peripheral lesions
▸▸ Size varies between 0.5 and 6.5 cm
▸▸ Tumors are typically gray-white nodules
▸▸ Pleural puckering may be present

Microscopic Findings

▸▸ Tumor cells growing in tufts or florets that lack fibrovascular cores
▸▸ These structures may be connected to alveolar walls or may be detached
▸▸ Ring-like glandular structures may float within alveolar spaces
▸▸ The tumor cells are usually small and cuboidal with variable nuclear atypia
▸▸ Psammoma bodies may be seen
▸▸ Vascular and stromal invasion is common; however, stromal invasion is not required for a diagnosis of micropapillary subtype
▸▸ May show spread through airspaces (STAS)
▸▸ Even small adenocarcinomas which show micropapillary pattern are more likely to have lymph node, intrapulmonary, brain, and bone metastases

Pathologic Differential Diagnoses

▸▸ Nonmucinous adenocarcinoma *in situ*
▸▸ Minimally invasive or lepidic predominant adenocarcinoma
▸▸ Papillary adenocarcinoma

INVASIVE MUCINOUS ADENOCARCINOMA

DIFFERENTIAL DIAGNOSES: MUCINOUS ADENOCARCINOMA *IN SITU*, METASTATIC MUCINOUS ADENOCARCINOMA FROM GASTROINTESTINAL TRACT OR FROM OVARY

Clinical Features

Invasive mucinous adenocarcinoma is a histologic subtype of invasive lung adenocarcinoma that shows tumor cells with goblet or columnar morphology with abundant intracytoplasmic mucin. Invasive mucinous adenocarcinoma was added to the 2011 IASLC/ATS/ERS Classification of Lung Adenocarcinoma and subsequent 2015 WHO Classification of Tumours of the Lung but was not in prior editions of the WHO Classification. In prior classifications, invasive mucinous adenocarcinoma would have been considered mucinous BAC. In the current WHO Classification, the lesions that were previously classified as BAC would be classified currently as AIS, MIA, LPA, adenocarcinoma, or invasive mucinous adenocarcinoma.

Initial smaller earlier studies had found that "mucinous BAC" is more commonly identified in smokers and in men. However, a 2018 review of the Surveillance, Epidemiology, and End Results (SEER) database by Moon et al. found that invasive mucinous adenocarcinoma was slightly more common in women (59% of cases) with a mean age of 66 years. Moon et al. found that invasive mucinous adenocarcinoma represented 0.2% of lung carcinomas and 1.5% of resected lung carcinomas.

Patients with invasive mucinous lung adenocarcinoma, like those with other lung carcinomas, may be asymptomatic or may have progressive shortness of breath, cough, chest pain, weight loss, or hemoptysis. However, more specifically, patients with invasive mucinous adenocarcinoma may have abundant mucoid secretions called bronchorrhea.

On imaging, invasive mucinous adenocarcinomas may show lobar or multilobar involvement, and may be multicentric and bilateral. Radiographically, tumors may range from nonsolid to solid and may show consolidation. Air bronchograms are common.

Pathologic Features

GROSS FINDINGS

Invasive mucinous adenocarcinoma typically occurs in the peripheral lung and grossly appears as a poorly circumscribed, soft, gelatinous tumor. Some tumors may show widely spread disseminated nodules or a diffuse pneumonia-like lobar consolidation. It typically lacks central desmoplastic fibrosis, anthracotic pigmentation, or pleural puckering.

MICROSCOPIC FINDINGS

Histologically, tumor cells characteristically show a goblet or columnar cell morphology with abundant intracytoplasmic mucin and small basally located nuclei (Fig. 11.28). Nuclear atypia is usually inconspicuous or absent. Surrounding alveolar spaces are often filled with mucin. The tumor cells may show a mixture of lepidic, acinar, papillary, and micropapillary growth patterns.

Ancillary Studies

The immunophenotype of mucinous adenocarcinoma of the lung may be quite different from nonmucinous

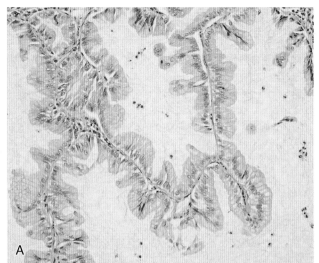
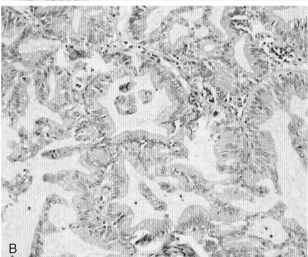

FIG. 11.28

A and **B,** Invasive mucinous adenocarcinoma. The tumor is composed of tall columnar cells with abundant apical mucin and basally located nuclei. The tumor has areas of micropapillary architecture (best seen in panel **B**) and is thus considered invasive. Mucin fills the alveolar spaces.

adenocarcinomas. Invasive mucinous adenocarcinomas are typically CK7 positive (83%–100% of cases) but also CK20 positive (25%–89% of cases). Invasive mucinous adenocarcinomas are less frequently positive for TTF-1 (27.5%–42% of cases) and Napsin A (32% of cases) in comparison with nonmucinous lung adenocarcinomas. They may also be positive for CDX-2 and villin (variably reported between 0% and up to 100% of cases in small studies).

While molecular studies are not necessary for diagnostic purposes, they may be important for therapeutic decisions. Invasive mucinous adenocarcinomas commonly have KRAS mutations (62%–86% of cases), but infrequently have been found to have EGFR mutation (0%–22% of cases).

In KRAS-negative cases, other mutations identified include gene fusions involving the NRG1, NTRK1, BRAF, and ALK and mutations within the ERBB2 and BRAF genes.

Differential Diagnosis

The differential diagnosis for invasive mucinous adenocarcinoma includes mucinous AIS, minimally invasive mucinous adenocarcinoma, and metastatic mucinous adenocarcinoma.

Mucinous AIS is rarely identified but differs from invasive mucinous adenocarcinoma (Fig. 11.29, Table 11.21) by showing all of the following criteria as defined by the 2015 WHO Classification: (1) small (less than or equal to 3 cm), localized adenocarcinoma with neoplastic cells growing along the pre-existing alveolar structures (lepidic growth); (2) no evidence of stromal, vascular, or pleural invasion; (3) no acinar, papillary, solid, or micropapillary growth patterns; and (4) no intra-alveolar tumor cells. In addition, if there are

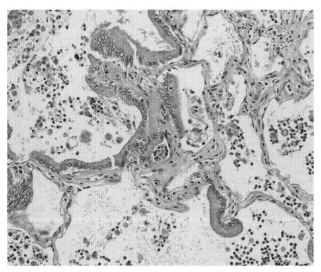

FIG. 11.29
Lepidic growth in mucinous adenocarcinoma. There is no papillary or micropapillary architecture in this area. If the entire tumor is less than or equal to 3 cm and shows pure lepidic growth, then the tumor would be best termed adenocarcinoma *in situ*.

multiple tumor foci, a tumor can only be considered AIS, if the tumors are favored to represent multiple separate primaries.

A minimally invasive mucinous adenocarcinoma, as defined by the 2015 WHO Classification, is small (less than or equal to 3 cm), localized adenocarcinoma showing predominantly lepidic growth with an invasive component measuring less than or equal to 0.5 cm in greatest dimension. A mucinous adenocarcinoma with more than 0.5 cm of an invasive pattern, such as acinar, papillary, solid, or micropapillary, would be classified as invasive mucinous adenocarcinoma (see Table 11.21).

The differential diagnosis of invasive mucinous adenocarcinoma of the lung includes metastatic mucinous adenocarcinoma from another location. In particular, differentiating from metastatic mucinous adenocarcinomas of gastrointestinal or pancreatic-biliary origin may be quite difficult. Primary invasive mucinous adenocarcinoma may have a similar immunophenotype which is positive for CK20, CDX2, and villin and negative for TTF-1 and Napsin A. In some cases, invasive mucinous adenocarcinoma of the lung can be differentiated from metastatic mucinous ovarian carcinoma by PAX8 staining which is positive in about one third of ovarian mucinous adenocarcinomas. Overall, immunostaining may not be helpful in identifying the primary site for mucinous adenocarcinomas, and clinical correlation may be necessary to differentiate.

Prognosis and Therapy

Although initial smaller studies had indicated that invasive mucinous adenocarcinomas have a worse prognosis than acinar or papillary types of nonmucinous lung adenocarcinomas, a 2018 review of the SEER database by Moon et al. found that for invasive mucinous adenocarcinoma, the 5-year lung cancer–specific survival was 69.3% and the median survival was 51.0 months. Invasive mucinous adenocarcinomas had an overall survival

TABLE 11.21
Histologic Features of Invasive Mucinous Adenocarcinoma Versus Nonmucinous Adenocarcinoma *In Situ* Versus Minimally Invasive Mucinous Adenocarcinoma

Invasive Mucinous Adenocarcinoma	Mucinous Adenocarcinoma *In Situ*	Minimally Invasive Mucinous Adenocarcinoma
• Any size	• Less than or equal to 3 cm	• Less than or equal to 3 cm
• Invasive component greater than 0.5 cm	• No evidence of stromal, vascular, or pleural invasion	• Invasive component less than or equal to 0.5 cm
• Invasive component may show a mixture of lepidic, acinar, papillary, and micropapillary growth patterns	• No evidence of lepidic, acinar, papillary, and micropapillary growth patterns	• Invasive component may show a mixture of lepidic, acinar, papillary, and micropapillary growth patterns
• Intra-alveolar tumor cells may be present	• No intra-alveolar tumor cells	• Intra-alveolar tumor cells may be present
• May show lobar or multilobar involvement • May be multicentric and bilateral	• Should be localized	• Should be localized

in some studies between lepidic predominant (which are considered low grade) and acinar or papillary predominant (which are considered intermediate grade) nonmucinous adenocarcinomas. For first-line treatment, they found that most patients were treated with surgery alone, but some received adjuvant or neoadjuvant chemotherapy and/or radiation therapy.

INVASIVE MUCINOUS ADENOCARCINOMA – DISEASE FACT SHEET

Definition
▸▸ Histologic subtype of invasive lung adenocarcinoma that shows tumor cells with goblet or columnar morphology with abundant intracytoplasmic mucin

Incidence and Location
▸▸ Represents 0.2% of lung carcinomas and 1.5% of resected lung carcinomas
▸▸ Usually located in the periphery of the lung

Age Distribution
▸▸ Slight female predominance with mean patient age 66 ± 12 years

Clinical Features
▸▸ Asymptomatic or may have progressive shortness of breath, cough, chest pain, or hemoptysis
▸▸ Bronchorrhea may be present

Radiologic Features
▸▸ Semi-solid or solid nodules
▸▸ Typically in the periphery of the lung

Prognosis and Therapy
▸▸ 5-year lung cancer–specific survival was 69.3% and the median survival was 51.0 months

---

INVASIVE MUCINOUS ADENOCARCINOMA – PATHOLOGIC FEATURES

Gross Findings
▸▸ Invasive mucinous adenocarcinoma typically occurs in the peripheral lung and grossly appears as a poorly circumscribed, soft, gelatinous tumor
▸▸ Some tumors may show widely spread disseminate nodules or a diffuse pneumonia-like lobar consolidation
▸▸ It typically lacks central desmoplastic fibrosis, anthracotic pigmentation, or pleural puckering

Microscopic Findings
▸▸ Tumor cells characteristically show a goblet or columnar cell morphology with abundant intracytoplasmic mucin and small basally located nuclei
▸▸ Nuclear atypia is usually inconspicuous or absent
▸▸ Surrounding alveolar spaces are often filled with mucin
▸▸ The tumor cells may show a mixture of lepidic, acinar, papillary, and micropapillary growth patterns

Pathologic Differential Diagnoses
▸▸ Mucinous adenocarcinoma *in situ*
▸▸ Minimally invasive mucinous adenocarcinoma
▸▸ Metastatic mucinous adenocarcinoma of gastrointestinal or ovarian origin

---

EPITHELIOID MESOTHELIOMA

DIFFERENTIAL DIAGNOSES: ADENOCARCINOMA, REACTIVE MESOTHELIAL HYPERPLASIA

Clinical Features

Epithelioid mesothelioma is a malignant tumor of mesothelial origin showing epithelioid morphology. These tumors occur over a wide age range, but the vast majority are seen in patients over the age of 60 years and are more common in men. The most common cause of mesothelioma is asbestos exposure. Other causes include therapeutic radiation for other tumors and in rare case genetic predisposition (germline mutation in BRCA1-associated protein-1 [BAP1]). Patients present with insidious onset of chest pain or dyspnea. Most classical radiologic findings include a diffuse circumferential rind of nodular pleura associated with effusion. Less commonly, malignant mesothelioma may present with isolated effusion without pleural nodularity. It is important to remember that none of the clinical symptoms or imaging findings are specific to mesothelioma.

Pathologic Features

GROSS FINDINGS

Early mesotheliomas may present with small nodules. With disease progression, the nodules coalesce to form a rind encasing the lung.

MICROSCOPIC FINDINGS

Epithelioid mesothelioma shows a wide range of histologic patterns, including solid, tubular, papillary, trabecular, micropapillary, microcystic, clear cell, and small cell. The neoplastic mesothelial cells are polygonal with moderate to abundant eosinophilic cytoplasm. The mitoses are variable. Demonstrating tissue invasion is essential in making the diagnosis of a malignant mesothelial process.

Ancillary Studies

Based on sensitivity and specificity, calretinin, cytokeratin 5/6, WT1, and D2-40 are the best positive markers to support mesothelial origin. In several recent studies, the finding of the loss of BAP1 by immunohistochemistry or the finding of homozygous deletion of p16 by fluorescence *in situ* hybridization (FISH) is present only in malignant mesothelioma and not in benign mesothelial proliferations.

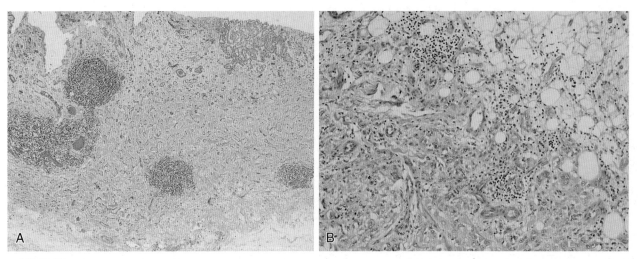

FIG. 11.30

A and **B,** Low-power and high-power view of epithelioid mesothelioma with overt infiltration into adipose and fibrous tissue.

Differential Diagnosis

The most common differential diagnosis for the epithelioid malignant mesothelioma is adenocarcinoma. There are many immunohistochemical markers that help in separating malignant mesothelioma from lung adenocarcinoma or metastatic adenocarcinoma from another site. It is important to remember that none of the markers are 100% specific. The International Mesothelioma Interest Group recommends the use of at least two mesothelial and two carcinoma markers to differentiate mesothelioma from adenocarcinoma. The best positive carcinoma markers are MOC31 and claudin 4, while the best mesothelioma markers are calretinin, cytokeratin 5/6, WT1, and D2-40.

When trying to differentiate between malignant mesothelioma and adenocarcinoma with a specific site of origin, an origin-specific marker (e.g., TTF-1 for lung adenocarcinoma) may be extremely helpful. However, GATA3 expression should be interpreted with caution, because in addition to being positive in metastatic breast carcinoma, it is expressed in up to one half of epithelioid mesotheliomas.

Exuberant reactive mesothelial proliferations may also mimic malignant mesothelioma. Overt tissue invasion is the key feature in making the diagnosis of malignant mesothelioma (Fig. 11.30, Table 11.22). Demonstration of the loss of BAP1 by immunohistochemistry or p16 deletion by FISH may be helpful in particularly challenging cases or in cytology specimens (Fig. 11.31).

Prognosis and Therapy

Overall, the long-term prognosis for mesothelioma is poor. The patients with epithelioid subtype of mesothelioma

TABLE 11.22

Comparison of Malignant Mesothelioma and Benign Mesothelial Proliferation

	Epithelioid Mesothelioma	Mesothelial Hyperplasia
Tissue invasion	Present	Absent
Necrosis	Helpful if present	Rare, if present, confined to the surface
BAP1	If lost, supports the diagnosis. Not very sensitive	Intact
Homozygous loss of p16 by FISH	70% of cases show loss	Intact

have the longest overall survival, approximately 14 months. There is no established histologic grading system; however, high nuclear grade and high mitotic activity are associated with worse prognosis. Chemotherapy and surgery are associated with improved survival.

EPITHELIOID MESOTHELIOMA – DISEASE FACT SHEET

Definition
▸▸ Malignant tumor of mesothelial origin with epithelioid morphology

Incidence and Location
▸▸ Tumor involves serosal membranes
▸▸ Right pleural involvement is more common than left (3:2)
▸▸ Bilateral involvement at diagnosis is unusual

Age Distribution
▸▸ Majority >60 years

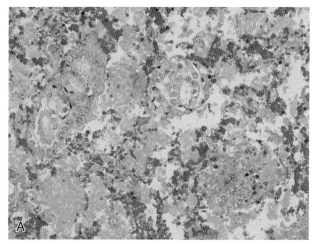

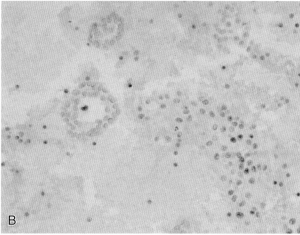

FIG. 11.31

A, Mesothelioma cells in effusion specimen showing loss of BAP1 by immunohistochemistry **(B)**. Note the staining in the background benign cells (internal positive control).

Clinical Features

▸▸ More common in men
▸▸ Etiology:
   ▸▸ Asbestos exposure
   ▸▸ Therapeutic radiation
   ▸▸ Inherited predisposition (germline mutation in BAP1)
▸▸ Insidious onset of chest pain and/or dyspnea

Radiologic Features

▸▸ Diffuse circumferential rind of nodular pleura
▸▸ Pleural effusion

Prognosis and Therapy

▸▸ Long-term prognosis is poor

EPITHELIOID MESOTHELIOMA – PATHOLOGIC FEATURES

Gross Findings

▸▸ Early disease presents with small nodules
▸▸ Later in disease progression nodule coalesce to form a rind encasing the lung

---

Microscopic Findings

▸▸ Wide range of histologic patterns (solid, tubular, papillary, trabecular, micropapillary, microcystic, clear cell, and small cell)
▸▸ Epithelioid cells with moderate to abundant cytoplasm
▸▸ Mitoses may be infrequent

Pathologic Differential Diagnoses

▸▸ Adenocarcinoma
▸▸ Reactive mesothelial hyperplasia

SARCOMATOID AND DESMOPLASTIC MESOTHELIOMA

DIFFERENTIAL DIAGNOSES: PLEURITIS, SARCOMATOID CARCINOMA, SARCOMA

Clinical Features

Sarcomatoid mesothelioma is a diffuse malignant spindle cell neoplasm of mesothelial origin involving serosal membranes. Desmoplastic malignant mesothelioma is characterized by malignant mesothelial cells involving dense collagenized tissue. Sarcomatoid type accounts for less than 10% and desmoplastic type for less than 2% of all mesotheliomas. Sarcomatoid mesothelioma is associated with frequent metastases and no effusion. Desmoplastic mesothelioma progresses rapidly and can metastasize to bone. Just like epithelioid mesotheliomas, sarcomatoid and desmoplastic mesotheliomas occur over a wide age range, but the vast majority are seen in patients over the age of 60 years and are more common in men. The most common cause of mesothelioma is asbestos exposure. Other causes include therapeutic radiation for other tumors and in rare case genetic predisposition (germline mutation in BAP1). Patients may present with insidious onset of chest pain or dyspnea. The most classical radiologic finding is a diffuse circumferential rind of nodular pleura.

Pathologic Features

GROSS FINDINGS

Tumor presents with diffuse pleural thickening or pleural-based mass.

MICROSCOPIC FINDINGS

Sarcomatoid mesothelioma is characterized by a proliferation of spindle cells with overt invasion into the fat, skeletal muscle, or lung parenchyma (Fig. 11.32). The neoplastic mesothelial cells are often deceptively bland, and the stromal invasion may be difficult to identify. In

FIG. 11.32
Sarcomatoid mesothelioma showing cellular proliferation with fat infiltration.

FIG. 11.33
Sarcomatoid mesothelioma with area of necrosis.

this case, a keratin stain, showing keratin-positive cells within the fat or skeletal muscle, is exceptionally helpful (see Ancillary Studies). In addition, the histologic finding of expansile nodules with sharp demarcation, bland necrosis (Fig. 11.33), and abrupt change in cellularity are of great diagnostic use. In some cases, sarcomatoid malignant mesothelioma may show frankly sarcomatous areas (e.g., osteosarcoma, chondrosarcoma).

Similar to sarcomatoid mesotheliomas, desmoplastic mesotheliomas are characterized by spindle cells; however, desmoplastic mesotheliomas typically have lower cellularity and show spindle cells embedded in hyalinized fibrous stroma, comprising at least 50% of the tumor.

Ancillary Studies

Sarcomatoid mesothelioma typically expresses keratin markers at least focally. However, approximately 5% of sarcomatoid mesotheliomas may be keratin negative. While keratin immunostain is not routinely used for the diagnosis of desmoplastic and sarcomatoid mesotheliomas, it is very useful in highlighting soft tissue invasion. The presence of cytokeratin-positive cells within the adipose tissue or skeletal muscle is essentially diagnostic of mesothelioma in the appropriate setting. Mesothelial markers that are used in epithelioid mesothelioma, such as WT1 and CK5/6, are not typically helpful, as most sarcomatoid and desmoplastic mesotheliomas do not express these markers. Calretinin and D2-40 may be expressed, with calretinin being the most common. Approximately 30% of sarcomatoid mesotheliomas demonstrate calretinin staining; however, the expression may be very focal. It is important to note that in the absence of cytokeratin expression, calretinin and D2-40 staining should not be interpreted as evidence of mesothelial differentiation. In particularly challenging cases, p16 FISH may be helpful, as homozygous deletion of p16 is seen in most sarcomatoid pleural mesotheliomas.

Differential Diagnosis

The differential diagnosis for sarcomatoid mesothelioma is broad and includes a wide variety of spindle cell proliferations, encompassing both benign and malignant processes. The neoplastic mesothelial cells are often deceptively bland and the stromal invasion may be difficult to identify, making it very challenging to differentiate sarcomatoid mesothelioma and some cases of organizing pleuritis. Demonstrating the presence of cytokeratin-positive cells within the adipose tissue or skeletal muscle is essentially diagnostic of mesothelioma in these cases. However, caution needs to be taken to not overinterpret fat-like spaces encountered in some cases of organizing pleuritis. Since those spaces are not formed by adipocytes, S100 immunostain may help to exclude true fat infiltration in mesothelioma cases. It should be noted, that keratin immunostain will show positive staining in both mesothelioma and pleuritis and it needs to be interpreted with caution. Horizontal cell growth parallel to the surface favors a diagnosis of organizing pleuritis (Table 11.23). In contrast, sarcomatoid or desmoplastic mesothelioma shows downward growth of haphazardly arranged keratin-positive neoplastic cells. Furthermore, the histologic finding of expansile nodules with sharp demarcation and abrupt change in cellularity favors the diagnosis of sarcomatoid mesothelioma, as this feature is usually not present in organizing pleuritis.

In organizing pleuritis, the vessels are oriented perpendicular to the surface and necrosis is typically absent (Figs. 11.34 and 11.35). In rare cases, if necrosis is seen, it is confined to the surface. Mitoses can be present in

TABLE 11.23

Comparison of Sarcomatoid Mesothelioma and Pleuritis

	Mesothelioma	Pleuritis
Soft tissue invasion	Present	Absent
Pattern of growth	Disordered	Sweeping parallel fascicles
Expansile nodules	Present	Absent
Bland necrosis	If present, very helpful	Absent
Zonation	Absent	Present
Capillaries	Few and disorganized	Perpendicular to the surface

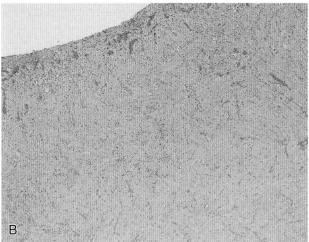

FIG. 11.35

Sarcomatoid mesothelioma **(A)** and organizing pleuritis **(B)**.

FIG. 11.34

Organizing pleuritis with zonation (i.e., cellularity greatest near the pleural surface) and capillaries arranged perpendicular to the surface.

both mesothelioma and organizing pleuritis; however, atypical forms should not be seen in benign proliferations. Unlike mesothelioma, organizing pleuritis shows increased cellularity at the surface with progressive decrease in cellularity away from the surface (zonation). In contrast, mesothelioma lacks zonation and shows haphazard arrangement of spindle cells throughout. The presence of cytologic atypia is not a helpful feature, unless severe. In some cases, sarcomatoid malignant mesothelioma may show frankly sarcomatous areas. Therefore, extensive sampling with a goal of identifying those areas may be useful. In particularly challenging cases, documenting homozygous loss of p16 by FISH technique may be helpful, as deletion of p16 is seen in most sarcomatoid pleural mesotheliomas.

The differential diagnosis for mesothelioma also includes sarcomatoid carcinomas which generally appear as circumscribed or localized lesions, but they can infiltrate or metastasize to serosal membranes and present as pleural thickening. Identification of an area of squamous or glandular differentiation would be diagnostic;

however, particularly in small samples, these areas may not be seen. If present, the expression of an origin-specific carcinoma marker, such as TTF-1 or Napsin A, would support the diagnosis of carcinoma rather than mesothelioma. To support mesothelial origin in malignancy with spindled morphology, calretinin and D2-40 immunostains are the most useful; however, the expression may be focal. Importantly, in the absence of cytokeratin expression, calretinin and D2-40 staining should not be interpreted as evidence of mesothelial differentiation. Markers that are used in epithelioid mesothelioma, such as WT1 and CK5/6, are not typically helpful, as they are lost in sarcomatoid and desmoplastic mesotheliomas. The use of GATA3 immunohistochemistry has been proposed for distinguishing sarcomatoid mesothelioma from sarcomatoid carcinoma of the lung, showing GATA3 to be a sensitive (100%) and specific (85%) marker for the diagnosis of mesothelioma.

Unlike sarcomatoid mesotheliomas, most sarcomas are keratin negative. Sarcomas showing keratin staining (e.g., epithelioid sarcomas, epithelioid angiosarcomas) present additional diagnostic challenge; however, they also show specific lineage markers or characteristic molecular changes in most cases.

Prognosis and Therapy

Sarcomatoid and desmoplastic mesotheliomas carry worse prognosis than epithelioid mesothelioma. Most patients succumb to the disease within 6 months.

SARCOMATOID AND DESMPLASTIC MESOTHELIOMA – DISEASE FACT SHEET

Definition
- ▸▸ Malignant tumor of mesothelial cells
- ▸▸ Diffuse pattern of growth
- ▸▸ Involving serosal membranes

Incidence and Location
- ▸▸ Serosal membranes

Age Distribution
- ▸▸ Majority > 60 years

Clinical Features
- ▸▸ More common in men
- ▸▸ Etiology:
  - ▸▸ Asbestos exposure
  - ▸▸ Therapeutic radiation
  - ▸▸ Inherited predisposition (germline mutation in BAP1)
- ▸▸ Insidious onset of chest pain and/or dyspnea

Radiologic Features
- ▸▸ Diffuse circumferential rind of nodular pleura

Prognosis and Therapy
- ▸▸ Worse than epithelioid mesothelioma (<6 months)

SARCOMATOID MESOTHELIOMA – PATHOLOGIC FEATURES

Gross Findings
- ▸▸ Early disease presents with small nodules
- ▸▸ Later in disease progression nodule coalesce to form a rind encasing the lung

Microscopic Findings
- ▸▸ Spindle cell proliferation with overt invasion into soft tissue or lung
- ▸▸ Bland necrosis
- ▸▸ Lack of zonation
- ▸▸ Disordered growth
- ▸▸ Expansile nodules
- ▸▸ Desmoplastic mesothelioma: at least 50% of the tumor is fibrous stroma

Pathologic Differential Diagnoses
- ▸▸ Pleuritis
- ▸▸ Sarcomatoid carcinoma
- ▸▸ Sarcoma

PULMONARY HAMARTOMA

DIFFERENTIAL DIAGNOSES: ADENOCARCINOMA, CHONDROMA, SARCOMA

Clinical Features

Pulmonary hamartomas are the most common benign neoplasms of the lungs. They are more common in men than in women and are typically identified in the fourth to sixth decades of life. About 90% of patients have peripheral pulmonary hamartomas which are asymptomatic and incidentally identified by chest radiology. About 10% of patients have endobronchial pulmonary hamartoma and present with symptoms of bronchial obstruction.

On chest radiographs, pulmonary hamartomas account for 8% of solitary, well-circumscribed nodules which are frequently referred to as "coin lesions." Multifocal pulmonary hamartomas are rare. Radiographically, popcorn calcification and adipose tissue may be identified.

Pathologic Features

GROSS FINDINGS

Pulmonary hamartomas are well-circumscribed, multilobulated, white-gray, glistening nodules. Most tumors are less than 4 cm.

MICROSCOPIC FINDINGS

Pulmonary hamartomas are composed of varying amounts of at least two mesenchymal elements including cartilage, fat, connective tissue, and smooth muscle (Fig. 11.36). Most hamartomas are composed predominantly of chondroid or chondromyxoid matrix. There are interspersed clefts lined by respiratory epithelium that are thought to represent entrapment of nonneoplastic epithelium by the mesenchymal tumor. Endobronchial tumors tend to show more adipose tissue and are less likely to contain the entrapped clefts of respiratory epithelium. The mesenchymal components show no significant atypia, minimal mitotic activity, and no necrosis.

Ancillary Studies

Immunohistochemical stains are not typically needed for diagnosis; however, mesenchymal markers including

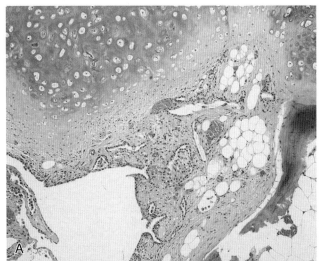

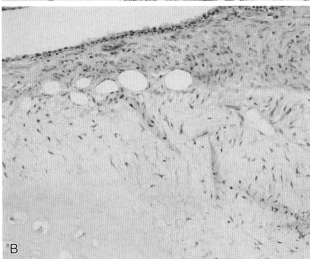

FIG. 11.36

A, Pulmonary hamartoma with slit-like spaces lined by respiratory epithelium, lobules of cartilage, adipose tissue, and bone. **B,** Higher-power view of pulmonary hamartoma with no cytologic atypia of the ciliated epithelium, adipose tissue, or cartilage.

vimentin are usually positive. Neither FISH nor molecular studies are typically necessary for diagnosis; however, there is a frequent translocation t(3;12)(q27-28;q14-15), which results in a fusion of the high-mobility group protein gene *HMGA2* and the *LPP* gene.

Differential Diagnosis

On small biopsy or cytology specimens, particularly if the mesenchymal components are scant, the entrapped respiratory epithelium may be predominant and could be mistaken for adenocarcinoma. However, careful examination for cilia on the epithelial cells and identification of chondroid matrix or adipose components are important for differentiating between pulmonary hamartoma and adenocarcinoma (Table 11.24).

TABLE 11.24

Comparison of Pulmonary Hamartoma and Adenocarcinoma

	Pulmonary Hamartoma	Adenocarcinoma
Radiographic appearance	• Coin lesions	• Coin lesion • Spiculated mass more frequently
Histologic findings	• At least two mesenchymal components, including cartilage, fat, connective tissue, and smooth muscle • Interspersed clefts of respiratory epithelium • No significant atypia	• Cytologic atypia, may contain nucleoli • No cilia • No mesenchymal component

TABLE 11.25

Comparison of Pulmonary Hamartoma and Carcinosarcoma

	Pulmonary Hamartoma	Carcinosarcoma
Radiographic appearance	• Coin lesions	• Irregular or spiculated mass more frequently
Histologic findings	• At least two mesenchymal components, including cartilage, fat, connective tissue, and smooth muscle • No significant atypia	• Heterologous sarcomatous components such as chondrosarcoma, rhabdomyosarcoma, and/or osteosarcoma • Rarely they may contain a component of liposarcoma or angiosarcoma • Mesenchymal components may show increased cytologic atypia, mitotic activity, and necrosis
	• Interspersed clefts of ciliated respiratory epithelium	• If adenocarcinoma component present, the tumor cells are not ciliated and may show increased cytologic atypia, mitotic activity, and overt invasion

The differential diagnosis for pulmonary hamartomas includes carcinosarcomas (Table 11.25), and the two may be confused particularly on small biopsies. Imaging features may be extremely helpful in differentiating these two entities, as pulmonary hamartomas are typically very slow-growing, well-circumscribed lesions, whereas carcinosarcomas typically have irregular or spiculated margins and may be rapidly growing. Carcinosarcomas are malignant tumors composed of a

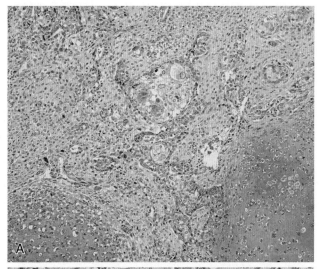

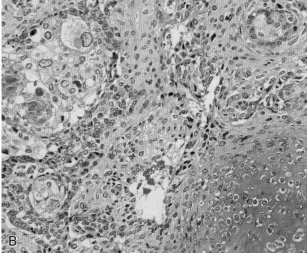

FIG. 11.37

A, Low-power view of carcinosarcoma with squamous cell carcinoma component (upper and center) and chondrosarcoma component (bottom left and right). **B,** High-power view of carcinosarcoma with squamous cell carcinoma component (left) and chondrosarcoma component (lower right). Note the nuclear enlargement, anisonucleosis, and irregular spacing of the cells in the chondrosarcoma component in comparison with pulmonary hamartoma.

TABLE 11.26

Comparison of Pulmonary Hamartoma and Chondroma

	Pulmonary Hamartoma	Chondroma
Age of patient	40–60 years	Less than 30 years
Sex of patient	Male > female	Female
Number of tumors	Solitary	Multiple (average 3)
Associated syndrome	None identified	Carney triad
Histologic findings	At least two mesenchymal components, including cartilage, fat, connective tissue, and smooth muscle.	Hyaline or myxohyaline cartilage, which is moderately cellular Surrounded by pseudocapsule Calcification and ossification is common
Mesenchymal components besides cartilage	Yes	No
Interspersed clefts of respiratory epithelium	Yes	No

mixture of non–small cell carcinoma (typically squamous cell carcinoma or adenocarcinoma) and heterologous sarcomatous components such as chondrosarcoma, rhabdomyosarcoma, and/or osteosarcoma (Fig. 11.37). Rarely they may contain a component of liposarcoma or angiosarcoma. The epithelioid component should show malignant features, such as cytologic atypia, increased mitotic activity, and possibly overt invasion. In cases with an adenocarcinoma component, the glandular tumor cells lack the cilia typically identified in pulmonary hamartomas. The sarcoma component usually also has malignant cytologic features and may show increased mitotic activity and necrosis.

Another major differential diagnosis is chondroma (Table 11.26), a benign neoplasm composed of hyaline or myxohyaline cartilage. Chondromas are usually found in young women (younger than 30 years of age) who have Carney triad (gastric stromal sarcoma, pulmonary chondroma, and extra-adrenal paragangliomas). In contrast to pulmonary hamartomas which are most commonly solitary, chondromas are often multiple in patients with Carney syndrome. Similar to pulmonary hamartomas, chondromas are well circumscribed and lobulated and lack cytologic atypia; however, chondromas do not have the entrapped respiratory epithelium or other mesenchymal components (e.g., adipose tissue) commonly identified in pulmonary hamartomas.

Sarcomas, in particular chondrosarcomas, are in the differential diagnosis (Table 11.27). Most sarcomas and chondrosarcomas in the lung represent metastases. However, chondrosarcoma has been rarely described to represent a primary lung tumor. Metastatic chondrosarcomas typically show increased cellularity, cytologic atypia, and may show increased mitotic activity and necrosis in comparison with pulmonary hamartoma (Fig. 11.38). The clefts of entrapped respiratory epithelium and other mesenchymal components are not typically seen in metastatic chondrosarcoma.

Prognosis and Therapy

Pulmonary hamartomas are slow-growing tumors with an excellent prognosis. Surgical resection is recommended for endobronchial, symptomatic, or growing parenchymal tumors. Recurrence or malignant transformation is rare.

TABLE 11.27

Comparison of Pulmonary Hamartoma and Chondrosarcoma

	Pulmonary Hamartoma	Chondrosarcoma
Histologic findings	At least two mesenchymal components, including cartilage, fat, connective tissue, and smooth muscle	Hyaline or myxohyaline cartilage, which is cellular Cytologic atypia Mitotic activity Necrotic chondrocytes
Mesenchymal components besides cartilage	Yes	No
Interspersed clefts of respiratory epithelium	Yes	No

PULMONARY HAMARTOMA – DISEASE FACT SHEET

Definition
▶▶ Most common benign neoplasm of lung
▶▶ Composed of varying amounts of at least two mesenchymal elements including cartilage, fat, connective tissue, and smooth muscle. Most hamartomas are composed predominantly of chondroid or chondromyxoid matrix.
▶▶ Contain interspersed clefts lined by respiratory epithelium that are thought to represent entrapment of non-neoplastic epithelium by the mesenchymal tumor

Incidence and Location
▶▶ Most lesions incidentally found and represent 8% of "coin lesions" on chest radiology
▶▶ 90% are peripheral and asymptomatic
▶▶ 10% are endobronchial and may present with obstructive symptoms

Age Distribution
▶▶ Fourth to sixth decades of life

Clinical Features
▶▶ Most often incidentally discovered

Radiologic Features
▶▶ Typically appear as "coin-lesions," which are solitary, well-circumscribed nodules
▶▶ Multifocal pulmonary hamartomas are rare
▶▶ Popcorn calcification and adipose tissue may be identified

Prognosis and Therapy
▶▶ Pulmonary hamartomas are slow-growing tumors with an excellent prognosis
▶▶ Surgical resection is recommended for endobronchial, symptomatic, or growing parenchymal tumors
▶▶ Recurrence or malignant transformation is rare

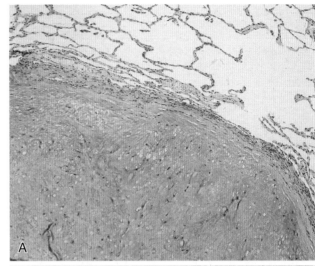
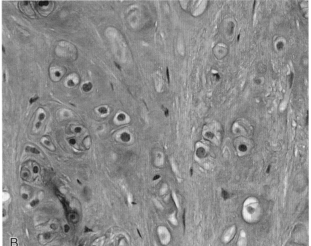

FIG. 11.38

A, Metastatic low-grade chondrosarcoma does not have additional mesenchymal elements (such as adipose tissue) and does not have slit-like spaces lined by respiratory epithelium. In this case, the nuclei are very bland with minimal cytologic atypia. In the absence of clinical history, differentiating between primary pulmonary chondroma and metastatic low-grade chondrosarcoma may be difficult histologically. **B,** Another example of metastatic chondrosarcoma with enlarged nuclei, increased nuclear hyperchromasia, and anisonucleosis. A rare binucleated cell is identified (left center). Some of the lacunae lack nuclei, consistent with necrosis.

PULMONARY HAMARTOMA – PATHOLOGIC FEATURES

Gross Findings
▶▶ Well-circumscribed, multilobulated, firm, white-gray, glistening nodule
▶▶ Most tumors are less than 4 cm

Microscopic Findings
▶▶ Composed of varying amounts of at least two mesenchymal elements including cartilage, fat, connective tissue, and smooth muscle
▶▶ Most hamartomas are composed predominantly of chondroid or chondromyxoid matrix
▶▶ There are interspersed clefts lined by respiratory epithelium that are thought to represent entrapment of non-neoplastic epithelium by the mesenchymal tumor

Continued

EPITHELIOID HEMANGIOENDOTHELIOMA

DIFFERENTIAL DIAGNOSES: AMYLOIDOSIS, HYALINIZED GRANULOMA, SCLEROSING PNEUMOCYTOMA, ADENOCARCINOMA, ANGIOSARCOMA

Clinical Features

Epithelioid hemangioendothelioma (EHE) is a low- to intermediate-grade malignant vascular tumor. It is more common in young women (median age is 38 years).

Approximately 10% of cases involve the lung alone and about 20% of cases have lung and liver involvement. Metastases are rare. Approximately half of the cases present with pain, which is the most common presenting symptom. On imaging, 60% of cases appear as multiple nodules and can mimic granulomatous or metastatic disease. Currently, there are no biomarkers to predict disease evolution.

Pathologic Features

GROSS FINDINGS

EHE presents with multiple circumscribed intraparenchymal nodules, typically measuring less than 2 cm. The nodules have gray, chondroid-appearing cut surface. Tumors that extend to the pleura may show pleural thickening.

MICROSCOPIC FINDINGS

EHE is frequently associated with vessels. At low power, the tumor forms round to oval nodule with eosinophilic sclerotic center. Focal necrosis can be seen. The stroma may be hyalinized, chondroid, or myxoid (Fig. 11.39).

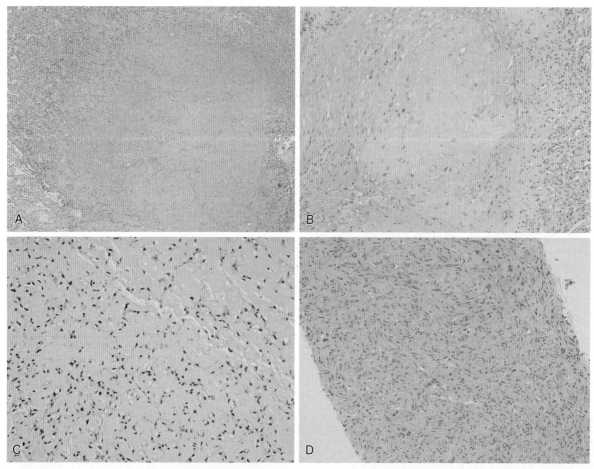

FIG. 11.39
Epithelioid hemangioendothelioma with hyalinized **(A and B)**, myxoid **(C)**, and with less significant stromal component **(D)**.

The tumor cells are round to slightly spindled with intracytoplasmic lumina containing red blood cells ("blister cells"). Occasionally tumors may show necrosis, increased mitotic activity, increased cellularity, and nuclear atypia.

Ancillary Studies

The tumor cells are positive for vascular markers (Fig. 11.40A and B). Focal cytokeratin expression is present in 25% to 35% of cases. Up to 50% of cases may show positive staining for CK7. Approximately 90% of EHEs contain fusion gene WWTR1-CAMTA1. Alternatively, a small subset of EHEs carry fusion oncogene involving YAP1 and TFE3.

Differential Diagnosis

Differential diagnosis is broad. If the tumor is extensively hyalinized, it may resemble amyloid deposition, hyalinized granuloma, or even organized infarct (Fig. 11.41).

Extensive sampling of the lesion away from the hyalinized center and the use of special stains (e.g., Congo red, silver stain, etc.) is needed in some cases.

The differential diagnosis also includes pneumocytoma, angiosarcoma, and adenocarcinoma.

Pneumocytoma (formerly known as sclerosing hemangioma) may enter the differential diagnosis, but it typically presents as a solitary mass at the periphery of the lung rather than multifocal bilateral lesions (Table 11.28). Pneumocytoma may show various architectural patterns, including solid, papillary, sclerotic, or a combination of the above, and is composed of two cells types: small cells with hobnail nuclei lining papillary structures and round cells with clear cytoplasm. Immunohistochemistry is of great value, because pneumocytoma, unlike EHE, demonstrates TTF-1 expression by immunohistochemistry, while EHE expresses vascular markers (see Fig. 11.40).

A major differential diagnosis consideration is angiosarcoma. EHEs are low- to intermediate-grade vascular tumors, whereas angiosarcomas are high-grade vascular tumors. Clinically, EHE occurs in younger patients and is more common in women, whereas angiosarcoma affects older patients and is more common in men. EHEs

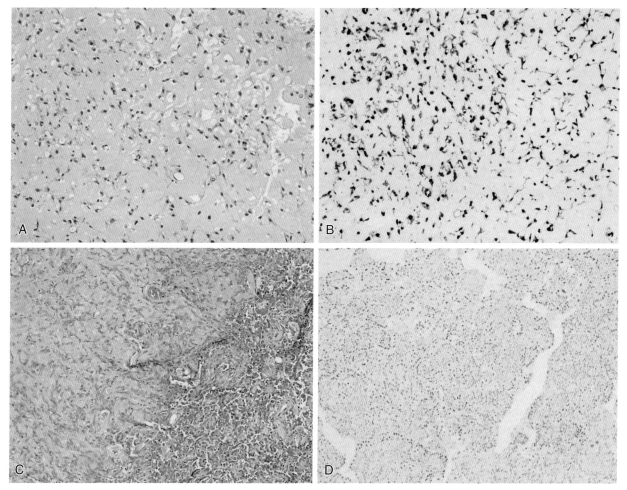

FIG. 11.40

Epithelioid hemangioendothelioma with myxoid stroma **(A)** and strong ERG expression **(B)**. Sclerosing pneumocytoma **(C)** showing TTF-1 expression **(D)**.

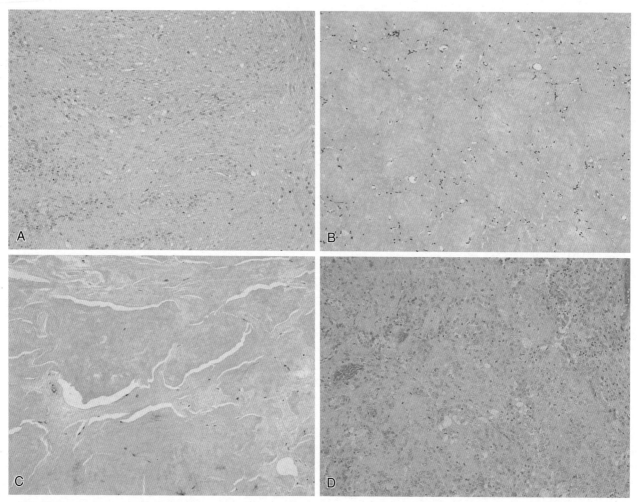

FIG. 11.41
Low-power view of epithelioid hemangioendothelioma **(A)**, hyalinized granuloma **(B)**, amyloidoma **(C)**, and sclerosing pneumocytoma **(D)**.

TABLE 11.28

Comparison of Epithelioid Hemangioendothelioma and Sclerosing Pneumocytoma

	Epithelioid Hemangioendothelioma	Sclerosing Pneumocytoma
Radiographic appearance	Multifocal disease with small bilateral nodules	Single peripheral mass
Immunohistochemical markers	Vascular markers	TTF-1

signet ring cell morphology. The lumina of EHE cells contains red blood cells rather than mucin in adenocarcinoma. EHE typically expresses vascular markers, but it is important to remember that a significant number of EHE cases may demonstrate cytokeratin expression. In addition, carcinomas rarely may focally express vascular markers. The characteristic WWTR1-CAMTA1 fusion is not seen in angiosarcoma or adenocarcinoma and the demonstration of this translocation can be useful in particularly challenging cases.

Prognosis and Therapy

EHE is a low- to intermediate-grade malignant neoplasm. It has a 60% 5-year survival rate. The prognosis is worse with prominent symptoms at the time of presentation, extensive intrapulmonary and pleural spread, and pleural effusion. Surgical excision is the treatment of choice if the disease is limited; however, it is often not feasible, given tumor multifocality. Radiation and chemotherapy are of little benefit.

are more likely to show intracytoplasmic vacuoles and contain myxoid, chondroid, or hyalinized stroma. Angiosarcomas are composed of anastomosing vascular channels with occasional papillary projections lined by atypical cells showing crowding, hobnailing, pleomorphism, and prominent mitotic activity (Fig. 11.42, Table 11.29).

On occasion, the differential diagnosis includes adenocarcinoma, especially poorly differentiated or with

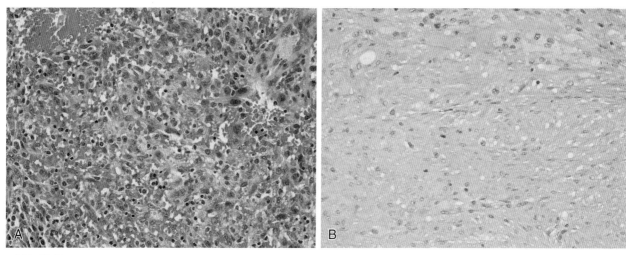

FIG. 11.42
Intermediate power of angiosarcoma with hemorrhage and large atypical cells **(A)** in contrast with epithelioid hemangioendothelioma **(B)**.

TABLE 11.29

Comparison of Epithelioid Hemangioendothelioma and Angiosarcoma

	Epithelioid Hemangioendothelioma	Angiosarcoma
Age of patient	Young	Older
Sex of patient	Female	Male
Tumor grade	Low to intermediate	High grade
Histologic findings	Sclerotic center Myxoid, chondroid, or hyaline stroma "Blister cells"	Anastomoses of vascular channels or papillary projections Pleomorphic cells Hobnailing Prominent mitotic activity

---

EPITHELIOID HEMANGIOENDOTHELIOMA – DISEASE FACT SHEET

Definition
▸▸ Low- to intermediate-grade malignant vascular tumor

Incidence and Location
▸▸ Most intraparenchymal and multifocal

Age Distribution
▸▸ 60%–80% are women
▸▸ 7–81 years

Clinical Features
▸▸ May present with pain and cough
▸▸ Often incidental finding

Radiologic Features
▸▸ Multiple small nodular lesions throughout both lungs
▸▸ Can mimic granulomatous or metastatic disease

Prognosis and Therapy
▸▸ No prognostic biomarkers
▸▸ 60% 5-year survival
▸▸ Does not respond to radiation or chemotherapy
▸▸ Worse with extensive intraparenchymal or pleural involvement

---

EPITHELIOID HEMANGIOENDOTHELIOMA – PATHOLOGIC FEATURES

Gross Findings
▸▸ Multiple well-circumscribed nodules with gray chondroid appearance
▸▸ Typically smaller than 2 cm

Microscopic Findings
▸▸ Associated with vessels
▸▸ Sclerotic center
▸▸ Hyalinized, chondroid, or myxoid stroma
▸▸ Epithelioid cells with cytoplasmic lumina containing red blood cells

Pathologic Differential Diagnoses
▸▸ Amyloidoma, hyalinized granuloma pneumocytoma, angiosarcoma, adenocarcinoma

LYMPHANGIOMYOMATOSIS

DIFFERENTIAL DIAGNOSES: ENDOMETRIAL STROMAL SARCOMA, BENIGN METASTASIZING LEIOMYOMA, CARCINOID TUMOR, SOLITARY FIBROUS TUMOR, CENTRILOBULAR EMPHYSEMA

Clinical Features

Lymphangiomyomatosis (LAM) is a chronic cystic lung disease characterized by proliferation of abnormal smooth muscle-like cells. It can be seen as sporadic disease or associated with tuberous sclerosis. Mutations in the tuberous sclerosis genes *TSC1* or *TSC2* are considered to be the cause of LAM. LAM affects predominantly women of childbearing age, and it is commonly seen in association with angiomyolipomas and lymphangiomyomas. The most common presenting symptom is dyspnea and over 50% of patients have a history of pneumothorax.

Pathologic Features

GROSS FINDINGS

LAM diffusely involves the lungs and may show cysts or small nodules.

MICROSCOPIC FINDINGS

LAM may be difficult to appreciate at low power. The disease typically shows extensive parenchymal involvement and histologically may demonstrate thin-walled cysts, nodules, or small cell clusters (Fig. 11.43). Frequently

smooth muscle–like LAM cells can grow along the airways and blood vessels. LAM cells are fusiform with a nucleus larger than other smooth muscle cells in the lung. They could be prominent or attenuated at the periphery of the cysts.

Ancillary Studies

LAM cells usually express markers of smooth muscle differentiation (e.g., desmin) and show expression of HMB-45 and MART-1 (Fig. 11.44). They are also positive for estrogen receptor and progesterone receptor.

Differential Diagnosis

Given that LAM is composed of cysts and clusters of smooth muscle–like cells, both cystic lung diseases and multifocal smooth muscle proliferations may enter the differential diagnosis (Table 11.30). Benign metastasizing leiomyomas are typically solid nodules; however,

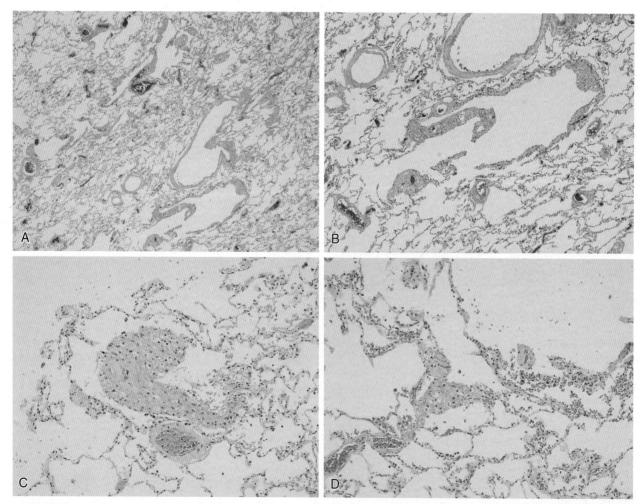

FIG. 11.43

Low-power view of lymphangiomyomatosis (LAM) with scattered cystic areas and small LAM cell clusters at the periphery of the cysts **(A and B)**. High-power view of LAM cells **(C)** with a more subtle example **(D)**.

the tumors may be extensively cystic. Pulmonary metastases of endometrial stromal sarcoma are uncommon but can be very challenging to diagnose. It is important to remember that lung is the most common location for distant metastasis of endometrial stromal sarcoma (Fig. 11.45). To work through this differential, the immunostains are of extreme importance. Neither metastatic endometrial stromal sarcoma nor benign metastasizing leiomyoma will react with HMB-45 or MART-1. Estrogen receptor and progesterone receptor immunostains may be positive in all discussed lesions and are not helpful in this case.

Occasionally, carcinoid tumor, especially with spindle cell morphology, or solitary fibrous tumors may enter the differential diagnosis, particularly in small biopsies. Unlike LAM cells, the neoplastic neuroendocrine cells should be positive for pancytokeratin and neuroendocrine markers. Solitary fibrous tumors demonstrate expression of CD34 and STAT6 by immunohistochemistry.

When compared with centrilobular emphysema, which affects predominantly upper lung zones, LAM cysts are uniformly distributed and are true cysts (Table 11.31).

Prognosis and Therapy

Conservative treatment is the initial approach. The mortality is estimated at 10% to 20%. Patients may undergo transplantation, although there are rare reports of disease recurrence. Sirolimus has been shown to improve quality of life. There is no evidence of improvement with estrogen antagonists.

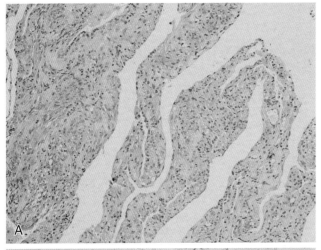
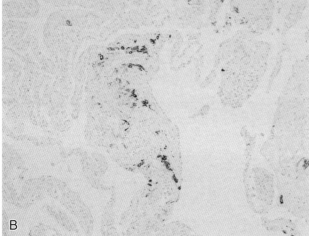

FIG. 11.44

Lymphangiomyomatosis **(A)** and HMB-45 immunostain **(B)**.

LYMPHANGIOMYOMATOSIS – DISEASE FACT SHEET

Definition
▶▶ Cystic lung disease
▶▶ Characterized by proliferation of abnormal smooth muscle–like cells

Incidence and Location
▶▶ Rare
▶▶ Diffuse lung involvement

Age Distribution
▶▶ Young women

Clinical Features
▶▶ Can be sporadic or associated with tuberous sclerosis

Radiologic Features
▶▶ Plain films may be normal in early disease or may show effusion or pneumothorax
▶▶ Reticular nodular pattern
▶▶ Well-circumscribed thin-walled cysts without lobar predominance

Continued

TABLE 11.30

Comparison of Lymphangiomyomatosis, Endometrial Stromal Sarcoma, and Benign Metastasizing Leiomyoma

	Lymphangiomyomatosis	Benign Metastasizing Leiomyoma	Endometrial Stromal Sarcoma
Presence of cysts	Present	Rare	Rare
Presence of smooth muscle	Yes	Yes	No
Presence of perivascular epithelioid cells	Yes	No	No

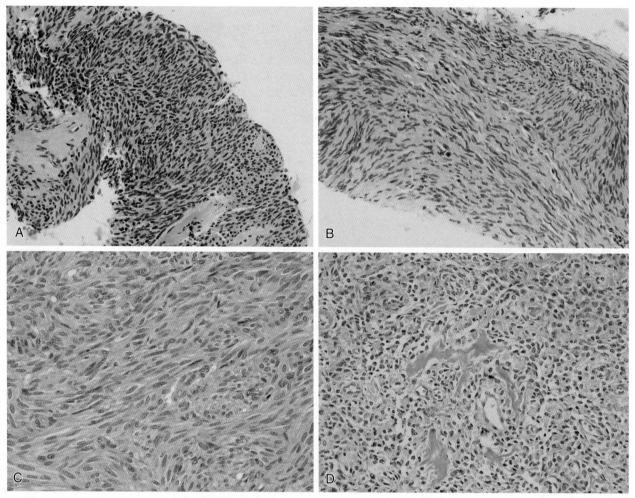

FIG. 11.45
Core biopsy of a benign metastasizing leiomyoma **(A and B)**, carcinoid tumor **(C)**, and endometrial stromal sarcoma **(D)**. Note the similarities in morphologic appearance. In these cases, immunohistochemistry is required.

TABLE 11.31

Comparison of Lymphangiomyomatosis and Centrilobular Emphysema

	Lymphangiomyomatosis	Centrilobular Emphysema
Sex of patient	Female	Male/Female
Location of cysts	Uniform	Upper lobe predominant
Associated tumors	Angiomyolipomas Lymphangiomyomas	No specific tumors
Histologic findings	Thin but discernable cyst wall	No cyst wall

LYMPHANGIOMYOMATOSIS – PATHOLOGIC FEATURES

Gross Findings
- ▶▶ Diffuse lung involvement
- ▶▶ Cysts and small nodules

Microscopic Findings
- ▶▶ Diffuse lung involvement
- ▶▶ Cysts, nodules, small clusters, or smooth muscle–like cells
- ▶▶ LAM cells are positive for smooth muscle markers, HMB-45, and MART-1

Pathologic Differential Diagnoses
- ▶▶ Benign metastasizing leiomyoma
- ▶▶ Metastatic endometrial stromal sarcoma
- ▶▶ Carcinoid tumor with spindle cell morphology
- ▶▶ Emphysema
- ▶▶ Solitary fibrous tumor

LYMPHANGIOMYOMATOSIS – DISEASE FACT SHEET—cont'd

Prognosis and Therapy
- ▶▶ No effective therapy
- ▶▶ Sirolimus improves quality of life
- ▶▶ Mortality is approximately 10%–20%
- ▶▶ Disease may recur after transplantation

SUGGESTED READINGS

Squamous Papilloma

Alagusundaramoorthy SS, Agrawal A. Respiratory papillomas. *Lung India.* 2016;33(5):522-527.

Flieder DB, Nicholson AG, Travis WD, Yatabe Y. Papillomas. In: Travis WD, Brambilla E, Burke AP, Marx A, Nicholson AG, eds. *WHO Classifications of Tumours of the Lung, Pleura, Thymus, and Heart.* 4th ed. Lyon: IARC; 2015:106-109.

Fortes HR, von Ranke FM, Escuissato DL, et al. Recurrent respiratory papillomatosis: a state-of-the-art review. *Respir Med.* 2017;126:116-121.

Go C, Schwartz MR, Donovan DT. Molecular transformation of recurrent respiratory papillomatosis: viral typing and p53 overexpression. *Ann Otol Rhinol Laryngol.* 2003;112(4):298-302.

Pham TT, Ongkeko WM, An Y, Yi ES. Protein expression of the tumor suppressors p16INK4A and p53 and disease progression in recurrent respiratory papillomatosis. *Laryngoscope.* 2007;117(2):253-257.

Carcinoid Tumors

Beasley MB, Brambilla E, Chirieac LR et al. Carcinoid tumor. In: Travis WD, Brambilla E, Burke AP, Marx A, Nicholson AG, eds. *WHO Classifications of Tumours of the Lung, Pleura, Thymus, and Heart.* 4th ed. Lyon: IARC; 2015:73.

De Palma A, Lorusso M, Di Gennaro F, et al. Pulmonary and mediastinal paragangliomas: rare endothoracic malignancies with challenging diagnosis and treatment. *J Thorac Dis.* 2018;10(9):5318-5327.

Duan K, Mete O. Algorithmic approach to neuroendocrine tumors in targeted biopsies: practical applications of immunohistochemical markers. *Cancer Cytopathol.* 2016;124(12):871-884.

Gorshtein A, Gross DJ, Barak D, et al. Diffuse idiopathic pulmonary neuroendocrine cell hyperplasia and the associated lung neuroendocrine tumors: clinical experience with a rare entity. *Cancer.* 2012;118:612-619.

Haynes CM, Sangoi AR, Pai RK. PAX8 is expressed in pancreatic well-differentiated neuroendocrine tumors and in extrapancreatic poorly differentiated neuroendocrine carcinomas in fine-needle aspiration biopsy specimens. *Cancer Cytopathol.* 2011;119(3):193-201.

Huang X, Liang QL, Jiang L, et al. Primary pulmonary paraganglioma: a case report and review of literature. *Medicine (Baltimore).* 2015;94(31):e1271.

Nassar AA, Jaroszewski DE, Helmers RA, et al. Diffuse idiopathic pulmonary neuroendocrine cell hyperplasia: a systematic overview. *Am J Respir Crit Care Med.* 2011;184:8-16.

Rekhtman N. Neuroendocrine tumors of the lung: an update. *Arch Pathol Lab Med.* 2010;134(11):1628-1638.

Rooper LM, Bishop JA, Westra WH. INSM1 is a sensitive and specific marker of neuroendocrine differentiation in head and neck tumors. *Am J Surg Pathol.* 2018;42(5):665-671.

Sangoi AR, Ohgami RS, Pai RK, Beck AH, McKenney JK, Pai RK. PAX8 expression reliably distinguishes pancreatic well-differentiated neuroendocrine tumors from ileal and pulmonary well-differentiated neuroendocrine tumors and pancreatic acinar cell carcinoma. *Mod Pathol.* 2011;24(3):412-424. doi:10.1038/modpathol.2010.176.

Srivastava A, Hornick JL. Immunohistochemical staining for CDX-2, PDX-1, NESP-55, and TTF-1 can help distinguish gastrointestinal carcinoid tumors from pancreatic endocrine and pulmonary carcinoid tumors. *Am J Surg Pathol.* 2009;33(4):626-632.

Zhang C, Schmidt LA, Hatanaka K, Thomas D, Lagstein A, Myers JL. Evaluation of napsin A, TTF-1, p63, p40, and CK5/6 immunohistochemical stains in pulmonary neuroendocrine tumors. *Am J Clin Pathol.* 2014;142(3):320-324.

Large Cell Neuroendocrine Carcinoma

Brambilla E, Beasley MB, Chirieac LR, et al. Large cell neuroendocrine carcinoma. In: Travis WD, Brambilla E, Burke AP, Marx A, Nicholson AG, eds. *WHO Classifications of Tumours of the Lung, Pleura, Thymus, and Heart.* 4th ed. Lyon: IARC; 2015:69.

Fasano M, Della Corte CM, Papaccio F, Ciardiello F, Morgillo F. Pulmonary large-cell neuroendocrine carcinoma: from epidemiology to therapy. *J Thorac Oncol.* 2015;10(8):1133-1141.

Fisseler-Eckhoff A, Demes M. Neuroendocrine tumors of the lung. *Cancers (Basel).* 2012;4(3):777-798.

Hiroshima K, Mino-Kenudson M. Update on large cell neuroendocrine carcinoma. *Transl Lung Cancer Res.* 2017;6(5):530-539. doi:10.21037/tlcr.2017.06.12.

Sholl LM, Nishino M, Pokharel S, et al. Primary pulmonary NUT midline carcinoma: clinical, radiographic, and pathologic characterizations. *J Thorac Oncol.* 2015;10(6):951-959.

Stelow EB. A review of NUT midline carcinoma. *Head Neck Pathol.* 2011;5(1):31-35.

Wang J, Ye L, Cai H, Jin M. Comparative study of large cell neuroendocrine carcinoma and small cell lung carcinoma in high-grade neuroendocrine tumors of the lung: a large population-based study. *J Cancer.* 2019;10(18):4226-4236.

Salivary Gland Neoplasms

Huo Z, Wu H, Li J, et al. Primary pulmonary mucoepidermoid carcinoma: histopathological and moleculargenetic studies of 26 cases. *PLoS One.* 2015;10(11):e0143169.

Ishikawa Y, Alvarez-Fernandez E, Aubry MC, et al. Salivary gland-type tumours. In: Travis WD, Brambilla E, Burke AP, Marx A, Nicholson AG, eds. *WHO Classifications of Tumours of the Lung, Pleura, Thymus, and Heart.* 4th ed. Lyon: IARC; 2015:99-105.

Komiya T, Perez RP, Yamamoto S, Neupane P. Primary lung mucoepidermoid carcinoma: analysis of prognostic factors using surveillance, epidemiology and end results program. *Clin Respir J.* 2017;11(6):847-853.

Molina JR, Aubry MC, Lewis JE, et al. Primary salivary gland-type lung cancer: spectrum of clinical presentation, histopathologic and prognostic factors. *Cancer.* 2007;110(10):2253-2259.

Pei J, Flieder DB, Patchefsky A, et al. Detecting MYB and MYBL1 fusion genes in tracheobronchial adenoid cystic carcinoma by targeted RNA-sequencing. *Mod Pathol.* 2019;32(10):1416-1420.

Resio BJ, Chiu AS, Hoag J, Dhanasopon AP, Blasberg JD, Boffa DJ. Primary salivary type lung cancers in the National Cancer Database. *Ann Thorac Surg.* 2018;105(6):1633-1639.

Roden AC, García JJ, Wehrs RN, et al. Histopathologic, immunophenotypic and cytogenetic features of pulmonary mucoepidermoid carcinoma. *Mod Pathol.* 2014;27(11):1479-1488.

Roden AC, Greipp PT, Knutson DL, et al. Histopathologic and cytogenetic features of pulmonary adenoid cystic carcinoma. *J Thorac Oncol.* 2015;10(11):1570-1575.

Yatabe Y, Brambilla E, Rekhtman N, et al. Adenosquamous carcinoma. In: Travis WD, Brambilla E, Burke AP, Marx A, Nicholson AG, eds. *WHO Classifications of Tumours of the Lung, Pleura, Thymus, and Heart.* 4th ed. Lyon: IARC; 2015:86-87.

Atypical Adenomatous Hyperplasia

Hu X, Fujimoto J, Ying L, et al. Multi-region exome sequencing reveals genomic evolution from preneoplasia to lung adenocarcinoma. *Nat Commun.* 2019;10(1):2978.

Mori M, Rao SK, Popper HH, Cagle PT, Fraire AE. Atypical adenomatous hyperplasia of the lung: a probable forerunner in the development of adenocarcinoma of the lung. *Mod Pathol.* 2001;14(2):72-84.

Noguchi M, Yatabe Y, Brambilla E, et al. Preinvasive lesions: atypical adenomatous hyperplasia and adenocarcinoma in situ. In: Travis WD, Brambilla E, Burke AP, Marx A, Nicholson AG, eds. *WHO Classifications of Tumours of the Lung, Pleura, Thymus, and Heart.* 4th ed. Lyon: IARC; 2015:46-50.

Sivakumar S, Lucas FAS, McDowell TL, et al. Genomic landscape of atypical adenomatous hyperplasia reveals divergent modes to lung adenocarcinoma. *Cancer Res.* 2017;77(22):6119-6130.

Suzuki K, Nagai K, Yoshida J, et al. The prognosis of resected lung carcinoma associated with atypical adenomatous hyperplasia: a comparison of the prognosis of well-differentiated adenocarcinoma associated with atypical adenomatous hyperplasia and intrapulmonary metastasis. *Cancer.* 1997;79(8):1521-1526.

Travis WD, Brambilla E, Noguchi M, et al. International Association for The Study of Lung Cancer/American Thoracic Society/European Respiratory Society International Multidisciplinary Classification of Lung Adenocarcinoma. *J Thorac Oncol.* 2011;6(2):244-285.

Micropapillary Adenocarcinoma

Amin MB, Tamboli P, Merchant SH, et al. Micropapillary component in lung adenocarcinoma: a distinctive histologic feature with possible prognostic significance. *Am J Surg Pathol.* 2002;26(3):358-364.

Austin JH, Garg K, Aberle D, et al. Radiologic implications of the 2011 classification of adenocarcinoma of the lung. *Radiology.* 2013; 266(1):62-71.

Cha MJ, Lee HY, Lee KS, et al. Micropapillary and solid subtypes of invasive lung adenocarcinoma: clinical predictors of histopathology and outcome. *J Thorac Cardiovasc Surg.* 2014;147(3):921-928.e2.

Dai C, Xie H, Kadeer X, et al. Relationship of Lymph Node Micrometastasis and micropapillary component and their joint influence on prognosis of patients with stage I lung adenocarcinoma. *Am J Surg Pathol.* 2017;41(9):1212-1220.

De Oliveira Duarte Achcar R, Nikiforova MN, Yousem SA. Micropapillary lung adenocarcinoma: EGFR, K-ras, and BRAF mutational profile. *Am J Clin Pathol.* 2009;131(5):694-700.

Lee JS, Kim EK, Kim M, Shim HS. Genetic and clinicopathologic characteristics of lung adenocarcinoma with tumor spread through air spaces. *Lung Cancer.* 2018;123:121-126.

Pyo JS, Kim JH. Clinicopathological significance of micropapillary pattern in lung adenocarcinoma. *Pathol Oncol Res.* 2018;24(3):547-555.

Roh MS, Lee JI, Choi PJ, Hong YS. Relationship between micropapillary component and micrometastasis in the regional lymph nodes of patients with stage I lung adenocarcinoma. *Histopathology.* 2004; 45(6):580-586.

Russell PA, Barnett SA, Walkiewicz M, et al. Correlation of mutation status and survival with predominant histologic subtype according to the new IASLC/ATS/ERS lung adenocarcinoma classification in stage III (N2) patients. *J Thorac Oncol.* 2013;8(4):461-468.

Sumiyoshi S, Yoshizawa A, Sonobe M, et al. Pulmonary adenocarcinomas with micropapillary component significantly correlate with recurrence, but can be well controlled with EGFR tyrosine kinase inhibitors in the early stages. *Lung Cancer.* 2013;81(1):53-59.

Travis WD, Brambilla E, Noguchi M, et al. International Association for the Study of Lung Cancer/American Thoracic Society/European Respiratory Society International Multidisciplinary Classification of Lung Adenocarcinoma. *J Thorac Oncol.* 2011;6(2):244-285.

Travis WD, Noguchi M, Yatabe Y, et al. Adenocarcinoma. In: Travis WD, Brambilla E, Burke AP, Marx A, Nicholson AG, eds. *WHO Classifications of Tumours of the Lung, Pleura, Thymus, and Heart.* 4th ed. Lyon: IARC; 2015:46-50.

Tsutsumida H, Nomoto M, Goto M, et al. A micropapillary pattern is predictive of a poor prognosis in lung adenocarcinoma, and reduced surfactant apoprotein A expression in the micropapillary pattern is an excellent indicator of a poor prognosis. *Mod Pathol.* 2007;20:638-647.

Yang X, Liu Y, Lian F, et al. Lepidic and micropapillary growth pattern and expression of Napsin A can stratify patients of stage I lung adenocarcinoma into different prognostic subgroup. *Int J Clin Exp Pathol.* 2014;7(4):1459-1468.

Yoshida Y, Nitadori JI, Shinozaki-Ushiku A, et al. Micropapillary histological subtype in lung adenocarcinoma of 2 cm or less: impact on recurrence and clinical predictors. *Gen Thorac Cardiovasc Surg.* 2017;65(5):273-279.

Yoshizawa A, Sumiyoshi S, Sonobe M, et al. Validation of the IASLC/ ATS/ERS lung adenocarcinoma classification for prognosis and association with EGFR and KRAS gene mutations: analysis of 440 Japanese patients. *J Thorac Oncol.* 2013;8(1):52-61.

Zhao ZR, To KF, Mok TS, Ng CS. Is there significance in identification of non-predominant micropapillary or solid components in early-stage lung adenocarcinoma? *Interact Cardiovasc Thorac Surg.* 2017;24(1): 121-125.

Zhang Y, Wang R, Cai D, et al. A comprehensive investigation of molecular features and prognosis of lung adenocarcinoma with micropapillary component. *J Thorac Oncol.* 2014;9(12):1772-1778.

Invasive Mucinous Adenocarcinoma

Boland JM, Maleszewski JJ, Wampfler JA, et al. Pulmonary invasive mucinous adenocarcinoma and mixed invasive mucinous/ nonmucinous adenocarcinoma-a clinicopathological and molecular genetic study with survival analysis. *Hum Pathol.* 2018;71:8-19.

Lee HY, Cha MJ, Lee KS, et al. Prognosis in resected invasive mucinous adenocarcinomas of the lung: related factors and comparison with resected nonmucinous adenocarcinomas. *J Thorac Oncol.* 2016;11(7):1064-1073.

Moon SW, Choi SY, Moon MH. Effect of invasive mucinous adenocarcinoma on lung cancer-specific survival after surgical resection: a population-based study. *J Thorac Dis.* 2018;10(6):3595-3608.

Shim HS, Kenudson M, Zheng Z, et al. Unique genetic and survival characteristics of invasive mucinous adenocarcinoma of the lung. *J Thorac Oncol.* 2015;10(8):1156-1162.

Sun F, Wang P, Zheng Y, et al. Diagnosis, clinicopathological characteristics and prognosis of pulmonary mucinous adenocarcinoma. *Oncol Lett.* 2018;15(1):489-494.

Travis WD, Yatabe Y, Brambilla E, et al. Variants of adenocarcinoma. In: Travis WD, Brambilla E, Burke AP, Marx A, Nicholson AG, eds. *WHO Classifications of Tumours of the Lung, Pleura, Thymus, and Heart.* 4th ed. Lyon: IARC; 2015:38-40.

Wu J, Chu PG, Jiang Z, Lau SK. Napsin A expression in primary mucin-producing adenocarcinomas of the lung: an immunohistochemical study. *Am J Clin Pathol.* 2013;139(2):160-166.

Yoshizawa A, Sumiyoshi S, Sonobe M, et al. Validation of the IASLC/ ATS/ERS lung adenocarcinoma classification for prognosis and association with EGFR and KRAS gene mutations: analysis of 440 Japanese patients. *J Thorac Oncol.* 2013;8(1):52-61.

Epithelioid Mesothelioma

Cigognetti M, Lonardi S, Fisogni S, et al. BAP1 (BRCA1-associated protein 1) is a highly specific marker for differentiating mesothelioma from reactive mesothelial proliferations. *Mod Pathol.* 2015;28(8):1043-1057. doi:10.1038/modpathol.2015.65.

Galateau-Salle F, Churg A, Roggli V, et al. Epithelioid mesothelioma. In: Travis WD, Brambilla E, Burke AP, Marx A, Nicholson AG, eds. *WHO Classifications of Tumours of the Lung, Pleura, Thymus, and Heart.* 4th ed. Lyon: IARC; 2015:156.

Facchetti F, Lonardi S, Gentili F, et al. Claudin 4 identifies a wide spectrum of epithelial neoplasms and represents a very useful marker for carcinoma versus mesothelioma diagnosis in pleural and peritoneal biopsies and effusions. *Virchows Arch.* 2007;451(3):669-680.

Husain AN, Colby TV, Ordóñez NG, et al. Guidelines for pathologic diagnosis of malignant mesothelioma: 2017 update of the consensus statement from the International Mesothelioma Interest Group. *Arch Pathol Lab Med.* 2018;142(1):89-108. doi:10.5858/arpa.2017-0124-RA.

Hwang HC, Sheffield BS, Rodriguez S, et al. Utility of BAP1 Immunohistochemistry and p16 (CDKN2A) FISH in the diagnosis of malignant mesothelioma in effusion cytology specimens. *Am J Surg Pathol.* 2016;40(1):120-126.

Miettinen M, McCue PA, Sarlomo-Rikala M, et al. GATA3: a multispecific but potentially useful marker in surgical pathology: a systematic analysis of 2500 epithelial and nonepithelial tumors. *Am J Surg Pathol.* 2014;38(1):13-22. doi:10.1097/PAS.0b013e3182a0218f.

Ordóñez NG. What are the current best immunohistochemical markers for the diagnosis of epithelioid mesothelioma? A review and update. *Hum Pathol.* 2007;38(1):1–16. doi:10.1016/j.humpath.2006.08.010.

Rosen LE, Karrison T, Ananthanarayanan V, et al. Nuclear grade and necrosis predict prognosis in malignant epithelioid pleural mesothelioma: a multi-institutional study. *Mod Pathol.* 2018;31(4):598-606. doi:10.1038/modpathol.2017.170.

Soini Y, Kinnula V, Kahlos K, Pääkkö P. Claudins in differential diagnosis between mesothelioma and metastatic adenocarcinoma of the pleura. *J Clin Pathol.* 2006;59(3):250-254. doi:10.1136/jcp.2005.028589.

Verma V, Ahern CA, Berlind CG, et al. Survival by histologic subtype of malignant pleural mesothelioma and the impact of surgical resection on overall survival. *Clin Lung Cancer.* 2018;19(6):e901-e912.

Sarcomatoid Mesothelioma

Berg KB, Churg A. GATA3 Immunohistochemistry for distinguishing sarcomatoid and desmoplastic mesothelioma from sarcomatoid carcinoma of the lung. *Am J Surg Pathol.* 2017;41(9):1221-1225. doi:10.1097/PAS.0000000000000825.

Chirieac LR, Pinkus GS, Pinkus JL, Godleski J, Sugarbaker DJ, Corson JM. The immunohistochemical characterization of sarcomatoid malignant mesothelioma of the pleura. *Am J Cancer Res.* 2011;1(1):14-24.

Churg A, Sheffield BS, Galateau-Salle F. New markers for separating benign from malignant mesothelial proliferations: are we there yet? *Arch Pathol Lab Med.* 2016;140(4):318-321. doi:10.5858/arpa.2015-0240-SA.

Husain AN, Colby TV, Ordóñez NG, et al. Guidelines for pathologic diagnosis of malignant mesothelioma: 2017 update of the consensus statement from the International Mesothelioma Interest Group. *Arch Pathol Lab Med.* 2018;142(1):89-108. doi:10.5858/arpa.2017-0124-RA.

Lucas DR, Pass HI, Madan SK, et al. Sarcomatoid mesothelioma and its histological mimics: a comparative immunohistochemical study. *Histopathology*. 2003;42(3):270-279.

Mangano WE, Cagle PT, Churg A, Vollmer RT, Roggli VL. The diagnosis of desmoplastic malignant mesothelioma and its distinction from fibrous pleurisy: a histologic and immunohistochemical analysis of 31 cases including p53 immunostaining. *Am J Clin Pathol*. 1998;110(2):191-199. doi:10.1093/ajcp/110.2.191.

Marchevsky AM, LeStang N, Hiroshima K, et al. The differential diagnosis between pleural sarcomatoid mesothelioma and spindle cell/pleomorphic (sarcomatoid) carcinomas of the lung: evidence-based guidelines from the International Mesothelioma Panel and the MESOPATH National Reference Center. *Hum Pathol*. 2017;67:160-168. doi:10.1016/j.humpath.2017.07.015.

Roggli V, Churg A, Chirieac LR, et al. Sarcomatoid, desmoplastic, and biphasic mesothelioma. In: Travis WD, Brambilla E, Burke AP, Marx A, Nicholson AG, eds. *WHO Classifications of Tumours of the Lung, Pleura, Thymus, and Heart*. 4th ed. Lyon: IARC; 2015:165.

Sheffield BS, Hwang HC, Lee AF, et al. BAP1 immunohistochemistry and p16 FISH to separate benign from malignant mesothelial proliferations. *Am J Surg Pathol*. 2015;39(7):977-982. doi:10.1097/PAS.0000000000000394.

Takeshima Y, Amatya VJ, Kushitani K, Kaneko M, Inai K. Value of immunohistochemistry in the differential diagnosis of pleural sarcomatoid mesothelioma from lung sarcomatoid carcinoma. *Histopathology*. 2009;54(6):667-676.

Pulmonary Hamartoma

Rogalla P, Lemke I, Kazmierczak B, Bullerdiek J. An identical HMGIC-LPP fusion transcript is consistently expressed in pulmonary chondroid hamartomas with t(3;12)(q27-28;q14-15). *Genes Chromosomes Cancer*. 2000;29(4):363-366.

Yasin JT, Daghlas SA, Hamid A, Gaballah AH. Primary pulmonary chondrosarcoma: a case report and literature review. *J Clin Imaging Sci*. 2020;10:3.

Elsayed H, Abdel Hady SM, Elbastawisy SE. Is resection necessary in biopsy-proven asymptomatic pulmonary hamartomas? *Interact Cardiovasc Thorac Surg*. 2015;21(6):773-776.

Thomashefski JF, Dacic S. Pulmonary hamartoma. In: Travis WD, Brambilla E, Burke AP, Marx A, Nicholson AG, eds. *WHO Classifications of Tumours of the Lung, Pleura, Thymus, and Heart*. 4th ed. Lyon: IARC; 2015:116.

Epithelioid Hemangioendothelioma

Antonescu CR, Le Loarer F, Mosquera JM, et al. Novel YAP1-TFE3 fusion defines a distinct subset of epithelioid hemangioendothelioma. *Genes Chromosomes Cancer*. 2013;52(8):775-784.

Cagle P, Dacic S. Epithelioid hemangioendothelioma. In: Travis WD, Brambilla E, Burke AP, Marx A, Nicholson AG, eds. *WHO Classifications of Tumours of the Lung, Pleura, Thymus, and Heart*. 4th ed. Lyon: IARC; 2015:123.

Gill R, O'Donnell RJ, Horvai A. Utility of immunohistochemistry for endothelial markers in distinguishing epithelioid hemangioendothelioma from carcinoma metastatic to bone. *Arch Pathol Lab Med*. 2009;133(6):967-972.

Hettmer S, Andrieux G, Hochrein J, et al. Epithelioid hemangioendotheliomas of the liver and lung in children and adolescents. *Pediatr Blood Cancer*. 2017;64(12). doi:10.1002/pbc.26675.

Keylock JB, Galvin JR, Franks TJ. Sclerosing hemangioma of the lung. *Arch Pathol Lab Med*. 2009;133(5):820-825.

Ren Y, Zhu M, Liu Y, Diao X, Zhang Y. Primary pulmonary angiosarcoma: three case reports and literature review. *Thorac Cancer*. 2016;7(5):607-613.

Sardaro A, Bardoscia L, Petruzzelli MF, Portaluri M. Epithelioid hemangioendothelioma: an overview and update on a rare vascular tumor. *Oncol Rev*. 2014;8(2):259. doi:10.4081/oncol.2014.259.

Shibuya R, Matsuyama A, Shiba E, Harada H, Yabuki K, Hisaoka M. CAMTA1 is a useful immunohistochemical marker for diagnosing epithelioid haemangioendothelioma. *Histopathology*. 2015;67(6):827-835.

Weissferdt A, Moran CA. Primary vascular tumors of the lungs: a review. *Ann Diagn Pathol*. 2010;14:296-308.

Lymphangiomyomatosis

Abbott GF, Rosado-de-Christenson ML, Frazier AA, Franks TJ, Pugatch RD, Galvin JR. From the archives of the AFIP: lymphangioleiomyomatosis—radiologic-pathologic correlation. *RadioGraphics*. 2005;25:803-828.

Aubry MC, Myers JL, Colby TV, Leslie KO, Tazelaar HD. Endometrial stromal sarcoma metastatic to the lung: a detailed analysis of 16 patients. *Am J Surg Pathol*. 2002;26:440-449. doi:10.1097/00000478-200204000-00005.

Choe YH, Jeon SY, Lee YC, et al. Benign metastasizing leiomyoma presenting as multiple cystic pulmonary nodules: a case report. *BMC Womens Health*. 2017;17(1):81. doi:10.1186/s12905-017-0435-6.

Dekeyzer S, Peters N, Smeets P, De Visschere P, Decaestecker K, Gosselin R. Lymphangioleiomyomatosis presenting with perirenal hemorrhage. *J Belg Soc Radiol*. 2015;99(1):46-49. doi:10.5334/jbr-btr.836.

Esteban JM, Allen WM, Schaerf RH. Benign metastasizing leiomyoma of the uterus: histologic and immunohistochemical characterization of primary and metastatic lesions. *Arch Pathol Lab Med*. 1999;123:960-962.

Harari S, Torre O, Moss J. Lymphangioleiomyomatosis: what do we know and what are we looking for? *Eur Respir Rev*. 2011;20(119):34-44. doi:10.1183/09059180.00011010.

Ki EY, Hwang SJ, Lee KH, et al. Benign metastasizing leiomyoma of the lung. *World J Surg Oncol*. 2013;11:279. Available at: https://doi.org/10.1186/1477-7819-11-279.

McCormack FX, Inoue Y, Moss J, et al. Efficacy and safety of sirolimus in lymphangioleiomyomatosis. *N Engl J Med*. 2011;364(17):1595-1606.

Moir LM. Lymphangioleiomyomatosis: current understanding and potential treatments. *Pharmacol Ther*. 2016;158:114-124.

Nicholson AG, Henske E, Travis WD. PEComatous Tumors. In: Travis WD, Brambilla E, Burke AP, Marx A, Nicholson AG, eds. *WHO Classifications of Tumours of the Lung, Pleura, Thymus, and Heart*. 4th ed. Lyon: IARC; 2015:117.

Pallisa E, Sanz P, Roman A, Majó J, Andreu J, Cáceres J. Lymphangioleiomyomatosis: pulmonary and abdominal findings with pathologic correlation. *Radiographics*. 2002;22 Spec No:S185-S198. doi:10.1148/radiographics.22.suppl_1.g02oc13s185.

Xu Y, Liang ZX, Guo JT, Su X, Lu YL, Guan XZ. Cystic and solitary nodular pulmonary metastases in a patient with low-grade endometrial stromal sarcoma: a case report and literature review. *Oncol Lett*. 2019;18(2):1133-1144. doi:10.3892/ol.2019.10409.

Zhang X, Travis WD. Pulmonary lymphangioleiomyomatosis. *Arch Pathol Lab Med*. 2010;134(12):1823-1828. doi:10.1043/2009-0576-RS.1.

TYPE A THYMOMA

DIFFERENTIAL DIAGNOSIS: SYNOVIAL SARCOMA

Clinical Features

Thymomas represent a morphologic spectrum of anterior mediastinal neoplasms derived from cortical and medullary epithelial cells of the thymus. They are typically encountered in the middle-aged patient; however, the age range at presentation is relatively broad. Thymoma can occur in the setting of myasthenia gravis and may rarely present with an accompanying pure red cell aplasia. Thymomas represent the most common epithelial neoplasm of the anterior mediastinum. Thymomas are considered malignant and can recur or metastasize. The malignant neoplastic cells are epithelial in nature, and the accompanying immature T-lymphocytes (thymocytes) are considered benign. There has been significant debate in the literature regarding the prognostic implications of subtyping thymomas based on the degree of epithelial and lymphoid elements. In this chapter, the focus will be differentiating the diagnosis of thymoma from other morphologic look-alike's, rather than histologic subtyping of the thymoma itself. For use in their reporting templates, the College of American Pathologists has adopted the World Health Organization (WHO) proposed system for thymoma subclassification (types A, AB, B1, B2, and B3 thymomas). Practical consideration has therefore been given to that system and it will be the only system referred to herein.

The WHO defines the type A thymoma as being composed of neoplastic cells with a spindle to oval morphology with correspondingly bland-appearing nuclei and inconspicuous nucleoli. By definition, these tumors lack significant numbers of immature T-cells. The type A thymoma is less frequently encountered than the so-called lymphocyte-rich thymomas (i.e., type B1 and B2). Patients may present with symptoms of myasthenia gravis or symptoms due to compression of the adjacent

mediastinal structures, including superior vena cava syndrome. Patients may present with cough, dysphagia, chest pain, or no symptoms at all.

Pathologic Features

GROSS FINDINGS

Type A thymomas are generally well circumscribed and encapsulated with tan-white cut surfaces. The grossly appreciable lobulations are usually less distinct than other thymoma subtypes. Cystic changes and dystrophic calcification are not uncommon findings. Like all thymomas, the type A thymoma has the capacity to invade the mediastinal soft tissue and adjacent organs; however, this has only rarely been reported. Care should be taken to orient en bloc resections that may include portions of pericardium and/or lung. Much like neoplasms of the thyroid, the capsule of the tumor should be extensively or entirely submitted in order to assess for invasion and establish proper pathologic staging.

MICROSCOPIC FINDINGS

Variable histologic findings can be observed in type A thymoma, but in general, these tumors are composed of spindled to oval cells with bland-appearing spindle-shaped nuclei, relatively fine chromatin, and inconspicuous nucleoli (Fig. 12.1). The tumor is usually surrounded by a fibrous capsule with thick fibrous septations. The tumor cells may grow in solid sheets, as short fascicles, or in a storiform pattern. Microcystic change is common and other architectural patterns include glandular structures, glomeruloid bodies, meningioma-like whirls, and rosettes. A synovial sarcoma–like pattern of growth with small round cells may also be present. Hemangiopericytoma-like thin-walled vessels are common. Perivascular clearing is infrequent compared with the lymphocyte-rich thymomas. By definition, background immature T-cells are inconspicuous. Mitoses are usually inconspicuous, and care should be taken not to over interpret mitotic figures corresponding to background immature T-cells.

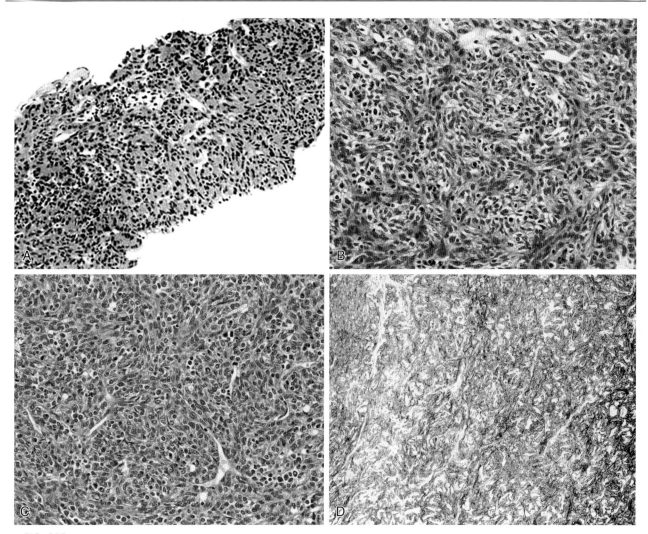

FIG. 12.1

Type A thymoma. **A,** Typical spindle cell pattern seen on core biopsy of a mediastinal mass. **B,** Combination of spindled to round cells seen in this resection specimen. **C,** Note the paucity of lymphocytes and lack of perivascular clearing. **D,** Tumor cells demonstrate uniform CK19 expression.

Ancillary Studies

Type A thymomas uniformly express cytokeratins including CK19, CK8/18, and somewhat variably AE1/3. The tumor cells are uniformly p63 positive and may express PAX8. The spindle cells may be focally CD20 positive; however, interpretation on small biopsy can be unreliable. The tumor cells are CD5 negative and lack expression of STAT6 and neuroendocrine markers. The background immature T-cells are TdT and CD1a positive.

Differential Diagnosis

The type A thymoma must be distinguished from other spindle cell neoplasms of the anterior mediastinum including synovial sarcoma, solitary fibrous tumor (SFT), and neuroendocrine tumors. Synovial sarcomas are often large at presentation and can present with a biphasic or monophasic histology composed of variable amounts of small round blue to spindled cells with interspersed glandular elements. Mediastinal synovial sarcomas are more often monophasic and demonstrate hemangiopericytoma-like vasculature, wiry collagen, alternating zones of hypercellularity and hypocellularity, and stromal mast cells (Fig. 12.2). Mediastinal synovial sarcomas often demonstrate high nuclear grade and elevated mitotic counts. Rhabdoid cells may also be encountered. A screening panel of immunohistochemical stains including cytokeratins, p63, STAT6, neuroendocrine markers, and TLE1 is of utility in this regard. Molecular confirmation of the diagnostic translocation t(X;18)(p11.2;q11.2) is also of utility in differentiating synovial sarcoma from type A thymoma (Table 12.1).

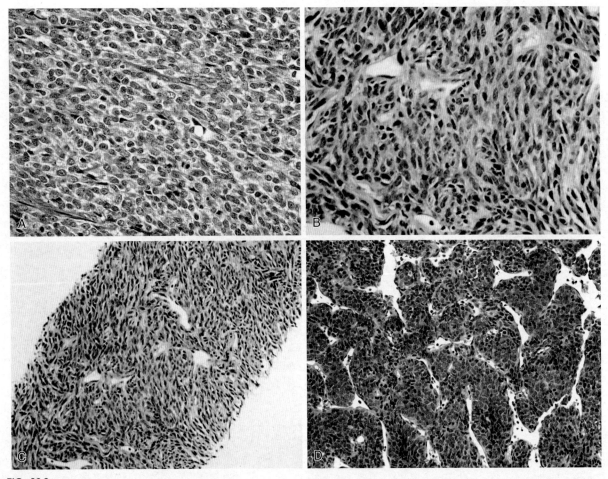

FIG. 12.2
Synovial sarcoma. **A,** Monomorphic hypercellular spindle cell proliferation with appreciable mitotic activity. **B** and **C,** Note the gaping hemangiopericytoma-like vascular spaces. **D,** Round to epithelioid-appearing tumor cells with typical hemangiopericytoma-like vessels.

TABLE 12.1

Histologic Features of Type A Thymoma Versus Synovial Sarcoma

Type A Thymoma	Synovial Sarcoma
• Spindled to oval cells • Microcystic change is common • Low nuclear grade, inconspicuous nucleoli	• Small round blue cell to spindled morphology • Variable degrees of glandular elements • High nuclear grade, elevated mitotic counts • Rhabdoid cells may be encountered
• Fibrous capsule with course septations	• Infiltrative boarders with destruction of the adjacent soft tissues
• Uniformly keratin and p63 positive • Benign background T-cells are TdT positive	• Variable keratin expression • TLE1 relatively sensitive and specific • Diagnostic translocation t(X;18)(p11.2;q11.2)

Prognosis and Therapy

Surgery is the mainstay of therapy for type A thymoma. Complete surgical resection (R0) portends the best prognosis. Overall survival has been reported to reach as high as 100% at 5 and 10 years with complete resection. With the exception of case reports, local recurrence and distant metastases are exceedingly rare. There is no clear link between prognosis and myasthenia gravis. Like all thymomas, prognosis is strongly linked to staging, which is defined pathologically by the extent of capsular invasion and/or invasion into the adjacent mediastinal soft tissues/organs and/or invasion into adjacent intrathoracic organs.

TYPE B1 THYMOMA

DIFFERENTIAL DIAGNOSIS: LYMPHOBLASTIC LEUKEMIA/LYMPHOMA

Clinical Features

The WHO defines the type B thymoma as an organotypic tumor being composed of polygonal-appearing neoplastic epithelial cells and varying degrees of immature T-cells. The so-called lymphocyte-rich thymomas include the types B1 and B2 with the type B1 generally composed of inconspicuous epithelial cells and abundant immature T-cells with some resemblance to normal thymus architecture in the form of pale-staining islands of medullary differentiation. The type B2 thymoma is generally composed of more conspicuous islands of neoplastic epithelial cells; however, it is very common to observe overlapping type B1 and B2 features in an otherwise lymphocytic-rich thymoma.

Collectively, the lymphocytic-rich thymomas are encountered much more frequently than the type A, AB, or B3 thymomas. The B2 thymoma is generally encountered more frequently than the B1 thymoma. The most common clinical manifestations are those of myasthenia gravis. Rarely encountered clinical complications include hypogammaglobulinemia (Good syndrome) and pure red cell anaplasia. Patients with type B thymomas, like patients with other types of thymomas, may also present with symptoms due to compression of the adjacent mediastinal structures, including superior vena cava syndrome. Patients may also present with cough, dysphagia, chest pain, or no symptoms at all.

Pathologic Features

GROSS FINDINGS

Type B1 thymomas are generally well encapsulated or circumscribed. The cut surfaces are firm to soft and generally have a tan-white coloration with nodular to lobulated growth patterns. These tumors can invade into adjacent mediastinal tissues and thoracic organs. While pericardial invasion is not common, adhesion to the pericardium is often encountered intraoperatively. Care should be taken to recognize the presence of adherent pericardial windows or other structures. In that regard, reading of the operative report or direct consultation with the attending surgeon prior to gross cutting is strongly advised. Similarly, direct consultation with the attending surgeon should be made prior to the gross cutting of un-oriented specimens. Much like neoplasms of the thyroid, the capsule of the tumor should be extensively or entirely submitted in order to assess for invasion and establish proper pathologic staging.

MICROSCOPIC FINDINGS

To the unaided eye, histologic sections of type B1 thymomas generally appear intensely blue with recognizable lobulations. At low magnification, thick fibrous capsules and septations become readily apparent with the intense blue staining owing to the numerous background immature T-lymphocytes. The tumor lobules are generally of irregular shape and size with associated fibrous septations. At high magnification, small collections of cells (generally 3 or less) with poorly defined pink cytoplasm can be recognized (Fig. 12.3). These neoplastic cells demonstrate round to oval nuclei with vesicular chromatin and small but appreciable nucleoli. Mitoses are usually indistinct among the tumor cells; however, brisk mitotic activity can be recognized among the background immature T-lymphocytes. A common feature among B1 thymomas is the presence of perivascular clearing, which is recognized as variably sized clear spaces surrounding small venules and containing variable amounts of proteinaceous fluid and/or small lymphocytes. Pale staining and vaguely nodular regions of decreased cellularity, termed medullary islands, are always present and may contain Hassall corpuscles. Variable numbers of lymphoid follicles may be scattered among or around the tumor lobules, particularly among patients experiencing myasthenia gravis. When invasive through the tumor capsule or into adjacent tissues or organs, the invasive front appears pushing and tumor cells generally retain a lobular architecture. Areas of type B2 and type B3 thymoma growth patterns can be encountered and should be described.

Ancillary Studies

The neoplastic epithelial cells typically demonstrate strong immunoreactivity to CK5/6, CK19, and p63. The

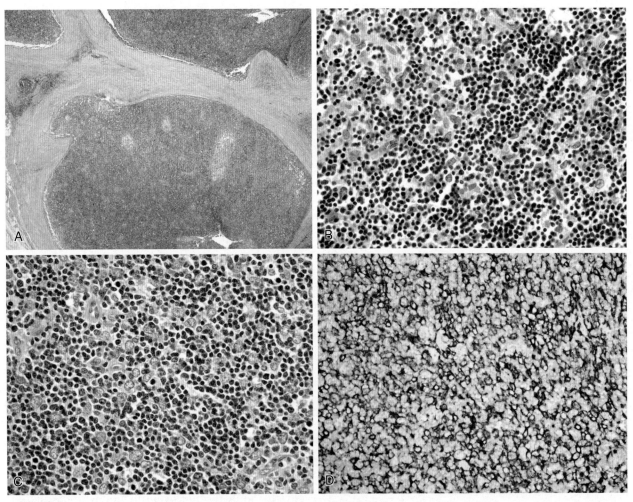

FIG. 12.3

Type B1 thymoma. **A,** At low magnification, pale stained medullary islands are seen on a background of coarsely septated tumor lobules composed of numerous small lymphocytes. **B** and **C,** At high magnification, the tumor cells demonstrate appreciable pink cytoplasm with round nuclei and central small nucleoli. **D,** Tumor cells are uniformly pancytokeratin positive.

neoplastic cells are commonly PAX8 positive and may demonstrate some CK8/18 and/or CK7 positivity. The neoplastic epithelial cells are epithelial membrane antigen (EMA), CK20, CD20, CD117, and CD5 negative. The intratumoral lymphocytes are CD3, CD5, TdT, CD1a, and CD99 positive with both CD4 and CD8 immunoreactivity, consistent with a cortical immature T-cell profile. The intratumoral lymphocytes will show a high proliferative index when interrogated with Ki-67 stains. The medullary islands generally contain few or no immature T-cells.

Differential Diagnosis

The lymphocyte-rich type B1 thymoma must be distinguished from other small lymphocyte-rich neoplasms, particularly lymphomas. In particular, T-cell lymphoblastic leukemia/lymphoma can mimic lymphocyte-rich thymomas. Robust keratin expression typically and readily delineates these two entities, but in order to avoid potential diagnostic pitfalls when individual keratins fail to express, panels of different epithelial antibodies including p63 should be employed. T-cell lymphoblastic lymphoma/leukemia is a malignancy of lymphoblasts characterized by small- to medium-size cells with scant cytoplasm, condensed chromatin, and inconspicuous nucleoli. Conspicuous mitotic activity and necrosis are commonly encountered. Like the intratumoral T-lymphocytes of the type B1 thymoma, the lymphoblasts are committed to the T-cell lineage and will display an immature cortical immunoprofile including TdT expression (Fig. 12.4). The lymphoblasts invariably demonstrate clonal rearrangement of the T-cell receptor genes. In addition, the malignant T-cells demonstrate much more infiltrative and destructive growth into the adjacent mediastinal adipose tissue. This is in comparison with the type B1 thymoma that demonstrates a thick capsule and course septations. Unlike the type B1 thymoma, regional lymph nodes are usually simultaneously involved (Table 12.2).

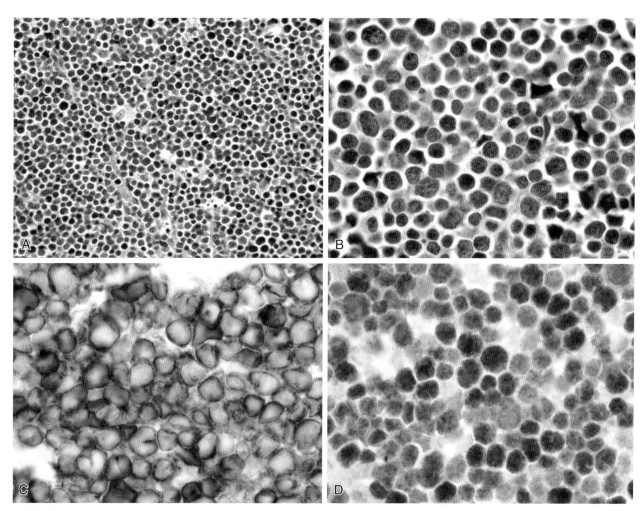

FIG. 12.4

T-lymphoblastic lymphoma/leukemia. **A,** At low magnification, this biopsy demonstrates densely packed small round cells with scant cytoplasm. **B,** At high magnification, the tumor cells demonstrate dispersed chromatin and small nucleoli. **C,** Tumor cells are uniformly CD3 positive. **D,** Tumor cells uniformly express terminal deoxynucleotidyl transferase.

TABLE 12.2
Histologic Features of Type B1 Thymoma Versus T-Lymphoblastic Leukemia/Lymphoma

Type B1 Thymoma	T-Lymphoblastic Leukemia/ Lymphoma
• Malignancy of thymic epithelial cells	• Malignancy of lymphoblasts
• Medullary differentiation is present	• Conspicuous mitotic activity and necrosis
• Tumor necrosis is uncommon	• Usually infiltrative and destructive growth into adjacent mediastinal adipose tissue
• Invasive front appears pushing and tumor cells generally retain a lobular architecture	• Simultaneously involve regional lymph nodes
• Uniformly keratin and p63 positive	• No keratin expression
• Benign background T-cells are TdT positive	• Malignant lymphoblasts are TdT positive
	• Clonal rearrangement of the T-cell receptor

Prognosis and Therapy

The prognosis for patients with thymomas depends largely on staging and resectability. Staging has been closely linked to the WHO histologic classification of thymomas. Patients with type A and AB thymomas tend to present as encapsulated lesions with lesser degrees of invasion into adjacent tissues and organs, and thus lower stage and better prognosis. The number of patients presenting with more locally invasive disease and therefore more advanced stage, increases slightly and gradually from types B1 to B2 to B3 thymomas, respectively. Thus, the prognosis for a patient with type B1 thymoma is slightly better than a patient with type B2 thymoma, wherein the prognosis is slightly better than a patient with type B3 thymoma. As stated earlier, surgery is the mainstay of therapy for thymomas; however, some success has been reported with adjuvant chemotherapy and/or radiation therapy.

TYPE B1 THYMOMA – DISEASE FACT SHEET

Definition
▶▶ Malignant epithelial neoplasm of the thymus composed of inconspicuous epithelial cells and abundant immature T-cells with some architectural resemblance to normal thymus architecture in the form of pale-staining islands of medullary differentiation

Incidence and Location
▶▶ Thymomas are relatively low-incidence tumors (in the United States estimated at 0.13–0.15 per 100,000 population at risk); however, collectively comprise about half of all mediastinal tumors

▶▶ Up to 15% of patients with established myasthenia gravis will develop a thymoma
▶▶ Tumors arise from the thymus and thus are typically located within the anterior mediastinum; though, significant extension into adjacent mediastinal structures or lung can occur

Age Distribution
▶▶ Exceedingly rare in children with a peak incidence in the sixth to seventh decade of life
▶▶ There is no well-defined age predilection

Clinical Features
▶▶ Commonly asymptomatic (discovered incidentally during chest imaging)
▶▶ Symptomatic patients may be due to compression of adjacent mediastinal structures
▶▶ Can manifest as an autoimmune disease, most commonly myasthenia gravis

Radiologic Features
▶▶ By computed tomography, tumors are typically rounded, smooth or lobulated masses of low soft tissue attenuation located between the sternum and great vessels
▶▶ Cystic change is common and calcification more frequent in lymphocyte-rich thymomas

Prognosis and Therapy
▶▶ Surgery is the mainstay of therapy for type B1 thymomas
▶▶ Prognosis depends largely on staging and resectability
▶▶ Some success has been reported with adjuvant chemotherapy and/or radiation therapy

TYPE B1 THYMOMA – PATHOLOGIC FEATURES

Gross Findings
▶▶ Generally well encapsulated or circumscribed
▶▶ Cut surfaces are nodular with an appreciable lobulated growth patterns
▶▶ Adhesion to the pericardium is often encountered intraoperatively

Microscopic Findings
▶▶ Thick fibrous capsules and septations readily apparent
▶▶ Intense blue staining owing to the numerous background immature T-lymphocytes
▶▶ High magnification shows small collections of ill-defined epithelial cells
▶▶ Cells have round to oval nuclei with vesicular chromatin and small but prominent nucleoli
▶▶ Pale staining and vaguely nodular regions of decreased cellularity, termed medullary islands, are always present and may contain Hassall corpuscles
▶▶ Invasive front appears pushing and tumor cells generally retain a lobular architecture
▶▶ Areas of type B2 and type B3 thymoma can be encountered and should be described

Pathologic Differential Diagnoses
▶▶ Must be distinguished from other small lymphocyte-rich neoplasms, particularly lymphomas

TYPE B3 THYMOMA

DIFFERENTIAL DIAGNOSIS: THYMIC CARCINOMA

Clinical Features

The WHO defines the type B3 thymoma as an epithelioid neoplasm derived from thymic epithelial cells and occurring with an incidence slightly lower than the incidence of type B1 and B2 thymomas. Like other thymomas, the most common clinical manifestations are those of myasthenia gravis. Rarely encountered clinical complications include hypogammaglobulinemia (Good syndrome) and pure red cell anaplasia. Patients may also present with symptoms due to compression of the adjacent mediastinal structures, including superior vena cava syndrome. Patients may also present with cough, dysphagia, chest pain, or no symptoms at all. There does not appear to be an age or sex predilection.

Pathologic Features

GROSS FINDINGS

Unlike other thymomas, type B3 thymomas are typically poorly circumscribed with seamless extension into the adjacent thymus and mediastinal adipose tissue. The tumors appear coarsely lobulated with fibrous septations. The cut surfaces are firm and tan-yellow in appearance. Hemorrhage and necrosis may be apparent.

MICROSCOPIC FINDINGS

Morphologically these tumors appear lobulated at low magnification. Thick fibrous septations are usually present, with or without a definable capsule. At higher magnification, these tumors are composed of relatively large cells with an epithelioid to polygonal cytoplasmic outline. The cytoplasm itself is pink to slightly hyalinized in appearance. The nuclei are round and typically centrally located. Nucleoli are typically conspicuous. There is a slight degree of monotony to the cells, which can be appreciated with some experience (Fig. 12.5). Intracellular bridges are not present. Immature lymphocytes are usually present among the tumor cells, but not to the extent seen in the lymphocyte-rich thymomas. The immature lymphocytes may be present in clusters or present singly among the malignant epithelial cells. Perivascular clearings, defined as spaces surrounding small venules or arterioles, are usually present. The perivascular clearings may be optically clear in

appearance, contain small lymphocytes, or contain proteinaceous pink fluid. Like other thymomas, the type B3 thymoma demonstrates a pushing growth front with preserved lobular architecture. Single cell or an infiltrative-appearing growth patterns are not present. Extensive microcytic change may also be observed. Mitoses may be conspicuous, but necrosis and frankly malignant cytologic atypia are rare. The type B3 thymoma can be encountered arising in a background lymphocyte-rich thymoma. Even when a minor component, the presence of a type B3 component should always be mentioned in the final pathology report. Type B3 thymomas can rarely demonstrate spindled or anaplastic-appearing morphologies. Such cases can generally be distinguished from thymic squamous cell carcinoma given the presence of TdT-positive T-lymphocytes and the lack of thymic squamous cell carcinoma markers (see Differential Diagnosis).

Ancillary Studies

Like other thymomas, the type B3 tumor cells are typically pancytokeratin positive. Other positive markers typically include CK19, CK5/6, p63, p40, and PAX8. The tumor cells are TTF-1 negative and lack evidence of neuroendocrine differentiation. Markers of thymic squamous cell carcinoma such as CD5, CD117, GLUT1, and MUC1 are usually negative, but can show focal expression in some cases. The intratumoral T-lymphocytes are TdT positive. Molecular testing and/or fluorescence *in situ* hybridization currently have no role in the diagnosis of type B3 thymomas.

Differential Diagnosis

The primary differential diagnostic consideration for a type B3 thymoma is thymic squamous cell carcinoma. It should be noted that thymic carcinoma is a blanket term defined anatomically as any form of carcinoma arising within the anterior mediastinum. The morphology of a thymic carcinoma can range from adenocarcinoma, neuroendocrine carcinoma, including small and large cell neuroendocrine carcinoma (LCNEC), salivary gland-type carcinomas, and germ cell–derived carcinomas. Most commonly, thymic carcinomas are of the squamous cell type. Given the somewhat squamous-like nature of the type B3 thymoma, differentiating between type B3 thymoma and thymic squamous cell carcinoma can be challenging, particularly on small biopsies. In contrast to the type B3 thymoma, thymic squamous cell carcinomas typically demonstrate frankly malignant cytologic atypia and may be keratinizing in nature (see Fig. 12.5). Intracellular bridges are often observed, and

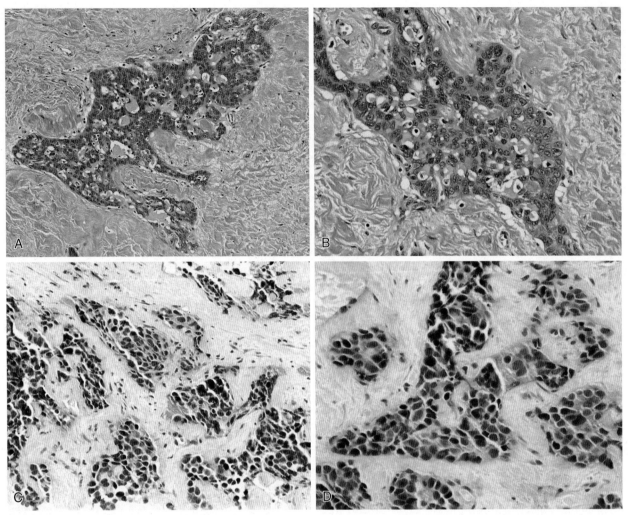

FIG. 12.5

Type B3 thymoma. **A,** At low magnification, the tumor cells are present in a background of collagenous fibrous stoma without an overt des-moplastic response. **B,** At high magnification, the tumor cells demonstrate typical eosinophilic cytoplasm with round nuclei and scattered admixed lymphocytes. Thymic squamous cell carcinoma. **C,** At low magnification, the tumor cells demonstrate high-grade features including enlarged and hyperchromatic nuclei with brisk mitotic activity. **D,** At high magnification, the cells demonstrate an angulated and infiltrative growth pattern. There is no keratinization in this example.

necrosis may be abundant. Unlike the type B3 thy-moma, there are no immature T-lymphocytes (thymo-cytes) present among the tumor cells. If lymphocytes are present, the cells are peripherally derived, TdT-negative, mature T-lymphocytes. Perivascular clearings are not present in thymic squamous cell carcinoma. If the afore-mentioned features are not present on small biopsy, evidence of a single cell or infiltrative growth pattern can be key to an accurate histologic interpretation. Fi-brous septations and lobular growth are not typical features of thymic squamous cell carcinoma. Immuno-histochemistry is of limited utility in differentiating between type B3 thymoma and thymic squamous cell carcinoma. Aside from the absence of TdT-positive, immature T-lymphocytes, thymic squamous cell carci-noma will typically stain positive for the same markers as a type B3 thymoma, that is, CK5/6, p40, p63, and PAX8. Thymic squamous cell carcinoma is typically CD5, C117, GLUT1, and MUC1 positive, whereas most,

but not all thymomas are typically negative for these markers. Thymic squamous cell carcinomas have been demonstrated to lack p16 expression by immunohisto-chemistry with subsequent homozygous gene loss observed by fluorescence *in situ* hybridization; however, this has not been thoroughly investigated among type B3 thymomas. Thymic squamous cell carcinoma can show focal immunohistochemical evidence of neuroen-docrine differentiation; however, this is not generally encountered in cases of type B3 thymoma (Table 12.3).

Prognosis and Therapy

As for all thymomas, prognosis depends largely on stag-ing and resectability. Staging has been closely linked to the WHO histologic classification of thymomas. When compared with other thymomas, type B3 thymomas

TABLE 12.3

Histologic Features of Type B3 Thymoma Versus Thymic Carcinoma

Type B3 Thymoma	Thymic Carcinoma
• Malignancy of thymic epithelial cells	• Blanket term, *most often thymic squamous cell carcinoma*, but may be salivary gland type, germ cell, neuroendocrine, etc.
• Perivascular clearing is common	• Frankly malignant cytologic atypia
• Tumor necrosis is uncommon	• Conspicuous mitotic activity and necrosis
• Fibrous septations and lobular growth	• Thymic squamous cell carcinoma maybe keratinizing with intracellular bridges
• Invasive front appears pushing and tumor cells generally retain a lobular architecture	• Usually infiltrative and destructive growth into adjacent mediastinal adipose tissue
• Immunohistochemistry is of limited utility	• No TdT positive T-lymphocytes
• Benign background T-cells are TdT positive	• Thymic squamous cell carcinoma typically CD5, CD117, GLUT1, and MUC1 positive
• Typically CD5 and CD117 negative	

generally present with a more advanced stage and thus poorer prognosis. In that regard, myasthenia gravis has been considered a favorable prognostic factor due to earlier tumor detection. Surgery is the mainstay of therapy for thymomas; however, recurrences have been reported among completely resected cases of advanced-stage type B3 thymomas. Some success has been reported with adjuvant chemotherapy and/or radiation therapy in unresectable or partially resected cases.

TYPE B3 THYMOMA – DISEASE FACT SHEET

Definition
▶▶ Malignant organotypic epithelial neoplasm of the thymus composed of relatively large cells with an epithelioid to polygonal cytoplasmic outline and somewhat eosinophilic appearing cytoplasm

Incidence and Location
▶▶ Thymomas are relatively low-incidence tumors (in the United States estimated at 0.13–0.15 per 100,000 population at risk); however, collectively comprise about half of all mediastinal tumors
▶▶ Up to 15% of patients with established myasthenia gravis will develop a thymoma
▶▶ Tumors arise from the thymus and thus are typically located within the anterior mediastinum; however, significant extension into adjacent mediastinal structures or lung can occur

Age Distribution
▶▶ Exceedingly rare in children with a peak incidence in the sixth to seventh decade of life
▶▶ There is no well-defined age predilection

Clinical Features
▶▶ Commonly asymptomatic (discovered incidentally during chest imaging)
▶▶ Symptomatic patients may be due to compression of adjacent mediastinal structures
▶▶ Can manifest as an autoimmune disease, most commonly myasthenia gravis

Radiologic Features
▶▶ By computed tomography, tumors are typically rounded, smooth or lobulated masses of low soft tissue attenuation located between the sternum and great vessels
▶▶ Cystic change is common and calcification may be present

Prognosis and Therapy
▶▶ Surgery is the mainstay of therapy for type B3 thymomas
▶▶ Prognosis depends largely on staging and resectability
▶▶ Some success has been reported with adjuvant chemotherapy and/or radiation therapy

TYPE B3 THYMOMA – PATHOLOGIC FEATURES

Gross Findings
▶▶ Typically poorly circumscribed with seamless extension into adjacent tissues
▶▶ Tumors appear coarsely lobulated with fibrous septations
▶▶ Cut surfaces are firm and tan-yellow in appearance
▶▶ Hemorrhage and necrosis may be apparent

Microscopic Findings
▶▶ Relatively large cells with an epithelioid to polygonal cytoplasmic outline
▶▶ Cytoplasm is pink to slightly hyalinized in appearance
▶▶ Nuclei are round and typically centrally located, whereas nucleoli are typically conspicuous
▶▶ Immature lymphocytes are usually present, but not to the extent of lymphocyte-rich thymomas
▶▶ Perivascular clearings are usually present

Pathologic Differential Diagnoses
▶▶ Must be distinguished from thymic carcinoma, particularly thymic squamous cell carcinoma

SMALL CELL CARCINOMA

DIFFERENTIAL DIAGNOSIS: LARGE CELL NEUROENDOCRINE CARCINOMA

Clinical Features

Small cell carcinoma (SmCC) of lung origin is more common than the extrapulmonary locations. Mediastinal small cell carcinomas (MSmCCs) are extremely rare and arise from the thymus in the anterior mediastinum. They account for up to 10% of all the thymic neuroendocrine tumors. Clinical symptoms include chest pain, cough, shortness of breath, weight loss, and possibly symptoms associated with compression of the superior vena cava. Invasion into the adjacent structures, lung, pericardium, pulmonary artery or aorta, and phrenic nerve has been described. Rarely, features of Cushing syndrome are seen due to the ectopic ACTH production. Despite the small number of cases, metastases to the lung, bone, brain, and liver are seen. Equal distribution of cases is seen in both men and women with a median age of 58 years (range, 37–63 years). In 2019, Dinter et al. proposed three major prognostic groups (Thy-NET G1, G2, and G3) for the thymic neuroendocrine tumors based on the copy number instability (CNI) score using low-coverage whole genomic sequencing data analysis. MSmCCs showed a high CNI score corresponding to the high-grade molecular group (NET G3).

Pathologic Features

GROSS FINDINGS

The tumors are large with a median diameter of 8.9 cm (largest reported 19 cm) associated with necrosis and hemorrhage. Scattered microcalcifications have been described.

MICROSCOPIC FINDINGS

Histologically MSmCCs are very similar to SmCC from other sites. The tumor cells are small, with round/oval nuclei with finely granular chromatin, inconspicuous/absent nucleoli, and scant cytoplasm. Some spindling of the nuclei can be seen (Figs. 12.6 and 12.7). Numerous mitoses > 10/10 HPFs along with apoptotic bodies are seen. Nuclear molding is better appreciated in cytology

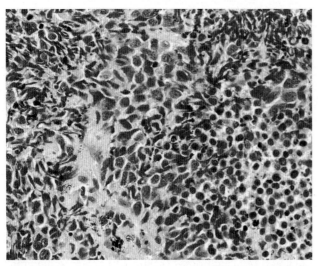

FIG. 12.6
Classic small cell carcinoma H&E morphology with sheets of small cells with finely granular nuclear chromatin with scant cytoplasm and inconspicuous nucleoli. Nuclear molding and crush artifacts are present.

smears. Crush artifacts with streaming of nuclei are frequently seen in small biopsies. Rare cases of combined MSmCCs with thymoma, squamous cell carcinoma, and adenosquamous carcinoma are reported in the literature.

Ancillary Studies

Immunohistochemistry with keratins (AE1/AE3 and CAM 5.2) shows a dot-like/perinuclear staining (Fig. 12.8) which helps in differentiating MSmCCs from lymphomas (positive for CD45, CD3 or CD20 or TdT) and other tumors such as melanomas (positive for HMB45/S100/Sox10). In addition to keratin studies, assessment of neuroendocrine markers such as synaptophysin, chromogranin, CD56 and INSM1 may prove useful. When keratins and neuroendocrine markers are nonreactive, more extensive workups to rule out less common small blue cell tumors such as rhabdomyosarcoma (desmin, myogenin), and PNET (CD99, EWSR1) may be warranted. Rare exceptions of keratin negativity have been documented. Similarly, positivity for neuroendocrine markers is not required for the diagnosis. Further, TTF-1 positivity is also seen in SmCC of lung origin, and hence cannot be used to determine the site of origin. The presence of clinical-radiological evidence of the thymic origin of the mass lesion would be extremely helpful in this scenario. An elevated Ki-67 (>50%) proliferation rate is usually seen. In 2021, in a study by Vrana et al., SATB2 expression was demonstrated in a small number of thymic SmCCs expanding the spectrum of SATB2 positivity outside of colorectal and appendiceal tumors.

Differential Diagnosis

In addition to excluding metastasis from lung SmCC (discussed earlier), the most important differential diagnosis is LCNEC (Table 12.4). Unlike the fine granular nuclear chromatin of MSmCCs, LCNEC shows vesicular nuclei with prominent nucleoli (Fig. 12.9). In addition to this, the tumor cells are larger with more abundant cytoplasm than cells of SmCC along with the neuroendocrine architecture (nests, trabeculae, and rosettes) which is extremely helpful in the distinction of these two entities. Extensive areas of necrosis are usually present. Positivity for at least one of the neuroendocrine markers (synaptophysin, chromogranin, INSM1, and CD56) along with morphologic features is enough for the diagnosis of LCNEC. Staining for CD5 and TTF-1 is generally negative. If any other carcinoma component (such as squamous cell carcinoma) constitutes ≥10%, then the tumor should be classified as a combined tumor.

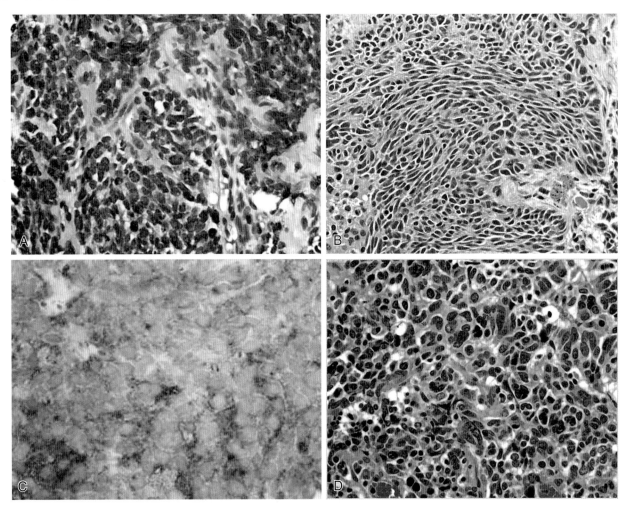

FIG. 12.7

Small cell carcinoma of the thymus (**A**) is similar to small cell carcinoma of the lung (**B**) with similar nuclear features and scant cytoplasm with cells often oval to spindle in shape. Strong immunoreactivity with synaptophysin is present (**C**). This is in comparison to large cell neuroendocrine carcinoma (**D**) with scattered larger cells, vesicular nucleoli and small prominent nucleoli, and abundant cytoplasm.

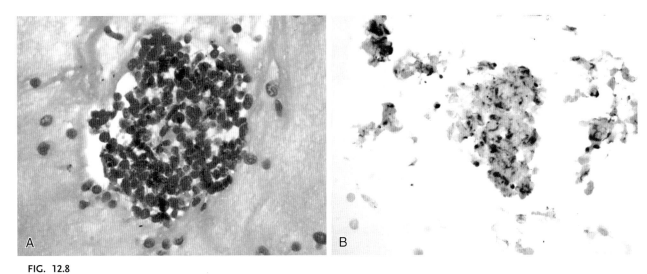

FIG. 12.8

Core biopsy of a mediastinal mass shows small cell carcinoma with the characteristic nuclear appearance (**A**) supported by delicate (perinuclear, dot-like) staining on keratin CAM 5.2 (**B**),

Continued

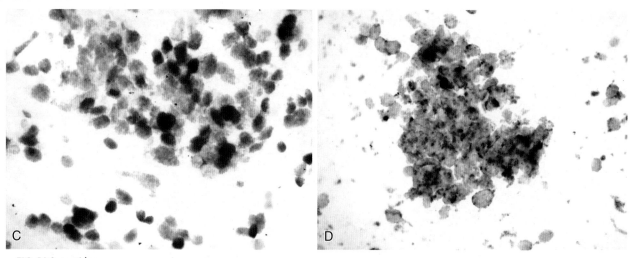

FIG. 12.8, cont'd
strong nuclear TTF-1 reactivity (**C**), and cytoplasmic granular synaptophysin reactivity (**D**).

TABLE 12.4

Histologic and Immunohistochemical Features of Mediastinal Small Cell Carcinoma Versus Mediastinal Large Cell Neuroendocrine Carcinoma

Small Cell Carcinoma	Large Cell Neuroendocrine Carcinoma
• Sheets of small epithelial cells with a distinct nuclear appearance	• Sheets of larger epithelial cells with neuroendocrine morphology
• Hyperchromatic nuclei with molding and overlapping	• Vesicular nuclei with prominent nucleoli
• Nuclear chromatin is finely granular with inconspicuous nucleoli	• Nuclear clearing with architectural nests, trabecular, and rosettes are present
• Scant amount of amphophilic cytoplasm	• Abundance of cytoplasm is seen
• Necrosis, mitoses, and nuclear breakdown seen	• Extensive necrosis and hemorrhage seen
• TTF-1 staining is positive similar to small cell carcinoma of the lung	• TTF-1 can be negative
• Presence of neuroendocrine marker positivity	• Any expression of neuroendocrine markers is sufficient if the morphology is supportive
• CD 5 and CD177 are negative	• CD 5 is negative and occasionally CD177 positive

---

Prognosis and Therapy

The 5-year survival rate for LCNEC is 30% to 66% versus a poorer rate of 0% for SmCC. In addition to radical surgery, temozolomide and platinum-based chemotherapy are used with distant metastases or in the case of incompletely resected tumors. Radiotherapy has proven useful in cases with local recurrences.

MEDIASTINAL SMALL CELL CARCINOMA – DISEASE FACT SHEET

Definition
▸▸ High-grade carcinoma of neuroendocrine origin
▸▸ Uncommon neoplasms of malignant behavior associated with poor prognosis

Incidence and Location
▸▸ Accounts for up to 10% of all the thymic neuroendocrine tumors
▸▸ Arise from the thymus in the anterior (prevascular) mediastinum

Age Distribution
▸▸ Equal distribution of cases seen in both men and women with a median age of 58 years (range, 37–63 years)

Clinical Features
▸▸ Invasion into the adjacent structures, lung, pericardium, pulmonary artery or aorta, and phrenic nerve and metastases to the lung, bone, brain, and liver are seen

Radiologic Features
▸▸ CT-imaging with contrast exhibits a mass lesion with infiltrative growth associated with moderate to intense enhancement due to its rich vasculature
▸▸ Fluorodeoxyglucose PET/CT identifies the tumor, lymph node involvement, and metastases

Prognosis and Therapy
▸▸ Surgery, chemotherapy, and radiotherapy have been used with variable success
▸▸ The 5-year survival rate is 0%, which carries the worse prognosis of all the neuroendocrine tumors

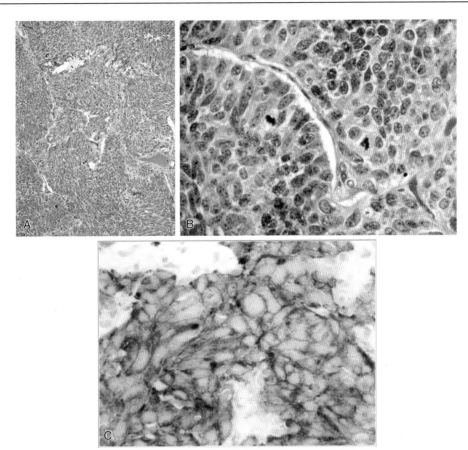

FIG. 12.9

A, A diagnosis of atypical carcinoid tumor was initially considered for this large cell neuroendocrine carcinoma. **B,** High-magnification microscopy confirms large cells with moderate amounts of amphophilic cytoplasm, nucleomegaly, prominent nucleoli, absence of nuclear molding and numerous mitoses, all features of large cell neuroendocrine carcinoma. **C,** Diffuse and strong synaptophysin immunoreactivity supports the morphologic impression.

MEDIASTINAL SMALL CELL CARCINOMA – PATHOLOGIC FEATURES

Gross Findings

▸▸ Large unencapsulated infiltrative mass lesions with a fleshy cut surface and punctate calcifications

▸▸ Examples with extensive necrosis and hemorrhage may mimic large cell neuroendocrine carcinoma

Microscopic Findings

▸▸ Presence of distinctive morphologic appearance

▸▸ Characteristic hyperchromatic nuclear appearance, with nuclear molding and overlapping

▸▸ Nuclear chromatin is finely granular with the absence of nucleoli

▸▸ Scant amounts of amphophilic cytoplasm and indistinct cell borders

▸▸ Nuclear streaming and spindling with crush artifact are commonly seen

▸▸ Numerous mitoses and apoptotic bodies are frequently seen

▸▸ Synaptophysin, chromogranin, INSM1, and CD56 positivity demonstrate neuroendocrine differentiation

▸▸ Ki-67 demonstrates a high proliferation rate usually >50% up to 100%

Pathologic Differential Diagnoses

▸▸ Pulmonary small cell carcinoma

▸▸ Large cell neuroendocrine carcinoma

SOLITARY FIBROUS TUMOR

DIFFERENTIAL DIAGNOSIS: NERVE SHEATH TUMOR

Clinical Features

Solitary fibrous tumor (SFT) is an intermediate (rarely metastasizing) mesenchymal neoplasm with a characteristic appearance on H&E stain, immunophenotype, and gene fusion involving *NAB2-STAT6* located on chromosome 12q13.3. Due to tremendous advancements in cytogenetics and immunohistochemistry, what was once thought of as two distinct entities, SFT and hemangiopericytoma, are now recognized as the same entity. The visceral pleura is the most common location within the thorax, followed by the lung, pericardium, and rarely the mediastinum. These tumors are incidentally discovered on chest imaging as they are slow-growing in most cases, but 10% of them behave aggressively. The larger tumors tend to cause symptoms such as cough, shortness of breath, and/or chest pain. A wide age range of involvement is seen with a peak incidence in the fifth to sixth decades of life.

Pathologic Features

GROSS FINDINGS

SFTs are large, well-circumscribed multinodular masses with a solid, firm and homogenous gray cut surfaces. Rarely hemorrhage, calcification, and minimal cystic necrosis are seen. If the borders are irregular and associated with extensive areas of necrosis, then a malignant transformation should be suspected.

MICROSCOPIC FINDINGS

Classic SFTs have a distinctive morphology, with spindled cells in a storiform pattern in a background of collagenous

(keloid-type) stroma (Fig. 12.10) and staghorn-shaped thin-walled large branching blood vessels (Figs. 12.11A–D). Ovoid cells with background stroma with focal or diffuse myxoid changes are also encountered. Cellular SFTs show less collagenization with a mixture of spindled to more rounded cells with ovoid and less elongated nuclei and condensed chromatin. Sometimes primitive appearing round cells are seen in markedly cellular SFTs. The blood vessels lack a connective tissue layer so that the endothelial cells come into contact with the surrounding tumor cells. Mitotic activity is generally minimal, and SFTs typically lack nuclear pleomorphism and/or necrosis.

There are several variants of SFTs which deserve special attention: fat-forming, giant cell-rich, and dedifferentiated types. The presence of abundant mature adipocytes in the stroma is seen in the fat-forming variant of SFT. These are usually seen in the deep soft tissues in the mediastinum, retroperitoneum, and several other sites. The presence of multinucleated stromal giant cells around the pseudovascular spaces seen in the giant cell variant often involves the periorbital soft tissue. However, the most relevant of these unusual variants is the dedifferentiated variant, which is seen in primary or recurrent tumors. Dedifferentiation is a histologic progression from a well-differentiated neoplasm to a high-grade sarcoma exhibiting various divergent components in the form of spindle cell sarcoma, undifferentiated pleomorphic sarcoma, osteosarcoma, or rhabdomyosarcoma. These high-grade sarcoma components are present adjacent to the conventional SFT and the transition from one to the other occurs abruptly.

Ancillary Studies

Historically, a combination of immunohistochemical studies including CD34, CD99, and BCL2 was used for diagnostic confirmation, until the advent and use of STAT6 in clinical settings. Currently, nuclear expression

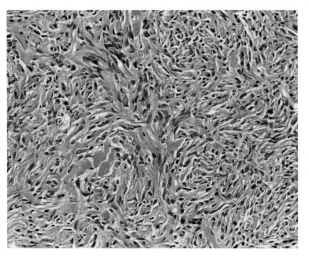

FIG. 12.10
Solitary fibrous tumor with uniform spindle cells exhibiting storiform pattern against a collagenous (keloidal-like) background.

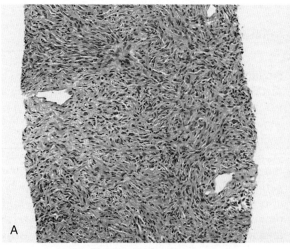
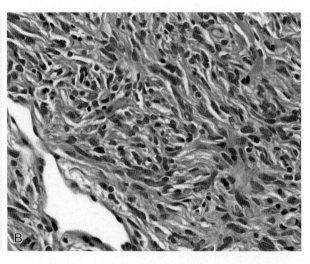

FIG. 12.11
Solitary fibrous tumor with varying cellularity, ranging from highly cellular (**A** and **B**) to paucicellular (**C** and **D**) with branching thin-walled staghorn blood vessels.

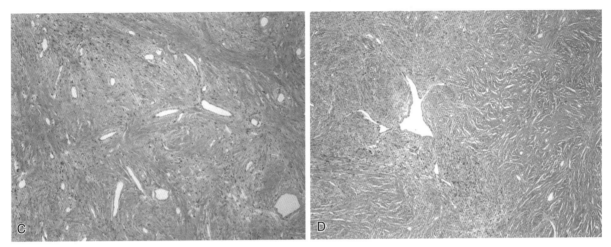

FIG. 12.11, cont'd

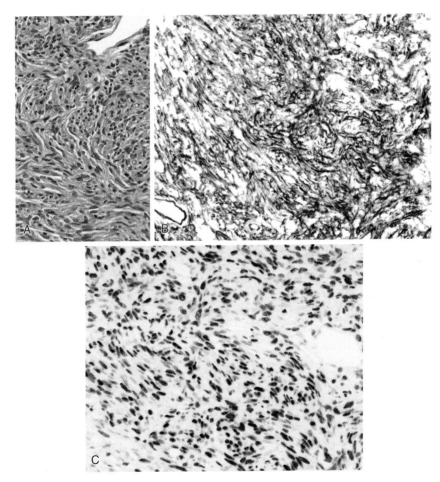

FIG. 12.12

Solitary fibrous tumor demonstrates the individual ovoid to spindle cells encircled by collagen (**A**) with diffuse strong predominantly membranous expression of CD34 by immunohistochemistry (**B**) which is less specific. A distinctive nuclear staining of STAT-6 immunohistochemistry (**C**) has emerged as a surrogate for NAB2-STAT6 gene fusion and shows excellent sensitivity and specificity.

of STAT6 has proved to be a sensitive and specific surrogate for *NAB2–STAT6* gene fusions with excellent sensitivity and specificity (Figs. 12.12A–C). The other markers such as CD34 are positive in 81% to 95% SFTs, whereas BCL2 shows a better sensitivity (>90%) than CD99 (75%) with low specificities due to their expression

in other soft tissue neoplasms. These markers may not be helpful in dedifferentiated SFTs due to loss in their expression. The expression of STAT6 is seen rarely in non-SFT mesenchymal tumors with both nuclear and cytoplasmic staining including well-differentiated/dedifferentiated liposarcoma, desmoid fibromatosis, unclassifiable sarcoma, neurofibroma, and others. Focal expression of keratins especially EMA, smooth muscle actin, beta-catenin, and glial fibrillary acidic protein (GFAP) is seen in few cases. However, no expression of desmin, CD31, and S100 is seen.

Differential Diagnosis

The presence of diverse histological growth patterns encountered in SFTs poses a diagnostic challenge as the list of soft tissue neoplasms in the differential diagnosis becomes long. Nerve sheath tumors including cellular schwannomas (Table 12.5) and malignant peripheral nerve sheath tumors (MPNSTs) form the bulk of the differential diagnosis. As cellular schwannomas are composed of fascicles of bland spindle cells in collagenous backgrounds along with thick-walled hyalinized blood vessels, schwannomas can be easily confused with SFTs. Few cases also show CD34 positivity. Careful examination for the presence of any fibrous capsule, wavy nuclei with tapered ends, and lymphocytic infiltrate with foamy macrophages, and more importantly S100 expression unlike STAT6 nuclear positivity would help in diagnosing cellular schwannomas. MPNST shows alternating hypercellular and hypocellular areas of spindle cells showing fascicular growth pattern with a branching hemangiopericytoma-like vascular pattern. Areas of palisading or rosette-like arrangements with areas of geographic necrosis are also present. Focal S100 expression is expected with few showing GFAP expression (Figs. 12.13A–F). S100 is not specific for nerve sheath tumors and has been reported in synovial sarcomas, leiomyosarcomas, and other mesenchymal neoplasms. When a higher-grade mesenchymal tumor arises in association with a coexisting benign neural tumor such as a neurofibroma or when there is a clinical history of neurofibromatosis, it is important to consider MPNST. Negative STAT6 along with the loss of the newer immunohistochemical stain, H3K27me3 are useful in addition to S100 expression in excluding the diagnosis of SFTs.

Prognosis and Therapy

Surgical resection with wide margins is the mainstay of management. Recurrence occurs in 10% to 25% of cases due to incomplete resection. Distant metastasis can occur in some cases and 75% of those patients who develop metastases die of the disease. Demicco et al. proposed, developed, and validated a risk stratification model for SFTs with the following variables: age, tumor size, mitotic count, and tumor necrosis to predict the development of metastasis in SFTs. A score of 0 or 1 is assigned for the patient's age (<55 or ≥55, respectively). A score of 0, 1, 2, or 3 is assigned for tumor size (<5 cm, 5 to <10 cm, 10 to <15, or ≥15, respectively). A score of 0, 1, or 2 is assigned for the mitotic count per 10 HPF (0, 1–3, or ≥4, respectively). A score of 0 or 1 is assigned based on the degree of tumor necrosis (<10% or ≥10%, respectively). The total cumulative score is then assigned a risk class of low (total score 0–3), intermediate (4–5), or high (6–7).

TABLE 12.5

Histologic and Immunohistochemical Features of Solitary Fibrous Tumor Versus Nerve Sheath Tumor

Solitary Fibrous Tumor	Nerve Sheath Tumor (Cellular Schwannoma)
• Classically with a pleural attachment	• Classically centered around the nerves
• Monomorphic spindle cells with variable cellularity	• Fascicles of bland spindle-shaped cells
• Wide histologic spectrum	• Wavy nuclei with tapered ends
• Branching thin-walled staghorn-type blood vessels	• Thick-walled and hyalinized blood vessels
• CD34 expression is seen in 81 to 95%	• Some cases show CD34 expression
• Nuclear STAT 6 expression is diagnostic	• No STAT-6 expression is reported
• S100 negativity is consistent	• Presence of S100 expression favors the diagnosis

---

SOLITARY FIBROUS TUMOR – DISEASE FACT SHEET

Definition

▸▸ An intermediate (rarely metastasizing) fibroblastic neoplasm with a characteristic appearance on H&E stain, immunophenotype, and gene fusion involving *NAB2-STAT6*

Incidence and Location

▸▸ Most commonly arises from the visceral pleura, accounting for 30% of cases. Less commonly lung parenchyma and pericardium and rarely mediastinum

Age Distribution

▸▸ No sex predilection. Pleural SFTs occur in somewhat older age, most frequently in the sixth decade of adult life

Clinical Features

▸▸ Usually asymptomatic. If symptoms present usually related to mass effect on the adjacent tissues/organs

Radiologic Features

▸▸ Can be incidentally discovered on imaging
▸▸ CT imaging shows sharply demarcated pleural-based soft tissue masses. Increased PET activity is seen in malignant tumors

Prognosis and Therapy

▸▸ Wide local excision is adequate. Recurrence is seen in cases with incomplete resection. No role for chemotherapy and radiotherapy
▸▸ Modified four-variable risk model by Demicco et al. predicts the metastatic risk of SFTs

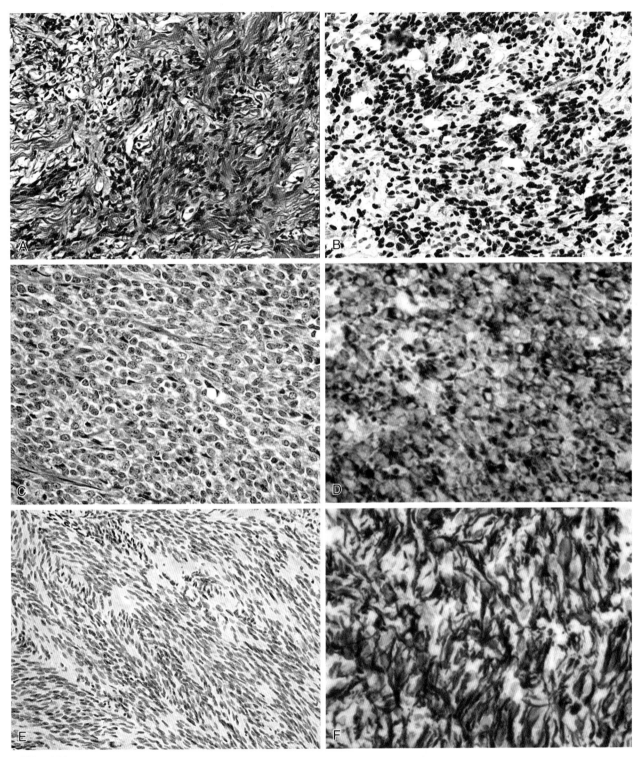

FIG. 12.13
Solitary fibrous tumor with sheets of small ovoid cells haphazardly present against fibrous stroma (**A**) supported by strong nuclear STAT-6 staining by immunohistochemistry (**B**). Monophasic synovial sarcoma with spindle to ovoid cell morphology in a sheet-like growth pattern (**C**) expressing strong Bcl-2 staining by immunohistochemistry (**D**) which can also be seen in solitary fibrous tumor. Hence, t(X;18)(p11.2;q11.2) molecular studies are confirmatory for synovial sarcoma. Cellular schwannoma composed of fascicles of bland spindle cells, wavy nuclei with tapered ends (**E**) showing strong GFAP expression by immunohistochemistry (**F**). S100 expression is also considered supportive of schwannoma which excludes a solitary fibrous tumor.

SOLITARY FIBROUS TUMOR – PATHOLOGIC FEATURES

Gross Findings

▸▸ Well-circumscribed, multinodular partially encapsulated masses with a white firm cut surface

▸▸ Pleural attachment is seen in a majority of cases

▸▸ Examples with necrosis, hemorrhage, and calcifications are occasionally present

▸▸ Aggressive tumors may show irregular infiltrative borders with areas of necrosis

Microscopic Findings

▸▸ Variably cellular tumors with diverse histologic features

▸▸ Uniform ovoid to spindle cells, patternless architecture, keloid-type collagenous stroma, branching staghorn thin-walled blood vessels

▸▸ Vascular channels lack a connective tissue layer and the surrounding tumor cells smudge with the endothelial cells

▸▸ Most tumors show low mitotic activity, minimal nuclear pleomorphism and/or necrosis

▸▸ Nuclear positivity by STAT6 immunohistochemical stain is a surrogate marker of NAB2-STAT6 gene fusion

▸▸ Positivity with CD34, BCL-2, and CD10 99 is common and less specific for SFTs

▸▸ Expression of immunohistochemical markers will be absent in dedifferentiated SFTs

Pathologic Differential Diagnoses

▸▸ Cellular schwannoma

▸▸ Malignant peripheral nerve sheath tumor (MPNST)

▸▸ Synovial sarcoma, monophasic

PARAGANGLIOMA

DIFFERENTIAL DIAGNOSIS: NEUROENDOCRINE TUMOR

Clinical Features

Paragangliomas arise from the chromaffin cells of the extra-adrenal sympathetic and parasympathetic paraganglia. Adrenal paragangliomas (pheochromocytomas) arise from the adrenal medulla. Knowledge of the exact anatomic location of a particular mass lesion may prove very useful in appropriately diagnosing a specific lesion as a paraganglioma. In the mediastinum, where paragangliomas are extremely rare, they constitute only 2% of all catecholamine-secreting tumors. The posterior mediastinum is the more common site than the anterior mediastinum. A female preponderance is known, and the median age of incidence seen is 45 years (range, 19–72 years). Unexplained hypertension may be the only presentation in functional tumors. Other symptoms like headaches, excessive diaphoresis, and palpitations are seen. The symptoms are due to the secretion of

norepinephrine and normetanephrine. The 24-hour urine elevated levels of norepinephrine and normetanephrine form the basis for the preoperative diagnosis. Nonfunctional tumors are less frequently seen. CT imaging with contrast media shows enhancement of the paraganglioma once biochemical evidence is present. ^{123}I-MIBG scanning by CT or MRI is highly specific for the assessment of single or multiple tumors. Paragangliomas are known to occur sporadically and also as part of several hereditary syndromes. Mutations in the succinate dehydrogenase (SDH) gene subunit (*SDHB*, *SDHD*, or *SDHC*) are seen in most familial paraganglioma cases. Further, the presence of *SDHB* mutations predisposes the patient to malignant transformation and metastasis. Paraganglioma along with gastrointestinal stromal tumor (GIST), and pulmonary chondromas may present as a part of the "Carney triad." In addition to these, von Hippel-Lindau (VHL) and multiple endocrine neoplasia (MEN) syndromes are the other associated hereditary syndromes.

Pathologic Features

GROSS FINDINGS

Mediastinal paragangliomas are partially or completely covered by a thin capsule and have a soft, heterogeneous, red-brown solid cut surface.

MICROSCOPIC FINDINGS

The polygonal chief cells are arranged in an organoid/nested pattern known as "zellballen" (Fig. 12.14). A wide range of varied histologic patterns such as trabecular, spindled, and angioma-like patterns are seen. These polygonal chief cells have abundant granular cytoplasm with bland round to oval nuclei. Arranged around the cell nests are the less conspicuous second type of spindled cells, called "sustentacular cells." The presence of a prominent delicate vascular network is seen in most tumors. Some cellular pleomorphism in most paragangliomas is reported (Fig. 12.15). Increased mitoses/Ki-67 index and necrosis are seen in metastatic paragangliomas.

Ancillary Studies

Immunohistochemical expression for neuroendocrine markers such as synaptophysin, chromogranin, and CD56 are well known (Fig. 12.16). These markers generally highlight the chief cells, while GFAP and S100 highlight the sustentacular cells (Fig. 12.17). Cytokeratin, TTF-1, and Napsin-A expression are negative in both types of cells. GATA-3 will be positive in a subset

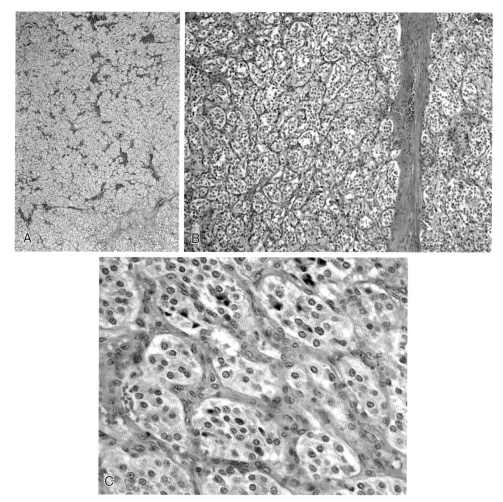

FIG. 12.14

Paraganglioma with the presence of organoid growth pattern and prominent vascular network (**A**). The tumor cells form small nests with rounded nuclei and eosinophilic cytoplasm (**B**) with the vascular network made up of capillaries (**C**).

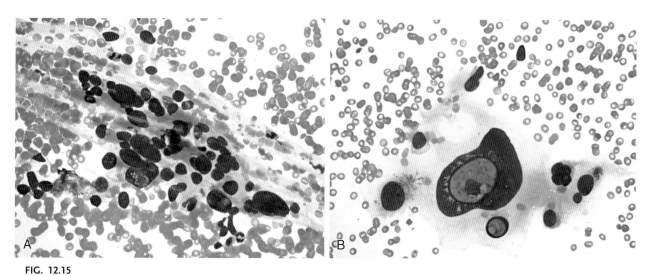

FIG. 12.15

Paraganglioma: Diff-Quik-stained cytology smears show ovoid cells in groups and clusters having fine granular nuclear chromatin (**A**), scattered bizarre pleomorphic nuclei and intranuclear inclusions (**B**).

Continued

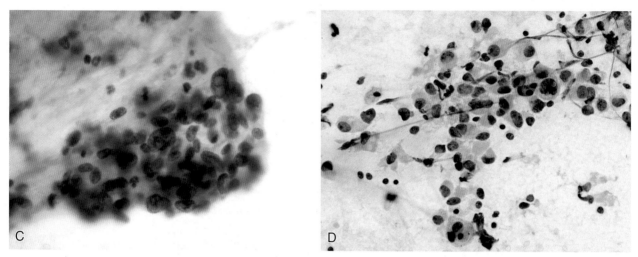

FIG. 12.15, cont'd
Pap-stained cytology smears show scattered spindle cells in addition to the round/ovoid cells in these loosely clustered groups (**C**) and **D**).

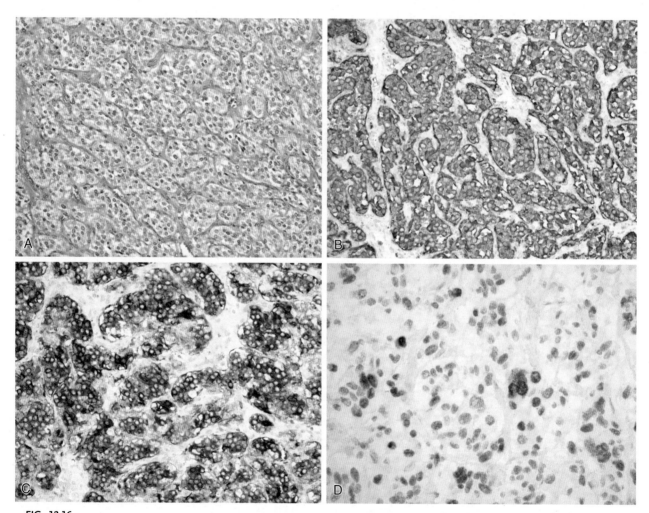

FIG. 12.16
Paraganglioma with the presence of organoid-nested pattern (**A**) showing a strong distinct cytoplasmic staining with neuroendocrine markers, such as synaptophysin (**B**), which is a sensitive marker for neuroendocrine differentiation but not as specific as chromogranin (**C**) with the subset of cases also staining for GATA-3 (**D**), showing a moderate, distinct nuclear staining.

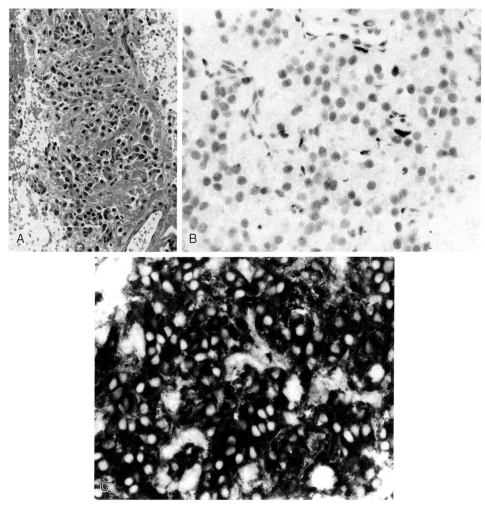

FIG. 12.17

Core biopsies of a mediastinal mass show organoid morphology with differential diagnosis of both paraganglioma and neuroendocrine tumor (**A**). S100 clinches the diagnosis of a paraganglioma with scattered staining of the spindle/sustentacular cells (**B**), while chromogranin (**C**) is positive in both the entities.

of cases (55%) (see Fig. 12.16D). The newer marker *SDHB* deserves a special mention. Immunohistochemical loss of SDHB protein acts as a surrogate marker for *SDHB* mutations. Patients with *SDHB* germline mutations develop metastases and tend to develop the disease earlier by 10 years compared to the patients with sporadic disease. Nuclear expression of *ATRX* is seen in patients with *ATRX* mutation. These somatic *ATRX* mutations are known to be associated with aggressive behavior.

Differential Diagnosis

The most important differential diagnosis for paraganglioma is a neuroendocrine tumor (carcinoid tumor) (Table 12.6). Others include medullary thyroid carcinoma metastatic to mediastinum and glomangioma. Morphologically, the neuroendocrine tumors demonstrate a nested, organoid, trabecular, or rosette-like growth pattern. Mostly the tumor cells tend to be small to medium, with moderate amounts of eosinophilic cytoplasm and the characteristic salt-and-pepper nuclear chromatin (Fig. 12.18). The classification as typical and atypical carcinoid is similar to lung carcinoid tumors. The mitotic rates are low (<2 mitoses per 2 mm^2) with no necrosis in a typical carcinoid tumor, while 2 to 10 mitoses per 2 mm^2 with/without necrosis are present in atypical carcinoid tumor. The neuroendocrine tumors are universally positive for pancytokeratin, synaptophysin, and chromogranin (see Fig. 12.18). TTF-1 is positive in a few cases (17%) while GATA-3 and Napsin-A are generally negative. Further, the lack of sustentacular cells and absent S100/GFAP staining is also useful in distinguishing them from paragangliomas. Amyloid deposits stained by Congo red stain and the presence of calcitonin point toward a medullary thyroid carcinoma. In cases of glomangioma, SMA is positive while the neuroendocrine markers are negative.

TABLE 12.6

Histologic and Immunohistochemical Features of Paraganglioma Versus Neuroendocrine Tumor (Fig. 12.17)

Paraganglioma	Neuroendocrine Tumor (Carcinoid)
• Classically has an organoid pattern with a prominent vascular network	• Mostly show trabecular and rosette growth pattern
• Two populations of cells: epithelioid and spindle	• One population of uniform appearing cells
• Often with endocrine atypia, bizarre pleomorphism	• A delicate vasculature between the tumor cells nests is seen
• Necrosis uncommon with sparse mitoses	• Mitoses and/or necrosis differentiate typical from atypical carcinoids
• Rarely shows spindled or angiomatoid morphology	• Rarely shows a wide variety of growth patterns
• Neuroendocrine markers positive	• Neuroendocrine markers positive
• S100 is positive in sustentacular cells	• No S100 positive cells seen
• Keratin is uniformly negative	• Ki-67 useful to differentiate from high-grade neuroendocrine carcinomas
	• Keratin staining is present

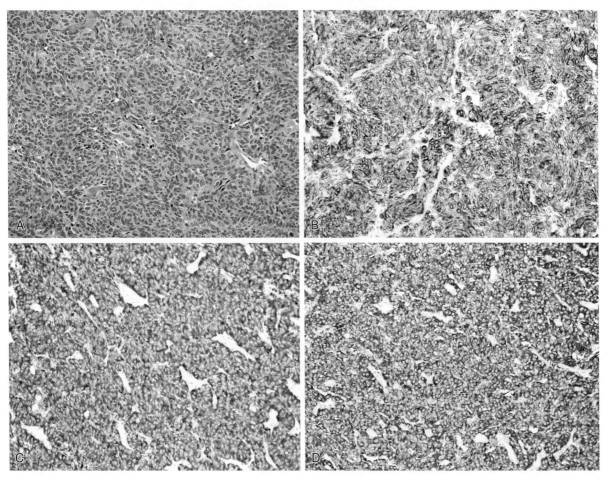

FIG. 12.18

Carcinoid tumor: Nests of uniform tumor cells having fine granular nuclear chromatin and moderate amounts of cytoplasm (**A**), strongly positive for pancytokeratin (AE1/3) (**B**), and neuroendocrine markers, such as synaptophysin (**C**) and chromogranin (**D**).

Prognosis and Therapy

In most centers, the current management practice for a diagnosis of paraganglioma is surgical excision as per consensus guidelines. Resections are often challenging in the mediastinum due to the close vicinity of the heart and the great vessels. Sometimes, resection of vital structures will be necessary. A recent study by Hsu et al. (2019) showed metastases to the bone, lung, lymph node, brain, and liver in 25% of cases. Also, a tendency for intraoperative bleeding was reported. Hence, the mediastinal paragangliomas do not always exhibit benign behavior as previously thought. They can be associated with significant morbidity and mortality. In incompletely resected tumors, adjuvant targeted therapies hold a place in the management. The presence of PD-L1 ≥1% expression in the tumor cells is seen in one fourth of cases with a fraction of them showing expression in 10% of cells. No data are available as to the response to anti-PD-L1 therapy. A comprehensive investigation to exclude an associated hereditary syndrome is important for follow-up of the patient and also genetic counseling of their families.

PARAGANGLIOMA – DISEASE FACT SHEET

Definition
▸▸ Neural crest neoplastic proliferation derived from chromaffin cells of the extra-adrenal sympathetic and parasympathetic paraganglia

Incidence and Location
▸▸ Extremely rare, 2% of all the catecholamine-secreting tumors and more common in the posterior mediastinum

Age Distribution
▸▸ Most common in women, the median age of 45 years (19–72 years)

Clinical Features
▸▸ Unexplained hypertension due to elevated norepinephrine and normetanephrine may be the only clinical symptom seen in the functional tumors

Radiologic Features
▸▸ CT or MRI are used to identify the location after biochemical evidence
▸▸ ^{123}I-MIBG scanning by CT or MRI offers the highest specificity for the detection of multiple tumors

Prognosis and Therapy
▸▸ Surgical excision is the standard management of care in most centers
▸▸ Intraoperative complications such as bleeding are associated with morbidity and mortality
▸▸ Metastases to the bone, lung, lymph node, brain, and liver in one fourth (25%) of the cases

---

PARAGANGLIOMA – PATHOLOGIC FEATURES

Gross Findings
▸▸ Well-circumscribed, encapsulated tumors with soft cut surfaces
▸▸ Adhesion or invasion into the adjacent structures in the mediastinum is common

Microscopic Findings
▸▸ Nests and sheets of polygonal tumor cells in a "zellballen" architecture
▸▸ Various histologic appearances like trabecular, cords, spindled, and angioma-like patterns are seen
▸▸ Rarely clear cell pattern with sclerotic stroma mimicking an infiltrative tumor seen can be seen
▸▸ Nests of the tumor cells are surrounded by spindled sustentacular cells

▸▸ The polygonal chief cells have abundant granular cytoplasm with bland round to oval nuclei
▸▸ Cellular pleomorphism and sparse mitoses may be seen
▸▸ The polygonal cells are positive for neuroendocrine markers, synaptophysin, chromogranin, and INSM1, while sustentacular cells are positive for S100 and GFAP

Pathologic Differential Diagnoses
▸▸ Neuroendocrine tumor (carcinoid tumor)
▸▸ Medullary thyroid carcinoma
▸▸ Glomangioma

PRIMARY MEDIASTINAL DIFFUSE LARGE B-CELL LYMPHOMA

DIFFERENTIAL DIAGNOSIS: CLASSICAL HODGKIN LYMPHOMA

Clinical Features

Primary mediastinal diffuse large B-cell lymphoma (PMDLBCL) is a distinct clinicopathologic entity with an aggressive behavior thought to arise from the B-cells in the thymus. It accounts for approximately 2% of non-Hodgkin lymphoma and up to 10% of diffuse large B-cell lymphomas (DLBCLs). In the United States, the annual incidence rate is approximately 0.4 per million. The disease is most commonly seen in young females and peaks at the third and fourth decades of life. In more than two thirds of cases, PMDLBCL presents with a rapidly enlarging anterior mediastinal mass that might give rise to local compressive symptoms (cough, dyspnea, dysphagia, and superior vena cava syndrome). Up to 80% of patients can have pulmonary, pleural, and pericardial involvement. During the initial disease, dissemination to extrathoracic organs is uncommon; however, relapse is often extrathoracic and involves the liver, gastrointestinal tract, kidneys, and ovaries. Involvement of the bone marrow is not typical. Elevated serum lactate dehydrogenase (LDH) and low beta-2 microglobulin levels are commonly seen. Radiologic features include an anterior mediastinal mass with or without unilateral elevation of the hemidiaphragm, pleural effusion, and pericardial effusion.

Pathologic Features

GROSS FINDINGS

PMDLBCL is not usually resected. Thus, characteristic gross morphologic features are not well described.

MICROSCOPIC FINDINGS

Typically, PMDLBCL shows diffuse growth of medium- to large-sized lymphocytes with variable degree of sclerosis. The nuclei can be round, pleomorphic, or multilobulated with abundant pale to clear cytoplasm (Fig. 12.19).

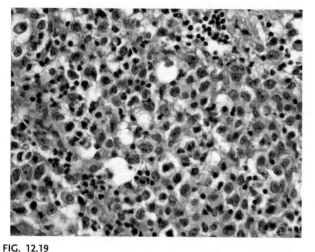

FIG. 12.19

Primary mediastinal diffuse large B-cell lymphoma showing medium- to large sized-lymphocytes with round to multilobed nuclei with prominent nucleoli and abundant pale to clear cytoplasm.

Occasional Reed–Sternberg-like cells might be seen. In some cases, prominent sclerosis with vague nodularity can be present.

Ancillary Studies

PMDLBCL expresses B-cell–related antigens (CD19, CD20, CD22, and CD79a) as well as PAX-5 and CD45 (Fig. 12.20). Surface and cytoplasmic immunoglobulin (Ig) expression is typically absent. In up to 80% of cases, positive CD30 staining is present. CD15 stain is usually negative. Other more frequently positive stains include IRF4/MUM1, with variable CD11c, MYC, BCL2, and BCL6 expression. Compared with other DLBCLs, the majority of PMDLBCL express CD23, MAL, PDL-1, PDL-2, and aberrant TNFAIP2 expression, whereas CD10 is typically negative. Other positive stains in PMDLBCL include CD54, CD95, BOB1, PU1, OCT2, and co-express TRAF1 and nuclear REL.

Genetic Abnormalities

Comparative genomic hybridization often shows gains in chromosomes 9p24.1 and 2p14–p16. The 9p24.1

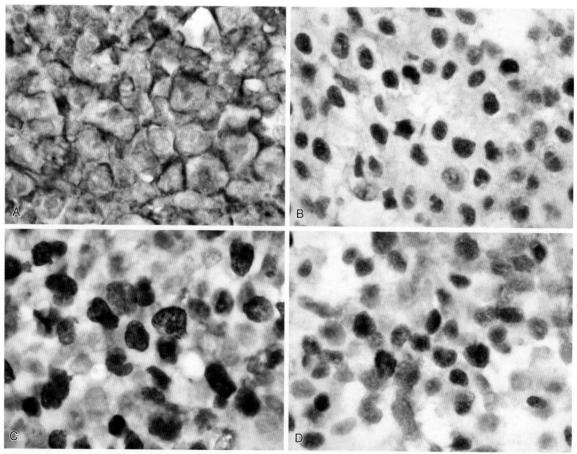

FIG. 12.20

Primary mediastinal diffuse large B-cell lymphoma. The tumor cells show membranous CD20 positivity (**A**) and nuclear BCL6 (**B**) and PAX-5 staining (**C**). The Ki-67 proliferation index is typically high (**D**).

rearrangement along with translocations involving the CIITA gene are unique to PMDLBCL. In more than half of the cases, rearrangements in the class II major histocompatibility complex (MHC) can be seen. Rearrangements of BCL2, BCL6, and MYC genes are uncommon. Other reported genetic abnormalities include NF-κB pathway (seen in approximately two thirds of cases) and STAT6 gene mutations.

Differential Diagnosis

The most important differential diagnosis for PMDLBL is classical Hodgkin lymphoma (CHL). Mediastinal involvement with CHL is common. However, B-symptoms (fever, night sweats, and weight loss) are seen more commonly in CHL, and LDH level is typically normal. Unlike PMDLBCL, CHL shows prominent granulocytic and histiocytic infiltration (Fig. 12.21). Although positive CD30 staining can be seen in both, in PMDLBCL it is usually heterogenous and weak. In addition, CHL expresses CD15 and is less likely to have a full set of B-cell markers (Fig. 12.22). In some cases, a significant morphologic and immunophenotypic overlap between PMDLBCL and CHL can be seen, and the term "mediastinal gray zone lymphoma" is applied (Fig. 12.23; Table 12.7).

Prognosis and Therapy

PMDLBCL carries a better prognosis than DLBCL, germinal center, and activated B-cell subtypes. Complete response after initial therapy is about 53% to 80%, with an overall 5-year survival rate of 50% to 65%. There is no widely accepted treatment protocol for PMDLBCL.

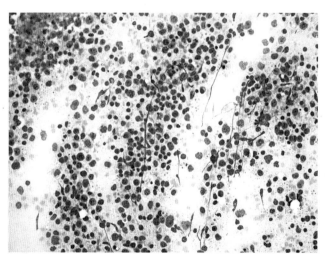

FIG. 12.21

Diff-Quick direct smears prepared from a fine-needle aspiration of a mediastinal mass with primary mediastinal diffuse large B-cell lymphoma. The lymphocytes are large with prominent nucleoli and abundant cytoplasm. Prominent lymphoglandular bodies are seen in the background.

R-CHOP (rituximab, cyclophosphamide, doxorubicin, oncovin, and prednisolone) as well as V/MACOP-B (methotrexate, doxorubicin, cyclophosphamide, oncovin, prednisone, and bleomycin) are typically administered in conjunction with consolidative radiation for the majority of patients.

PRIMARY MEDIASTINAL DIFFUSE LARGE B-CELL LYMPHOMA – DISEASE FACT SHEET

Definition
▸▸ An aggressive mature B-cell lymphoma thought to arise from B-cells in the thymus

Incidence and Location
▸▸ Almost always arise in the anterior mediastinum
▸▸ Accounts for approximately 2% of non-Hodgkin lymphoma and up to 10% of diffuse large B-cell lymphomas
▸▸ The annual incidence rate in the United States is approximately 0.4 per million

Age Distribution
▸▸ Most frequently in young females and peaks at the third and fourth decades of life

Clinical Features
▸▸ Rapidly enlarging and bulky anterior mediastinal mass
▸▸ Local compressive symptoms including cough, dyspnea, dysphagia, and superior vena cava syndrome might be seen
▸▸ Elevated serum LDH and low beta-2 microglobulin

Radiologic Features
▸▸ Large anterior mediastinal mass with or without a unilateral elevation of hemidiaphragm, pleural effusion, and pericardial effusion

Prognosis and Therapy
▸▸ Complete response after initial therapy is 53%–80%. Overall 5-year survival rate is 50%–65%
▸▸ Typically, patients are treated with rituximab plus chemotherapeutic regimen with or without radiotherapy

---

PRIMARY MEDIASTINAL DIFFUSE LARGE B-CELL LYMPHOMA – PATHOLOGIC FEATURES

Gross Findings
▸▸ Characteristic gross morphologic features are not well described (a nonsurgical disease)

Microscopic Findings
▸▸ Diffuse growth of medium- to large-sized lymphocytes with variable degree of sclerosis
▸▸ The nuclei can be round, pleomorphic, or multilobulated with abundant pale to clear cytoplasm
▸▸ Occasional Reed–Sternberg-like cells might be seen
▸▸ Prominent sclerosis with vague nodularity with or without necrosis can be present

Ancillary Studies
▸▸ Positive B-cell–related antigens (CD19, CD20, CD22, and CD79a) as well as PAX-5 and CD45

▶▶ Absent surface and cytoplasmic immunoglobulin (Ig) expression
▶▶ CD30 is frequently expressed, but CD15 stain is usually negative
▶▶ Positive IRF4/MUM1 with variable CD11c, MYC, BCL2, and BCL6 expression
▶▶ CD23, MAL, PDL-1, PDL-2, and aberrant TNFAIP2 expression

▶▶ Other less commonly used stains: CD54, CD95, BOB1, PU1, OCT2, co-expression of TRAF1 and nuclear REL

Pathologic Differential Diagnoses

▶▶ Classical Hodgkin lymphoma
▶▶ Diffuse large B-cell lymphoma, NOS

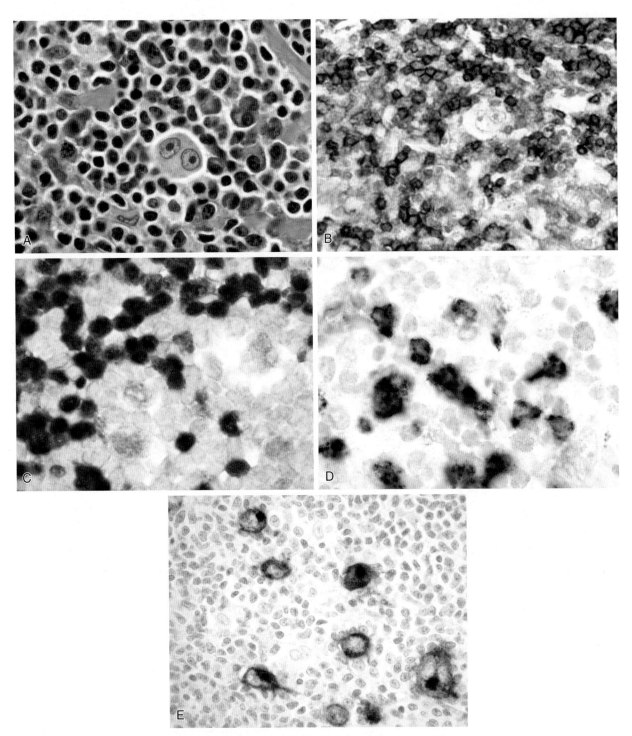

FIG. 12.22

Classical Hodgkin lymphoma. Binucleated Reed-Sternberg (RS) cell is seen in the center with prominent eosinophilic nucleoli. The background shows mixed inflammatory cells containing small lymphocytes, histiocytes, and plasma cells (**A**). The RS cells are negative for CD45 (**B**) and show weak PAX-5 staining (**C**) with only background lymphocytes are staining. CD15 (**D**) and CD30 (**E**) are typically positive.

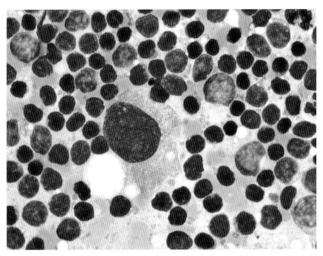

FIG. 12.23

Diff-Quick direct smear prepared from a fine-needle aspiration of a mediastinal mass with classical Hodgkin lymphoma. A mononuclear Reed-Sternberg cell with multiple prominent nucleoli is present in the center.

TABLE 12.7

Clinical, Histologic, and Immunohistochemical Features of Primary Mediastinal Diffuse Large B-Cell Lymphoma (PMDLBCL) Versus Classical Hodgkin Lymphoma (CHL)

PMDLBCL	CHL
• Almost always occurs in the anterior mediastinum	• Mediastinal involvement occurs in up to 80% of cases
• B-symptoms less common	• B-symptoms more common
• Elevated serum LDH	• Normal serum LDH
• Typically lacks granulocytes and histiocytes	• Prominent granulocytic and histiocytic infiltration
• Reed–Sternberg-like cells (occasionally) with positive CD30	• Reed-Sternberg cells with positive CD30
• Positive pan B-cell markers and CD45. Negative CD15	• Negative pan B-cell markers and CD45. Positive CD15

SEMINOMATOUS GERM CELL TUMOR

DIFFERENTIAL DIAGNOSIS: NON-SEMINOMATOUS GERM CELL TUMORS

Clinical Features

Germ cell tumors are relatively uncommon neoplasms that most frequently arise in the gonads. However, they can also arise in other locations including the retroperitoneum, anterior mediastinum, and the pineal gland. Primary mediastinal germ cell tumors (PMGCTs) are

histologically, immunophenotypically, and serologically identical to their gonadal counterparts. They represent approximately 15% of anterior mediastinal tumors and occur at a median age of 40 years. PMGCTs can be classified into seminomatous germ cell tumor (SGCT) and non-seminomatous germ cell tumors (NSGCTs). Only 20% to 30% of PMGCTs are pure seminoma (SGCT). NSGCTs constitute the majority of PMGCTs; these include teratoma (mature or immature), yolk sac tumor (YST), embryonal carcinoma (EC), choriocarcinoma, or mixed tumors. Chest pain and dyspnea are the most common clinical symptoms for patients with PMGCTs. Large tumors might compress the superior vena cava causing superior vena cava syndrome (hoarseness of voice, hemoptysis, and swelling of the face or upper body). The most common elevated serum markers include alpha-fetoprotein (AFP), human chorionic gonadotropin (HCG), and LDH. AFP is almost always elevated in pure YSTs or mixed germ cell tumors with YST component, but AFP is unlikely to be elevated in patients with pure seminomas. HCG elevations can be seen in both seminoma and NSGCTs and are related to the presence of trophoblastic-like giant cells in pure seminoma. Serum LDH and placental alkaline phosphatase (PLAP) might also be elevated in seminoma.

Pathologic Features

GROSS FINDINGS

Seminomas are characteristically described as well-circumscribed, homogenous, lobulated gray masses. NSGCTs can have variable macroscopic appearances depending on the variable proportions of different components. Teratomas usually present as solid and cystic heterogenous masses with mucoid material. Hair, cartilage, or bone might also be seen. Choriocarcinomas are most often described as hemorrhagic masses with variable amounts of necrosis. YSTs usually form smooth gelatinous masses with variably cystic cut surfaces. ECs form gray-white masses with variable areas of hemorrhage and necrosis.

MICROSCOPIC FINDINGS

Seminoma classically forms nests and sheets of polygonal cells separated by thin fibrous bands with distinct cell borders and clear cytoplasm (Fig. 12.24). The nuclei are relatively regular with vesicular chromatin and conspicuous nucleoli. The fibrous bands are typically associated with a brisk lymphocytic infiltrate with occasional granulomatous reaction. Scattered multinucleated syncytiotrophoblast giant cells can also be seen. YST has a wide range of morphologic growth patterns. The reticular or microcystic pattern is the most common pattern seen.

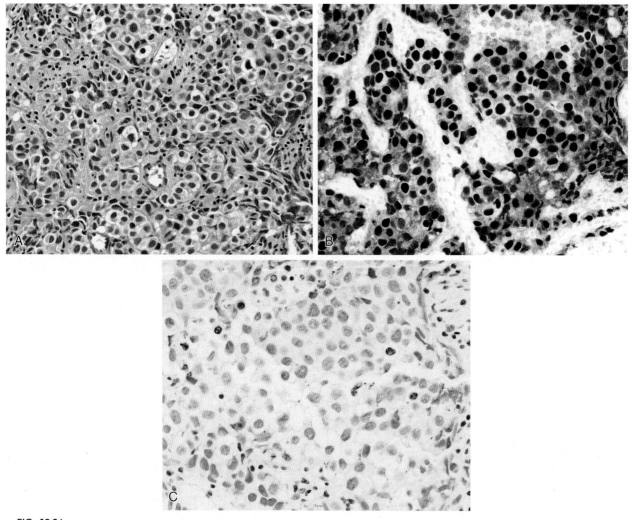

FIG. 12.24
Classic seminoma showing fairly uniform cells with distinct cell borders, clear to eosinophilic cytoplasm in a vaguely nested growth pattern. Scattered lymphocytes can be seen in the background (**A**). OCT3/4 shows positive nuclear staining (**B**) with only focal/weak pancytokeratin staining (**C**).

The tumor cells form a meshwork of thin-walled cysts lined by vacuolated cuboidal or flattened cells embedded in a myxoid loose stroma (Fig. 12.25). Eosinophilic globules might also be present. Other patterns that YST can show include glandular-alveolar, papillary, solid, macrocystic, hepatoid, endodermal sinus, and polyvesicular vitelline patterns. EC grows in solid, glandular, and tubulopapillary configurations. The cells show a minimal degree of differentiation with large nuclei, vesicular chromatin, prominent nucleoli, and indistinct cell borders. Occasional cells with smudged nuclei can be seen. The cytoplasm can be basophilic, eosinophilic, or amphophilic. Teratoma can be mature or immature. Mature teratoma can show variable somatic tissues including skin, cartilage, muscle as well as neural, thyroid, respiratory, gastrointestinal, or genitourinary epithelia (Fig. 12.26). Immature teratoma is characterized by the presence of primitive neuroectodermal tissue or blastemal elements. Choriocarcinoma consists of haphazardly arranged cytotrophoblasts, syncytiotrophoblasts, and intermediate trophoblasts present in an extensive hemorrhagic and necrotic background (Fig. 12.27). Syncytiotrophoblasts are multinucleated with large irregular nuclei and eosinophilic cytoplasm. Cytotrophoblasts are large with single round nuclei and pale to clear cytoplasm. Intermediate trophoblasts are larger than cytotrophoblasts with irregular smudged nuclei (Table 12.8).

Ancillary Studies

Classical seminoma shows nuclear immunoreactivity for SALL4 and OCT3/4. PLAP, D2-40, and CD117 stains show diffuse membranous and cytoplasmic reactivity with only focal and weak cytokeratin expression. In addition to SALL4, OCT3/4, PLAP, and cytokeratin, EC is typically positive for CD30, and CD117 is usually

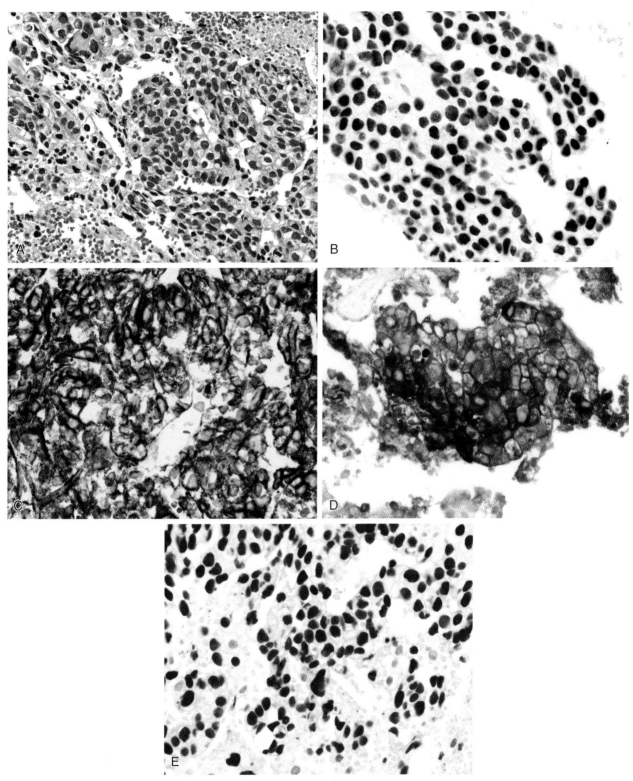

FIG. 12.25

Microcystic pattern of yolk sac tumor. The cells are cuboidal with relatively bland nuclei. The cytoplasm is vacuolated with distinct cell borders (**A**). The tumor cells are positive for SALL4 (**B**), pancytokeratin (**C**), and PLAP (**D**). TTF-1 stain can be positive (**E**), a diagnostic pitfall for primary lung malignancy.

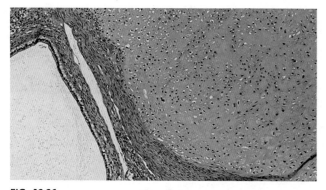

FIG. 12.26

Mature teratoma. Mixture of cartilage (*right*) and ciliated columnar epithelium (*left*).

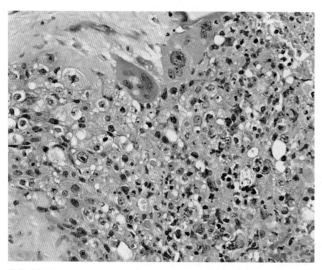

FIG. 12.27

Choriocarcinoma. Admixed cytotrophoblasts (single nuclei with pale cytoplasm) and syncytiotrophoblasts (multinucleated with eosinophilic cytoplasm) are present with extensive hemorrhage.

TABLE 12.8

Comparison of Histologic Features of Various Germ Cell Tumors

SEMINOMA	EMBRYONAL CARCINOMA
• Fairly uniform polygonal cells with nested growth pattern	• Prominent nuclear pleomorphism with glandular, papillary, and solid patterns
GLANDULAR YST	**EMBRYONAL CARCINOMA**
• Evenly spaced nuclei with minimal cytologic atypia.	• Markedly atypical cells with nuclear overlapping.
SEMINOMA WITH SYNCYTIOTROPHOBLASTS	**CHORIOCARCINOMA**
• Lacks the cytotrophoblastic component, prominent necrosis and hemorrhage	• Syncytiotrophoblasts, cytotrophoblasts, and intermediate trophoblasts with prominent necrosis and hemorrhage

negative. The majority of YSTs stain positively with AFP and low-molecular-weight cytokeratin. Glypican-3, CD117, and PLAP can also be positive in YSTs, whereas OCT3/4 and CD30 are usually negative. The syncytiotrophoblasts of choriocarcinoma are positive for HCG, inhibin, EMA, and human placental lactogen (HPL) and negative for SALL4. In contrast, cytotrophoblasts are usually positive for SALL4, while HCG and HPL are negative (Table 12.9). Teratoma has no specific markers; however, immunohistochemical studies can aid in recognizing and differentiating any form of somatic malignancy that may arise.

Differential Diagnosis

The morphologic features of seminoma might overlap with EC. Unlike seminoma, cells of EC show significant degree of nuclear pleomorphism with formation of glandular, papillary, and solid structures. EC lacks the lymphomatous background and the granulomatous inflammation that is characteristic of seminoma. In challenging cases, negative cytokeratin and CD30 stains along with CD117 expression strongly suggest seminoma rather than EC. As previously mentioned, EC can have solid and glandular areas which might raise the possibility of glandular and solid patterns of YST. YST shows evenly spaced nuclei with no significant cytologic atypia compared with EC. Immunophenotypically, YST is positive for AFP and glypican-3 and negative for CD30 and OCT3/4. The syncytiotrophoblasts seen in choriocarcinoma can also be seen in seminoma. However, seminoma lacks the cytotrophoblastic component and typically does not show the characteristic necrosis and hemorrhage seen in choriocarcinoma. Serum HCG level can be elevated in both (although markedly elevated in choriocarcinoma). Unlike choriocarcinoma, seminoma cells are positive for OCT3/4 and CD117.

Prognosis and Therapy

Primary mediastinal seminoma carries a significant better survival than NSGCTs with up to 90% overall survival. The survival rate for NSGCTs is 40% to 50% and falls to 20% when there is a metastatic disease. In some institutions, pure mediastinal seminoma can be treated with only radiation or chemotherapy with no surgical intervention needed. Mature teratoma is treated with surgery with no role for chemotherapy. The recommended treatment regimen for other NSGCTs includes neoadjuvant chemotherapy followed by surgical resection.

TABLE 12.9

Immunohistochemical Profiles of Seminoma and Non-Seminomatous Germ Cell Tumors

	Cytokeratin	SALL4	OCT 3/4	PLAP	CD117	D2-40	CD30	AFP	Glypican-3	HCG
Seminoma	−/focal	+	+	+	+	+	−/focal	−	−	+ (syncytiotrophoblasts)
YST	+	+	−	+/−	+/−	−	−	+	+	−
EC	+	+	+	+/−	−	+/focal	+	−	−/+	−
Choriocarcinoma	+	+ (cytotrophoblasts)	−	+/−	−	−	−	−	+ (syncytiotrophoblasts)	+ (syncytiotrophoblasts)

PRIMARY MEDIASTINAL GERM CELL TUMORS (SGCT VS. NSGCT) – DISEASE FACT SHEET

Definition
▸▸ Relatively rare group of tumors that are histologically and serologically identical to their gonadal counterparts

Incidence and Location
▸▸ Primary mediastinal germ cell tumors account for 1%–3% of germ cell tumors and represent approximately 15% of anterior mediastinal tumors

Age Distribution
▸▸ Most frequently in the adolescent/young adult age group, median age of 40 years

Clinical Features
▸▸ Chest pain and dyspnea are the most common clinical symptoms
▸▸ Large tumors might cause compressive symptoms, including superior vena cava syndrome (hoarseness of voice, hemoptysis, and swelling of the face or upper body)

Radiologic Features
▸▸ Seminoma shows homogeneous lobulated mass that can appear very similar to lymphoma
▸▸ Non-seminomatous germ cell tumors (NSGCTs) are usually large with variable mixed solid and cystic areas. Calcifications, necrosis, and hemorrhage might be present

Prognosis and Therapy
▸▸ Pure seminoma carries an excellent prognosis with up to 90% overall survival. Typically, they are treated with only radiation or chemotherapy without surgical intervention
▸▸ The survival rate for NSGCTs is 40%–50% and falls to 20% when there is a metastatic disease. With the exception of teratoma (only surgery if needed), NSGCTs are treated with neoadjuvant chemotherapy followed by surgical resection.

PRIMARY MEDIASTINAL GERM CELL TUMORS (SGCT VS. NSGCT) – PATHOLOGIC FEATURES

Gross Findings
▸▸ Seminomas form well-circumscribed homogeneous lobulated gray masses

▸▸ Gross morphology of NSGCTs is variable and depends on proportions of different components:
  ▸▸ YST: smooth gelatinous mass with variably cystic areas
  ▸▸ EC: gray white mass with variable areas of hemorrhage and necrosis
  ▸▸ Choriocarcinoma: hemorrhagic mass with variable amount of necrosis
  ▸▸ Teratoma: solid and cystic heterogenous mass, mucus, hair, cartilage, or bone possible

Microscopic Findings
▸▸ **Seminoma:**
  ▸▸ Nests and sheets of polygonal cells with distinct cell borders and clear cytoplasm
  ▸▸ Nests and sheets separated by thin fibrous bands
  ▸▸ Nuclei relatively regular with vesicular chromatin and conspicuous nucleoli
  ▸▸ Fibrous bands associated with lymphocytic infiltrate with occasional granulomata
▸▸ **NSGCT:**
  ▸▸ YST: Multiple patterns. Reticular or microcystic pattern most common with meshwork of thin-walled cysts lined by vacuolated cuboidal or flattened cells embedded in myxoid loose stroma
  ▸▸ EC: Solid, glandular and tubulopapillary patterns. Cells are pleomorphic with large nuclei, vesicular chromatin, prominent nucleoli, and indistinct cell borders
  ▸▸ Choriocarcinoma: Haphazardly arranged cytotrophoblasts, syncytiotrophoblasts, and intermediate trophoblasts present in hemorrhagic and necrotic backgrounds
  ▸▸ Teratoma: Mature: Mixture of mature epithelial and mesenchymal elements, including squamous epithelium, neural tissue, and glandular tissues. Virtually all tissue types can be present. Immature teratoma: Primitive neuroectodermal tissue or blastemal elements.

Ancillary Testing
▸▸ Seminoma: positive for SALL4, OCT3/4, PLAP, D2-40 and CD117 stains. Negative/weak cytokeratin staining
▸▸ YST: positive AFP, low-molecular-weight cytokeratin, glypican-3, and variable CD117 and PLAP staining. Negative OCT3/4 and CD30
▸▸ EC: positive SALL4, OCT3/4, PLAP, cytokeratin, and CD30. Negative CD117
▸▸ Choriocarcinoma: syncytiotrophoblasts positive for HCG, inhibin, EMA, glypican-3, and HPL while negative SALL4. Cytotrophoblasts are positive for SALL4 while negative HPL and HCG
▸▸ Teratoma: No specific markers

SARCOIDOSIS

DIFFERENTIAL DIAGNOSIS: HISTOPLASMOSIS

Clinical Features

Sarcoidosis is a multisystem granulomatous disease characterized by the presence of non-necrotizing granulomatous inflammation, most commonly affecting the lungs and mediastinal lymph nodes. In the United States, the annual incidence of sarcoidosis is more than three times higher in African-Americans (35.5 per 100,000) than in White Americans (10.9 per 100,000). The diagnosis of sarcoidosis requires clinicopathologic correlation, after excluding other potential etiologic causes of granulomatous inflammation. Sarcoidosis has a wide spectrum of manifestations ranging from an asymptomatic early presentation (discovered incidentally) to a life-threatening progressive and relapsing disease. Symptomatic patients usually have fatigue, anorexia, weight loss, fever, and chronic cough. Other symptoms depend on the severity and involvement of other organ(s). Löfgren syndrome represents an acute presentation consisting of bilateral hilar adenopathy, arthritis, and erythema nodosum and occurs in up to 34% of patients. Currently, CT scan represents the gold standard method for disease detection. Typical radiologic findings for sarcoidosis include symmetric bilateral hilar and/or mediastinal lymphadenopathy and parenchymal lung nodules along the vessels, fissures, and septa.

Pathologic Features

GROSS FINDINGS

The involved lymph nodes are usually enlarged, yellowish, and might be calcified. In an advanced disease, multiple masses/nodules can be seen measuring up to several centimeters in diameter (nodular sarcoidosis).

MICROSCOPIC FINDINGS

The hallmark of sarcoidosis is the presence of multiple small granulomas (Fig. 12.28). Classic sarcoidal granulomas are non-necrotizing; however, small foci of necrosis can be seen in up 39% of cases. Occasional giant cell formation can be present. Some granulomas may contain asteroid bodies (star-shaped crystals) and/or Schaumann bodies (laminated calcifications). Senescent granulomas are usually hyalinized with dense fibrosis.

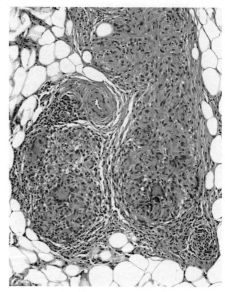

FIG. 12.28

Sarcoidosis. Multiple small non-necrotizing granulomas with scattered multinucleated giant cells. The AFB and GMS stains are negative for mycobacterial and fungal organisms, respectively (not shown).

Ancillary Studies

No light microscopic or slide-based ancillary tests are known to specifically confirm a diagnosis of sarcoidosis. Special stains for fungal and acid-fast organisms should be negative by definition. Assessment of serum markers such as serum amyloid A (SAA), soluble interleukin-2 receptor (sIL-2R), lysozyme, angiotensin-converting enzyme (ACE), C-reactive protein, and the glycoprotein KL-6 may be useful in the diagnosis and follow-up of some patients.

Differential Diagnosis

The most important differential diagnoses for sarcoidosis are infections, particularly fungal and mycobacterial infections. Histoplasmosis is an opportunistic fungal infection caused by the dimorphic fungus *Histoplasma capsulatum* and is seen more commonly in immunocompromised patients. Compared with sarcoidal granulomas, those seen in histoplasmosis are typically larger, more necrotizing, and often with peripheral palisading of histiocytes. GMS and PAS are often required to illustrate the characteristic small, narrow-base budding intracellular yeasts (2–4 microns in diameter) (Fig. 12.29; Table 12.10).

Prognosis and Therapy

Treatment of early sarcoidosis is often supportive, and spontaneous resolution may occur. In up to 30% of

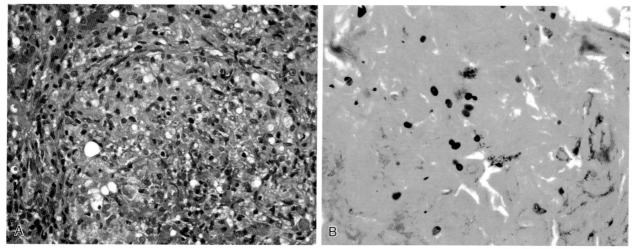

FIG. 12.29

Histoplasmosis. **A,** Large epithelioid granuloma with focal central necrosis. **B,** GMS stain highlights small narrow-base budding intracellular yeasts.

TABLE 12.10

Histologic Features of Sarcoidosis Versus Histoplasmosis

Sarcoidosis	Histoplasmosis
• Small non-necrotizing granulomas	• Granulomas are usually larger and more necrotizing
• Peripheral palisading of histiocytes rare	• Peripheral palisading of histiocytes common
• Negative GMS and PAS stains for fungal organisms	• GMS and PAS stains show small (2–4 microns) narrow-base budding intracellular yeasts

---

Clinical Features

▸▸ Most commonly asymptomatic (discovered during routine chest radiograph)

▸▸ Symptomatic patients usually have fatigue, anorexia, weight loss, fever, and chronic cough

Radiologic Features

▸▸ Symmetric bilateral hilar and/or mediastinal lymphadenopathy

▸▸ Parenchymal lung nodules along the vessels, fissures, and septa

Prognosis and Therapy

▸▸ Treatment for early sarcoidosis is often supportive and spontaneous resolution may occur

▸▸ In more advanced disease, patients are typically treated with steroids and/or other immunomodulatory agents

---

cases, a more progressive clinical course might follow. Fatality usually results from pulmonary, neurologic, or cardiovascular disease. Corticosteroids remain the mainstay of treatment. Other lines of treatments include methotrexate, leflunomide, azathioprine, and other biologic agents.

SARCOIDOSIS – DISEASE FACT SHEET

Definition

▸▸ A multisystem granulomatous disease characterized by the presence of non-necrotizing granulomas

Incidence and Location

▸▸ In the United States the disease is more than three times higher in African-Americans (35.5 per 100,000) than in White-Americans (10.9 per 100,000)

▸▸ Most commonly involves the lungs and mediastinal lymph nodes, but virtually any other organ can be involved

Age Distribution

▸▸ Usually affects middle-age people with a slight female predilection

---

SARCOIDOSIS – PATHOLOGIC FEATURES

Gross Findings

▸▸ The involved lymph nodes are usually enlarged, yellowish, and might be calcified

▸▸ Multiple masses/nodules can be seen in an advanced disease measuring several centimeters in diameter (nodular sarcoidosis)

Microscopic Findings

▸▸ Multiple small non-necrotizing granulomas with/without focal necrosis

▸▸ Asteroid bodies (star-shaped crystals) and/or Schaumann bodies (laminated calcifications) might be seen

Pathologic Differential Diagnoses

▸▸ Infectious granulomatous disease (histoplasmosis, mycobacterial infection, and others)

▸▸ Berylliosis

▸▸ Wegener granulomatosis

SUGGESTED READINGS

Type A Thymoma/Synovial Sarcoma

Weissferdt A, Kalhor N, Bishop JA, et al. Thymoma: a clinicopathological correlation of 1470 cases. *Hum Pathol.* 2018;73:7-15.

Oramas DM, Moran CA. Thymoma: challenges and pitfalls in biopsy interpretation. *Adv Anat Pathol.* 2021;28(5):291-297.

Weissferdt A, Moran CA. The histomorphologic spectrum of spindle cell thymoma. *Hum Pathol.* 2014;45(3):437-445.

den Bakker MA, Roden AC, Marx A, Marino M. Histologic classification of thymoma: a practical guide for routine cases. *J Thorac Oncol.* 2014; 9(9 suppl 2):S125-S130.

WHO Classification of Tumours Editorial Board. *Thoracic Tumors.* Lyon: IARC Press; 2021.

Terra SBSP, Aesif SW, Maleszewski JJ, Folpe AL, Boland JM. Mediastinal synovial sarcoma: clinicopathologic analysis of 21 cases with molecular confirmation. *Am J Surg Pathol.* 2018;42(6):761-766.

Syred K, Weissferdt A. Primary mediastinal synovial sarcoma. *Mediastinum.* 2020;4:13.

Amary MF, Berisha F, Bernardi Fdel C, et al. Detection of SS18-SSX fusion transcripts in formalin-fixed paraffin-embedded neoplasms: analysis of conventional RT-PCR, qRT-PCR and dual color FISH as diagnostic tools for synovial sarcoma. *Mod Pathol.* 2007;20(4):482-496.

Yano M, Toyooka S, Tsukuda K, et al. SYT-SSX fusion genes in synovial sarcoma of the thorax. *Lung Cancer.* 2004;44(3):391-397.

WHO Classification of Tumours Editorial Board. *Tumors of Soft Tissue and Bone.* Lyon: IARC Press; 2020.

Type B1 Thymoma/T-Lymphoblastic Leukemia/Lymphoma

Weissferdt A, Kalhor N, Bishop JA, et al. Thymoma: a clinicopathological correlation of 1470 cases. *Hum Pathol.* 2018;73:7-15.

Oramas DM, Moran CA. Thymoma: challenges and pitfalls in biopsy interpretation. *Adv Anat Pathol.* 2021;28(5):291-297.

den Bakker MA, Roden AC, Marx A, Marino M. Histologic classification of thymoma: a practical guide for routine cases. *J Thorac Oncol.* 2014; 9(9 suppl 2):S125-S130.

WHO Classification of Tumours Editorial Board. *Thoracic Tumors.* Lyon: IARC Press; 2021.

Boddu P, Thakral B, Alhuraiji A, et al. Distinguishing thymoma from T-lymphoblastic Leukaemia/Lymphoma: a case-based evaluation. *J Clin Pathol.* 2019;72(3):251-257.

Jevremovic D, Roden AC, Ketterling RP, Kurtin PJ, McPhail ED. LMO2 is a specific marker of T-lymphoblastic leukemia/lymphoma. *Am J Clin Pathol.* 2016;145(2):180-190.

Pina-Oviedo S. Mediastinal lymphoproliferative disorders. *Adv Anat Pathol.* 2021;28(5):307-334.

Roden AC, Fang W, Shen Y, et al. Distribution of mediastinal lesions across multi-institutional, international, radiology databases. *J Thorac Oncol.* 2020;15(4):568-579.

Wang X, Wang W, Vega F, Quesada AE. Aggressive mediastinal lymphomas. *Semin Diagn Pathol.* 2021:S0740-2570(21)00049-6. https://doi.org/10.1053/j.semdp.2021.06.010

Aljudi A, Weinzierl E, Elkhalifa M, Park S. The hematological differential diagnosis of mediastinal masses. *Clin Lab Med.* 2021;41(3):389-404.

Type B3 Thymoma/Thymic Carcinoma

Weissferdt A, Kalhor N, Bishop JA, et al. Thymoma: a clinicopathological correlation of 1470 cases. *Hum Pathol.* 2018;73:7-15.

Oramas DM, Moran CA. Thymoma: challenges and pitfalls in biopsy interpretation. *Adv Anat Pathol.* 2021;28(5):291-297.

Weissferdt A, Moran CA. The histomorphologic spectrum of spindle cell thymoma. *Hum Pathol.* 2014;45(3):437-445.

den Bakker MA, Roden AC, Marx A, Marino M. Histologic classification of thymoma: a practical guide for routine cases. *J Thorac Oncol.* 2014;9(9 suppl 2):S125-S130.

WHO Classification of Tumours Editorial Board. *Thoracic Tumors.* Lyon: IARC Press; 2021.

Roden AC, Szolkowska M. Common and rare carcinomas of the thymus. *Virchows Arch.* 2021;478(1):111-128.

Weissferdt A, Moran CA. Staging of thymic epithelial neoplasms: thymoma and thymic carcinoma. *Am J Clin Pathol.* 2019;151(6):593-597.

Aesif SW, Aubry MC, Yi ES, et al. Loss of p16INK4A expression and homozygous CDKN2A deletion are associated with worse outcome and younger age in thymic carcinomas. *J Thorac Oncol.* 2017;12(5):860-871.

Weissferdt A, Wistuba II, Moran CA. Molecular aspects of thymic carcinoma. *Lung Cancer.* 2012;78(2):127-132.

Zettl A, Ströbel P, Wagner K, et al. Recurrent genetic aberrations in thymoma and thymic carcinoma. *Am J Pathol.* 2000;157(1):257-266.

Small Cell Carcinoma

Wick MR, Scheithauer BW. Oat-cell carcinoma of the thymus. *Cancer.* 1982;49(8):1652-1657.

Wick MR, Scheithauer BW, Weiland LH, et al. Primary thymic carcinomas. *Am J Surg Pathol.* 1982;6(7):613-630.

Kuo TT, Chang JP, Lin FJ, et al. Thymic carcinomas: histopathological varieties and immunohistochemical study. *Am J Surg Pathol.* 1990; 14(1):24-34.

Travis WD, Marchevsky AM, Nicholson AG, et al. Small cell carcinoma of the thymus. In: *WHO Classification of Thoracic Tumours.* 5th ed. Lyon: International Agency for Research on Cancer; 2021.

Dacic S, Ströbel P. Challenges in lung and thoracic pathology. *Virchows Arch.* 2021;478:1-3.

Tiffet O, Nicholson AG, Ladas G, et al. A clinicopathologic study of 12 neuroendocrine tumors arising in the thymus. *Chest.* 2003;124(1): 141-146.

Dinter H, Bohnenberger H, Beck J, et al. Molecular classification of neuroendocrine tumors of the thymus. *J Thorac Oncol.* 2019;14(8):1472-1483.

Li J, Xia T, Zhang W, et al. Primary small cell neuroendocrine carcinoma of the mediastinum: computed tomography and histopathological correlation. *J Comput Assist Tomogr.* 2014;38(2):174-178.

Ströbel P, Zettl A, Shilo K, et al. Tumor genetics and survival of thymic neuroendocrine neoplasms: a multi-institutional clinicopathologic study. *Genes Chromosomes Cancer.* 2014;53(9):738-749.

Crona J, Björklund P, Welin S, et al. Treatment, prognostic markers and survival in thymic neuroendocrine tumours. A study from a single tertiary referral centre. *Lung Cancer.* 2013;79(3):289-293.

Li J, Xia T, Zhang W, et al. Primary small cell neuroendocrine carcinoma of the mediastinum: computed tomography and histopathological correlation. *J Comput Assist Tomogr.* 2014;38(2):174-178.

Vrana JA, Boland JM, Terra SBSP, et al. SATB2 is expressed in a subset of pulmonary and thymic neuroendocrine tumors. *Am J Clin Pathol.* 2021;156(5):853-865. doi:10.1093/ajcp/aqab038.

Solitary Fibrous Tumor/Nerve Sheath Tumor

Witkin GB, Rosai J. Solitary fibrous tumor of the mediastinum. A report of 14 cases. *Am J Surg Pathol.* 1989;13(7):547-557.

England DM, Hochholzer L, McCarthy MJ. Localized benign and malignant fibrous tumors of the pleura. A clinicopathologic review of 223 cases. *Am J Surg Pathol.* 1989;13(8):640-658. Erratum in: Am J Surg Pathol. 1991;15(8):818. doi:10.1097/00000478-198908000-00003.

Zhou C, Li W, Shao J, Zhao J. Thoracic solitary fibrous tumors: an analysis of 70 patients who underwent surgical resection in a single institution. *J Cancer Res Clin Oncol.* 2020;146(5):1245-1252.

Singh N, Collingwood R, Eich ML, et al. NAB2-STAT6 gene fusions to evaluate primary/metastasis of hemangiopericytoma/solitary fibrous tumors. *Am J Clin Pathol.* 2021;156(5):906-912. doi:10.1093/ajcp/aqab045.

Fletcher CD, Bridge JA, Lee JC. Extrapleural solitary fibrous tumour. In: Fletcher CD, ed. *WHO Classification of Tumours of Soft Tissue and Bone.* 4th ed. Lyon: IARC; 2013:80-82.

Rao N, Colby TV, Falconieri G, et al. Intrapulmonary solitary fibrous tumors: clinicopathologic and immunohistochemical study of 24 cases. *Am J Surg Pathol.* 2013;37(2):155-166.

Demicco EG, Park MS, Araujo DM, et al. Solitary fibrous tumor: a clinicopathological study of 110 cases and proposed risk assessment model. *Mod Pathol.* 2012;25(9):1298-1306.

Demicco EG, Wagner MJ, Maki RG, et al. Risk assessment in solitary fibrous tumors: validation and refinement of a risk stratification model. *Mod Pathol.* 2017;30(10):1433-1442.

Demicco EG, Fritchie KJ, Han A. Solitary fibrous tumour. In: WHO Classification of Tumours Editorial Board, ed. *World Health Organisation Classification of Soft Tissue and Bone Tumours.* 5th ed. Lyon: IARC Press; 2019:104-108.

Hanau CA, Miettinen M. Solitary fibrous tumor: histological and immunohistochemical spectrum of benign and malignant variants presenting at different sites. *Hum Pathol.* 1995;26(4):440-449.

Tavora F, Calabrese F, Demicco EG, et al. Solitary fibrous tumor of the thorax. In: *WHO Classification of Thoracic Tumours.* 5th ed. Lyon: International Agency for Research on Cancer; 2021:284-285.

Tariq MU, Din NU, Abdul-Ghafar J, et al. The many faces of solitary fibrous tumor; diversity of histological features, differential diagnosis and role of molecular studies and surrogate markers in avoiding misdiagnosis and predicting the behavior. *Diagn Pathol.* 2021;16(1):32.

Ronchi A, Cozzolino I, Zito Marino F, et al. Extrapleural solitary fibrous tumor: a distinct entity from pleural solitary fibrous tumor. An update on clinical, molecular and diagnostic features. *Ann Diagn Pathol.* 2018;34:142-150.

Lecoutere E, Creytens D. Multifocal cytokeratin expression in pleural and abdominal malignant solitary fibrous tumors: an unusual diagnostic pitfall. *Virchows Arch.* 2015;467(1):119-121.

Paraganglioma

Neumann HPH, Young Jr WF, Eng C. Pheochromocytoma and paraganglioma. *N Engl J Med.* 2019;381(6):552-565.

Erickson D, Kudva YC, Ebersold MJ, et al. Benign paragangliomas: clinical presentation and treatment outcomes in 236 patients. *J Clin Endocrinol Metab.* 2001;86(11):5210-5216.

Brown ML, Zayas GE, Abel MD, et al. Mediastinal paragangliomas: the Mayo Clinic experience. *Ann Thorac Surg.* 2008;86(3):946-951.

Young Jr WF. Adrenal medulla, catecholamines, and pheochromocytoma. In: Goldman L, Ausiello D, eds. *Cecil Medicine.* 23rd ed. Philadelphia, PA; Saunders Elsevier: 2008;1721-1727.

Hsu YR, Torres-Mora J, Kipp BR, et al. Clinicopathological, immunophenotypic and genetic studies of mediastinal paragangliomas. *Eur J Cardiothorac Surg.* 2019;56(5):867-875.

Weissferdt A, Kalhor N, Liu H, et al. Thymic neuroendocrine tumors (paraganglioma and carcinoid tumors): a comparative immunohistochemical study of 46 cases. *Hum Pathol.* 2014;45(12):2463-2470.

Moran CA, Suster S, Fishback N, Koss MN. Mediastinal paragangliomas. A clinicopathologic and immunohistochemical study of 16 cases. *Cancer.* 1993;72(8):2358-2364.

Chen H, Sippel RS, O'Dorisio MS, et al. The North American Neuroendocrine Tumor Society consensus guideline for the diagnosis and management of neuroendocrine tumors. *Pancreas.* 2010;39(6):775-783.

Lenders JWM, Eisenhofer G, Mannelli M, Pacak K. Phaeochromocytoma. *Lancet.* 2005;366(9486):665-675.

Brink I, Hoegerle S, Klisch J, Bley TA. Imaging of pheochromocytoma and paraganglioma. *Fam Cancer.* 2005;4(1):61-68.

Primary Mediastinal Large B-Cell Lymphoma

Zinzani PL, Piccaluga PP. Primary mediastinal DLBCL: evolving biologic understanding and therapeutic strategies. *Curr Oncol Rep.* 2011;13: 407-415.

Pfau D, Smith DA, Beck R, et al. Primary mediastinal large B-Cell lymphoma: a review for radiologists. *AJR Am J Roentgenol.* 2019;213(5): W194-W210.

Martelli M, Ferreri A, Di Rocco A, Ansuinelli M, Johnson PWM. Primary mediastinal large B-cell lymphoma. *Crit Rev Oncol Hematol.* 2017;113:318-327.

Sukswai N, Lyapichev K, Khoury JD, Medeiros LJ. Diffuse large B-cell lymphoma variants: an update. *Pathology.* 2020;52(1):53-67.

Shi QY, Feng X, Chen H, et al. Primary mediastinal large B-cell lymphoma: a clinicopathologic study of 27 cases. *Zhonghua Bing Li Xue Za Zhi.* 2017;46(9):607-612.

Lees C, Keane C, Gandhi MK, Gunawardana J. Biology and therapy of primary mediastinal B-cell lymphoma: current status and future directions. *Br J Haematol.* 2019;185(1):25-41.

Bhatt VR, Mourya R, Shrestha R, Armitage JO. Primary mediastinal large B-cell lymphoma. *Cancer Treat Rev.* 2015;41(6):476-485.

Grant C, Dunleavy K, Eberle FC, Pittaluga S, Wilson WH, Jaffe ES. Primary mediastinal large B-cell lymphoma, classic Hodgkin lymphoma presenting in the mediastinum, and mediastinal gray zone lymphoma: what is the oncologist to do? *Curr Hematol Malig Rep.* 2011;6(3):157-163.

Lees C, Keane C, Gandhi MK, Gunawardana J. Biology and therapy of primary mediastinal B-cell lymphoma: current status and future directions. *Br J Haematol.* 2019;185(1):25-41.

Twa DD, Steidl C. Structural genomic alterations in primary mediastinal large B-cell lymphoma. *Leuk Lymphoma.* 2015;56(8):2239-2250.

Mediastinal Germ Cell Tumors

Moran CA, Suster S. Primary germ cell tumors of the mediastinum: I. Analysis of 322 cases with special emphasis on teratomatous lesions and a proposal for histopathologic classification and clinical staging. *Cancer.* 1997;80(4):681-690.

Bokemeyer C, Nichols CR, Droz JP, et al. Extragonadal germ cell tumors of the mediastinum and retroperitoneum: results from an international analysis. *J Clin Oncol.* 2002;20(7):1864-1873.

Rosti G, Secondino S, Necchi A, Fornarini G, Pedrazzoli P. Primary mediastinal germ cell tumors. *Semin Oncol.* 2019;46(2):107-111.

Wood DE. Mediastinal germ cell tumors. *Semin Thorac Cardiovasc Surg.* 2000;12(4):278-289.

Albany C, Einhorn LH. Extragonadal germ cell tumors: clinical presentation and management. *Curr Opin Oncol.* 2013;25(3):261-265.

Wong V, Geynisman DM. Incidentally discovered primary mediastinal germ cell tumor. *JAAPA.* 2020;33(4):35-37.

Ronchi A, Cozzolino I, Montella M, et al. Extragonadal germ cell tumors: not just a matter of location. A review about clinical, molecular and pathological features. *Cancer Med.* 2019;8(16):6832-6840.

Chetaille B, Massard G, Falcoz PE. Mediastinal germ cell tumors: anatomopathology, classification, teratomas and malignant tumors. *Rev Pneumol Clin.* 2010;66(1):63-70.

Knapp RH, Hurt RD, Payne WS, et al. Malignant germ cell tumors of the mediastinum. *J Thorac Cardiovasc Surg.* 1985;89(1):82-89.

Montresor E, Nifosì F, Lupi A, et al. Primary germinal tumors of the mediastinum: our experience in 9 cases. *Chir Ital.* 1994;46(3): 46-52.

Sham JS, Fu KH, Choi PH, Lau WH, Khin MA, Choy D. Primary mediastinal seminoma. *Oncology.* 1990;47(2):124-127.

Niehans GA, Manivel JC, Copland GT, Scheithauer BW, Wick MR. Immunohistochemistry of germ cell and trophoblastic neoplasms. *Cancer.* 1988;62(6):1113-1123.

Chahoud J, Zhang M, Shah A, Lin SH, Pisters LL, Tu SM. Managing seminomatous and nonseminomatous germ cell tumors. *Curr Opin Oncol.* 2018;30(3):181-188.

Sarcoidosis/Histoplasmosis

Soto-Gomez N, Peters JI, Nambiar AM. Diagnosis and management of sarcoidosis. *Am Fam Physician.* 2016;93(10):840-848.

Crouser ED, Maier LA, Wilson KC, et al. Diagnosis and detection of sarcoidosis. An Official American Thoracic Society Clinical Practice Guideline. *Am J Respir Crit Care Med.* 2020;201(8):e26-e51.

Iannuzzi MC, Rybicki BA, Teirstein AS. Sarcoidosis. *N Engl J Med.* 2007; 357(21):2153-2165.

Silva M, Nunes H, Valeyre D, Sverzellati N. Imaging of sarcoidosis. *Clin Rev Allergy Immunol.* 2015;49(1):45-53.

Llanos O, Hamzeh N. Sarcoidosis. *Med Clin North Am.* 2019;103(3): 527-534.

English JC III, Patel PJ, Greer KE. Sarcoidosis. *J Am Acad Dermatol.* 2001;44(5):725-743; quiz 744-746.

Wheat LJ, Azar MM, Bahr NC, Spec A, Relich RF, Hage C. Histoplasmosis. *Infect Dis Clin North Am.* 2016;30(1):207-227.

Baughman RP. Treatment of sarcoidosis. *Panminerva Med.* 2013;55(2): 175-189.

Erbay M, Özsu S, Ayaydın Mürtezaoğlu ES, et al. Causes of mediastinal/hilar granulomatous lymphadenitis. *Tuberk Toraks.* 2018;66(3):212-216.

Costabel U. Sarcoidosis: clinical update. *Eur Respir J Suppl.* 2001;32: 56s-68s.

Arkema EV, Cozier YC. Epidemiology of sarcoidosis: current findings and future directions. *Ther Adv Chronic Dis.* 2018;9(11):227-240.

HYPERTROPHIC LICHEN PLANUS

DIFFERENTIAL DIAGNOSIS: SQUAMOUS CELL CARCINOMA

Clinical Features

Lichen planus is a T-cell–mediated autoimmune disease affecting the skin or mucosal surfaces. It has several clinical and pathologic variants, one of which is hypertrophic lichen planus (HLP). HLP typically occurs on the lower extremities, particularly the shins and the ankles. Unlike classic lichen planus which presents as flat-topped purple papules, HLP manifests as thick, hyperkeratotic, and erythematous plaques or nodules, commonly raising clinical concern for squamous cell carcinoma (SCC). Patients with HLP often present with multiple lesions and may also have lesions of classic lichen planus and oral lichen planus.

Pathologic Features

GROSS FINDINGS

Lesions of HLP are most commonly encountered in shave or punch biopsies, where the skin surface is keratotic and/or erythematous.

MICROSCOPIC FINDINGS

Histopathologically, HLP is characterized by moderate to marked epidermal acanthosis and hyperkeratosis associated with lichenoid inflammation. Notably, the lichenoid infiltrate is accentuated at the base of the elongated and broadened rete ridges (Figs. 13.1–13.3). Evidence of interface change including basal epidermal vacuolation and cytoid bodies is readily appreciated in these areas (see Figs. 13.1C and 13.3B). The infiltrate is composed of predominantly lymphocytes. Eosinophils, while typically absent in classic lichen planus, are not uncommon in HLP. Keratinocytes in HLP are enlarged

with abundant eosinophilic cytoplasm; however, nuclear atypia or pleomorphism is absent or minimal (see Fig. 13.3B). Hyperkeratosis is present, but atypical parakeratosis (crowded large retained nuclei in stratum corneum) is usually absent. Overall, the epidermal changes are those of reactive pseudoepitheliomatous hyperplasia. Wedge-shaped hypergranulosis may be present.

Ancillary Studies

Ancillary studies are usually not needed for the diagnosis of HLP. Demonstration of absence of perforating elastic fibers by elastic stains such as Verhoeff-van Gieson may help distinguish HLP from keratoacanthoma or well-differentiated SCC.

Differential Diagnosis

Histologic distinction of HLP and well-differentiated SCC can be challenging, especially when there is robust pseudoepitheliomatous hyperplasia or when the base of the lesion is not visualized in a partial biopsy (see Fig. 13.2). Clinically, the presence of multiple lesions or a history of lichen planus would favor a diagnosis of HLP, although biopsies are frequently performed to exclude SCC arising in HLP. Microscopically, the presence of a lichenoid infiltrate concentrated at the base of the elongated rete ridges would support HLP, whereas inflammation in SCC, when present, does not usually show the same affinity for the base of the rete ridges (Figs. 13.4 and 13.5). It is also more common to see lichenoid dermatitis involving the surrounding skin in HLP than in SCC. Significant architectural complexity, such as multiple angulated squamous nests infiltrating the dermis, should warrant a diagnosis of SCC (see Figs. 13.4 and 13.5), as HLP should not demonstrate compelling dermal invasion. Paradoxic differentiation, in which the squamous nests present at the base of the lesion are more eosinophilic than those in the superficial aspect (see Fig. 13.4B), is another feature of SCC. Cytologic atypia and nuclear pleomorphism would also favor SCC (see Fig. 13.5B). As mentioned above, presence

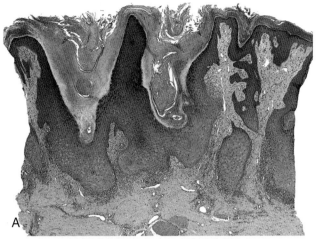

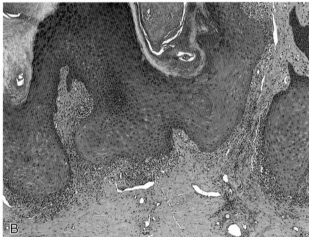

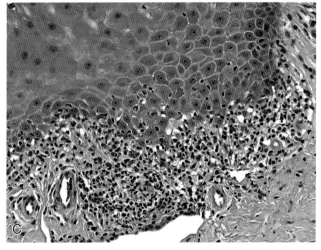

FIG. 13.1

An example of hypertrophic lichen planus showing pseudoepitheliomatous hyperplasia of the epidermis with a lichenoid infiltrate concentrated at the base of the broadened and elongated rete ridges (**A**). The infiltrate is composed of predominantly lymphocytes (**B**). Degeneration of the basal epidermis is evidenced by infiltration of lymphocytes and presence of cytoid bodies. No significant keratinocytic atypia is appreciated (**C**).

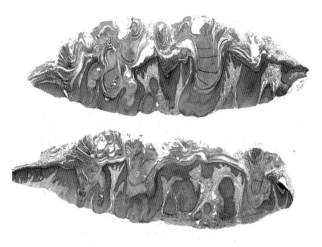

FIG. 13.2

Shave biopsy of another hypertrophic lichen planus illustrates the diagnostic challenge in its distinction from squamous cell carcinoma when the base of the lesion is not visualized.

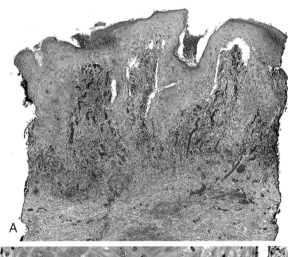

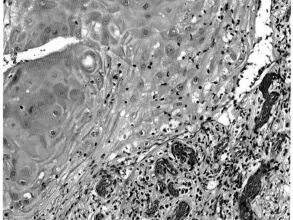

FIG. 13.3

This example of hypertrophic lichen planus reveals a more eosinophilic epidermis associated with lichenoid inflammation (**A**). Higher magnification reveals abundant eosinophilic cytoplasm in the keratinocytes without nuclear atypia or pleomorphism (**B**). Cytoid bodies are present.

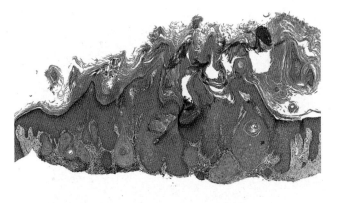

A

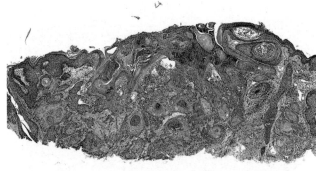

A

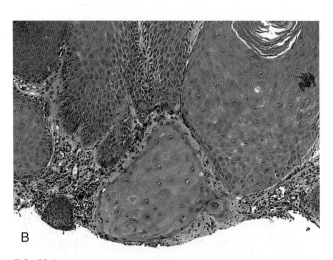

B

FIG. 13.4

A superficially invasive well-differentiated squamous cell carcinoma demonstrates a more complex architecture including several irregular nests in the dermis (**A**). The squamous nests at the base of the lesion appear more eosinophilic, consistent with paradoxic differentiation (**B**).

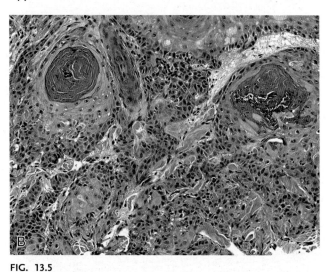

B

FIG. 13.5

A moderately differentiated squamous cell carcinoma shows a significantly more complex architecture with clear infiltration of the dermis (**A**). Cytologic atypia and pleomorphism are readily appreciated at high magnification (**B**).

of perforating elastic fibers in the hyperplastic epidermis has been shown in many well-differentiated SCCs, and less commonly in HLP. Perineural or lymphovascular invasion would also support a diagnosis of SCC (Table 13.1). In the setting of a superficial shave biopsy where a definitive diagnosis is not possible, however, a diagnosis of "atypical squamous proliferation" with a comment explaining the considerations for both HLP and SCC is most appropriate and should prompt additional sampling if clinically indicated.

Prognosis and Therapy

HLP is a benign condition, although chronic cases may rarely undergo malignant transformation to SCC. Treatment options include topical or intralesional steroids and acitretin. In cases demonstrating significant histopathologic overlap with SCC, it is advisable to treat with steroids or acitretin before re-biopsy or excision of any persistent lesions to exclude SCC.

TABLE 13.1

Histologic Features of Hypertrophic Lichen Planus Versus Squamous Cell Carcinoma

Hypertrophic Lichen Planus	Squamous Cell Carcinoma
• Variable elongation and broadening of rete ridges	• Irregular and complex epidermal hyperplasia and dermal squamous nests
• Lichenoid inflammation concentrated at the base of the elongated rete ridges	• Lichenoid inflammation, if present, is not concentrated at the base of the rete ridges
• No significant squamous atypia	• Squamous atypia is present
• Hyperkeratosis without atypical parakeratosis	• Atypical parakeratosis is frequently present
• No perineural or lymphovascular invasion	• Perineural or lymphovascular invasion may be present

TRICHOEPITHELIOMA

DIFFERENTIAL DIAGNOSIS: BASAL CELL CARCINOMA

Clinical Features

Trichoepitheliomas classically present as small papules on the central face, either as solitary or multiple tumors. Solitary lesions may be classic trichoepithelioma (cribriform trichoblastoma) or desmoplastic trichoepithelioma (columnar trichoblastoma). Desmoplastic trichoepitheliomas have an annular appearance with a central dell. Sporadic trichoepitheliomas arise in adulthood.

Multiple trichoepitheliomas may be associated with inherited conditions (multiple familial trichoepithelioma,

Brooke-Spiegler syndrome, or Rombo syndrome). Multiple trichoepitheliomas can merge into plaques. Rare presentations include linear forms or hemifacial plaques. In Brooke-Spiegler syndrome, trichoepitheliomas are accompanied by cylindromas and spiradenomas. In Rombo syndrome, trichoepitheliomas arise in childhood, and are accompanied by vermiculate atrophoderma, milia, hypotrichosis, basal cell carcinoma (BCC), and peripheral vasodilation.

Pathologic Features

GROSS FINDINGS

Trichoepithelioma is most commonly biopsied by shave method, in which the skin surface shows a skin-colored, dome-shaped papule.

MICROSCOPIC FINDINGS

Trichoepithelioma is a biphasic tumor consisting of follicular germinative epithelium accompanied by follicular stroma (Fig. 13.6A). Small basaloid tumor cells are arranged in thin interanastomosing cords and small nests. Horn cysts (infundibulocystic differentiation), variably sized keratinizing cysts lined by infundibular epithelium (Fig. 13.6B), are often present and can be numerous. Giant cell reaction and calcification encountered in many tumors are likely secondary changes to horn cysts. The associated follicular stroma is characterized by small fibroblasts and delicate collagen fibrils organized around tumor islands (see Fig. 13.6B). Papillary mesenchymal bodies (rudimentary follicular structures, characterized by a condensation of ovoid mesenchymal cells cupped by follicular epithelium) can often be identified (Fig. 13.6C). Mitoses are sparse to absent. Cytologic atypia is absent.

In desmoplastic trichoepithelioma (columnar trichoblastoma), follicular germinative cells are arranged in thin strands within a sclerotic stroma (Fig. 13.6E). Horn cysts are usually present. Other evidence of follicular differentiation can be subtle. Similar to classic trichoepithelioma, desmoplastic trichoepithelioma lacks significant atypia or proliferative activity.

Ancillary Studies

IMMUNOHISTOCHEMISTRY

As with other benign follicular tumors, CK20 decorates scattered small colonizing Merkel cells in most trichoepitheliomas (see Fig. 13.6E). Other reported immunohistochemical markers include diffuse PHLDA1, peripheral BCL2, and stromal CD10.

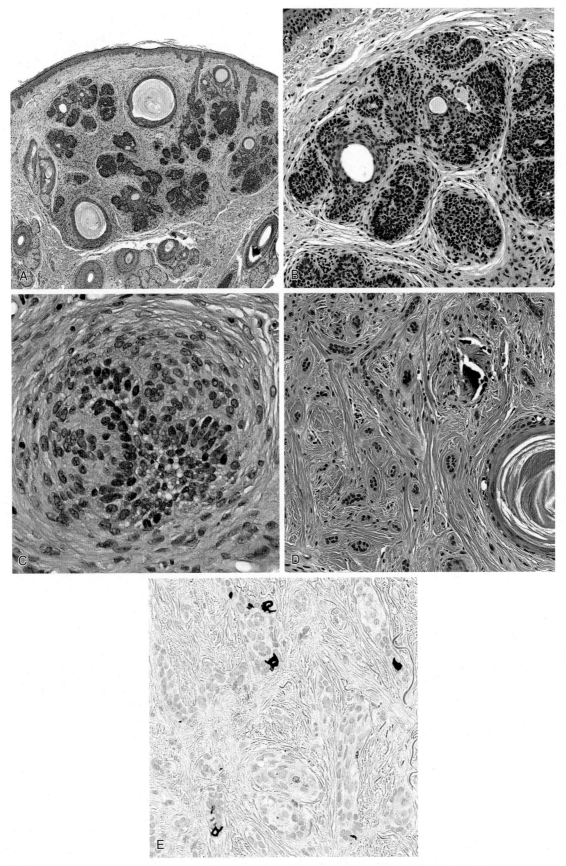

FIG. 13.6

Trichoepithelioma. Circumscribed dermal tumor with horn cysts (**A**). Germinative follicular epithelium with characteristic fine stroma (**B**). Papillary mesenchymal body, with ovoid mesenchymal cells cupped by follicular epithelium (**C**). Desmoplastic trichoepithelioma, characterized by horn cysts and strands of small basaloid cells in sclerotic stroma (**D**). Cytokeratin-20 decorates colonizing Merkel cells in trichoepithelioma (**E**).

MOLECULAR STUDIES

Molecular changes in sporadic lesions are not well characterized. A minority of cases have *PTCH1* mutations (predicted to result in Hedgehog pathway activation, similar to BCC) or *CTNNB1* mutations (predicted to activate the Wnt/beta-catenin pathway). Familial/syndromic forms are associated with germline inactivation of the *CYLD* gene, encoding a negative regulator of the nuclear factor kappa-B pathway. The exception is Rombo syndrome, which does not have a known germline mutation.

Differential Diagnosis

The main differential diagnosis is with BCC (Table 13.2). Features of BCC can include peripheral palisading, cleft retraction, cytologic atypia, numerous mitoses, myxoinflammatory stroma, and infiltrative growth (Fig. 13.7). Mucin can be observed in association with either trichoepithelioma or BCC. Horn cysts are rare in BCC with the exception of infundibulocystic BCC (see Fig. 13.7). Papillary mesenchymal bodies can be identified in many trichoepitheliomas and are rare in BCC. As with other benign follicular tumors, CK20+ colonizing Merkel cells are present in most trichoepitheliomas (see Fig. 13.6E) and are absent in BCC. Androgen receptor expression is absent in trichoepithelioma and present in BCC; however, expression in BCC can be weak and focal. Additional proposed

TABLE 13.2

Histologic Features of Trichoepithelioma Versus Basal Cell Carcinoma

Trichoepithelioma	Basal Cell Carcinoma
Small basaloid cells, may have peripheral palisading	Large basaloid cells with prominent peripheral palisading
Limited or no connection to epidermis	Can have broad connection to epidermis
Circumscribed	Asymmetric, infiltrative
No cleft between tumor and stroma	Cleft retraction between tumor and stroma
Follicular differentiation—follicular stroma, papillary mesenchymal bodies	Myxoinflammatory stroma No papillary mesenchymal bodies
Horn cysts	Horn cysts rare (exception: infundibulocystic basal cell carcinoma)
No perineural invasion	Can be perineural invasion
No atypia	Atypia
CK20 decorates colonizing Merkel cells	Absence of CK20+ colonizing Merkel cells

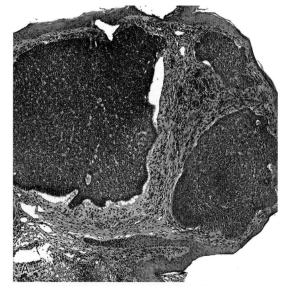

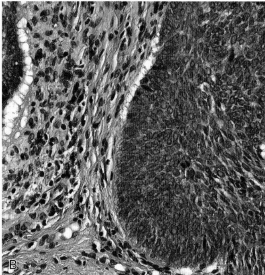

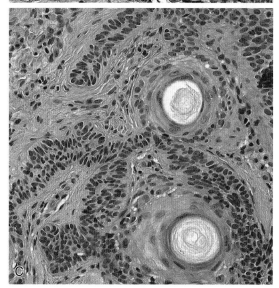

FIG. 13.7

BCC demonstrates cleft retraction and inflammatory stroma (**A**). Crowded enlarged atypical nuclei, mitotic activity, and peripheral palisading with inflammatory stroma (**B**). Horn cysts in infundibulocystic BCC accompanied by cytologic atypia and dermal mucin (**C**).

markers include PHLDA1 (positive in trichoepithelioma, negative in BCC with the possible exception of micronodular BCC) and CD10 (stromal expression in trichoepithelioma, tumor expression in BCC). Markers that may be less sensitive and specific include CD34 (stromal expression in trichoepithelioma, tumor expression in BCC) and BCL2 (peripheral tumor expression in trichoepithelioma, diffuse tumor expression in BCC). However, no single marker is completely sensitive and specific.

Trichoepithelioma may also raise a differential diagnosis for other benign follicular tumors. Trichoblastoma characteristically displays less horn cyst formation and has a more primitive appearance with larger tumor cell nodules. However, there is substantial morphologic overlap with trichoepithelioma, and most texts consider trichoepithelioma to be a variant of trichoblastoma. Trichoadenoma (a follicular tumor with a predominance of horn cysts) may also represent a variant of trichoblastoma/trichoepithelioma. Basaloid follicular hamartoma also contains horn cysts; unlike trichoepithelioma, there is broad connection to the epidermis, with follicular epithelium that is more often infundibular than germinative in appearance.

Desmoplastic trichoepithelioma must be distinguished from other sclerosing cutaneous tumors, including microcystic adnexal carcinoma (MAC), syringoma, and morpheaform BCC. Morpheaform BCC can be distinguished from desmoplastic trichoepithelioma by features described above. Of note, classic stromal changes, cleft retraction, and atypia may be less prominent in morpheaform BCC. Additional details on diagnostic evaluation of sclerosing tumors are provided in the Microcystic Adnexal Carcinoma section.

Prognosis and Therapy

Prognosis is excellent. Malignant progression is exceedingly rare.

TRICHOEPITHELIOMA – DISEASE FACT SHEET

Definition
- Follicular germinative tumor with follicular stroma, often with horn cysts

Incidence and Location
- Uncommon to rare
- Predominantly arises on face, with infrequent presentation on trunk or extremities

Age Distribution
- Adult (familial forms may manifest at puberty; Rombo-associated tumors may emerge in childhood

---

Clinical Features
- Solitary papule on face (desmoplastic trichoepithelioma will have central dell)
- Multiple trichoepitheliomas: tumors may coalesce into plaques

Prognosis and Therapy
- Benign course; malignant progression is exceedingly rare

TRICHOEPITHELIOMA – PATHOLOGIC FEATURES

Microscopic Findings
- Biphasic tumor: follicular germinative epithelium and follicular stroma
- Follicular germinative epithelium: small basaloid cells without atypia; fine interanastomosing strands and nodules with horn cysts
- Follicular stroma: fine collagen and small fibroblasts, organized around epithelial strands/nodules
- Papillary mesenchymal bodies: Ovoid mesenchymal cells cupped or surrounded by rim of follicular epithelium

Pathologic Differential Diagnoses
- Basal cell carcinoma, other follicular and sweat gland tumors

MICROCYSTIC ADNEXAL CARCINOMA

DIFFERENTIAL DIAGNOSES: SYRINGOMA, DESMOPLASTIC TRICHOEPITHELIOMA

Clinical Features

The classic presentation for MAC is a firm plaque on the face (especially the nasolabial fold or lip) of a middle-aged or older individual. Younger patients can also present with MACs. Other than head and neck, rare anatomic sites include the trunk and extremities. Tumors have an average size of 2 cm but can be much larger. Local sensory symptoms may be reported, likely in association with perineural invasion. MAC might clinically resemble other non-melanoma skin cancers, cyst, or scar. The subtle clinical appearance and slow growth can lead to long delays in diagnosis.

Pathologic Features

GROSS FINDINGS

A firm tumor with involvement of deep tissues may be observed.

MICROSCOPIC FINDINGS

MAC is a sclerosing sweat gland carcinoma with a component of follicular differentiation. Follicular differentiation

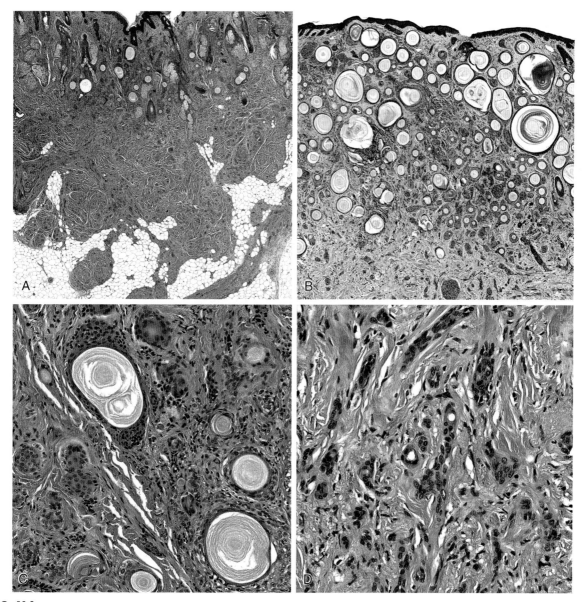

FIG. 13.8

Microcystic adnexal carcinoma shows superficial horn cysts and subtle deep infiltrative growth into subcutits (**A**). Horn cysts can be numerous (**B**). Horn cysts with inflammation and sclerosis (**C**). Deep infiltrating strands with small tumor cells (**D**). Luminal spaces may be numerous or rare.

manifests as small infundibular cysts (horn cysts) that may be scattered or numerous in the superficial dermis (Fig. 13.8A–C). Giant cell reaction and calcification can occur. The deeper component displays characteristic features of a sclerosing sweat gland carcinoma, with deceptively bland deeply infiltrating strands of small cuboidal cells associated with a sclerotic stroma (see Fig. 13.8A and D). Some strands display two-layered ductal differentiation (see Fig. 13.8D), although this finding can be focal. The tumor can infiltrate skeletal muscle and bone. Perineural invasion is a frequent finding. Mitoses are rare to absent, and there is no cytologic atypia. The solid carcinoma variant of MAC displays small infiltrative epithelial aggregates. Rare findings include predominance of stroma, with isolated small cell nests; single filing; clear cell change; or focal divergent adnexal differentiation.

Ancillary Studies

IMMUNOHISTOCHEMISTRY

The immunophenotype is non-specific. CK5/6 and p63 are expressed. Lumina can be highlighted by CEA and EMA. Variable results have been described for PHLDA1. GCDFP-15 and Ber-EP4 are negative.

MOLECULAR STUDIES

There is molecular heterogeneity among MACs. A fraction of cases demonstrates molecular features similar to other carcinomas, including UV mutations and *TP53* mutation. Another subset of tumors harbors frame-preserving insertions of the *JAK1* kinase, associated with increased phospho-STAT3 expression. Amplification of other oncogenes can also be observed.

Differential Diagnosis

Definitive diagnosis can be challenging in limited samples. The differential diagnosis most frequently involves other sclerosing neoplasms (Fig. 13.9–13.11), which can appear identical on limited samples. Morpheaform (sclerosing) BCC (see Fig. 13.9) lacks ductal structures and might show areas of more classic BCC with peripheral palisading and cleft retraction; tumors are typically BerEp4+ and lack lumina. Syringomas display similar tadpole-like structures in sclerotic stroma, but lack infiltrative growth (see Fig. 13.10; Table 13.3). Desmoplastic trichoepitheliomas have follicular germinative features such as papillary mesenchymal bodies that are absent in MAC. Unlike MAC, desmoplastic trichoepithelioma lacks infiltrative growth, perineural invasion, and ductal differentiation (see Fig. 13.11; Table 13.4). Rarely, superficial biopsy of lesions with numerous horn cysts (see Fig. 13.8B) might raise consideration for other benign follicular tumors such as trichoadenoma.

Horn cysts and minimal atypia distinguish MAC from other sclerosing eccrine carcinomas (squamoid

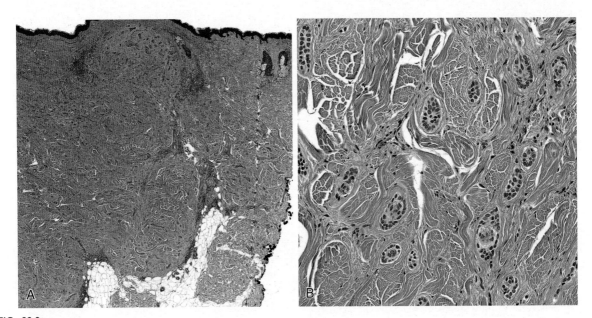

FIG. 13.9

Morpheaform basal cell carcinoma (BCC) shows subtle deep infiltration (**A**). More conventional BCC may be identified superficially. Basaloid islands and strands with subtle peripheral palisading in sclerotic stroma (**B**).

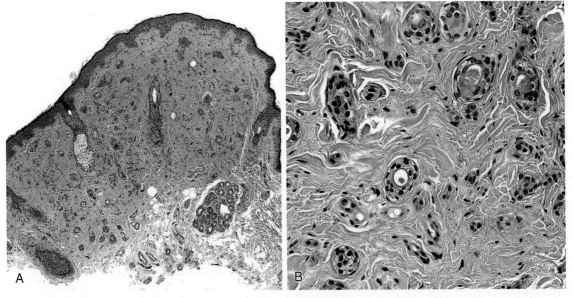

FIG. 13.10

Syringomas display circumscribed growth without deep extension (**A**). Tadpole-shaped ductal structures in a sclerotic stroma (**B**).

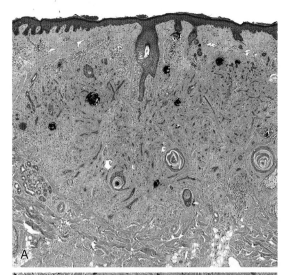

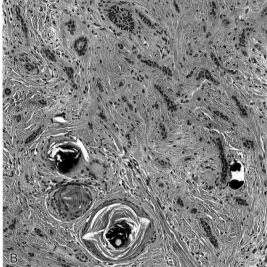

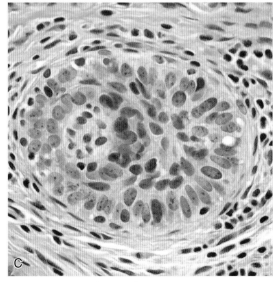

TABLE 13.3

Histologic Features of Microcystic Adnexal Carcinoma Versus Syringoma

Microcystic Adnexal Carcinoma	Syringoma
Horn cysts, strands of bland tumor cells, sclerotic stroma	Strands of bland tumor cells, sclerotic stroma; horn cysts can occur but are not classic
Deep infiltrative growth	Circumscribed growth, usually confined to upper dermis (rare extension to deep dermis, subcutis)
Glandular differentiation—small lumina (might be restricted to deeper component and focal)	Glandular differentiation predominates, with dilated lumina in a tadpole configuration
Perineural invasion	No perineural invasion
Limited to no atypia	No atypia

TABLE 13.4

Histologic Features of Microcystic Adnexal Carcinoma Versus Desmoplastic Trichoepithelioma

Microcystic Adnexal Carcinoma	Desmoplastic Trichoepithelioma
Horn cysts (superficially), strands of bland tumor cells, sclerotic stroma	Horn cysts, strands of bland tumor cells, sclerotic stroma
Deep infiltrative growth	Circumscribed
Glandular differentiation in deeper component (may be focal, or not apparent in superficial biopsies)	Follicular differentiation—follicular stroma, papillary mesenchymal bodies
Perineural invasion	No perineural invasion
Limited or no atypia	No atypia
CK20 negative	CK20 decorates colonizing Merkel cells

FIG. 13.11

Desmoplastic trichoepithelioma is a sclerotic tumor with circumscribed base, horn cysts, and calcifications (**A**). Horn cysts and strands of basaloid cells in sclerotic stroma (**B**). A papillary mesenchymal body consists of follicular epithelium surrounding a focus of mesenchymal cells with rounded nuclei (**C**).

eccrine ductal carcinoma, syringoid carcinoma). The solid carcinoma variant of MAC is distinguished from porocarcinoma by horn cysts, and absence of significant cytologic atypia. Similar lesions on the nipple are classified as syringomatous adenoma. A rare condition similar to Nicolau-Balus syndrome can be associated with multifocal lesions resembling MACs.

Prognosis and Therapy

Excision is the mainstay of treatment but may be challenging and disfiguring due to deep tumor growth that can involve bone. Recurrences are frequent after incomplete excision. Metastasis is exceedingly rare. Options are limited for inoperable disease; most tumors are resistant to radiotherapy, and targeted therapies are lacking.

MERKEL CELL CARCINOMA

DIFFERENTIAL DIAGNOSES: BASAL CELL CARCINOMA, METASTATIC NEUROENDOCRINE CARCINOMA

Clinical Features

Merkel cell carcinoma (MCC) typically presents as a rapidly growing nodule on the head, neck, or extremity of an elderly individual. MCC presents more frequently and at a younger age in immunosuppressed individuals. Less than 5% of patients are under 50 years old. There is a slight male predominance. The most frequent site of involvement is the head and neck, followed by extremities. Although relatively rare, the incidence of MCC is increasing, possibly due to increased diagnostic recognition and/or as part of a larger trend for non-melanoma skin cancers. MCC classically presents as a rapidly growing violaceous nodule that can clinically resemble basal cell carcinoma, squamous cells carcinoma, amelanotic melanoma, lymphoma, or cyst. A minority of cases presents in the parotid or lymph nodes as metastatic disease of unknown primary.

Pathologic Features

GROSS FINDINGS

Usually a nonspecific fleshy tumor centered in the dermis that can extend into the subcutis and deeper structures. Ulceration and necrosis may be present.

MICROSCOPIC FINDINGS

MCC is a poorly differentiated neuroendocrine carcinoma of the small cell type. At scanning magnification, MCC is usually centered in the dermis (Fig. 13.12A), with potential involvement of the subcutis, and infrequent intraepidermal spread. Ulceration can be present. Tumor cells may form large nodules or infiltrate through collagen. At higher magnification, tumor cells display powdery chromatin, numerous mitoses, and minimal cytoplasm (Fig. 13.12B). Cell morphologies can be defined by size, including small cell (potentially resembling lymphoma), intermediate, and large. Multiple morphologies often coexist in the same tumor. Nuclear molding and crush artifact can be prominent. Tumor stroma can display variable degrees of fibrosis, mucin, and inflammatory change (Fig. 13.12C). Angiolymphatic invasion is a common finding and can be extensive. A minority are associated with overlying squamous cell carcinoma in situ (SCCIS), or more rarely invasive SCC. Metaplastic change can occur in a minority of tumors, most frequently characterized by squamous morulae; rare forms of metaplastic differentiation include eccrine, neuroblastic, or sarcomatoid. Pleomorphism and clear cell change are rare findings.

Cutaneous MCC metastases (satellite/in transit, or rarely distant) can be histologically identical to primary tumors. Therefore, correlation with clinical history is essential for distinguishing primary from metastatic MCC. Occasionally, MCC can metastasize to sites of other locoregional skin tumors such as SCC or BCC (see Fig. 13.12), highlighting the need for increased scrutiny of skin biopsies in the draining skin of MCC.

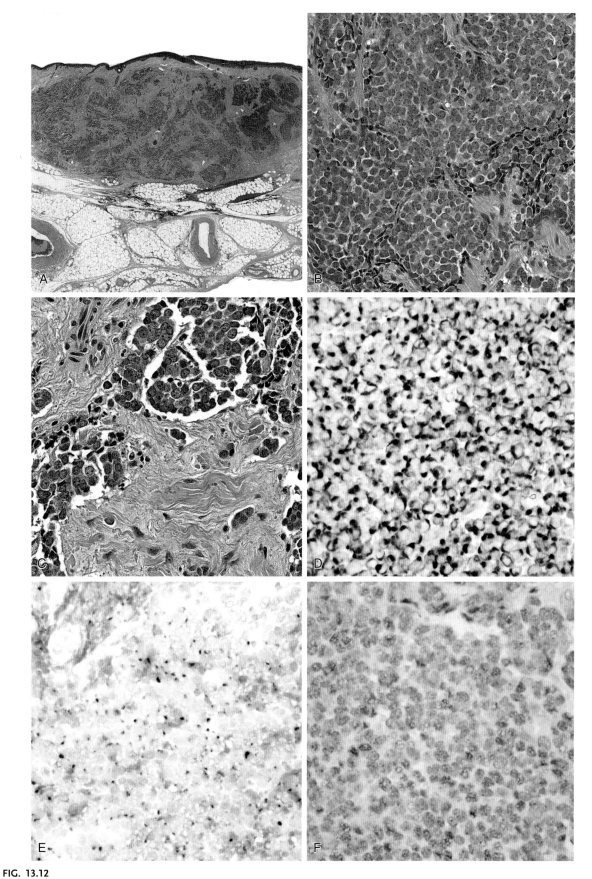

FIG. 13.12

Merkel cell carcinoma. Large dermal tumor with infiltrative border (**A**). Round tumor cells with powdery neuroendocrine chromatin, minimal cytoplasm, crush artifact, and mitoses (**B**). Stromal mucin and associated irregular tumor clefts (**C**). Paranuclear dot pattern of CK20 (**D**). Paranuclear dot pattern of neurofilament (**E**). Nuclear staining for Merkel cell polyomavirus (MCPyV) large T antigen (**F**).

Ancillary Studies

IMMUNOHISTOCHEMISTRY AND OTHER CHROMOGENIC STUDIES

Immunohistochemistry is key to confirming the diagnosis. Broad-spectrum cytokeratins and CK20 stain most tumors in a characteristic perinuclear dot pattern (see Fig. 13.12D). Cytoplasmic and dot staining often coexist, imparting a signet-ring staining pattern. Occasional tumors display pure cytoplasmic staining. In ~10% of cases, CK20 can be focal or absent. Neuroendocrine and neural markers (chromogranin A, synaptophysin, neuron-specific enolase, CD56, and neurofilament) are expressed (see Fig. 13.12E), although no single marker is completely sensitive. TTF1 expression is absent in most cases. A majority of cases express Merkel cell polyomavirus (MCPyV) large T antigen detectable by immunohistochemistry (see Fig. 13.12F), with nuclear or nuclear and cytoplasmic staining. MCPyV T antigen expression can also be detected by RNA *in situ* hybridization. Additional markers expressed in most MCC include SATB2, CD99, and ATOH1. In a minority, TdT and PAX5 expression is detectable.

MOLECULAR STUDIES

Two molecular subclasses of MCC exist: MCPyV positive and MCPyV negative (UV-associated). MCPyV-positive MCC is characterized by expression of oncogenic MCPyV T antigens, and low tumor mutation burden. MCPyV-negative MCC displays high tumor mutation burden, UV mutation signature, and recurrent *TP53* and *RB1* mutation. Heterogeneous oncogene activation events (*PIK3CA* mutation, *MYCL* amplification, and others) occur in a minority of tumors.

Differential Diagnosis

The primary differential diagnosis is with metastatic small cell carcinoma (SmCC) from a non-cutaneous site (Table 13.5). Immunophenotyping can assist with this distinction, although clinical correlation is essential as no immunohistochemical stain is completely sensitive and specific. Non-cutaneous SmCCs display limited to absent CK20 expression; no significant neurofilament or MCPyV large T expression; and positive TTF1 expression (pulmonary and cervical SmCC). Parotid SmCC can be immunophenotypically identical to MCC, and distinction from metastatic MCC of unknown primary can be impossible in this context. Location in deep soft tissue is more characteristic of metastasis than primary MCC. MCPyV-negative MCC can display immunophenotypic aberrancy (such as CK20 negativity, and TTF1 focal/weak positive), which raise challenges with distinction from SmCC.

TABLE 13.5

Histologic Features of Merkel Cell Carcinoma versus Metastatic Neuroendocrine Carcinoma

Merkel Cell Carcinoma	Metastatic Neuroendocrine Carcinoma
Small blue cell tumor	Small blue cell tumor
Dermal +/– subcutaneous extension, with infrequent involvement of epidermis	Dermal or subcutaneous; location in deep tissue favors metastasis; intraepidermal involvement very rare
IHC: Cytokeratin: dot or cytoplasmic CK7: can be expressed (18%) CK20: dot-like, diffuse in most (expressed in 88%) Neurofilament with dot-like pattern (80%) MCPyV: positive (majority) TTF1: negative (weak focal positive in <10%) HPV: negative TdT: positive in minority (25%) PAX5: positive in minority	IHC: Cytokeratin: cytoplasmic (focal dot in some cases) CK20: focal or absent (exceptions: salivary, cervical) Neurofilament: negative (exceptions: cervical, salivary) MCPyV: negative (possible exception: parotid) TTF1: positive (lung, cervical) HPV: negative (exception: cervical) TdT: negative PAX5: positive or negative
Molecular: MCPyV DNA, RNA OR UV-signature mutations	Molecular: MCPyV– (possible exception: parotid) No UV-signature mutations SCLC may show tobacco signature mutations

IHC, immunohistochemistry; *SCLC*, small cell lung cancer; *UV*, ultraviolet.

Other small cell neoplasms of the skin may enter the differential diagnosis. Small cell melanoma expresses melanocytic markers (SOX10, Melan-A, HMB45) that are not expressed in MCC.

Lymphoma expresses CD45 and CD3 or CD20/CD79a, unlike MCC. PAX5 and TdT may be expressed in MCC. As individuals with lymphoma are at higher risk of MCC, sentinel lymph node examination for MCC can demonstrate involvement by chronic lymphocytic leukemia that may have been previously undetected.

Ewing sarcoma is negative for MCPyV and demonstrates *EWSR1* translocation. CK20 expression has not been rigorously examined in Ewing sarcoma. Both Ewing sarcoma and MCC can express CD99, FLI1, and NSE.

MCC can be mistaken for BCC (Table 13.6). MCC lacks peripheral palisading and myxoinflammatory stroma classic for BCC (Fig. 13.13). MCC tumor clefts are irregular (see Fig. 13.12C), in contrast to the smooth peripheral clefting of BCC (see Fig. 13.13). BCC should not display a true small cell morphology. BCC is CK20 negative and strongly expresses CK5/6 and p63, unlike MCC. Neuroendocrine marker expression, BerEP4, and stromal mucin do not distinguish MCC from BCC.

Rarely, MCC with squamous metaplasia might raise diagnostic confusion with basaloid SCC (CK20 negative, MCPyV negative, CK5/6 positive, p63 strongly

TABLE 13.6

Histologic Features of Merkel Cell Carcinoma Versus Basal Cell Carcinoma

Merkel Cell Carcinoma	Basal Cell Carcinoma
Low power: "blue" or basaloid appearance, nodular or infiltrative growth, may be prominent trabecular growth	Low power: "blue" or basaloid appearance, nodular or infiltrative growth, palisading and clefting may be apparent
Stroma may have increased mucin or inflammatory host response but lacks full features of BCC such as prominent fibroblasts	Classic stromal changes (mucin intermingled with fibrosis and prominent fibroblasts, with variable inflammation)
Irregular clefting within and around edges of tumor	Clefting at stroma-tumor interface, with smooth tumor borders along cleft
Small to large round cells with crush artifact	Large basaloid cells
No palisading	Peripheral palisading
Angiolymphatic invasion frequently observed	Angiolymphatic invasion very rare
IHC: Cytokeratins dot-like +/-cytoplasmic CK20 positive (88%) MCPyV positive (60%–80%) ATOH1 positive p63 and CK5/6 usually weak or negative Markers with overlap: Neuroendocrine: positive Ber-EP4: positive	IHC: Cytokeratins: cytoplasmic CK20 negative MCPyV negative ATOH1 negative p63 and CK5/6 strongly positive Markers with overlap: Neuroendocrine: +/– Ber-EP4: positive
Molecular: UV signature with *TP53* and *RB1* mutations OR MCPyV	Molecular: UV signature with mutations of HH pathway and/or *TP53* No MCPyV

HH, hedgehog; *IHC*, immunohistochemistry; *UV*, ultraviolet.

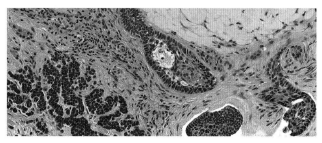

FIG. 13.13

Metastatic Merkel cell carcinoma (*left*) with incidental adjacent basal cell carcinoma (*right*). Basal cell carcinoma displays prominent peripheral palisading and smooth clefts around tumor borders.

positive) or poorly differentiated adnexal carcinoma (CK20 negative).

Well-differentiated neuroendocrine tumors of the skin (carcinoid) are exceedingly rare, and lack expression of SATB2 and CK20. Endocrine mucin-producing sweat gland carcinoma is an eyelid tumor that lacks morphologic similarity to MCC.

Prognosis and Therapy

MCC displays a 33% to 46% disease-specific mortality rate in some studies, although other studies report a less aggressive course; 26% of patients present with regional metastases, and 8% present with distant metastases. The most important prognostic parameters (tumor diameter and the presence/pattern of metastatic disease) form the basis for AJCC staging of MCC. Metastasis to regional lymph nodes can occur even for small tumors. Excision and sentinel lymph node mapping are mainstays of therapy. Immunohistochemistry is recommended for pathologic evaluation of sentinel lymph nodes. Evidence suggests that larger lymph node deposits are more prognostically significant, although this has not been incorporated into staging. Radiotherapy is applied to the primary tumor site (sometimes reserved for larger tumors) and positive nodal basins. Checkpoint inhibitor immunotherapy is approved for stage IV disease and investigational in the adjuvant setting. Chemotherapy is palliative.

MERKEL CELL CARCINOMA – DISEASE FACT SHEET

Definition
▶▶ Poorly differentiated primary cutaneous neuroendocrine carcinoma

Incidence
▶▶ 0.79 cases per 100,000 (USA, 2011)

Age Distribution
▶▶ Predominantly elderly (rarely <50 years old)

Clinical Features
▶▶ Rapidly growing violaceous cutaneous nodule, usually on sun-exposed skin

Prognosis and Therapy
▶▶ Tumor size and presence/pattern of metastatic disease are major prognostic factors
▶▶ Metastases may be satellite/in-transit, regional nodal, or distant
▶▶ Excision and radiotherapy are mainstays
▶▶ Immunotherapy (checkpoint inhibitor) is approved for distant disease, and under investigation as adjuvant therapy
▶▶ Chemotherapy is palliative

MERKEL CELL CARCINOMA – PATHOLOGIC FEATURES

Gross Findings
▶▶ Fleshy dermal tumor, often large and with deep extension

Microscopic Findings
▶▶ Nodular or infiltrative tumor, usually centered in dermis; may involve epidermis or subcutis
▶▶ Small round blue cells with neuroendocrine chromatin and minimal cytoplasm
▶▶ Mitoses, nuclear molding, and crush
▶▶ Perinuclear dot staining with CK20, pan-keratin, and neurofilament

Continued

MERKEL CELL CARCINOMA – PATHOLOGIC FEATURES—cont'd

▸▸ Neuroendocrine and neural marker expression: chromogranin A, synaptophysin, CD56 (NCAM), neurofilament
▸▸ Other positive stains: Ber-EP4, ATOH1, CD99, CK7 (minority), TdT (minority), PAX5 (minority)
▸▸ Negative or weak expression of TTF1, CK5/6

Pathologic Differential Diagnoses

▸▸ Basal cell carcinoma, basaloid squamous cell carcinoma, poorly differentiated adnexal carcinoma, small cell melanoma, lymphoma, metastatic neuroendocrine carcinoma, other small cell tumors

EXTRAMAMMARY PAGET DISEASE

DIFFERENTIAL DIAGNOSES: SQUAMOUS CELL CARCINOMA *IN SITU*, MELANOMA *IN SITU*

Clinical Features

Extramammary Paget disease (EMPD) is a rare disorder defined as intraepithelial adenocarcinoma at an anatomic location other than the breast. Postmenopausal white women and older Asian men (typical age 60–80, average age 65) are the age groups most commonly affected. EMPD occurs most commonly at anatomic locations with prominent apocrine sweat glands (genital skin, anus, and axillae) but can affect a wide array of sites. Vulva is the most common site of involvement, followed by the perianal region. The scrotum is the most commonly involved anatomic location in male patients.

EMPD can be classified as either primary (not associated with internal malignancy) or secondary (resulting from the spread of an underlying colorectal, prostatic, or other invasive carcinoma). Primary EMPD, the more common type, is thought to arise from skin adnexal structures. EMPD tends to develop gradually over time, and pruritus is often the presenting symptom. Consequently, the correct diagnosis is frequently delayed for long periods of time after the patient's initial presentation. EMPD can be mistaken for a number of more common dermatologic entities such as lichen sclerosus, dermatophytosis, candidiasis, contact dermatitis, eczema, or psoriasis, among many others.

Pathologic Features

GROSS FINDINGS

Lesions of EMPD are typically encountered as punch or shave biopsy specimens. The skin surface is typically erythematous, often with surface alteration (scaly or ulcerated).

MICROSCOPIC FINDINGS

The cell of origin in EMPD is disputed but could be the result of a proliferation of adnexal or epidermal stem cells. Malignant transformation of Toker cells, which reside in mammary-type glands of the vulva, has been proposed. Histologic evaluation reveals a proliferation of atypical intraepidermal cells that are present as single cells or may form groups or nests. Epidermal hyperplasia is often present (Fig. 13.14A) and can resemble fibroepithelioma of Pinkus (Fig. 13.14B) or rarely syringofibroadenomatous change. Parakeratosis is common; however, atypical parakeratosis is not typically seen. An "eyeliner" sign, which represents a layer of normal keratinocytes underneath tumor cells, may be visible, as tumor cells of EMPD characteristically reside in the lower half of the epidermis but slightly above the dermal-epidermal junction (Fig. 13.15). The neoplastic cells are cytologically distinct from background keratinocytes, often displaying

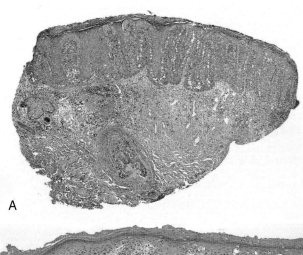

A

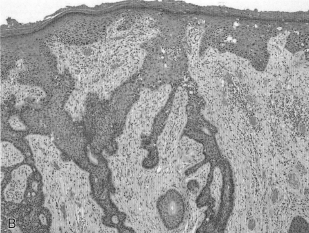

B

FIG. 13.14

Low-magnification image of a case of extramammary Paget disease (EMPD) on the scrotum of a 77-year-old man demonstrates a confluent proliferation of pale, epithelioid cells along the dermal-epidermal junction (**A**). Reactive acanthosis and hyperkeratosis of the epidermis is also visualized. The background epidermal hyperplasia of this case of EMPD resembles fibroepithelioma of Pinkus, which can be a helpful diagnostic clue (**B**).

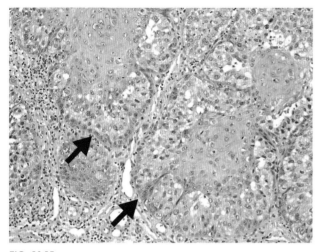

FIG. 13.15

An "eyeliner" sign (conserved placement of normal basal layer keratinocytes denoted by the *arrows*) can often be seen in extramammary Paget disease and can help distinguish this disorder from melanoma *in situ*. This case also shows prominent involvement of adnexal structures which should be distinguished from dermal invasion, which has prognostic significance.

clear to palely eosinophilic, vacuolated cytoplasm and different nuclear features such as hyperchromasia or occasionally prominent nucleoli (Fig. 13.16A and B). Architecturally, lesional cells show varying levels of elevation above the basement membrane, termed pagetoid spread, a phenomenon which can also be observed in the main histologic mimics of EMPD. Formation of intraepithelial glandular structures may be evident. Extension down adnexal structures can be prominent, which should not be mistaken for dermal invasion, which carries prognostic significance.

Ancillary Studies

IMMUNOHISTOCHEMISTRY

Immunohistochemistry is usually helpful in establishing the diagnosis of EMPD. Low-molecular-weight keratins such as cytokeratin 7 (CK7; Fig. 13.16C) and

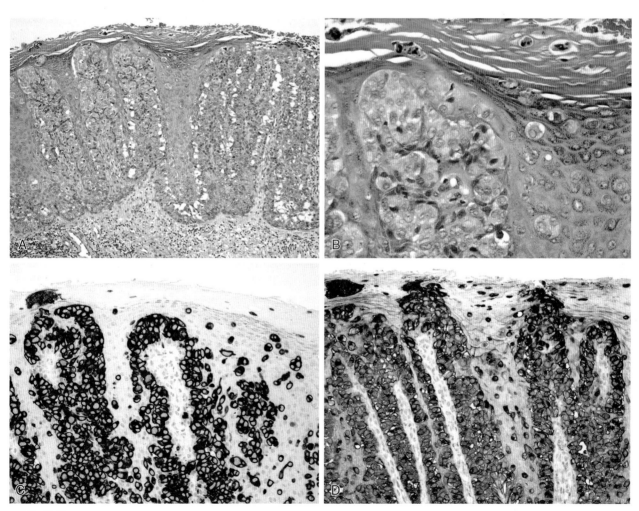

FIG. 13.16

An intermediate-power image of the case shown in Fig. 13.14 revealing upward migration of neoplastic cells within the epidermis (**A**). High-power image showing the cytologic detail of tumor cells with abundant palely eosinophilic cytoplasm and vesicular chromatin disposed in nests and as single cells. Many of the cells show cytoplasmic vacuolization (**B**). Immunohistochemistry for cytokeratin 7 demonstrating strong cytoplasmic reactivity in tumor cells without expression in the background normal epidermis (**C**). Immunohistochemistry for CEA demonstrating cytoplasmic expression in neoplastic cells, again without significant staining in the background epidermis (**D**).

CAM5.2 will typically (but not always) strongly stain EMPD cells, which may also show expression of polyclonal CEA (Fig. 13.16D) and EMA. Low-molecular-weight keratins are typically negative in background squamous epithelium/epidermis (see Fig. 13.16C), which tend to express high-molecular-weight keratins such as CK5/6 and 34βE12. EMPD commonly expresses GCDFP15. Expression of CK20 is indicative of secondary EMPD from a colorectal or genitourinary primary. GATA3 has been reported as a sensitive marker for primary EMPD and positivity does not imply origin from an underlying urothelial carcinoma. Mucicarmine can be used to highlight intracytoplasmic mucin, while PAS positivity with diastase resistance is also commonly seen.

MOLECULAR STUDIES

HER2/neu (ERBB2) activating mutations or amplification are seen in a minority (approximately 10%) of EMPD, potentially representing a therapeutic target.

Differential Diagnosis

Several entities can show pagetoid spread of atypical cells within the epidermis, the most commonly encountered being SCCIS (Table 13.7) and melanoma in situ (MIS) (Table 13.8). Although the diagnosis of SCCIS is often straightforward with clear demonstration of full-thickness epidermal atypia topped by confluent parakeratosis, lesions with prominent single cell pagetoid spread are occasionally encountered (Fig. 13.17). Immunohistochemistry can be utilized to resolve the differential diagnosis, as SCCIS is typically positive for high-molecular-weight keratins such as CK5/6, CK903 (34βE12), and MNF116. SCCIS is also typically positive for p63 (see Fig. 13.17C), and generally (though not in all cases) lacks expression of CK7 and CAM5.2 (see Fig. 13.17D). Squamous neoplasia at genital sites (vulvar squamous intraepithelial neoplasia, penile squamous intraepithelial neoplasia, and anal intraepithelial neoplasia) are often HPV-associated and hence overexpress p16, which can also be assayed immunohistochemically (see Fig. 13.17F).

MIS is an additional frequently encountered mimic (Fig. 13.18). The growth pattern for MIS differs, however, in that most of the lesional cells tend to be positioned at the dermal-epidermal junction rather than slightly above it. Pagetoid spread, though, can be prominent. Tumor cells of MIS usually contain gray to amphiphilic cytoplasm, sometimes with dusty melanin pigment. Nuclei are often hyperchromatic with prominent nucleoli. MIS nearly always demonstrates expression of SOX10 as well as specific melanocytic markers such as Melan-A/MART-1 (Table 13.8). Rare cases of pigmented EMPD require a high degree of suspicion to differentiate from MIS.

Prognosis and Therapy

A thorough evaluation for an underlying malignancy is warranted in most cases prior to definitive surgery. The mainstay for treatment of EMPD is surgical excision. Mohs micrographic surgery may be superior to simple excision but is not uniformly performed. Although the 5-year survival rate is high for patients without invasive disease (>90%), local recurrences are frequent. Invasive disease is associated with a poorer prognosis. The depth of dermal invasion is associated with a number of prognostic indicators including lymph node involvement, decreased disease-free survival, and decreased overall survival. Tumors that invade to a depth of less than 1 mm are considered microinvasive, as lesions that invade deeper than 1 mm are associated with a higher risk of adverse outcome.

EXTRAMAMMARY PAGET DISEASE – DISEASE FACT SHEET

Definition
▶▶ Primary cutaneous in situ (intraepidermal) adenocarcinoma that occurs at an anatomic location other than the breast

Incidence and Location
▶▶ Rare
▶▶ Most common at anatomic locations with prominent apocrine glands (vulva, perianal, scrotum, etc.)

Age Distribution
▶▶ Older adults (average age 65)
▶▶ Most commonly postmenopausal women and Asian men

Clinical Features
▶▶ Pruritis or pain with an insidious presentation
▶▶ Erythematous plaques that may have surface alteration (ulceration, scaliness)
▶▶ Correct diagnosis may be delayed several years after presentation due to non-specificity of symptoms

Prognosis and Therapy
▶▶ Surgical therapy is the mainstay of treatment
▶▶ Mohs micrographic surgery may offer superior outcomes in terms of tissue preservation and margin control
▶▶ Local recurrence is common
▶▶ Dermal invasion carries prognostic significance

EXTRAMAMMARY PAGET DISEASE – PATHOLOGIC FEATURES

Gross Findings
▶▶ Erythematous plaques, often with surface alteration (scaly or ulcerated)
▶▶ Often mistaken for other more common dermatologic entities such as dermatophytosis, candidiasis, eczema, contact dermatitis, or psoriasis, among others

Microscopic Findings
▶▶ Intraepidermal proliferation of atypical epithelioid cells with palely eosinophilic cytoplasm that exhibit pagetoid spread
▶▶ Can form ductal structures or show cytoplasmic vacuolization

EXTRAMAMMARY PAGET DISEASE – PATHOLOGIC FEATURES—cont'd

▸▸ Nuclei often contain vesicular chromatin
▸▸ Epidermal hyperplasia which can resemble fibroepithelioma of Pinkus or syringofibroadenoma
▸▸ Parakeratosis is often present, but is not atypical

▸▸ An "eyeliner" sign of normal keratinocytes is often seen
▸▸ Dermal invasion may be present

Pathologic Differential Diagnoses

▸▸ Squamous cell carcinoma *in situ*
▸▸ Melanoma *in situ*

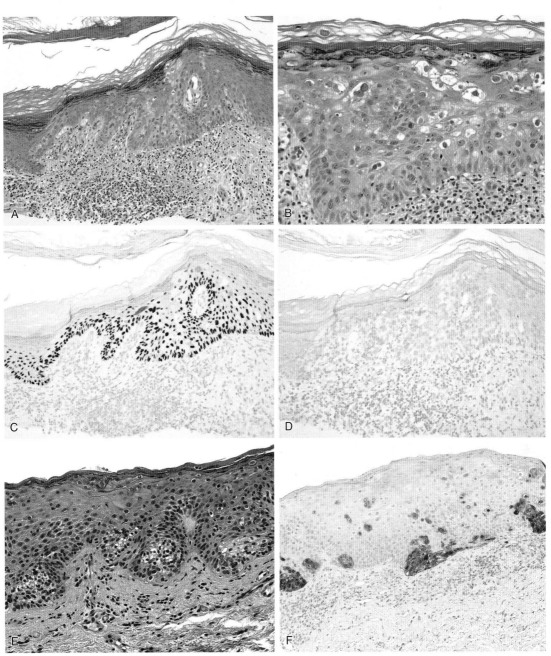

FIG. 13.17

This case of squamous cell carcinoma *in situ* (SCCIS) demonstrates prominent upward intraepidermal spread of neoplastic cells. Although areas of more conventional SCCIS are often present, this histologic appearance can cause diagnostic confusion with extramammary Paget disease or melanoma *in situ* (**A**). Higher-power image demonstrating the cytologic characteristics with some neoplastic keratinocytes showing formation of intracytoplasmic granules as they enter the stratum granulosum. Atypical parakeratosis is often present above lesions (**B**). A p63 immunostain demonstrating positive reactivity in larger, atypical nuclei in addition to background normal keratinocytes (**C**). A CAM5.2 stain in this case is negative in tumor cells (**D**). Note that some cases of SCCIS can show expression of low-molecular-weight keratins such as CAM5.2 and CK7; therefore, a panel of immunostains that includes other markers such as EMA and CEA are recommended for high diagnostic accuracy. CK20 expression may be seen in secondary EMPD, and p63 staining can be observed in secondary EMPD arising from urothelial carcinoma. Case of vulvar intraepithelial neoplasia mimicking Paget disease with nest formation by atypical keratinocytes (**E**). Immunohistochemistry for p16 demonstrates strong positivity in lesional cells, indicative of human papillomavirus infection (**F**).

TABLE 13.7

Histologic Features of Extramammary Paget Disease Versus Squamous Cell Carcinoma *In Situ*

Extramammary Paget Disease	Squamous Cell Carcinoma *In Situ*
• Clear to palely eosinophilic, vacuolated cytoplasm	• Eosinophilic cytoplasm with keratin bridges between atypical cells
• Typically lacks atypical parakeratosis, and lesions often show epidermal hyperplasia that can resemble fibroepithelioma of Pinkus or rarely syringofibroadenoma	• Atypical parakeratosis is a common finding
• No significant squamous atypia	• Squamous atypia is present
IHC:	IHC:
• Primary EMPD tends to be positive for CEA, EMA, low-molecular-weight keratins (CK7, CAM5.2)	• Typically positive for high-molecular-weight keratins (CK5/6, 34βE12), p63
• Secondary EMPD can show expression of CK20 if disease arose from an underlying colorectal or genitourinary primary	• Most (though not all) cases are negative for CK7 and CAM5.2
• GCDFP15 often positive	• Negative for GCDFP15

EMPD, extramammary Paget disease; *IHC*, immunohistochemistry.

TABLE 13.8

Histologic Features of Extramammary Paget Disease Versus Melanoma *In Situ*

Extramammary Paget Disease	Melanoma *In Situ*
• Pale, vacuolated cytoplasm	• Gray to amphiphilic cytoplasm, sometimes with dusty melanin pigment
• The majority of cells are situated slightly above the dermal-epidermal junction, often with an "eyeliner" sign of normal basal layer keratinocytes just below neoplastic cells	• The majority of cells are present at the dermal-epidermal junction with no "eyeliner" sign
• Nuclei most commonly contain vesicular chromatin	• Chromatin is often hyperchromatic with prominent nucleoli
• Glandular differentiation sometimes present	• Glandular differentiation not seen
IHC:	IHC:
• Primary EMPD tends to be positive for CEA, EMA, low-molecular-weight keratins (CK7, CAM5.2)	• Positive for S100, SOX-10, Melan-A, and HMB45
• Secondary EMPD can show expression of CK20 if from a colorectal or genitourinary primary	• Negative for cytokeratins, GATA3, and GCDFP15
• GATA3 and GCDFP15 often positive	

EMPD, extramammary Paget disease; *IHC*, immunohistochemistry.

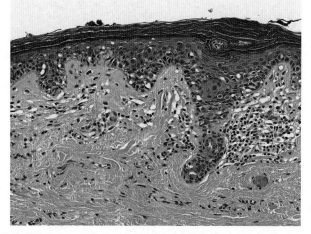

FIG. 13.18

Melanoma *in situ* of the vulva. Atypical single melanocytes with hyperchromatic chromatin and demonstrating prominent pagetoid spread. Immunohistochemistry for SOX-10 or Melan-A can be used to confirm the diagnosis.

DESMOPLASTIC MELANOMA

DIFFERENTIAL DIAGNOSES: SCAR, NEUROFIBROMA

Clinical Features

Desmoplastic melanoma (DM) typically occurs on sun-damaged skin of elderly patients, most commonly the head and neck region. It is most commonly associated with lentigo maligna–type melanoma (approximately 75% of cases); however, DM can also be found associated with superficial spreading type and acral lentiginous melanoma. DM has also been described at mucosal sites.

Pathologic Features

GROSS FINDINGS

A range of gross appearances can be observed for DM. A pigmented plaque with dermal induration is common; however, lesions may also present as a dermal nodule resembling a cyst. DM is usually seen in a shave biopsy specimen.

MICROSCOPIC FINDINGS

The histopathologic features of DM can be notoriously subtle. Histologic sections show a dermal proliferation of bland spindled cells in a collagenous background, classically with a patchy lymphoid infiltrate (Fig. 13.19A). Cellularity is typically low, in contrast to spindle cell melanoma. The epidermis often contains an atypical junctional component diagnostic of MIS (Fig. 13.19B); however, solely intradermal DMs have been described, which either represent primary

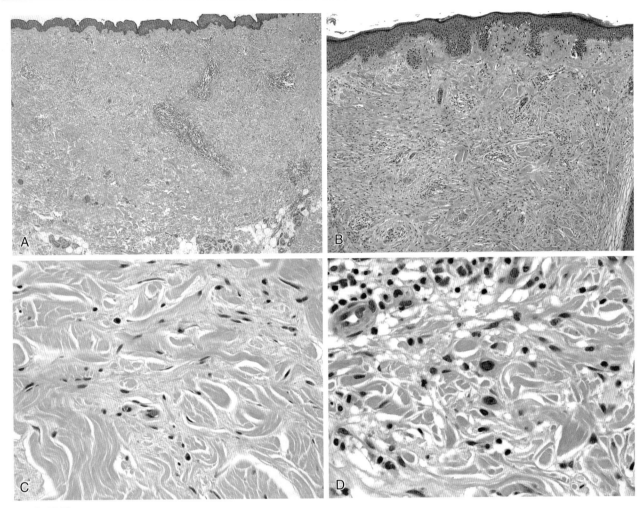

FIG. 13.19

Low-power view of desmoplastic melanoma (DM) showing a characteristic patchy lymphoid infiltrate (**A**). An atypical nested and lentiginous junctional melanocytic proliferation is seen over a dermal proliferation of spindle cells arranged in a storiform appearance within a collagenous stroma (**B**). This tumor demonstrates Schwannian cytomorphology with bland spindle cells containing wavy, hyperchromatic nuclei. Scattered mast cells can be seen in the background (**C**). Upon close inspection, many cases of DM reveal occasional highly atypical cells with enlarged nuclei and prominent nucleoli (**D**).

dermal lesions or tumors in which the junctional component has entirely regressed. Local and metastatic recurrences also often contain only a dermal component. The low-power impression of involved dermis often gives an impression that the normal collagenous architecture is somehow disrupted, which can increase suspicion. Tumor cells may be arranged in fascicles or in a storiform configuration. Perineural invasion is a common feature, and lymphovascular invasion may also infrequently be observed.

Cytologically, tumor cells can show considerable variation, and can resemble Schwannian forms with curved hyperchromatic nuclei (Fig. 13.19C). Cells with eosinophilic cytoplasm with elongated nuclei, resembling normal fibroblasts, can also be seen, in addition to forms with basophilic cytoplasm and large, irregular and hyperchromatic nuclei. Upon close inspection, highly atypical forms with prominent nucleoli can often be seen (Fig. 13.19D), which can increase suspicion for the diag-

nosis. Additionally, occasional mitoses can commonly be observed; however, brisk mitotic activity is usually not a feature. DM often penetrates deep into the skin and subcutis and can show a prominent myxoid background (Fig. 13.20A). There may be invasion of the subcutaneous tissue or even underlying skeletal muscle or other deep structures. DM can and often does exist with other cytologic variants of invasive melanoma such as epithelioid or spindle cell invasive melanoma. Tumors that contain greater than 90% DM within the invasive component are often referred to as "pure desmoplastic" melanomas.

Ancillary Studies

IMMUNOHISTOCHEMISTRY

SOX10 and S100 protein are typically expressed diffusely throughout the tumor (Fig. 13.20B and C); however,

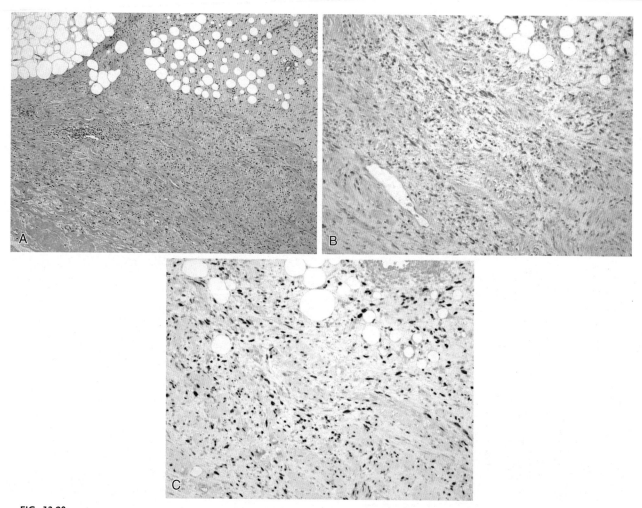

FIG. 13.20

This tumor, which shows a prominent myxoid stroma, is seen extending deep into the subcutaneous tissue (**A**). Tumor cells are strongly and diffusely for S100 protein (**B**) and SOX-10 (**C**).

expression of specific melanocytic markers such as Melan-A and HMB-45 is typically absent. Immunohistochemistry for p16 can be useful; however, as a minority of melanomas harbor homozygous loss of the *CDKN2A* locus, staining for p16 has limited sensitivity, including in DM. A number of additional markers have been employed to distinguish DM from histologic mimics, including p53, which has been shown to be expressed in DM, as well as CD34 (see Differential Diagnosis section later). PRAME, a newer immunohistochemical marker that stains many melanomas, is unfortunately expressed only in a minority of DMs.

MOLECULAR STUDIES

Aberrations involving the various components of the MAPK and PI3K pathways are most common; however, *BRAF* and *NRAS* mutations, commonly found in conventional melanomas, are infrequent. Generally, DM has a much higher mutational burden than other variants of melanoma (approximately tenfold). A UV signature is characteristic. Mutations in *NF1*, a protein

involved in the MAPK pathway, are a common feature of DMs and are found in greater than 90% of tumors.

Differential Diagnosis

Definitive diagnosis can be challenging when presented with a small biopsy or a specimen lacking a sufficiently atypical junctional melanocytic proliferation to enable designation as MIS. Scar tissue can closely resemble DM, as activated fibroblasts within scar often grow in a fascicular arrangement. However, scar typically shows parallel orientation of collagen fibers to the epidermis, in contrast to the haphazard arrangement characteristic of DM (Fig. 13.21A). Vertically oriented blood vessels are another common finding in scars. Adnexal structures are often absent. Additionally, if early in the repair process, granulation tissue may be present. Upon close inspection, the highly atypical cells seen in DM, such as those seen in Fig. 13.19D, are not apparent, and the predominant cell type is the activated fibroblast that shows fine chro-

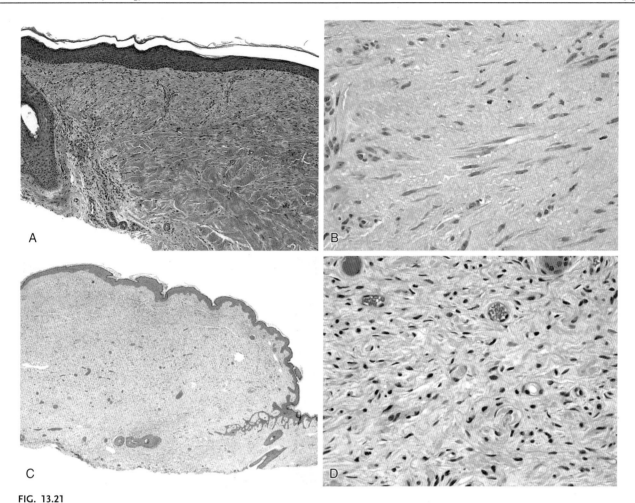

FIG. 13.21

Low-power image of a dermal scar showing parallel orientation of collagen fibers to the overlying epidermis with vertically oriented vessels present (**A**). Note the lack of adnexal structures within the scarred area. High-power image showing activated fibroblasts: uniform bland spindle cells with vesicular chromatin and punctate nucleoli within a collagenous background (**B**). Low-power image of a neurofibroma revealing a polypoid appearance (**C**). High-power image demonstrating a polymorphous population of bland spindle cells ranging from somewhat plump but with banal cytologic features to slender with wavy, hyperchromatic nuclei (**D**). Numerous mast cells can be seen in the background.

matin, regular nuclear outlines, and small nucleoli (Fig. 13.21B and Table 13.9). The use of immunohistochemistry for S100 and SOX10 can be misleading, as resident dendritic cells, which are often present in increased numbers in scar tissue, can express S100 protein as well as SOX10. Although sometimes difficult for a pathologist to elicit, particularly in the setting of consultative practice, a clinical history of a procedure at the site can be helpful in establishing a diagnosis of scar.

DM may also be mistaken for a neurotized nevus or neurofibroma, particularly if the tumor shows Schwannian cytomorphology. Additionally, neurofibroma can show ancient change with hyperchromatic, smudgy chromatin, which can be misinterpreted as atypia. Neurofibromas are often polypoid in appearance, in contrast to the plaque-like or architecture of DM (Fig. 13.21C). Mast cells, which commonly colonize neurofibromas (Fig. 13.21D), may also be present in DM (see Fig. 13.19C). At high power, neurofibromas reveal a polymorphous population of bland spindle cells ranging from somewhat plump but with banal cytologic features to slen-

der with wavy, hyperchromatic nuclei. Numerous mast cells can be seen in the background. Thickened collagen fibers that resemble shredded carrot are a common feature of neurofibromas but are not present in all cases, particularly in dermal-based tumors. S100 and SOX10 are of little value in distinguishing DM from neurofibroma, as both entities strongly express both markers. However, other immunohistochemical stains may be helpful in resolving this differential diagnosis. These include p53, which has been shown to be frequently overexpressed in DM but not in neurofibroma. Additionally, CD34 characteristically shows a diffuse "fingerprint" pattern in most neurofibromas, which is usually not seen in DM (Table 13.10). In some cases, DM can be confused with dermatofibrosarcoma protuberans (DFSP) or dermatofibroma, particularly in biopsies lacking an atypical junctional component. Malignant peripheral nerve sheath tumor (MPNST) is another potential histologic mimic; however, MPNST typically shows only multifocal and weak positivity for S100 protein and SOX10 when present.

TABLE 13.9
Histologic Features of Desmoplastic Melanoma Versus Scar

Desmoplastic Melanoma	Scar
• Patchy lymphoid infiltrate at low power	• Infiltrate often contains numerous histiocytes and multinucleated giant cells
• Perturbation of the normal collagen pattern with random orientation	• Collagen fibers are often arranged parallel to the overlying epidermis with vertically oriented blood vessels
• An atypical junctional melanocytic component can often be demonstrated and will usually show confluent growth and pagetoid spread	• Reactive junctional melanocytic hyperplasia can occur over and around scars but does not show confluent growth or pagetoid spread
• Upon close scrutiny, highly atypical cells with prominent nucleoli as well as dermal mitoses can usually be found	• Composed of bland fibroblasts that can have an activated appearance with regular nuclear outlines, vesicular chromatin, and small nucleoli
• Adnexal structures usually intact	• Adnexal structures usually absent or distorted

TABLE 13.10
Histologic Features of Desmoplastic Melanoma Versus Neurofibroma

Desmoplastic Melanoma	Neurofibroma
• Usually a flat lesion or subtle plaque, often with an irregular pigmented macule	• Often polypoid
• Perturbation of the normal collagen pattern with prominent desmoplasia	• "Carrot shred" collagen sometimes seen
• Patchy lymphoid infiltrate at low power	• Typically no significant inflammatory infiltrate present, unless traumatized
• Upon close scrutiny, highly atypical cells with prominent nucleoli as well as occasional dermal mitoses can usually be found	• Dermal proliferation of bland spindle cells with wavy, hyperchromatic nuclei; however, cells can show senescent changes with smudgy nuclear hyperchromasia
• An atypical junctional melanocytic component can often be demonstrated and will usually show confluent growth and pagetoid spread	• No atypical junctional melanocytic hyperplasia, unless on sun-damaged skin (solar melanocytosis can be present)

Prognosis and Therapy

Surgical management is the mainstay of treatment. As many tumors present at a locally advanced stage, margin control can be particularly challenging. Local recurrences are frequent. If a lesion is unable to be cleared by excision, radiation therapy can be used as an adjunctive treatment. Sentinel lymph node biopsy is typically performed in melanomas greater than 1.0 mm in depth; however, tumors with a pure desmoplastic invasive component have a lower chance of giving rise to regional lymph node involvement.

DESMOPLASTIC MELANOMA – DISEASE FACT SHEET

Definition
▸▸ A histologic variant of melanoma composed of bland spindle cells in a collagenous stroma

Incidence and Location
▸▸ Uncommon
▸▸ Most commonly occurs on the head and neck in association with lentigo maligna melanoma

Age Distribution
▸▸ Older adults

Clinical Features
▸▸ Most commonly presents as a pigmented macule or plaque on sun-damaged skin with dermal induration

Prognosis and Therapy
▸▸ Surgery is the mainstay of treatment
▸▸ Sentinel lymph node biopsy is often performed for melanomas of >1.0 mm thickness; however, pure desmoplastic melanomas tend not to metastasize to lymph nodes
▸▸ Radiation can be used as an adjunctive treatment for local control

DESMOPLASTIC MELANOMA – PATHOLOGIC FEATURES

Gross Findings
▸▸ Dermal plaque associated with an irregularly shaped pigmented macule
▸▸ Dermal nodule or plaque on sun-damaged skin

Microscopic Findings
▸▸ Patchy lymphocytic infiltrate with disrupted collagen at low magnification
▸▸ Collagenous to myxoid stroma
▸▸ Fascicles or storiform arrangement of bland spindled cells that can resemble Schwann cells or normal fibroblasts
▸▸ Highly atypical cells with prominent nucleoli as well as occasional mitoses can usually be found at high power

Pathologic Differential Diagnoses
▸▸ Scar
▸▸ Neurofibroma
▸▸ Dermatofibroma
▸▸ Dermatofibrosarcoma protuberans
▸▸ Malignant peripheral nerve sheath tumor

SPITZ NEVUS

DIFFERENTIAL DIAGNOSES: ATPYICAL SPITZ TUMOR, SPITZOID MELANOMA

Clinical Features

Spitz nevi represent 1% to 2% of all biopsied nevi. Spitz nevi usually present in younger individuals and are rare after the fourth decade of life. Clinically, Spitz nevi are 6 to 8 mm in diameter, circumscribed, and symmetric. The classic appearance is a pink papule or nodule; however, pigment can be observed. There is some predilection for the face in children and extremities in adults.

The pigmented spindle cell nevus of Reed is a variant of Spitz nevus that classically presents on the thigh of women in the third decade of life.

Rare presentations of Spitz nevus include agminated (grouped) and eruptive/disseminated. Some published reports of multiple Spitz nevi likely represent BAP1-inactivated melanocytic tumors (see later); other cases demonstrate lesions with classic morphology of Spitz nevi.

Pathologic Features

GROSS FINDINGS

Gross findings are similar to the clinical presentation: a well-circumscribed papule or nodule, with pigmentation that can vary from absent to dark.

MICROSCOPIC FINDINGS

Spitzoid melanocytes are large, spindled or epithelioid melanocytes with abundant cytoplasm and a prominent nucleolus (Fig. 13.22). The cytoplasm is lightly amphophilic in most cases but can be pigmented.

Spitz nevi can be junctional, compound, or dermal. At scanning magnification, there is circumscription and symmetry (see Fig. 13.22A). The junctional component is accompanied by epidermal hyperplasia, most prominent in the center of the nevus. Junctional nests are large and interanastomosing, with prominent clefting at the edges of nests (Fig. 13.22B). Melanocytes may display vertical orientation in nests ("raining down"). Single intraepidermal melanocytes are more frequently encountered than in conventional nevi. Both nests and single melanocytes can display transepithelial elimination resembling high-level pagetoid scatter. Kamino bodies (intraepidermal round pink concretions proposed to be derived from basement membrane material) are often present (see Fig. 13.22B).

The dermal component of Spitz nevi consists of nests and single cells. There is a decrease in cell size with descent, although small cells at the base can retain nucleoli and a minimal amount of cytoplasm. Superficial dermal mitoses can be encountered but should not be numerous. Expansile dermal growth is absent.

Variant morphologies exist. Desmoplastic Spitz nevus consists of melanocytes dispersed in a sclerotic stroma (see Fig. 13.22C). In the pigmented spindle cell nevus of Reed, heavily pigmented spindled melanocytes are present in junctional nests (see Fig. 13.22D). Angiomatoid Spitz nevus is a desmoplastic Spitz variant with prominent vasculature. Pagetoid Spitz nevus displays large pagetoid cells with minimal nesting; unlike MIS, there is limited to absent cytologic atypia. Combined Spitz nevi demonstrate morphologic features of Spitz nevus and another nevus type, such as ordinary, dysplastic, or blue nevi. The category of plexiform Spitz nevus has been proposed to describe nevi with ALK or ROS1 fusions (described later) (see Fig. 13.22E and F).

Ancillary Studies

IMMUNOHISTOCHEMISTRY

Spitz nevi express standard melanocytic markers including Melan-A, S100, and SOX10. Expression of the tumor suppressor p16 is retained in all but rare cases. Dermal proliferative index (Ki-67) is low. HMB45 expression is stratified. PRAME overexpression is uncommon but has been described. ALK can be detected by high-sensitivity immunohistochemistry in lesions bearing the ALK fusion (see Fig. 13.22F).

MOLECULAR STUDIES

Amplification of the HRAS gene (chromosome 11p) is an oncogenic driver in 20% of Spitz nevi, especially desmoplastic Spitz. Activating HRAS mutation can occur in association with amplification or as an isolated finding. Chromosome 7q is a rare site of recurrent copy gain. Tetraploidy occurs in 5% to 10%. Heterozygous loss of chromosome 9p21 (CDKN2A) is rare, and homozygous loss is not observed. BRAF V600E mutations are absent.

Kinase fusions occur in some Spitz nevi, atypical Spitz tumors, and spitzoid melanoma. ALK and ROS1 fusions are associated with plexiform growth pattern. Pigmented spindle cell nevi of Reed frequently harbor NTRK3 and MYO5A fusions. Numerous other kinase genes have also been implicated in oncogenic fusions in spitzoid neoplasms.

Melanocytic tumors with BAP1 loss are discussed under Differential Diagnosis.

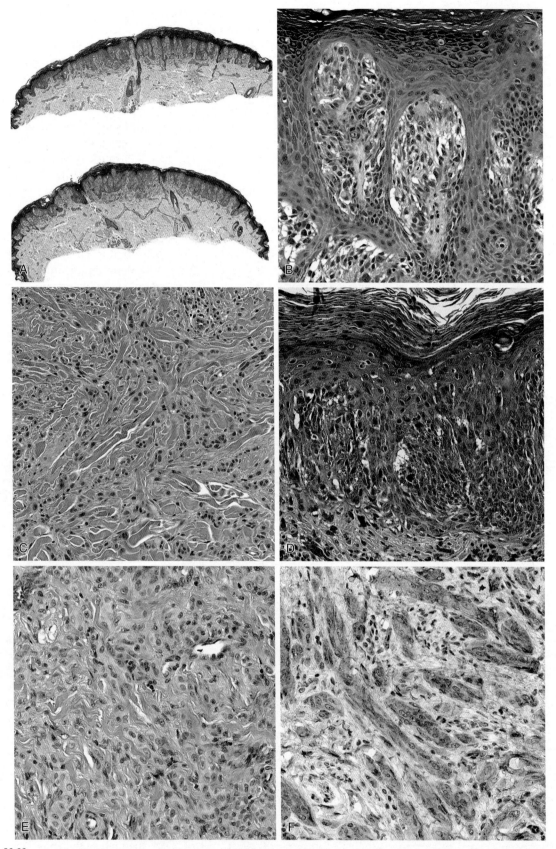

FIG. 13.22

Spitz nevus with circumscription, symmetry, and associated epidermal acanthosis (**A**). Spitz nevus with large junctional nests displaying cleft-ing and Kamino bodies (**B**). Desmoplastic Spitz nevus with characteristic sclerotic stroma (**C**). Pigmented spindle cell nevus of Reed (**D**). Plexiform growth associated with ALK rearrangement (**E**). ALK immunohistochemical expression associated with ALK rearrangement (**F**).

Differential Diagnosis

Spitzoid melanocytic neoplasms occupy a spectrum including benign (Spitz nevi), borderline, and malignant (spitzoid melanoma/malignant Spitz tumor) forms. The boundaries between these categories are in flux, as morphologic and molecular investigations advance knowledge regarding which lesions are predicted to behave in an indolent or aggressive manner.

Atypical Spitz tumors are borderline tumors exhibiting dermal growth that deviates significantly from a nevus, especially expansile growth without maturation (Fig. 13.23A and B; Table 13.11). Constituent melanocytes may be epithelioid or spindled (see Fig. 13.23B). Mitoses might be readily identifiable. The junctional

TABLE 13.11

Histologic Features of Spitz Nevus Versus Atypical Spitz Tumor

Spitz Nevus	Atypical Spitz Tumor
Size usually <6 mm	Size may be >10 mm
Circumscribed, symmetric	Usually symmetric and circumscribed, but may have small nests extending away from main tumor laterally or at base
No ulceration	May be ulcerated
Enlarged epithelioid or spindled cells with abundant amphophilic cytoplasm, prominent nucleoli	Enlarged epithelioid or spindled cells with abundant amphophilic cytoplasm, prominent nucleoli
Junctional, dermal, or compound	Dermal or compound
Regular nuclear membrane contours; mild variability in nuclear size; hyperchromasia mild or absent	May have atypia (irregular nuclear membrane contours, pleomorphism, hyperchromasia)
Large junctional nests with peripheral clefting; minor component of single melanocytes (for nevi with a junctional component)	Junctional component may be similar to Spitz nevi, or display small irregular nests and single-unit basal layer melanocytes over the dome of the dermal proliferation
Pagetoid scatter not prominent (exception: pagetoid Spitz nevus)	Pagetoid scatter not prominent in most cases; no melanoma in situ
Dermal growth patterns: nests or single cells; low dermal cellularity	Dermal growth patterns: nested, expansile/sheet-like, fascicular, plexiform; high dermal cellularity
Dermal mitoses more common than in ordinary nevi, but infrequent and superficial	Dermal mitoses may be numerous Deep or peripheral/marginal mitoses are a feature of high-risk tumors
Dermal maturation with diminished cell size toward base; small cells at base may retain cytoplasm and nucleoli, unlike ordinary nevi	Dermal maturation may be present (similar to Spitz nevus) or absent
IHC: p16: retained Low dermal proliferative index BRAF-V600E: negative BAP1: retained	IHC: p16: loss (minority) May have elevated dermal proliferative index BRAF-V600E: positive (in BAPoma) BAP1: lost (in BAPoma)

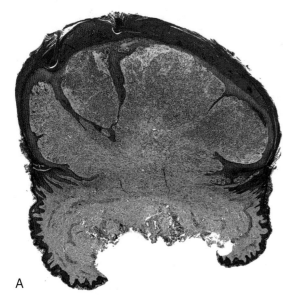

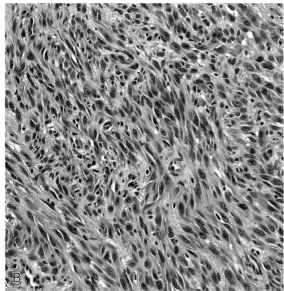

FIG. 13.23

Atypical Spitz tumor shows expansile dermal growth (**A**). Enlarged spindled cells displaying fascicular growth in hypercellular nodules (**B**).

component may be absent, nested, or disorganized. MIS should not be present. Atypical Spitz tumors can display an indolent or aggressive course. Concerning findings include numerous mitoses, deep/peripheral or atypical mitoses, high-grade cytologic atypia, asymmetry, or ulceration. Molecular studies are often pursued for risk stratification (see later).

Markedly atypical spitzoid proliferations that lack deep dermal growth, raising a differential diagnosis with MIS or thin invasive melanoma, also occur.

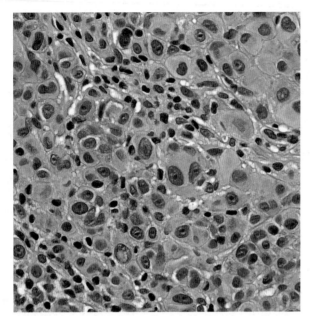

FIG. 13.24

Epithelioid atypical melanocytes in an atypical spitzoid neoplasm associated with BAP1 loss. An ordinary nevus component is often present (not shown).

Melanocytic tumors with inactivation of the *BAP1* gene display morphologic overlap with Spitz neoplasms and were historically grouped among combined nevi (Spitz and ordinary) or atypical Spitz tumors. These are now designated as a distinct class of melanocytic tumor, with proposed names including Wiesner nevus, melanocytic BAP1-inactivated intradermal tumor, BAPoma, or epithelioid atypical Spitz tumor. These tumors can arise sporadically or in association with germline *BAP1* mutation. The classic appearance is a biphenotypic dermal tumor, with an ordinary dermal nevus that transitions to nodules of enlarged atypical epithelioid cells accompanied by inflammation (Fig. 13.24). Both components label for BRAF V600E, whereas BAP1 expression is retained in the ordinary component and lost in the epithelioid component. It has been proposed that a significant junctional component favors a syndromic tumor over a sporadic tumor. Some lesions contain only epithelioid melanocytes and lack the ordinary component. In some cases, there is increased mitotic activity, expansile growth, and/or cytologic atypia, warranting classification as a borderline tumor. Frankly malignant features can be identified, and warrant designation as melanoma.

Spitzoid melanomas are melanomas that display some cytologic and/or architectural features of Spitz nevus (Fig. 13.25A and B; Table 13.12). As such, this is a heterogeneous category, including malignant tumors with molecular similarity to other spitzoid neoplasms (such as kinase fusions), as well as conventional melanoma with incidental morphologic similarity to Spitz nevi. Alternative designations (malignant Spitz tumor,

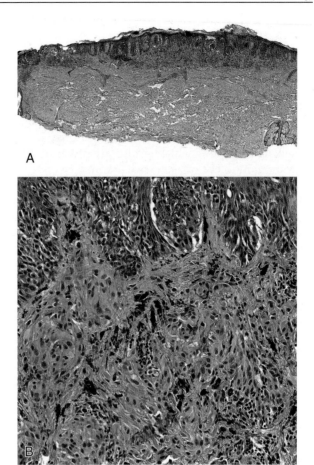

FIG. 13.25

A spitzoid melanoma shows asymmetry on scanning magnification, combined with spitzoid architectural features including clefting around large junctional nests (**A**). Severe cytologic atypia and poor nesting (**B**).

TABLE 13.12

Histologic Features of Spitz Nevus Versus Spitzoid Melanoma

Spitz Nevus	Spitzoid Melanoma (Malignant Spitz Tumor)
Enlarged epithelioid or spindled cells with abundant amphophilic cytoplasm, prominent nucleoli	Enlarged epithelioid or spindled cells with abundant amphophilic cytoplasm, prominent nucleoli
Regular nuclear membrane contours; mild variability in nuclear size; hyperchromasia mild or absent	Irregular nuclear membrane contours, marked pleomorphism, prominent hyperchromasia
Size usually <6 mm	Size may be >10 mm
Circumscribed, symmetric	May be asymmetric, poorly circumscribed
No ulceration	May be ulcerated
Large junctional nests with peripheral clefting; minor component of single melanocytes (for nevi with a junctional component)	Predominance of single melanocytes over nests; may have a component of large nests with clefting

Continued

TABLE 13.12
Histologic Features of Spitz Nevus versus Spitzoid Melanoma—cont'd

Spitz Nevus	Spitzoid Melanoma (Malignant Spitz Tumor)
Upward ascent of nests and few individual melanocytes (exception: pagetoid Spitz nevus)	High-level pagetoid scatter of individual melanocytes
Kamino bodies may occur	Kamino bodies rare but have been reported
Dermal mitoses more common than in ordinary nevi, but infrequent and superficial	Dermal mitoses may be numerous, atypical, deep
Dermal growth patterns: nests or single cells; low dermal cellularity	Dermal growth patterns: nested, expansile/sheet-like; high dermal cellularity
Dermal maturation with diminished cell size toward base; small cells at base may retain cytoplasm and nucleoli	Dermal maturation absent, although there may be decreased cell size at base due to pseudomaturation
Dermal inflammation often more prominent than ordinary nevi; halo phenomenon is rare	May have changes of inflammatory regression
IHC: p16: no diffuse loss Ki-67: low dermal proliferative index HMB45: stratified (superficial staining with deep loss) BRAF-V600E: negative	IHC: p16: loss (minority) Ki-67: may have elevated dermal proliferative index HMB45: variable (stratified, lost, or overexpressed) BRAF-V600E: positive or negative

SPITZ NEVUS – DISEASE FACT SHEET

Definition
- ▸▸ Nevus with characteristic cytomorphologic and architectural features

Incidence
- ▸▸ Approximately 1%–2% of all biopsied nevi

Age Distribution
- ▸▸ Average age 21 years; often in childhood; most are in patients <30 years

Clinical Features
- ▸▸ 6–8 mm in diameter, circumscribed, and symmetric
- ▸▸ Papule or nodule; pink, lightly pigmented, or darkly pigmented
- ▸▸ Anatomic site is variable (more frequently on face in children, and extremities in adults)

Prognosis and Therapy
- ▸▸ Managed by removal
- ▸▸ Benign course

SPITZ NEVUS – PATHOLOGIC FEATURES

Gross Findings
- ▸▸ Circumscribed papule with variable pigmentation

Microscopic Findings
- ▸▸ Spitzoid morphology: large spindled or epithelioid melanocytes with light-staining cytoplasm, large nucleus, prominent nucleolus
- ▸▸ Scanning: circumscribed, symmetric
- ▸▸ Junctional architecture: large interanastomosing nests with peripheral clefting; increased single melanocytes; transepithelial elimination of nests and single melanocytes; Kamino bodies
- ▸▸ Dermal architecture: altered maturation with retained cytoplasm and nucleoli at base; may be desmoplastic/sclerotic stroma; lacks expansile/sheet-like growth or high proliferative activity

Pathologic Differential Diagnoses
- ▸▸ Atypical Spitz tumor, spitzoid melanoma

Spitz melanoma) imply more specific similarity to Spitz nevi.

Molecular features associated with aggressive course in spitzoid neoplasms, supporting classification as melanoma, include homozygous 9p21 deletion affecting the *CDKN2A* tumor suppressor, *TERT* promoter mutation, and numerous (>3) copy number aberrations. However, although there is a role for molecular analysis in borderline tumors, these techniques are generally unnecessary for predicting the clinical course of overtly benign Spitz nevi.

Prognosis and Therapy

Complete removal is the usual management for Spitz nevi. The risk of malignant progression for Spitz nevi is low to absent.

NEVOID MELANOMA

DIFFERENTIAL DIAGNOSIS: MELANOCYTIC NEVUS

Clinical Features

Nevoid melanoma is a melanoma subtype that is often difficult to recognize clinically. It may present as an exophytic papillomatous lesion simulating a polypoid intradermal nevus, or as a largely flat or shallow dome-shaped papule. The mean age of patients is between fifth and sixth decades, although a wide age range may be affected. The trunk and extremities are the most common sites, except the exophytic papillomatous lesions of which up to 40% occur on the head.

Pathologic Features

GROSS FINDINGS

The majority of nevoid melanomas are shallow dome-shaped lesions visible on the skin surface. A small subset of cases displays an exophytic, papillomatous and polypoid configuration with the epicenter protruding above the skin surface. Most lesions are pigmented, and more than one color may be present. The borders of the lesions are usually well defined.

MICROSCOPIC FINDINGS

Lesions with an exophytic papillomatous configuration are characterized by a predominantly intradermal melanocytic proliferation, in which the dermal melanocytes are often compartmentalized into lobules by thin and elongated rete ridges (Fig. 13.26A and B). Other lesions commonly comprise an atypical junctional component similar to superficial spreading MIS, and a dermal component with a nested growth pattern (Fig. 13.27A–C). Some of the dermal nests may be abnormally large, consisting of >100 cells. Regardless of the overall configuration, the melanoma cells are relatively small and display "pseudomaturation," that is, diminution in nest size and cell size with depth (see Figs. 13.26C and 13.27D). Although these cells appear small and uniform, close inspection would reveal subtle nuclear pleomorphism, irregularities, and hyperchromasia (Fig. 13.27E). Nucleoli may be visible even in the deepest and smallest melanocytes. Mitoses are often present and are more frequent in the exophytic papillomatous lesions (see Fig. 13.27E).

Ancillary Studies

IMMUNOHISTOCHEMISTRY

A multitude of immunohistochemical stains may be helpful in confirming the diagnosis of nevoid melanoma. In benign ordinary nevi, HMB45 typically shows a stratified staining pattern: strong staining of the junctional melanocytes, and graded (progressively weaker to absent) staining in the superficial to deep dermal melanocytes. Deviation from this stratified pattern, such as patchy or stronger HMB45 staining in deeper nests, would be concerning for melanoma (Fig. 13.28A). Ki-67 proliferation index of the dermal melanocytes, best appreciated when coupled with MART1 staining, is also informative in that it is usually elevated (>1%) in nevoid melanoma (Fig. 13.28B). Loss of p16 expression in a diffuse or patchy/zonal pattern may be indicative of homozygous loss of *CDKN2A* (a tumor suppressor gene) which is worrisome for melanoma (Fig. 13.28C). PRAME immunostain has been increasingly used in distinguishing melanoma from nevus. Diffuse and strong PRAME expression would support a diagnosis of melanoma (Fig. 13.28D).

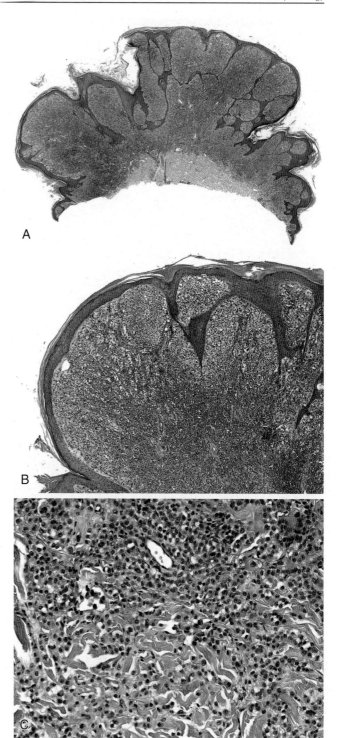

FIG. 13.26

A nevoid melanoma with an exophytic papillary silhouette. Closely packed dermal nests are compartmentalized into lobules by elongated, thin rete ridges (**A**). There is diminution in nest size and cell size with depth, imparting the appearance of maturation at low and medium magnifications (**B**). However, close inspection reveals that the deepest melanocytes remain to be small epithelioid with moderate amount of cytoplasm and visible nucleoli, consistent with "pseudomaturation." (**C**).

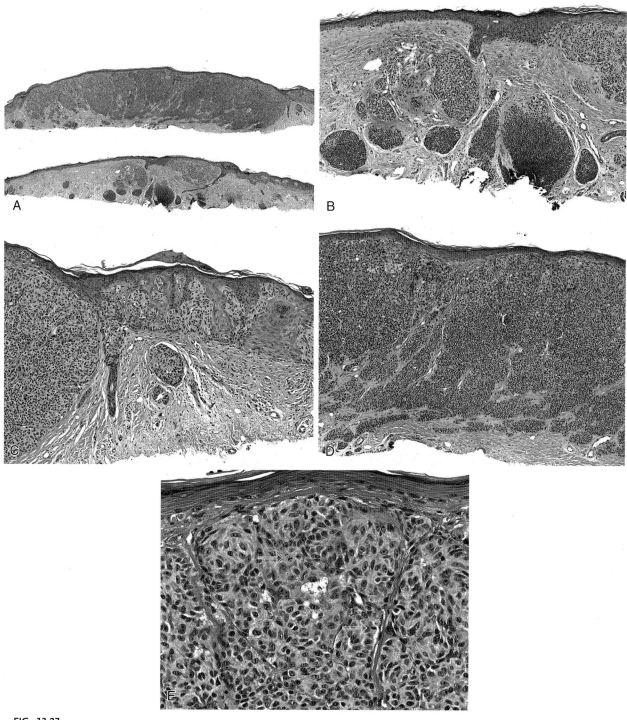

FIG. 13.27

This nevoid melanoma demonstrates a plaque-like architecture (**A**). The deepest melanocytes remain in nests despite diminution in cell size (**B**). Melanoma *in situ* is present at the periphery of this lesion (**C**). The dermal nests are abnormally large and fused (**D**). Two mitoses are identified in this field *(arrows)*.

MOLECULAR STUDIES

Fluorescence *in situ* hybridization (FISH) using probes that target chromosomes 6p25 (*RREB1*), 6q23 (*MYB*), 8q24 (*MYC*), 9p21 (*CDKN2A*), and 11q13 (*CCND1*) demonstrates aberrations in the majority of nevoid melanomas. The largest study to date (Yelamos et al.) reported a sensitivity of 74%. The most frequent abnormality was gain of *RREB1* at 6p25 (49%), although aberrancy at any of the above loci may be seen in nevoid melanoma. Array comparative genomic hybridization (aCGH) also appears highly sensitive for nevoid melanoma. Mutational analyses suggest frequent *NRAS* activating mutation and *TERT* promoter mutation.

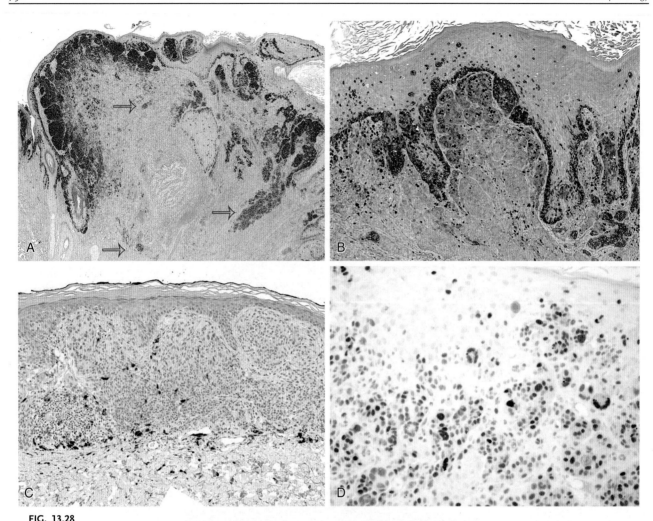

FIG. 13.28

Immunohistochemical findings in nevoid melanoma. HMB45 shows a non-stratified staining pattern, with patchy areas of staining beyond the superficial aspect *(arrows)* (**A**). Ki-67/MART1 shows a high Ki-67 proliferation index *(brown)* in the superficial dermal nests (**B**). Expression for p16 is lost in this nevoid melanoma (**C**). PRAME is diffusely positive in the neoplastic melanocytes (**D**).

Differential Diagnosis

Because nevoid melanoma by definition mimics melanocytic nevus, its distinction from a benign nevus is notoriously challenging (Table 13.13). Unlike nevoid melanoma which is often asymmetric, a benign nevus should demonstrate a symmetric silhouette (Fig. 13.29A). The dermal nests in a nevus are evenly sized and separated by collagen fibers rather than being back-to-back. Expansile growth should be absent in a nevus. The dermal nests in a nevus should also display appropriate maturation with depth, in that the deepest melanocytes are small with scant cytoplasm, uniform condensed nuclei, and inconspicuous nucleoli (Fig. 13.29B). Mitoses are rare and, when present, are found in the upper portion of a nevus. Atypical mitoses should be absent. By immunohistochemistry, most benign nevi show nuclear Ki-67 staining in <1% of the dermal melanocytes. Immunostain for p16 typically reveals diffuse or

"checkerboard" staining throughout the lesion (Fig. 13.29C). As mentioned above, HMB45 staining should be stratified in an ordinary nevus. PRAME is negative in the majority of benign nevi (Fig. 13.29D). Melanocytic nevi commonly harbor *BRAF* mutation but lack other genetic abnormalities.

Prognosis and Therapy

Pathology report of a nevoid melanoma should at least include Breslow depth and presence/absence of ulceration for proper pathologic tumor staging. Thin melanomas (<1.0 mm in depth) are associated with better prognosis than intermediate and thick melanomas. All nevoid melanomas should be completely excised. Sentinel lymph node biopsy may be considered in tumors staged pT1b (≥0.8 mm in depth) and above due to increased risk for regional metastasis.

TABLE 13.13

Histologic Features of Nevoid Melanoma Versus Melanocytic Nevus

Nevoid Melanoma	Melanocytic Nevus
• Melanoma *in situ* may be present	• Absence of melanoma *in situ*
• Dermal melanocytic nests may be abnormally large and closely packed, often compartmentalized into lobules by elongated rete ridges	• Dermal melanocytic nests are evenly sized and separated by collagen fibers
• "Pseudomaturation" of dermal melanocytes	• Complete maturation of dermal melanocytes
• Increased mitotic/proliferative activity	• Mitoses are rare or absent; Ki-67 proliferation index is usually <1%
• HMB45 staining may be non-stratified	• Stratified HMB45 staining
• PRAME immunostain may be positive	• PRAME immunostain is negative
• FISH and aCGH commonly show copy number aberrations	• FISH and aCGH are negative
• Frequent *NRAS* activating mutation and *TERT* promoter mutation	• Commonly harbor *BRAF* mutation but lack *NRAS* and *TERT* promoter mutations

aCGH, Array comparative genomic hybridization; *FISH,* fluorescence *in situ* hybridization.

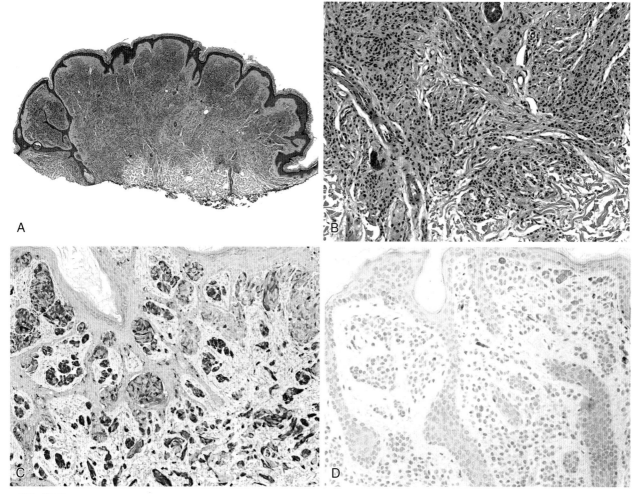

FIG. 13.29

An exophytic intradermal nevus demonstrates a symmetry silhouette without expansile growth or thinning of rete ridges (**A**). The melanocytes mature completely with depth, lacking cytologic atypia (**B**). Immunohistochemistry for p16 displays solid or "checkerboard" staining in all melanocytic nests (**C**). PRAME, a nuclear marker, is diffusely negative (**D**).

RECURRENT NEVUS PHENOMENON

DIFFERENTIAL DIAGNOSIS: MELANOMA

Clinical Features

Recurrent nevus phenomenon (RNP; also "persistent melanocytic nevus," "regenerating nevus," or "pseudomelanoma") occurs in the setting of benign nevi that have previously undergone incomplete removal, typically within 6 months from the initial procedure. The impetus to biopsy is clinically concerning repigmentation or otherwise atypical appearance (asymmetry, variable coloration, or irregular borders) at the site of a previously biopsied nevus. RNP can also occur at sites where nevi have been completely excised, suggesting regrowth from cutaneous adnexal structures or from adjacent epidermis. RNP has a slight female predominance and most commonly occurs in the third decade of life. The most common location is on the back, which could reflect the anatomic distribution of biopsied nevi.

Pathologic Features

GROSS FINDINGS

Typically, RNP presents as repigmentation at the site of a previously biopsied or incompletely excised nevus. Irregular shape and pigmentation lead to concern for melanoma, particularly if the previously biopsied nevus was classified as atypical or dysplastic. Background pallor is often present, representative of dermal scar, and may be interpreted clinically as regression. Pigment does not usually extend beyond the confines of the scar.

MICROSCOPIC FINDINGS

The previously biopsied nevus may be of a number of types, including ordinary (most common; can be classified as junctional, compound, or intradermal), dysplastic, congenital, blue, or rarely other histologic types such as Spitz nevi. Recurrent nevi usually have a symmetric appearance at low power. Characteristically, dermal scar is present with numerous pigmented macrophages and an overlying proliferation of junctional epithelioid melanocytes that can show near-confluent growth (Fig. 13.30A–C). Background lymphohistiocytic inflammation is often present. The junctional proliferation usually does not extend beyond the lateral confines of the underlying dermal scar. The rete ridges are typically effaced, as in Fig. 13.30, but a minority of cases (up to 15%) can show a retiform epidermis. Cytologic atypia can be present, depending on the degree of atypia of the previously incompletely excised nevus. High-level pagetoid spread and confluent growth are typically not features but can be present in a minority of cases, leading to considerable diagnostic overlap with MIS. Significant cytologic atypia can also be seen in the recurrent dermal component, if present, with rare mitotic activity. Background intradermal or junctional nevus can often be seen at the periphery of the lesion outside of the central scar. The residual melanocytes show features typical of the previously incompletely removed nevus (such as in Fig. 13.30D); however, rare normal mitoses and cytologic atypia can be observed in the residual nevomelanocyte population as well within areas in close proximity to scar. Review of the previously excised lesion is warranted in such challenging cases showing histologic overlap with melanoma.

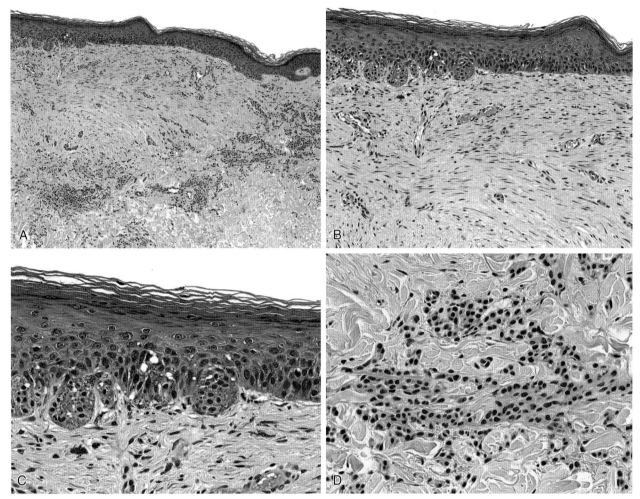

FIG. 13.30

Recurrent nevus phenomenon. Low-power image demonstrating an area of scar within the superficial dermis surrounded by an intradermal nevus (**A**). A junctional melanocytic proliferation can be seen in the overlying epidermis, and the rete ridges are effaced. Near-confluent growth of atypical melanocytes arranged in a nested and lentiginous configuration with abundant dusty cytoplasm but with small nuclei and without prominent pagetoid spread (**B**). Scar is seen in the dermis, characterized by activated fibroblasts and collagen fibers oriented parallel to the overlying epidermis, lymphocytic inflammation, and scattered pigment-laden macrophages. High-power view of the atypical junctional component showing mild to moderate cytologic atypia including nuclear hyperchromasia with near-confluent growth of melanocytes disposed in nests and as single cells (**C**). High-level pagetoid spread is not evident in this example, which is true in most cases. High-power image of residual intradermal nevomelanocytes showing bland nuclear characteristics without tumorigenic growth or conspicuous mitoses (**D**).

Ancillary Studies

IMMUNOHISTOCHEMISTRY

The use of immunohistochemical markers such as SOX10 will typically highlight a basally oriented melanocytic proliferation of melanocytes, usually without high-level pagetoid spread. A Ki-67 immunostain, most helpful when performed as part of a duplex protocol along with Melan-A/MART-1 to ensure exclusion of background inflammatory cells, will reveal a low proliferative index in dermal recurrent melanocytes. A p16 stain will reveal retention of expression. Prominent HMB45 expression is often observed in RNP and should not be a cause for concern.

MOLECULAR STUDIES

FISH using a multiprobe panel as well as aCGH can be used to exclude melanoma in difficult cases.

Differential Diagnosis

RNP can show a high degree of overlap with melanoma, especially in cases with late-stage regression consisting of extensive dermal fibrosis without the prominent inflammation characteristic of early changes of regression. Partial biopsies can also cause diagnostic confusion if both scar and atypical melanocytes extend to margin and/or residual benign nevus is not represented in histologic

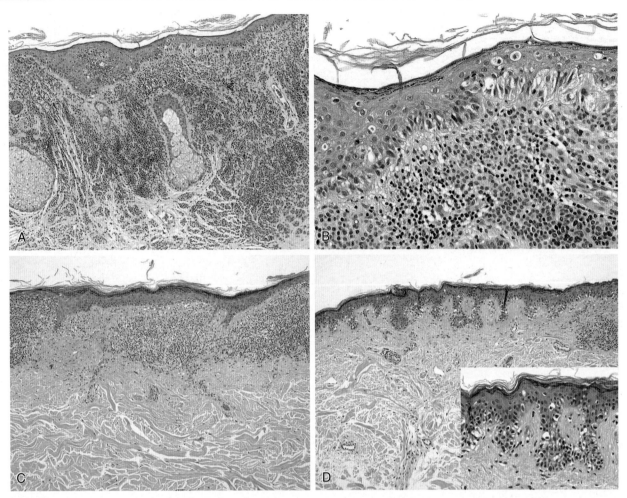

FIG. 13.31

Melanoma arising in association with a nevus. At low power, an atypical intradermal melanocytic proliferation can be seen arising over a benign-appearing intradermal nevus that demonstrates convincing histologic evidence of maturation with descent into the dermis (**A**). At high power, the junctional melanocytes display confluent growth, high-level pagetoid spread, and severe cytologic atypia with nuclear pleomorphism and abundant gray, dusty cytoplasm (**B**). Low-power image of an area of early to mid-stage regression within melanoma (**C**). Melanoma *in situ* extends beyond the lateral confines of the area of regression. Cytologic atypia and architectural disarray characteristic of melanoma *in situ* can be seen *(inset)* (**D**).

sections. In some cases, it is not possible to histologically reliably distinguish melanoma with regression from RNP. MIS can occur in association with an intradermal nevus (Fig. 13.31A). Additionally, melanoma that is incompletely excised can contain in the dermis an area of scarring, the atypical cells of malignant melanoma will generally extend beyond the confines of the scar. However, again, this determination can prove challenging in partial biopsies. In contrast to the morphologic features of RNP, the junctional component of melanoma often shows a higher degree of cytologic pleomorphism with prominent high-level pagetoid spread (Fig. 13.31B and Table 13.14). In cases of melanoma with regression, MIS will typically extend beyond the area of regression (Fig. 13.31C and D). Correlation with the clinical history, which can be difficult to elucidate if the patient has seen multiple providers, can confirm a prior biopsy at the site and help firmly establish a diagnosis. Review of the prior case to confirm benignity is often required and is the best discriminator in difficult cases.

Prognosis and Therapy

Complete excision of a recurrent nevus is curative.

RECURRENT NEVUS PHENOMENON – DISEASE FACT SHEET

Definition
▸▸ Atypical proliferation of melanocytes at the site of a previously incompletely removed benign or atypical nevus

Incidence and Location
▸▸ Uncommon, but may occur in any benign nevus that has been incompletely removed
▸▸ Most common site is the back, which may reflect the anatomic distribution of biopsied nevi

Age Distribution
▸▸ May occur in any age but tends to occur in younger patients (third decade)

TABLE 13.14

Histologic Features of Recurrent Nevus Phenomenon Versus Melanoma

Recurrent Nevus Phenomenon	Melanoma
• Symmetric at low power	• Asymmetry at low power
• Atypical melanocytic proliferation usually does not extend beyond the lateral confines of the scar	• Atypical melanocytic proliferation usually extends beyond lateral border of regression if present
• Effacement of rete ridges is commonly seen	• Effacement of rete ridges typically only seen in lentigo maligna melanoma or melanoma with late-stage (densely fibrotic) regression
• Usually mild to moderate cytologic atypia	• Severe cytologic atypia in many cases
• Low mitotic rate within dermis	• Often contains dermal mitoses
• Most cases do not show prominent pagetoid spread or confluent growth	• Prominent pagetoid spread and confluent growth are often features
• Prior specimen (from previous biopsy or excision) shows a benign or atypical nevus	• Prior specimen (from previous biopsy or excision) shows melanoma

RECURRENT NEVUS PHENOMENON – DISEASE FACT SHEET—cont'd

Clinical Features
▸▸ Slight female predominance
▸▸ Typically occurs within 6 months of the initial procedure
▸▸ Impetus to biopsy is repigmentation within the scar or otherwise atypical clinical appearance

Prognosis and Therapy
▸▸ Complete excision is curative

RECURRENT NEVUS PHENOMENON – PATHOLOGIC FEATURES

Gross Findings
▸▸ Atypical repigmentation at the site of a previously biopsied nevus, often with pigment irregularity and areas of pallor

Microscopic Findings
▸▸ Symmetric appearance at low power
▸▸ Atypical melanocytic proliferation confined to scar
▸▸ May be surrounded by background nevus resembling prior lesion that was incompletely removed
▸▸ Effacement of the rete ridges in most cases (minority of cases, up to 15%, show a retiform epidermis)
▸▸ Typically no high-level pagetoid spread or true confluent growth, but these features can be seen in some cases
▸▸ Review of the prior biopsy is crucial for difficult cases that resemble melanoma or are incompletely sampled with scar at margins

Pathologic Differential Diagnoses
▸▸ Melanoma, in particular cases with regression or recurrence after excision

NODAL NEVUS

DIFFERENTIAL DIAGNOSIS: NODAL METASTATIC MELANOMA

Clinical Features

Nodal melanocytic nevus is a histopathologic finding that is typically without clinical manifestation (lymphadenopathy). It is usually an incidental finding during examination of lymph nodes for metastatic carcinoma or melanoma. The involved lymph node may be found in the draining nodal basin of a congenital nevus, or of a melanoma occurring in association with a nevus, although such association is not always present. Nodal nevi are also not detected by imaging studies.

Pathologic Features

GROSS FINDINGS

Nodal nevi are typically small and only appreciable microscopically.

MICROSCOPIC FINDINGS

Most nodal nevi are confined to the nodal capsule, sometimes juxtaposed to or protruding into the lymphatic channels within the capsule (Fig. 13.32A). The nevus cells are small and uniform, with scant cytoplasm, bland nuclei, and inconspicuous nucleoli (Fig. 13.32B). Mitoses are absent. Occasional nodal nevi are more cellular, consisting of larger aggregates of more plump melanocytes expanding the nodal capsule. Although plump, these melanocytes remain uniform and resemble "type A" nevus cells in cutaneous ordinary nevi (Fig. 13.33A and B). Rarely, nodal blue nevus may be seen in which the lesional cells are spindle with hyperpigmented dendritic processes.

Nodal nevi may sometimes track along the nodal trabeculae. Nevus cells may be occasionally found in the nodal parenchyma, posing significant diagnostic challenge. Regardless of location, however, the cytomorphology of nevus cells should be bland, with scant cytoplasm, small nuclei, and inconspicuous nucleoli. When found in patients with history of melanoma, comparison of the cytologic features with those of the primary melanoma would be helpful in excluding a metastatic melanoma.

Ancillary Studies

IMMUNOHISTOCHEMISTRY

Numerous studies have examined the utility of different immunohistochemical stains in differentiating nodal

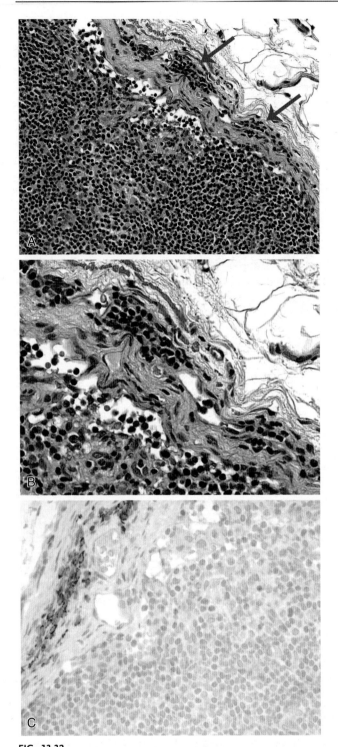

FIG. 13.32

A nodal nevus is confined to the capsule (**A**). The nevus cells are small and bland (**B**). PRAME/MART1 demonstrates red cytoplasmic staining for MART1 in these cells without concurrent brown nuclear PRAME staining (**C**).

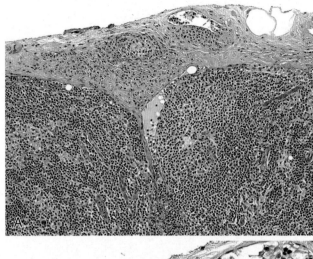

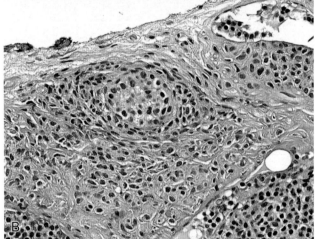

FIG. 13.33

Another nodal nevus is found adjacent to lymphatics in the nodal capsule (**A**). Some of these melanocytes are nested and display a plumper morphology resembling "type A" nevus cells; however, nuclear atypia and pleomorphism is absent (**B**).

nevus from nodal metastatic melanoma. Various markers for melanocytic differentiation such as S100, Melan-A (MART1), tyrosinase, and SOX10 highlight nodal nevi but do not distinguish them from melanoma. Nevertheless, once highlighted by a cytoplasmic marker (such as Melan-A), examination for nuclear atypia on the counter

stain is possible (see Fig. 13.32C). HMB45 is typically negative in nodal nevi, although it can be positive in a subset of the nevus cells, similar to what is seen in some cutaneous nevi especially when type A cells are present. Expression of p16 is essentially always retained. Nodal nevi are negative for PRAME; a double PRAME/MART1 immunostain is preferred due to background PRAME staining of nodal histiocytes (see Fig. 13.32C). 5-hMC, an epigenetic marker, is expressed in nodal nevi. Ki-67 is typically completely negative in nodal nevi, although rarely larger nevi may display a low proliferation index (<1%). Other potential useful immunostains include fatty acid synthase and acetyl-CoA carboxylase, both of which should be negative in nodal nevus.

MOLECULAR STUDIES

The majority of nodal nevi harbor *BRAF* activating mutation. FISH using probes that target chromosomal loci 6p25 (*RREB1*), 6q23 (*MYB*), and 11q13 (*CCND1*) is expected to yield negative results in nodal nevi.

Differential Diagnosis

Distinction between nodal nevus and nodal metastatic melanoma can be notoriously difficult especially when the primary melanoma demonstrates nevoid features. Metastatic melanomas most commonly involve the subcapsular sinuses, followed by the nodal parenchyma (Fig. 13.34A). Confinement to the nodal capsule is very

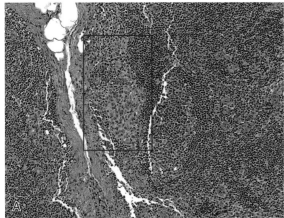

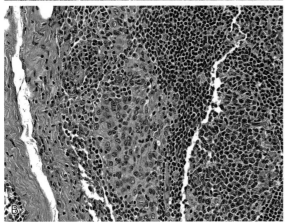

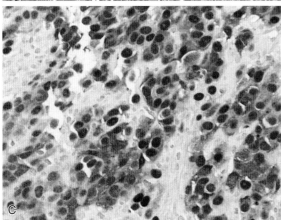

FIG. 13.34

A focus of metastatic melanoma in the parenchyma of a lymph node *(square)* (**A**). These cells are large, epithelioid, and pleomorphic with conspicuous nucleoli (**B**). A double PRAME/MART1 stain on another metastatic melanoma demonstrates nuclear PRAME staining in the MART1 positive melanocytes (**C**).

TABLE 13.15

Histologic Features of Nodal Nevus Versus Nodal Metastatic Melanoma

Nodal Nevus	Nodal Metastatic Melanoma
• Typically confined to nodal capsule and trabeculae	• Typically involves subcapsular sinuses and nodal parenchyma
• Small oval to spindle melanocytes with scant cytoplasm, uniform nuclei, and inconspicuous nucleoli	• Large epithelioid melanocytes with ample amount of cytoplasm, enlarged nuclei, coarse chromatin, and prominent nucleoli
• Mitoses are absent	• Mitoses may be found
• Low to absent Ki-67 staining ($<$1%)	• Elevated Ki-67 proliferation index ($>$1%)
• Negative for PRAME	• Positive for PRAME
• Retained p16 staining	• Expression for p16 may be lost
• Negative fluorescence *in situ* hybridization	• Fluorescence *in situ* hybridization frequently demonstrates copy number aberrations

unusual. Most metastatic melanomas display cytologic atypia such as large epithelioid morphology, ample amount of cytoplasm, enlarged and pleomorphic nuclei, coarse chromatin, and prominent nucleoli (Fig. 13.34B). Mitoses may be observed. As mentioned above, immunohistochemical markers may help discriminate nodal nevi from nodal metastatic melanoma. Ki-67 proliferation index is typically elevated ($>$1%) in metastatic melanoma. Diffuse and strong HMB45 expression, loss of p16, and positive PRAME staining (Fig. 13.34C) would further support a diagnosis of metastatic melanoma (Table 13.15). Other reported immunohistochemical findings in metastatic melanoma include loss of 5-hMC expression, and positive staining for fatty acid synthase and acetyl-CoA carboxylase. The majority of metastatic melanoma should demonstrate copy number aberrations by FISH.

When found in lymph nodes obtained from carcinoma patients (most frequently breast carcinoma), the differential diagnosis may include metastatic carcinoma. The capsular location, bland cytomorphology, and when necessary, expression for melanocytic markers as opposed to cytokeratin, should clinch the diagnosis of nodal nevus.

Prognosis and Therapy

Nodal nevi are benign and do not require treatment or follow-up. Malignant transformation of nodal nevus has not been reported, although it has been speculated that some nodal metastatic melanomas of unknown primary may have arisen from pre-existing nodal nevi. This latter hypothesis remains unproven. The presence of nodal nevus does not affect the prognosis of melanoma patients.

NODAL NEVUS – DISEASE FACT SHEET

Definition
▸▸ Benign melanocytic rests in lymph nodes

Incidence and Location
▸▸ 0.017%–22%
▸▸ Most commonly found in axillary lymph nodes, followed by inguinal and cervical nodes

Age Distribution
▸▸ Most commonly found in patients aged 30–60 years

Clinical Features
▸▸ None

Prognosis and Therapy
▸▸ Benign finding which does not require therapy

NODAL NEVUS – PATHOLOGIC FEATURES

Gross Findings
▸▸ Typical not appreciable on gross examination

Microscopic Findings
▸▸ Aggregates of melanocytes found in the nodal capsule or along nodal trabeculae
▸▸ May protrude into lymphatic space
▸▸ Small and bland melanocytes with scant cytoplasm, small nuclei, and inconspicuous nucleoli

Pathologic Differential Diagnoses
▸▸ Nodal metastatic melanoma or carcinoma

CELLULAR DERMATOFIBROMA

DIFFERENTIAL DIAGNOSIS: DERMATOFIBROSARCOMA PROTUBERANS

Clinical Features

Cellular dermatofibroma (CDF), also known as cellular benign fibrous histiocytoma, often presents as a subcutaneous nodule with a clinical diagnosis of a cyst. Lesions most commonly occur on the extremities and head and neck, and young males are most commonly affected. The vast majority of cases behave in a benign fashion.

Pathologic Features

GROSS FINDINGS

Gross examination reveals a dermal-based nodule.

MICROSCOPIC FINDINGS

Scanning magnification typically reveals a dermal-based neoplasm that is unencapsulated but relatively circumscribed (Fig. 13.35A). The tumor may extend into the superficial subcutis; however, broad infiltration of subcutaneous tissue is not seen. Entrapment of collagen is often identified at the periphery (Fig. 13.35B). The tumor is composed of a heterogeneous population of spindle cells ranging from plump to fusiform but with bland nuclei (Fig. 13.35C). The growth pattern is usually fascicular or storiform. Mitoses are often present, which can be a disconcerting feature. Necrosis may also be present in a minority of cases. If fat necrosis is present at the interface of the deep dermis and subcutis, accompanying lymphocytic inflammation is generally seen (Fig. 13.35D). Epidermal hyperplasia, sometimes with hyperpigmentation, is often present above the lesion, a characteristic also seen in typical dermatofibroma.

Ancillary Studies

IMMUNOHISTOCHEMISTRY

Smooth muscle actin is expressed weakly in the majority of cases. However, other markers of smooth muscle differentiation, such as desmin and H-caldesmon, are negative. Membranous CD34 positivity, which is characteristic of DFSP, is seen in a minority of cases but is typically limited to the outer rim of the tumor (Fig. 13.35E) as opposed to diffuse expression seen in DFSP.

Differential Diagnosis

The principal alternative diagnostic consideration is DFSP (Table 13.16). DFSP typically presents as a multinodular, slowly growing mass or plaque on the trunk or proximal lower extremities of younger adults, but can occur at the distal extremities and even at acral sites. DFSP is characterized by a dermal proliferation of bland, monomorphic fibroblast-like cells typically arranged in a storiform growth pattern (Fig. 13.36). Cytologic pleomorphism is not a feature. Irregular infiltration of subcutaneous adipose tissue in a honeycomb-like pattern is characteristic (see Fig. 13.36A), and adnexal structures are usually entrapped with preservation of their normal morphology. Tumor cells of DFSP often spread along the subcutaneous fibrous septae, resulting in difficulty in

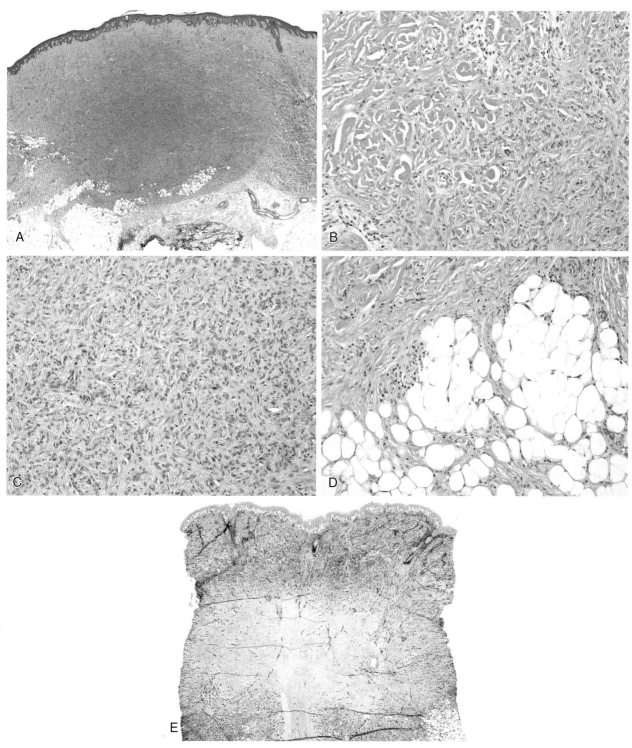

FIG. 13.35

Microscopic findings of cellular dermatofibroma (CDF). Scanning magnification image showing a vaguely circumscribed but unencapsulated cellular dermal proliferation that involves the superficial subcutis (**A**). Collagen entrapment can often be seen at the periphery (**B**). Higher-power image demonstrating a storiform arrangement of tumor cells with variable cytologic features ranging from plump to fusiform but with bland nuclear characteristics (**C**). A focus of fat necrosis seen at the dermal/subcutaneous interface which is associated with lymphocytic inflammation (**D**). A rim of peripheral CD34 expression is seen in this example of CDF, which is a common occurrence (**E**).

TABLE 13.16

Histologic Features of Cellular Dermatofibroma Versus Dermatofibrosarcoma Protuberans

Cellular Dermatofibroma	Dermatofibrosarcoma Protuberans
• Vaguely circumscribed	• Typically shows an infiltrative growth pattern
• Usually limited to the dermis but can show focal infiltration of the subcutaneous fat	• Characterized by broad infiltration of the subcutaneous fat
• Fascicular to loosely storiform architecture	• Typically diffusely storiform; fibrosarcomatous (high-grade) examples show a herringbone architecture
• Epidermal hyperplasia and hyperpigmentation often present above the lesion	• Epidermis is typically unaltered
• Polymorphous population of spindle cells ranging from fusiform to plump	• Highly monomorphic yet bland cytology
IHC: • Diffuse, weak expression of smooth muscle actin • CD34 may show a peripheral rim of staining	IHC: • Diffusely positive for CD34 • Lacks expression of smooth muscle actin
• Molecular: Some tumors may show abnormal cytogenetic findings but lack the t(17;22) translocation	• Molecular: >90% of cases harbor t(17;22) resulting in a COL1A1-PDGFB fusion gene that can be detected by FISH or PCR

eosinophilic cytoplasm. Although CDF is usually weakly but diffusely positive for smooth muscle actin, tumors do not express desmin or H-caldesmon.

Spindle cell xanthogranuloma, a histologic variant of juvenile xanthogranuloma commonly located on the head and neck or upper trunk, can also enter into the differential diagnosis. Such lesions typically diffusely express histiocytic markers such as CD163 and PU.1. CD68 is also typically positive; however, this marker lacks specificity. Spindle cell granuloma often contains at least a few foamy macrophages and/or Touton-type giant cells and lack epidermal hyperplasia often seen in cases of CDF or typical dermatofibroma.

Other variants of dermatofibroma may enter into the differential diagnosis. Aneurysmal dermatofibroma is also highly cellular and contains large pools of red blood cells that are not lined by endothelial cells. Epithelioid dermatofibroma (epithelioid fibrous histiocytoma) is a biologically distinct variant that harbors translocations involving the *ALK* gene resulting in overexpression of a fused protein product that can be detected using ALK immunohistochemistry. Histologically, epithelioid dermatofibroma often shows an epidermal collarette and typically does not show collagen entrapment. Composite cells are more rounded and epithelioid than seen in other variants of dermatofibroma and often show occasional multinucleation with distinct nucleoli. Atypical dermatofibroma (formerly known as "dermatofibroma with monster cells") is also usually highly cellular but shows marked cytologic pleomorphism with cells containing bizarre nuclei. As in CDF, numerous mitoses as well as necrosis can be seen.

Prognosis and Therapy

Approximately 20% of cases of CDF can recur locally and non-destructively following incomplete removal. Accordingly, conservative complete excision of these lesions is preferred. Clinicians may opt for observation at anatomically sensitive sites such as the head and neck. Regional or distant metastasis is exceedingly rare but has been described.

local control; hence, wide excision is preferred. Despite the tendency to recur locally, conventional DFSP rarely metastasizes. However, a high-grade variant, referred to as DFSP with fibrosarcomatous transformation, which is characterized by a herringbone architectural pattern with increased cellularity (see Fig. 13.36D), does have the potential for distant metastatic spread (up to 23% in some series). Immunohistochemistry for CD34 can be helpful for excluding DFSP, as most cases show strong and diffuse expression of this marker (see Fig. 13.36E). CD34 expression can, however, be lost in fibrosarcomatous DFSP. Additionally, the presence of fat necrosis without an associated lymphoid infiltrate is common in DFSP. Alternatively, in CDF, fat necrosis is instead usually accompanied by a lymphocytic infiltrate. Entrapment of collagen fibers is typically seen at the periphery of CDF; however, this finding can be focally seen in some cases of DFSP. Greater than 90% of cases of DFSP harbor a t(17;22) translocation resulting in a COL1A1-PDGFB fusion gene. An alternative, less commonly seen fusion partner is *PDGFD*.

CDF can also be mistaken for leiomyosarcoma, particularly in small biopsies. Leiomyosarcoma, which grows in a fascicular pattern, contains cells with blunt-ended nuclei resembling a cigar as well as brightly

CELLULAR DERMATOFIBROMA – DISEASE FACT SHEET

Definition
▸▸ One of many variants of dermatofibroma that is highly cellular and usually larger than typical dermatofibroma

Incidence and Location
▸▸ Uncommon
▸▸ Most commonly occurs on the extremities and head and neck area

Age Distribution
▸▸ Young adults, particularly males

Continued

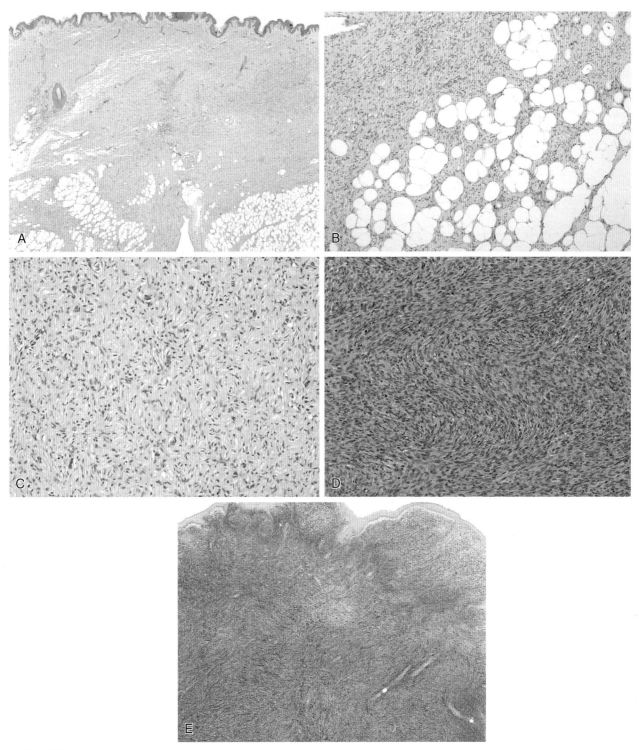

FIG. 13.36

Microscopic findings of dermatofibrosarcoma protuberans (DFSP). Scanning magnification image showing a dermal spindle cell population with broad involvement of the underlying subcutaneous adipose tissue (**A**). A honeycomb-like pattern of infiltration of the subcutaneous adipose tissue is characteristic of DFSP (**B**). The majority of the tumor cells show a storiform arrangement and monotonous cytology with bland nuclear features (**C**). A case demonstrating fibrosarcomatous transformation with a herringbone architecture and increased cellularity and mitotic activity (**D**). DFSP typically strongly and diffusely expresses CD34, in contrast to the peripheral rim of staining often seen in cellular dermatofibroma (**E**).

CELLULAR DERMATOFIBROMA – DISEASE FACT SHEET—cont'd

Clinical Features

▸▸ Presents as a dermal/subcutaneous nodule that is often mistaken for a cyst

Prognosis and Therapy

▸▸ Approximately 20% of cases recur locally and non-destructively if not completely removed
▸▸ Conservative complete excision is preferred; observation is an option at sensitive anatomic locations

---

CELLULAR DERMATOFIBROMA – PATHOLOGIC FEATURES

Gross Findings

▸▸ Dermal/subcutaneous nodule

Microscopic Findings

▸▸ Vaguely circumscribed but unencapsulated
▸▸ Fascicular to storiform arrangement of polymorphous spindle cells ranging from fusiform to plump
▸▸ Collagen entrapment at the periphery
▸▸ Can involve superficial subcutaneous tissue with fat necrosis containing a lymphoid infiltrate
▸▸ Polymorphous population of tumor cells ranging from plump to fusiform

Pathologic Differential Diagnoses

▸▸ Dermatofibrosarcoma protuberans
▸▸ Smooth muscle neoplasms
▸▸ Spindle cell xanthogranuloma
▸▸ Other variants of dermatofibroma (DF), including aneurysmal, epithelioid, and atypical DF

ATYPICAL FIBROXANTHOMA

DIFFERENTIAL DIAGNOSIS: SARCOMATOID SQUAMOUS CELL CARCINOMA, PLEOMORPHIC DERMAL SARCOMA

Clinical Features

Atypical fibroxanthoma (AFX) presents as an isolated nodule, often ulcerated, on sun-damaged skin of the elderly. There is a strong predilection for the head and neck. Presentation at younger age and other anatomic sites may occur in the setting of xeroderma pigmentosum or Li-Fraumeni syndrome.

Pathologic Features

GROSS FINDINGS

There are no specific gross findings.

MICROSCOPIC FINDINGS

Scanning magnification reveals a circumscribed dermal tumor in a nodular or plaque-like configuration (Fig. 13.37A). The tumor often broadly abuts the epidermis and may be ulcerated, but lacks an epidermal component. There is no squamous or melanocytic precursor. Ulceration is frequently observed. There is sheet-like growth of markedly atypical spindled and/or epithelioid cells, with scattered multinucleated cells (Fig. 13.37B). Perineural invasion and angiolymphatic invasion are absent. Tumor necrosis is absent (some definitions allow for focal necrosis). There is no substantial involvement of the subcutis. Unusual findings include myxoid stroma, sclerotic stroma, keloidal collagen (Fig. 13.37C), clear cells (Fig. 13.37D), granular cells, or pseudoangiomatous features.

Ancillary Studies

IMMUNOHISTOCHEMISTRY

AFX is negative for specific differentiation markers. Specifically, there is no expression of melanocytic markers (S100, SOX10, Melan-A, HMB45), epithelial markers (cytokeratins, p63), specific muscle markers (desmin or caldesmon), or specific vascular markers (ERG). Smooth muscle actin may label cells in a membranous pattern. CD10 and vimentin are usually diffusely positive, but do not reliably distinguish AFX from other tumors on the differential diagnosis. CD68, CD163, and MiTF can be expressed. Unusual cases express EMA, CD31, or CD34. In rare cases, the giant cell component labels with Melan-A and HMB45.

MOLECULAR STUDIES

UV-pattern mutations are present. Similar to cutaneous SCC, AFX have highly recurrent *TP53* mutations, often accompanied by *CDKN2A* mutation (less frequently deletion). *TERT* promoter mutations have been described. A minority have mutations in the kinase *PIK3CA*.

Differential Diagnosis

Immunohistochemistry, and microscopic evaluation of the entire lesion, are essential for definitive diagnosis. The differential diagnosis includes sarcomatoid SCC, DM, leiomyosarcoma, angiosarcoma, pleomorphic dermal sarcoma (PDS; previously undifferentiated pleomorphic sarcoma), and other spindle cell malignances that can involve the dermis. Of these, angiosarcoma and leiomyosarcoma can be excluded by morphology in many cases.

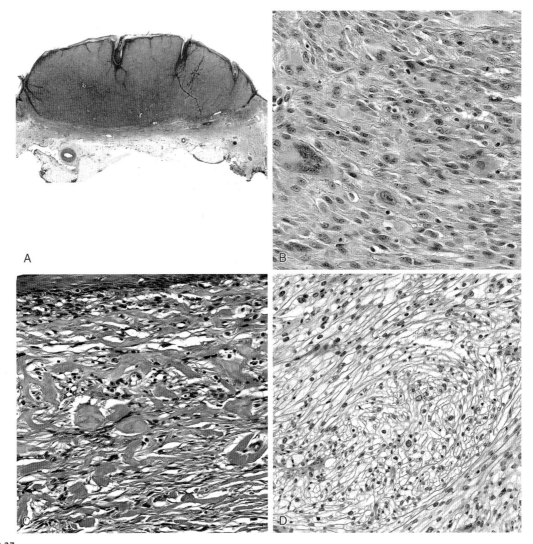

FIG. 13.37

An atypical fibroxanthoma filling the dermis without involvement of subcutis (**A**). Atypical epithelioid and spindled cells with multinucleated forms (**B**). (**C**) Zones of keloidal collagen with interspersed atypical cells may be present (**C**). Clear cell atypical fibroxanthoma (rare variant) (**D**).

PDS (Fig. 13.38; Table 13.17) cannot be excluded without evaluation of the tumor in its entirety. Features that warrant a diagnosis of PDS rather than AFX include significant subcutaneous extension (see Fig. 13.38A), perineural invasion, angiolymphatic invasion, or tumor necrosis. Of note, the proper classification for tumors with some subcutaneous extension (greater than focal) can be unclear, as there is no quantitative threshold for the degree of subcutaneous involvement that warrants a diagnosis of PDS over AFX. There is disagreement among classification schema regarding whether tumors >2 cm in size (that otherwise meet criteria for AFX) should be classified as AFX or PDS.

Sarcomatoid SCC (Table 13.18) can also enter the differential diagnosis. Expression of epithelial markers (cytokeratins, p63/p40) distinguishes sarcomatoid SCC from AFX. Multiple immunohistochemical stains are required for this distinction because epithelial marker expression can be variably lost in sarcomatoid SCC, including some or all cytokeratins. Cytokeratin-negative/p63-positive (or rarely cytokeratin-positive/p63-negative)

immunophenotypes can be observed in sarcomatoid SCC. (Of note, some propose that cytokeratin-negative/p63-positive tumors should be classified as AFX.) CD10 can be expressed in both AFX and SCC.

Desmoplastic/spindle melanoma displays expression of melanocytic markers, although HMB45 and Melan-A expression can be lost in a subset. DM can have minimal to absent *in situ* component in a significant fraction of cases. MiTF and CD10 can be expressed in both AFX and melanoma. S100+ dendritic cells can be abundant in AFX, and these may be a source of diagnostic challenge in limited biopsies. The rare occurrence of HMB45+/Melan-A+ giant cells in AFX also represents a diagnostic pitfall.

Atypical fibrous histiocytoma is the atypical variant of dermatofibroma, displaying atypical cells interspersed among more conventional dermatofibroma. In contrast, AFX lacks features of dermatofibroma. Atypical fibrous histiocytoma occurs on the extremities of younger patients, without evidence of severe photodamage, unlike AFX.

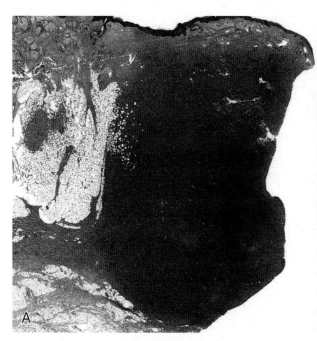

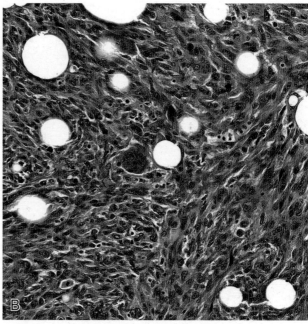

FIG. 13.38

Pleomorphic dermal sarcoma is an infiltrative tumor with extensive subcutaneous extension (**A**). Malignant cells including multinucleate forms, similar to those observed in atypical fibroxanthoma (**B**).

TABLE 13.17

Histologic Features of Atypical Fibroxanthoma Versus Pleomorphic Dermal Sarcoma

Atypical Fibroxanthoma	Pleomorphic Dermal Sarcoma
Dermal spindle cell proliferation with high-grade atypia	Spindle cell proliferation with malignant atypia involving dermis and often deeper tissues
Size usually <2 cm (some approaches define tumors >2 cm as pleomorphic dermal sarcoma)	Size may exceed 2 cm
Minimal or no involvement of subcutis	One or more of the following: Substantial involvement of subcutis
No perineural invasion	Perineural invasion
No angiolymphatic invasion	Angiolymphatic invasion
No tumor necrosis	Tumor necrosis
	Size >2 cm (per some studies)
IHC: negative for specific lineage markers (epithelial, melanocytic, muscle, etc.)	IHC: negative for specific lineage markers (epithelial, melanocytic, muscle, etc.)
Molecular:	Molecular:
TP53 mutation	*TP53* mutation
CDKN2A mutation (less frequently deletion)	*CDKN2A* deletion
PIK3CA mutation (minority)	PIK3CA mutations rare to absent
RAS mutations rare to absent	RAS mutations (minority)

TABLE 13.18

Histologic Features of Atypical Fibroxanthoma Versus Sarcomatoid Squamous Cell Carcinoma

Atypical Fibroxanthoma	Sarcomatoid Squamous Cell Carcinoma
Dermal spindle cell proliferation with high-grade atypia	Spindle cell proliferation with high-grade atypia, involving dermis and possibly deeper tissue
No connection to epidermis (but may closely abut the epidermis)	May connect to overlying actinic keratosis or SCCIS
No morphologic evidence of specific differentiation	May have component of conventional SCC
No tumor necrosis, perineural invasion, angiolymphatic invasion, deep subcutaneous involvement	May have tumor necrosis, perineural invasion, angiolymphatic invasion, deep subcutaneous involvement
IHC:	IHC:
Epithelial marker (CK, p63/p40): negative	Epithelial marker (CK, p63/p40): positive
GATA3: negative	GATA3: positive (may be less sensitive than p63)
CD10: positive	CD10: +/−
Smooth muscle actin membranous or negative	Smooth muscle actin membranous or negative
Melanocytic markers negative	Melanocytic markers negative
Molecular:	Molecular:
TP53 mutation	*TP53* and *CDKN2A* mutation
CDKN2A mutation (less frequently deletion)	PIK3CA mutation (minority)
PIK3CA mutation (minority)	RAS mutation (minority)
RAS mutations rare to absent	

IHC, immunohistochemistry; *SCC*, squamous cell carcinoma; *SCCIS*, squamous cell carcinoma in situ.

Cutaneous metastases from internal malignancy often present on the scalp. Clinical history is essential. Metastatic renal cell carcinoma expresses CD10 and may not show reliable keratin expression, but typically demonstrates strong PAX8 expression. The possibility of PAX8 expression in AFX has not yet been examined.

Prognosis and Therapy

Metastasis is rare. Excision is typically curative. Recurrences are infrequent, and usually related to incomplete excision.

ATYPICAL FIBROXANTHOMA – DISEASE FACT SHEET

Definition
▸▸ Atypical dermal spindle cell proliferation on sun-exposed skin without specific differentiation

Incidence
▸▸ Rare

Age Distribution
▸▸ Middle-aged to elderly (may occur in younger patients with xeroderma pigmentosum or Li-Fraumeni)

Clinical Features
▸▸ Sun-exposed skin (especially head and neck) of elderly individuals
▸▸ In xeroderma pigmentosum and Li-Fraumeni, can present at younger age and with broader anatomic distribution

Prognosis and Therapy
▸▸ Risk of recurrence is low with complete excision
▸▸ Progression, metastasis is rare

ATYPICAL FIBROXANTHOMA – PATHOLOGIC FEATURES

Gross Findings
▸▸ No specific gross findings

Microscopic Findings
▸▸ Dermal tumor with limited/no subcutaneous extension, and no epidermal connection
▸▸ Frequently ulcerated
▸▸ Striking cytologic atypia of spindled and/or epithelioid cells, with multinucleated forms
▸▸ Mitoses: frequent, may be atypical
▸▸ By definition, there is no perineural invasion, angiolymphatic invasion, or significant tumor necrosis
▸▸ No morphologic or immunohistochemical evidence of specific differentiation

Pathologic Differential Diagnoses
▸▸ Sarcomatoid squamous cell carcinoma, pleomorphic dermal sarcoma, leiomyosarcoma, desmoplastic melanoma, (rarely) angiosarcoma, atypical fibrous histiocytoma

---

EPITHELIOID SARCOMA

DIFFERENTIAL DIAGNOSES: GRANULOMA ANNULARE, RHEUMATOID NODULE

Clinical Features

Epithelioid sarcoma (ES) is a rare malignancy that can be divided into two subtypes: the conventional (distal) type, which will be the focus of this section, typically occurs on the distal extremities of adolescents and young adults. Males are more commonly affected. The second subtype, the proximal type preferentially affects the groin, trunk, axilla, or proximal extremities and shows characteristic histopathologic features detailed below. However, the age range and anatomic distribution of both subtypes are wide. ES typically presents as a large, dermal or subcutaneous slow-growing mass. Unlike most other sarcomas, metastasis to lymph nodes is common, and cutaneous satellite nodules may be observed. Spread to lungs is also frequent.

Pathologic Features

GROSS FINDINGS

Gross examination reveals a dermal or subcutaneous tumor that can be ulcerated.

MICROSCOPIC FINDINGS

Microscopic evaluation reveals a dermal or subcutaneous proliferation which is often multinodular. An infiltrative growth pattern is common, with spread along fascial planes often observed. Central necrosis resembling that seen in granulomatous diseases is a typical finding (Fig. 13.39A and B). Areas of the tumor can also show background fibrosis (Fig. 13.39C) or myxoid change. The tumor is composed of epithelioid to spindled cells with palely eosinophilic cytoplasm and vesicular chromatin (see Fig. 13.39C and D). Mitoses are typically rare. Perineural and lymphovascular invasion, however, are often present.

Proximal-type ES is typically composed of larger, monomorphic-appearing epithelioid cells with prominent nucleoli that typically grow in diffuse sheets of cells (Fig. 13.40). Rhabdoid intracytoplasmic inclusions are common, and the mitotic rate is often high. Tumors of the proximal type typically do not show granuloma-like features. Hybrid tumors with features of proximal and conventional (distal) type have also been described.

Ancillary Studies

Immunohistochemistry is a useful adjunct as cytokeratin expression can be demonstrated in most cases (see Fig. 13.39E). Additionally, approximately 60% of cases are positive for CD34. A minority of cases are positive for smooth muscle actin. Recurrent genetic abnormalities are seen in the 22q11.2 region, resulting in loss of INI1 (SMARCB1) protein expression in most (greater than 90%) cases (see Fig. 13.39F). INI1 is a

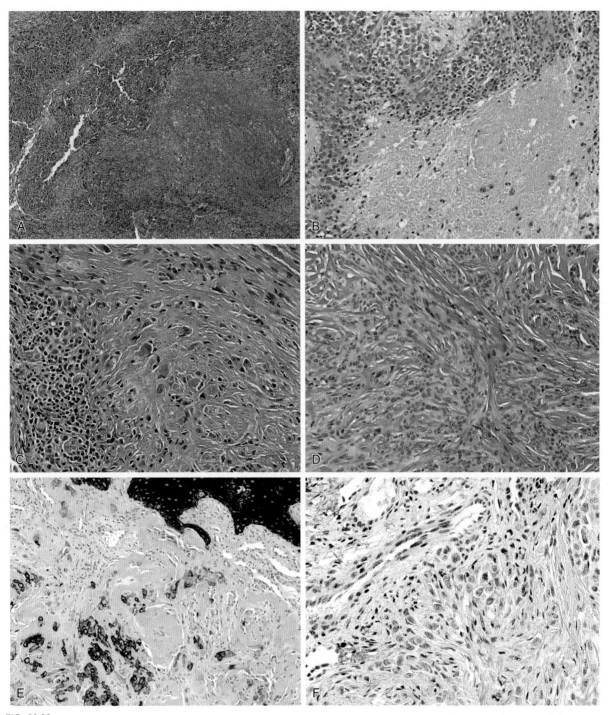

FIG. 13.39

(**A, B**) Conventional (distal)-type epithelioid sarcoma characteristically shows areas of central necrosis within sheets of tumor (**A, B**). Tumor cells can be epithelioid in appearance with palely eosinophilic cytoplasm within a fibrotic stroma (**C**). Tumor cells can also have a spindled morphology within the same tumor (**D**). Cytokeratin expression (in this case, AE1/AE3) is seen in most examples (**E**). INI1 loss is seen in greater than 90% of cases and can be a highly useful diagnostic adjunct (**F**). Retained expression of this nuclear protein is seen in background endothelial and inflammatory cells.

member of the SWI/SNF chromatin remodeling complex and is also recurrently mutated or deleted in malignant rhabdoid tumor, among other neoplasms. As this genetic abnormality is common to both subtypes of ES, the tumors are thought to exist along a morphologic spectrum.

Differential Diagnosis

Conventional (distal)-type ES can be mistaken for a granulomatous process such as granuloma annulare (GA) (Fig. 13.41) or rheumatoid nodule (Fig. 13.42; often histologically indistinguishable from deep GA).

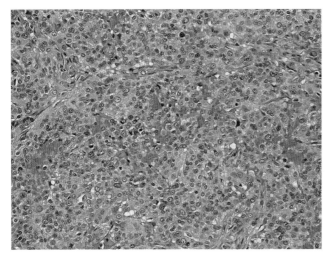

FIG. 13.40

Proximal-type epithelioid sarcoma typically grows in diffuse sheets of cells. Tumor cells are typically larger than those of conventional (distal)-type epithelioid sarcoma and have prominent nucleoli. In contrast to conventional (distal)-type epithelioid sarcoma, granuloma-like features are not commonly seen.

In contrast to granulomatous processes, the cytologic characteristics of the tumor cells of ES tend to be larger with different nuclear features. Palisading of lesional cells can be observed in both ES and GA and is not a useful distinguishing feature. Although cytologically similar to ES tumor cells, the histiocytes of granulomatous processes tend to have oval nuclei which are often folded with fine chromatin and punctate nucleoli (see Fig. 13.41C). The cells of ES characteristically show considerable cytologic atypia well beyond what is seen in cases of GA. A perivascular lymphoid infiltrate is usually encountered in GA, often with conspicuous eosinophils. The use of a histiocytic immunohistochemical marker such as CD163 or CD68 as well as broad-spectrum cytokeratin and INI1 immunostains will usually resolve any diagnostic confusion, particularly in instances where reliable clinical history is lacking (Table 13.19). Other tumors that can be mistaken for conventional (distal)-type ES include angiosarcoma (particularly due to CD34 reactivity) and metastatic carcinoma (which typically expresses cytokeratins).

Proximal-type ES can be mistaken for a large number of entities such as extrarenal rhabdoid tumor (which also shows loss of INI1 expression), melanoma, rhabdomyosarcoma, and undifferentiated carcinoma, among others. Other tumors that show loss of INI1 expression include a subset of epithelioid MPNSTs, myoepithelial carcinomas, and extraskeletal myxoid chondrosarcomas.

Prognosis and Therapy

Prognosis is poor for both subtypes of ES. Nearly one third of patients present with nodal involvement, while

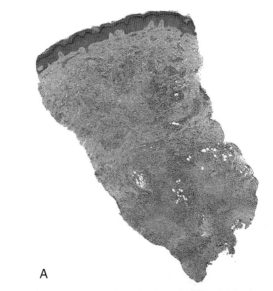

A

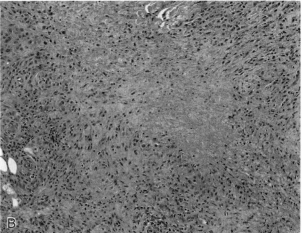

B

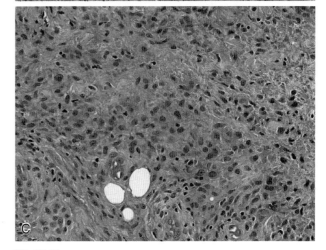

C

FIG. 13.41

Low-power view of granuloma annulare (**A**). Similar to epithelioid sarcoma (ES), central necrosis is often seen in granulomatous processes, which often show peripheral palisading of histiocytes (**B**). The histiocytes seen in granulomatous dermatitides are cytologically similar to those of ES (**C**). However, the cytoplasm of the histiocytes of granuloma annulare tend to be amphiphilic, and the cell nuclei are usually oval and often folded with small and sometimes multiple nucleoli. High-grade cytologic atypia is lacking. The use of a histiocytic marker such as CD163 or CD68 as well as broad-spectrum cytokeratin and INI1 immunostains will usually resolve any diagnostic confusion.

approximately 20% have evidence of metastatic disease at the time of initial presentation. Although the 5-year survival rate is approximately 70%, the 20-year survival is dismal at approximately 25%. Proximal-type ES appears to behave more aggressively. Tumor size and status of metastatic disease both appear to be independent predictors of clinical outcome. As ES has a propensity for nodal involvement, like clear cell sarcoma and synovial sarcoma, the use of sentinel lymph node biopsy has been proposed as a prognostic tool. Results of small studies suggest that the incidence of occult lymph node metastases is fairly low; however, larger clinical trials are needed. The mainstay of treatment for ES is wide surgical excision, with radiation and chemotherapy used as adjuncts.

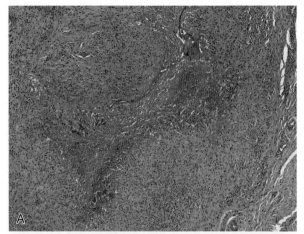

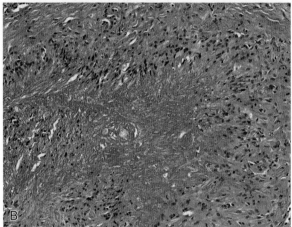

FIG. 13.42

Rheumatoid nodule (histologically identical to deep granuloma annulare) shows subcutaneous necrotizing granulomas (**A**). Closer inspection reveals prominent peripheral palisading of histiocytes with central fibrinoid necrosis (**B**).

TABLE 13.19

Histologic Features of Epithelioid Sarcoma Versus Granuloma Annulare

Epithelioid Sarcoma	Granuloma Annulare
• Infiltrative growth along fascial planes	• Although borders can be ill-defined, aggressive growth along facial planes is not seen
• Tumor cells are palely eosinophilic with vesicular chromatin	• Composite histiocytes generally have amphiphilic to gray cytoplasm with oval, folded nuclei and small, often multiple, nucleoli
• Cytologic atypia present	• Minimal cytologic atypia
IHC: Positive for cytokeratins with loss of nuclear expression of INI1 in the vast majority of cases. CD34 positive in approximately 60%. Smooth muscle actin positive in a minority of cases.	IHC: Positive for histiocytic markers such as CD163 and CD68

IHC, immunohistochemistry.

EPITHELIOID SARCOMA – DISEASE FACT SHEET

Definition
▶▶ Aggressive soft tissue sarcoma of undetermined histologic differentiation

Incidence and Location
▶▶ Rare
▶▶ Deep soft tissue of the distal extremities, especially hand and wrist, are the most common sites
▶▶ Often extends into the dermis

Age Distribution
▶▶ Adolescents and young adults, preferentially male

Clinical Features
▶▶ Presents as single or multiple grouped soft tissue masses that are often ulcerated

Prognosis and Therapy
▶▶ Up to one third of patients with nodal involvement with 20% having evidence of metastatic disease at initial presentation
▶▶ 5-year survival approximately 70%, 20-year survival approximately 25%

EPITHELIOID SARCOMA – PATHOLOGIC FEATURES

Gross Findings
▶▶ Subcutaneous mass that is often ulcerated

Microscopic Findings
▶▶ Often multinodular
▶▶ Central necrosis within tumor islands
▶▶ Epithelioid to spindled cells with palely eosinophilic cytoplasm and vesicular chromatin
▶▶ Mitoses usually not numerous
▶▶ Lymphovascular or perineural invasion common

Pathologic Differential Diagnoses
▶▶ Granulomatous processes such as granuloma annulare and rheumatoid nodule, angiosarcoma, metastatic carcinoma

ATYPICAL VASCULAR LESION

DIFFERENTIAL DIAGNOSIS: LOW-GRADE ANGIOSARCOMA

Clinical Features

Atypical vascular lesion (AVL) is a benign vascular lesion arising 2 to 3 years after radiation therapy. The typical presentation is small (<5 mm) solitary or multiple well-circumscribed papules, vesicles, or plaques, arising in irradiated skin, most commonly on the breast or axilla.

Pathologic Features

GROSS FINDINGS

Single or multiple well-circumscribed papules or nodules are present.

MICROSCOPIC FINDINGS

AVL is usually confined to the upper and mid dermis (Fig. 13.43A) with occasional extension to the deeper dermis. The subcutis is spared. Rare cases involve breast parenchyma. There is symmetric, circumscribed wedge-shaped architecture. The most common form (the lymphatic type) is composed of irregular, angulated thin-walled vessels (Fig. 13.43B). There may be focal interanastomosis and back-to-back growth. Small intraluminal papillations can be present. Endothelial nuclei are enlarged and dark, and may protrude into the vascular lumina (see Fig. 13.43B). However, definitive cytologic atypia (pleomorphism, multilayering, nucleoli) is rare in AVL, and mitoses are not identified.

The vascular type of AVL resembles microvenular hemangioma or hobnail hemangioma. There is occasional mild cytologic atypia and rare mitoses. Malignant endothelial atypia, including endothelial multilayering, is absent.

Ancillary Studies

IMMUNOHISTOCHEMISTRY

For lymphatic-type AVL, immunohistochemical stains demonstrate expression of vascular and lymphatic markers including D2-40, ERG, and CD31, with variable CD34. The vascular variant expresses CD31, CD34, and ERG, but not D2-40. Myc is negative, or displays focal weak staining (Fig. 13.43C).

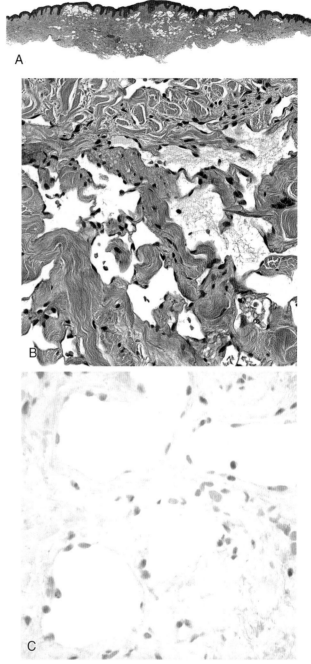

FIG. 13.43

Atypical vascular lesion consists of dilated, ectatic vessels, predominantly in the superficial dermis (**A**). Enlarged hyperchromatic endothelial nuclei can protrude into the lumen (**B**). Other atypical features (nucleoli, multilayering, mitoses) are absent. Stroma protrudes into luminal spaces. Myc immunohistochemistry is negative or shows weak focal positivity (**C**).

MOLECULAR STUDIES

Proposed etiologies include lymphatic obstruction or radiation-induced vascular proliferation; therefore, it is unclear whether AVL represents a neoplastic or reactive phenomenon. *MYC* and *FLT4* amplifications are absent in AVL, unlike angiosarcoma. *TP53* variants have been described in AVLs but are predominantly single nucleotide polymorphisms or variants of uncertain significance.

Differential Diagnosis

The major diagnostic distinction is with radiation-induced angiosarcoma (Table 13.20, Fig. 13.44). Clinical history can be critical to determine whether the lesion appears similar to AVL (small circumscribed papules) or angiosarcoma (poorly defined bruise-like lesion). Angiosarcoma and AVL may appear identical on a partial biopsy. Furthermore, AVL and angiosarcoma can coexist. Microscopically, angiosarcoma displays an infiltrative growth pattern and can display deep extension (see Fig. 13.44A), unlike AVL. Blood lakes and extensive collagen dissection are also features of angiosarcoma. Angiosarcomas display mitotic activity and elevated Ki-67 proliferative index (>10%) and cytologic atypia (hyperchromasia, nucleoli, pleomorphism, coarse chromatin, and nuclear multilayering) (see Fig. 13.44B). Some areas of angiosarcoma can lack atypia. Myc is strongly expressed in the majority of post-radiation angiosarcomas (see Fig. 13.44C) and is weak or negative in AVL (see Fig. 13.43C). FISH demonstrates *MYC* amplification in post-radiation angiosarcoma, but not AVL. PROX1 immunohistochemistry (variable in AVL, positive in angiosarcoma) has also been proposed to be diagnostically useful.

The differential diagnosis for AVL can also include chronic radiation dermatitis, hobnail hemangioma, lymphangioma circumscriptum, lymphangioendothelioma, and Kaposi sarcoma.

Benign lymphangiomatous papules on irradiated skin have been proposed to be a superficial variant of AVL, although some consider these to be a distinct diagnostic entity.

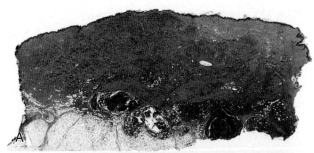
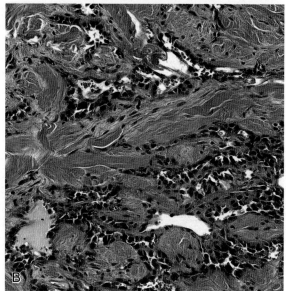
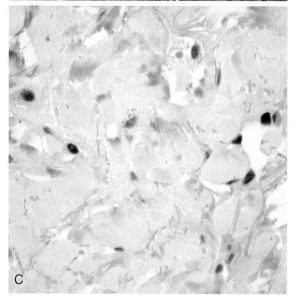

FIG. 13.44

Angiosarcoma with deep extension, high cellularity, and blood lake (**A**). Atypical endothelial cells display hyperchromasia, nucleoli, mitoses, and multilayering (**B**). Myc expression in angiosarcoma by immunohistochemistry (**C**).

TABLE 13.20

Histologic Features of Atypical Vascular Lesion Versus Low-Grade Angiosarcoma

Atypical Vascular Lesion	Low-Grade Angiosarcoma
Circumscribed and V-shaped (but may appear infiltrative in partial sampling), predominantly or entirely in the superficial-mid dermis	Infiltrative Superficial, deep, or both
Architecture: thin-walled interconnecting ectatic vessels (lymphatic type) or well-defined narrow vessels (vascular type)	Architecture: irregular interanastomosing channels dissecting through collagen Blood lakes
Inter-anastomosis is less prominent than in angiosarcoma	
Thin projections of endothelium-covered stroma into vascular lumina	
Smooth muscle surrounds vessel walls	
Endothelial cells: variably enlarged, hyperchromatic; may be hobnailing; atypia is mild except in rare cases	Endothelial cells: enlargement, hyperchromasia, hobnailing; also pleomorphism, nucleoli, multilayering, mitoses
IHC: Myc: focal weak staining in minority Prox1: weak, focal	IHC: Myc: strong staining is sensitive, specific Prox1: positive

Prognosis and Therapy

AVL is managed by excision and monitoring, although complete excision can be challenging for patients with a high burden of lesions. AVL displays a benign course, with rare malignant progression.

ATYPICAL VASCULAR LESION – DISEASE FACT SHEET

Definition
▶▶ Benign vascular proliferation arising in irradiated skin

Incidence
▶▶ Restricted to irradiated skin

Age Distribution
▶▶ Adults (similar to age distribution for breast cancer)

Clinical Features
▶▶ Well-defined, single or multiple vesicles, papules, or plaques

Prognosis and Therapy
▶▶ Benign course (malignant progression is exceptional)
▶▶ Managed by excision, monitoring

ATYPICAL VASCULAR LESION – PATHOLOGIC FEATURES

Gross Findings
▶▶ Single or multiple well-circumscribed papules or nodules, usually <5 mm

Microscopic Findings
▶▶ Wedge-shaped, circumscribed lesion confined to the dermis (usually upper/mid dermis)
▶▶ Lymphatic type (resemblance to lymphangioma) or vascular type (resemblance to hemangioma)
▶▶ Angulated thin-walled vessels lined by enlarged hyperchromatic endothelial cells
▶▶ Interanastomosis and collagen dissection are limited or absent
▶▶ Nucleoli, pleomorphism, mitoses are rare to absent

Pathologic Differential Diagnoses
▶▶ Post-radiation angiosarcoma, radiation dermatitis, hobnail hemangioma (and other hemangiomas), lymphangioma circumscriptum, lymphangioendothelioma, and Kaposi sarcoma

---

CUTANEOUS B-CELL LYMPHOID HYPERPLASIA

DIFFERENTIAL DIAGNOSES: PRIMARY CUTANEOUS FOLLICLE CENTER LYMPHOMA, PRIMARY CUTANEOUS MARGINAL ZONE LYMPHOMA

Clinical Features

Cutaneous lymphoid hyperplasia refers to a robust reactive lymphoid infiltrate of the skin secondary to various stimuli. Clinically these lesions are solitary or multiple, and may present as erythematous papules, nodules, or plaques. Pruritus is not uncommon. The head and neck region is most frequently involved, followed by the extremities and trunk. Common culprits include drugs, arthropod bites, hair dyes, tattoos, localized trauma (such as ear piercing), and viral infections, although in many cases the causative trigger is not clearly identified.

Pathologic Features

GROSS FINDINGS

Most cases are punch biopsies without significant gross findings.

MICROSCOPIC FINDINGS

Cutaneous lymphoid hyperplasia is also referred to as "pseudolymphoma" of the skin because the dense lymphoid infiltrate often raises concern for a cutaneous lymphoma. The infiltrate is typically mixed, although in many cases it may be classified as a T-cell predominant or B-cell predominant process. While the histopathologic findings of cutaneous lymphoid hyperplasia are protean, two major patterns have been described. The first pattern is a plaque-like infiltrate with epidermotropism or folliculotropism. This pattern typically involves a T-cell predominant reactive infiltrate and closely mimics mycosis fungoides, in which Pautrier microabscesses and/or lymphocyte tagging of the basal layer may be present.

The second pattern is a multinodular or diffuse lymphoid infiltrate involving primarily the dermis (Fig. 13.45A). Such infiltrate is typically B-cell predominant, in which nodular B-cell aggregates are admixed with and surrounded by T-cells. Germinal centers may be found within the nodular B-cell aggregates. The germinal centers are usually small and are not expansile or markedly irregular (Fig. 13.45B). Polarization, tingible body macrophages, and a surrounding mantle zones can be appreciated in well-formed germinal centers (Fig. 13.46C). Plasma cells are usually found at the periphery of the infiltrate (Fig. 13.45C). Scattered eosinophils and histiocytes may also be present. The epidermis and adnexal epithelia are usually spared. The majority of the lymphocytes outside of the germinal centers are small, although scattered large activated lymphocytes may also be present.

Ancillary Studies

IMMUNOHISTOCHEMISTRY

Immunohistochemistry is crucial in evaluating cutaneous lymphoid hyperplasia. CD3 and CD20 provide information on the predominant cell type. In B-cell lymphoid hyperplasia, there are nodular aggregates of

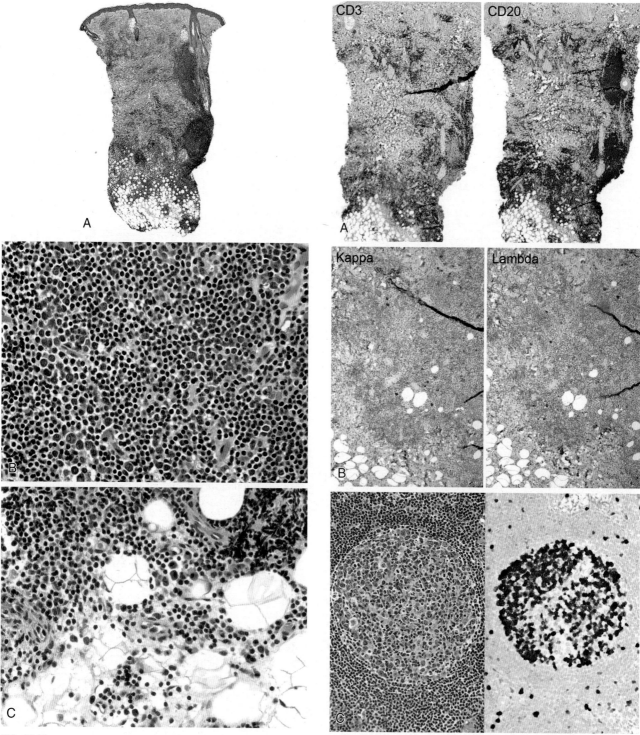

FIG. 13.45

A case of cutaneous B-cell lymphoid hyperplasia shows a multinodular dense lymphoid infiltrate in the dermis and superficial subcutis (**A**). Small aggregates of germinal center cells (large centroblasts) are surrounded by small lymphocytes in the nodular areas (**B**). Plasma cells and eosinophils are present at the periphery of the infiltrate (**C**).

FIG. 13.46

Immunohistochemical finding in cutaneous B-cell lymphoid hyperplasia. The infiltrate is a mixture of CD20+ B-cells and CD3+ T-cells (**A**). The B-cells form nodular aggregates which are surrounded by T-cells. The plasma cells demonstrate polytypic kappa and lambda light chain expression (**B**). A well-formed reactive lymphoid follicle is polarized, contains some tingible body macrophages, and is surrounded by a mantle zone (**C**, *left*). Ki-67 reveals a high proliferation index in the germinal center cells (**C**, *right*).

CD20-positive B cells surrounded by CD3-positive T-cells. CD21 often reveals the presence of follicular dendritic meshworks within the B-cell nodules. Germinal center cells within these meshworks express Bcl-6 and CD10 but not Bcl-2. Ki-67 proliferation index in the germinal centers should be high (>90%) (see Fig. 13.46C). Plasma cells, when present, should demonstrate polytypic kappa and lambda light chain expression (Fig. 13.46B). CD43 should mark the T-cells only. CD30 may highlight scattered activated cells without significant clustering.

MOLECULAR STUDIES

Clonality testing is frequently employed when histomorphology and immunohistochemistry are inconclusive. Clonality may be assessed by polymerase chain reaction (PCR) or next-generation sequencing. For B-cell infiltrates, it is most common to look for clonal rearrangement of the immunoglobulin heavy chain (IGH) and/or kappa light chain (IGK) by PCR. It should be noted that while most cases of cutaneous lymphoid hyperplasia should result in a polyclonal (negative) result, it is not uncommon to detect a monoclonal population in a reactive process ("pseudoclonality"). As such, a positive clonality test is not synonymous with malignancy. When multiple lesions are present at different anatomic sites in a patient, consideration may be given to performing an identical clonality test on different lesions to compare clones across these biopsies. Detection of an identical clone would serve as strong evidence of a neoplastic process, whereas different pseudoclones or absence of clones in these biopsies would support a reactive process.

Differential Diagnosis

The most common B-cell lymphomas of the skin are primary cutaneous follicle center lymphoma (PCFCL) and primary cutaneous marginal zone lymphoma (PCMZL), both of which may closely mimic cutaneous B-cell lymphoid hyperplasia clinically and histopathologically.

PCFCL mostly frequently presents as erythematous papules or nodules in the head and neck region or the trunk. Microscopically, there is a dense multinodular lymphoid infiltrate in the dermis. Multiple germinal centers are usually discernible on hematoxylin-eosin stain. These germinal centers may be abnormally large and expansile, and irregularly shaped (Fig. 13.47A and C). CD21 helps outline these abnormal lymphoid follicles. Polarization of centroblasts and centrocytes is usually absent, as are tingible body macrophages (Fig. 13.48). These germinal centers may lack a mantle zone. The neoplastic follicles often display an abnormally low Ki-67 proliferation index (<90%) (Fig. 13.47B). The neoplastic follicles can be highlighted by Bcl-6 and CD10 (see Fig. 13.48A). Unlike systemic/nodal follicular lymphoma, however, the neoplastic cells in PCFCL are typically negative for Bcl-2. Plasma cells, when present, are reactive in nature and are therefore expected to be polytypic. Clonal rearrangement of IGH and/or IGK would support a diagnosis of PCFCL over cutaneous lymphoid hyperplasia (Table 13.21).

PCMZL typically presents as erythematous papules or nodules on the upper extremities or the trunk. In PCMZL, there is a dense lymphoid infiltrate with perivascular and periadnexal accentuation in the dermis (Fig. 13.49). Germinal centers are often present and may be expanded by colonizing marginal zone cells. This feature is best appreciated on CD21 immunostain, which would demonstrate fragmentation of the follicular dendritic meshwork (see Fig. 13.49E). The neoplastic cells may be "monocytoid" with moderate amount of pale cytoplasm and indented nuclei (marginal zone cells), lymphoplasmacytic, or plasmacytic (Figs. 13.49

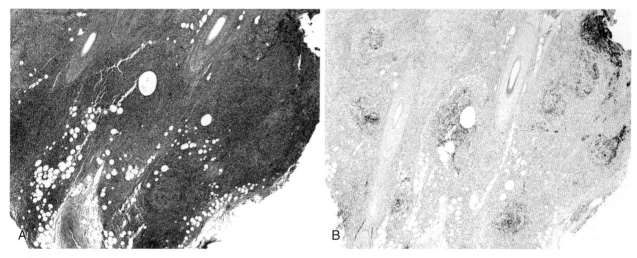

FIG. 13.47

A case of primary cutaneous follicle center lymphoma shows a diffuse to vaguely nodular lymphoid infiltrate in the deep dermis and superficial subcutis (**A**). Multiple germinal centers are highlighted by CD21, some of which are abnormally large (**B**).

Continued

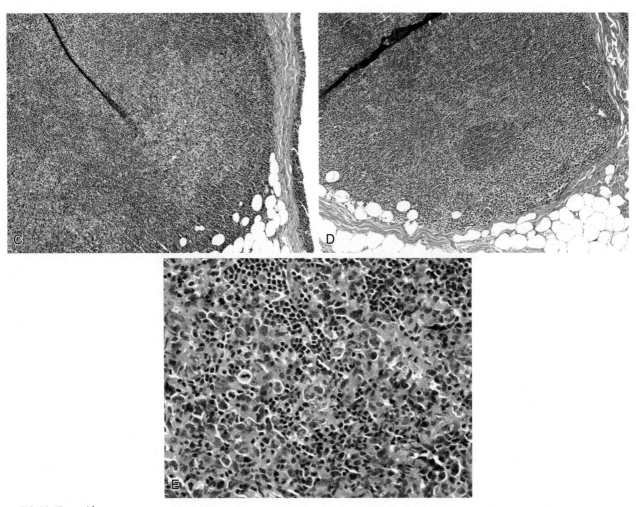

FIG. 13.47, cont'd
Some neoplastic lymphoid follicles are highly irregular and lack mantle zones (**C, D**). Atypical germinal center cells in an irregular follicle (**E**).

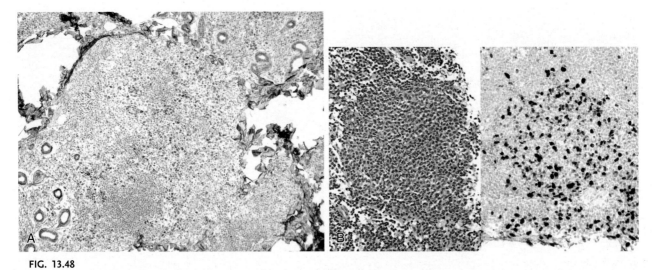

FIG. 13.48
Immunohistochemical findings in primary cutaneous follicle center lymphoma. Bcl-6 immunostain highlights the highly irregular germinal centers. A neoplastic lymphoid follicle lacking polarization, tingible body macrophages, and mantle zone (**B**, *left*) reveals an abnormally low Ki-67 proliferation index (<90%) (**B**, *right*).

TABLE 13.21

Histologic Features of Cutaneous B-cell Lymphoid Hyperplasia Versus Primary Cutaneous Follicle Center Lymphoma

Cutaneous B-Cell Lymphoid Hyperplasia	Primary Cutaneous Follicle Center Lymphoma
• Germinal centers are not expansile or highly irregular	• Germinal centers are abnormally large and irregular
• Mantle zones, polarization of centroblasts and centrocytes, and tingible body macrophages may be appreciated	• Mantle zones, polarization of germinal centers, and tingible body macrophages may be absent
• High Ki-67 proliferation index (>90%) in reactive lymphoid follicles	• Abnormally low Ki-67 proliferation index (<90%) in neoplastic lymphoid follicles
• Clonality studies are usually negative	• Clonality detected by IGH and IGK gene rearrangement studies

and 13.50). There is usually a combination of these cells, although occasional cases may display an overwhelming predominance of one cell type. For example, a plasmacytic variant consisting of mostly plasma cells may resemble a plasmacytoma (see Fig. 13.50). The neoplastic lymphocytes are positive for Bcl-2 while negative for Bcl-6 and CD10. Some cases also demonstrate CD43 positivity (Fig. 13.51). The plasma cells in PCMZL are usually monotypic (kappa- or lambda-restricted) with rare exceptions (see Fig. 13.51). Dutcher bodies may be observed in the neoplastic plasma cells (Fig. 13.50C). Clonal rearrangement of IGH and/or IGK would support a diagnosis of PCMZL over cutaneous lymphoid hyperplasia (Table 13.22). Alteration of the FAS gene has been reported as a recurrent finding in PCMZL.

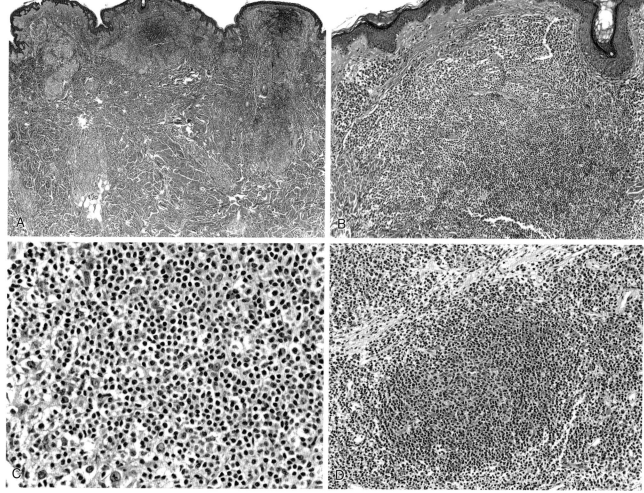

FIG. 13.49

A case of primary cutaneous marginal zone lymphoma shows a multinodular dense lymphoid infiltrate in the dermis (**A**). The infiltrate is composed of predominantly small lymphocytes and plasma cells (**B**). Many of the small lymphocytes contain pale cytoplasm, imparting a monocytoid appearance (**C**). Occasional lymphoid follicles are found (**D**).

Continued

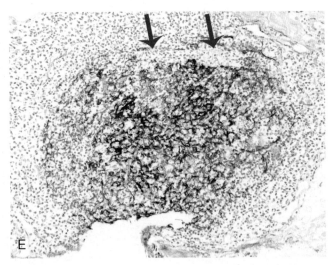

FIG. 13.49, cont'd
CD21 reveals fragmentation of a follicular dendritic meshwork *(arrows)* due to colonization of the germinal centers by marginal zone cells (**E**).

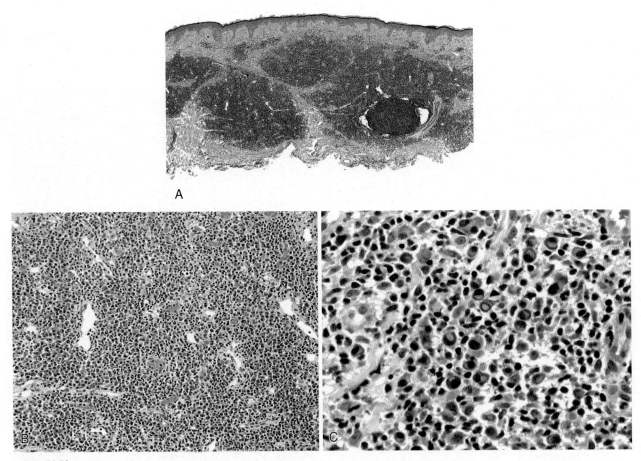

FIG. 13.50
A plasmacytic variant of primary cutaneous marginal zone lymphoma also demonstrates a multinodular lymphoid infiltrate in the dermis (**A**). Numerous plasma cells are present in a mixture with small lymphocytes (**B**). Some atypical plasma cells contain Dutcher bodies (**C**).

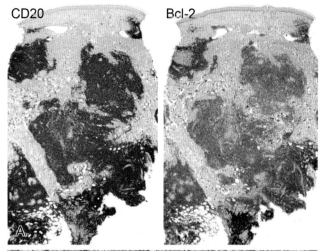

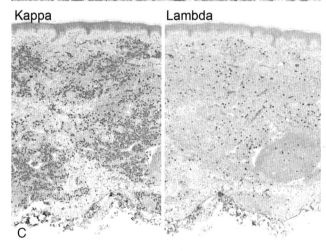

FIG. 13.51

Primary cutaneous marginal zone lymphoma is composed of CD20+ B-cells co-expressing Bcl-2, supporting marginal zone differentiation (**A**). The infiltrate is also positive for CD43 (**B**). The plasma cells are kappa-restricted (**C**).

TABLE 13.22

Histologic Features of Cutaneous B-Cell Lymphoid Hyperplasia Versus Primary Cutaneous Marginal Zone Lymphoma

Cutaneous B-Cell Lymphoid Hyperplasia	Primary Cutaneous Marginal Zone Lymphoma
• Mixtures of cell types	• May demonstrate proliferation of monocytoid (marginal zone), lymphoplasmacytic, or plasma cells
• Germinal centers do not display colonization by neoplastic marginal zone cells	• Germinal centers display colonization by neoplastic marginal zone cells, evidenced by fragmentation of follicle dendritic meshworks on CD21 immunostain
• Plasma cells are polytypic and lack cytologic atypia	• Plasma cells are monotypic and may display cytologic atypia including Dutcher bodies
• No CD43 expression by B-cells	• Neoplastic B-cells may express CD43
• Clonality studies are usually negative	• Clonality detected by IGH and IGK gene rearrangement studies

Prognosis and Therapy

The outcome of cutaneous lymphoid hyperplasia varies depending on the triggering events. Most lesions resolve over time upon withdrawal of the inciting factor. Localized treatment such as intralesional steroid injection or modest excision may be needed for more persistent cases. Other lesions may persist despite treatment and require re-biopsy to exclude progression to lymphoma.

CUTANEOUS B-CELL LYMPHOID HYPERPLASIA – DISEASE FACT SHEET

Definition
▸▸ Robust reactive B-cell infiltrate in the skin simulating cutaneous lymphoma

Incidence and Location
▸▸ Incidence is unknown
▸▸ Most commonly head and neck, followed by extremities and trunk

Age Distribution
▸▸ Usually adults but any age group may be affected

Clinical Features
▸▸ Erythematous papules, nodules, or plaques
▸▸ Pruritus common

Prognosis and Therapy
▸▸ May persist for variable duration before spontaneous resolution
▸▸ May recur upon repeated trigger

SUBCUTANEOUS PANNICULITIS-LIKE T-CELL LYMPHOMA

DIFFERENTIAL DIAGNOSIS: LUPUS ERYTHEMATOSUS PANNICULITIS

Clinical Features

Subcutaneous panniculitis-like T-cell lymphoma (SPTCL) is a cytotoxic T-cell lymphoma involving primarily the subcutaneous fat. It affects adults of any age; pediatric cases are rare. The lesions are solitary or multiple erythematous nodules or plaques without surface changes. The lesions are most commonly located on the lower extremities. Other body sites are less frequently involved. The clinical features of SPTCL resemble many panniculitides and hence the name. A small number of cases are associated with hemophagocytic syndrome.

Pathologic Features

GROSS FINDINGS

Most cases of SPTCL are evaluated by punch biopsies without particular gross findings.

MICROSCOPIC FINDINGS

There is a dense, diffuse atypical lymphoid infiltrate involving the subcutaneous fat (Fig. 13.52A). The overlying dermis and epidermis are largely unremarkable. The subcutaneous lymphocytes tend to percolate between adipocytes, resulting in a "rimming" pattern (Fig. 13.52B). The majority of these lymphocytes are small to medium in size, admixed with occasional large cells. They contain scant to moderate amount of cytoplasm and pleomorphic nuclei. Mitoses are readily found. Germinal centers are not seen. "Grungy" tumor necrosis is common (Fig. 13.52C). Lipomembranous fat necrosis may also be observed in some cases. On the other hand, hyaline fat necrosis typical of lupus erythematosus panniculitis (LEP) is a rare finding in SPTCL. Plasma cells are usually sparse.

Ancillary Studies

IMMUNOHISTOCHEMISTRY

The neoplastic T-cells in SPTCL demonstrate a CD4–/CD8+ and cytotoxic (TIA+/granzyme+) immunophenotype (Fig. 13.52D). They usually retain pan-T-cell markers CD3, CD2, and CD5. They are α/β T-cells which express TCR βF1 but not TCR γ/δ. CD30 is negative. Demonstration of adipocyte rimming by Ki-67 positive lymphocytes is highly specific for the diagnosis of SPTCL when compared with LEP (see Fig. 13.52D). CD123 may highlight scattered individual plasmacytoid dendritic

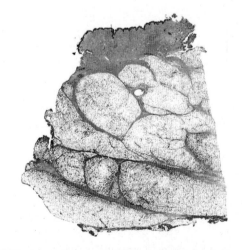

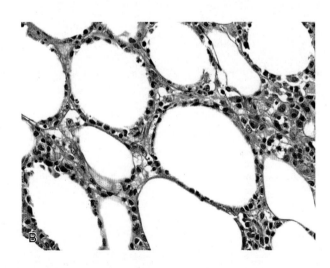

FIG. 13.52
A subcutaneous lymphocytic infiltrate diffusely percolating between adipocytes in a case of subcutaneous panniculitis-like T-cell lymphoma (SPTCL) (**A**). There is rimming of individual adipocytes by atypical and pleomorphic lymphocytes (**B**).

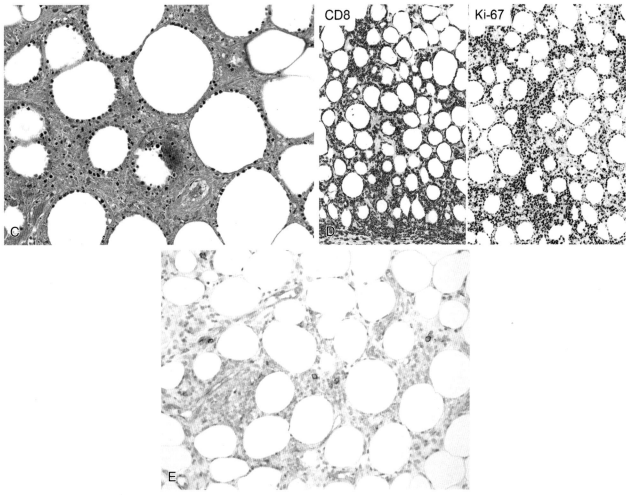

FIG. 13.52, cont'd

Grungy necrosis is common (**C**). The neoplastic cells are CD8+ cytotoxic T-cells (**D**, *left*), the majority of which are also Ki-67 positive (**D**, *right*). Adipocyte rimming by numerous Ki-67 positive cells is typical of SPTCL. CD123 immunostain reveals only rare single plasmacytoid dendritic cells in the infiltrate (**E**).

cells; however, clusters of >15 plasmacytoid dendritic cells are typically absent in SPTCL (see Fig. 13.52E).

MOLECULAR STUDIES

T-cell clonality may be demonstrated by T-cell receptor gene rearrangement studies. High-throughput sequencing has identified a few candidate gene mutations (*ARID1B*, *KMT2D*, and *PLCG1*), but no recurrent mutations have been identified to date.

Differential Diagnosis

Distinction between SPTCL and LEP is notoriously difficult. Clinically LEP is characterized by recurrent erythematous nodules on the extremities. The lesion may resolve with lipoatrophy. Histopathologically, LEP is a lobular lymphocytic panniculitis with or without overlying epidermal and dermal changes typically seen in cutaneous lupus erythematosus—namely, vacuolar interface dermatitis, periadnexal and perivascular lymphoplasmacytic infiltrate, and dermal mucin (Fig. 13.53A and E). The lymphocytic infiltrate in the subcutis often includes nodular paraseptal aggregates which may contain germinal centers (Fig. 13.53B). Other lymphocytes percolate between adipocytes and may simulate adipocyte rimming seen in SPTCL; however, these lymphocytes demonstrate minimal cytologic atypia (Fig. 13.53C) and a lower Ki-67 proliferation index when compared with those in SPTCL. Plasma cells are readily identified, often in small clusters, in the subcutaneous fat. Hyaline fat necrosis is characteristic (Fig. 13.53D). The T-cells in LEP are a mixture of CD4+ helper cells and CD8+ cytotoxic cells. They express TCR βF1 and pan-T-cell markers. CD123 would highlight an increased number of plasmacytoid dendritic cells frequently forming clusters in the skin and/or subcutis (Fig. 13.53F and Table 13.23).

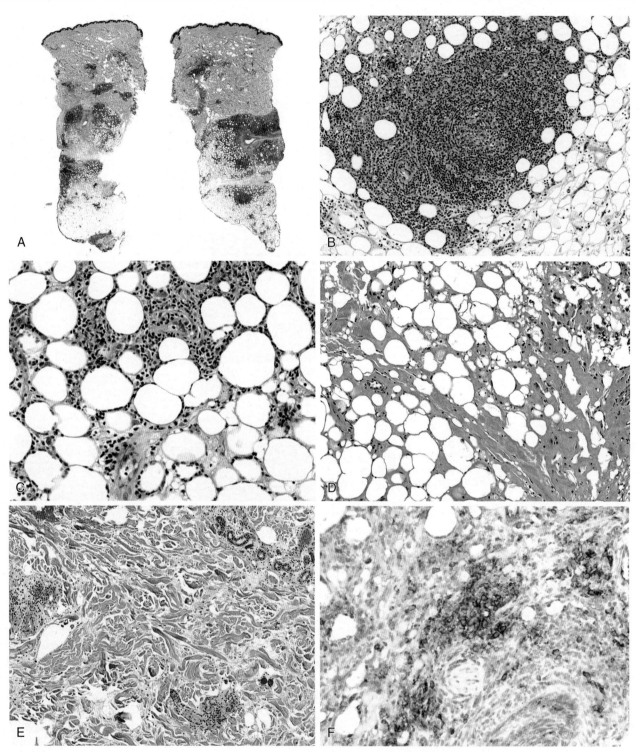

FIG. 13.53

Lupus erythematosus panniculitis is characterized by a subcutaneous lymphocytic infiltrate with paraseptal lymphoid nodules (**A**). Some of the paraseptal nodules contain lymphoid follicles (**B**). Adipocyte rimming is seen in areas; however, the degree of cytologic atypia is much less than that seen in subcutaneous panniculitis-like T-cell lymphoma (**C**). Hyaline fat necrosis is often present (**D**). The overlying dermis shows a perivascular and periadnexal lymphocytic infiltrate, and increased dermal mucin typical of cutaneous lupus erythematosus (**E**). CD123 immunostain reveals aggregates of plasmacytoid dendritic cells in the infiltrate (**F**).

TABLE 13.23

Histologic Features of Subcutaneous Panniculitis-Like T-Cell Lymphoma Versus Lupus Erythematosus Panniculitis

Subcutaneous Panniculitis-Like T-Cell Lymphoma	Lupus Erythematosus Panniculitis
• No epidermal or dermal changes	• Epidermis and dermis may demonstrate classic features of cutaneous lupus erythematosus
• Paraseptal B-cell-rich lymphoid nodules absent	• Paraseptal B-cell-rich lymphoid nodules may be present
• Adipocyte rimming by atypical pleomorphic CD8+/Ki-67+ lymphocytes	• Absence of adipocyte rimming by CD8+/Ki-67+ atypical lymphocytes
• Grungy tumor necrosis common; hyaline fat necrosis uncommon	• Hyaline fat necrosis
• Plasma cells are sparse or absent	• Plasma cells readily found
• Absence of CD123+ plasmacytoid dendritic cell clusters	• CD123+ plasmacytoid dendritic cell clusters commonly present
• T-cell clonality may be detected	• T-cell clonality studies usually negative

Prognosis and Therapy

Most cases of SPTCL show a protracted course. A minority of cases, especially those associated with hemophagocytic syndrome, behave more aggressively. Systemic steroids, radiotherapy, and systemic chemotherapy may be used to treat SPTCL.

SUBCUTANEOUS PANNICULITIS-LIKE T-CELL LYMPHOMA – DISEASE FACT SHEET

Definition
▸▸ Cytotoxic α/β T-cell lymphoma involving the subcutis

Incidence and Location
▸▸ Relatively rare lymphoma
▸▸ Most commonly involves the lower extremities; other sites are involved less frequently

Age Distribution
▸▸ Adults of any age

Clinical Features
▸▸ Erythematous nodules or plaques without skin surface changes
▸▸ Clinically indistinguishable from panniculitides

Prognosis and Therapy
▸▸ Most cases follow a protracted course
▸▸ Systemic steroids, radiotherapy, or chemotherapy

SUBCUTANEOUS PANNICULITIS-LIKE T-CELL LYMPHOMA – PATHOLOGIC FEATURES

Gross Findings
▸▸ No particular gross findings on skin biopsies

Microscopic Findings
▸▸ Diffuse lymphocytic infiltrate in subcutaneous fat
▸▸ Adipocyte rimming by atypical, pleomorphic lymphocytes
▸▸ Grungy tumor necrosis
▸▸ Paucity of B-cells and plasma cells
▸▸ Neoplastic T-cells demonstrate an α/β cytotoxic phenotype: TCR βF1+/CD3+/CD4−/CD8+/TIA+/granzyme+
▸▸ High Ki-67 proliferation index
▸▸ Paucity of CD123+ plasmacytoid dendritic cells

Pathologic Differential Diagnoses
▸▸ Lupus erythematosus panniculitis

SUGGESTED READINGS

Hypertrophic Lichen Planus

Totonchy MB, Leventhal JS, Ko CJ, Leffell DJ. Hypertrophic lichen planus and well-differentiated squamous cell carcinoma: a diagnostic conundrum. *Dermatol Surg.* 2018;44(11):1466-1470.

Alomari A, McNiff JM. The significance of eosinophils in hypertrophic lichen planus. *J Cutan Pathol.* 2014;41(4):347-352.

Levandoski KA, Nazarian RM, Asgari MM. Hypertrophic lichen planus mimicking squamous cell carcinoma: the importance of clinicopathologic correlation. *JAAD Case Rep.* 2017;3(2):151-154.

Bowen AR, Burt L, Boucher K, Tristani-Firouzi P, Florell SR. Use of proliferation rate, p53 staining and perforating elastic fibers in distinguishing keratoacanthoma from hypertrophic lichen planus: a pilot study. *J Cutan Pathol.* 2012;39(2):243-250.

Shah K, Kazlouskaya V, Lal K, Molina D, Elston DM. Perforating elastic fibers ("elastic fiber trapping") in the differentiation of keratoacanthoma, conventional squamous cell carcinoma and pseudocarcinomatous epithelial hyperplasia. *J Cutan Pathol.* 2014;41(2):108-112.

Dietert JB, Rabkin MS, Joseph AK. Squamous cell carcinoma versus hypertrophic lichen planus; a difficult differential diagnosis of great significance in approach to treatment. *Dermatol Surg.* 2017;43(2):297-299.

Knackstedt TJ, Collins LK, Li Z, Yan S, Samie FH. Squamous cell carcinoma arising in hypertrophic lichen planus: a review and analysis of 38 cases. *Dermatol Surg.* 2015;41(12):1411-1418.

Trichoepithelioma

Hile G, Harms PW. Update on molecular genetic alterations of cutaneous adnexal neoplasms. *Surg Pathol Clin.* 2021;14(2):251-272.

Elder DE, Massi D, Scolyer RA, Willemze R, eds. *WHO Classification of Skin Tumors.* 4th ed. Lyon, France: International Agency for Research on Cancer; 2018.

Stanoszek LM, Wang GY, Harms PW. Histologic mimics of basal cell carcinoma. *Arch Pathol Lab Med.* 2017;141(11):1490-1502.

Kazakov D, McKee P, Michal M, Kacerovska D. *Cutaneous Adnexal Tumors.* Philadelphia, Lippincott Williams and Wilkins; 2012.

Hu G, Onder M, Gill M, et al. A novel missense mutation in CYLD in a family with Brooke-Spiegler syndrome. *J Invest Dermatol.* 2003;121(4):732-734.

Vorechovsky I, Unden AB, Sandstedt B, Toftgard R, Stahle-Backdahl M. Trichoepitheliomas contain somatic mutations in the overexpressed PTCH gene: support for a gatekeeper mechanism in skin tumorigenesis. *Cancer Res.* 1997;57(21):4677-4681.

Rasmussen JE. A syndrome of trichoepitheliomas, milia, and cylindromas. *Arch Dermatol.* 1975;111(5):610-614.

Microcystic Adnexal Carcinoma

Hile G, Harms PW. Update on molecular genetic alterations of cutaneous adnexal neoplasms. *Surg Pathol Clin.* 2021;14(2):251-272.

Chan MP, Plouffe KR, Liu CJ, et al. Next-generation sequencing implicates oncogenic roles for p53 and JAK/STAT signaling in microcystic adnexal carcinomas. *Mod Pathol.* 2020;33(6): 1092-1103.

Worley B, Owen JL, Barker CA, et al. Evidence-based clinical practice guidelines for microcystic adnexal carcinoma: informed by a systematic review. *JAMA Dermatol.* 2019;155(9):1059-1068.

King BJ, Tolkachjov SN, Winchester DS, et al. Demographics and outcomes of microcystic adnexal carcinoma. *J Am Acad Dermatol.* 2018;79(4):756-758.

Elder DE, Massi D, Scolyer RA, Willemze R, eds. *WHO Classification of Skin Tumors.* 4 ed. Lyon, International Agency for Research on Cancer; 2018.

Stanoszek LM, Wang GY, Harms PW. Histologic mimics of basal cell carcinoma. *Arch Pathol Lab Med.* 2017;141(11):1490-1502.

Cardoso JC, Calonje E. Malignant sweat gland tumours: an update. *Histopathology.* 2015;67(5):589-606.

Kazakov D, McKee P, Michal M, Kacerovska D. *Cutaneous Adnexal Tumors.* Philadelphia, Lippincott Williams and Wilkins; 2012.

Merkel Cell Carcinoma

Tetzlaff MT, Harms PW. Danger is only skin deep: aggressive epidermal carcinomas. An overview of the diagnosis, demographics, molecular-genetics, staging, prognostic biomarkers, and therapeutic advances in Merkel cell carcinoma. *Mod Pathol.* 2020;33(suppl 1):42-55.

Kervarrec T, Tallet A, Miquelestorena-Standley E, et al. Diagnostic accuracy of a panel of immunohistochemical and molecular markers to distinguish Merkel cell carcinoma from other neuroendocrine carcinomas. *Mod Pathol.* 2019;32(4):499-510.

Harms PW, Harms KL, Moore PS, et al. The biology and treatment of Merkel cell carcinoma: current understanding and research priorities. *Nat Rev Clin Oncol.* 2018;15(12):763-776.

Harms PW. Update on Merkel Cell Carcinoma. *Clin Lab Med.* 2017;37(3): 485-501.

Harms KL, Healy MA, Nghiem P, et al. Analysis of prognostic factors from 9387 Merkel Cell carcinoma cases forms the basis for the new 8th edition AJCC staging system. *Ann Surg Oncol.* 2016;23(11):3564-3571.

Goh G, Walradt T, Markarov V, et al. Mutational landscape of MCPyV-positive and MCPyV-negative Merkel cell carcinomas with implications for immunotherapy. *Oncotarget.* 2016;7(3):3403-3415.

Wong SQ, Waldeck K, Vergara IA, et al. UV-associated mutations underlie the etiology of MCV-negative Merkel cell carcinomas. *Cancer Res.* 2015;75(24):5228-5234.

Harms PW, Vats P, Verhaegen ME, et al. The distinctive mutational spectra of polyomavirus-negative Merkel cell carcinoma. *Cancer Res.* 2015;75(18):3720-3727.

Feng H, Shuda M, Chang Y, Moore PS. Clonal integration of a polyomavirus in human Merkel cell carcinoma. *Science.* 2008;319(5866): 1096-1100.

Extramammary Paget Disease

Asel M, LeBoeuf NR. Extramammary Paget's disease. *Hematol Oncol Clin North Am.* 2019;33:73-85.

Chang J, Prieto VG, Sangueza M, et al. Diagnostic utility of p63 expression in the differential diagnosis of pagetoid squamous cell carcinoma in situ and extramammary Paget disease: a histopathologic study of 70 cases. *Am J Dermatopathol.* 2014;36:49-53.

Goldblum JR, Hart WR. Vulvar Paget's disease: a clinicopathologic and immunohistochemical study of 19 cases. *Am J Surg Pathol.* 1997;21:1178-1187.

Hatta N, Yamada M, Hirano T, et al. Extramammary Paget's disease: treatment, prognostic factors and outcome in 76 patients. *Br J Dermatol.* 2008;158:313-318.

Herrel LA, Weiss AD, Goodman M, et al. Extramammary Paget's disease in males: survival outcomes in 495 patients. *Ann Surg Oncol.* 2015; 22:1625-1630.

Kiavash K, Kim S, Thompson AD. "Pigmented extramammary Paget disease"-a potential mimicker of malignant melanoma and a pitfall in diagnosis: a case report and review of the literature. *Am J Dermatopathol.* 2019;41:45-49.

Ohnishi T, Watanabe S. The use of cytokeratins 7 and 20 in the diagnosis of primary and secondary extramammary Paget's disease. *Br J Dermatol.* 2000;142:243-247.

Perrotto J, Abbott JJ, Ceilley RI, et al. The role of immunohistochemistry in discriminating primary from secondary extramammary Paget disease. *Am J Dermatopathol.* 2010;32:137-143.

Shaco-Levy R, Bean SM, Vollmer RT, et al. Paget disease of the vulva: a histologic study of 56 cases correlating pathologic features and disease course. *Int J Gynecol Pathol.* 2010;29:69-78.

Simonds RM, Segal RJ, Sharma A. Extramammary Paget's disease: a review of the literature. *Int J Dermatol.* 2019;58:871-879.

Tanaka R, Sasajima Y, Tsuda H, et al. Human epidermal growth factor receptor 2 protein overexpression and gene amplification in extramammary Paget disease. *Br J Dermatol.* 2013;168:1259-1266.

Thomas CJ, Wood GC, Marks VJ. Mohs micrographic surgery in the treatment of rare aggressive cutaneous tumors: the Geisinger experience. *Dermatol Surg.* 2007;33:333-339.

Zhao M, Zhou L, Sun L, et al. GATA3 is a sensitive marker for primary genital extramammary Paget disease: an immunohistochemical study of 72 cases with comparison to gross cystic disease fluid protein 15. *Diagn Pathol.* 2017;12:51.

Desmoplastic Melanoma

Behrens EL, Boothe W, D'Silva N, et al. SOX-10 staining in dermal scars. *J Cutan Pathol.* 2019;46:579-585.

Blokhin E, Pulitzer M, Busam KJ. Immunohistochemical expression of p16 in desmoplastic melanoma. *J Cutan Pathol.* 2013;40:796-800.

Busam KJ. Desmoplastic melanoma. *Surg Pathol Clin.* 2009;2:511-520.

Elsensohn A, Shiu J, Grove N, et al. Distinguishing neurofibroma from desmoplastic melanoma: the value of p53. *Am J Surg Pathol.* 2018; 42:372-375.

Hawkins WG, Busam KJ, Ben-Porat L, et al. Desmoplastic melanoma: a pathologically and clinically distinct form of cutaneous melanoma. *Ann Surg Oncol.* 2005;12:207-213.

Lezcano C, Jungbluth AA, Nehal KS, et al. PRAME expression in melanocytic tumors. *Am J Surg Pathol.* 2018;42:1456-1465.

Plaza JA, Bonneau P, Prieto V, et al. Desmoplastic melanoma: an updated immunohistochemical analysis of 40 cases with a proposal for an additional panel of stains for diagnosis. *J Cutan Pathol.* 2016;43: 313-323.

Shain AH, Garrido M, Botton T, et al. Exome sequencing of desmoplastic melanoma identifies recurrent NFKBIE promoter mutations and diverse activating mutations in the MAPK pathway. *Nat Genet.* 2015; 47:1194-1199.

Wiesner T, Kiuru M, Scott SN, et al. NF1 mutations are common in desmoplastic melanoma. *Am J Surg Pathol.* 2015;39:1357-1362.

Yeh I, McCalmont TH. Distinguishing neurofibroma from desmoplastic melanoma: the value of the CD34 fingerprint. *J Cutan Pathol.* 2011; 38:625-630.

Spitz Nevus

Alomari AK, Miedema JR, Carter MD, et al. DNA copy number changes correlate with clinical behavior in melanocytic neoplasms: proposal of an algorithmic approach. *Mod Pathol.* 2020;33(7):1307-1317.

Hillen LM, van den Oord J, Geybels MS, Becker JC, Zur Hausen A, Winnepenninckx V. Genomic landscape of spitzoid neoplasms impacting patient management. *Front Med (Lausanne).* 2018;5:344.

Harms KL, Lowe L, Fullen DR, Harms PW. Atypical Spitz tumors: a diagnostic challenge. *Arch Pathol Lab Med.* 2015;139(10):1263-1270.

Busam KJ, Kutzner H, Cerroni L, Wiesner T. Clinical and pathologic findings of Spitz nevi and atypical Spitz tumors with ALK fusions. *Am J Surg Pathol.* 2014;38(7):925-933.

Wiesner T, He J, Yelensky R, et al. Kinase fusions are frequent in Spitz tumours and spitzoid melanomas. *Nat Commun.* 2014;5:3116.

Gerami P, Busam K, Cochran A, et al. Histomorphologic assessment and interobserver diagnostic reproducibility of atypical spitzoid melanocytic neoplasms with long-term follow-up. *Am J Surg Pathol.* 2014;38(7):934-940.

Wiesner T, Murali R, Fried I, et al. A distinct subset of atypical Spitz tumors is characterized by BRAF mutation and loss of BAP1 expression. *Am J Surg Pathol.* 2012;36(6):818-830.

Wiesner T, Obenauf AC, Murali R, et al. Germline mutations in BAP1 predispose to melanocytic tumors. *Nat Genet.* 2011;43(10):1018-1021.

Nevoid Melanoma

Zembowicz A, McCusker M, Chiarelli C, et al. Morphological analysis of nevoid melanoma: a study of 20 cases with a review of the literature. *Am J Dermatopathol*. 2001;23(3):167-175.

Magro CM, Crowson AN, Mihm MC. Unusual variants of malignant melanoma. *Mod Pathol*. 2006;19 suppl 2:S41-S70.

Cook MG, Massi D, Blokx WAM, et al. New insights into naevoid melanomas: a clinicopathological reassessment. *Histopathology*. 2017;71(6):943-950.

Cabrera R, Recule F. Unusual clinical presentations of malignant melanoma: a review of clinical and histologic features with special emphasis on dermatoscopic findings. *Am J Clin Dermatol*. 2018;19(suppl 1):15-23.

Newman MD, Lertsburapa T, Mirzabeigi M, Mafee M, Guitart J, Gerami P. Fluorescence in situ hybridization as a tool for microstaging in malignant melanoma. *Mod Pathol*. 2009;22(8):989-995.

Yelamos O, Busam KJ, Lee C, et al. Morphologic clues and utility of fluorescence in situ hybridization for the diagnosis of nevoid melanoma. *J Cutan Pathol*. 2015;42(11):796-806.

Mesbah Ardakani N, Singh S, Thomas C, et al. Mitotically active nevus and nevoid melanoma: a clinicopathological and molecular study. *Am J Dermatopathol*. 2021;43(3):182-190.

Jackett LA, Colebatch AJ, Rawson RV, et al. Molecular profiling of noncoding mutations distinguishes nevoid melanomas from mitotically active nevi in pregnancy. *Am J Surg Pathol*. 2020;44(3):357-367.

O'Rourke EA, Balzer B, Barry CI, Frishberg DP. Nevic mitoses: a review of 1041 cases. *Am J Dermatopathol*. 2013;35(1):30-33.

Lezcano C, Jungbluth AA, Nehal KS, Hollmann TJ, Busam KJ. PRAME expression in melanocytic tumors. *Am J Surg Pathol*. 2018;42:1456-1465.

Shain AH, Yeh I, Kovalyshyn I, et al. The genetic evolution of melanoma from precursor lesions. *N Engl J Med*. 2015;373:1926-1936.

Recurrent Nevus Phenomenon

King R, Hayzen BA, Page RN, et al. Recurrent nevus phenomenon: a clinicopathologic study of 357 cases and histologic comparison with melanoma with regression. *Mod Pathol*. 2009;22:611-617.

Kornberg R, Ackerman AB. Pseudomelanoma: recurrent melanocytic nevus following partial surgical removal. *Arch Dermatol*. 1975;111:1588-1590.

Miedema J, Andea AA. Through the looking glass and what you find there: making sense of comparative genomic hybridization and fluorescence in situ hybridization for melanoma diagnosis. *Mod Pathol*. 2020;33:1318-1330.

Park HK, Leonard DD, Arrington JH III, et al. Recurrent melanocytic nevi: clinical and histologic review of 175 cases. *J Am Acad Dermatol*. 1987;17:285-292.

Sommer LL, Barcia SM, Clarke LE, et al. Persistent melanocytic nevi: a review and analysis of 205 cases. *J Cutan Pathol*. 2011;38:503-507.

Vilain RE, McCarthy SW, Scolyer RA. The regenerating naevus. *Pathology*. 2016;48:108-112.

Nodal Nevus

Bowen AR, Duffy KL, Clayton FC, Andtbacka RH, Florell SR. Benign melanocytic lymph node deposits in the setting of giant congenital melanocytic nevi: the large congenital nodal nevus. *J Cutan Pathol*. 2015;42(11):832-839.

Piana S, Tagliavini E, Ragazzi M, et al. Lymph node melanocytic nevi: pathogenesis and differential diagnoses, with special reference to p16 reactivity. *Pathol Res Pract*. 2015;211(5):381-388.

Kim HJ, Seo JW, Roh MS, Lee JH, Song KH. Clinical features and prognosis of Asian patients with acral lentiginous melanoma who have nodal nevi in their sentinel lymph node biopsy specimen. *J Am Acad Dermatol*. 2018;79(4):706-713.

Holt JB, Sangueza OP, Levine EA, et al. Nodal melanocytic nevi in sentinel lymph nodes. Correlation with melanoma-associated cutaneous nevi. *Am J Clin Pathol*. 2004;121(1):58-63.

Lezcano C, Pulitzer M, Moy AP, Hollmann TJ, Jungbluth AA, Busam KJ. Immunohistochemistry for PRAME in the distinction of nodal nevi from metastatic melanoma. *Am J Surg Pathol*. 2020;44(4):503-508.

Saab J, Santos-Zabala ML, Loda M, Stack EC, Hollmann TJ. Fatty acid synthase and acetyl-CoA carboxylase are expressed in nodal metastatic melanoma but not in benign intracapsular nodal nevi. *Am J Dermatopathol*. 2018;40(4):259-264.

Lohmann CM, Iversen K, Jungbluth AA, Berwick M, Busam KJ. Expression of melanocyte differentiation antigens and ki-67 in nodal nevi and comparison of ki-67 expression with metastatic melanoma. *Am J Surg Pathol*. 2002;26(10):1351-1357.

Dalton SR, Gerami P, Kolaitis NA, et al. Use of fluorescence in situ hybridization (FISH) to distinguish intranodal nevus from metastatic melanoma. *Am J Surg Pathol*. 2010;34(2):231-237.

Taube JM, Begum S, Shi C, Eshleman JR, Westra WH. Benign nodal nevi frequently harbor the activating V600E BRAF mutation. *Am J Surg Pathol*. 2009;33(4):568-571.

de Beer FSA, van Diest PJ, Sigurdsson V, El Sharouni M. Intra-nodal nevi in sentinel node-negative patients with cutaneous melanoma does not influence survival. *J Eur Acad Dermatol Venereol*. 2019;33(12):2291-2295.

Cellular Dermatofibroma

Doyle LA, Fletcher CD. Metastasizing "benign" cutaneous fibrous histiocytoma: a clinicopathologic analysis of 16 cases. *Am J Surg Pathol*. 2013;37:484-495.

Doyle LA, Mariño-Enriquez A, Fletcher CD, et al. ALK rearrangement and overexpression in epithelioid fibrous histiocytoma. *Mod Pathol*. 2015;28:904-912.

Nakamura Y, Nakamura A, Muto M. Solitary spindle cell xanthogranuloma mimicking a Spitz nevus. *Am J Dermatopathol*. 2013;35:865-867.

Schechter SA, Bresler SC, Patel RM. Fat necrosis with an associated lymphocytic infiltrate represents a histopathologic clue that distinguishes cellular dermatofibroma from dermatofibrosarcoma protuberans. *J Cutan Pathol*. 2020;47:913-916.

Shah KK, McHugh JB, Folpe AL, et al. Dermatofibrosarcoma protuberans of distal extremities and acral sites: a clinicopathologic analysis of 27 cases. *Am J Surg Pathol*. 2018;42:413-419.

Volpicelli ER, Fletcher CDM. Desmin and CD34 positivity in cellular fibrous histiocytoma: an immunohistochemical analysis of 100 cases. *J Cutan Pathol*. 2012;39:747-752.

Zelger BW, Staudacher C, Orchard G, et al. Solitary and generalized variants of spindle cell xanthogranuloma (progressive nodular histiocytosis). *Histopathology*. 1995;27:11-19.

Atypical Fibroxanthoma

Miller TI, Zoumberos NA, Johnson B, et al. A genomic survey of sarcomas on sun-exposed skin reveals distinctive candidate drivers and potentially targetable mutations. *Hum Pathol*. 2020;102:60-69.

Koelsche C, Stichel D, Griewank KG, et al. Genome-wide methylation profiling and copy number analysis in atypical fibroxanthomas and pleomorphic dermal sarcomas indicate a similar molecular phenotype. *Clin Sarcoma Res*. 2019;9:2.

Elder DE, Massi D, Scolyer RA, Willemze R, eds. *WHO Classification of Skin Tumors*. 4th ed. Lyon, International Agency for Research on Cancer; 2018.

Griewank KG, Wiesner T, Murali R, et al. Atypical fibroxanthoma and pleomorphic dermal sarcoma harbor frequent NOTCH1/2 and FAT1 mutations and similar DNA copy number alteration profiles. *Mod Pathol*. 2017;31(3):418-428.

Griewank KG, Schilling B, Murali R, et al. TERT promoter mutations are frequent in atypical fibroxanthomas and pleomorphic dermal sarcomas. *Mod Pathol*. 2014;27(4):502-508.

Ha Lan TT, Chen SJ, Arps DP, et al. Expression of the p40 isoform of p63 has high specificity for cutaneous sarcomatoid squamous cell carcinoma. *J Cutan Pathol*. 2014;41(11):831-838.

Miller K, Goodlad JR, Brenn T. Pleomorphic dermal sarcoma: adverse histologic features predict aggressive behavior and allow distinction from atypical fibroxanthoma. *Am J Surg Pathol*. 2012;36(9):1317-1326.

Mirza B, Weedon D. Atypical fibroxanthoma: a clinicopathological study of 89 cases. *Australas J Dermatol*. 2005;46(4):235-238.

Epithelioid Sarcoma

Elsamna ST, Amer K, Elkattawy O, et al. Epithelioid sarcoma: half a century later. *Acta Oncol*. 2020;59:48-54.

Guillou L, Wadden C, Coindre JM, et al. "Proximal-type" epithelioid sarcoma, a distinctive aggressive neoplasm showing rhabdoid features. Clinicopathologic, immunohistochemical, and ultrastructural study of a series. *Am J Surg Pathol*. 1997;21:130-146.

Hollmann TJ, Hornick JL. INI1-deficient tumors: diagnostic features and molecular genetics. *Am J Surg Pathol*. 2011;35:e47-e63.

Hornick JL, Dal Cin P, Fletcher CD. Loss of INI1 expression is characteristic of both conventional and proximal-type epithelioid sarcoma. *Am J Surg Pathol*. 2009;33:542-550.

Maduekwe UN, Hornicek FJ, Springfield DS, et al. Role of sentinel lymph node biopsy in the staging of synovial, epithelioid, and clear cell sarcomas. *Ann Surg Oncol*. 2009;16:1356-1363.

Atypical Vascular Lesion

Ronen S, Ivan D, Torres-Cabala CA, et al. Post-radiation vascular lesions of the breast. *J Cutan Pathol*. 2019;46(1):52-58.

Elder DE, Massi D, Scolyer RA, Willemze R, eds. *WHO Classification of Skin Tumors*. 4th ed. Lyon, International Agency for Research on Cancer; 2018.

Shon W, Billings SD. Cutaneous malignant vascular neoplasms. *Clin Lab Med*. 2017;37(3):633-646.

Udager AM, Ishikawa MK, Lucas DR, McHugh JB, Patel RM. MYC immunohistochemistry in angiosarcoma and atypical vascular lesions: practical considerations based on a single institutional experience. *Pathology*. 2016;48(7):697-704.

Mentzel T, Schildhaus HU, Palmedo G, Buttner R, Kutzner H. Postradiation cutaneous angiosarcoma after treatment of breast carcinoma is characterized by MYC amplification in contrast to atypical vascular lesions after radiotherapy and control cases: clinicopathological, immunohistochemical and molecular analysis of 66 cases. *Mod Pathol*. 2012;25(1):75-85.

Fernandez AP, Sun Y, Tubbs RR, Goldblum JR, Billings SD. FISH for MYC amplification and anti-MYC immunohistochemistry: useful diagnostic tools in the assessment of secondary angiosarcoma and atypical vascular proliferations. *J Cutan Pathol*. 2012;39(2):234-242.

Manner J, Radlwimmer B, Hohenberger P, et al. MYC high level gene amplification is a distinctive feature of angiosarcomas after irradiation or chronic lymphedema. *Am J Pathol*. 2010;176(1):34-39.

Weaver J, Billings SD. Postradiation cutaneous vascular tumors of the breast: a review. *Semin Diagn Pathol*. 2009;26(3):141-149.

Cutaneous B-Cell Lymphoid Hyperplasia

Bergman R, Khamaysi K, Khamaysi Z, Ben Arie Y. A study of histologic and immunophenotypical staining patterns in cutaneous lymphoid hyperplasia. *J Am Acad Dermatol*. 2011;65(1):112-124.

Choi ME, Lee KH, Lim DJ, et al. Clinical and histopathological characteristics of cutaneous lymphoid hyperplasia: a comparative study according to causative factors. *J Clin Med*. 2020;9(4):1217.

Bergman R, Khamaysi K, Khamaysi Z, Ben Arie Y. A study of histologic and immunophenotypical staining patterns in cutaneous lymphoid hyperplasia. *J Am Acad Dermatol*. 2011;65(1):112-124.

Hristov AC, Comfere NI, Vidal CI, Sundram U. Kappa and lambda immunohistochemistry and in situ hybridization in the evaluation of atypical cutaneous lymphoid infiltrates. *J Cutan Pathol*. 2020;47(11):1103-1110.

Schafernak KT, Variakojis D, Goolsby CL, et al. Clonality assessment of cutaneous B-cell lymphoid proliferations: a comparison of flow cytometry immunophenotyping, molecular studies, and immunohistochemistry/in situ hybridization and review of the literature. *Am J Dermatopathol*. 2014;36(10):781-795.

Evans PA, Pott C, Groenen PJ, et al. Significantly improved PCR-based clonality testing in B-cell malignancies by use of multiple immunoglobulin gene targets. Report of the BIOMED-2 Concerted Action BHM4-CT98-3936. *Leukemia*. 2007;21:207-214.

Scheijen B, Meijers RWJ, Rijntjes J, et al. Next-generation sequencing of immunoglobulin gene rearrangements for clonality assessment: a technical feasibility study by EuroClonality-NGS. *Leukemia*. 2019;33(9):2227-2240.

Skala SL, Hristov B, Hristov AC. Primary cutaneous follicle center lymphoma. *Arch Pathol Lab Med*. 2018;142(11):1313-1321.

Cho-Vega JH, Vega F, Rassidakis G, Medeiros LJ. Primary cutaneous marginal zone B-cell lymphoma. *Am J Clin Pathol*. 2006;125 Suppl:S38-S49.

Maurus K, Appenzeller S, Roth S, et al. Panel sequencing shows recurrent genetic FAS alterations in primary cutaneous marginal zone lymphoma. *J Invest Dermatol*. 2018;138(7):1573-1581.

Subcutaneous Panniculitis-Like T-Cell Lymphoma

Willemze R, Jansen PM, Cerroni L, et al. Subcutaneous panniculitis-like T-cell lymphoma: definition, classification, and prognostic factors: an EORTC Cutaneous Lymphoma Group Study of 83 cases. *Blood*. 2008;111:838-845.

Rutnin S, Porntharukcharoen S, Boonsakan P. Clinicopathologic, immunophenotypic, and molecular analysis of subcutaneous panniculitis-like T-cell lymphoma: a retrospective study in a tertiary care center. *J Cutan Pathol*. 2019;46(1):44-51.

Arps DP, Patel RM. Lupus profundus (panniculitis): a potential mimic of subcutaneous panniculitis-like T-cell lymphoma. *Arch Pathol Lab Med*. 2013;137(9):1211-1215.

LeBlanc RE, Tavallaee M, Kim YH, Kim J. Useful parameters for distinguishing subcutaneous panniculitis-like T cell lymphoma from lupus erythematosus panniculitis. *Am J Surg Pathol*. 2016;40:745-754.

Sitthinamsuwan P, Pattanaprichakul P, Treetipsatit J, et al. Subcutaneous panniculitis-like T-cell lymphoma versus lupus erythematosus panniculitis: distinction by means of the periadipocytic cell proliferation index. *Am J Dermatopathol*. 2018;40(8):567-574.

Chen SJT, Tse JY, Harms PW, Hristov AC, Chan MP. Utility of CD123 immunohistochemistry in differentiating lupus erythematosus from cutaneous T cell lymphoma. *Histopathology*. 2019;74(6):908-916.

Fernandez-Pol S, Costa HA, Steiner DF, et al. High-throughput sequencing of subcutaneous panniculitis-like T-cell lymphoma reveals candidate pathogenic mutations. *Appl Immunohistochem Mol Morphol*. 2019;27(10):740-748.

Page numbers followed by "*f*" indicate figures, "*t*" indicate tables, and "*b*" indicate boxes.